HANDBOOK OF DEVELOPMENTAL RESEARCH METHODS

HANDBOOK OF DEVELOPMENTAL RESEARCH METHODS

Edited by

BRETT LAURSEN

TODD D. LITTLE

NOEL A. CARD

THE GUILFORD PRESS

New York London

A Division of Guilford Publications, Inc.
72 Spring Street, New York, NY 10012
www.guilford.com

Printed in the United States of America

This book is printed on acid-free paper.

Last digit is print number: 9 8 7 6 5 4 3 2 1

Library of Congress Cataloging-in-Publication Data

Handbook of developmental research methods / edited by Brett Laursen, Todd D. Little, Noel A. Card.

p. cm.

Includes bibliographical references and index.

ISBN 978-1-60623-609-3 (hardcover)

1. Developmental psychology—Research—Methodology. 2. Developmental psychology—Longitudinal studies. I. Laursen, Brett Paul. II. Little, Todd D. III. Card, Noel A.

BF713.H3643 2012

155.072′1—dc23

2011019742

Preface

Many handbooks claim to be essential. This one truly is. If you study development, it is unlikely that you have been able to keep up with the rapid changes in analytic methodologies. Even if your job title includes "advanced methodologist," it is unlikely that you have been able to stay abreast of the latest offerings from your colleagues.

There are plenty of handbooks on research methods, but none are aimed specifically at developmental scholars. This is a difference with a distinction. To study development is to study change. Each of the chapters in this volume is focused on applying a methodological tool to the measurement of change. Some tools were specifically designed to measure change. Other tools have been adapted to incorporate the demands of developmental research. Developmental scholars no longer have to make do with figuring out how static approaches can be applied to dynamic data, because the world's leading developmental methodologists have applied themselves to this task.

The results are pleasantly overwhelming. Not long ago, developmental scientists needed only to be conversant in repeated-measures analyses of variance and stepwise regression. There are now dozens of alternatives to these techniques, most of which are more flexible and more powerful. Unlike their predecessors, these new techniques continue to evolve and improve. Powerful new software drives many of these advances. But keeping up with the pace of change in developmental research methods requires more than software upgrades. One must understand the fundamentals at the heart of each method in order to understand how change is measured and represented.

Lars Bergman, the wise Swedish methodologist, often reminds us to examine the assumptions of an analytic procedure. One need not be able to conduct complicated analyses in order to understand them. Unfortunately, many statistical packages make the analyses easy and the assumptions opaque to the point that it can sometimes be difficult to examine the assumptions. Each contributor to this handbook was tasked with the challenge of explaining the assumptions of a developmental method in accessible nontechnical language. The reader should come away from each chapter understanding the basic purpose of a procedure and the principles that animate that procedure. If we have been successful, the relevance of each method to your own research should be apparent.

The volume is more than a primer, however. Methodologists will be pleased to hear that expositions of assumptions are followed by a careful explication of recent technical advances. This is not an abstract exercise. In most cases, the summary of cutting-edge practices is accompanied by a specific research example that concretizes the procedure. These illustrations should prove useful to readers hoping to apply the technique to their own data. Many authors have helpfully provided scripts and data samples to facilitate the application process. These supplemental materials are available online at *www.crmda.ku.edu/Guilford/HDRM.*

The volume is divided into seven sections. The opening section on measurement and design is followed by a section on approaches to data collection. These chapters are devoted to issues that concern the design and implementation of developmental research. The next three sections concern interindividual longitudinal analysis, intraindividual longitudinal analysis, and analyses that combine the two. These chapters describe cutting-edge analytic practices designed specifically for developmental data. The section that follows addresses the burgeoning topic of nonindependent data with a unique collection of chapters devoted to developmental applications. The volume closes with a section on special topics in data analysis, a heading that encompasses important research methods that tend to be underutilized by developmental scholars. All but the last section open with a unique chapter on foundational issues written by eminent developmental methodologists. We gave these scholars free rein in defining the material covered, instructing them only to provide an expansive overview of the field. Except for those addressing foundational issues, the chapters in the handbook follow a similar outline: (1) central issues; (2) conceptual principles and statistical assumptions; (3) developmental applications; (4) illustration; and (5) future directions.

In keeping with the admonition of our esteemed colleague, let us be specific about our assumptions. We consider change to be central to the study of development. Contemporary students might be amazed to learn that within their lifetimes, cross-sectional data were used to gauge developmental trends and the presence of statistically significant differences in one age group and that the absence of such differences in another was thought to constitute a developmental finding of note. This sort of methodology is no longer tenable; development cannot be measured in the absence of data from multiple time points. The chapters in this volume take as their starting point the assumption that development is synonymous with change and that longitudinal data are a prerequisite for the study of change.

Change can be measured at the level of the variable or at the level of the individual. Longitudinal change can be examined between and within individuals using interindividual and intraindividual procedures, respectively. The assumptions of each are quite different. Studies that demonstrate change at the level of the variable assume that the developmental trends illustrated apply equally well to all members of the sample or population. Studies that demonstrate change at the level of the individual assume that the unique developmental patterns shared across subgroups of individuals do not apply to the population as a whole. Some have described these approaches as antithetical, but we prefer to think of them as complementary. Both approaches are well represented in this book.

We assume the high standard of best methodological practices. Scholars have long known of biases arising from samples of convenience, statistical nonindependence, demand characteristics, recall load, attrition, and measurement and scaling variance. There was once a good excuse for sweeping these problems aside, namely, the absence of a remedy. This is no longer the case, and those who ignore these biases do so at their own peril. This handbook contains several chapters that identify and explain sources of bias in developmental research. Importantly, each chapter also describes methods for assessing and addressing the challenges that arise in developmental research. Forewarned is forearmed: Many methodological problems can be avoided or mitigated with appropriate design strategies. Look for tips on strengthening developmental research with designs that anticipate potential sources of bias.

Finally, we assume that research methods are tools designed to aid the scholar in identifying developmental change. Important implications follow from this assumption. Different tools can be selected for the same job. Holes can be made with hammers, and holes can be made with drills. The choice of the appropriate tool depends on the aims of the investigator. Some tools are clearly inappropriate for the task at hand. One cannot install a window with tools designed to dig ditches. Thus research questions must be matched to developmental methods. We strongly believe that an investigator cannot make an informed choice without a working knowledge of how each research method works. Research questions often carry hidden assumptions. Developmental questions are informed by the models and ontogenetic theories of the investigator. Hypotheses usually call for certain types of methodologies. Because the assumptions of methodological tools differ, similar data or even the same data may yield different depictions of change. Put another way, research questions drive the selection of developmental methods, which can foreshadow whether and how developmental changes are described. The chapters in this handbook will help to clarify the unappreciated link between research questions, methods, and developmental change by illuminating the assumptions inherent in each.

A volume of this magnitude requires enormous effort from many parties. Todd Little and Noel Card are as knowledgeable as they are congenial; I could not ask for better collaborators. Shalynn Howard cheerfully compiled and organized the chapters. Jeff Friedrich assisted with proofreading. The Center for Research Methods and Data Analysis at the University of Kansas (Todd D. Little, Director) graciously agreed to host and maintain the website dedicated to the ancillary materials from this volume at *wwwcrmda.ku.edu/Guilford/HDRM*. C. Deborah Laughton and Seymour Weingarten of The Guilford Press convinced us of the merits of this project and worked to meet what must have seemed like unreasonable demands. Thanks to our families (Erika, Kirsten, and Erik; Patty; Jeanet, Gabby, and Angie), whose love and forbearance were tested but never found lacking. We are gratified by the cooperation we received from our methodological colleagues; most of those who were invited to participate agreed to do so. Our contributors were, for the most part, a timely and responsive bunch. Their collective wisdom is humbling.

BRETT LAURSEN
Fort Lauderdale, Florida
January 2011

Contents

The companion website *www.crmda.ku.edu/Guilford/HDRM* includes data files and syntax for the examples in the book as well as additional support materials.

PART I

Measurement and Design

CHAPTER 1

Foundational Issues of Design and Measurement in Developmental Research

SCOTT M. HOFER
VALGEIR THORVALDSSON
ANDREA M. PICCININ

Attention to study design and measurement is essential for developmental lifespan research because of the complexity of maturational and aging processes influencing within-person change and variation across the lifespan and in different historical and cultural contexts. A variety of research designs have been used within the broad enterprise of lifespan developmental science, ranging from cross-sectional and longitudinal quasi-experimental designs to controlled experiments. Quasi-experimental studies are the most typical because many hypothesis tests of interest are not possible to conduct within the contexts of controlled experimental designs for practical and ethical reasons.

A majority of theoretical propositions related to the human lifespan are based on cross-sectional evidence of between-person age differences. However, inferences about age-related changes from these studies are confounded by birth cohort effects (e.g., Rönnlund & Nilsson, 2008; Schaie, 2008) and mortality selection (e.g., Kurland, Johnson, Egleston, & Diehr, 2009), and for a variety of additional reasons greatly limit the opportunities to draw inferences about individual and population change (Hofer, Flaherty, & Hoffman, 2006; Hofer & Sliwinski, 2001; Kraemer, Yesavage, Taylor, & Kupfer, 2000; Molenaar, 2008; Molenaar, Huizenga, & Nesselroade, 2003; Sliwinski, Hoffman, & Hofer, 2010a; Wohlwill, 1970, 1973).

Advances in understanding development and aging require obtaining and analyzing data on within-person change. Longitudinal designs are essential for the quantification of individual differences in patterns and rates of within-person change. Such data provide important opportunities for examining the interdependency among developmental processes and the influences of risk and protective factors across the lifespan. Longitudinal data can also be used to facilitate understanding of how between-person differences at a particular age or time period arise through change processes (e.g., Hofer et al., 2006). In this chapter we discuss a variety of issues concerning designs, measurements, and analysis of data from quasi-experimental studies with the main aim of identifying and explaining individual differences in developmental processes.

Analytical Aims of Developmental Research

The study of development and aging comprises research across different levels of analysis: population average patterns of change, individual differences in function and rate of change, and within-person dynamics across different temporal intervals. Each level provides complementary information about population trends, individual differences, and individual effects. These levels of analysis are based on successively disaggregated effects and temporal sampling frames that are important to consider when interpreting and comparing effects across longitudinal studies (Hofer & Piccinin, 2010; Hofer & Sliwinski, 2006). Taken together, the pattern of mean trends and the structure of individual differences in change and variation provide a basis for understanding the relative independence or interdependence of time-related processes.

Population Average Rates of Change

Estimating average trends, conditional on birth cohort, culture, and other population differences, provides important comparative evidence for differential change. For example, an important distinction between types of intelligence is based on differential patterns of lifespan change (i.e., fluid ability begins to decline at an earlier age and at a steeper rate than crystallized knowledge). Historical cohort differences permit a window on how different contexts can have lasting effects on maturational and aging-related outcomes.

Correlated Rates of Change

Multivariate growth models provide estimates of associations in rates of change across variables. Estimates of correlated rates of change (i.e., between-person analysis of correlated change) can answer the question of whether individuals who change more rapidly on one variable also change more rapidly on another. For example, Hofer and colleagues (2009) evaluated the structure of change in emotional and behavioral disturbance from adolescence to young adulthood—correlated baseline levels, linear rates of change, and time-specific variation—and reported moderate magnitudes of interdependence among change and variation.

The structure of between-person differences in rate of change has been frequently evaluated in the area of cognitive aging. Longitudinal studies suggest that, although cognitive changes across different domains are correlated, these associations are relatively weak (e.g., Anstey, Hofer, & Luszcz, 2003; Hultsch, Hertzog, Small, McDonald-Miszczk, & Dixon, 1992; Johansson et al., 2004; Lindenberger & Ghisletta, 2009; Sliwinski & Buschke, 1999; Sliwinski, Hofer, & Hall, 2003; Wilson et al., 2002; Zimprich & Martin, 2002) compared with cross-sectional results of high amounts of shared age-related variance (Lindenberger & Baltes, 1994; Verhaeghen & Salthouse, 1997). These findings bring into question theoretical claims that a common aging factor drives most of the cognitive loss experienced by aging adults. Common factor models account for the covariance in cross-sectional data because multivariate analyses of age-heterogeneous data are confounded by average age differences. This confound spuriously inflates the estimated age-related associations (e.g., Hofer et al., 2006; Hofer & Sliwinski, 2001).

Coupled Within-Person Processes

In longitudinal studies on aging with widely spaced assessments, short-term variations are assumed to be small relative to long-term changes. If short-term temporal variability is moderate to high, however, single assessments will produce imprecise estimates of an individual's characteristic level of functioning. This imprecision has important implications for estimates of individual change. Figure 1.1 shows how a repeated series of measurements can be decomposed into population average trend, individual deviation from the trend, and time-specific variation about the individual-level slope as distinct from error. In most designs, the error is indistinguishable from time-specific variation. Most studies emphasize estimates of long-term change and not short-term variation, which is typically modeled as a nuisance parameter. Short-term intraindividual variability can, however, be an interesting predictor or outcome in itself. Sufficient evidence now exists to establish intraindividual cognitive variability as a reliable source of information embedded in between-person differences (Almeida & Kessler, 1998; Almeida & McDonald, 1998). The reliability of cognitive variability is especially noteworthy among older adults (Eizenman, Nesselroade, Featherman, & Rowe, 1997; Horn, 1972; Martin & Hofer, 2004; Neiss & Almeida, 2004; Nesselroade, 2001, 2004) and encourages greater emphasis on within-person dynamics in modeling of aging data.

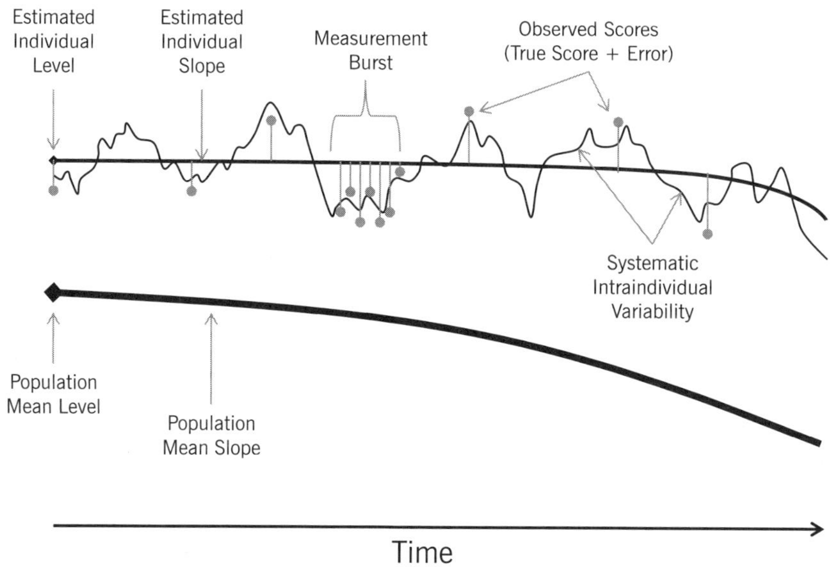

FIGURE 1.1. Theoretical decomposition of an individual's observed scores. From Hofer and Piccinin (2010). Copyright 2010 by Oxford University Press. Reprinted with permission.

Although a measurement burst design that includes sets of closely spaced measurements separated by wider intervals would facilitate the study of intraindividual variation, typical longitudinal designs with widely spaced intervals (i.e., 2 years) also permit tests of influences on intraindividual variation. These focus on the occasion-specific residuals after accounting for the individual and population trajectories (see, e.g., Sliwinski et al., 2003). Different time-sampling schedules will yield patterns of variability that result from different influences on the individual. For example, we might consider sampling over seconds or minutes (e.g., attentional lapses), within test (e.g., practice), within session (e.g., fatigue, order effects, motivation), within day (e.g., time of day effects), across days or weeks (e.g., environmental perturbations, physical health, practice), or across months or years (e.g., maturation, aging).

Longitudinal Designs and Issues for Describing and Explaining Developing Processes

Research designed to capture features of development and aging involves a number of decisions regarding the sampling of individuals and of times and types of measurements. Depending on the questions of interest, individuals can be drawn from different populations of birth cohorts, cultures, and nations; at different historical periods; with short- or long-term intervals between assessments; and with measures that are time invariant or time varying within individuals. Longitudinal studies vary in a number of elements (e.g., Lerner, Schwartz, & Phelps, 2009), such as differences in samples (e.g., age homogeneous vs. age heterogeneous; representativeness), number of occasions (e.g., few vs. many), spacing between assessments (e.g., widely spaced panel designs, single session learning experiment), and whether new samples of individuals are obtained at subsequent measurement occasions (e.g., sequential designs). These features can be combined in a number of ways to create study designs that are particularly suitable for answering research questions that vary in scope from regarding population change across birth cohorts to focusing on the dynamics of short-term within-person processes.

An essential consideration of all longitudinal study designs is their sensitivity for detecting key events, predictors, and processes. These include the dynamics of biological and social processes and measurements of critical events that cause change in functional status of the individual. In particular, sufficient data within individuals must be collected in order to permit understanding of both rapid and gradual decline. Next we highlight issues that we see as foremost in the design of longitudinal studies that focus on within-person processes.

Identifying Within-Person Change and Variation

Measurement of time-specific factors permits statistical control of within-person variation and provides greater statistical power for detecting within-person change. The measurement burst design (Sliwinski, 2008; Walls, Barta, Stawski, Collyer, & Hofer, Chapter 4, this volume) features bursts of measurements that are spaced over longer intervals. An important feature of this design is the separation of (1) short-term (day-to-day) within-person variability, (2) long-term (year-to-year) within-person variation and change, and (3) stable between-person individual differences. Because most intensive measurement designs (e.g., daily diary studies, ecological momentary assessment) measure behavior over a short time window (e.g., 1 week), they will confound short-term variability, change that transpires over long intervals, and stable individual differences. Measurement burst designs have been used to separate short-term retest effects from long-term age-related cognitive change (Sliwinski, Hoffman, & Hofer, 2010a) and to evaluate how within-person emotional reactivity to stress (across a week of repeated measures) is related to decreases in cognitive performance (Sliwinski, Smyth, Hofer, & Stawski, 2006). These types of analyses are limited to data that are collected in measurement burst designs.

Most developmental theory strives to describe and explain characteristics of changes that occur within individuals at different periods of the lifespan. This emphasis on within-person causal processes is, however, not well represented in designs and analyses of current studies in the field of developmental psychology. A major limitation of many of the current longitudinal studies is that they feature designs with widely spaced intervals, potentially limiting the formulation and test of hypotheses about influences on intraindividual variation and change as a result of not having sufficient information about the processes and events (i.e., interval censoring).

An increasing number of measurement burst, daily diary, and event-linked design studies (e.g., Moskowitz, Russell, Sadikaj, & Sutton, 2009) have been initiated in recent years. Such studies have the potential to improve the reliability of measurement and permit a better understanding of within-person dynamics. The availability of a greater number of measurements provides a valuable opportunity to identify and measure factors that may be related to changes in the individual's behavior (e.g., daily stress, health event), and permits the modeling of learning effects and intraindividual variability. Differences in temporal sampling across longitudinal studies will also lead to opportunities to test a given hypothesis from different angles, because the measurements will tap into different sources of change and fluctuation that result from different exogenous influences (Martin & Hofer, 2004; Newell, Liu, & Meyer-Kress, 2001).

The crux of the challenge is to identify a within-person change point (i.e., deviation from an established within-person normative trajectory) in the context of within-person variation. Recent research has focused on optimizing the design and analysis features of cognitive assessments that will permit reliable and sensitive assessment of cognitive functioning and identification of key causal factors underlying short-term and long-term change in functioning (Pavel et al., 2008). An important consideration is that of sampling time in longitudinal studies, particularly measuring causal variables within the time frame in which they have the greatest effects on the outcome variables (Gollob & Reichardt, 1987).

In general, longitudinal observational studies pose a number of challenges for causal inference, including the potential mismatch of the temporal sampling and the causal model (e.g., Boker, Molenaar, & Nesselroade, 2009; Gollob & Reichardt, 1987); differences in the reliability of measurement instruments and emphasis on relative shifts in between-person differences over time (Rogosa, 1980); unmodeled simultaneous associations between cause and effect in the evaluation of lagged effects; exclusion of other causal variables (regression misspecification; Morgan & Winship, 2007); and bias due to confounds among levels of analysis, such as unmodeled nonlinear trends (i.e., age–slope interaction; see Bauer & Cai, 2009; Hofer et al., 2006).

Retest and Reactivity Effects in Longitudinal Studies

Identification of individual differences in a developmental change trajectory is obtained with analyses of repeated measurements of the same individuals over time. To maintain measurement invariance, researchers rely on the same types of measurements across the subsequent testing occasions, permitting study participants to respond differently to the repeated measurements due to learning test-taking strategy or better acquaintance within the context of the measurement. These types of retest effects are a threat to the internal validity of longitudinal studies (e.g., Schaie & Hofer, 2001). The problem is to determine whether the observed within-person change is due to retest effects or to change in the constructs under study.

Several solutions have been proposed to adjust for retest effects in the cognitive aging literature. Retest effects can be identified as between-group difference across the previous participants and a nonpreviously measured representative sample of the same age and cohort (Rönnlund, Nyberg, Bäckman, & Nilsson, 2005; Schaie, 1988). Chronological age and other important demographic variables are generally held constant in these comparisons, as the validity of the retest adjustment relies on the equality of the groups. The main focus in this approach is on the group mean differences; individual differences and within-person variability in retest effects are not identified (Thorvaldsson, Hofer, Berg, & Johansson, 2006). Another approach relies on systematic manipulation of temporal intervals between occasions in a planned missing time-lag design (McArdle & Woodcock, 1997). An implicit assumption of this approach is that retest effects are reduced by the passage of time. Yet another approach has been proposed that does not rely on manipulation of the sampling design in the longitudinal study (McArdle, Ferrer-Caja, Hamagami, & Woodcock, 2002; Rabbitt, Diggle, Smith, Holland, & McInnes, 2001). In this approach, within-person change is estimated as a partial effect after adjustment for a participant's number of previous measurement occasions. However, when parameterization of the retest effect covaries with "time in the study," in the presence of cohort effects, the resulting estimates can be seriously biased (Sliwinski et al., 2010a).

In fact, it is difficult to argue that any of the previously mentioned approaches can sufficiently separate retest effects from developmental trends at the individual level. Retest effects most likely vary across individuals, as well as within individuals over time. The assumptions of these approaches are therefore unlikely to hold. As a consequence, the between-person comparisons become poor approximations. The essential problem is that quantification of the retest effect and the developmental trend is conducted within the same measurement procedure. There is therefore no index with which to separate the two in the design of most longitudinal studies. This problem can be partly circumvented by collecting information about retest effects from other measurements, as is done in the measurement burst design (Nesselroade, 1991; Sliwinski, 2008), in which the time index for learning effects (e.g., days) is different from the time index for long-term aging effects (e.g., years). This design may permit separation of learning (i.e., retest effects), learning decay, and long-term within-person change (i.e., aging). By modeling learning within sets of closely spaced measurements, repeated at longer intervals, one can statistically decompose learning and decay functions that overlay normative maturation and aging in order to reveal change in an individual's asymptotic performance over longer periods of time (months or years).

Although retest effects are often regarded as the critical limitation of longitudinal designs (e.g., Salthouse, 2009), such learning effects are embedded in the processes under study (e.g., memory). Because performance under the same "novel" conditions can never be observed repeatedly, relative individual differences within each study must provide the basis for inferring relative change conditional on design effects (i.e., number of test items, test exposure; Hofer & Sliwinski, 2006; Thorvaldsson et al., 2006; Thorvaldsson, Hofer, Hassing, & Johansson, 2008). The alternative, however—cross-sectional design—in which different people are measured only once, provides little to no basis for valid inferences about individual differences in aging-related change.

Optimizing Measurement for Developmental Research

Longitudinal designs require careful consideration of the phenomenon under study, choice of time sampling, validity of measurement instruments, and statistical analysis. Age and cohort heterogeneous samples vary in terms of population selection effects related to attrition and mortality and amount of gains from repeated testing exposure. Statistical analyses must take into account these design and sampling characteristics in order to make meaningful inferences to the population. To account for these characteristics requires an analysis that adjusts for (i.e., conditions on) population characteristics such as age, birth cohort, and mortality in such a way as to permit conditional inferences to defined and accessible populations (e.g., change in individuals of a particular age and surviving to a particular age; see, e.g., Kurland et al., 2009).

The following sections consider a range of additional issues for research on development and aging. Inherent in our discussion is the fundamental requirement that scientific progress is based on replication. Confirmation of previous findings can be based on patterns of results but, in a more rigorous use, features the evaluation of quantitative differences in individual and population change. To achieve a higher level of rigor requires that tests used in one study map sufficiently onto the same construct in another study. In the section on measurement issues, we describe the evaluation of measurement invariance, with reference to key resources and applications.

Measurement Invariance over Time

The main goals of developmental research are usually not achievable without careful assessment and modeling of individual change and variation over time. In order to model individual change over time, it is essential that measurements obtained at different times and across groups have the same measurement properties—that is, that the measurements are factorially invariant and permit valid quantitative comparisons. Factorial invariance is a foundational aspect of empirical research (e.g., Meredith, 1993; Meredith & Horn, 2001; Widaman & Reise, 1997). The importance of factorial invariance is especially true in the social sciences, in which important objects of study are latent constructs whose nature and validity are derived from consideration of interrelationships with other latent and observed constructs. Factorial invariance is essential for studies that implicitly require the comparability of constructs across samples differing in age, birth cohort, and country and over time.

Any study making comparisons across time or groups assumes measurement invariance. Within the framework of structural equation modeling it is possible to test this assertion. A logical hierarchy of constraints are implemented in factor models, beginning with configural invariance, which requires the same number of factors and pattern of salient factor loadings across groups. The factor model is identified by fixing the factor estimates (i.e., mean, variance) in one group and propagating this identification by constraining the corresponding parameters (i.e., intercept, loading) of the respective indicators across groups or occasions. Using this model as a baseline, Meredith's (1993; see also Hofer, Horn, & Eber, 1997; Little, 1997; Widaman & Reise, 1997) hierarchy of constraints is fit to the data: (1) weak factorial invariance (also known as "metric" invariance) involves equivalence of factor-variable regressions (i.e., factor loadings), (2) strong factorial invariance adds constraints on manifest intercept (mean) terms and requires that one factor mean be fixed to specify the metric of the latent variables, and (3) strict factorial invariance further constrains unique variances to be equivalent (however, this latter constraint is not generally considered necessary for factorial invariance to be supported; Little, 1997; Little, Card, Slegers, & Ledford, 2007). Factor-level variances, covariances, and means must be freely estimated because factorial invariance concerns only the measurement model. Bontempo and Hofer (2007) describe and demonstrate methods for assessing factorial invariance with continuous and categorical indicators in cross-sectional and longitudinal samples. A sequence of nested models from least to most constrained is recommended. For multi-occasion models in the context of considerable age-based change, bias in the factor structure (i.e., due to mean trends related to age heterogeneity within occasion) may result unless age heterogeneity is small compared with the amount of change expected (Meredith & Horn, 2001).

Factor models with polytomous (ordered categorical) indicators and robust procedures for item-level invariance tests are important extensions of factorial invariance testing procedures. Recent software enhancements relax the assumption of continuous and normally distributed indicators and permit direct analysis of binary and ordinal (polytomous) indicators (e.g., Millsap & Yun-Tein, 2004; Muthén & Asparouhov, 2002).

Item Response Models

Item response theory (IRT) provides a formal model of the individual's response to items that make up a scale. It offers many advantages in the development and refinement of psychometric instruments. One major benefit of an IRT framework is that the placement of items onto a continuum of difficulty (severity) facilitates comparably scaled construct scores from two measures with overlapping but disjoint item sets. There is a close relationship between IRT and certain classes of factor models (see Reise, Widaman, & Pugh, 1993; Takane & de Leeuw, 1987). Factor-analytic models are preferable when constructs are multidimensional (e.g., somatic, cognitive, emotion dimensions of depression) and items are factorially complex, which is often the case. Factor models also readily extend to first- and second-order latent constructs, whereas IRT models focus on first-order unidimensional latent constructs and estimate an item's measurement parameters in the context of one such construct at a time.

Replication and Generalizability: Considering Measurement and Design

Replication and extension of results across studies are essential for cumulative theory building in the developmental sciences. Study and cohort comparisons of models and results provide an important platform for evaluating hypotheses at all levels of analysis. Comparison across studies additionally provides an opportunity to understand how differences in research design, sample composition, measurements, and statistical analysis influence inferences regarding developmental and aging-related outcomes. A primary challenge is the comparability of outcomes and covariates based on measurement instruments that may differ in language, difficulty, number of items, type of items, range of measurement, and other properties. Comparison difficulties are further compounded by differences in sample composition (including different birth cohorts, cultures, and social systems), representativeness, and study quality.

For example, it can be difficult to gauge differences across studies from different historical periods, based on samples of different birth cohorts or countries, because the measures themselves differ. However, a majority of longitudinal studies permit comparison at the construct level. Measures can vary at a number of levels, and within a single nation large operational differences can be found (e.g., Wiener, Hanley, Clark, & Van Nostrand, 1990). These differences can be magnified in cross-cultural or cross-national data: Variation is inevitably introduced due to differences in language, administration, and item relevance. Furthermore, sampling characteristics can be strikingly different, such that results reflect expectations for different sections of the population. A balance must be found between optimal similarity of administration, similarity of meaning, and significance of meaning while at the same time avoiding unreasonable loss of information or lack of depth. These challenges must be addressed in a collaborative endeavor, but they are also critical to general development of the field, for without some means for comparing findings, research products lack validation (e.g., Curran & Hussong, 2009; Hofer & Piccinin, 2009).

Measurement Harmonization

An important aspect of quantitative comparison of results across studies that use different measures involves the harmonization of such measures. When measures are identical or sufficiently comparable across studies, direct analysis of raw data permits inferences regarding influences associated with rare events (i.e., incidence of diseases), provides increased power for the detection of associations and interactions, provides more reliable estimates of population-level change, and permits the test of hypotheses regarding possible sources of mixed findings (e.g., education differences) across studies.

For any harmonization procedure, a first step is to identify commonalities and develop rules or scoring criteria to permit quantitative comparison of estimates from the affiliated studies. In rule-based harmonization, scoring protocols are developed based on careful analysis of the question-and-response format (e.g., Fortier et al., 2010). For multiple-item measures, such as cognitive and personality constructs, psychometric harmonization procedures such as factorial invariance and IRT models are typically used (e.g., Curran et al., 2008; McArdle, Grimm, Hamagami, Bowles, & Meredith, 2009).

When identical measures are not available and harmonization is not possible because of insufficient item overlap, data may be compared at the level of a latent construct with an emphasis on pattern and magnitude of standardized effects (see, e.g., Thorvaldsson et al., 2011). Standardization to pseudocorrelation or *t*-scores may also be used (e.g., Tisak & Meredith, 1989), but this does not necessarily make measures quantitatively comparable. This type of harmonization can facilitate synthesis of results, permit sensitivity analysis within and across studies, and provide a basis for reconciliation of study differences.

Challenges and Future Directions

In this chapter, we outlined some of the challenges researchers face as they seek to describe and explain individual differences in patterns, predictors, and consequences of within-person change. Theoretically based decisions about measurement and design are essential for integrative lifespan developmental research with focus on nomothetic and idiosyncratic individual change over time. Identifying early life determinants of middle and later adulthood outcomes requires very long studies of the same individuals. Understanding within-day and day-to-day variation in cognition, stress, and health requires an intensive measurement design. The successive assessment of such bursts of measurements can provide the researcher opportunities to evaluate changes in within-person processes and intraindividual variability over long periods of time (e.g., Walls et al., Chapter 4, this volume). In all such cases, the integration of theory, design, measurement, and statistical analysis is foundational.

Future research will be strengthened by the use of intensive but minimally obtrusive measurements of individual behavior and physiology over long periods of time in order to permit sensitive detection of change from an individual's normative performance (level and variation about characteristic level). As discussed earlier, one approach to assessment is based on the measurement burst design, permitting statistical decomposition of learning and decay functions that overlie normative aging and that will be sensitive for detecting accelerated change due to pathological processes. The demands on the participants for such an intensive measurement study will be facilitated by self-administered assessments performed in the participants' homes, permitting intensive longitudinal data collection in large probability samples that are not constrained by geographical proximity to clinics and labs. Internet-based surveys and testing may also serve to minimize problems associated with an individual's relocation and help to circumvent the interval censoring problem endemic in more typical longitudinal assessments. The central objective is to optimize the design and analysis features for particular developmental research questions that will permit reliable and sensitive assessment of functioning, change in functioning, and key causal factors underlying short-term variation and long-term change.

Acknowledgments

This chapter was supported by National Institutes of Health Grant No. AG026453 and the Swedish Research Council.

References

Almeida, D. M., & Kessler, R. C. (1998). Everyday stressors and gender differences in daily distress. *Journal of Personality and Social Psychology, 75*, 670–680.

Almeida, D. M., & McDonald, D. (1998). Weekly rhythms of parents' work stress, home stress, and parent–adolescent tension. In A. C. Crouter & R. Larson (Eds.), *Temporal rhythms in adolescence: Clocks, calendars, and the coordination of daily life* (pp. 53–67). San Francisco: Jossey-Bass.

Anstey, K. J., Hofer, S. M., & Luszcz, M. A. (2003). A latent growth curve analysis of late life cognitive and sensory function over eight years: Evidence for specific and common factors underlying change. *Psychology and Aging, 18*, 714–726.

Bauer, D. J., & Cai, L. (2009). Consequences of unmodeled nonlinear effects in multilevel models. *Journal of Educational and Behavioral Statistics, 34*, 97–114.

Boker, S. M., Molenaar, P. C. M., & Nesselroade, J. R. (2009). Issues in intraindividual variability: Individual differences in equilibria and dynamics over multiple time scales. *Psychology and Aging, 24*, 858–862.

Bontempo, D. E., & Hofer, S. M. (2007). Assessing factorial invariance in cross-sectional and longitudinal studies. In A. D. Ong & M. H. M. van Dulmen (Eds.), *Oxford handbook of methods in positive psychology* (pp. 153–176). New York: Oxford University Press.

Curran, P. J., & Hussong, A. M. (2009). Integrative data analysis: The simultaneous analysis of multiple data sets. *Psychological Methods, 14*, 81–100.

Curran, P. J., Hussong, A. M., Cai, L., Huang, W., Chassin, L., Sher, K. J., et al. (2008). Pooling data from multiple prospective studies: The role of item response theory in integrative analysis. *Developmental Psychology, 44*, 365–380.

Eizenman, D. R., Nesselroade, J. R., Featherman, D. L., & Rowe, J. W. (1997). Intraindividual variability in perceived control in an older sample: The MacArthur Successful Aging Studies. *Psychology and Aging, 12*, 489–502.

Fortier, I., Burton, P. R., Robson, P. J., Ferretti, V., Little, J., L'Heureux, F., et al. (2010). Quality, quantity and harmony: The DataSHaPER approach to integrating data across bioclinical studies. *International Journal of Epidemiology, 39*, 1383–1393.

Gollob, H. F., & Reichardt, C. S. (1987). Taking account of time lags in causal models. *Child Development, 58*, 80–92.

Hofer, S. M., Flaherty, B. P., & Hoffman, L. (2006). Cross-sectional analysis of time-dependent data: Problems of mean-induced association in age-heterogeneous samples and an alternative method based on sequential narrow age-cohorts. *Multivariate Behavioral Research, 41*, 165–187.

Hofer, S. M., Gray, K. M., Piccinin, A. M., Mackinnon, A., Bontempo, D. E., Einfeld, S. L., et al. (2009). Correlated and coupled within-person change in emotional and behavioral disturbance in individuals with intellectual disability. *American Journal on Intellectual and Developmental Disabilities, 114*(5), 307–321.

Hofer, S. M., Horn, J. L., & Eber, H. W. (1997). A robust five-factor structure of the 16PF: Evidence from independent rotation and confirmatory factorial invariance procedures. *Personality and Individual Differences, 23*, 247–269.

Hofer, S. M., & Piccinin, A. M. (2009). Integrative data analysis through coordination of measurement and analysis protocol across independent longitudinal studies. *Psychological Methods, 14*, 150–164.

Hofer, S. M., & Piccinin, A. M. (2010). Toward an integrative science of life-span development and aging. *Journals of Gerontology: Series B. Psychological Sciences and Social Sciences, 65B*(3), 269–278.

Hofer, S. M., & Sliwinski, M. J. (2001). Understanding ageing: An evaluation of research designs for assessing the interdependence of ageing-related changes. *Gerontology, 47*, 341–352.

Hofer, S. M., & Sliwinski, M. J. (2006). Design and analysis of longitudinal studies of aging. In J. E. Birren & K. W. Schaie (Eds.), *Handbook of the psychology of aging* (6th ed., pp. 15–37). San Diego, CA: Academic Press.

Horn, J. (1972). State, trait and change dimensions of intelligence. *British Journal of Educational Psychology, 42*, 159–185.

Hultsch, D. F., Hertzog, C., Small, B. J., McDonald-Miszczk, L., & Dixon, R. A. (1992). Short-term longitudinal change in cognitive performance in later life. *Psychology and Aging, 7*, 571–584.

Johansson, B., Hofer, S. M., Allaire, J. C., Maldonado-Molina, M., Piccinin, A. M., Berg, S., et al. (2004). Change in memory and cognitive functioning in the oldest-old: The effects of proximity to death in genetically related individuals over a six-year period. *Psychology and Aging, 19*, 145–156.

Kraemer, H. C., Yesavage, J. A., Taylor, J. L., & Kupfer, D. (2000). How can we learn about developmental processes from cross-sectional studies, or can we? *American Journal of Psychiatry, 157,* 163–171.

Kurland, B. F., Johnson, L. L., Egleston, B. L., & Diehr, P. H. (2009). Longitudinal data with follow-up truncated by death: Match the analysis method to research aims. *Statistical Science, 24,* 211–222.

Lerner, R. M., Schwartz, S. J., & Phelps, E. (2009). Problematics of time and timing in the longitudinal study of human development: Theoretical and methodological issues. *Human Development, 52,* 44–68.

Lindenberger, U., & Baltes, P. B. (1994). Sensory functioning and intelligence in old age: A strong connection. *Psychology and Aging, 9,* 339–355.

Lindenberger, U., & Ghisletta, P. (2009). Cognitive and sensory declines in old age: Gauging the evidence for a common cause. *Psychology and Aging, 24,* 1–16.

Little, T. D. (1997). Mean and covariance structures (MACS) analyses of cross-cultural data: Practical and theoretical issues. *Multivariate Behavioral Research, 32,* 53–76.

Little, T. D., Card, N. A., Slegers, D. W., & Ledford, E. C. (2007). Representing contextual effects in multiple-group MACS models. In T. D. Little, J. A. Bovaird, & N. A. Card (Eds.), *Modeling contextual effects in longitudinal studies* (pp. 121–147). Mahwah, NJ: Erlbaum.

Martin, M., & Hofer, S. M. (2004). Intraindividual variability, change, and aging: Conceptual and analytical issues. *Gerontology, 50,* 7–11.

McArdle, J. J., Ferrer-Caja, E., Hamagami, F., & Woodcock, W. (2002). Comparative longitudinal structural analyses of growth and decline of multiple intellectual abilities over life span. *Developmental Psychology, 38,* 115–142.

McArdle, J. J., Grimm, K. J., Hamagami, F., Bowles, R. P., & Meredith, W. (2009). Modeling life-span growth curves of cognition using longitudinal data with multiple samples and changing scales of measurements. *Psychological Methods, 14,* 126–149.

McArdle, J. J., & Woodcock, R. W. (1997). Expanding test–retest designs to include developmental time-lag components. *Psychological Methods, 4,* 403–435.

Meredith, W. (1993). Measurement invariance, factor analysis and factorial invariance. *Psychometrika, 58*(4), 525–543.

Meredith, W., & Horn, J. (2001). The role of factorial invariance in modeling growth and change. In L. M. Collins (Ed.), *New methods for the analysis of change* (pp. 203–240). Washington, DC: American Psychological Association.

Millsap, R. E., & Yun-Tein, J. (2004). Assessing factorial invariance in ordered-categorical measures. *Multivariate Behavioral Research, 39,* 479–515.

Molenaar, P. C. M. (2008). Consequences of the ergodic theorems for classical test theory, factor analysis, and the analysis of developmental processes. In S. M. Hofer & D. F. Alwin (Eds.), *Handbook of cognitive aging* (pp. 90–104). Thousand Oaks, CA: Sage.

Molenaar, P. C. M., Huizenga, H. M., & Nesselroade, J. R. (2003). The relationship between the structure of interindividual and intraindividual variability: A theoretical and empirical vindication of developmental systems theory. In U. M. Staudinger & U. Lindenberger (Eds.), *Understanding human development: Dialogues with lifespan psychology* (pp. 339–360). Dordrecht, The Netherlands: Kluwer Academic.

Morgan, S. L., & Winship, C. (2007). *Counterfactuals and causal inference.* New York: Cambridge University Press.

Moskowitz, D. S., Russell, J. J., Sadikaj, G., & Sutton, R. (2009). Measuring people intensively. *Canadian Psychology, 50,* 131–140.

Muthén, B. O., & Asparouhov, T. (2002, December 9). Latent variable analysis with categorical outcomes: Multiple-group and growth modeling in Mplus [Mplus Web Notes: No. 4, Version 5]. Retrieved January 20, 2004, from *www.statmodel.com/mplus/examples/webnotes/CatMGLong.pdf.*

Neiss, M., & Almeida, D. M. (2004). Age differences in the heritability of mean and intraindividual variation of psychological distress. *Gerontology, 50*, 22–27.
Nesselroade, J. R. (1991). The warp and woof of the developmental fabric. In R. Downs, L. Liben, & D. S. Palermo (Eds.), *Visions of aesthetics, the environment, and development: The legacy of Joachim F. Wohwill* (pp. 213–240). Hillsdale, NJ: Erlbaum.
Nesselroade, J. R. (2001). Intraindividual variability in development within and between individuals. *European Psychologist, 6*, 187–193.
Nesselroade, J. R. (2004). Intraindividual variability and short-term change. *Gerontology, 50*, 44–47.
Newell, K., Liu, Y., & Meyer-Kress, G. (2001). Time scales in motor learning and development. *Psychological Review, 108*, 57–82.
Pavel, M., Jimison, H. B., Hayes, T. L., Kaye, J., Dishman, E., Wild, K., et al. (2008). Continuous, unobtrusive monitoring for the assessment of cognitive function. In S. M. Hofer & D. F. Alwin (Eds.), *Handbook of cognitive aging: Interdisciplinary perspectives* (pp. 524–543). Thousand Oaks, CA: Sage.
Rabbitt, P., Diggle, P., Smith, D., Holland, F., & McInnes, L. (2001). Identifying and separating the effects of practice and of cognitive ageing during a large longitudinal study of elderly community residents. *Neuropsychologia, 39*, 532–543.
Reise, S. P., Widaman, K. F., & Pugh, R. H. (1993). Confirmatory factor analysis and item response theory: Two approaches for exploring measurement invariance. *Psychological Bulletin, 114*(3), 552–566.
Rogosa, D. R. (1980). A critique of cross-lagged correlation. *Psychological Bulletin, 88*, 245–258.
Rönnlund, M., & Nilsson, L. G. (2008). The magnitude, generality, and determinants of Flynn effects on forms of declarative memory and visuospatial ability: Time-sequential analyses of data from a Swedish cohort study. *Intelligence, 36*, 192–209.
Rönnlund, M., Nyberg, L., Bäckman, L., & Nilsson, L. G. (2005). Stability, growth, and decline in adult life span development of declarative memory: Cross-sectional and longitudinal data from a population-based study. *Psychology and Aging, 20*, 3–18.
Salthouse, T. A. (2009). When does age-related cognitive decline begin? *Neurobiology of Aging, 30*, 507–514.
Schaie, K. W. (1988). Internal validity threats in studies of adult cognitive development. In M. L. Howe & C. J. Brainerd (Eds.), *Cognitive development in adulthood: Progress in cognitive development research* (pp. 241–272). New York: Springer-Verlag.
Schaie, K. W. (2008). Historical processes of patterns of cognitive aging. In S. M. Hofer & D. F. Alwin (Eds.), *Handbook of cognitive aging* (pp. 368–383). Thousand Oaks, CA: Sage.
Schaie, K. W., & Hofer, S. M. (2001). Longitudinal studies in aging research. In J. E. Birren & K. W. Schaie (Eds.), *Handbook of the psychology of aging* (5th ed., pp. 53–77). San Diego, CA: Academic Press.
Sliwinski, M. J. (2008). Measurement-burst designs for social health research. *Social and Personality Psychology Compass, 2*(1), 245–261.
Sliwinski, M., & Buschke, H. (1999). Cross-sectional and longitudinal relationships among age, memory and processing speed. *Psychology and Aging, 14*, 18–33.
Sliwinski, M. J., Hofer, S. M., & Hall, C. (2003). Correlated and coupled cognitive change in older adults with and without clinical dementia. *Psychology and Aging, 18*, 672–683.
Sliwinski, M. J., Hoffman, L., & Hofer, S. M. (2010a). Evaluating convergence of within-person change and between-person age differences in age-heterogeneous longitudinal studies. *Research in Human Development, 7*, 45–60.
Sliwinski, M. J., Hoffman, L., & Hofer, S. M. (2010b). Modeling retest and aging effects in a measurement-burst design. In P. C. M. Molenaar & K. M. Newell (Eds.), *Individual pathways of change: Statistical models for analyzing learning and development* (pp. 37–50). Washington, DC: American Psychological Association.

Sliwinski, M. J., Smyth, J., Hofer, S. M., & Stawski, R. (2006). Intraindividual coupling of daily stress and cognition. *Psychology and Aging, 21*, 545–557.

Takane, Y., & de Leeuw, J. (1987). On the relationship between item response theory and factor analysis of discretized variables. *Psychometrika, 52*, 393–408.

Thorvaldsson, V., Hofer, S. M., Berg, S., & Johansson, B. (2006). Effects of repeated testing in a longitudinal age-homogeneous study of cognitive aging. *Journal of Gerontology: Psychological Sciences, 61B*, P348–P354.

Thorvaldsson, V., Hofer, S. M., Hassing, L., & Johansson, B. (2008). Cognitive change as conditional on age heterogeneity in onset of mortality-related processes and repeated testing effects. In S. M. Hofer & D. F. Alwin (Eds.), *Handbook on cognitive aging: Interdisciplinary perspectives* (pp. 284–297). Thousand Oaks, CA: Sage.

Thorvaldsson, V., MacDonald, S. W. S., Fratiglioni, L., Winblad, B., Kivipelto, M., Laukka, E. J., et al. (2011). Onset and rate of cognitive change before dementia diagnosis: Findings from two Swedish population-based longitudinal studies. *Journal of the International Neuropsychological Society, 17*, 154–162.

Tisak, J., & Meredith, W. (1989). Exploratory longitudinal factor analysis in multiple populations. *Psychometrika, 54*, 261–281.

Verhaeghen, P., & Salthouse, T. A. (1997). Meta-analyses of age–cognition relations in adulthood: Estimates of linear and nonlinear age effects and structural models. *Psychological Bulletin, 122*, 231–249.

Widaman, K. F., & Reise, S. P. (1997). Exploring the measurement invariance of psychological instruments: Applications in the substance use domain. In K. J. Bryant & M. Windle (Eds.), *The science of prevention: Methodological advances from alcohol and substance abuse research* (pp. 281–324). Washington, DC: American Psychological Association.

Wiener, J. M., Hanley, R. J., Clark, R., & Van Nostrand, J. F. (1990). Measuring the activities of daily living: Comparisons across national surveys. *Journal of Gerontology: Social Sciences, 45*(6), S229–S237.

Wilson, R. S., Beckett, L. A., Barnes, L. L., Schneider, J. A., Bach, J., Evans, D. A., et al. (2002). Individual differences in rates of change in cognitive abilities of older persons. *Psychology and Aging, 17*, 179–193.

Wohlwill, J. (1970). Methodology and research strategy in the study of developmental change. In L. R. Goulet & P. B. Baltes (Eds.), *Life-span developmental psychology: Research and theory* (pp. 149–191). New York: Academic Press.

Wohlwill, J. F. (1973). *The study of behavioral development*. New York: Academic Press.

Zimprich, D., & Martin, M. (2002). Can longitudinal changes in processing speed explain longitudinal age changes in fluid intelligence? *Psychology and Aging, 17*, 690–695.

CHAPTER 2

Causal Inference, Identification, and Plausibility

E. MICHAEL FOSTER

Causal inference involves inferring cause-and-effect relationships from associations in observational data (i.e., outside of randomization). Causal inference lies at the heart of developmental science (Foster, 2010a; Rutter, 2007). Many developmentalists seek not only to understand but also to foster children's development. Although noble, this aim poses an enormous scientific challenge. In particular, achieving this goal requires knowledge of cause-and-effect relationships. The question is not whether a risk is associated with an outcome but whether changing or manipulating the risk will alter the outcome. This issue is especially challenging because many developmental questions involve putative risks, exposures, conditions, or characteristics that vary from one child to the next but to which individuals cannot be randomly assigned.

For example, a key developmental question involves the effect on children's development of growing up in a single-parent family (e.g., Foster & Kalil, 2007; McLanahan & Sandefur, 1994). Clearly, growing up in such circumstances is associated with worse developmental outcomes. Whether that relationship is causal—whether the child would have actually fared better had the father been at home—is much less certain (Foster & Kalil, 2007). It depends on a "counterfactual," a state of the world that did not occur.

The reader will quickly recognize that many proxies are available for the counterfactual outcome. These might include developmental outcomes for otherwise similar children living with both parents. Or one might consider how the child was faring during a period when the child's father was in the household. Comparisons across time or children—that is, associations—represent a substitute for the comparisons of interest across potential outcomes. Other possibilities are more subtle—we might compare children living in different states in which the penalties for marriage (e.g., reductions in welfare payments) differ and affect the likelihood of marriage. The methodology of causal inference considers the assumptions required to move from these associations to questions of cause and effect.

Central Issues

Causal inference is a set of tools for distinguishing associations from cause-and-effect relationships or, rather, inferring the latter from the former. Researchers across a range of fields have made considerable progress in developing methodology for causal inference. To some extent, improvements in causal inference involve better statistical tools (e.g., propensity scores). To a large degree, these improvements also reflect and require better causal thinking—for example, conceptualization of the nature of causal inference. For example, researchers now better understand how an idiosyncratic sample compromises not only external but also internal validity. Causal inference based on such samples is damaged in ways that are difficult to repair (Hernan, Hernandez-Diaz, & Robins, 2004). Researchers also better understand the nature of some important questions. As discussed later, for example, researchers now better understand the challenges of mediation in a causal inference framework (Sobel, 2008).

These improvements reflect the two-pronged nature of causal inference. To move from association to causal relationships involves both careful thinking and sound statistical methodology (Pearl, 2009). Using an advanced statistical tool in an analysis with the wrong set of covariates still produces bad causal inference.

Causal thinking is essential to causal inference because the fundamental problem of causal inference is really a matter of reasoning—or, more specifically, "identification" (Greenland & Morgenstern, 2001; Heckman & Vytlacil, 2007; Rubin, 2005). That problem reflects the fact that a child will experience different outcomes depending on the level of exposure, yet only one exposure and one outcome are observed. In the simplest case, there are two potential outcomes corresponding to whether the individual is exposed or not—how the child will fare (1) if living with his or her father or (2) if not. The effect of exposure is the difference between the two, but of course we observe only one of these at a point in time for a given child. In other words, we have one known and two unknowns (the two potential outcomes); in such situations, the statistical model is said to be "underidentified."

One needs to add enough logical structure to the problem to identify the model. One possibility is to identify a group of individuals not exposed who are "otherwise comparable" and to compare the two groups. Another possibility is to examine the individual's outcome prior to being exposed. The key point is that even such a within-person comparison involves an assumption—such as that the individual's outcome would not have changed in the absence of exposure.

This chapter reviews methods old and new in terms of the underlying assumptions required for causal inference. The focus is on the issue of identification: What are the assumptions required to produce an estimate of the effect of an exposure or treatment? The chapter devotes relatively little space to differences in alternative methodologies; that information is available elsewhere. (For a review, see Heckman & Vytlacil, 2007, or, in a more psychologist-friendly format, Foster, 2010a.) The chapter emphasizes one key assumption, ignorability or exchangeability, that differentiates alternative approaches. For that reason, the chapter largely ignores technical details of estimation.

Conceptual Principles and Statistical Assumptions

Potential Outcomes Framework

The counterfactual lies at the heart of causal inference: What would happen to an individual or entity if we changed his or her exposure? This perspective defines the effect of interest: the difference between what did happen and what would have happened had the individual not experienced the treatment. A comparison of these "potential outcomes" determines the effect of exposure. Only one potential outcome is observed, and the others represent "counterfactuals."

Even in instances in which the exposure cannot be manipulated (a person's race or gender), causal inference is still possible, and it rests on the existence of a counterfactual. To capture the effect of a child's race, one has to assess how that child would have fared if he or she had been born black instead of white, for instance. Researchers are not in complete agreement about this point. Some would argue that causal inference is not possible if a treatment cannot be manipulated (Holland, 1986). On the other hand, some experts such as Pearl clearly take it as a given that one could look at the effects of gender (Pearl, 2000).

We can express the counterfactual more formally using the potential outcomes framework (Holland, 1986; Rubin, 2005). In that framework, one is interested in a treatment (or exposure or characteristic) (D) and some outcome (Y). $D = 1$ or 0 for the treated and untreated groups, respectively. For each individual, one can think of him or her as having two possible outcomes Y_1 and Y_0, corresponding to his or her outcomes if treated or not. (In some instances, researchers refer to $Y_{0,i}$ as $Y_i(0)$. We use notation of this sort when we address mediation later.)

One can characterize each individual by three variables (Y_0, Y_1, D)—the outcome if treated, if not treated, and the treatment status. The fundamental problem is that we do not observe (the joint distribution of) all three random variables. Rather, we observe D for each individual (was he or she treated or not) and either Y_1 or Y_0 for the treated ($D = 1$) and untreated ($D = 0$), respectively. One can write that $Y_{obs} = (D^*Y_1)+((1-D)^*Y_0)$, where Y_{obs} is the observed outcome.

We have omitted a person subscript to this point, but these outcomes differ across individuals, both because individuals differ in the treatment they receive and because of other factors (differentiating even those who receive the same treatment). What we would like to know is the treatment effect—that is, $\tau_i = Y_{1,\mathrm{i}} - Y_{0,i}$—ideally for every individual i. We cannot calculate this term for a given person because we observe only one of them.

Can we get traction on this problem if we reduce our goal? What if we wanted to know the mean of the distribution of effects, $\tau = E[Y_{1,i} - Y_{0,i}] = E[Y_{1,i}] - E[Y_{0,i}]$? The problem is that neither of the two terms is observed even if we have multiple individuals who are and are not exposed. In particular, we observe not $E[Y_{1,i}]$ but $E[Y_{1,i}|D_i = 1]$ and not $E[Y_{0,i}]$ but $E[Y_{0,i}|D_i = 0]$. One sees the outcome under treatment only for those treated and the converse for untreated individuals. The difference between these two terms is an association.

These quantities are related to the terms of interest,

$$E[Y_{1,i}] = p(D_i = 1)E[Y_{1,i}|D_i = 1] + p(D_i = 0)\mathbf{E}[\mathbf{Y}_{1,\mathrm{i}}|\mathbf{D}_\mathrm{i} = \mathbf{0}]. \quad \mathbf{(2.1)}$$

The average outcome for all individuals, were they all treated, is the weighted average of the treated outcome for those who received treatment and for those who did not. The weights are the proportions of the sample that do and do not receive treatment. The emboldened term is unobserved; it is the average of a counterfactual value, the outcome in the treated state for those who were not actually treated. That expectation and the expression as a whole cannot be calculated without some additional assumptions. *This problem is the fundamental problem of causal inference.*

Similarly,

$$E[Y_{0,i}] = p(D_i = 1)\mathbf{E[Y_{0,i}|D_i = 1]} + p(D_i = 0)E[Y_{0,i}|D_i = 0]. \quad \textbf{(2.2)}$$

The emboldened term is again unobserved—we do not know the average untreated outcome for the individuals who received treatment.

Given these two terms, one can rewrite τ as

$$\begin{aligned}\tau = (&p(D_i = 1)E[Y_{1,i}|D_i = 1] + p(D_i = 0)\mathbf{E[Y_{1,i}|D_i = 0]}) - \\ (&p(D_i = 1)\mathbf{E[Y_{0,i}|D_i = 1]} + p(D_i = 0)E[Y_{0,i}|D_i = 0]).\end{aligned} \quad \textbf{(2.3)}$$

One can rewrite this term as

$$\begin{aligned}\tau = (&p(D_i = 1)\big[E[Y_{1,i}|D_i = 1] - \mathbf{E[Y_{1,i}|D_i = 1]}\big] + \\ &p(D_i = 0)\big[\mathbf{E[Y_{1,i}|D_i = 0]} - E[Y_{0,i}|D_i = 0]\big].\end{aligned} \quad \textbf{(2.4)}$$

The treatment effect is the weighted sum of the treatment effects for those treated and those not treated. We label the first the "average effect of treatment for the treated" (ATT) and the second "average effect of treatment on the untreated" (ATU). τ is labeled the "average treatment effect" (ATE).

If one were interested in the effect of family structure on a child's development, the ATT would represent the effect of living in a female-headed family for those children living in such families. For these children, the counterfactual represents life in a two-parent family. Conversely, the ATU is the effect for children living in two-parent families. The two effects might differ depending on the presence or absence of factors that amplify or dampen the effect of family structure. For example, the ATT would be smaller than the ATU if (1) the benefits of a father are especially great for children of less educated mothers and (2) less educated women are more likely to form single-parent families. An important issue is whether the decision to form a single-parent family reflects the likely impact on the child—additional challenges arise if decisions about family structure reflect the consequences.

The ATE is "not identified." Equation 2.4 represents one equation but includes two unknowns; it is not possible to generate a unique estimate of the treatment effect. This problem would exist no matter the sample size; it is a problem of logic rather than an empirical problem per se.

At this point, we have reached a dead end unless we add more structure to the problem. Such structure will involve one or more additional assumptions about treatment assignment and perhaps more data. Such data are likely especially useful when they are collected from a study design tailored to answer the causal question of interest.

Before proceeding, we want to make clear three assumptions we have made implicitly so far. The first assumption is the stable unit treatment value assumption (SUTVA;

Rubin, 1980). This assumption requires that one's counterfactual states ($Y_{0,i}$ and $Y_{1,i}$) do not depend on the treatment status of other individuals. One can note that in the preceding math, there is no "interference" among individuals: an individual's outcome Y_i does not depend on the treatment received by person j. As discussed later, many problems in developmental science may not fit this assumption.

The second assumption is positivity. This assumption requires that the probability that a given individual receives *each* level of treatment is positive for every combination of treatment and covariates. This assumption eliminates illogical possibilities, such as men developing uterine cancer. As discussed later, this assumption has an empirical counterpart.

A third assumption is consistency (Cole & Frangakis, 2008). This assumption implies that the outcome of treatment does not depend on the assignment mechanism. For example, this assumption means that the returns from enrolling a child in daycare are the same for all, regardless of the mix of incentives that led to that choice. Some families may enroll their children because of a government subsidy. On the other hand, others may enroll because they perceive large benefits. Consistency means that the benefits of early childhood education do not depend on the mix of incentives.

Next we consider two specific methodological approaches (random assignment and ordinary regression) and highlight the value of these approaches from the perspective of identification—that is, the features of a design or an analysis that allow one to estimate the effect of treatment.

The Value of Random Assignment

What if we could randomly assign exposure? Random assignment solves the identification problem (Rosenberger & Lachin, 2002). We can replace the unknowns in the preceding with terms we can calculate. In particular, in our equations, we can freely substitute $E[Y_{0,i}|D_i = 0]$ for $E[Y_{0,i}|D_i = 1]$ and $E[Y_{1,i}|D_i = 1]$ for $E[Y_{1,i}|D_i = 0]$. The only remaining uncertainty is statistical uncertainty stemming from sampling. The uncertainty due to the treatment mechanism no longer exists; that mechanism can be effectively ignored.

The essence of random assignment is exchangeability—we can exchange the experiences of individuals not receiving the treatment (which are observed) for those of individuals currently receiving treatment were they not to receive treatment (which is not observed). We can be confident that no confounding occurs—no possibility exists of confusing the effect of treatment with preexisting differences among individuals actually receiving different treatments. This lack of confounding is true for both the variables *we can measure and those we cannot or have not* (Rosenberger & Lachin, 2002). The latter involves unobserved confounding, and removing it is among the principal benefits of randomization.

Regression and Causal Inference

As noted, in many instances, one cannot randomize individuals to exposures of interest. The solution is to make stronger *assumptions* about treatment assignment. One such assumption is ignorability, or the ignorable treatment assumption. Ignorability *assumes* that—among individuals with an equivalent profile of covariates—treatment assignment is *as if* random assignment spontaneously occurred. A key point is that ignorability is now an assumption rather than a feature of the design, as it would be in random assignment.

As discussed in detail later, ordinary regression represents a package of assumptions, but at its most basic level, it is a form of matching or stratification. One essentially calculates the effect of an exposure within strata or matched groups and then obtains an overall estimate of the effect of that exposure by combining the different estimates. For example, suppose one had a regression with an outcome explained by exposure (living in a single-parent family or not) and a covariate such as family income. In that case, regression calculates the difference between the exposed and not exposed among those in a given income category. It then combines these estimates into an overall estimate of the effect of family structure. It is in that sense that regression controls for a covariate.

From a causal inference perspective, the key feature of regression is the ignorability assumption. Regression embodies this assumption by assuming that the covariates (including exposure) are uncorrelated with the unobserved determinants of the outcome (i.e., the error term). This assumption is referred to in several ways, such as "no unobserved confounding" or "selection on the observables (only)" (Angrist & Pischke, 2008; Lee, 2005). These assumptions are effectively equivalent to ignorability and exchangeability. In the case of family structure, the regression is assuming that from the perspective of children's outcomes, family structure is as if randomly assigned among those at the same income level. That is, within an income stratum, the association between family structure and children's outcomes reflects only the effect of the former on the latter.

The ignorability assumption can be written in different ways, but in our framework, the assumption stipulates that

$$E[Y_{1,i}|X_i = x, d_i = 0] = E[Y_{1,i}|X_i = x, d_i = 1]. \quad \textbf{(2.5)}$$

Conditional on the set of covariates, X, the value of the outcome at a level of treatment is unrelated to treatment chosen. In essence, we can exchange the expectation we do not observe (the left-hand side) with one we do observe (the right-hand side).

Note that the specific form of ignorability depends on the treatment effect of interest. Equation (2.5) is enough to identify the ATU (i.e., to provide a unique estimate). On the other hand, an analogous equality

$$E[Y_{0,i}|X_i = x, d_i = 0] = E[Y_{0,i}|X_i = x, d_i = 1] \quad \textbf{(2.6)}$$

is required to estimate ATT. Both are required to estimate ATE.

How specifically does ordinary regression handle these assumptions? At this point, regression adds assumptions that give the model a specific structure. In particular, it specifies the expectations in equations such as (2.6) as a linear function of the covariates included. In doing so, it handles several potential problems seamlessly. For example, suppose there are some values of the X variable for which there are few or even no observations in the exposed or comparison group. In that case, regression effectively fits a line to the available observations and extrapolates the counterfactual expectation along that line.

Regression also effectively combines the stratum-specific estimates of the effect of the exposure. In particular, the regression estimate is the weighted within-strata between-group difference. The weights reflect not only the distribution of cases across the strata (as they would to estimate one of the three treatment effects of interest) but also an added factor—the variance of the treatment within strata. Strata in which the observations are split equally between the treatment and comparison groups have greater weight. This feature of the model is useful for explaining the variance in the outcome but has implications for understanding the effect of treatment.

As a result, the regression estimate can differ quite a bit from the ATE, ATT, and ATU. In some instances, the results might be quite surprising or even undesirable. For example, consider the effect of family structure on child outcomes controlling for family income. In that case, low-income strata in which single-parent families are the norm would contribute little to the overall estimated effect of family structure. These are just the families of greatest interest in many instances.

Alternatives to Regression and the Propensity Score

One might form conditional expectations (such as Equation 2.5) in any of several ways, such as matching. If one can find cases that have similar values for the covariates, one can assume that individuals experiencing the exposure would look like their matches among those not exposed (and vice versa). To estimate the effect of exposure, we can calculate the difference between the matched cases. One then can average those effects to compute the overall effect of treatment.

Suppose that boys were more likely to be exposed to a treatment of interest. In that case, gender is potentially confounded with the effect of the exposure. As a remedy, one might match exposed and comparison cases on gender and calculate treatment effects among boys and girls separately. One then could combine these estimates into an overall effect of exposure.

Matching has several advantages, such as the absence of any presumed relationship between the outcome and the variables used to match. Problems arise, however, when we want to match on multiple variables and/or in samples of moderate size. Seldom is a sample large enough to match individuals on exact values of a large number of variables. In that case, matching involves finding cases that are "close" to each other, and the wrinkle involves a definition of "close." The latter involves specifying a weight function that combines differences across variables into a measure of closeness.

The propensity score is the predicted probability of exposure, and it is here that one can see the benefits of methodology that incorporates it. The propensity score is a statistical convenience, no more and no less, and its key properties are mechanical. The propensity score is the predicted probability of receiving the treatment or exposure. One can calculate the propensity score in a variety of ways, but most common is using a parametric model (such as logistic regression). The propensity score is a weighted sum of the covariates in which the weighting reflects the strength of the association between the covariates and treatment status—that is, the potential for the covariates to confound the relationship between exposure and the outcome. When conditioning on the propensity score, any remaining between-group variation in the covariates included is due to chance alone (Rosenbaum & Rubin, 1983).

A major advantage of the propensity score is that it eliminates the practical problem of matching on multiple variables. It also has other benefits in terms of diagnosing potential problems with regression. For example, regression essentially extrapolates the counterfactual for individuals whose profile of covariates makes them unique or nearly so to the exposed or comparison group. Regression generally accomplishes this task without alerting the researcher. In contrast, the propensity score makes these cases easy to identify—the propensity score for these individuals is close to 0 or 1. In such an instance, there are several alternatives, such as dropping these cases and describing them separately (Rosenbaum & Rubin, 1985). However one resolves the problem, the ability to identify such cases is a key contribution of the propensity score. (For a fuller discussion of the benefits of the propensity score, see Foster, 2010a; Morgan & Winship, 2007.)

In sum, although propensity score methods have advantages over regression, the key is that these methods all assume ignorability.

Replacing Ignorability

Is ignorability reasonable? Because this assumption primarily involves the behavior of unobserved characteristics—how they influence the exposure and the outcome—the assumption cannot be assessed empirically. However, one can gauge its plausibility based on what one knows about the exposure and its determinants. For example, research on the effects of breastfeeding often does not include mother's IQ as a covariate (Jiang & Foster, in press). Such an omitted variable seems likely to influence many outcomes of interest, and in that case, IQ represents an omitted confounder; ignorability is violated. If ignorability is unreasonable, one cannot simply relax the assumption. From an identification perspective, one can see that it can be replaced only with another assumption(s). One strategy is instrumental variables estimation.

Instrumental variables estimation (IVE) has a long history in statistics and econometrics and allows one to estimate the effect of a treatment even with unobserved confounding. The key feature of the instrumental variable is that it influences exposure but does not influence the outcome directly—that is, the effect of the instrumental variable on the outcome is fully mediated.

Consider again the effect of living in a single-parent family. Suppose that after adjusting for many potential confounders, one still suspects that unobserved confounding affects comparisons of children living in single- and two-parent families. A possible strategy would involve finding a potential determinant of marital decisions that does not influence child outcomes directly, such as elimination of the marriage penalty in the tax code. Suppose one has two waves of data involving families of both types—one collected when the marriage penalty was in force, the other after its repeal. IVE would involve comparing child outcomes before and after the marriage penalty *without regard to their family structure*. Similarly, one might compare family structure before and after the repeal. The IVE is the ratio of these two effects.

Suppose that prior to the repeal, the average score on a test of academic performance in our sample was 108; after repeal, 110. Suppose that in the first year of the study, 42% of the sample lived with single parents; after repeal, 38%. The implied IVE is (110 – 108)/(.38 – .42) = –2/.04 = 50 points. Whether this result is large or small depends on other factors, such as the standard deviation of the scores. This calculation depends critically on the assumed structure of the relationships—namely, that the effect of the repeal is fully mediated. This means that for those families in which there was no change in family structure, there was no effect of the repeal. In that case, 96% of the sample would experience no change in score; 4% would experience the effect of family structure, and the overall effect would be 2 points. The implied relationship is

$$(.96*0)+(.04*\begin{bmatrix}\text{Effect of}\\ \text{family structure}\end{bmatrix})=2\cdot$$

One also can see that the model assumes that the reduction from 42% to 38% involves only 4% of the sample actually changing exposure.[1]

How is the effect of interest identified? This approach does not assume that ignorability applies to family structure. However, the model does assume that comparisons before and after the repeal do reveal the effect of the repeal itself—that there are no unobserved confounders affecting that comparison. In the case at hand, such confounding might involve other changes in children's environment that occurred coincident with the repeal of the marriage penalty.

More Challenging Identification Problems: Mediation

Identification poses challenges for causal inference, and more complex causal questions pose greater challenges of identification. Mediation is an instance in which one is interested not only in the effect of an exposure but also in understanding the mechanism by which it exerts its influence. For example, living in a single-parent family may influence adolescents' behavior through monitoring; two parents may be better able to sanction undesirable behavior (McLanahan & Sandefur, 1994). Another possible mechanism or mediator could be poverty. Single-parent families often live in poverty, and that fact alone will shape children's outcomes. The extent to which monitoring and poverty status "explain" or account for the effect of family structure may be of interest.

Mediation, however, poses identification challenges of its own. In effect, the mediator defines a new layer of counterfactuals. For each child, only one exposure and one value of the mediator is observed; as a result, one must think about how the child would have fared not just in a different type of family structure but also at a different value for the mediator. For example, one might be interested in how a child living with a poor single mother would have fared were he or she living in a (1) nonpoor single-parent family or (2) a poor two-parent family. Comparisons of the child's actual status with the latter would indicate the "direct" effect of family structure (i.e., the effect of exposure with the mediator unchanging). In this framework, one can see that there are multiple direct effects of interest. For example, one might consider the effect of family structure either for the poor or the nonpoor (Vanderweele, 2008). Comparisons with the former would reveal the effect of the mediator itself. Combined with the effect of family structure on poverty status, one could calculate an indirect effect of family structure mediated by poverty status.

Using regression to tackle this problem will be familiar to many readers. One simply would include family structure and poverty status as regressors. The literature in psychology and elsewhere is filled with studies of mediation of this sort, and a seminal article by Baron and Kenny has been cited over 18,000 times (Baron & Kenny, 1986). Over time, this literature has grown to include tests with better statistical properties and a broader array of data structures (such as multilevel models) (Bauer, Preacher, & Gil, 2006).

[1]The data reveal a net change of only 4%, but 6% of the sample might have moved into a two-parent family and 2% moved the other way. IVE assumes that the instrumental variable makes exposure more (or less) likely for all sample members. This assumption is known as monotonicity (Imbens & Rubin, 1996).

This literature, however, makes a key, implicit assumption—that the mediator itself does not suffer from unobserved confounding (Sobel, 2008).[2] A regression analysis of poverty status as a mediator of family structure would assume that poverty is not correlated with unobserved determinants of the outcome. This assumption is clearly not self-evident; researchers have considered the degree to which poverty per se (i.e., the lack of material resources) is correlated with other, unmeasured qualities of the family (Mayer, 1997). If such unobserved confounding exists, the estimated effect of poverty status is biased, and the resulting direct and indirect effects of family structure are also incorrect.

Researchers analyzing data from intervention studies recognized this problem earlier than did those examining other exposures in observational data (Sheiner & Rubin, 1995). For example, the former might be interested in the mediating role of compliance with an intervention's requirements. That the mediator is not randomized—that is, it is affected potentially by unobserved confounding—stands in stark contrast to the exposure itself, which is randomly assigned.

To address this problem more formally, one can expand the counterfactual framework to include the mediator. One solution involves *principal strata*, a set of four counterfactual states defined by exposure and the mediator. In this case, the mediator is assumed to be dichotomous (Barnard, Frangakis, Hill, & Rubin, 2003; Frangakis & Rubin, 2002; Vanderweele, 2008). (See Table 2.1.) These four groups have been labeled to reflect the fact that they were developed in applications in which the mediator was compliance, but the basic statistical structure extends to any exposure and mediation. (In the case of family structure, poverty can be interpreted as "compliance"—i.e., as exposed to the presumed causal mechanism.)

As illustrated in Table 2.1, the first group is labeled "always"—those who comply whether they are exposed or not. In the case of family structure, these are children who are poor whether they live in single-parent or two-parent families. Similarly, one might define the "never" group as those who would not comply whether they are exposed or not. In the case of family structure, these would be children who would not be poor whether they lived in single- or two-parent households. Similarly, one can think of "compliers" as individuals who would comply—that is, they are exposed to the mediator if they are treated but not

TABLE 2.1. Principal Strata

	Probabilities		Potential outcomes	
Principal strata	Treated	Comparison	Treated	Comparison
Always	P_A	Q_A	$Y(1,1)_A$	$Y(0,1)_A$
Compliers	P_C	Q_C	$Y(1,1)_C$	$Y(0,0)_C$
Defiers	P_D	Q_D	$Y(1,0)_D$	$Y(0,1)_D$
Never	P_N	Q_N	$Y(1,0)_N$	$Y(0,0)_N$

Note. P_A refers to the probability of being treated (or exposed) and a member of the "always" strata. Q_A refers to the probability of not being treated and a member of that stratum.

[2] This approach makes an additional assumption as well that the mediating variable does not moderate the effect of the exposure or treatment. If it does, the standard strategy does not produce a decomposition of direct and indirect effects (Kaufman, MacLehose, & Kaufman, 2004).

otherwise. These are analogous to children who are poor in single-parent families but who would escape poverty if they lived in two-parent families. "Defiers" are those who comply if not exposed but do not if exposed. In our illustration, these are individuals who are poor in two-parent families but not in single-parent families. The principal strata define seven probabilities and eight expected values. (One can determine the eighth probability in the table from the other seven, as they sum to 1.) The expected values are denoted as $Y(E,M)$—the value of the outcome defined by exposure status and the mediator.

Two features of the table are evident. First, if all of these parameters could be estimated from the data, one could define the effects of interest. For example, one might use information on the "always" and "never" groups to examine the direct effects of the treatment (Vanderweele, 2008). One might ascertain indirect effects by comparing values of potential outcomes defined by both the exposure and the mediator *within subgroups defined by the principal strata*. For example, $Y(1,1)_A$ is the value of the outcome for individuals who were exposed and who experienced the mediator. The subscript A indicates that they are in the "always" group. Because these individuals always experience the mediator, the relevant comparison involves $Y(1,1)_A$ and $Y(0,1)_A$. Reflecting their status in the "always" group, the second term in the parentheses denoting mediator status is 1 in both instances. For these individuals, the only effects of exposure involve direct effects. One might compare potential outcomes for a different stratum in a similar manner. In the case of the compliers, the relevant terms are $Y(1,1)_C$ and $Y(0,0)_C$. The difference between these values reflects both direct and indirect effects of the exposure.

Second, once we recognize the available data (Table 2.2), one can see that the model is underidentified. We observe only seven pieces of data pertaining to a 2-by-2 table of Compliance × Exposure. Each cell has a mean and contains a proportion of the sample. Of course, one probability is again redundant: all individuals are in one of the four possible table cells.

The elements in the two tables are related, and those relationships are equations. For example:

$$Y_a = \frac{P_A}{P_A + P_C} Y(1,1)_A + \frac{P_C}{P_A + P_C} Y(1,1)_C$$

This equation reveals that the observed mean for treated (or exposed) individuals who comply is actually an average of two means for two groups, Always and Compliers (when treated). Without an additional assumption (such as randomization), there is no reason to assume that the two means involved are equal. This highlights a broader point: One has only 7 of these equations and 15 unknowns. *Without additional information, our model is underidentified. Indeed, we are in worse shape than the standard problem—we are "short" seven equations.*

TABLE 2.2. Observed Data

	Probabilities		Expected values	
	Comply	Not	Comply	Not
Exposed	P_a	P_b	Y_a	Y_b
Comparison	P_c	P_d	Y_c	Y_d

As with exposure itself, one can identify the model by adding information about the problem; that is, about the relationship between exposure, the mediator, and the outcome. For example, one might assume that there are no defiers—there are no children who are poor in two-parent families who would not be poor if in a single-parent family. This effectively deletes one row of Table 2.1 and eliminates four unknowns (P_D, Q_D, $Y(1,0)_D$ and $Y(0,1)_D$). The model now contains 11 unknowns.

This assumption is part of the standard solution in the clinical trials literature (labeled "principal stratification"). One also eliminates two parameters by assuming randomization. After eliminating the defiers, the left-hand panel of Table 2.1 represents a 3×2 contingency table. That table has 5 unique probabilities. With randomization (i.e., independence of the principal strata and the probability of exposure), one can characterize that table with the margins alone (that is, three probabilities). That eliminates two additional parameters. The model now includes only nine unknowns but still two more than we have pieces of data.

Finally, this solution assumes that the effect of the intervention is fully mediated by compliance; that is, if the intervention does not change compliance, then the intervention has no effect. That assumption implies that $Y(1,1)_A = Y(0,1)_A$ and $Y(1,0)_N = Y(0,0)_N$ and eliminates two parameters. Taken together, these assumptions eliminate eight unknowns, leaving seven equations, corresponding to the seven knowns. The former can be solved for the latter, and the model is identified.

Discussion

This chapter presents identification as the fundamental problem of causal inference. However, identification is not the only step. For example, ignorability can identify key parameters, but the validity of the assumption depends on the sensible choice of covariates to include (and exclude). Even before that stage of the analysis, careful consideration of the treatment or exposure of interest is essential. For example, one might want to distinguish among single- and two-parent families according to the presence of other relatives, such as a grandmother.

Identification and other decisions about the analysis choices are related and perhaps in conflict. Differentiating the exposure (as with grandparents) might make conceptual sense. However, as one considers more differentiated exposures, the exposure may involve more and more choices by the families involved. For example, one would have to consider why a grandmother had moved into the household in the first place. Perhaps that choice reflected unobserved factors influencing the child or even the child's behavior. Such possibilities make ignorability harder to justify.

Outside of random assignment, one cannot infer causal relationships from associations without additional assumptions. These should be tailored to the specifics of the problem of interest. Some would argue that the simpler the assumptions the better (Manski, 2007), but the tradeoff between simplicity and plausibility varies across disciplines. What seems clear is that the more complex the processes determining the treatment or exposure, the more carefully the trade-off between plausibility and complexity must be considered. Simple, plausible analyses may not be possible for very complex processes, such as exposures that evolve over time in response to the outcome of interest (Robins, 1997, 1999a, 1999b).

In many instances, developmental theory argues for exposures that are complex. In general, however, methodology in developmental psychology has lagged far behind the complexity of developmental thinking. For example, many developmental theories involve interactions among individuals; on the other hand, the vast majority of analyses assume linear relationships. Adding an interaction term only scratches the surface in terms of addressing the fundamental nonlinearities implied by theory. Similarly, causal inference is central to developmental psychology, yet very little of modern methodology has been applied. In many instances, the old methodology does not provide a less preferred answer. Rather, as in the case of time-varying confounding, standard methodology provides the wrong answer.

The complexity of the assumptions on which causality rests cannot be considered apart from the overall complexity of the analysis. A very elaborate measurement model may not be possible in IVE of nonlinear relationships. In that sense, the overall complexity of an analysis is constrained, and one must balance the costs and benefits of deploying complexity in alternative aspects of the model. Currently, one could argue that developmentalists are using complexity in the wrong places. Many models include elaborate specifications of latent classes or factors yet assume the simplest linear relationships among these constructs. These simple relationships are often quite structured in their timing and allow for no unobserved confounding anywhere in the model (Foster, 2010b).

In sum, careful thinking about identification represents the first step in better causal inference, and better causal inference offers the promise of better matching the results of analyses with the key questions in human development.

References

Angrist, J. D., & Pischke, J.-S. (2008). *Mostly harmless econometrics: An empiricist's companion.* Princeton, NJ: Princeton University Press.

Barnard, J., Frangakis, C. E., Hill, J. L., & Rubin, D. B. (2003). Principal stratification approach to broken randomized experiments: A case study of school choice vouchers in New York City. *Journal of the American Statistical Association, 98*, 299–323.

Baron, R. M., & Kenny, D. A. (1986). The moderator–mediator variable distinction in social psychological research: Conceptual, strategic, and statistical considerations. *Journal of Personality and Social Psychology, 51*(6), 1173–1182.

Bauer, D. J., Preacher, K. J., & Gil, K. M. (2006). Conceptualizing and testing random indirect effects and moderated mediation in multilevel models: New procedures and recommendations. *Psychological Methods, 11*(2), 142–163.

Cole, S. R., & Frangakis, C. E. (2008). *On the consistency statement in causal inference: A definition or an assumption.*Unpublished manuscript.

Foster, E. (2010a). Causal inference and developmental psychology. *Developmental Psychology, 46*(6), 1454–1480.

Foster, E. M. (2010b). The U-shaped relationship between complexity and usefulness. *Developmental Psychology, 46*(6), 1760–1766.

Foster, E. M., & Kalil, A. (2007). Living arrangements and children's development in low-income white, black, and Latino families. *Child Development, 78*(6), 1657–1674.

Frangakis, C. E., & Rubin, D. B. (2002). Principal stratification in causal inference. *Biometrics, 58*(1), 21–29.

Greenland, S., & Morgenstern, H. (2001). Confounding in health research. *Annual Review of Public Health, 22*(1), 189–212.

Heckman, J. J., & Vytlacil, E. J. (2007). Econometric evaluation of social programs: Part I. Causal models, structural models and econometric policy evaluation. *Handbook of Econometrics, 6*, 4779–4874.

Hernan, M. A., Hernandez-Diaz, S., & Robins, J. M. (2004). A structural approach to selection bias. *Epidemiology, 15*(5), 615–625.

Holland, P. W. (1986). Statistics and causal inference. *Journal of the American Statistical Association, 81*(396), 945–960.

Imbens, G. W., & Rubin, D. B. (1996). *Estimating outcome distributions for compliers in instrumental variables models*. Cambridge, MA: Harvard University Press.

Jiang, M., & Foster, E. M. (in press). Breastfeeding and the children's cognitive outcomes: A propensity score matching approach. *Maternal and Child Health Journal*.

Kaufman, J. S., MacLehose, R. F., & Rubin, D. B. (2004). A further critique of the analytic strategy of adjusting for covariates to identify biologic mediation. *Epidemiologic Perspectives and Innovations, 1*(1), 4.

Lee, M. (2005). *Micro-econometrics for policy, program, and treatment effects*. Oxford, UK: Oxford University Press.

Manski, C. F. (2007). *Identification for prediction and decision*. Cambridge, MA: Harvard University Press.

Mayer, S. E. (1997). *What money can't buy: Family income and children's life chances*. Cambridge, MA: Harvard University Press.

McLanahan, S., & Sandefur, G. D. (1994). *Growing up with a single parent: What hurts, what helps*. Cambridge, MA: Harvard University Press.

Morgan, S. L., & Winship, C. (2007). *Counterfactuals and causal inference: Methods and principles for social research*. New York: Cambridge University Press.

Pearl, J. (2000). *Causality: Models, reasoning, and inference*. Cambridge, UK: Cambridge University Press.

Pearl, J. (2009). *Causality: Models, reasoning, and inference* (2nd ed.). Cambridge, UK: Cambridge University Press.

Robins, J. M. (1997, August). *Marginal structural models*. Paper presented at the annual meeting of the American Statistical Association, Section on Bayesian Statistical Science, Washington, DC.

Robins, J. M. (1999a). Association, causation, and marginal structural models. *Synthese, 121*(1), 151–179.

Robins, J. M. (1999b). Marginal structural models versus structural nested models as tools for causal inference. *Statistical Models in Epidemiology: The Environment and Clinical Trials, 16*, 95–134.

Rosenbaum, P. R., & Rubin, D. B. (1983). The central role of the propensity score in observational studies for causal effects. *Biometrika, 70*(1), 41–55.

Rosenbaum, P. R., & Rubin, D. B. (1985). The bias due to incomplete matching. *Biometrics, 41*(1), 103–116.

Rosenberger, W. F., & Lachin, J. M. (2002). *Randomization in clinical trials: Theory and practice*. New York: Wiley.

Rubin, D. B. (1980). Randomization analysis of experimental data: The Fisher randomization test: Comment. *Journal of the American Statistical Association, 75*, 591–593.

Rubin, D. B. (2005). Causal inference using potential outcomes: Design, modeling, decisions. *Journal of the American Statistical Association, 100*, 322–331.

Rutter, M. (2007). Proceeding from observed correlation to causal inference: The use of natural experiments. *Perspectives on Psychological Science, 2*(4), 377–395.

Sheiner, L. B., & Rubin, D. B. (1995). Intention-to-treat analysis and the goals of clinical trials. *Clinical Pharmacology and Therapeutics, 57*(1), 6–15.

Sobel, M. E. (2008). Identification of causal parameters in randomized studies with mediating variables. *Journal of Educational and Behavioral Statistics, 33*(2), 230–251.

Vanderweele, T. J. (2008). Simple relations between principal stratification and direct and indirect effects. *Statistics and Probability Letters, 78*, 2957–2962.

CHAPTER 3

Accelerated Longitudinal Designs

SUSAN C. DUNCAN
TERRY E. DUNCAN

Central Issues

Age-related behavior can be studied with either longitudinal or cross-sectional data (Baltes, 1968). When attempting to advance knowledge about development across the lifespan, longitudinal designs clearly have many advantages over comparable cross-sectional methods. In particular, a true longitudinal design is able to study the same person at different time points, thus permitting within-individual analyses of change. Cross-sectional designs allow only the study of variations between individuals, whereas longitudinal designs permit the study of both changes within individuals and variations between individuals. Unfortunately, true (single, long-term) longitudinal designs often present practical problems related to time constraints, subject attrition, and the cost of continual and multiple subject assessments. Given these problems, researchers have long sought alternative approaches that retain the advantages and minimize the disadvantages of the true longitudinal design.

Bell (1953) introduced an alternative method to accelerate the collection of longitudinal information based on the idea of convergence. The Bell method consisted of collecting limited repeated measurements of independent age cohorts and temporally overlapping the cohort data. More recently, this technique has gained popularity as the accelerated longitudinal design (Nesselroade & Baltes, 1979).

The accelerated longitudinal design offers numerous ways to analyze data. Historically, such methods included multiple regression and analysis of variance (ANOVA). But traditional fixed-effects analytic methods were limited in their treatment of repeated-measures and other nested designs. They analyzed only mean-level changes and treated random differences among individuals as a nuisance parameter, or error variance. Analytic methods better suited to nested data structures have subsequently emerged under labels such as *multilevel* or *hierarchical linear models, mixed-effects models, random-effects models*, and *random coefficient models* (e.g., Aitkin & Longford, 1986; de Leeuw & Kreft, 1986; Duncan, Duncan, Hops, & Stoolmiller, 1995; Goldstein, 1986; Raudenbush & Bryk, 1988).

Structural equation modeling (SEM) methodology has been extended to analyze data from accelerated designs. Latent growth curve analyses are particularly useful. Rao (1958) and Tucker (1958) conducted formative work to provide a means of modeling a developmental function as a factor of repeated observations. Their approach focuses on within-individual data and analyses to determine how behaviors change over time. In the past two decades, research has demonstrated the utility of the accelerated longitudinal study design in conjunction with latent growth modeling (LGM) analysis (e.g., T. E. Duncan, Duncan, & Strycker, 2006; McArdle, 1988; Meredith & Tisak, 1990).

Conceptual Principles and Statistical Assumptions

The accelerated longitudinal research design links adjacent segments of limited longitudinal data from different age cohorts to create a common long-term developmental trend, or growth curve. Thus researchers can approximate a long-term longitudinal study by conducting several simultaneous short-term longitudinal studies of different age cohorts.

An advantage of the accelerated longitudinal study design over the single-cohort longitudinal design is the shorter total follow-up period, which reduces problems of cumulative testing effects and attrition. Results can be produced more quickly. Another advantage is that following several cohorts, rather than one, increases confidence in the generalizability of the results. Researchers can corroborate trends observed in the repeated measures for each age cohort.

The main disadvantage of the accelerated longitudinal design, compared with the single-cohort longitudinal design, is the shorter amount of time available for collecting data to track within-individual developmental sequences. As a result, some researchers question whether the accelerated longitudinal design provides a valid and effective means of constructing the full longitudinal growth curve. The accelerated longitudinal approach also may not fully assess the impacts of important events and intervening variables on the course of development. For instance, known predictors of long-term change may not be found across the short-term segments of the accelerated design. In addition, accelerated designs limit the conclusions that may be drawn about onset and termination of behaviors at points with little or no cohort overlap (Raudenbush & Chan, 1992).

Features of the Accelerated Longitudinal Design: Age, Period, and Cohort Effects

A single longitudinal study of one sample followed across time has many advantages over a comparable cross-sectional study of different individuals. Longitudinal studies also have disadvantages. One problem is the distinction between aging, period, and cohort effects. In developmental research, a *cohort* is defined as a group of individuals experiencing the same event (often, birth) during the same time period (often, 1 year). *Cohort effects* follow from membership in one cohort rather than another. *Period effects* refer to influences within a specific time or historical period. *Aging effects* refer to changes that occur with age.

Cross-sectional data confound aging and cohort effects, whereas longitudinal data confound aging and period effects. In cross-sectional data, cohorts may differ in their composition and in the changes that can be attributed to age. In longitudinal data, individuals may differ because of historical events that influence development and because of changes that accompany aging. To draw viable conclusions from longitudinal data about age-related changes, one must disentangle aging and period effects (Tonry, Ohlin, & Farrington, 1991).

An advantage of the accelerated design is that aging effects may be studied independently of period and cohort effects. Different cohorts of the same ages in different periods can be linked together to represent a longitudinal trend. Subjects in the cohorts should be as comparable as possible. Researchers must determine the appropriate number of cohorts, the total number of years for follow-up, and the overlap between cohorts. Tonry and colleagues (1991) argue that the follow-up period should be long in order to gain the key advantages of longitudinal research, but recommend a 7- or 8-year maximum follow-up period to avoid problems of continuity of research organization and funding and to minimize subject attrition. The number of different cohorts should not be too great, as each cohort may require separate analysis. Each cohort must contain a minimum number of subjects in order to draw valid conclusions and to estimate population parameters with relative power and narrow confidence intervals and margins of error (Tonry et al., 1991).

The period of overlap between cohorts should be as long as possible to facilitate the disentangling of aging effects and the linkage of different cohorts. Tonry et al. (1991) suggest that the period of overlap should equal the total follow-up period minus the intercohort interval. For example, using a maximum follow-up period of about 8 years and a minimum intercohort interval of 2 years (e.g., 10-year-old cohort and 12-year-old cohort), the maximum period of overlap would be 6 years (ages 12–17 years).

As with true longitudinal designs, researchers using accelerated designs must be able to assess the impact of important events and life transitions on the course of development. The follow-up period must be long enough before and after important events to establish effects on development. In an accelerated design with multiple cohorts, the total length of the follow-up period in years and the interval in years between each cohort determine the minimum follow-up time before and after any given age, assuming that the event and its causal impact occurs at a particular age (Tonry et al., 1991).

The accelerated longitudinal design (Tonry et al., 1991) allows researchers to analyze data and disseminate findings sooner than in a true longitudinal study. Additional analyses can then validate earlier findings and extend conclusions. The length of the developmental period of interest dictates how many cohorts and follow-up periods are necessary and the amount of overlap required between cohorts.

Accelerated Longitudinal Designs and Missing Data

Longitudinal data sets typically suffer from some form of missing data. In an accelerated design, most missing data arise from planned missingness. Because planned missingness is under the researcher's control, the missing data generally can be considered missing at random (MAR). Beyond some loss of statistical power, planned missingness poses minimal threats to statistical conclusions.

The strategy for handling missing data within the accelerated longitudinal design consists of expanding the SEM to include means or regression intercepts and then partitioning the sample into subgroups with distinct patterns of missing data (e.g., different cohorts with different segments of the overall curve). Equality constraints across the groups representing distinct patterns of missingness are imposed in a multiple-sample analysis to obtain unbiased and consistent parameter estimates. These equality constraints across the missing data subsamples are not of substantive interest, but, because the hypothesized model is assumed to be invariant across cohorts or groups, they function to ensure correct estimation of model parameters. To permit an appropriate large-sample chi-square test of model fit, one must obtain the likelihood values for restricted H_0 and unrestricted H_1 model hypotheses.

Under the unrestricted H_1 hypothesis, the parameters of interest are the variances, covariances, and means of the observed variables. The H_1 hypothesis tests equality of the moment matrices, with equality constraints for common parameters imposed across the groups. The unrestricted H_1 model also tests whether the data are missing completely at random (MCAR). When the pattern of missingness is completely random, different subsamples can be regarded as distinct random samples from the same population. Even if the data are found to be MCAR, a suitable H_0 substantive model may not exist. Therefore, the subsequent test of the more restricted H_0 model is statistically warranted.

The H_0 model (e.g., the hypothesized accelerated LGM in which the parameters of interest are assumed to be invariant across groups) imposes equality restrictions across the groups representing various missing data patterns for common parameters. The parameters are regression coefficients, variances, and covariances of the independent variables and the regression intercepts, or means, of the dependent variables. The difference in chi-square values and degrees of freedom for the two analyses gives a correct test of H_0 against H_1. Even if the data are not MCAR and the test of H_0 against H_1 is rejected, analyses may proceed under a less restrictive assumption that the missing data are MAR and that the missing-data mechanism is "ignorable" (Rubin, 1976). When the assumptions of MCAR or MAR are tenable, the maximum-likelihood estimations generated from the structural equation analyses exhibit no large-sample bias.

Through the use of maximum-likelihood (ML) estimation procedures, SEM programs can provide estimates for planned missingness (as in the accelerated design), as well as for other types of missing data. Both model- and imputation-based missing-data approaches can produce parameter estimates under a particular model of nonresponse (Rubin, 1987). Most standard SEM programs now allow the estimation of the ML function at the level of the individual. This approach to the analysis of partially missing data is an extension of the multiple-group method previously described but calculates the log-likelihood of the data for each observation (raw ML or full information maximum-likelihood [FIML] estimation). With this procedure, parameters can be estimated in missing-data models (including accelerated designs) without resorting to multiple-group analyses. In conducting missing-data analyses, the inclusion of variables potentially associated with the MAR process increases the validity and generalizability of results. Graham (2003) outlined a method for including auxiliary variables in LGM models to aid in estimating the model's missingness (also see Graham, 2003, for a technical explanation).

Developmental Applications

The use of an accelerated longitudinal study design with LGM analyses has increased over the past 10 years, but it is not widespread. Studies demonstrating the utility of the accelerated design for investigating individual change over time have been conducted in a variety of areas of human development, including youth substance use (Duncan, Duncan, & Hops, 1994, 1996; Tildesley & Andrews, 2008), family and individual processes (Anderson, 1993, 1995; Baer & Schmitz, 2000; Watt, 2008), intellectual abilities (McArdle, Ferrer-

Caja, Hamagami, & Woodcock, 2002), and health-related behaviors such as physical activity (Duncan, Duncan, Strycker, & Chaumeton, 2007).

McArdle and Hamagami (1991) and others (Raudenbush & Chan, 1992, 1993; Tonry et al., 1991) have raised questions about the viability of the accelerated longitudinal design in approximating a true longitudinal growth curve. To address these concerns, Duncan and colleagues (1996) compared an accelerated LGM (four different age cohorts, each measured at 1-year intervals over a 3-year period) forming a developmental trajectory of alcohol use spanning 12–17 years of age with data collected from the same study sample on a single cohort over six annual assessments (ages 12–17). The models did not differ significantly in their representation of alcohol-use trajectories and effects of covariates on these trajectories. Results from this study and from the Study 1 illustration that follows support the viability of the accelerated longitudinal design.

Illustration

This section details two examples of the accelerated longitudinal design. Both studies examine change in youth alcohol use. The first study compares findings from an accelerated LGM to a true longitudinal LGM. The second study examines change in alcohol use (use vs. nonuse) from ages 9 to 16 years using an accelerated LGM approach.

Study 1: Comparison of Accelerated LGM and True Longitudinal LGM

Using LGM, Study 1 (T. E. Duncan et al., 2006) tested an accelerated design against a true longitudinal design (using data assessed from a single age cohort). The accelerated design modeled the development of alcohol use from 12 to 16 years of age over a 3-year period; the true longitudinal model spanned a 5-year period. Data were taken from the National Youth Survey (Elliott, 1976).

For the accelerated longitudinal model, data came from three different age cohorts (12, 13, and 14 years of age at the initial assessment) that were measured three times at approximately 1-year intervals (time 1 to time 3), representing an overall age range of 12–16 years. This choice of age cohorts ensured that the time of measurement and age of testing were approximately staggered (McArdle & Anderson, 1989). That is, the average age of the first cohort at the second measurement period was about the same as the average age of the second cohort at the initial measurement, and so forth. The sample sizes for the three cohorts were 248, 250, and 231, respectively ($N = 729$). An additional 11-year-old cohort ($N = 215$) represented data from a true longitudinal design. Data for the 11-year-old cohort came from five assessments (time 2 to time 6; 12–16 years of age), allowing a comparison of the developmental trends for similar age spans from two different designs.

Figure 3.1 shows the LGM designs that were tested. Groups 1, 2, and 3 represent the accelerated LGM. The same developmental model is assumed in each cohort, allowing for hypothesis testing of convergence across separate groups and of the feasibility of specifying a common growth trajectory over the 5 years represented by the design.

The accelerated model serves as a proxy for the true longitudinal model (Group 4 in Figure 3.1), which uses data from yearly assessments of the 11-year-old cohort (Group 4) over a 5-year period beginning at 12 years of age. The basic model tests the hypothesized linear growth in alcohol use with fixed parameter restrictions.

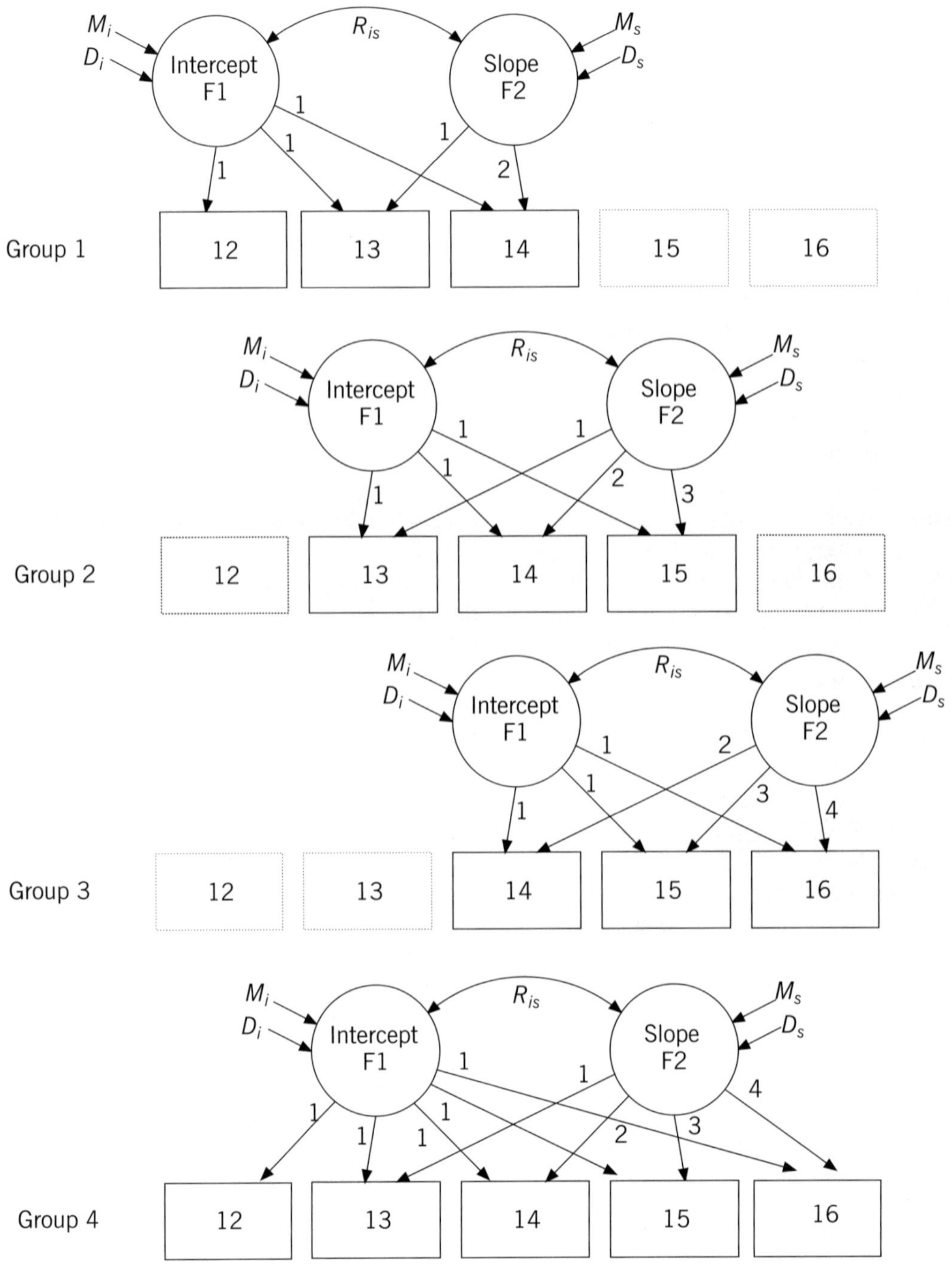

FIGURE 3.1. Representation of the multiple-sample combined accelerated and true longitudinal LGM.

F1 represents factor 1, the intercept, and F2 represents factor 2, the slope. The basis terms (factor loadings) of the intercept are fixed at 1. To identify the model, at least two slope loadings must be fixed to two different values. In this example, the model specifications fix the loadings at 0, 1, 2, 3, and 4 to represent a linear trajectory of alcohol use. The model constrains the mean of the intercept, M_i, to 0. The model estimates the slope mean, M_s, and variances of the intercept, D_i, and slope, D_s, as well as the correlation, R_{is}, between the intercept and slope.

The overlap in ages in the accelerated longitudinal design creates a quasi-longitudinal study of 5 years spanning ages 12–16. Moreover, because each age cohort, representing a different pattern of missingness due to design, contributes a different section to the overall developmental curve, the complete curve can be constructed using information from all cohorts simultaneously. The model specifications assume that a common linear trajectory characterizes the set of staggered age group curves and that this trajectory accurately approximates the developmental trend generated from the 11-year-old cohort data within the true longitudinal design.

The models compared trends in the accelerated and true longitudinal models under the assumption of linear growth. Model fit was assessed using the chi-square goodness of fit test, comparative fit index (CFI; Bentler, 1990), and root mean square error of approximation (RMSEA; Browne & Cudeck, 1993). Fit indices for the accelerated model were $\chi^2(17, N = 729) = 65.746, p < .001$, CFI = .978, and RMSEA = .063. The true longitudinal model fit indices were: $\chi^2(10, N = 215) = 60.171, p < .001$, CFI = .953, and RMSEA = .153. Significant slope means indicate that growth in alcohol use occurred over the 5 adolescent years approximated by the accelerated longitudinal model, as well as in the true longitudinal model. Significant variances indicate substantial variation in individuals in initial status and change in alcohol use.

Lagrange multiplier (LM) tests assisted in determining whether any of the constraints imposed on the common parameter estimates across the three age cohort groups resulted in statistically significant differences in those common estimates across the three cohorts. The LM test (Aitchison & Silvey, 1958) evaluates the effect of adding free parameters to a restricted model (i.e., reducing restrictions placed on the model). Lee and Bentler (1980) adopted the LM principle for covariance structure analysis and made the LM test available for all distributional assumptions, as well as for evaluation of cross-group equality constraints in multiple-sample models. The LM test and the chi-square difference test (D), which is based on separate estimation of two nested models, are asymptotically equivalent chi-square tests (Bentler & Dijkstra, 1985). Thus the LM test can be interpreted as if a D test had been done, and it represents an approximate decrease in model goodness-of-fit chi-square resulting from freeing previously fixed parameters and eliminating equality restrictions. Because LM statistics are conveniently obtained in a single computer run, the LM test can easily provide guidance on modifications to cross-group constraints to improve model fit to the data (Bentler & Chou, 1986).

With three groups and two degrees of freedom, two single-degree-of-freedom LM tests were conducted for each parameter estimate in the model. Examination of the LM statistics between the cohorts in the accelerated model revealed that no cross-group constraints, if released, would represent statistically significant differences in the estimates for the same parameters in the three cohorts.

Next, a combined multiple-sample LGM analysis with all four groups (three cohorts in the accelerated model and the single cohort assessed over 5 years in the true longitudinal model) tested whether significant differences existed between estimates from the two designs. Model specifications constrained the latent means, latent variances, latent covariances, and residual errors to be equal across the cohorts. Model fitting procedures for the combined multiple-sample LGM specifying linear growth resulted in the following indices of fit: $\chi^2(37, N = 944) = 139.150$, $p < .001$, CFI = .962, and RMSEA = .054. Generally, a value of .90 or greater on the CFI (Bentler, 1990) represents acceptable model fit, and RMSEA values between .05 and .08 indicate fair fit (Browne & Cudeck, 1993). Thus the multiple-sample model adequately fit the data.

Examination of the means, variances, and reproduced means indicated considerable similarity in estimates across the accelerated and true longitudinal models. These similarities can be seen in Figure 3.2, which shows the trajectory of alcohol use for each cohort over time in the accelerated design model, the estimated linear trajectory for the accelerated design, and the trajectory of alcohol use for the true longitudinal model cohort.

LM tests again showed that no cross-group constraints, if released, would represent 'statistically significant differences between the same parameters in the different models. The LM results give further evidence of the generalizability of the accelerated design to adequately approximate parameters estimated within a true longitudinal design.

Study 2: An Accelerated LGM of Youth Alcohol Use

Study 2 (S. C. Duncan, Duncan, & Strycker, 2006) examined growth in alcohol use among youths from ages 9 to 16 years and aimed to determine the influence of hypothesized covariates on change in alcohol use. An accelerated LGM modeled dichotomous alcohol use (use versus nonuse) over time and accounted for demographic variables and contextual covariates.

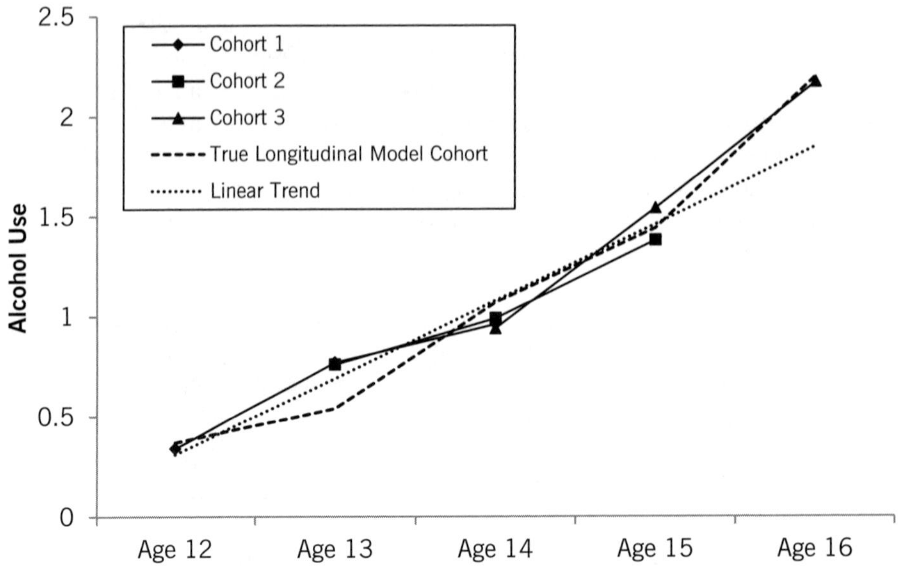

FIGURE 3.2. The trajectory of alcohol use by cohort over time in the accelerated design model, the estimated linear trajectory for the accelerated design, and the trajectory of alcohol use for the true longitudinal model cohort. The alcohol use scale ranged from never (0) to more than once a day (5).

Until recently, most applications of LGM have modeled normally distributed continuous outcome variables. Some behaviors, such as youth substance use, are not normally distributed because of the population's generally low base rates of use. Recent advances now allow the modeling of categorical data in LGM. Study 2 modeled alcohol use as a binary variable, distinguishing between any alcohol use (coded 1) and nonuse (coded 0). The model specifications regressed use versus nonuse on the growth factors using a probit model within a random-effects growth-modeling framework. Detailed specifications for the modeling of ordered categorical dependent variables are described in Muthén (2001). Analyses were conducted using Mplus software (Muthén & Muthén, 2004).

Data were collected across 4 years (1999–2003) from residents of a large metropolitan area in the Northwest. The sample comprised 405 youths and their families. Youths were 48.4% female, 50.4% African American, and 49.6% white. Detailed recruitment information is in Duncan, Strycker, Duncan, He, and Stark (2002).

The three age cohorts (N = 139 9-year-olds; N = 138 11-year-olds; N = 128 13-year-olds) were part of an accelerated longitudinal study. By temporally overlapping short-term longitudinal studies of the three cohorts, a common developmental trajectory spanning ages 9–16 could be created with only 4 years of data collection.

Figure 3.3 depicts the accelerated LGM. Cohort 1 represents the 9-year-old cohort with data for ages 9, 10, 11, and 12 years at time 1 (T1), time 2 (T2), time 3 (T3), and time 4 (T4), respectively. Cohort 2 represents the 11-year-old cohort with data for ages 11, 12, 13, and 14 years. Cohort 3 represents the 13-year-old cohort with data for ages 13, 14, 15, and 16 years. F1 represents factor 1, the intercept, and F2 represents factor 2, the slope. The basis terms (factor loadings) of the intercept are fixed at 1. The basis terms of the slope are fixed (0–7) to represent a linear growth trend from ages 9 to 16 years. The mean of the intercept, M_i, is constrained to 0. The slope mean, M_s, and variances of the intercept, D_i, and slope, D_s, are estimated, as well as the correlation, R_{is}, between the intercept and slope.

For the categorical y variables, the model specifies τ's (threshold parameters), rather than e's (measurement errors), which are typically modeled for continuous normally distributed outcome variables, to represent category intervals. In the case of a dichotomous outcome, one threshold is specified for alcohol use at each time point (T1 to T4). The model imposes across-time measurement invariance by specifying $\tau_1 = \tau_2 = \tau_3 = \tau_4$. Although the model involves categorical dependent variables, the latent variables (growth parameters F1 and F2) are continuous in nature, as in the case of continuous normally distributed repeated-measures variables.

The accelerated LGM was estimated within a multiple-sample (multiple-group) context and used a robust weighted least squares estimator. The model placed cross-group (cohort) equality constraints for all free parameters, including the latent slope means, latent variances for the intercept and slope, the latent covariances between the intercept and slope, and threshold parameters of the observed variables. The model fixed the mean intercept at 0 for each cohort and fixed the linear trend using basis terms from 0 to 7. Assuming the same developmental model in each group, the model tests convergence across separate cohorts, as well as the feasibility of specifying a common "true longitudinal" growth trajectory over the 8 years.

Fitting a linear accelerated LGM to the data for alcohol use produced an acceptable chi-square test statistic, $\chi^2(11, N = 405) = 16.153$, $p = .135$, and fit indices, CFI = .994, and RMSEA = .059. These fit statistics indicate that the accelerated LGM provides an

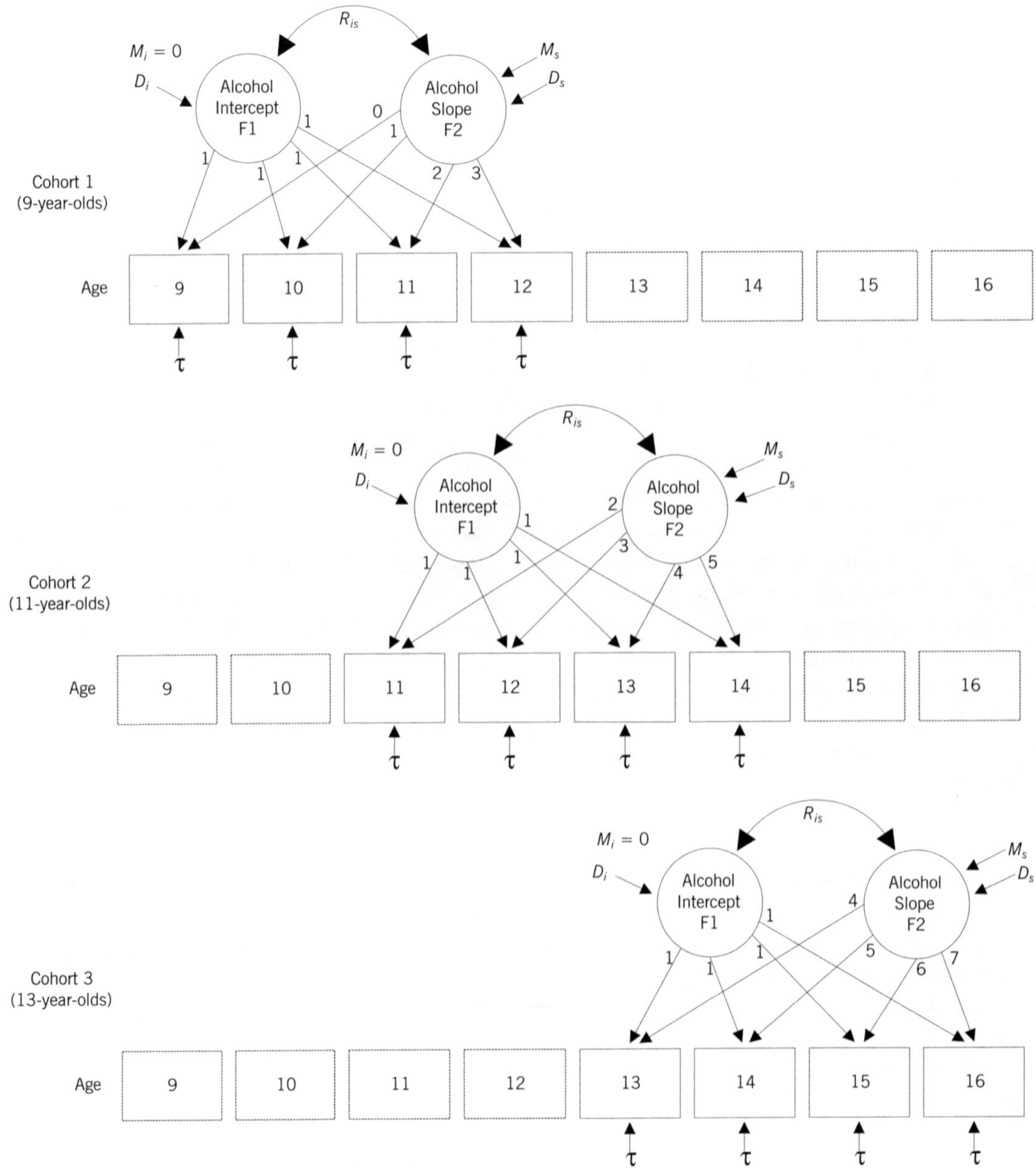

FIGURE 3.3. Representation of the cohort-sequential latent growth model (LGM) for change in adolescent alcohol use from ages 9–16 years.

adequate fit to the data (Bentler, 1990; Browne & Cudeck, 1993). An examination of the model's modification indices suggested no differences in the growth parameters of interest across cohorts. Similar to the LM test (Bentler, 1986), modification indices (Sörbom, 1989) can be used to approximate the noncentrality parameter for each restriction (1 degree of freedom) imposed on the model (Satorra, 1989). For a given fixed parameter of an equality constraint in a model, a modification index can be computed to predict the reduction in the model's chi-square that would accompany the freeing of a fixed parameter of the release of an equality constraint. The relationship between the LM and modification index tests are asymptotically equivalent (Satorra, 1989). The modification index results justify the use of an accelerated longitudinal model to approximate a true longitudinal curve in these data and suggest that the three cohorts were sampled from the same true longitudinal population.

The linear model resulted in a significant mean slope, $M_S = .105$, $t = 2.757$, $p < .01$, indicating a steady increase in the prevalence of alcohol use from ages 9 to 16 years, according to the accelerated longitudinal model. The M_S value of .105 can be interpreted as the increase in use per unit of time (i.e., $.105 \times 3$ [T4 – T1 = 3 units of time] = .315), which corresponds to the actual increase in proportion of users from ages 9 to 16 years (i.e., .442 [proportion of users at T4 for cohort 3] – .129 [proportion of users at T1 for cohort 1] = .313). The variances for the intercept and slope were $D_i = 1.050$, $t = 5.610$, $p < .001$, and $D_s = .104$, $t = 2.483$, $p < .05$, respectively, indicating substantial variation across individuals in initial alcohol use and in change in alcohol use over time. The results of the model fit, modification indices, and significant slope mean and variance support the study hypotheses regarding the use of the accelerated model and the linear developmental trajectory of alcohol use. Figure 3.4 shows the trajectory of alcohol use for each cohort over time and the estimated linear trajectory from the accelerated model of alcohol use from ages 9 to 16 years.

Although the separate cohort slopes in Figure 3.4 may not appear to follow the same linear trend, it is important to remember that the function of the accelerated design is to piece the cohort slopes together to form a "true" longitudinal curve that best represents the slope of alcohol use from ages 9 to 16 years. Overall, results indicate an upward linear trend in the proportion of young alcohol users in this 8-year period. A subsequent conditional model with covariates was also tested and is described in S. C. Duncan and colleagues (2006).

In this example, LGM and an accelerated design estimated longitudinal curves spanning 8 years from ages 9 to 16 years using only 4 years of data. This study, along with other research (e.g., S. C. Duncan et al., 1996; McArdle & Hamagami, 1992; Raudenbush & Chan, 1992), demonstrates that the accelerated design is an efficient method for examining longitudinal data.

Future Directions

The search continues for the best methods to address complex issues in longitudinal studies of human development. As the field continues to expand, new and more complex research questions will be posed, and these questions will prompt the development of new statistical methods. Accelerated longitudinal designs, in conjunction with LGM, benefit the field in a number of ways. For example, these strategies allow researchers to (1) reduce the number of cohorts and assessments needed to examine change over time, reducing costs, subject

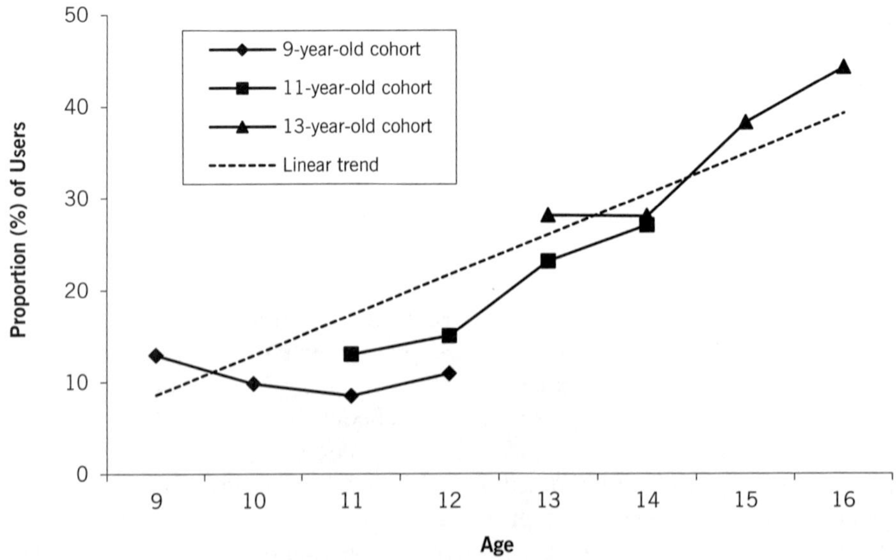

FIGURE 3.4. Proportion of alcohol users by cohort (9, 11, and 13 years), joined together to form a trajectory of alcohol use from ages 9–16 years.

burden, and attrition; (2) estimate the mean trajectory of the individual growth curves for a given population; (3) examine variability in individual trajectories about the mean growth curve; (4) study the fit of linear and nonlinear growth functions; (5) assess the psychometric properties of individual indicators of status and change; and (6) use these indicators as outcomes, which can be predicted by between- or within-subjects covariates, or as predictors of subsequent between- or within-subjects outcomes. The accelerated longitudinal design allows data to be linked from overlapping cohorts as a valid and efficient means of mapping development over long time spans—and of testing the integrity of models based on these accelerated curves.

Despite guidance from some researchers (e.g., Tonry et al., 1991), questions remain about the optimal number of time points per subject, points of overlap across adjacent cohorts, and subjects per cohort (Raudenbush & Chan, 1992). Generally, to increase the likelihood of convergence in fitting the accelerated longitudinal model, cohorts should overlap as much as possible, sample sizes within each cohort should be relatively large, and cohorts should be as comparable as possible (T. E. Duncan et al., 2006; Tonry et al., 1991).

Accelerated longitudinal designs do not approximate true longitudinal designs in all situations. For example, results are likely to differ if the cross-sectional aspects of the accelerated design do not adequately reflect historical or other intervening processes. In such cases, researchers must determine whether important information might be lost or estimates biased in an accelerated longitudinal design. If so, then a true longitudinal design is needed.

The field would benefit from more studies comparing accelerated longitudinal designs with true longitudinal designs. Duncan and colleagues (S. C. Duncan et al., 1996; T. E. Duncan et al., 2006) are the only studies of which we are aware that directly compared the two designs using LGM analyses. Both studies employed adolescent alcohol use data.

Comparisons in other substantive areas and with other analytic techniques would help determine whether similar conclusions about the viability of accelerated longitudinal designs can be drawn under different assumptions.

Acknowledgments

This research was supported by Grant No. AA11510 from the National Institute on Alcohol Abuse and Alcoholism and Grant No. HD35873 from the National Institute of Child Health and Human Development. Partial support in preparing this chapter was provided by Grant No. DA018760 from the National Institute on Drug Abuse.

References

Aitchison, J., & Silvey, D. C. (1958). Maximum likelihood estimation of parameters subject to restraints. *Annals of Mathematical Statistics, 29*, 813–828.

Aitkin, M., & Longford, N. (1986). Statistical modeling issues in school effectiveness studies. *Journal of the Royal Statistical Society, Series A, 149*, 1–43.

Anderson, E. R. (1993). Analyzing change in short-term longitudinal research using cohort-sequential designs. *Journal of Consulting and Clinical Psychology, 61*, 929–940.

Anderson, E. R. (1995). Accelerating and maximizing information from short-term longitudinal research. In J. M. Gottman (Ed.), *The analysis of change* (pp. 139–163). Hillsdale, NJ: Erlbaum.

Baer, J., & Schmitz, M. F. (2000). Latent growth curve modeling with a cohort sequential design. *Social Work Research, 24*, 243–247.

Baltes, P. (1968). Longitudinal and cross-sectional sequences in the study of age and generation effects. *Human Development, 11*, 145–171.

Bell, R. Q. (1953). Convergence: An accelerated longitudinal approach. *Child Development, 24*, 145–152.

Bentler, P. M. (1986). *Lagrange Multiplier and Wald tests for EQS and EQS/PC*. Los Angeles: BMDP Statistical Software.

Bentler, P. M. (1990). Comparative fit indices in structural models. *Psychological Bulletin, 107*, 238–246.

Bentler, P. M., & Chou, C.-P. (1986, April). *Statistics for parameter expansion and contraction in structural models*. Paper presented at the American Educational Research Association Meeting, San Francisco.

Bentler, P. M., & Dijkstra, T. (1985). Efficient estimation via linearization in structural models. In P. R. Krishnaiah (Ed.), *Multivariate analysis—VI* (pp. 9–42). Amsterdam: North-Holland.

Browne, M., & Cudeck, R. (1993). Alternative ways of assessing model fit. In K. A. Bollen & J. S. Long (Eds.), *Testing structural equation models* (pp. 136–162). Newbury Park, CA: Sage.

de Leeuw, J., & Kreft, I. (1986). Random coefficient models for multilevel analysis. *Journal of Educational Statistics, 11*, 57–85.

Duncan, S. C., Duncan, T. E., & Hops, H. (1996). Analysis of longitudinal data within accelerated longitudinal designs. *Psychological Methods, 1*, 236–248.

Duncan, S. C., Duncan, T. E., & Strycker, L. A. (2006). Alcohol use from ages 9–16: A cohort-sequential latent growth model. *Drug and Alcohol Dependence, 81*, 71–81.

Duncan, S. C., Duncan, T. E., Strycker, L. A., & Chaumeton, N. R. (2007). A cohort-sequential latent growth model of physical activity from ages 12 to 17 years. *Annals of Behavioral Medicine, 33*, 80–89.

Duncan, S. C., Strycker, L. A., Duncan, T. E., He, H., & Stark, M. (2002). Telephone recruitment of a random stratified African American and white family study sample. *Journal of Ethnicity in Substance Abuse, 1*, 57–73.

Duncan, T. E., Duncan, S. C., & Hops, H. (1994). The effects of family cohesiveness and peer encouragement on the development of adolescent alcohol use: A cohort-sequential approach to the analysis of longitudinal data. *Journal of Studies on Alcohol, 55*, 588–599.

Duncan, T. E., Duncan, S. C., Hops, H., & Stoolmiller, M. (1995). Analyzing longitudinal substance use data via generalized estimating equation methodology. *Multivariate Behavioral Research, 30*, 317–339.

Duncan, T. E., Duncan, S. C., & Strycker, L. A. (2006). *An introduction to latent variable growth curve modeling: Concepts, issues, and applications* (2nd ed.). Mahwah, NJ: Erlbaum.

Elliott, D. S. (1976). *National Youth Survey [United States]: Wave 1* [ICPSR version, computer file]. Boulder, CO: University of Colorado, Behavioral Research Institute [producer]; Ann Arbor, MI: Inter-University Consortium for Political and Social Research [distributor].

Goldstein, H. (1986). Multilevel mixed linear model analysis using iterative generalized least squares. *Biometrika, 73*, 43–56.

Graham, J. W. (2003). Adding missing-data-relevant variables to FIML-based structural equation models. *Structural Equation Modeling, 10*, 80–100.

Lee, S. Y., & Bentler, P. M. (1980). Some asymptotic properties of constrained generalized least squares estimation in covariance structure models. *South African Statistical Journal, 14*, 1221–1236.

McArdle, J. J. (1988). Dynamic but structural equation modeling of repeated measures data. In R. B. Cattell & J. Nesselroade (Eds.), *Handbook of multivariate experimental psychology* (2nd ed., pp. 561–614). New York: Plenum Press.

McArdle, J. J., & Anderson, E. R. (1989). Latent growth models for research on aging. In L. E. Biren & K. W. Schaie (Eds.), *The handbook of the psychology of aging* (3rd ed., pp. 21–44). San Diego, CA: Academic Press.

McArdle, J. J., Ferrer-Caja, E., Hamagami, F., & Woodcock, R. W. (2002). Comparative longitudinal structural analyses of the growth and decline of multiple intellectual abilities over the life span. *Developmental Psychology, 38*, 115–142.

McArdle, J. J., & Hamagami, F. (1991). Modeling incomplete longitudinal and cross-sectional data using latent growth structural models. In L. M. Collins & J. C. Horn (Eds.), *Best methods for the analysis of change* (pp. 276–304). Washington, DC: American Psychological Association.

McArdle, J. J., & Hamagami, F. (1992). Modeling incomplete longitudinal and cross-sectional data using latent growth structural models. *Experimental Aging Research, 18*, 145–166.

Meredith, W., & Tisak, J. (1990). Latent curve analysis. *Psychometrika, 55*, 107–122.

Muthén, B. (2001). Second-generation structural equation modeling with a combination of categorical and continuous latent variables: New opportunities for latent class/latent growth modeling. In L. M. Collins & A. Sayer (Eds.), *New methods for the analysis of change* (pp. 291–322). Washington, DC: American Psychological Association.

Muthén, L. K., & Muthén, B. O. (2004). *Mplus user's guide* (3rd ed.). Los Angeles: Authors.

Nesselroade, J. R., & Baltes, P. B. (1979). *Longitudinal research in the study of behavior and development*. San Diego, CA: Academic Press.

Rao, C. R. (1958). Some statistical methods for comparison of growth curves. *Biometrics, 14*, 1–17.

Raudenbush, S., & Bryk, A. (1988). Methodological advances in studying effects of schools and classrooms on student learning. In E. Z. Roth (Ed.), *Review of research in education* (pp. 423–475). Washington, DC: American Educational Research Association.

Raudenbush, S. W., & Chan, W. (1992). Growth curve analysis in accelerated longitudinal designs. *Journal of Research on Crime and Delinquency, 29*, 387–411.

Raudenbush, S. W., & Chan, W. (1993). Application of a hierarchical model to the study of adolescent deviance in an overlapping cohort design. *Journal of Consulting and Clinical Psychology, 61*, 941–951.

Rubin, D. B. (1976). Inference and missing data. *Biometrika, 61*, 581–592.

Rubin, D. B. (1987). *Multiple imputation for nonresponse in surveys*. New York: Wiley.

Satorra, A. (1989). Alternative test criteria in covariance structure analysis: A unified approach. *Psychometrika, 54*, 131–151.

Sörbom, D. (1989). Model modification. *Psychometrika, 54*, 371–384.

Tildesley, E. A., & Andrews, J. A. (2008). The development of children's intentions to use alcohol: Direct and indirect effects of parent alcohol use and parenting behaviors. *Psychology of Addictive Behaviors, 22*, 326–339.

Tonry, M., Ohlin, L., & Farrington, D. P. (1991). *Human development and criminal behavior: New ways of advancing knowledge*. New York: Springer-Verlag.

Tucker, L. R. (1958). Determination of parameters of a functional relation by factor analysis. *Psychometrika, 23*, 19–23.

Watt, H. M. (2008). A latent growth curve modeling approach using an accelerated longitudinal design: The ontogeny of boys' and girls' talent perceptions and intrinsic values through adolescence. *Educational Research and Evaluation, 14*, 287–304.

CHAPTER 4

Time-Scale-Dependent Longitudinal Designs

THEODORE A. WALLS
WILLIAM D. BARTA
ROBERT S. STAWSKI
CHARLES E. COLLYER
SCOTT M. HOFER

Over the last several years, researchers have employed an increasing variety of intensive longitudinal research designs. The phenomenon under investigation may be a time-varying outcome, such as the number of instances of a given behavior in a given time frame. One question might be whether concurrent continuous or discontinuous factors underlie the manifestation of a behavior. Intensive measures referring to one time scale (such as days) are obtained over the course of a predetermined time frame (which may be measured in terms of weeks or months). The latter is referred to as an epoch or burst. For various scientific or practical reasons, when data on two or more epochs are collected, the researcher decides to incorporate a gap in time between epochs when data are not collected. This approach has been referred to as a "measurement burst design" (e.g., Martin & Hofer, 2004; Nesselroade & Schmidt-McCollam, 2000; Sliwinski, 2008). Examples of the design are appearing in the literature with increasing frequency (e.g., Sliwinski, Almeida, Smyth, & Stawski, 2009; Weinstein, Mermelstein, & Shiffman, 2008).

The term "measurement burst design" appears to have originated in a passage in Nesselroade's (1991) theoretical paper addressing key issues in the study of intraindividual variability. As Nesselroade framed the issue, "longitudinal research designs need to be planned around successive 'bursts' of measurement rather than merely successive ones" (p. 235). As is discussed, the measurement burst design offers certain important advantages to the researcher beyond intensive longitudinal designs that do not vary time scales (c.f., Collins, 2006; Walls & Schafer, 2006). One benefit is the ability to examine a lengthy period of time intensively without obtaining intensive measures continuously over the entire course of the study. A second benefit is the ability to integrate information that is specific to the time scale of measurement. That is, even if the object of one's investigation remains the same, the time scale of measurement will have an important impact on the information that is obtained. For example, if the number of hours a student spends studying is aggregated over the span of a semester, the researcher may fail to observe variability in the number of hours spent studying during the last few days before final exams begin. In this example, data aggregated by semester and data aggregated by week may each provide complementary insights on the phenomenon under investigation, and reveal important differences between students who distribute their studying hours over the semesters and those who "cram" toward the end of the semester.

The measurement burst design is a special case of the interrupted time series design. An interrupted time series design includes a time-registered independent variable such as a planned manipulation(s) or a naturalistic occurrence(s) that results in a change in the parameters describing the series following the time of registration (Campbell & Stanley, 1966; Cook & Campbell, 1979; see also Schmitz, Klug, & Hertel, Chapter 11, this volume). In the burst design, the assignment of measurement periods is based on theoretical and empirically based decisions about the time scale at which a process or phenomenon is optimally captured, as well as consideration of how particular aspects of the process (e.g., intraindividual variance or asymptote) may change over longer periods. From this standpoint, many possible designs could be considered, not only the relatively straightforward design involving equally spaced measurement bursts (e.g., at 6-month intervals), each comprising multiple assessments (e.g., daily for several days). In this chapter, we consider alternative temporal sampling designs within the interrupted time series family and explore other potential designs based on decisions about sufficient or optimal time scales for capturing particular processes. We refer to this framework as time-scale-dependent longitudinal design (TDLD). A key objective is to provide a basis for researchers to develop studies of process that effectively utilize multiple time scales and intensive measurements. The chapter is organized in five sections: central issues, conceptual principles and statistical assumptions, developmental applications, an illustration, and future directions.

Central Issues

The interrupted time series design and its more recent instantiation in the multiple measurement burst study warrant a brief review. Interest in time series designs in a developmental context emerged in the 1930s (cf. Fiske & Rice, 1955).

Origins of the Design: Interrupted Time Series

The interrupted time series (ITS) design was first described by Campbell and Stanley (1963) and was further elaborated in several subsequent publications, including, notably, Campbell (1969a, 1969b) and Cook and Campbell (1979) (see also Schmitz, Klug, & Hertel, Chapter 11, this volume). The original conception of the design involved a single series, such as that resulting from seismic aftershocks over time in one region. They saw potential extensions to the study of causal sequences in social experimentation. The main statistical approach was limited to inspection of differences between epochs in the mean or slope of a univariate series. This was later extended to formal time series analysis and was frequently employed in the classic ABAB design in studies of operant conditioning (Barlow, Nock, & Hersen, 2009; Box & Jenkins, 1970). ABAB refers to the four-step sequence: baseline, treatment, return to baseline, treatment. The purpose of the return-to-baseline step is to verify that any change in the outcome measure coincident with the treatment can plausibly be attributed to treatment as opposed to some extraneous influence.

A sequence of repeated measures is obtained and, at one or more points in the sequence, there is a gap in measurement. The rationale for obtaining multiple pre- and posttest measures is that the criterion variable is likely to exhibit systematic, context-sensitive intraindividual variation. Therefore, in order to determine that a posttreatment increase in the criterion variable is in fact the result of treatment, the researcher will look for an average increase or change in relation to the local maximum. When parameters reflecting information within one period of measurement are considered from period to period, whether the parameters are simple descriptive statistics or more complex indicators of a process, the resulting analysis necessarily occurs at a higher time scale. Hence, a formal definition of a measurement burst design from an ITS perspective is: an ITS in which interest in the evolution of lower time scale processes (such as minute to minute) is considered over higher time scales (such as day to day). By contrast, an approach that simply views bins of minute-to-minute information as equivalent slices without a decision about a higher time-scale-design motivation would fall outside of our definition, or minimally within it. Relevant consideration of the role of time scale in longitudinal studies can be found in Bertenthal (2007) and Newell (1990).

Although it may seem obvious that the measurement burst design is a special case of the ITS, details of the design as a special case have not received careful consideration. Designs in psychophysics (e.g., Swets, 1964) and motor control (e.g., Rosenbaum & Collyer, 1998) may in fact have been early instances of the design, without being explicitly named as such. The motivation for many studies of perceptual and motor processes has been to intensively study the abilities of individuals, and practical considerations naturally lead to multiple sessions or bursts of data collection. Contemporary cases of the design in use have been in extensions of daily diary studies, with epochs of days spaced by several months. Substantively, these studies have focused on "daily hassles" and, to a lesser extent, addiction. The motivation for these studies has often been an interest in micro-level processes in cases in which continuous measurement may have been difficult or impossible. Challenges in these cases include difficulties with participant compliance with burdensome protocols, as well as potential problems with reactivity and validity (Hufford, Shields, Shiffman, Paty, & Balabanis,, 2002; cf. Campbell & Stanley, 1963; Varkey, Pompili, & Walls, 2011).

Campbell and Stanley (1963) stated that "the essence of the time-series design is the presence of a periodic measurement process on some group or individual and the introduction of an experimental change into this time series of measurements, the results of which are indicated by a discontinuity in the measurements recorded in the time series" (p. 37). However, the source of the discontinuity is not always an experimental manipulation. The researcher may, for example, wish to undertake an observational study of naturally occurring events, such as the effect of a flood on local employment (McDowall, McCleary, Meidinger, & Hay, 1980). Such a situation could also be repeatedly interrupted at a calendar time scale, as in the case of sequential events of neighborhood violence, resulting in a naturalistic but nonetheless time-scale-dependent design.

Interest in ITS designs within psychology can be traced back at least as far as the 1930s (cf. Fiske & Rice, 1955). Social and behavioral sciences at this point in time were influenced by learning theory. Learning theorists initially studied organisms' typical responses to overt stimuli before and after exposures to positive and negative reinforcements. As their field progressed, they considered the temporal processes by which complex patterns of behaviors are shaped. Members of the organismic school of developmental psychology were also interested in intraindividual processes. The term *microgenesis*, a translation of the German *Aktualgenese* or "genetic realization," is a concept that can be traced back to Werner's work at the University of Hamburg in the 1920s (Rosenthal, 2004). Microgenesis refers to "the temporal period between the presentation of a stimulus and the formation of a single, relatively stabilized cognitive response to this stimulus" (Flavell & Draguns, 1957, p. 197). This temporal period may be fleetingly small. What distinguishes a microgenetic process is its explicit attention to prior stimulus exposure on subsequent motivational, behavioral, and/or cognitive processes.

In summary, the utility of ITS designs as a means by which to interrupt an ongoing process and thereby draw inferences about that process is not new. However, the recognition that processes may evolve over higher order time scales is a relatively recent innovation from which to devise (or observe) interruption of a process. A few concomitant themes warrant attention in regard to consideration of processes in general; we cover these in the later section on developmental applications.

Conceptual Principles and Statistical Assumptions

Conceptually, the burst designs demand a careful consideration of the processes that are of interest to the researcher. A useful image may be that of a long wall with windows spaced along it and a process going on in a corridor on the other side. The process can be observed (in detail) at the windows, but not between the windows. That is, even if there are gaps in observation, an overall pattern of increase or decline may still be discerned. This is the premise of any longitudinal design, but here emphasis is placed on intensive designs that are capable of achieving a high level of granularity. The benefits of increased granularity include, first, the potential to reveal patterned, recurring temporal shapes embedded within a larger trajectory and, second, an increased ability to detect the presence of discrete, disruptive events that alter the course of the trajectory.

The focus of this chapter includes mapping intraindividual variation and change at two (or more) time scales and the possibility of discontinuous change (i.e., change processes triggered by disruptive events, resulting in a state of disequilibrium) or of stability of processes over longer time intervals. Note that this design is not limited to scenarios in which "days" or within-day processes in the lives of individuals are the smallest unit of analysis. One could look instead at weekly or yearly bursts and at the behavior of cohorts or other aggregated groupings. The sampling of different temporal units will yield different patterns of within-person variation and change that result from different internal states and influences on the individual (e.g., Bertenthal, 2007; Boker, Molenaar, & Nesselroade, 2009; Martin & Hofer, 2004).

Naturalistic Time-Scale-Dependent Time Series

This design reflects processes at different time scales or the evolution of a process studied at one time scale when measured at time points over a higher time scale.

[O1 O2 O3 ...] DELAY [O1 O2 O3] DELAY [O1 O2 O3] . . . .

Note: O = Observations; Observations may be evenly spaced (fixed interval), or they may be unevenly spaced, as in event or location contingent measurements.

Experimental Time-Scale-Dependent Time Series

An elaboration of this design involves study of change in processes via an experiment or randomization to groups, where X denotes the intervention point on the longer time scale:

R G1 [O1 O2 O3 ...] DELAY [O1 O2 O3] X DELAY [O1 O2 O3] . . .
G2 [O1 O2 O3 ...] DELAY [O1 O2 O3] DELAY [O1 O2 O3] . . . .

Another elaboration of the design can be interruption within the lower time scale, such as when traditional ITS designs are replicated over time:

[O1 X O2 O3 . . .] DELAY [O1 X O2 O3] DELAY [01 X O2 O3] . . . .

Whether the design is naturalistic or experimental, the spacing of measurements can be even or uneven. Uneven spacing can be produced either by event-driven measurements or the experimenter's randomization. Finally, of course, additional levels of time, additional groups, or interruptions/interventions at multiple time scales can be employed. This prospect may become increasingly plausible as lower time-scale information on biological and motoric signals is tracked continuously, such as when blocks or nested blocks of time for contexts, marker variables, and developmental epochs are considered.

An interesting question is whether Cook and Campbell's (1979) classic enumeration of threats to internal and external validity for experimental designs is complete with respect to this elaborated form of the design or whether other issues arise. For example, in comparing multiple epochs in which intensive measures have been obtained, a risk is that the passage of time will allow the participant to change to the extent that he or she will answer the same questions through a "different lens," or calibrate his or her responses differently. Whereas practical benefits of the design (e.g., reduced participant burden, possibly lower reactivity, reduced costs) are compelling, further questions can be raised in the following regards. First, in the case of a naturalistic multiple time point interruption, is it clear that the interruptions are occurring purely as a result of the criterion selection variable, or could other factors confound this variable? For example, neighborhood violence could be highly correlated with political or economic shifts, and these changes may remain unchanged even after violent behavior has subsided. Second, can the shape of the primary outcome be assessed well over short time bursts, and is this shape likely to be comparable from epoch to epoch as the overall higher order time course influences phenomena? For example, the epochs reflecting the shape of electrocardiogram signals before, during, and after some calendar time level disease onset, treatment, and remission may be very different both theoretically and in practice. Statistical tests of differences from epoch to epoch of differently shaped phenomena are likely to be very challenging to deploy.

Third, some concerns about selectivity in the case of the experimental time-scale-dependent design are worth considering. The nature of time scale as a criterion for selection of observation/planned missingness periods can be a double-edged sword. On one hand, reducing the number of intensive reporting intervals should reduce reporting burdens and thereby increase self-report validity. On the other hand, temporal undersampling may miss important features of all or some intraindividual change and variation or the events that cause such variation, as some individuals may manifest rapid or other interesting changes between epochs that would be undetected. This is a particularly important consideration when inference to particular individuals is of interest.

From a population perspective, it may not be necessary to capture the process fully in each individual, within overall inferences drawing from all available data and assuming exchangeability. Such a design is one of planned missingness with respect to the time element (e.g., McArdle, 1994). These concerns lead to the need for consideration of contemporary longitudinal concepts regarding time series. For example, an expectation that a series will reflect stationarity would enable the process to be modeled with a number of informative multivariate within-subject approaches, such as dynamic factor analysis or state-space modeling (Chow, Ho, Hamaker, & Dolan, 2010; Zhang, 2010). By contrast, if a specific pattern is expected within each burst, nonparametric functional forms or diverse parameterizations may be needed (Fok & Ramsay, 2006). In this case, the comparability from burst to burst can become much more challenging. Our later example in this chapter handles levels of time scale in the case of pain measurements with multilevel modeling; substantive questions levied at this database at this time did not require consideration of these more challenging modeling issues.

Developmental Applications

The distinction between nomothetic and idiographic approaches has a long history (Allport, 1937; Cattell, 1946, 1966; Lamiell, 1998). Nomothetic researchers seek to delineate broadly generalizable phenomena, whereas idiographic researchers seek to delineate empirically verifiable events and processes that contribute to within-person description and explanation. Although nomothetic research goals can sometimes be achieved using cross-sectional or panel designs, it is difficult to conceive of idiographic research goals that can be achieved without considering the effects of the passage of time. Idiographic methods are generally applied to studying the influence of prior experiences and events on subsequent behaviors and sometimes with continuities or discontinuities of behavior as the individual transitions from one setting to another.

In this tradition, Nesselroade and Jones (Jones & Nesselroade, 1990; Nesselroade & Jones, 1991) proposed what they called a *multivariate, replicated, single-subject, repeated-measures design*. One feature of this design is the use of repeated measures to empirically validate a hypothesized intraindividual temporal sequence. A second feature is the replication of the observed temporal sequence using observations drawn from multiple research participants as a means of establishing generalizability.

Nesselroade and Jones also noted the potential utility of incorporating successive "measurement bursts," giving the example of studies of therapeutic change in the context of interactions between clients and mental health professionals. In this example, a series of intensive measurements can be obtained prior to treatment for comparison with a series of intensive measurements obtained following the completion of treatment. This approach thereby incorporates almost all of the elements of the TDLDs that are the focus of this chapter, except multiple manipulations invoking interruptions.

Research may either focus on a planned interruption consisting of some form of treatment or it may focus on naturalistically occurring events. The latter—for example, fluctuations in daily stress—are, in theory, linked to corresponding fluctuations in behavior. Grzywacz and Almeida (2008) found support for a same-day association between stress and risk of binge drinking both within and between persons; they also found that a "pile up" of stress across at least 3 successive days accounted for additional variability in drinking behavior.

Grzywacz and Almeida's (2008) study may be regarded as an ex post facto design in that the distinction between high stress and low stress days is derived by categorizing the data after they have been collected. It differs from traditional ex post facto designs because the focus is on intraindividual change. This design seeks to simulate quasi-experimental designs by establishing, in retrospect, measures of variables both before and after exposure to the critical stimulus (i.e., "treatment").

Context Dependency

Taking Grzywacz and Almeida's (2008) study as an example, "high stress days" and "low stress days" represent two sets of conditions during which patterns of drinking behavior are expected to differ. The within-day stress–alcohol relationship and the between-day stress–alcohol relationship may be conceptualized as operating at two separate time scales. This leads to a broader point about the range of applications of TDLD.

People who are able to accurately report changes in their social or physical context may nonetheless fail to observe the relationship between changes in context and changes in their own behavior. A researcher may nonetheless be able to note these changes by sampling the individual's behavior in a range of contexts. Hence, diary-based event sampling may mitigate the effects of *consistency bias*, defined as the belief that one's past attitudes and behavior are more consistent with current attitudes and behavior than is actually the case (Jaspers, Lubbers, & De Graaf, 2009). For example, people provide different explanations of their motives for getting divorced when asked before and after the divorces (De Graaf & Kalmijn, 2006).

People overestimate the degree to which their future behavior will match their current intentions. Intentions to practice a health-protective behavior (e.g., safer sex) are at best moderately associated with subsequent behavior (Fishbein, Hennessy, Yzer, & Douglas, 2003). Similarly, *preference reversals* refer to discrepancies between goals and actions; an example is the individual who pays monthly dues at a gym that he or she never attends or who plans to avoid high-calorie snacks but nevertheless fails to resist the urge (Berns, Laibson, & Loewenstein, 2007).

Age-related changes in the ability to accurately identify the contextual determinants of one's own past behavior and to accurately predict one's future behavior remain understudied in the field of developmental psychology. These changes are nonetheless key indicators of an individual's functional capacity to exercise self-regulated behavior.

A benefit of an intensive longitudinal approach, then, is the unique perspective that it affords the researcher. Participants' self-report accuracy is likely more reliable with respect to currently experienced contexts as compared with self-reports of behavior in past or future contexts. A researcher, however, can accumulate "in context" data from multiple contexts and attempt to ascertain the degree to which the same experiences—being offered an alcoholic beverage, having an opportunity to engage in unprotected sex, or more generally having the opportunity to behave in an intention-congruent or intention-incongruent manner—will lead to different outcomes depending on the presence of identifiable contextual cues.

Ecological Constraints and Facilitators

Using TDLD also can afford the opportunity to arrive at more precise understanding of the factors influencing a behavior. For example, if the goal is to test the effect of alcohol use reduction treatments on drinking behavior, it is important to recognize that some individuals—for example, children under close parental supervision—may exhibit reduced drinking that is not attributable to the treatment. Other treatment recipients may face unusually high exposure to cues that elicit drinking behavior. An increase in drinking among these individuals does not necessarily cast doubt on the efficacy or effectiveness of the treatment; rather, it may simply impose a parameter (a certain level of exposure to drinking cues) at which reductions in drinking behavior are more or less likely to occur following treatment. Hypotheses implicating context-sensitive treatment-related change in behavior and hypotheses implicating context-sensitive differences in the maintenance or deterioration of treatment-related behavior change over time are amenable to being evaluated using a TDLD approach.

Classifying Contextual Influences

In documenting the occurrence of transitions by the individual from one context to another, the researcher may be concerned with either *marker* or *process* variables. A marker variable is a discrete point in time at which a psychologically meaningful change has occurred. Examples are marriage, giving birth, being transferred to a new school, and being deployed to combat. A process variable has "antecedents, durations, contexts, and outcomes" (Reese & Smyer, 1983, p. 2). So, for example, the transition to a new job may involve an increase in stress that is either abrupt or gradual, depending on the circumstances, and an eventual decline in stress as the individual adapts. These time-varying factors may be characterized either as dynamically stable or as reflective of developmental change. An example of the former is a hypothetical relationship between stress and impulsive behaviors such as binge drinking. As noted earlier, Grzywacz and Almeida (2008) found a significant difference between days on which high perceived stress was reported and days on which relatively low stress was reported. If the propensity to engage in binge drinking episodes is consistent—elevated on high stress days and reduced on low stress days—this illustrates dynamic stability and in a sense demonstrates replicability.

The distinction between a dynamically stable process and a developmental process may depend on the time scale one chooses to adopt. If the window of observation is a week or a month or even a year, the relationship between stress and binge drinking may appear to be stable. However, if the window of observation is several years, one may find that the more frequent binge drinkers exhibit a steady increase in overall alcohol consumption (Maggs & Schulenberg, 2004–2005). In this scenario, collecting intensive data on binge drinking on successive occasions—let us say, intensive data collected on occasions that are separated by 6 months or a year—will provide data on the changes in the day-to-day association between stress and binge drinking that arise over the course of several months. It is plausible that early in the onset of problem drinking behavior, stress is related to drinking, but that as drinking becomes more habitual and routine, the association with stress declines.

Examples of Marker Variables

Havighurst (1948) developed the concept of developmental tasks. These refer to the "demands, constraints, and opportunities provided by the social environment" as they influence the individual's goal of achieving optimal adaptation (p. 9). Havighurst theorized that failure to achieve a developmental task—for example, attaining an age-appropriate level of education—would adversely affect the individual's chances of mastering subsequent tasks. This may be represented as a marker variable—for example, nonattainment of a high-school diploma as a predictor of subsequent vocational outcomes.

This basic idea has been extended to encompass sequential discrete events. This is referred to as *cumulative disadvantage* (cf. Ross & Wu, 1996). Formal education is an often cited correlate of healthy lifestyle (e.g., abstinence from smoking, moderate alcohol use, etc.). Yet, as Ross and Wu point out, that healthy lifestyle is already evident prior to enrollment among individuals who attend college. One may speculate, then, that the protective effects of education will affect individuals differently depending on their prior status. The sociodemographic factors that predict college attendance also predict alcohol use.

If sociodemographic factors are in fact important determinants of behavior, personological accounts of problem drinking, which rely on constructs such as "low self-control," convey a misleading picture. That is, low self-control is not merely an attribute of persons, but is an effect of the individual's exposure to stressful environments. The marker variable, in this case, may consist of the point in time at which a transition from one environment to another has occurred. One may conjecture that improving an individual's environment will lead to reductions in problem behavior—indeed, evidence suggests that altering living environments is a powerful means of reducing the reinstatement of drug use among abstinent individuals (Solinasi, Chauvet, Thiriet, El Rawas, & Jaber, 2008). A key question from the standpoint of treatment planning is to arrive at a better understanding of the likely speed, peak level, and stability of behavior change based on duration of exposure to an improved environment. This is another example of a type of question that can be addressed using a TDLD approach.

Marker Variables in Ecological Momentary Assessment

In the naturalistic study of behavior, researchers sometimes examine the effects of so-called daily hassles on subsequent behavior. Events—for example, having an argument with a spouse or coworker—are used as markers indicating the onset of increased stress or negative affect (NA). Stress and NA are, in turn, recognized to be proximate antecedents of occasions of cigarette smoking, alcohol use, and other health-compromising self-regulatory behaviors. Ecological momentary assessment (EMA) describes a subset of diary studies in which, typically, multiple measures are collected within a single day, and the goal is to assess intraindividual fluctuations in affective and motivational states such as NA and craving. EMA has been facilitated by advances such as handheld computers, which permit the convenient capture of momentary data (Stone & Shiffman, 1994, 2002).

As a practical matter, it is difficult to establish the moment at which a hassle or disturbing event has inflected a change in affective state. The marker event (e.g., an argument with a coworker) may signal the onset of increased NA, or increased NA may have led to the argument. A reciprocal process might exist, such that increasing NA directly contributes to the escalation of the argument and vice versa. The individual providing self-report data may fail to recognize this as it is happening. Hence, situations arise in which markers may be present but are difficult to localize.

A practical solution to this problem is to regard markers not as a single point in time but as a meaningful pattern of successive measurements. Along these lines, Shiffman and Waters (2004) compared different time scales for analyzing EMA data on smoking lapses. They observed that, prior to lapse events, successive measures of within-day NA showed a pattern of increase. So a "marker" may not consist of a single point but instead of a point at which a change in trajectory can be observed across successive observations.

Illustration

In this short example, we wish both to share the form of data that result from a TDLD and to develop a sense of the questions and analyses that can be pursued with the design. Our data, involving burst reports on pain over calendar time, may not be truly developmental in nature; however, the course of pain over the study period is directly analogous to many developmental studies (e.g., vocabulary growth at intervals within a developmental stage). Our model would be deployed in the same manner for typical developmental data.

The data for the current example come from 116 older adults (mean age = 80, *SD* = 6, range = 66–95, 72% female, mean education = 15 years, *SD* = 2) who participated in a longitudinal study of health and cognition. Participants completed self-report measures of physical pain and daily stress on each of six daily sessions for a 14-day period. These bursts of six daily measurements were repeated every 6 months for a 2-year period, yielding up to five bursts of 30 daily assessments (see Sliwinski, Smyth, Hofer, & Stawski, 2006, for more details on study specifics).

Individuals were required to rate how much pain they had experienced during the previous 24 hours on a continuous scale ranging from 0 (no pain) to 100 ("the most pain you could imagine"). Additionally, participants completed a version of the Daily Inventory of Stressful Events (DISE; Almeida, Wethington, & Kessler, 2002). The version of the DISE included in this study consisted of a stem, "During the past 24 hours," followed by five questions: (1) Did you have an argument or disagreement with anyone? (2) Did anything else happen that you could have argued or disagreed about, but you decided to let it pass? (3) Did anything happen to a close friend or relative that turned out to be stressful for you? (4) Did anything stressful happen regarding your personal health? (5) Did anything else happen that most people would consider stressful?

Participants rated the severity of each of each of these stressors using a 4-point scale (0 = *not at all* to 3 = *very*). Individuals were then probed regarding the specific content of experienced stressors. For the current example, we used the subjective severity appraisals as our index of daily stress by calculating the average severity of the events reported across each day. Other quantifications of stress could be used in this context (e.g., peak stress) and may make appropriate theoretical sense for certain hypotheses. However, individuals in the current study typically reported only one stressful event per day, rendering peak stress and average daily stress almost perfectly collinear, and considering the benefits of alternative quantifications of stress is beyond the scope of this example.

Applying the Multilevel Model to Time-Scale-Dependent Longitudinal Data

For the purposes of the current illustration, we used multilevel or hierarchical linear modeling (Laird & Ware, 1982; Raudenbush & Bryk, 2002). This analytic framework allowed us to decompose variability in pain ratings, to model shorter- and longer-term trends in the data, and to consider associations between variables at three different levels of analysis (i.e., across days, bursts, and people). An unconditional multilevel model was used to decompose total variability in pain into three components: day-to-day variability, burst-to-burst variability, and between-person variability. A three-level model was fit to the pain data in which level 1 reflected within-person variability across days, level 2 reflected within-person variability across biannual bursts, and level 3 reflected between-persons variability. A pedagogical treatment of this overall approach with a similar three-level model can be reviewed in Walls, Jung, and Schwartz (2006). The first two levels both describe within-person sources of variability, but over different time scales. Variability at level 3 describes between-person variability in level of pain, averaged across all sessions and bursts. The following model served as the basis for these analyses:

$$\text{Pain}_{ijk} = \pi_{0jk} + \pi_{1jk}\text{Session}_{ijk} + e_{ijk} \qquad \text{(Level 1)}$$

$$\pi_{0jk} = \beta_{00k} + \beta_{01k}\text{Burst}_{.jk} + \beta_{02k}\text{Burst*Burst}_{.jk} + U_{0jk} \qquad \text{(Level 2)}$$

$$\pi_{1jk} = \beta_{10k} + U_{1jk}$$

$$\beta_{00k} = \gamma_{000} + \gamma_{001}\text{Age}_{..k} + V_{00k} \qquad \text{(Level 3)}$$

$$\beta_{01k} = \gamma_{010} + V_{01k}$$

$$\beta_{10k} = \gamma_{100} + V_{10k} \qquad \textbf{(4.1)}$$

where Pain_{ijk} is the pain score for session i, burst j, and person k. The variance components for the level 1 residuals, $\text{Var}(e_{ijk})$, and the level 2 residuals, $\text{Var}(U_{0jk})$, both reflect within-person variability, but each with its own cadence. Level 1 residuals reflect within-person day-to-day variability, and level 2 residuals reflect within-person variability observed across 6-month intervals. Variance in the level 3 residuals, $\text{Var}(V_{0k})$, indicates the amount of stable variability (i.e., individual differences) in affect that exists between persons (averaged across all sessions and bursts). Computing the ratio of any single variance to the sum of all three ($\text{Var}(e_{ijk}) + \text{Var}(U_{0jk}) + \text{Var}(V_{00k})$) will provide an index of the ratio of the total variability that exists at each level (i.e., the day level, the burst level, and the person level). Equation 4.1 also allows the session (i.e., testing reactivity) effects to vary randomly from burst to burst (U_{1jk}) and from person to person (V_{10k}). The effect of burst (or long-term change) is allowed to vary randomly from person to person (V_{01k}). There are also fixed, or average, effects that reflect the average pain score (γ_{000}), the average session effect (γ_{100}) and the average burst effect (γ_{010}). The fixed effect of baseline age (γ_{001}) was also estimated. Age was centered at 80, which was the average age at the first assessment. Estimates of parameters were estimated using SAS Proc Mixed under full information maximum likelihood using all available data (under the assumption of missing at random) with all random effects (i.e., variances and covariances) freely estimated.

Additionally, we examined the associations between daily stress and pain reports at the three levels of analysis—within person across days, within person across bursts, and between persons. Three variables were created to include in the statistical models, corresponding to the stress effects at each level of analysis. At level 1, the stress × day_{ijk} variable refers to the self-reported stress severity for day i during burst j for person k. At level 2, the stress × burst_{jk} variable refers to the average daily stress for person k during burst j, and at level 3, the stress × person_k variable represents the average daily stress for person k aggregated across all days and bursts. The stress variables were grand-mean centered (e.g., Hoffman & Stawski, 2009) but were not further centered within persons or within bursts. We chose to use the grand-mean-centered raw stress values in order to maintain a consistent meaning of the daily stress values across individuals and bursts. The stress variables, centered in this fashion, can be interpreted as such: stress × day_{ijk} is the average within-person day-level stress slope, stress × $\text{burst}_{.jk}$ is the *difference* between the within-person day-level and within-person burst-level slopes, and stress × $\text{person}_{..k}$ is the *difference* between the within-person burst level and the (between-person) person-level slopes (Snijders & Bosker, 1999). We used the ESTIMATE command from SAS Proc Mixed to produce burst-level (stress × day_{ijk} + stress × $\text{burst}_{.jk}$) and person-level (stress × day_{ijk} + stress × $\text{burst}_{.jk}$ + stress × $\text{person}_{..k}$) reactivity slope estimates and their standard errors.

Within this statistical framework, we are able to examine associations at three levels of analysis (i.e., within persons across days, within persons across bursts, and between persons) simultaneously. The association within person across days indicates the extent to which pain ratings were higher on days individuals rated experiencing more severe stress. The association within person across bursts indicates the extent to which pain ratings were higher during bursts (6-month epochs) in which individuals rated experiencing more severe stress. The between-person association indicates the extent to which pain ratings were higher for individuals who reported experiencing more severe stress. Thus, the first two types of associations reflect the extent to which stress and pain ratings are coupled within persons over two different temporal intervals (i.e., days and bursts), whereas the last type of association reflects the extent to which individual differences in stress and pain ratings are associated.

Results

The first model we estimated was a fully empty model, simply to decompose variability in daily pain ratings across the three levels of analysis. As can be seen in Table 4.1 (Model 1), the intraclass correlation coefficient (ICC) was .37 (135.44/(135.44 + 92.84 + 135.97)), indicating that 37% of the variability in pain ratings reflected between-persons differences. The remaining 63% of the variability reflected within-person variability across the two different temporal scales, across days (37%) and semiannual bursts (25%). Thus the vast majority of variability in pain ratings reflected within-person variation.

Next, we sought to expand Model 1 to consider cross-sectional and longitudinal aging trends in physical pain reports. This was accomplished by employing equation 4.1. Figure 4.1 displays the mean pain ratings across sessions and bursts for the duration of the study. Visual inspection of Figure 4.1 suggests a couple of noteworthy points. First, there is noticeable variability in pain ratings across days within a burst, with evidence of pain ratings decreasing across the successive 6 days of assessments. Second, there is noticeable variability in pain ratings across bursts (average pain across the six assessments), with some evidence suggesting that pain ratings are increasing across successive bursts of assessment.

TABLE 4.1. Multilevel Model Estimates for Pain across Days, Bursts, and Persons

	Model 1			Model 2			Model 3		
	Estimate	*SE*	*p*	Estimate	*SE*	*p*	Estimate	*SE*	*p*
Fixed effects									
Intercept	14.26	0.98	< .01	9.07	2.14	< .01	5.56	2.17	0.01
Session				–0.82	0.14	< .01	–0.79	0.14	< .01
Burst				4.46	1.46	< .01	4.18	1.45	< .01
Burst*Burst				–0.55	0.24	0.03	–0.47	0.24	0.05
Baseline Age				–0.08	0.03	< .01	–0.02	0.03	0.49
Stress (WP Day)							0.43	0.12	< .01
Stress (WP Burst)							1.57	1.54	0.31
Stress (BP)							2.38	0.45	< .01
Variance components									
Person level									
Intercept	135.44	18.46	< .01	122.48	34.25	< .01	100.36	32.08	< .01
Cov I.S.				–5.69	3.16	0.07	–5.04	3.06	0.09
Session				0.66	0.48	0.09	0.63	0.47	0.09
Cov I.B.				0.11	8.06	0.98	0.76	7.79	0.92
Cov S.B.				0.49	0.77	0.53	0.54	0.76	0.48
Burst				6.27	2.54	< .01	6.64	2.56	< .01
Burst level									
Intercept	92.84	7.69	< .01	105.31	15.97	< .01	103.04	15.89	< .01
Cov I.S.				–7.74	2.89	< .01	–7.74	2.86	< .01
Session				2.04	0.68	< .01	2.05	0.68	< .01
Session level									
Residual	135.97	3.3	< .01	124.55	3.52	< .01	123.95	3.49	< .01

Note. Cov, covariance; I, intercept; S, session; B, burst.

As can be seen in Model 2 in Table 4.1, the fixed effects of the model revealed that pain reports significantly decreased across days within a burst (estimate = –0.82, *SE* = 0.14). Importantly, the burst effect, which captures more durable longitudinal changes in pain ratings, was significant and positive (estimate = 4.46, *SE* = 1.46), indicating that pain ratings were increasing by about 4.5 points per year of aging. Furthermore, the quadratic burst term was also significant and negative (estimate = –0.55, *SE* = 0.24), indicating that the rate of increase in pain ratings was decelerating. In contrast to the evidence for longitudinal increases in pain ratings, the cross-sectional age effect was significant and negative (estimate = –0.08, *SE* = 0.03), indicating that the participants who were older on entry into the study reported having lower pain on average. Thus, the longitudinal and cross-sectional age trends tell opposing stories, with the former indicating that *getting* older is associated with increasing pain, whereas *being* older is associated with decreased pain. We did test whether baseline age moderated the longitudinal burst effect and found no evidence to suggest such

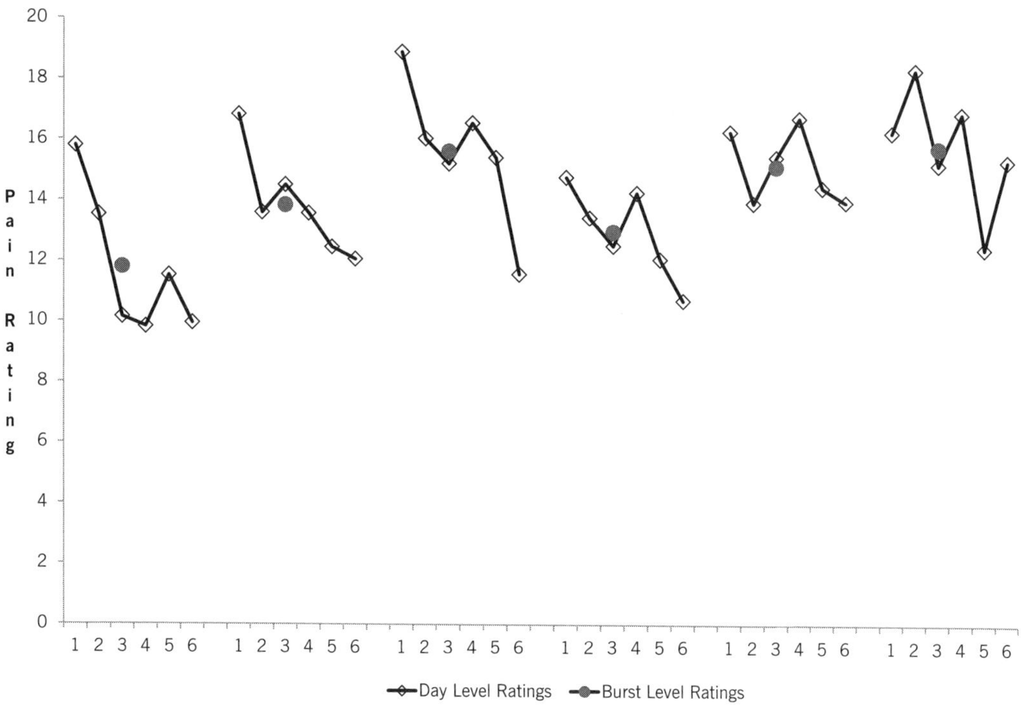

FIGURE 4.1. Average pain levels across days and bursts. Diamonds reflect sample average pain ratings for a given day; circles reflect sample average pain for burst.

moderation. Additionally, it is worth noting that the random effect for burst, which allows for individual differences in the growth trajectory for pain, was significant, indicating evidence of heterogeneity in the rate of change in pain ratings.

The opposing directions of the cross-sectional and longitudinal effects could reflect a selectivity bias, whereby older pain-ridden individuals are underrepresented in the sample, or differential age-related thresholds for pain ratings. Nonetheless, these opposing effects provide strong evidence that the effects of *being* older and of *getting* older are not equivalent. This finding echoes Robinson's (1950) caveat of the ecological fallacy, whereby the use of aggregate statistics of a sample to make inferences about any given individual in the sample can often lead to incorrect conclusions, and indicates that appropriately nuanced and circumspect conclusions regarding cross-sectional versus longitudinal trends and between-person versus within-person associations, given the available data, are necessary.

Finally, we wanted to consider whether daily stress was associated with pain at three levels of analysis (i.e., within-persons across days, within-persons across bursts, and between persons). To test these associations, the $stress\_day_{ijk}$, $stress\_burst_{.jk}$, and $stress\_person_{..k}$ variables were added to equation 4.1 at levels 1, 2, and 3, respectively. The results of these stress analyses can be seen in Model 3 in Table 4.1. At the day level, the stress effect was significant (estimate = 0.43, SE = 0.12), indicating that on days on which participants reported their stressors to be more severe, they also rated their bodily pain on that day as being worse. At the burst level, stressor severity ratings and pain ratings were not significantly associated (estimate = 1.57, SE = 1.54), indicating that there was no reliable association between the average severity of a participant's stressors at a given burst of measurement and his or her average pain levels during that burst. Finally, at the person level, we did see a significant association between stressor severity and pain ratings such that participants who reported their stressors to be more severe on average also reported having worse pain (estimate = 2.38, *SE* = 0.45). Furthermore, we did explore whether the day-level (level 1) or person-level (level 3) stress effects interacted with cross-sectional age or the longitudinal growth trajectories and did not find any such evidence. Thus stressor severity and pain ratings do exhibit significant positive associations between persons, as well as within persons over time. This latter effect, however, appears to be more specific to a faster temporal cadence, day-to-day coupling of stress and pain levels, rather than to a slow temporal cadence, coupling of stress and pain levels over semiannual assessments.

A few important limitations to our illustration should be noted. First, we have not explored the possibility of different error covariance structures carefully for this example. It could be that an autoregressive process of the residuals would be theoretically most appropriate; however, some aspects of the substantive measurements made us cautious about this assumption. Moreover, within the multilevel modeling framework it is not clear how to anticipate a covariance structure for burst-to-burst intervals or possibly higher levels of a TDLD.

Future Directions

This chapter presents a discussion of TDLDs, consisting of specific variations of an ITS design in which time-varying processes are sampled across at least two different time scales. A researcher might wish to examine temporal trends in the amount of time students spend studying during the days or weeks leading up to an exam and compare these trends on successive semesters to determine whether students' studying habits improve over time as a function of increasing commitment, emotional maturity, or the demands imposed by increasingly challenging material. In that the exam constitutes a discrete reference point, it functions as a marker variable, and the amount of time remaining until the day of the exam functions as a process variable that is (one may predict) inversely related to amount of time spent studying. An important feature of these designs is that they permit an evaluation of between-person differences in model parameters obtained within the burst (e.g., time spent studying, pattern of study) that are related to other individual characteristics (e.g., stress, health) and to external outcomes measured within the burst (scores on examination, course grade).

Proceeding from this basic idea, a wide range of practical applications present themselves. One may consider, for example, a habitual response that is dynamically stable at one time scale (e.g., drinking to reduce stress) but that exhibits a directional trend (e.g., increasing alcohol dependence) on another time scale. A related example is the sampling of self-reported quality of marital interactions before and after a treatment aimed at improving communication skills. The value of obtaining preintervention and postintervention data at multiple time points is that instances of marital discord are unevenly distributed over time. Furthermore, retrospective accounts may be biased by the effects of subsequent events on the accuracy of recall.

Used prospectively, a TDLD may offer a useful alternative to a randomized controlled design when randomization is not feasible. If a treatment is structured so that the starting date varies by participant but the duration of treatment is constant, one may observe whether a change that is plausibly attributable to treatment replicates itself for different persons and under varying historical circumstances (Hawkins, Sanson-Fisher, Shakeshaft, D'Este, & Green, 2007). If this multiple baseline approach is merged with TDLD, one may monitor the interaction between treatment dosage and change in treatment-related outcomes, based on comparisons between measures obtained from the same participant before, during, and following treatment. This mitigates many of the threats to validity that have traditionally been addressed using randomization procedures and can rigorously evaluate the question of whether change in behavior has occurred, whether this change is likely attributable to treatment, and whether the change is significant.

Another important feature of the TDLD is that it provides a design-based approach for dealing with reactivity or retest effects, a confound in typical widely spaced longitudinal designs that can limit comparison of results across studies. For example, in the area of cognitive functioning, the application of measurement burst designs permits the modeling of change in asymptotic performance, estimated within each burst, over longer periods of time across burst measurements.

The selection of temporal intervals for a particular application is challenging. The selection of temporal sampling is critical, with oversampling better than undersampling the process of interest (e.g., Boker & Nesselroade, 2002). Replication, generalizability, and comparisons across studies that use different sampling frames will have to be considered, as studies using different sampling intervals are likely to require different interpretations of within- and between-person processes (Martin & Hofer, 2004). Gollob and Reichardt (1987) discuss this issue in terms of measuring causal predictors when they have their maximal effect and the problems in typical studies when this is not a consideration. Also important is the related issue of interval censoring and the temporal resolution by which particular time-varying events can be modeled and compared across studies, although subgroup analyses can be performed on the individuals experiencing a common event. We expect that with increased empirical data, useful temporal sampling frames will be better understood.

The TDLD provides many opportunities to understand individual processes and model the continued development of individuals over time. The design itself is by definition an efficient design in that temporal sampling of different temporal resolutions is performed to capture important aspects of individual functioning across both short-term and long-term periods. There are numerous analytical opportunities for directly modeling within-person processes but also for an increased understanding of between-person differences in a variety of potential parameters that capture the within-person level, change, and variation. The inclusion of more intensive measurements within typical widely spaced longitudinal designs has the potential to enhance measurement of between-person differences but, more important, to permit a basis for understanding long-term change in intraindividual processes.

Acknowledgments

Theodore A. Walls was supported by a research scholar grant from the American Cancer Society (No. MRSG-07-015-01) and Scott M. Hofer was supported by National Institutes of Health Grant No. G026453. We would like to thank Martin Sliwinski for use of the data (supported by National Institutes of Health Grant No. R01 AG12448) that served as the example for this chapter.

References

Allport, G. (1937). *Personality: A psychological interpretation*. New York: Henry Holt.

Almeida, D. M., Wethington, E., & Kessler, R. C. (2002). The Daily Inventory of Stressful Experiences (DISE): An interview-based approach for measuring daily stressors. *Assessment, 9*, 41–55.

Barlow, D. H., Nock, M. K., & Hersen, M. (2009). *Single case experimental designs: Strategies for studying behavior change*. Boston: Pearson.

Berns, G. S., Laibson, D., & Loewenstein, G. (2007). Intertemporal choice: Toward an integrative framework. *Trends in Cognitive Sciences, 11*(11), 482–488.

Bertenthal, B. I. (2007). Dynamical systems: It's all about time. In S. Boker & M. Wenger (Eds.), *Data analytic techniques for dynamical systems* (pp. 1–24). Mahwah, NJ: Erlbaum.

Boker, S. M., Molenaar, P., & Nesselroade, J. R. (2009) Issues in intraindividual variability: Individual differences in equilibria and dynamics over multiple time scales. *Psychology and Aging, 24*, 858–862.

Boker, S. M., & Nesselroade, J. R. (2002). A method for modeling the intrinsic dynamics of intraindividual variability: Recovering the parameters of simulated oscillators in multi-wave panel data. *Multivariate Behavioral Research, 37*, 127–160.

Box, G., & Jenkins, G. (1970). *Time series analysis: Forecasting and control*. San Francisco: Holden-Day.

Campbell, D. T. (1969a). From description to experimentation: Interpreting trends as quasi-experiments. In C. W. Harris (Ed.), *Problems in measuring change* (pp. 212–242). Madison: University of Wisconsin Press.

Campbell, D. T. (1969b). Reforms as experiments. *American Psychologist, 24*, 409–429.

Campbell, D. T., & Stanley, J. C. (1963). Experimental and quasi-experimental designs for research on teaching. In N. L. Gage (Ed.), *Handbook of research on teaching* (pp. 171–246). Chicago: Rand McNally.

Campbell, D. T., & Stanley, J. C. (1966). *Experimental and quasiexperimental designs for research*. Chicago: Rand McNally.

Cattell, R. B. (1946). Personality structure and measurement: I. The operational determination of trait unities. *British Journal of Psychology, 36*, 159–174.

Cattell, R. B. (1966). The data box: Its ordering of total resources in terms of possible relational systems. In R. B. Cattell (Ed.), *Handbook of multivariate experimental psychology* (p. 67–128). Chicago: Rand McNally.

Chow, S.-M., Ho, M. R., Hamaker, E. L., & Dolan, C. V. (2010). Equivalence and differences between structural equation modeling and state-space modeling techniques. *Structural Equation Modeling, 17*, 303–332.

Collins, L. M. (2006). Analysis of longitudinal data: The integration of theoretical model, temporal design, and statistical model. *Annual Review of Psychology, 57*, 505–528.

Cook, T. D., & Campbell, D. T. (1979). *Quasi-experimentation: Design and analysis issues for field settings*. Chicago: Rand McNally.

De Graaf, P. M., & Kalmijn, M. (2006). Divorce motives in a period of rising divorce: Evidence from a Dutch life-history survey. *Journal of Family Issues, 27*, 483–505.

Fishbein, M., Hennessy, M., Yzer, M., & Douglas, J. (2003). Can we explain why some people do and some people do not act on their intentions? *Psychology, Health, and Medicine, 8*, 3–18.

Fiske, D. W., & Rice, L. (1955). Intra-individual response variability. *Psychological Bulletin, 3*, 217–250.

Flavell, J. H., & Draguns, J. (1957). A microgenetic approach to perception and thought. *Psychological Bulletin, 54*(3), 197–217.

Fok, C.C.-T., & Ramsay, J. O. (2006). Periodic trends, non-periodic trends and their interactions in longitudinal or functional data. In T. A. Walls & J. L. Schafer (Eds.), *Models for intensive longitudinal data* (pp. 109–122). New York: Oxford University Press.

Gollob, H. F., & Reichardt, C. S. (1987). Taking account of time lags in causal models. *Child Development, 58*, 80–92.

Grzywacz, J. G., & Almeida, D. M. (2008). Stress and binge drinking: A daily process examination of stressor pile-up and socioeconomic status in affect regulation. *International Journal of Stress Management, 15*(4), 364–380.

Havighurst, R. J. (1948). *Developmental tasks and education*. New York: McKay.

Hawkins, N. G., Sanson-Fisher, R. W., Shakeshaft, A., D'Este, C., & Green, L. W. (2007). The multiple baseline design for evaluating population-based research. *American Journal of Preventative Medicine, 33*(2), 162–168.

Hoffman, L., & Stawski, R. S. (2009). Persons as contexts: Evaluating between-person and within-person effects in longitudinal analysis. *Research in Human Development, 6*, 97–120.

Hufford, M. R., Shields, A. L., Shiffman, S., Paty, J., & Balabanis, M. (2002). Reactivity to ecological momentary assessment: An example using undergraduate problem drinkers. *Psychology of Addictive Behaviors, 16*(3), 205–211.

Jaspers, E., Lubbers, M., & De Graaf, N. D. (2009). Measuring once twice: An evaluation of recalling attitudes in survey research. *European Sociological Review, 25*(3), 287–301.

Jones, C. J., & Nesselroade, J. R. (1990). Multivariate, replicated, single-subject designs and P-technique factor analysis: A selective review of intraindividual change studies. *Experimental Aging Research, 16*, 171–183.

Laird, N., & Ware, J. (1982). Random-effects models for longitudinal data. *Biometrics, 38*, 963–974.

Lamiell, J. T. (1998). "Nomothetic" and "idiographic": Contrasting Windelband's understanding with contemporary usage. *Theory and Psychology, 8*, 23–38.

Maggs, J. L., & Schulenberg, J. E. (2004–2005). Trajectories of alcohol use during the transition to adulthood. *Alcohol Research and Health, 28*(4), 195–201.

Martin, M., & Hofer, S. M. (2004). Intraindividual variability, change, and aging: Conceptual and analytical issues. *Gerontology, 50*, 7–11.

McArdle, J. J. (1994). Structural factor analysis experiments with incomplete data. *Multivariate Behavioral Research, 29*(4), 409–454.

McDowall, D., McCleary, R., Meidinger, E. E., & Hay, R. A. (1980). *Interrupted time series analysis*. Beverly Hills, CA: Sage.

Nesselroade, J. R. (1991). The warp and the woof of the developmental fabric. In R. M. Downs & L. S. Liben (Eds.), *Visions of aesthetics, the environment and development: The legacy of Joachim F. Wohlwill* (pp. 213–240). Hillsdale, NJ: Erlbaum.

Nesselroade, J. R., & Jones, C. J. (1991). Multi-modal selection effects in the study of adult development: A perspective on multivariate, replicated, single-subject, repeated measures. *Experimental Aging Research, 11*, 21–27.

Nesselroade, J. R., & Schmidt-McCollam, K. M. (2000). Putting the process in developmental processes. *International Journal of Behavioral Development, 24*, 295–300.

Newell, A. (1990). *Unified theories of cognition*. Cambridge, MA: Harvard University Press.

Raudenbush, S. W., & Bryk, A. S. (2002). *Hierarchical linear models: Applications and data analysis methods* (2nd ed.). Thousand Oaks, CA: Sage.

Reese, H. W., & Smyer, M. A. (1983). The dimensionalization of life events. In E. J. Callahan & K. McCluskey (Ed.), *Life-span developmental psychology: Non-normative life events*. New York: Academic Press.

Robinson, W. S. (1950). Ecological correlations and the behavior of individuals. *American Sociological Review, 15*, 351–357.

Rosenbaum, D. A., & Collyer, C. E. (Eds.). (1998). *Timing of behavior: Neural, psychological, and computational perspectives*. Cambridge, MA: MIT Press.

Rosenthal, V. (2004). Microgenesis, immediate experience, and visual processes in reading. In A. Carsetti (Ed.), *Seeing, thinking and knowing: Meaning and self-organisation in visual cognition and thought* (pp. 221–244). Norwell, MA: Kluwer.

Ross, C. E., & Wu, C.-L. (1996). Education, age, and the cumulative advantage in health. *Journal of Health and Social Behavior, 37*(1), 104–120.

Shiffman, S., & Waters, A. J. (2004). Negative affect and smoking lapses: A prospective analysis. *Journal of Consulting and Clinical Psychology, 72*, 192–201.

Sliwinski, M. J. (2008). Measurement-burst designs for social health research. *Social and Personality Psychology Compass, 2*, 245–261.

Sliwinski, M. J., Almeida, D. M., Smyth, J. M., & Stawski, R. S. (2009). Intraindividual change and variability in daily stress processes: Findings from two measurement-burst diary studies. *Psychology and Aging, 24*, 828–840.

Sliwinski, M. J., Smyth, J. M., Hofer, S. M., & Stawski, R. S. (2006). Intraindividual coupling of daily stress and cognition. *Psychology and Aging, 21*(3), 545–557.

Snijders, T., & Bosker, R. (1999). *Multilevel analysis: An introduction to basic and advanced multilevel modeling*. London: Sage.

Solinasi, M., Chauvet, C., Thiriet, N., El Rawas, R., & Jaber, M. (2008). Reversal of cocaine addiction by environmental enrichment. *Proceedings of the National Academy of Sciences of the United States of America, 105*(44), 17145–17150.

Stone, A. A., & Shiffman, S. (Eds.). (1994). Ecological momentary assessment (EMA) in behavioral medicine [Special issue]. *Annals of Behavioral Medicine, 16*.

Stone, A. A., & Shiffman, S. (2002). Capturing momentary, self-report data: A proposal for reporting guidelines. *Annals of Behavioral Medicine, 24*, 236–243.

Swets, J. A. (Ed.). (1964). *Signal detection and recognition by human observers: Contemporary readings*. New York: Wiley.

Varkey, J. P., Pompili, D., & Walls, T. A. (2011). Human motion recognition using a wireless sensor-based wearable system. *ACM/Springer Journal of Personal and Ubiquitous Computing* [Special issue: Sensor-driven Computing and Applications for Ambient Intelligence], pp. 1–14.

Walls, T. A., Jung, H., & Schwartz, J. (2006). Multilevel models and intensive longitudinal data. In T. A. Walls & J. S. Schafer (Eds.), *Models for intensive longitudinal data* (pp. 3–37). New York: Oxford University Press.

Walls, T. A., & Schafer, J. S. (2006). *Models for intensive longitudinal data*. New York: Oxford University Press.

Weinstein, N. D. (2007). Misleading tests of health behavior theories. *Annals of Behavioral Medicine, 33*(1), 1–10.

Weinstein, S. M., Mermelstein, R., & Shiffman, S. (2008). Mood variability and cigarette smoking escalation among adolescents. *Psychology of Addictive Behaviors, 22*(4), 504–513.

Zhang, G. (2010). Dynamic factor analysis with ordinal variables. In S.-M. Chow, E. Ferrer, & F. Hsieh (Eds.), *Statistical methods for modeling human dynamics: An interdisciplinary dialogue*. New York: Taylor & Francis.

CHAPTER 5

Event Frequency Measurement

BRETT LAURSEN
JAAP DENISSEN
DAVID F. BJORKLUND

How many times were you intoxicated during the last month?

How many meals did you eat at home with your parents during the last week?

How much time did you spend on the Internet yesterday?

How often do you feel sad or depressed?

In this chapter we discuss the measurement of event frequencies. We focus on the cognitive underpinnings of frequency reports. Questions about the frequency of an event require the respondent to interpret the request and retrieve the information. Age differences in processing and retrieval abilities and in beliefs about the efficacy of retrieval strategies shape responses to questions about the rate and number of times an event is experienced. This has important implications for our understanding of developmental phenomena, because age differences in reports of event frequencies may not be a product of changes in the occurrence of an event but rather a reflection of changes in strategies used or an artifact of the questions asked.

Developmental scientists tend to take event frequency reports at face value. Poor internal or interrater reliability and marginal stability are usually attributed to one of two sources of error. Perceptual biases are a product of systematic differences in the information received about events or in the interpretation of events. Recounting biases are a product of systematic differences in the willingness to recount events or in the presentation of recounted events. Consider the well-established finding that adolescent self-reports of antisocial behavior are higher than maternal reports of their adolescent child's antisocial behavior (Verhulst & van der Ende, 1992). Perceptual biases may arise because mothers lack direct information about delinquent acts or because children encode deviant behaviors as harmless horseplay. Recounting biases may arise because mothers are embarrassed to acknowledge the shortcomings of a child or because children exaggerate participation in deviant acts to promote an oppositional identity.

In this chapter we focus on a third source of reporting bias, that arising from the cognitive demands of the task and the cognitive abilities of the respondent. Different respondents with different cognitive capabilities may use different retrieval strategies that give rise to different reporting biases. It follows that mothers and children may recount different rates of delinquent acts because one estimates events and the other attempts to count them.

Our chapter is divided into five sections. In the first section we illustrate the confusion that arises when different studies solicit information about event frequencies with questions that differ in subtle but important ways. In the second section we review memory retrieval strategies and discuss the quality of the frequency estimates that each produces. In the third section we summarize developmental differences in memory abilities, with an eye toward understanding how age-related changes in cognitive functions may affect retrieval strategy usage and event frequency estimates. In the fourth section we turn to the statistical consequences of reporting biases. Error variance and construct stability vary as a function of retrieval strategies, which, in turn, alter associations with outcome variables. In the fifth section we present a strategy for attenuating differential patterns of association arising from measurement differences in error variance and construct stability.

Central Issues

Measuring Frequencies

Measurement approaches may be divided into those that measure the frequency of events from the past, the recent past, and the present. Distinctions rest largely on the degree to which memory factors into the report. Retrospective reports measure events that occurred from the past week up to the past year; memory load is assumed to be highest in these reports. Recent reports assess events from the same or previous day; some memory load is required but minimal interference is assumed. Contemporary reports describe events occurring at the moment of assessment; minimal memory is required for these reports. Empirical examples will illustrate how conclusions differ with measurement practices.

Retrospective Reports

Retrospective assessments that span 1 week to 1 month are common. When justification is offered, it centers on the dual notion that this period is long enough for reports to be representative and short enough for events to be remembered. Examples include the Issues Checklist (Prinz, Foster, Kent, & O'Leary, 1979; Robin & Foster, 1984), in which parents and children identify all issues discussed during the past month or 2 weeks and rate the emotional intensity of each, and the Children's Depression Inventory, a survey of depressive symptoms during the previous 2 weeks (Kovacs, 1985). Time frames of 6–12 months are not unusual, however. Participants in Monitoring the Future report the frequency of drug, cigarette, and alcohol use during the past 12 months (Wallace et al., 2003), and respondents to the Child Behavior Checklist and the Youth Self-Report describe the relative frequency of specific problem behaviors during the previous 6 months (Achenbach, 1991). Longer assessment periods are not recommended. Comparisons of retrospective reports of hyperactivity, internalizing symptoms, delinquency, and arrests at age 18 with concurrent reports during childhood and adolescence revealed few associations that were statistically significant after corrections for chance agreement (Henry, Moffitt, Caspi, Langley, & Silva, 1994).

Unfortunately, it is not simply the case that one type of retrospective report is superior to another. Memory errors tend to increase with each week added to the time frame for recall, so the validity of reports decreases as the retrospective period lengthens (Thompson, 1982). Variance ascribed to individual differences in personality traits, relationship history, and cognitive schemas grows in proportion to the length of recall (Laursen & Collins, 2009). But longer time frames provide data on more events. The principle of aggregation holds that stability and reliability increase as the number of measurement points increases, which gives longer retrospective periods a decided advantage (Rushton, Brainerd, & Pressley, 1983). This suggests that the investigator who uses retrospective reports must balance concerns about validity with concerns about reliability when making decisions about recall periods.

Recent Reports

In response to concerns about retrospective reports, same-day or single-day reports have grown in popularity. Although technically retrospective, reports of events for the current or preceding day are distinguished from those of longer time frames because recent memory traces are assumed to be less biased and more accessible when interference is reduced (Robinson & Clore, 2002). Interval contingent diary studies require participants to record events at fixed time periods, such as every evening. To recount target events, participants may be asked to reconstruct all events of the previous day in chronological order, or they may be asked about the frequency of various forms of the target event. Reports may be recorded for several consecutive days and aggregated across the recording period.

Consistent with the principle of aggregation, single-day assessments of conflict frequency have lower internal reliability and stability than reports collected and aggregated across several consecutive days (Burk, Denissen, van Doorn, Branje, & Laursen, 2009). As was the case with retrospective reports, the advantages of recent report techniques that maximize reliability and stability must be weighed against threats to validity. Too many requests for information may introduce reporter fatigue, which can threaten the accuracy (and therefore the validity) of reports gathered over a period of successive days (Bolger, Davis, & Rafaeli, 2003).

Contemporary Reports

There are two types of contemporary reports: event sampling and time sampling. Both require participants to carry data recording devices or paper-and-pencil questionnaires at all times. With event-contingent sampling, participants complete an inventory each time a specific event occurs. With time-based sampling, participants complete an inventory on a fixed or random schedule throughout the day. When cued, participants describe the activities in which they are currently engaged or those that transpired since the last reporting time. Time-based and event-contingent strategies may be combined such that participant reports focus on target behaviors or activities described at random or fixed intervals.

Single responses from contemporary reports are not very reliable, but aggregated responses tend to be both stable and consistent (Diener & Larsen, 1984). Contemporary reports minimize retrospective bias. Validity is generally good, but reports from certain times and reports about certain events are unlikely to be obtained because participants are loath to stop what they are doing to complete a survey. Obtaining a representative sample is probably the biggest threat to the validity of contemporary reports, because the procedure places an extraordinary burden on participants.

Divergent Methods Produce Divergent Results

Research practices reflect the absence of a consensus on reporting practices. This lack of uniformity almost guarantees a confusing array of divergent results. The problem is illustrated here with a selective summary of parent–adolescent conflict. In one pair of studies, adolescents and parents reviewed a list of discussion topics and reported four to five (Steinberg, 1988) or five to seven (Smetana, Daddis, & Chuang, 2003) conversations that were not "very calm" during the preceding 2 weeks. In another study, adolescents reviewed a list of conflict topics and reported that during the past year disagreements over each of the 11 topics arose fewer than "a couple of times" per year and more than "not at all," which works out to be about one conflict per month (Shanahan, McHale, Osgood, & Crouter, 2007). Two studies asked adolescents to identify the number of conflicts arising during the previous day from a list of conflict topics (Adams & Laursen, 2007; Laursen, 1995). In both cases adolescents reported between two and three daily conflicts with mothers and about one daily conflict with fathers. A final set of studies asked participants to recount all social interactions during the previous day and indicate which involved conflict (Burk et al., 2009; Jensen-Campbell & Graziano, 2001). Across 7 consecutive days, adolescents reported one disagreement with parents every other day.

What is the frequency of parent–adolescent conflict? It is difficult to draw conclusions from studies whose estimates range from one conflict per month to three or four conflicts per day. Frequency estimates appear to vary as a function of the measurement practices. The evidence suggests that different reporting methods pull for different cognitive retrieval strategies that may heighten or lessen estimates of event frequency, a claim we review in the next section.

Conceptual Principles

Consider the request for a frequency estimate from an information processing perspective. The individual must (1) perceive the event, (2) label the event, (3) encode the event in memory, and (4) retrieve the event from memory. Variations in these processes influence frequency estimates, but these factors are beyond the control of most investigators. The selection of retrieval strategies, however, is often determined by the investigator. Cognitive retrieval strategies are sensitive to assessment methods, because the information requested determines the strategy employed. Put another way, different types of inquiry carry different cognitive demands, which suggests that the questions shape answers.

Cognitive Retrieval Strategies and Their Influence on Event Frequency Reports

Memory researchers typically divide event cognitive retrieval strategies into three broad categories (Blair & Burton, 1987; Brown, 1995): (1) experiential strategies, which involve identifying concurrent or recent experiences; (2) enumerative strategies, which involve some form of remembering and counting; and (3) semantic strategies, which involve some form of direct recall. Table 5.1 summarizes each.

TABLE 5.1. Retrieval Strategies and Their Implications for Event Frequency Estimation

Retrieval strategy	Examples and implications
Experiential	*Are you currently listening to music?*
Minimal retrieval required. Participants record contemporaneous events. Event frequency must be aggregated across reports from different times.	Difficult to capture rare events. Underreporting is a risk for events that participants are disinclined to interrupt.
Enumeration	*How many times were you afraid this week?*
Episodic. Participants retrieve specific events from memory and count the number of events recalled.	Accurate for events that are distinctive, atypical, and recent. Underreporting is a risk for frequent or mundane events and longer periods of recall.
Extrapolation from limited episodic recall. Participants estimate the number of events, retrieving from memory specific events arising during representative or recent time periods and extrapolating to longer time periods.	Accurate for events that are scheduled or recurrent. Underreporting and overreporting are risks for rare or clustered events. Reporting errors can occur when limited frequency counts are inaccurately extrapolated into total frequency counts because of faulty math.
Semantic	
Direct retrieval of tally or rate information.	*How much time did you spend in vigorous physical activity this week?*
Participants retrieve from memory the specific number of events or the specific rate of event occurrence.	Tally information is accurate for important events that are automatically tabulated as running totals. Underreporting is a risk as event frequencies increase. Rate information is accurate for events whose occurrence is invariant. Reporting errors can occur when the encoded rate is incorrectly mapped onto the recall period.
Conversion of beliefs and qualitative impressions. Participants retrieve from memory a subjective label describing the rate of event occurrence and use it to estimate event frequency.	Most accurate for low-frequency responses (e.g., converting "none" or "rarely" into specific event frequencies). Overreporting is a risk for high-frequency responses because participants tend to select large round numbers.

Experiential

Individuals use experiential strategies to describe experiences that are recent or ongoing. All responses to inquiries about event participation require some information retrieval, but requests concerning current or recent events are assumed to require the least cognitive effort because the experience is still fresh in the mind. Memory interference is presumed to be negligible because immediate responses leave little time for forgetting. Recall biases are minimized, although participants may still reflect on events when prompted by a signal or question.

Experiential strategies are not without bias. Affective arousal may introduce reporting error that might otherwise be eliminated with the benefit of calm reflection. Respondents complete reports in context, which means in the company of interaction partners. Responses may be intentionally inaccurate out of concern that interaction partners could access reports. The setting or the presence of a particular individual may be a source of unintentional bias; global feelings and impressions about particular people and places may be difficult to disentangle from actual events, particularly when the event is incongruous with the surroundings. Finally, reporting lags are confounded with events. Participants rarely complete reports while driving motorcycles, playing sports, or having sex. It is not known whether discrepancies between reports made in vivo and reports made minutes or hours later are greater for some particular events than for others. If so, there is considerable potential for systematic bias.

Enumeration

To enumerate is to count. In this case, events are recalled from memory, and a tally is reported. Enumeration retrieval strategies take two forms: episodic recall and episode-based estimation. Episodic recall involves a search of the memory for all instances that match the category of event requested (Williams & Durso, 1986). Remembered events are counted and reported. Episode-based estimation, also known as enumeration and extrapolation (Brown, 2002), involves the recollection of a subset of events, which are used to estimate a total. Respondents may remember events from a specific unit of time (e.g., counting text messages sent this afternoon and extrapolating to estimate text messages sent during the previous 24 hours), from a representative unit of time (e.g., tallying disagreements with parents for a typical day and extrapolating to a weekly total), or from a subordinate category of events (e.g., counting conversations with one friend and extrapolating to all friends).

Enumeration is accurate when participants are asked to recount events that are salient and infrequent. The more events there are to remember, the greater the chances that some will be forgotten, which suggests that underreporting is a risk for frequent events (Burton & Blair, 1991). The same is true for events that are mundane or that lack distinguishing features. Recent events are more apt to be recalled than distant events. Enumeration and extrapolation carry additional risks. Extrapolation works best for recurrent events that arise at fixed intervals (Brown, 1995). Atypical events and events that are punctuated or clustered together tend to be misestimated. Math errors pose a unique hazard because extrapolation usually requires mental multiplication.

Semantic

Other strategies access event frequency information from memory without enumeration. Direct retrieval involves recalling the number of events or their rate of occurrence. In some cases, direct retrieval is available because frequency information was automatically encoded (Hasher & Zacks, 1979). In other cases, direct retrieval is available because event totals were previously enumerated. Finally, some event totals are directly accessible because participants keep a running tally of occurrences.

Other forms of semantic retrieval are less precise. In some cases, participants have access only to beliefs or qualitative impressions about event frequency. Belief- or impression-based strategies entail the retrieval of labels that describe the rate of occurrence (e.g., rarely or sometimes), which are then used as the basis of quantitative estimates of event frequencies (Conrad, Brown, & Cashman, 1998). Thus subjective opinions are converted into seemingly objective frequency counts. The availability heuristic (Tversky & Kahneman, 1973) suggests that the ease with which events are recalled influences beliefs about quantity. The easier it is to recall instances or exemplars, the higher the estimate of event frequency. Thus salience may be confounded with frequency estimation when impression-based strategies are employed.

Direct retrieval can be remarkably accurate for infrequent, prominent events. But the risk of zooming or telescoping (projecting events into or out of the time frame for recall) is considerable because event dates are often not encoded or recalled (Sudman & Bradburn, 1974). Running tallies may get muddled with the passage of time, particularly as the number of events grows. Yet these risks pale when compared with those associated with the conversion of qualitative impressions into quantitative frequency estimates. Terms describing events that never occur are readily converted into zero, but accuracy declines as event frequencies increase because of the arbitrary conversion of descriptive labels to numbers (Brown, 2002). For common events, respondents usually convert labels into round numbers, which inflates frequencies.

Factors That Influence Strategy Selection

Faced with a request for a frequency count, most respondents initially check to see if a number can be retrieved directly from memory. If not, enumeration is usually the first strategy considered (Menon, Raghubir, & Schwarz, 1995). What determines whether enumeration will be pursued or abandoned in favor of qualitative impressions? Effort is typically balanced against accuracy; specifically, respondents attempt to minimize effort and maximize accuracy (Burton & Blair, 1991). Enumeration requires more time and more mental effort than the conversion of beliefs, which often amount to little more than educated guesses. When the task of counting events is deemed to be burdensome and time-consuming, participants opt for the faster and easier strategy of converting impressions. Respondents also evaluate different retrieval strategies for accuracy and select the strategy that is most likely to provide the correct answer. Respondents will favor the conversion of impressions over enumeration if the latter is perceived to be too much work or if they have reason to doubt the accuracy of their event counts. Otherwise, enumeration is preferred as the more accurate approach.

In addition to effort and accuracy, strategy selection varies according to characteristics of respondents and the content of the question. We consider each in turn.

Respondent Attributes

Highly motivated participants are more willing to invest effort in responses and are more concerned about the accuracy of their responses than are unmotivated participants. As a result, highly motivated participants tend to use enumeration, and unmotivated participants tend to use estimates derived from qualitative impressions. Systematic biases follow, because underestimation tends to accompany enumeration and overestimation tends to accompany qualitative impressions. Motivation is probably confounded with attributes such as education and personality, raising the prospect that educated, diligent participants select retrieval strategies biased toward underreporting and that uneducated, indifferent participants will select retrieval strategies biased toward overreporting.

There are gender differences in retrieval strategy selection. Consider the finding that males report more average lifetime sexual partners than females do. Braggadocio and evolutionary predispositions have been invoked as explanations, but recent findings suggest a more parsimonious interpretation: Men tend to provide estimates based on qualitative impressions, whereas women are more apt to respond using episodic recall (Brown & Sinclair, 1999).

Questionnaire Content

Respondents look to the questionnaire for clues about event frequencies, particularly if they are seeking to minimize mental effort or are concerned about the accuracy of their reports. Reliance on questionnaire clues varies with retrieval strategies. Frequencies derived from enumeration are little influenced by questionnaire content, but the effect on frequencies derived from the conversion of qualitative impressions is pronounced.

Questionnaire instructions point respondents toward retrieval strategies. Explicit directions to recall and count specific events pull for enumeration, whereas instructions to estimate rates or frequencies pull for conversion of impressions (Schimmack, 2002). Instructions alerting respondents to the difficulty of the task and reminders about the importance of accurate reports increase the use of enumeration (Schwarz et al., 1991).

The time interval selected for recall also points respondents toward retrieval strategies. As a general rule, shorter time frames are more amenable to enumeration than longer time frames because there are fewer events to count (Blair & Burton, 1987). Participants also look to time frames for clues concerning investigator expectations about frequency. Long time frames imply rare events, and short time frames imply common events; as the time frame for recall increases, respondents report fewer events per unit of time (Winkielman, Knäuper, & Schwarz, 1998). This effect may be attenuated somewhat when the same time period is adopted in multiple successive questions (Igou, Bless, & Schwarz, 2002).

The type of event to be recalled shapes the recall strategy. Rare and significant events may be accessed through direct retrieval or enumeration; frequent and mundane events cannot. Emotions are particularly hard to enumerate because they are encoded in terms of the triggering event, not the emotion experienced.

Question formats shape retrieval strategies. To aid with recall, investigators may decompose questions, breaking behavioral frequency reports for a broad category down into separate frequency reports for subcategories (e.g., replacing one question about dining in restaurants with separate questions about dining in Italian restaurants, seafood restaurants, fast food restaurants, and so on). Decomposition tends to encourage elaboration by providing memory cues, but frequent, mundane events are overreported because estimation procedures place the same event in multiple subcategories (Belli, Schwarz, Singer, & Talarico, 2000). Decomposition by companions and location is more effective in facilitating recall than decomposition by time. Hurried respondents avoid enumeration (Brown, 1995). It follows that interviews pull for estimation because of the implicit time constraints imposed by a waiting interviewer. Time limits on the completion of questionnaires do the same. Respondents confronting lengthy or multiple questionnaires may also perceive time pressures. Overestimation is likely in these conditions.

Response scales shape retrieval strategies. Participants are more likely to enumerate when they are required to fill in a blank (e.g., How many sodas did you drink last week? ______) than when response options are delimited by frequency scales, because participants may use the scales to shape estimates of their own behavior. Respondents (particularly unmotivated ones) may be tempted to select the scale midpoint, in the belief that this represents a typical response. Other respondents will look to the scale range, particularly the high end of the scale, for cues about response tendencies (Schwarz, Bless, Bohner, Harlacher, & Kellenbenz, 1991). Frequency scales with a low upper bound imply rare events that pull for enumeration. Response scales with a high upper bound imply common events that pull for conversion of impressions. Response scales with vague quantifiers as endpoints worsen the problem, because the same anchors mean different things to different people (Wright, Gaskell, & O'Muircheartaigh, 1994). The addition of anchor labels to frequency scales can change the number of events reported.

Developmental Applications

Children's accuracy in recounting the frequency of past events is influenced by a host of cognitive factors. None is more important than memory. Few developmental studies explicitly assess children's frequency estimates of important behavior, although studies have investigated children's frequency estimates of recently presented items (e.g., "Keep track of how many times each word is presented in this list"). These studies capture differences in automatic processing, which occurs without initiation and requires few mental resources. In an early study, 8-, 10-, and 12-year-old children and college adults were asked to keep track of the number of times each word appeared in a word list (Hasher & Chromiak, 1977). Half of the participants at each age were told that some of the words might be presented more than once and that they would later be asked how many times they saw each word. The remaining participants were simply told to remember the words so that they could answer some questions about them later on. Following the list presentation, all participants were asked to estimate how many times each word had been presented. Performance was greater for the informed than the uninformed participants, but, importantly, estimates were generally accurate and did not vary significantly with age. Subsequent research similarly reported no age differences in frequency estimation between children in kindergarten and in third grade (Hasher & Zacks, 1979), although other studies suggest small but significant differences between children in kindergarten and in fifth grade (e.g., Lund, Hall, Wilson, & Humphreys, 1983).

Most investigations into children's frequency estimations are not concerned with how many times a certain word was presented in a list, but with events that have occurred. Here, the concern is with explicit (deliberate) and effortful memory, which, unlike implicit and automatic memory, displays substantial improvement with age (see Schneider, 2010, for a review). Deliberate memory encompasses event memory, which is a form of autobiographical memory. Event memory is memory for things that happen to us during the course of everyday life. Memory for daily events increases over the preschool and early school years, as children learn to form narratives to tell a story so that another person can understand it. Event memory is constructive, with children recalling the gist of the event and in the process transforming what was actually said or done.

There are a host of age-related factors that influence how much children remember about past events (Schneider, 2010), including the use of strategies, children's knowledge of the workings of their memories (metamemory), their ability to monitor the source of their knowledge (source monitoring), and what they know about the events they are remembering (knowledge base). Older children are more likely than younger children to use strategies both to organize their experiences at input and to retrieve information at output (Bjorklund, Dukes, & Brown, 2009). Children's metamemory abilities also show substantial improvements with age. For example, preschool and early school-age children overestimate their ability to remember specific items and events (Shin, Bjorklund, & Beck, 2007). Young children seem unaware that strategies are available that can aid their recall of information or of the connection between using a strategy and improving memory performance (Justice, Baker-Ward, Gupta, & Jannings, 1997).

Another important factor that influences the accuracy of children's event memory is source monitoring, which refers to being aware of the origins of information one remembers. Although we all occasionally confuse knowledge sources, young children are more apt to incorrectly recall performing an action themselves that was actually performed by another person and are especially more likely to confuse imagined versus actual events (Foley, Ratner, & Gentes, 2010; Foley, Santini, & Sopasakis, 1989). Such source monitoring errors produce frequency overestimation.

Similar overestimation errors arise among young children who confuse witnessing an event with hearing about an event. In one set of studies (Principe, Haines, Adkins, & Guiliano, 2010; Principe, Kanaya, Ceci, & Singh, 2006), preschool children witnessed a magic show in which a magician failed to pull a rabbit out of his hat. Following the show, some children overheard an unfamiliar adult say that the trick failed because the rabbit escaped and was in the classroom eating carrots. When interviewed 1 week later, a majority of children who had heard the rumor reported that the rabbit had escaped and was loose in the classroom; many professed seeing the runaway bunny, often providing vivid descriptions of the (non)event. Older children and adults are less susceptible to this type of reconstructive memory error.

Perhaps the most potent factor affecting children's recall of events is background knowledge, or knowledge base, which typically increases with age (see Schneider, 2010, for a review). The more knowledge children have about what they are trying to remember, the more likely they are to use strategies effectively, and the more likely they are to remember information even in the absence of apparent strategies (Bjorklund & Zeman, 1982; Schwenck, Bjorklund, & Schneider, 2009). For example, children who know more about stressful and invasive medical procedures subsequently remember more accurate information and recall less inaccurate information than less knowledgeable children (Goodman, Quas, Batterman-Faunce, Riddlesberger, & Kuhn, 1994; Ornstein et al., 2006).

Familiarity increases memory accuracy for typical events, but it may decrease accuracy for atypical events. In one study 4- and 6-year-old children were given a mock physical examination and asked to recall specific aspects of the exam both immediately and 12 weeks later (Ornstein et al., 1998). Children recalled fewer specific actions at the 12-week than at the immediate assessment, but patterns of recall differed as a function of whether the events under question were typical for a physical exam (e.g., the doctor listening to the children's hearts with a stethoscope) or atypical (e.g., the doctor using alcohol to wipe their belly buttons). Some expected procedures were omitted from the exams (e.g., measuring blood pressure). Both 4- and 6-year-old children recalled more typical than atypical events, reflecting the positive role of knowledge base on event memory. However, at the 12-week assessment, correct denials (i.e., stating correctly that an event did not happen) were significantly greater for atypical events that did not happen than for typical events that did not happen. False alarms (i.e., reporting that an event happened when it did not) were also higher for typical events than for atypical events. Knowing what usually happens caused children to falsely remember what did happen.

Statistical Assumptions

One statistical problem that arises when assessing age differences in event frequencies is that it is usually difficult to disentangle the person who rates the events from the person who is being rated. For example, if members of a family provide self-ratings of hostility and parents report behaving hostilely more frequently than children do, this difference could reflect the fact that interactions with parents are more contentious, but it could also be a product of a recollection bias by certain reporters. By the same token, differences between children in hostility may reflect real differences in roles or reporting biases that are a product of differences in cognitive maturity.

Round-robin studies disentangle the characteristics of the person who is rated from the characteristics of the person who is providing the ratings. In round-robin studies, every member of the group rates every other member, making each individual both a rater and a target (Warner, Kenny, & Stoto, 1979). We use this statistical approach to illustrate how rater characteristics such as age and social role can be disentangled from features of the persons who are rated.

We begin by distinguishing reliability from validity using a hierarchical measurement model (see Figure 5.1). Reliability refers to fluctuations in scores that are a function of random variance due to item content, time-specific measurement error, or rating source. Validity refers to associations between endogenous elements of the measurement model and theoretically related exogenous variables outside of the model. These associations occur at both the manifest and the latent levels. At the manifest level, specific frequency reports (e.g., hostile behaviors during the past hour) may be compared with objective measures (e.g., videotaped interactions). On the latent level, scale scores may be linked to theoretically related constructs (e.g., reports of hostile behavior correlated with a measure of trait hostility).

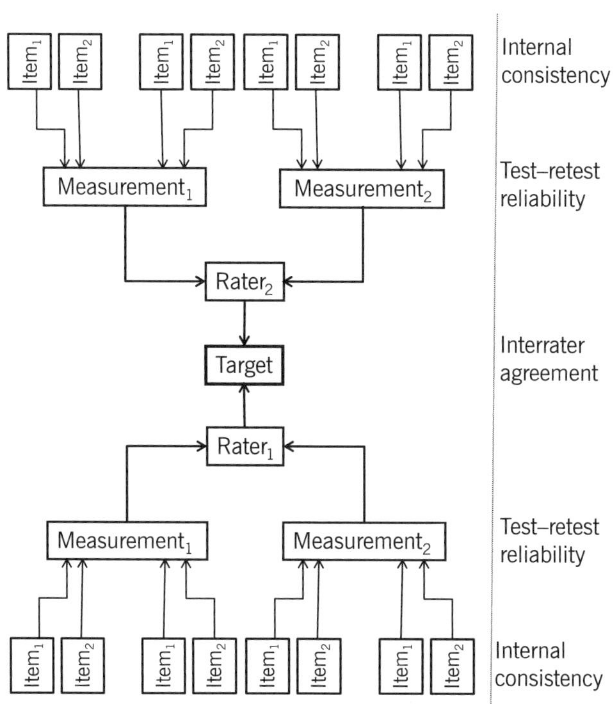

FIGURE 5.1. Distinguishing reliability from validity using a hierarchical measurement model.

The assessment and interpretation of reliability involves assumptions that are not usually made explicit. In essence, reliability increases with the correlation between interchangeable indices of an underlying latent construct. In the case of perfect reliability, indices correlate perfectly, and the loading of each index on a general latent factor is 1. In such a case, targets would not differ in their rank order on the different indices. Behaviors that are perfectly exchangeable indices of an underlying construct are rare, particularly when a trait has different behavioral correlates but the expression of one behavior suppresses the likelihood of the expression of the other behaviors. In addition, some behaviors are genuinely singular (e.g., suicide), in which case it is impossible to establish reliability at the item level. Finally, there are limits to the use of single behaviors (e.g., symptoms) as expressions of underlying latent variables (Borsboom, Mellenbergh, & Van Heerden, 2003).

Calculating the reliability of a measure across different assessments basically assumes that the true stability of the underlying construct is perfect (i.e., a test–retest correlation of 1.0). For highly stable constructs measured repeatedly at short intervals (e.g., intelligence tests 2 weeks apart), it may be reasonable to assume perfect stability. But if developmental processes are the focus, this assumption removes potentially meaningful changes in rank-order position.

Illustration

To illustrate how frequency reports differ according to the age and social role of participants, we describe results from the Family and Personality Project (Haselager & van Aken, 1999), a three-wave longitudinal study of 288 intact families with two adolescent children (mean ages at the first measurement wave = 14.5 and 12.4 for the older and younger child). We focus on three ratings of hostile behavior frequency ("threatening me," "insulting me," and "being aggressive toward me"). Responses on a Likert-type scale (1 = *never* to 5 = *very often*) were highly skewed so reports were dichotomized as the presence or absence of hostile behavior.

Item-level reliability was calculated separately as conventional Cronbach alpha for all of the 36 multilevel cells (see Table 5.2). An analysis of variance (ANOVA) was conducted with Fisher-transformed reliabilities as the dependent variable. There was a significant main effect of rater, $F(3,32) = 2.89$, $p = .05$, which was a product of the lower alpha of mothers when compared with other raters. Mothers also reported less hostile behavior than other raters, and their ratings had less variance, suggesting that mothers may have underreported hostility (leniency bias), leading to a suppression of variance and a reduction in item consistency.

There was a main effect for target, $F(3, 32) = 4.09$, $p = .01$, with higher reliabilities for assessments of children ($M = .82$) compared with assessments of parents ($M = .68$). There were corresponding differences in mean levels of targets, with higher values for children ($M = .95$, $SD = .61$) than for parents ($M = .63$, $SD = .52$). The main effect of wave (change over time) did not reach statistical significance, $F(2, 33) = 2.02$, $p = .15$, but wave was correlated with reliability ($r = .33$), indicating improved reliability during later assessments (when children were older). A post hoc general linear model analysis tested whether this increase in reliability differed between raters or targets, but wave did not interact with either, suggesting age-related changes were not specific to children or parents as raters or targets.

The analysis of rater-, target-, and time-specific differences in reliability inform the interpretation of results from the multilevel analyses. For example, the higher reliabilities

TABLE 5.2. Alpha Reliabilities, Means, and Standard Deviations by Raters, Targets, and Waves

		Rater											
		Father			Mother			Older child			Younger child		
Target	Wave	Alpha	*M*	*SD*	Alpha	*M*	*SD*	Alpha	*M*	*SD*	Alpha	*M*	*SD*
Father	1				0.53	0.44	0.72	0.56	0.92	0.99	0.56	0.85	0.96
	2				0.48	0.43	0.70	0.61	0.86	1.00	0.55	0.73	0.90
	3				0.55	0.41	0.71	0.70	0.92	1.08	0.62	0.72	0.95
Mother	1	0.55	0.57	0.83				0.53	0.60	0.85	0.60	0.62	0.90
	2	0.64	0.60	0.89				0.65	0.60	0.91	0.53	0.49	0.79
	3	0.66	0.65	0.93				0.68	0.56	0.91	0.50	0.39	0.71
Older child	1	0.62	0.80	0.96	0.57	0.63	0.86				0.76	1.47	1.19
	2	0.69	0.89	1.05	0.63	0.70	0.93				0.74	1.38	1.17
	3	0.73	0.87	1.06	0.60	0.64	0.89				0.74	1.28	1.17
Younger child	1	0.63	0.69	0.92	0.47	0.53	0.78	0.73	1.57	1.16			
	2	0.69	0.80	1.01	0.55	0.54	0.81	0.75	1.55	1.18			
	3	0.69	0.80	1.02	0.69	0.53	0.88	0.77	1.35	1.19			
Mean		0.66	0.74	0.96	0.57	0.54	0.81	0.67	0.99	1.03	0.63	0.88	0.97

for children as targets increases the chances (on psychometric grounds) of finding more differences between oldest and youngest targets than between mother and father targets.

A model was specified with sum scores specified at level 1, which were allowed to vary between three waves and targets. Results from the baseline model indicated that the reliability of the level 2 intercept (across waves) was 0.76, suggesting a moderate degree of temporal consistency between measurements. The reliability of the level 3 intercept (across raters) was 0.43, indicating a somewhat lower degree of agreement between raters. Random variations across both intercepts was highly significant ($p < .001$), with 44% of the variance occurring between waves and 15% between raters, whereas the remaining variance was random variance.

A model was specified that included target and rater age as predictors at level 1 (as age varied across waves). Rater gender and parent status (a dummy with a value of 1 if the rater was a parent) was included at level 2, and gender and parent status of the targets were included at level 3. Finally, cross-level interactions specified parent status as a predictor of the level 1 association between behavior reports and raters' and targets' ages.

Results are reported in terms of unstandardized regression coefficients. The overall intercept was 1.99, which refers to the average number of hostile interaction behaviors for a participant with a value of zero on all predictors. Less hostility was reported for female targets, $b = -.189, p < .01$, and parent targets, $b = -.631, p = .03$. There was a corresponding leniency bias in raters, with lower ratings provided by females, $b = -.228, p < .01$, and parents, $b = -1.092, p < .01$.

Reports of hostile behaviors were negatively associated with raters' age, $b = -.021$, $p = .02$, on level 1. This negative association was qualified by a cross-level interaction with rater parent status, $b = .028, p < .01$. Because parents were coded 1, the negative association between rater age and hostility frequency was restricted to children ($-.021 + .028 = .007$ and thus negligible). In other words, children reported fewer hostile interactions when they got older, whereas reports by parents did not vary with age. Findings for target age and hostile behaviors and for the cross-level interaction with target category did not reach statistical significance.

This example illustrates analyses that determine whether there are age-related changes in event frequencies and event frequency reliability and whether age-related changes in the latter are responsible for age-related changes in the former.

Future Directions

We know that children's memories improve with age, so we assume that they should be able to provide more accurate recollections of the frequencies of recent events. Children's greater familiarity with events, however, may cause them to construct a false reality, assuming that actions that usually occur during an event likely occurred in a specific episode they are trying to remember. It is not clear that this problem dissipates with age.

An even bigger unknown concerns the possibility of developmental differences in the use of specific retrieval strategies. The cognitive strategies elicited by different types of inquiries may also vary as a function of cognitive maturation. Schwarz (2003) suggested that there may be age-related differences in the degree to which respondents are influenced by characteristics of surveys, such that the very old may be most susceptible to questionnaire content bias because they are least certain about their memory for events. To this we add that the very young might be the least susceptible to content bias because they hold an unrealistic faith in their powers of recollection. But this is speculation. The difficult task ahead involves disentangling age-related changes in mean level behavioral frequencies from changes in the use of particular retrieval strategies in response to specific requests for information.

Greater attention must be paid to the prospect that instrument reliability may vary across reports and ages. But this is only a start. Round-robin designs are impractical for most longitudinal endeavors. Furthermore, reliability fixes do not address the fundamental problem that the same question may mean different things to participants of different ages. One solution may involve coaching participants in the use of specific retrieval strategies prior to answering questionnaires to reduce variance associated with strategy preference.

Acknowledgment

Brett Laursen received support for the preparation of this chapter from the U.S. National Science Foundation (Grant No. 0923745 and 0909733).

References

Achenbach, T. M. (1991). *Integrative guide for the 1991 CBCL/4-18, YSR, and TRF profiles*. Burlington: University of Vermont.

Adams, R., & Laursen, B. (2007). The correlates of conflict: Disagreement is not necessarily detrimental. *Journal of Family Psychology, 21*, 445–458.

Belli, R. F., Schwarz, N., Singer, E., & Talarico, J. (2000). Decomposition can harm the accuracy of behavioural frequency reports. *Applied Cognitive Psychology, 14*, 295–308.

Bjorklund, D. F., Dukes, C., & Brown, R. D. (2009). The development of memory strategies. In M. L. Courage & N. Cowan (Eds.), *The development of memory in infancy and childhood* (pp. 145–175). New York: Psychology Press.

Bjorklund, D. F., & Zeman, B. R. (1982). Children's organization and metamemory awareness in the recall of familiar information. *Child Development, 53*, 799–810.

Blair, E., & Burton, S. (1987). Cognitive processes used by survey respondents to answer behavioral frequency questions. *Journal of Consumer Research, 14*, 208–288.

Bolger, N., Davis, A., & Rafaeli, E. (2003). Diary methods: Capturing life as it is lived. *Annual Review of Psychology, 54*, 579–616.

Borsboom, D., Mellenbergh, G. J., & Van Heerden, J. (2003). The theoretical status of latent variables. *Psychological Review, 110*, 203–219.

Brown, N. R. (1995). Estimation strategies and the judgment of event frequency. *Journal of Experimental Psychology: Learning, Memory, and Cognition, 21*, 1539–1553.

Brown, N. R. (2002). Encoding, representing, and estimating event frequencies: A multiple strategy perspective. In P. Sedlmeier & T. Betsch (Eds.), *Etc. frequency processing and cognition* (pp. 37–53). New York: Oxford University Press.

Brown, N. R., & Sinclair, R. C. (1999). Estimating number of lifetime sexual partners: Men and women do it differently. *Journal of Sex Research, 36*, 292–297.

Burk, W. J., Denissen, J., van Doorn, M. D., Branje, S. J. T., & Laursen, B. (2009). The vicissitudes of conflict measurement: Stability and reliability in the frequency of disagreements. *European Psychologist, 14*, 153–159.

Burton, S., & Blair, E. (1991). Task conditions, response formulation processes, and response accuracy for behavioral frequency questions in surveys. *Public Opinion Quarterly, 55*, 50–79.

Conrad, F. G., Brown, N. R., & Cashman, E. (1998). Strategies for answering behavioral frequency questions. *Memory, 6*, 339–366.

Diener, E., & Larsen, R. J. (1984). Temporal stability and cross-situational consistency of affective, cognitive, and behavioral responses. *Journal of Personality and Social Psychology, 47*, 871–883.

Foley, M. A., Ratner, H. H., & Gentes, E. (2010). Helping children enter into another's experiences: The look and feel of it. *Journal of Cognition and Development, 11*, 217–239.

Foley, M. A., Santini, C., & Sopasakis, M. (1989). Discriminating between memories: Evidence for children's spontaneous elaborations. *Journal of Experimental Child Psychology, 48*, 146–169.

Goodman, G. S., Quas, J. A., Batterman-Faunce, J. M., Riddlesberger, M. M., & Kuhn, J. (1994). Predictors of accurate and inaccurate memories of traumatic events experienced in childhood. *Consciousness and Cognition, 3*, 269–294.

Haselager, G. J. T., & van Aken, M. A. G. (1999). *Family and personality: Vol. 1. First measurement wave*. Nijmegen, The Netherlands: University of Nijmegen.

Hasher, L., & Chromiak, W. (1977). The processing of frequency information: An automatic mechanism? *Journal of Verbal Learning and Verbal Behavior, 16*, 173–184.

Hasher, L., & Zacks, R. T. (1979). Automatic and effortful processes in memory. *Journal of Experimental Psychology: General, 108*, 356–388.

Henry, B., Moffitt, T. E., Caspi, A., Langley, J., & Silva, P. A. (1994). On the "remembrance of things past": A longitudinal evaluation of the retrospective method. *Psychological Assessment, 6*, 92–101.

Igou, E. R., Bless, H., & Schwarz, N. (2002). Making sense of standardized survey questions: The influence of reference periods and their repetition. *Communication Monographs, 69*, 179–187.

Jensen-Campbell, L. A., & Graziano, W. G. (2001). Agreeableness as a moderator of interpersonal conflict. *Journal of Personality, 69*, 323–362.

Justice, E. M., Baker-Ward, L., Gupta, S., & Jannings, L. R. (1997). Means to the goal of remembering:

Developmental changes in awareness of strategy use–performance relations. *Journal of Experimental Child Psychology, 65*, 293–314.
Kovacs, M. (1985). The Children's Depression Inventory (CDI). *Psychopharmacology Bulletin, 21*, 995–998.
Laursen, B. (1995). Conflict and social interaction in adolescent relationships. *Journal of Research on Adolescence, 5*, 55–70.
Laursen, B., & Collins, W. A. (2009). Parent–child relationships during adolescence. In R. Lerner & L. Steinberg (Eds.), *Handbook of adolescent psychology: Vol. 2. Contextual influences on adolescent development* (3rd ed., pp. 3–42). New York: Wiley.
Lund, A. M., Hall, J. W., Wilson, K. P., & Humphreys, M. S. (1983). Frequency judgment accuracy as a function of age and school achievement (learning disabled versus non-learning-disabled) patterns. *Journal of Experimental Child Psychology, 35*, 236–247.
Menon, G., Raghubir, P., & Schwarz, N. (1995). Behavioral frequency judgments: An accessibility–diagnosticity framework. *Journal of Consumer Research, 22*, 212–228.
Ornstein, P. A., Baker-Ward, L., Gordon, B. N., Pelphrey, K. A., Tyler, C. S., & Gramzow, E. (2006). The influence of prior knowledge and repeated questioning on children's long-term retention of the details of a pediatric examination. *Developmental Psychology, 42*, 332–344.
Ornstein, P. A., Merritt, K. A., Baker-Ward, L., Furtado, E., Gordon, B. N., & Principe, G. F. (1998). Children's knowledge, expectation, and long-term retention. *Applied Cognitive Psychology, 12*, 387–405.
Principe, G. F., Haines, B., Adkins, A., & Guiliano, S. (2010). False rumors and true belief: Memory processes underlying children's errant reports of rumored events. *Journal of Experimental Child Psychology, 107*, 407–422.
Principe, G. F., Kanaya, T., Ceci, S. J., & Singh, M. (2006). Believing is seeing: How rumors can engender false memories in preschoolers. *Psychological Science, 17*, 243–248.
Prinz, R. J., Foster, S. L., Kent, R. N., & O'Leary, K. D. (1979). Multivariate assessment of conflict in distressed and non-distressed mother–adolescent dyads. *Journal of Applied Behavior Analysis, 12*, 691–700.
Robin, A. L., & Foster, S. L. (1984). Problem-solving communication training: A behavioral family systems approach to parent–adolescent conflict. In P. Karoly & J. J. Steffen (Eds.), *Adolescent behavior disorders: Foundations and contemporary concerns* (pp. 195–240). Lexington, MA: Heath.
Robinson, M. D., & Clore, G. L. (2002). Belief and feeling: Evidence for an accessibility model of emotional self-report. *Psychological Bulletin, 128*, 934–960.
Rushton, J. P., Brainerd, C. J., & Pressley, M. (1983). Behavioral development and construct validity: The principle of aggregation. *Psychological Bulletin, 94*, 118–138.
Schimmack, U. (2002). Frequency judgments of emotions: The cognitive basis of personality assessment. In P. Sedlmeier & T. Betsch (Eds.), *Etc. frequency processing and cognition* (pp. 189–204). New York: Oxford University Press.
Schneider, W. (2010). Memory development in childhood. In U. Goswami (Ed.), *Blackwell handbook of childhood cognitive development* (2nd ed., pp. 236–256). London, UK: Blackwell.
Schwarz, N. (2003). Self-reports in consumer research: The challenge of comparing cohorts and cultures. *Journal of Consumer Research, 29*, 588–594.
Schwarz, N., Bless, H., Bohner, G., Harlacher, U., & Kellenbenz, M. (1991). Response scales as frames of reference: The impact of frequency range on diagnostic judgments. *Applied Cognitive Psychology, 5*, 37–49.
Schwarz, N., Bless, H., Strack, F., Klumpp, G., Rittenauer-Schatka, H., & Simons, A. (1991). Ease of retrieval as information: Another look at the availability heuristic. *Journal of Personality and Social Psychology, 61*, 195–202.
Schwenck, C., Bjorklund, D. F., & Schneider, W. (2009). Developmental and individual differences in

young children's use and maintenance of a selective memory strategy. *Developmental Psychology, 45*, 1034–1050.

Shanahan, L., McHale, S. M., Osgood, W., & Crouter, A. C. (2007). Conflict frequency with mothers and fathers from middle childhood to late adolescence: Within- and between-families comparisons. *Developmental Psychology, 43*, 539–550.

Shin, H.-E., Bjorklund, D. F., & Beck, E. F. (2007). The adaptive nature of children's overestimation in a strategic memory task. *Cognitive Development, 22*, 197–212.

Smetana, J. G., Daddis, C., & Chuang, S. S. (2003). "Clean your room!": A longitudinal investigation of adolescent–parent conflict and conflict resolution in middle-class African American families. *Journal of Adolescent Research, 18*, 631–650.

Steinberg, L. (1988). Reciprocal relation between parent–child distance and pubertal maturation. *Developmental Psychology, 24*, 122–128.

Sudman, S., & Bradburn, N. M. (1974). *Response effects in surveys: A review and synthesis*. Chicago: Aldine.

Thompson, C. P. (1982). Memory for unique personal events: The roommate study. *Memory and Cognition, 10*, 324–332.

Tversky, A., & Kahneman, D. (1973). Availability: A heuristic for judging frequency and probability. *Cognitive Psychology, 5*, 207–232.

Verhulst, F. C., & van der Ende, J. (1992). Agreement between parents' reports and adolescents' self-reports of problem behavior. *Journal of Child Psychology and Psychiatry, 33*, 1011–1023.

Wallace, J. M., Jr., Bachman, J. G., O'Malley, P. M., Schulenberg, J. E., Cooper, S. M., & Johnston, L. D. (2003). Gender and ethnic differences in smoking, drinking and illicit drug use among American 8th, 10th and 12th grade students, 1976–2000. *Addiction, 98*, 225–234.

Warner, R. M., Kenny, D. A., & Stoto, M. (1979). A new round robin analysis of variance for social interaction data. *Journal of Personality and Social Psychology, 37*, 1742–1757.

Williams, K. W., & Durso, F. T. (1986). Judging category frequency: Automaticity or availability? *Journal of Experimental Psychology: Learning, Memory, and Cognition, 12*, 387–396.

Winkielman, P., Knäuper, B., & Schwarz, N. (1998). Looking back at anger: Reference periods change the interpretation of emotion frequency questions. *Journal of Personality and Social Psychology, 75*, 719–728.

Wright, D. B., Gaskell, G. D., & O'Muircheartaigh, C. A. (1994). How much is "quite a bit"?: Mapping absolute values onto vague quantifiers. *Applied Cognitive Psychology, 8*, 479–496.

CHAPTER 6

The Impact of Scaling and Measurement Methods on Individual Differences in Growth

SUSAN E. EMBRETSON
JOHN POGGIO

Studying individual differences in growth or change is a defining aspect of longitudinal studies in psychology. Individual differences in growth may be due to genetic differences, to varying exposure to environments that affect development, or to an interaction of genes and environments. Growth may differ not only in absolute amount between individuals but also in the nature of the trend over time or age. For some individuals, growth may be linear, whereas for other individuals it may be nonlinear. Plateaus or sudden accelerations are, in theory, also possible aspects of growth.

Advances in methods for longitudinal data analysis can increase the validity of inferences about individual differences in growth. Powerful modeling techniques, including both longitudinal models and multilevel models, have been applied to analyze data on growth. McArdle and Bell (2000), for example, used special formulations of structural equation models to estimate individual differences in growth. Little, Lindenberger, and Maier (2000) combined structural equation modeling and multilevel modeling to address issues about sample selectivity and growth.

However, all analyses depend on the quality of the measurements that represent the dependent variable(s) of interest. Unfortunately, individual differences in the amount of growth and the shape of the growth curves can be due to scaling artifacts rather than to substantive sources of individual differences. Conversely, individual differences in growth can be masked by scaling artifacts. That is, results on individual differences in growth can be due to the measurement scale level that is achieved by the measures, as well as to measurement error and bias. Similar effects can be expected on group comparisons of growth (Embretson, 1996).

This chapter explicates the various sources of scaling artifacts that can affect the results in growth. Possible solutions are discussed and illustrated. The chapter begins with the classic consideration of measurement scale levels and the relationship of psychological data and test theory models to scale level. Then, after we elaborate the various sources of artifacts, an example is presented to illustrate some of the various artifacts.

Measurement Scale Level

Traditional Scaling Concepts

Stevens's (1946) taxonomy is the most well-known and frequently cited source of measurement scale levels in psychology. Although the validity of the taxonomy has often been disputed (e.g., Gaito, 1980; Lord, 1953; Michell, 1986, 1990) and alternative taxonomies have been proposed (e.g., see Coombs, 1950; Torgerson, 1958), Stevens's taxonomy remains influential. In Stevens's (1946) taxonomy, four scale levels are distinguished. These scale levels differ from one another in the number of axioms that hold for the numerical values of variables. The axioms concern the relationship between scale scores in terms of identity, order, additivity, and origin. The appropriateness of the axioms within each scale level determines how the scaled values can be compared and treated statistically (McDonald, 1999; Torgerson, 1958).

Nominal Scale

The nominal scale of measurement is the most basic of the four levels. Two objects measured on a nominal scale can be compared only in terms of whether or not they fall into the same or different categories (equality/sameness and inequality/difference, respectively). The values represent the latent variable by exhaustive and mutually exclusive categories. Examples of observed nominal variables include gender, ethnicity, and treatment type, as well as other properties. Some latent variables are also categorical (e.g., Piaget's theory has several variables measuring conservation, and on each variable a person would either be a conserver or a nonconserver or possibly in a third category called transitional).

The nominal scale provides limited information about individual differences. For example, all persons in a given category (e.g., females, treatment group, personality type) are interpreted as being equivalent to one another in terms of the psychological property value, but all the individuals in one category are different (in assigned value) from persons in another category (e.g., males are different from females). Nominal variables are also described as "qualitative" in the sense that the variables reflect qualities rather than amounts of a characteristic. Nevertheless, the limited information results in greater flexibility when attempting to transform variable values. In fact, numbers need not be involved until coding is needed for the purposes of multiple regression or other statistical models (e.g., Cohen, Cohen, West, & Aiken, 2003).

Ordinal Scale

In ordinal scales, values can be ordered along a continuum, where the continuum corresponds to the psychological trait. Being measured as the first, second, third, tenth, and so on. in a group represents measurement at the ordinal scale level. The ordinal scale differs from the nominal scale primarily in that the categories are ordered. As a result, transformations must be monotonic. However, the size of the difference between any given contiguous values is unknown. Thus parametric statistics can be regarded as inappropriate because these statistics require arithmetic operations that presume equal intervals between scores. However, ordinal scales are flexible because the original values can be squared or logged, or any operation that *is monotonic* (order preserving) can be performed on them without violating the relationship between any two values.

Interval Scale

In interval scales, the order of values and the distance between each set of values represents the psychological continuum. That is, the *distance* (i.e., differences) between any two values can be compared with the difference between any other two values based on magnitude. Because equal differences imply equal scale distances, the numbers can be mathematically manipulated by combining, concatenating, or adding them to one another. Parametric statistics, such as commonly used in growth modeling, are appropriate for this scale level.

Given the additional information about the relations among values on an interval scale of measurement, transformations of original values are more limited in flexibility than for ordinal and nominal variable values. Specifically, only linear transformations are permissible because they preserve the interval-level information in the data. However, there is no fixed origin or natural zero on the continuum for an interval scale. Rather, an origin is selected arbitrarily.

Ratio Scale

In the Stevens system, relations among values at the ratio scale level contain the richest quantitative information. Numbers with an underlying ratio scale lie along the real, continuous number line. In particular, a natural and absolute zero is part of the scale, thus providing a true, fixed origin about which all other values vary. Any movement (or variation) of a given value or number from this origin occurs via units of 1. The greater the distance from the origin, the greater the property value due to a greater accumulation of unit distances from the origin.

Substantially more variety in mathematical and statistical modeling can be performed on these types of data due to the extensive information available. However, the advantage of greater information is accompanied by a greater restriction in transformation methods compared with the previous scale levels. Namely, the original value x can be multiplied only by a constant c to create a transformed y value: $y = cx$.

Scale Level and Psychological Data

The types of inferential statistical tests that can be performed on data vary according to scale level; parametric tests are considered more appropriate for interval and ratio-level data, whereas nominal and ordinal data are best approached with nonparametric tests. Although this point has been disputed, as noted earlier, longitudinal studies in which individuals in growth are a primary focus are particularly influenced by scale level.

Thus an important issue is whether commonly used psychological measures and tasks meet the requirements of at least the interval scale level. For example, counts of behaviors in terms of reported incidents in some defined context or number of items passed or endorsed on a test are quite commonplace as psychological data. If the interpretations to be made from the data are limited to the specifically defined context or the specific test, raw counts could be regarded as ratio scaled because there is a natural zero for persons who never exhibit the behavior or who get all items wrong. However, it is rare that such specific contexts are of interest in psychology. That is, typically the task context or test is assumed to represent a broader domain of behavior, and the purpose is to generalize from the specific task to the broader domain. Responses are presumed to depend on a latent variable that represents a tendency to respond in a certain way to the broader domain of interest. Although behavior counts may sometimes be regarded as ratio scale, most psychological data are interpreted as depending on latent variables, which probably are *not linearly related* to a specific behavioral count. Thus, most observed psychological data probably achieve only ordinal scale properties.

However, test theory models can be applied to achieve higher level scale properties. As shown next, some test theory models may be justified as achieving interval level scales.

Test Theory Models and Scale Level

Item Response Theory Models

In item response theory (IRT), item performance (or endorsement) can be used to locate items and persons on a latent trait continuum (hence its synonymy with "latent trait theory"). Both unidimensional and multidimensional IRT models are available (Embretson & Reise, 2000; Reckase, 2009), with a variety of structural forms (DeBoeck & Wilson, 2004; van der Linden & Hambleton, 1997).

In applying IRT models, it is assumed that responses to items are locally independent. That is, after controlling for trait levels of persons, there is no additional relationship between the items. Error is accounted for in the model in the probability of endorsing the item.

The most simple IRT model is the Rasch (1960) model, which gives the probability of person s endorsing (or accurately responding to) item I as follows:

$$P(X_{is} = 1 | \theta_s, \beta_i) = e^{\theta_s - \beta_i} / 1 + e^{\theta_s - \beta_i} \quad \textbf{(6.1)}$$

where the probability is a logistic function of the simple difference between the person's trait location, θ_s, and the location of item i on the same latent trait continuum, β_i. The Rasch model can be justified as obtaining interval-level scores for both items and persons, according to Luce and Tukey's (1964) theory of conjoint measurement, because the model can be transformed so that the outcome is an additive combination of the parameters. That is, the Rasch model can also be expressed as follows:

$$\ln(P_{is}/1 - P_{is}) = \theta_s - \beta_i, \quad \textbf{(6.2)}$$

where the outcome variable (expressed here as log odds) is an additive function of two other variables (i.e., the item and person parameters).

Another feature of Rasch models is the invariant meaning of person and item calibrations, a property referred to as specific objectivity. That is, it can be shown that for any pair of trait level scores, say θ_1 and θ_2, the difference in log odds for solving *any* item β_i is given by the simple difference in the trait levels as follows:

$$\ln[P(X_{i1} = 1)/(1 - P(X_{i1} = 1)] - \ln[P(X_{i2} = 1)/(1 - P(X_{i2} = 1)] = \theta_1 - \theta_2 \quad \textbf{(6.3)}$$

This relationship is often shown as justifying interval-level scale properties of trait levels when scaled as θ_s in the Rasch model. Conversely, for any pair of items, it can be shown that the difference in log odds that *any* person will respond positively is the difference in their difficulty values. In combination, these two general relationships constitute a property that is termed *specific objectivity*. That is, the difference between any two abilities has invariant meaning with respect to the items, and the difference between any two items has invariant meaning with respect to ability. Specific objectivity is a property that is unique to the Rasch IRT model.

Although other IRT models, such as the two-parameter (2PL) or three-parameter (3PL) logistic models, do not meet specific objectivity as does the Rasch model, interval scaling can still be justified. Consider the 2PL model, as follows:

$$P(X_{is} = 1|\theta_s, \beta_i) = e^{\alpha_i(\theta_s - \beta_i)}/1 + e^{\alpha_i(\theta_s - \beta_i)}, \quad \textbf{(6.4)}$$

where θ_s and β_i are defined as in equation 6.1, and α_i is a slope parameter for item discrimination. In this case, the difference between the log odds for any two persons on an item with difficulty β_i will depend on the item discrimination parameter, α_i, as follows:

$$\ln[P(X_{i1} = 1)/(1 - P(X_{i1} = 1)] - \ln[P(X_{i2} = 1)/(1 - P(X_{i2} = 1)] = \alpha_i(\theta_1 - \theta_2). \quad \textbf{(6.5)}$$

Notice that invariant meaning of *score* differences for a particular item requires an additional parameter, α_i. However, the same item parameter is applied to all levels of θ_s such that score differences have a constant meaning with respect to a particular item. This phenomenon also provides a justification for interval-level measurement. Item differences in log odds for the same person will depend on both item discrimination and item difficulty, however. Nonetheless, items still can be compared with other items without relying on population-specific, contextual information (i.e., as in norm-referenced measurement).

Classical Test Theory Models

The basic classical test theory (CTT) model does not include item differences. That is, observed test scores, X_{sk}, on test k are a function of true score, X_t, and error, e_{sk}, as follows:

$$X_{sk} = X_t + e_{sk}. \quad \textbf{(6.6)}$$

Notice that no parameters are included to represent differences between items. Thus obtaining comparable measures from different test forms requires careful balancing of items for difficulty and discrimination. Furthermore, most CTT applications assume equal error variances between persons to compute classical reliability statistics.

True scores and their linear transformations do not have score intervals that have invariant meaning for item performance, as shown in equation 6.2 and equation 6.4 for IRT scores. The distribution of scores and the meaning of the test score intervals depend critically on the match of item difficulty level to the trait level of the population.

To illustrate this relationship and other relationships to be considered subsequently, data were simulated. The total simulation included (1) three groups of 1,000 cases each that show low, moderate, and high levels on the latent trait; (2) three 30-item tests with easy, moderate, and hard item difficulty levels, and (3) five time points, in which the mean true trait level increased linearly for each group but individual differences in change also were simulated. The true trait parameters of the simulators within the three groups were randomly selected *z*-scores from three normally distributed populations that differed in means. Item responses were generated from the true person and item parameters by comparing the IRT predicted probabilities to randomly selected probabilities in a uniform distribution (0,1).

For the current example, the moderate population was used to study the impact of test difficulty level. As expected, the distribution of CTT total scores on the moderate test was nearly normal, whereas the easy test and the hard test scores were substantially positively skewed for the easier test and negatively skewed for the easier measure.

The CTT scores on the three tests that differ in difficulty are not linearly related, even though they represent the same true latent trait scores. Figure 6.1 presents a scatterplot of

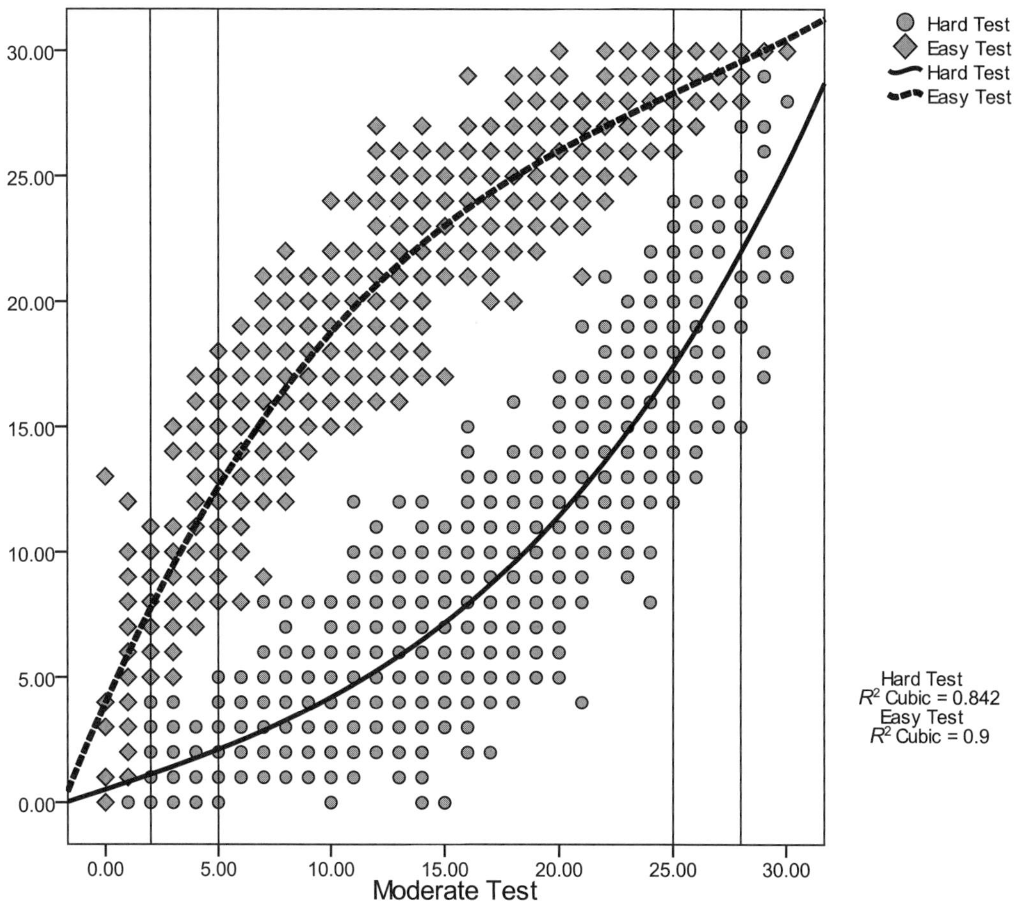

FIGURE 6.1. Regression of hard and easy test scores on moderate test scores in population.

the relationship of total scores on the easy test and the hard test to scores on the moderate test. It can be seen that the meaning of score intervals on the moderate test varies across score levels on the other two tests. For example, for scores of 25 and 28 on the moderate test, the predicted scores on the hard test are 17.21 and 22.5, respectively. Thus a difference of 3 points on the moderate test becomes a difference of more than 5 points on the hard test. However, on the low end of the moderate test, the scores of 2 and 5 have predicted scores of 1.3 and 1.8, respectively, on the hard test. Thus, in this case, a difference of 3 points becomes a difference of 0.5. Similar comparisons could be made from the moderate to the easy test.

It should be noted that, although IRT was used to generate scores, similar results for CTT test equating over varying test difficulty levels could be observed. For example, in equipercentile equating, scores are equated from their percentile ranks in the same population. A result similar to Figure 6.1 would be observed if the two equated tests differed in difficulty levels. *Thus the meaning of the score differences depends on the level of the scores and the difficulty of the test.*

Sources of Scaling Artifacts in Analyzing Growth

Test Theory Model

The choice of a test theory model can have a significant impact on the results from a study on individual differences in growth. Figure 6.2 shows the mapping of total scores on IRT trait level for a test of moderate difficulty. The relationship is clearly nonlinear, with the most rapid changes in score level occurring for moderate trait levels. At the low end and at the high end of the trait level scale, test scores change more slowly.

Suppose that the researcher is interested in comparing changes over time among three individuals who differ in initial score levels. Suppose, further, that each individual gains 1 point on the total score at each time period. On the total score scale, change would be linear over time, with the same slope for all three persons. However, a rather different result would be obtained using the latent trait scale equivalents for each total score from Figure

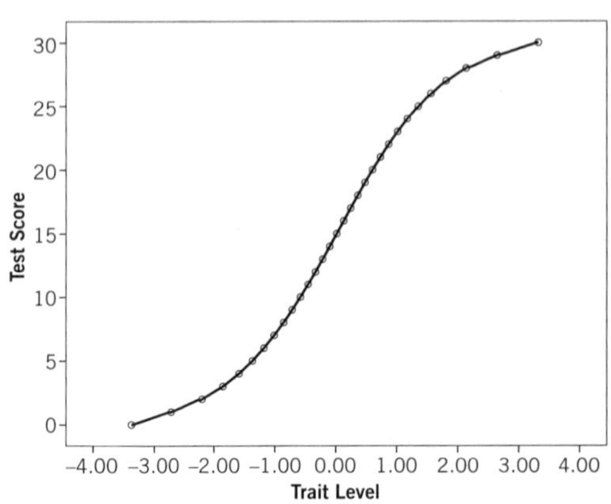

FIGURE 6.2. Mapping of total test score on trait level for test of moderate difficulty.

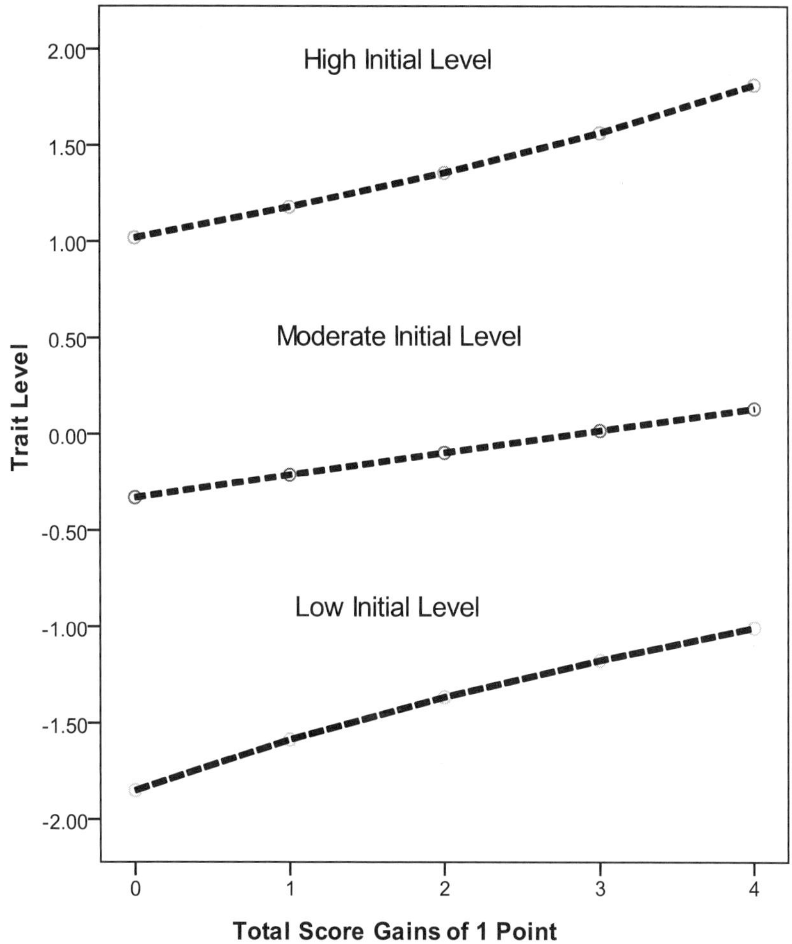

FIGURE 6.3. Change in trait level associated with 1-point gain in total score at three initial levels.

6.2. Figure 6.3 presents the curves on the latent trait scale for the three persons. Notice that the change appears fairly linear for the person who had a moderate initial score level, but not for the other two persons. For the person with the high initial score level, change appears to be accelerating over time, and for the person with the low initial score level, trait levels seem to be decelerating. In brief, a change of 1 point on the total score scale has different meaning, depending on the level of the score.

A similar impact on growth curves on the CTT scale scores can be observed from tests of different difficulty levels. Figure 6.4 presents growth curves for the same person based on three different test difficulty levels. Although the same true trait level generated these results and true trait level increased linearly over time, it can be seen that these growth curves differ substantially. On the easy test (1), little gain is observed, and it appears to be decelerating over time. On the moderate test (2) and hard test (3), greater gain is observed. Although the scores are influenced somewhat by measurement error, it is not clear that these curves could be fit with the same test form.

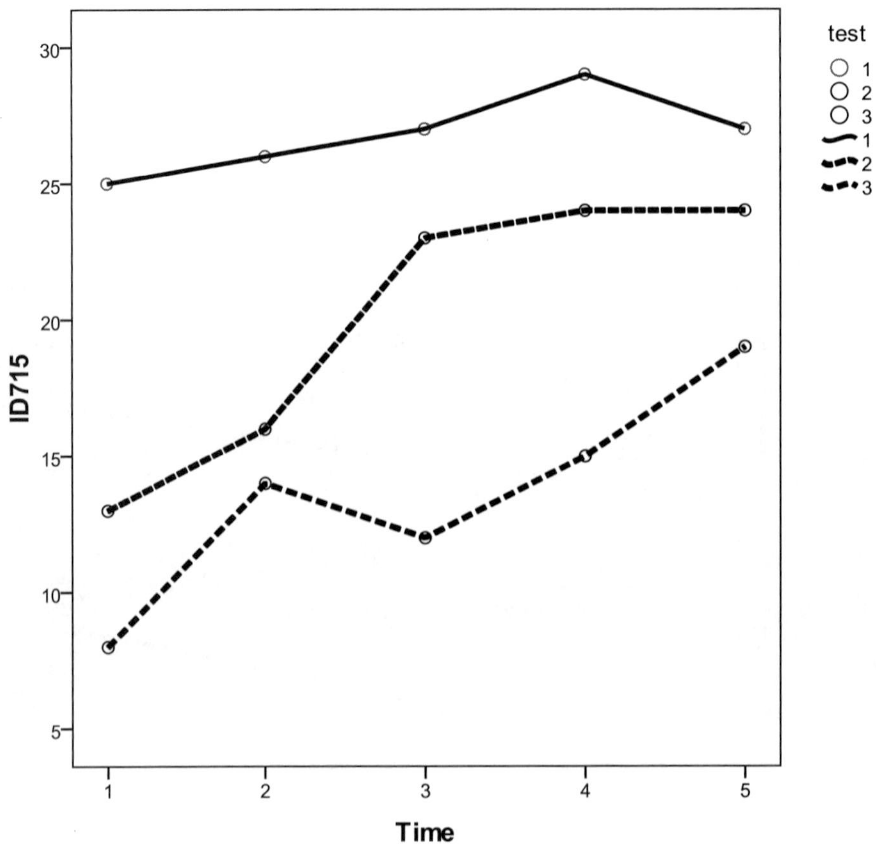

FIGURE 6.4. Growth curves for one person at three different test difficulty levels.

Similar effects of test difficulty level occur for population growth curves. Figure 6.5 presents results on test difficulty for a population growth curve. It can be seen that the trend on the moderate test appears to be linear, which corresponds to the true trait level. However, for the easy test, scores appear to be decelerating over time, whereas for the hard test, scores are accelerating over time.

Which results are most accurate? Because the IRT latent trait scales do have a basis for justifying interval level properties and the CTT scores do not, the results based on the IRT scale scores are more justifiable. Thus applying CTT scale scoring when IRT trait scoring can be used leads to artifacts in understanding growth.

Measurement Error and Bias

The desirable properties of IRT latent trait scores that were described previously pertain to the true trait scale score. In practice, latent trait scores must be estimated from responses to items on tests. The psychometric properties of the items on the test can lead to other sources of scaling artifacts. Differences in item difficulty, item discrimination, and guessing can have an impact on measurement error and bias.

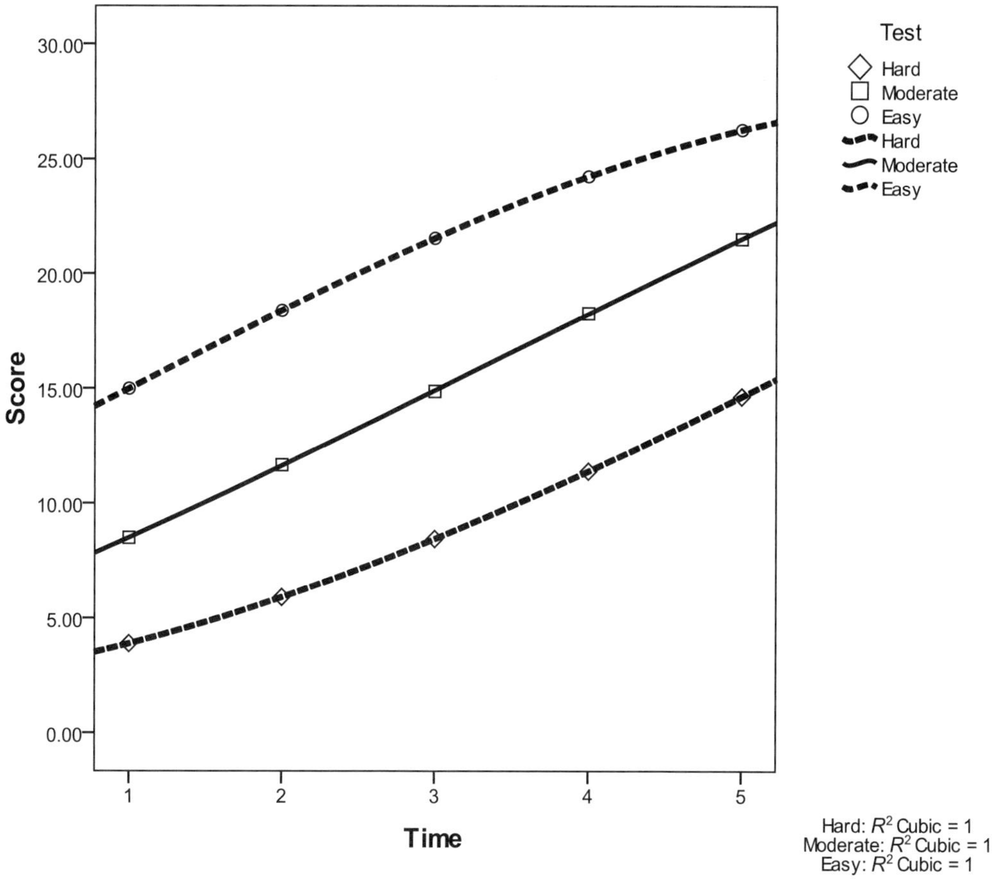

FIGURE 6.5. Population growth curve means and test difficulty levels.

Measurement Error

In IRT, measurement error depends on the amount of information that is available for a particular score level. If the item difficulties are mostly clustered to yield a probability of .40–.60 in the population, more information is available for scores near the mean. For extreme scores, there are fewer appropriate items and hence greater measurement errors. Figure 6.6 shows a relationship of latent trait level and measurement error in a Rasch model. Differences in item discrimination, which is estimated in many IRT models, also affect measurement error. That is, measurement error increases as item discrimination decreases.

In CTT, unlike IRT, it is assumed that measurement errors are equal across score scale. Thus a single standard error of measurement is applied to all scores, typically computed from a reliability estimate (e.g., Cronbach's alpha) and the standard deviation of scores. Methods to estimate differing measurement errors at different score levels have been developed (Feldt & Brennan, 1989). However, most applications of CTT utilize uniform standard errors across score levels.

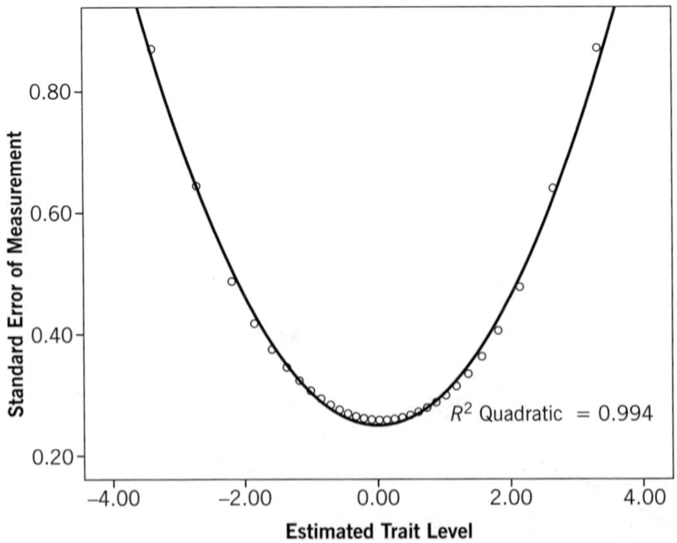

FIGURE 6.6. Relationship of standard error of measurement to IRT trait level on moderate test.

Varying measurement errors across trait levels can complicate the estimation of individual growth curves. If some points have greater unreliability, such points could affect the fit of various growth curves disproportionately, that is, differentially.

Bias

In IRT, extreme trait levels will be poorly estimated because there are too few appropriate items. Thus insufficient information is available for such scores. In fact, for perfect scores at either end of the scale, trait levels cannot be estimated by simple maximum likelihood.

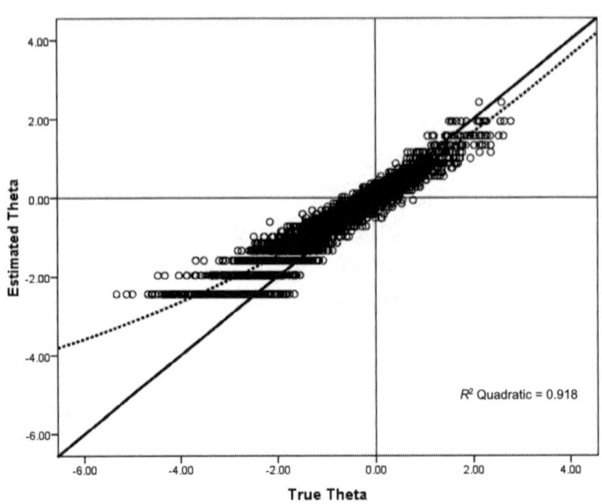

FIGURE 6.7. Regression of estimated latent trait level on true trait level.

To compensate for the insufficient information, a prior distribution is used in estimating trait levels in the *expected a posteriori* (EAP) method. Essentially, EAP results in regressing extreme estimates toward the population mean. This method would lead to bias at the extremes, especially for data from mixed populations or from populations with more uniform distributions.

Figure 6.7 shows the regression of EAP trait level estimates from a test with moderate difficulty on true trait level estimates. Shown on Figure 6.7 is a reference line that denotes perfect prediction and a fitted quadratic regression line. By comparing the two lines, it can be seen that high trait levels are underestimated and that low trait levels are overestimated. The data are from the simulation described previously, and all three groups are included. When the test provides the most information for the group with moderate trait levels, the group with lower true trait levels will be overestimated, and the group with higher true trait levels will be underestimated.

Impact on Growth Curves with Repeated Measures

Measurement error and bias, especially in combination, can seriously affect the fitting of individual growth curves. If the same or parallel tests are administered over time, the measurement error and bias will vary as a function of the appropriateness of the test for the person at the particular time period.

Figure 6.8 shows the true and estimated trait levels for two different cases over time, along with a 98% confidence interval. On the left side of Figure 6.8, the trait levels over time are well estimated and fairly close to the true trait level over time. Furthermore, the measurement error bands are moderate in size. No particular problem would be involved in fitting a growth curve to this case because the trait levels over time are well estimated by a test with moderate difficulty level.

However, the case on the right side shows that true trait level is consistently higher than estimated trait level and that the difference increases over time. Furthermore, the error bands are much broader than for the person on the right side, yet true trait level is not

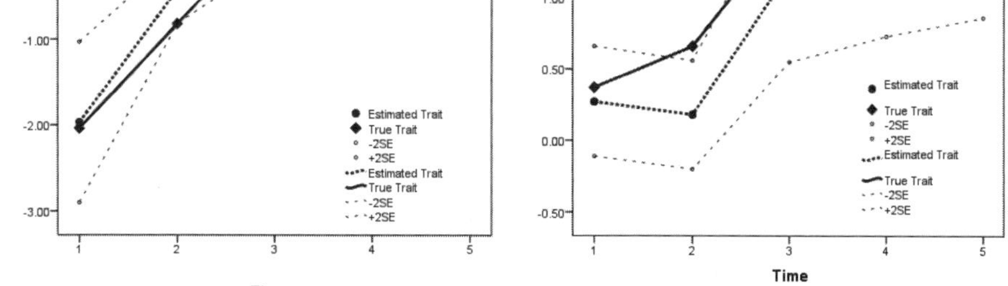

FIGURE 6.8. Impact of measurement error and bias on individual growth curves.

consistently contained within the boundaries. This person's trait level is not well estimated by a test of moderate difficulty level. Trait level at time 1 is reasonably well estimated, as the person's trait level is only slightly above the difficulty level of the moderate test. However, the available information in the moderate test for estimating trait level becomes increasingly poor as trait level increases over time. Thus the trait estimates at the later times have not only greater measurement error but also more bias.

Curve fitting for the second person reflects the impact of measurement error and bias. The true trait level over time is well fit by a linear relationship to time ($R^2 = .940$). However, the estimated trait level is less well fit by the linear relationship ($R^2 = .862$). Also, the slope of the curve for estimated trait level ($b = .372$) indicates lesser growth than obtained from the true trait level ($b = .481$). Furthermore, better fit is observed with a different curve for the estimated trait levels, namely, a cubic growth curve ($R^2 = .925$). Thus neither the shape of the growth curve nor the amount of growth, given a common curve, corresponds well between the estimated and true trait levels.

Construct Shift

Item Change to Accommodate Increased Trait Levels

If examinee performance levels are increasing, more difficult items may be needed. However, increased item difficulty could result in shifted constructs. For example, Reckase and McKinley (1991) found that the harder items on a paragraph comprehension test involved greater impact of a second dimension (vocabulary level) than easier items. For personality and attitude measures, more extreme items may also be affected by secondary dimensions.

If secondary dimensions are involved for more difficult items, change at different levels will have different meaning, even if interval-level measurement is formally achieved. That is, increasing scores from lower trait levels will involve change on the originally intended trait 1 (e.g., comprehension), whereas increasing scores at higher levels could be primarily due to a shifted or altered construct trait 2 (e.g., comprehension *plus* vocabulary).

Thus it is important to evaluate dimensionality of the measures. Two basic methods are available. First, in full-information factor analysis, a multidimensional IRT model is applied to the item response data (e.g., Bock, Gibbons, & Muraki, 1991). Second, exploratory or confirmatory factor analysis can be applied with structural equation modeling of appropriate item intercorrelations, such as tetrachoric or polychoric (Jöreskog, 1994) correlations. The two methods typically produce similar results.

If more than one dimension is supported in the data, a method must be selected to accommodate the data. If the secondary dimension is not considered to be theoretically interesting, then a bifactor model can be applied to either full-information or confirmatory factor analysis to obtain better estimates for the central dimension of growth. If the secondary dimensions are theoretically interesting, however, then individual differences in growth would require tracking both the central and auxiliary dimensions.

Practice Effects

Item familiarity leads to increased scores. If the same test is repeated, earlier responses may be memorized and repeated without the person fully processing item content again. Scores may increase on repeated cognitive measures due mainly to the efficiency of responding to previously considered items that were missed. Even if alternative test forms with different item content are available for the repeated measurements, scores on cognitive measures may increase presumably *because strategies for handling the item type are developed*. Thus the original test score reflects individual differences in test-taking strategy, in addition to the construct levels. In the case of personality and attitude measurements, repeated test administration can lead to differing emphasis on the test context in item responses (Tourangeau, 2000). For example, scores could become more homogeneous as test context becomes more salient.

Thus practice can also shift the construct over time. Trait scores at later measurement periods may depend more on automated performance mechanisms than performance at earlier measurement periods. For cognitive measures, scores may increase due to increased automaticity. Thus the impact of strategy change will be confounded with time effects.

Measurement Design and Scaling Artifacts

The test design affects how scaling artifacts may influence growth and trend estimates. Features of test design that affect the role of scaling artifacts include: (1) the relationship between the psychometric properties of the multiple measures (constant or varied), (2) the score reporting format (continuous or categorical), and (3) test theory model (CTT or IRT). The role of test theory model has already been considered, so this section focuses on the other two features of test design. The features are analyzed assuming IRT scaling, but similar effects would be observed with CTT scaling.

Design of Multiple Measures

There are two basic test designs for the psychometric properties of multiple measures used repeatedly over time: constant psychometric properties versus varied psychometric properties. These designs have different sources of susceptibility to scaling artifacts. In this section, the two measurement designs and their vulnerability to various scaling artifacts are discussed.

Constant Psychometric Properties

For multiple measures with constant psychometric properties, there are two basic designs: (1) repeated measurements with the same test and (2) repeated measures with parallel tests. For these tests, the items are repeated or matched so that the construct(s) measured by the tests are presumably held constant by design.

Nonetheless, a major artifact for growth assessment is construct shift. That is, the construct(s) involved in examinees' performance may vary across measurements, due to changes in the manner in which examinees approach the items. Practice effects can occur in two ways, as discussed previously. First, scores on the repeated measurements may increase due to memory of items when one test form is used. Second, scores may increase on either the same form or alternative forms due to practice effects for the item type. For cognitive measures, practice effects can lead to score increases, whereas for self-report personality and attitude measurements the impact of response style or context effects could increase.

The constant test design is also particularly vulnerable to measurement error and bias effects. The constant test difficulty level becomes especially problematic when large amounts of change are observed over time. Figure 6.9 shows the impact of test difficulty level for the populations with low and high mean trait levels, based on the test of moderate difficulty administered repeatedly over time. Shown are estimated and true trait level means for both groups over time. Notice that change may be either underestimated or overestimated, depending on whether the test is too easy or too hard relative to the trait levels at a particular time. For the high group, trait level is underestimated at the last time periods, as the moderate test becomes increasingly uninformative about the higher ability levels. For the low group, trait level is overestimated during the earlier time periods, as the moderate test is particularly uninformative for the trait levels at that time.

Varied Psychometric Properties

For repeated measurements with varied difficulty levels, the tests are designed to be appropriate when levels of the construct(s) change across the measurement period. For example, achievement scores across school grade show increasing difficulty levels to reflect the

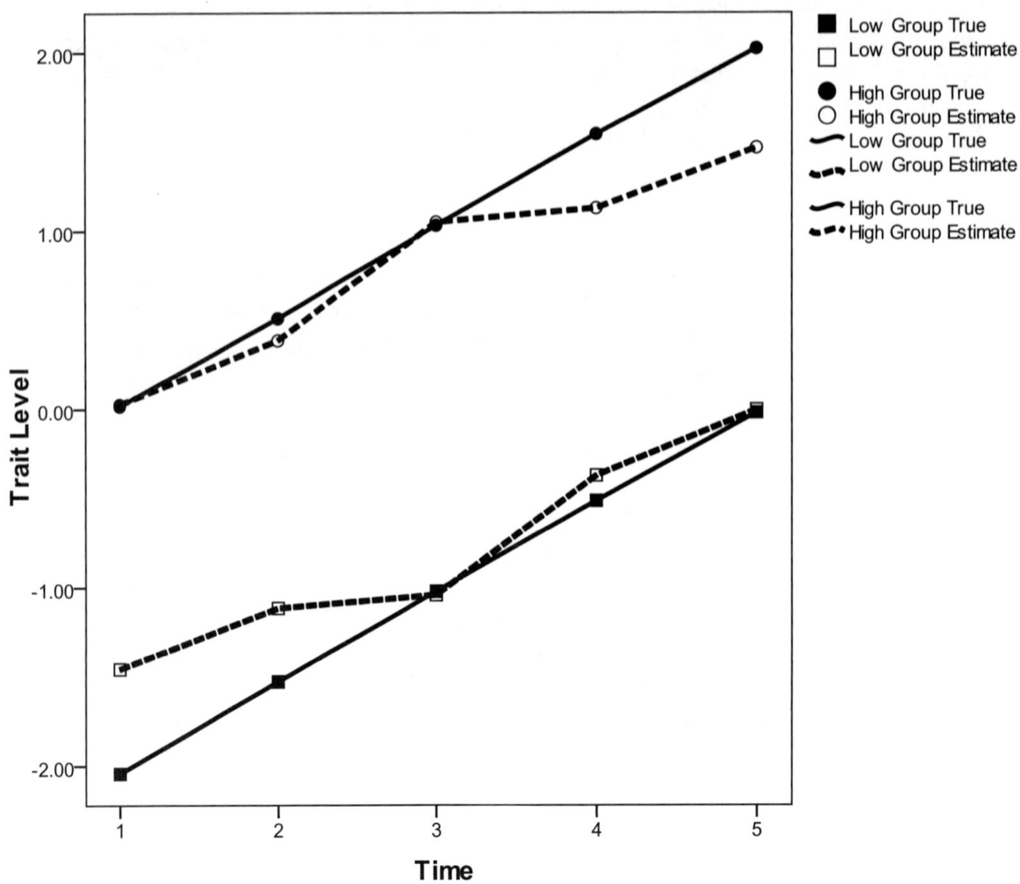

FIGURE 6.9. Growth curves for high and low groups on moderate test.

impact of instruction. Or, for example, some ability tests have multiple levels across ages. There are several types of test designs in this category: (1) multiple measures with partial overlap, (2) multiple measures with no overlap, and (3) adaptive tests, with individualized test forms at each measurement.

There are several potential issues in measuring growth with measures designed to vary in difficulty level. First, the construct may shift across measures as new item content is introduced to reflect increased performance levels. This same source of artifact was reviewed earlier with constant measures. Second, the items must be linked so that performance levels may be compared. Several different methods for test equating are available, such as random group equating, anchor items, and linear equating (see du Toit, 2003, pp. 532–537). These methods have various limitations, which are beyond the scope of this discussion. Third, the tests with systematically varied difficulty levels may not be sufficient or appropriate to counter the increased measurement error and bias that results from the changing trait levels of examinees.

Nonetheless, the impact of differential measurement error and bias can be mitigated when the appropriate test is selected for the various levels. Figure 6.10 presents growth curves for the same two populations as shown on Figure 6.9, except that an appropriate multilevel test was selected to estimate trait levels. That is, the easy test was selected for

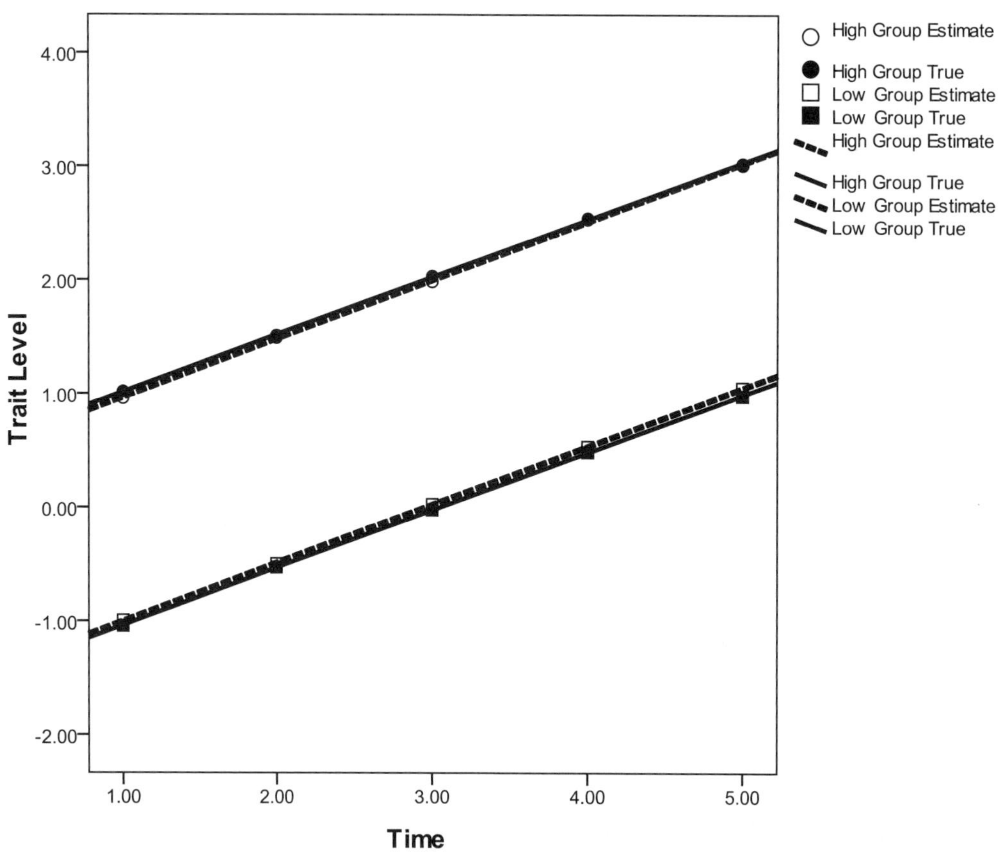

FIGURE 6.10. Growth curves for high and low groups on multilevel test.

the low group and the hard test was selected for the high group. These tests were linked with a randomly equivalent group design. Notice that the estimated trait growth curve and the true trait growth curve are now indistinguishable. There is no longer any overestimation or underestimation of trait levels.

The value of multilevel tests depends on selecting the appropriate test for the various groups or individuals to be studied. This design is not feasible if no previous estimates of initial trait level are available and if the growth trajectory is unknown, which is probably the case for many longitudinal studies. However, the fully adaptive test design (Lord, 1980), in which the most informative item is selected to measure the individual after each item response, requires no prior estimates to provide effective measurements for each person at each time. The rapidly increasing computerization of test administration makes this more adequate test design increasingly practical for measuring over a wide range of trait levels.

Score Reporting Format

The score reporting formats also affect the nature of reporting change over time. For the continuous score formats, the goal is to measure a construct accurately over a broad range of individual differences. Interval-level measurement is needed so that changes in scores reflect equal changes in the construct at all levels. If not, growth cannot be compared.

In contrast, if scores are reported as category membership, changes in classifications would be the primary focus of growth studies. For example, categorical variables that may be important in longitudinal research are proficiency versus nonproficiency and normality versus abnormality. In this case, the score reporting format is nominal level measurement.

Although the score report format is not continuous, measurement error is still relevant. Assume that categories are ordered on a continuum on which individuals vary. Accurate classification depends on having sufficient information at some threshold level to distinguish between categories. Thus, if the category threshold is low, items that are relatively easy are needed to provide maximum information. If the item information is focused too high, the measurement error surrounding the lower threshold would be higher, resulting in less accurate classifications.

Similarly, construct shift can provide complications for the categorical score reporting format. That is, if more than one construct is involved in items near a threshold, the classification into the category could be due to varying patterns of trait levels. Construct shift can be assessed by the same methods as indicated earlier when the focus was on trait level. Also, theoretical considerations will be important to determine how to treat construct shift when it does occur near a category threshold.

Example of Longitudinal Study of Growth

The development of mathematical thinking is a socially important topic, in that United States children lag behind children in many other countries (Programme for International Student Assessment, 2010). Especially crucial to developing mathematical competency are the middle school years, in which the foundations for algebra should be established (National Mathematics Advisory Panel, 2008). Furthermore, there are important individual differences in mathematical competency; namely, gender and socioeconomic differences

(U.S. Department of Education, 2009). Gender differences remain an important focus of research (Spelke, 2005), particularly because men are more heavily represented in careers involving mathematics. Gender differences may be especially important during the crucial period in which the foundations for algebra are introduced. Both genetic factors, such as the slower maturation of boys, and environmental factors, such as the greater emphasis on conformity for girls, may affect the growth of mathematical thinking in the middle school years. Similarly, socioeconomic background is another important individual-differences variable associated with mathematical achievement (U.S. Department of Education, 2001). The critical middle school period may be associated with differential growth by socioeconomic background.

In the current study, mathematical achievement test scores for the middle school/junior high school years were available for a large random sample of students in a state measured over time. This sample can be used to study individual differences in the development of mathematical competency in the middle school years.

Method

Test

Item response data and scores on the year-end state accountability test for mathematical competency were obtained for a large random sample of students in a state. For this sample, scores on the sixth-, seventh-, and eighth-grade tests were available. The measurement design is multilevel, as the tests are geared to assess the mathematical standards at the different grade levels. The items assess increasingly complex aspects of mathematics, which leads to grade-level differences in item difficulty and different content by grade.

Examinees

The examinees are 1,330 students selected at random. Students in sixth grade were randomly sampled from state records and then matched to their seventh- and eighth-grade records. These students took the same form of the state mathematics test at each grade. Background data on gender and lunch status were also available from the student records. Lunch status (i.e., qualifying for free lunch) depends on socioeconomic factors and can be used to represent low socioeconomic status.

Results

Overall Statistics and Comparisons: CTT

Descriptive statistics on the tests at the grades are shown in Table 6.1. Proportion correct scores are important for scoring reporting on standards-based tests. Although test items fulfill a blueprint, proportion correct scores still must be regarded as raw scores when comparing across tests because item difficulties can vary substantially. Thus proportion correct scores were converted into standard scores ($M = 100$, $SD = 20$) within each grade and then summed cumulatively at each grade to represent growth.

Another type of CTT scaled score shown in Table 6.1 is estimated domain proportion correct. In this analysis, the domain was defined as the 256 items on the tests across

TABLE 6.1. Descriptive Statistics on Proportion Correct and Estimated Domain Probabilities by Grade

	N	Mean	*SD*
Prop. correct grade 6	1,330	0.7479	0.16504
Prop. correct grade 7	1,330	0.6851	0.17885
Prop. correct grade 8	1,330	0.7064	0.17205
Domain grade 6	1,330	0.6827	0.19085
Domain grade 7	1,330	0.7650	0.16212
Domain grade 8	1,330	0.7686	0.16064
Valid *N* (listwise)	1,330		

grades. Expected probabilities of solving items in the domain were estimated at each grade using IRT estimates (multidimensional Rasch model for learning and change; see the next subsection). Although the domain estimates are derived from IRT, the score scaling of proportion correct is a CTT metric.

Proficiency categories are another type of CTT score. In education testing, a very common way to monitor performance change of students is to set an annual performance target at each grade and then to evaluate the extent of growth by studying the amount of change or shift in pupil standing over time. Grade-level performance targets, termed performance standards, are thoughtfully, though not altogether or always empirically, determined in consideration of societal expectations and grade-level performance goals. Proficiency categories are a type of CTT score in these data because the proficiency score cutlines are based on percentage correct scores. For these tests (same unique grade tests in mathematics) at these grades (6, 7, 8) over years (2006–2008) for these students (n = 1330), Table 6.2 reports the performance standing over time by grade and gender. The first three rows in Table 6.2 report the independent performance standings (percent proficient) at each measured grade and for gender. It can be seen that proficiency rates are relatively constant across grades, although item difficulty (see Table 6.1) changes over grade level.

Construct shift was examined by a series of exploratory factor analyses. We examined these same data (n = 1,330 students measured at grades (6, 7, 8) on the same tests. Although we studied a variety of factor analytic approaches, results from these data were altogether consistent. Factoring (principal axes) of these three items for the distinct measures (grade 6, 7, and 8 examinations) or simultaneously (256 items in all) led to a single dominant factor accounting for approximately 15% of the variance. Extraction of factors varied very slightly by grade, suggesting four or five factors (scree test), but never accounted for more than 25% of the observed score variance. Correlation between regression-based factor scores on the first unrotated principal axis dimension over grades ranged from .80 to .85. When all items were factored simultaneously, a single emerging factor correlated .92–.94 with the within-grade unrotated principal factors. Rotated factor score correlations (orthogonal or oblique solutions) across grades were consistently low, averaging .00 to .20, suggesting unique factor composites linked to item features and specific skills being evaluated.

Overall Statistics and Comparisons: IRT

The three multilevel tests also were calibrated with both the Rasch and the 2PL models. First, separate calibrations were conducted within each test. A goodness-of-fit test conducted on the composite likelihoods indicated that the 2PL model fit the data significantly better than the Rasch model ($\Delta\chi^2_{562}$ = 8,090, $p < .001$). Goodness-of-fit tests were also conducted on items within each analysis by comparing expected versus observed responses within varying levels of the latent trait. The results indicated that the mean ratio of chi square to degrees of freedom was much smaller for the 2PL model ($M_{\chi^2/df} = 1.874$) than for the Rasch model ($M_{\chi^2/df} = 5.377$). Thus an IRT model that includes varying item discrimination parameters provides the best fit to the data.

Two multidimensional IRT growth models were then fit to the data. First, the multidimensional Rasch model for learning and change (MRMLC; Embretson, 1991) was fit to the data. In this model, growth is modeled over time using a quasi-Weiner simplex structure to define latent dimensions. The model parameters include estimates of individuals' initial status and modifiabilities, as well as item difficulty parameters. Estimates of effective ability at each time point also may be computed. For the current analysis, item parameter estimates for MRMLC were obtained using the Bock–Aiken expectation-maximization algorithm for maximum likelihood with multidimensional quadrature, using a beta version of the IRT-PRO2 software. Constraints were set in the item discrimination parameter matrix according to the Weiner simplex pattern. Individual initial status and modifiabilities were estimated using the EAP method with the estimated item parameters. Table 6.3 presents the means for initial status and the modifiabilities. It can be seen that both modifiability 1 and modifiability 2 are positive, indicating growth in competency. Also shown in Table 6.3 are the MRMLC weighted estimates of overall competency by grade level. It can be seen that the greatest change in MRMLC competency level occurs between Grade 6 and Grade 7.

TABLE 6.2. Change in Proficiency Categories across Grades by Gender

	Total % proficient	% female proficient	% male proficient
Separate grades			
Grade 6	77	78	77
Grade 7	77	80	74
Grade 8	77	78	76
Pattern (6–7–8)			
P–P–P	66	68	64
P–P–NP	4	4	4
P–NP–NP	4	4	4
NP–NP–NP	12	11	14
NP–NP–P	3	3	3
NP–P–P	4	5	4
NP–P–NP	3	2	3
P–NP–P	4	2	5

Note. P, proficient; NP, not proficient.

Second, a 2PL version of the IRT growth model, the structured latent trait model (SLTM; Embretson, 1997), was fit to the data. In this model of growth, like MRMLC, a quasi-Weiner simplex pattern is postulated for the involvement of latent dimensions over time. However, items may differ in discrimination on both initial status and modifiability. Table 6.3 presents the initial status and modifiabilities estimated from SLTM. As for MRMLC, estimates for both modifiabilities are positive. Although modifiability 1 is about the same as estimated from MRMLC, modifiability 2 is substantially greater from SLTM. Finally, Table 6.3 also shows the overall SLTM competency estimates by grade level.

Consistent with the within-grade comparisons of fit for IRT models, it was expected that the 2PL version of the growth model would provide the best fit. A likelihood ratio goodness-of-fit test indicated that SLTM fit significantly better than MRMLC ($\Delta\chi^2_{509}$ = 13,324, $p < .001$), as expected. Thus, on the basis of fit, SLTM is the preferred IRT growth model. However, to provide a comparison of scaling effects, the impact of gender and socioeconomic differences on mathematical achievement was examined using both models.

Gender Differences

First, CTT standard scores were analyzed for overall gender effects. The Wilks' lambda test for a multivariate analysis of Gender yielded no significant effect ($F_{3,1326} = 1.256$, $p = .288$). Standard scores were also examined cumulatively over time with a repeated measures design, Time (3) by Gender (2). The Wilks' lambda multivariate test in the repeated-measures design indicated a significant effect of Time ($F_{2,1327} = 17{,}830.139$, $p < .001$) but no significant interaction of Gender and Time ($F_{2,1327} = 1.442$, $p = .237$). Furthermore, Gender had no significant main effect ($F_{1,1328} = .995$, $p = .319$) in the between-subjects analysis.

Figure 6.11 presents the estimated domain proportion correct across grade levels by gender. Although there appears to be an interaction of time and gender, the Wilks' lambda

TABLE 6.3. IRT Growth Scores by Grade

	N	Mean	*SD*
MRMLC Estimates			
Initial status	1,330	–.02768	1.556785
Modif. 1	1,330	1.19476	1.063532
Modif. 2	1,330	.06280	.835672
Grade 6	1,330	–.0177	.99634
Grade 7	1,330	.4602	1.01014
Grade 8	1,330	.4847	1.01166
SLTM Estimates			
Initial status	1,330	.01008	1.609831
Modif. 1	1,330	1.17932	1.112929
Modif. 2	1,330	.59458	.940491
Grade 6	1,330	.0067	1.07698
Grade 7	1,330	.5431	1.12388
Grade 8	1,330	.6173	1.14463

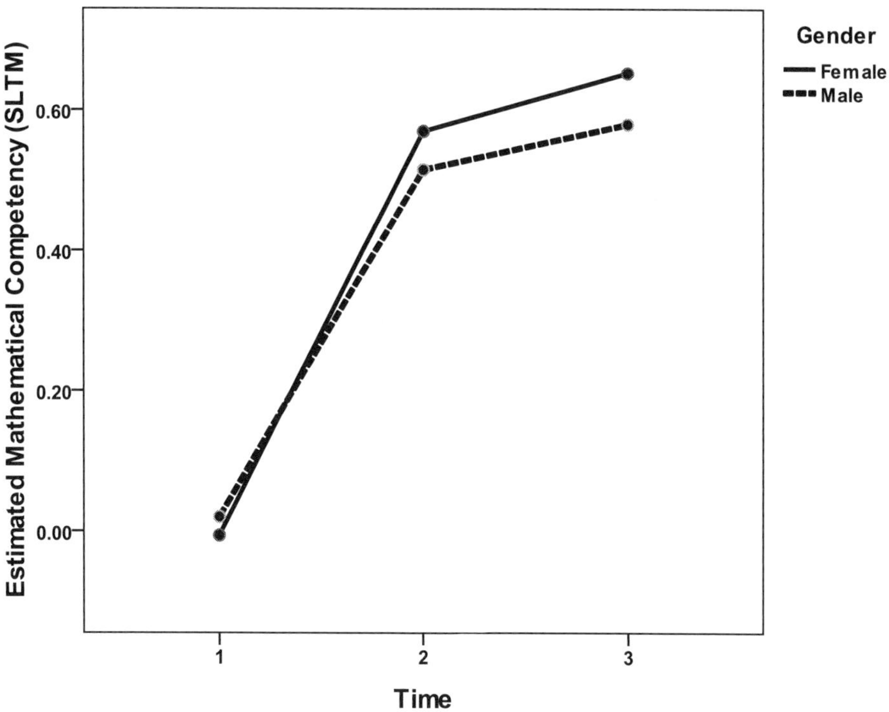

FIGURE 6.11. Growth in mathematical achievement over time by gender.

multivariate test from a repeated-measures analysis indicated that Time-by-Gender interaction was not significant ($F_{2,1327} = 1.014, p = .363$). However, Time was significantly associated with increases in mathematical competency ($F_{2,1327} = 577.393, p < .001$). Finally, the between-subjects analysis indicated that Gender was not significantly related to mathematical competency ($F_{1,1328} = .987, p = .321$). The last eight rows in Table 6.2 show the conjoint patterns observed, for example, the percentage of students (and then separately for females and males) scoring Proficient (P) on all three grade tests (P–P–P), the percentage of all students (and for each gender) evaluated based on test score as Not Proficient (NP) on each of the three tests over grades (NP–NP–NP), and so forth. Seen as independent groups over time, the passing percentages are equivalent over grades examined. Studied by gender, females are observed to outperform males over grades but not in a consistent form; that is, grade 7 females do notably better than their male peers. When these data are studied by their dependency—how the individual does over time—a somewhat discernable pattern emerges: females in the main outperform males, though the groups perform only modestly (64–68% Proficient), and males are found to display the more inconsistent or aberrant patterns—P–NP–P or NP–P–NP—that largely account for their lower overall performance.

To examine trend in proficiency categorization, we moved to a logistic regression, treating the grade 8 Proficient–Not Proficient classification as the criterion and the independent variables or predictors being grade 6 and grade 7 proficiency standing, gender, and the respective interactions. Results matched the CTT findings: Each succeeding grade forecast grade 8 classification with greater accuracy ($R^2 = 51.9\%$, and 86% grade 8 classification accuracy with a very slight tendency to predict Not Proficient students as Proficient).

Gender was not observed to offer discrimination, and gender-by-grade-classification interactions were not significant. The grade 6-by-grade 7 skill interaction was significant (p = .003, R^2 increase = 1%). Given this pattern of findings largely matching the CTT results but not the 2PL approach, and when coupled with the loss of precision and potential diagnosis by factor measurement (approximately 15% common variance over items and very distinct rotated factors), this methodology offers little if anything over the preceding approaches and is not endorsed for studying growth.

Next, MRMLC overall trait levels at each time were analyzed in a repeated-measures design. For Gender, although the Wilks' lambda multivariate test indicated that the Time main effect was highly significant ($F_{2,1327} = 850.818, p < .001$), Time did not interact significantly with Gender ($F_{2,1327} = .356, p = .701$). Furthermore, the between-subjects analysis indicated that the Gender main effect was not significant ($F_{1,1328} = .667, p = .414$).

However, the results from fitting SLTM had a different pattern in the repeated-measures analysis. Importantly, the Wilks' lambda multivariate test for interaction of Time and Gender ($F_{2,1327} = 5.390, p = .005$) was statistically significant. Furthermore, like MRMLC, the Wilks' lambda multivariate test indicated that Time was significant ($F_{2,1327} = 857.972$, $p < .001$), and the between-subjects analysis indicated that the overall impact of Gender was not significant ($F_{1,1328} = .325, p = .568$). Figure 6.12 presents the resulting growth curves by gender. It can be seen that, although mathematical competency is approximately equal between girls and boys at grade 6, the growth trajectory for girls is flatter across the subsequent grade levels.

In summary, gender differences were not observed when achievement was scaled in CTT metric, either by scale scores or by expected domain proportion correct. That is,

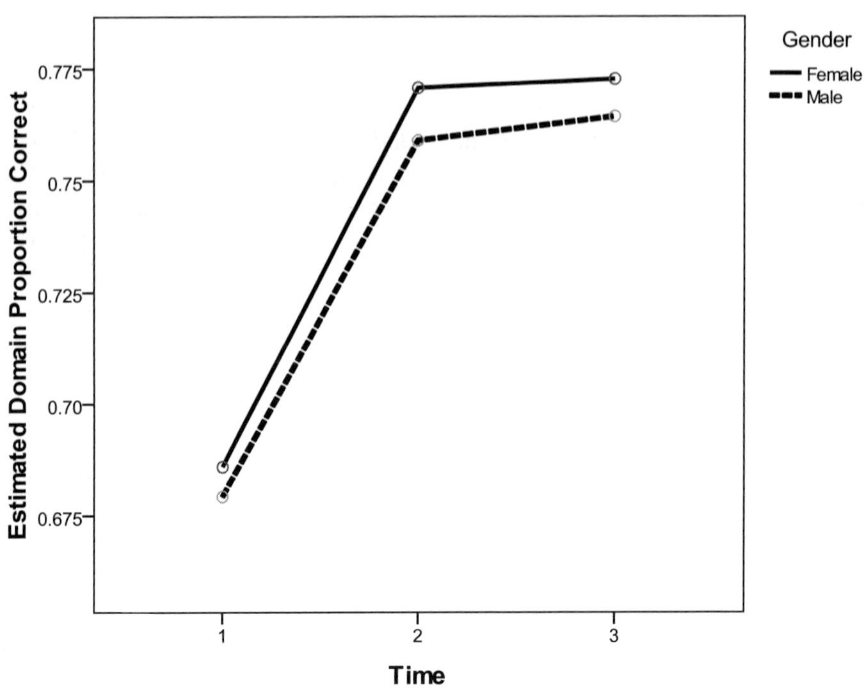

FIGURE 6.12. Gender differences in estimated true domain scores.

neither overall differences nor interactions of gender with time was observed. The IRT results showed a different pattern. If achievement level was estimated with MRMLC, gender was unrelated to competency levels, as for the CTT scale scores. Thus scaling differences alone are not a source of differences between the various analyses. However, when achievement level was estimated with SLTM, a highly significant interaction of gender and growth of achievement was found. It should be noted that based on goodness of fit, SLTM could be justified as giving the most appropriate results.

SES Differences

CTT scores also were analyzed for socioeconomic differences in mathematical achievement. The Wilks' lambda multivariate test in an overall multivariate comparison yielded a highly significant effect of SES ($F_{3,1181} = 84.554$, $p < .001$) on standard scores. Standard scores were then examined cumulatively over time with a repeated-measures design, SES (2) by Time (3). The Wilks' lambda multivariate test indicated a highly significant interaction of SES and Time ($F_{2,1182} = 119.873$, $p < .001$) and a highly significant effect for Time ($F_{2,1182} = 16{,}893.453$, $p < .001$). The between-subjects analysis yielded a highly significant main effect for SES ($F_{1,1183} = 251.443$, $p < .001$). An analysis of CTT domain scores was also performed for SES in a similar manner as for Gender. The Wilks' lambda multivariate test indicated a highly significant main effect of Time ($F_{2,1182} = 521.830$, $p < .001$) and highly significant interaction of SES and Time ($F_{2,1182} = 7.579$, $p < .001$). The between-subjects analysis also yielded a highly significant main effect for SES ($F_{1,1183} = 253.541$, $p < .001$).

Next, MRMLC overall trait estimates were analyzed in a repeated-measures analysis design. Time was significantly associated with increases in mathematical competency ($F_{2,1182} = 707.353$, $p < .001$), but Time did not interact significantly with SES ($F_{2,1182} = .742$, $p = .476$). Furthermore, the between-subjects analysis indicated that SES had a significant main effect ($F_{1,1183} = 242.204$, $p < .001$). Similarly, the repeated-measures analysis from SLTM trait estimates also indicated that both Time ($F_{2,1182} = 741.125$, $p < .001$) and SES ($F_{1,1183} = 232.673$, $p < .001$) had significant impact on mathematical competency. Importantly, however, the interaction of Time and SES ($F_{2,1182} = .182$, $p = .834$) was not statistically significant.

In summary, the CTT scale score analysis supported significant main effects of SES and Time, with positive growth in mathematical competency occurring over time and generally lower levels of competency associated with low SES. However, the CTT scale score analyses also included a highly significant interaction of SES and Time, with the students from lower SES backgrounds gaining more. In contrast, although both IRT growth models also found a significant main effect for SES and Time, neither MRMLC nor SLTM estimates yielded a significant SES-by-Time interaction. Thus the CTT- and IRT-based analyses lead to different conclusions about the impact of socioeconomic background on the growth of mathematical competency in the middle school years.

Discussion

The preceding results on gender and socioeconomic differences clearly indicate that scaling makes a difference in results on individual differences in growth. However, which scaling method, CTT-based or IRT-based, led to significant differences in the growth trajectory over time depended on the analysis. How can these results be interpreted, and which analysis yields the most accurate assessment of growth differences?

For gender, differences in growth were not detected with any method except the SLTM IRT growth model. That is, neither the analyses based on CTT scaled scores nor the analyses based on MRMLC scaled scores detected any significant gender differences. Thus the scaling intervals alone cannot account for the different findings, as both MRMLC and SLTM are based on IRT scaling. It could be expected that score intervals are less important in these analyses because the test difficulty level is equally appropriate for both groups (i.e., mean performance did not differ by gender). As Figure 6.2 shows, the regression of IRT score on CTT total score is nearly linear for moderate score levels (i.e., –1.0–1.0).

The explanation for the significant differences in growth based on SLTM scores resides in the varying item discriminations in the model. That is, the scale scores in SLTM, unlike the other three scale scores, are based on item responses that are weighted by discrimination on the common dimensions, like factor scores. The factor analysis results indicated that mathematical competency within grade levels consists of a composite of a common factor and several specific skill factors. Thus the interpretation of gender differences in growth of mathematical competency is restricted to the general factors across grades.

The results on SES, in contrast, are due to scale intervals. That is, low-SES students gain more across grades when mathematical achievement is based on CTT scale scores. However, when competency is measured with IRT scale scores, both MRMLC scores and SLTM scores, no significant differences in growth are found. The explanation is the differential appropriateness test difficulty level. Small changes in IRT-based scores are associated with larger changes in item solving probability for detecting score changes when item difficulty level is most appropriate. The items in the tests are relatively easy (see Table 6.1) and hence more appropriate for estimating changes in low competency levels than for changes in higher competency levels. The mean mathematical competency is substantially lower for students from low-SES backgrounds, which leads to their apparently larger growth when based on CTT scores. Consequently, the significantly greater growth in CTT scale scores for low-SES students can be attributed to a scaling artifact.

Summary

This chapter has examined the impact of scaling on studies of individual differences in growth. The theoretical properties of scale levels were considered in the context of the available test theory models for scoring psychological tests. IRT leads to more theoretically justifiable scaling of test scores than CTT. Simulation examples were presented to show that CTT scaling, in which score intervals cannot be regarded as equal, can lead to inaccurate estimates of individual differences in growth.

However, test design is also crucial to providing accurate estimates of growth. Measurement error and bias in estimating trait levels will lead to inaccurate estimates of growth. This effect occurs when test difficulty level is not optimal for the particular individual or group. Multilevel and adaptive tests, in contrast, can lead to more justifiable measures of growth. Another artifact, construct shift, can also affect estimates of growth. Methods for assessing construct shift were considered, but how to handle construct shift when estimating growth depends, in part, on the theoretical nature of the construct being studied.

A longitudinal study on mathematical competency was presented as a real example to illustrate the effects of scaling and measurement error. Two important individual-differences variables, gender and socioeconomic status, were examined for impact on growth in the middle school years. It was found that different conclusions about growth were related to the scaling technique. Analyses based on classical test theory scores found more growth in mathematical competency for students from low socioeconomic backgrounds than for students from higher socioeconomic backgrounds. This finding can be regarded as an artifact of the scale level achieved with CTT scores because (1) the scores based on IRT scaling show no significant differences between socioeconomic groups in growth and (2) the differences in findings are readily explainable from the varying appropriateness of test difficulty level for students from the two socioeconomic groups.

Gender differences in growth, in contrast, were found only with one of two IRT growth models. That is, girls gained more in competency over the middle school years than boys. The CTT-based scores yielded no significant differences in growth by gender. The model for which gender differences in growth were observed, SLTM (Embretson, 1997), differed from the other IRT model and the CTT models in that items were weighted by discrimination on the common dimensions. Thus the SLTM scale scores had less measurement error and less impact of small specific factors on the test. In this case, the IRT-based scaling led to a more powerful test of individual differences in growth.

References

Bock, R. D., Gibbons, R., & Muraki, E. J. (1988). Full-information item factor analysis. *Applied Psychological Measurement,12*, 261–280.

Cohen, J., Cohen, P., West, S., & Aiken, L. S. (2003). *Applied multiple regression/correlation analysis for the behavioral sciences* (3rd ed.). Mahwah, NJ: Erlbaum.

Coombs, C. H. (1950). Psychological scaling without a unit of measurement. *Psychological Review, 57,* 145–158.

DeBoeck, P., & Wilson, M. (2004). *Explanatory item response models: A generalized linear and nonlinear approach*. New York: Springer-Verlag.

du Toit, M. (2003). *IRT from SSI.* Chicago: Scientific Software International.

Embretson, S. E. (1991). A multidimensional latent trait model for measuring learning and change. *Psychometrika, 56,* 495–516.

Embretson, S. E. (1996). Item response theory models and inferential bias in multiple group comparisons. *Applied Psychological Measurement, 20,* 201–212.

Embretson, S. E. (1997). Structured ability models in tests designed from cognitive theory. In M. Wilson, G. Engelhard, & K. Draney (Eds.), *Objective measurement III* (pp. 223–236). Norwood, NJ: Ablex.

Embretson, S. E., & Reise, S. P. (2000). *Item response theory for psychologists*. Mahwah, NJ: Erlbaum.

Feldt, L. S., & Brennan, R. L. (1989). Reliability. In R. L. Linn (Ed.), *Educational measurement* (3rd ed., pp. 105–146). New York: Macmillan.

Gaito, J. (1980). Measurement scales and statistics: Resurgence of an old misconception. *Psychological Bulletin, 87,* 564–567.

Joreskog, K. G. (1994). On the estimation of polychoric correlations and their asymptotic covariance matrix. *Psychometrika, 59*(3), 381–389.

Little, T. D., Lindenberger, U., & Maier, H. (2000). Selectivity and generalizability in longitudinal

research: On the effects of continuers and dropouts. In T. D. Little, K. U. Schnabel, & J. Baumert (Eds.), *Modeling longitudinal and multilevel data* (pp. 187–200). Mahwah, NJ: Erlbaum.
Lord, F. M. (1953). On the statistical treatment of football numbers. *American Psychologist, 8*, 750–751.
Lord, F. M. (1980). *Applications of item response theory to practical testing problems*. Hillsdale, NJ: Erlbaum.
Luce, R. D., & Tukey, J. W. (1964). Simultaneous conjoint measurement: A new type of fundamental measurement. *Journal of Mathematical Psychology, 1*, 1–27.
McArdle, J. J., & Bell, R. Q. (2000). An introduction to latent growth curve models for developmental data analysis. In T. D. Little, K. U. Schnabel, & J. Baumert (Eds.), *Modeling longitudinal and multilevel data* (pp. 57–94). Mahwah, NJ: Erlbaum.
McDonald, R. P. (1999). *Test theory: A unified treatment*. Mahwah, NJ: Erlbaum.
Michell, J. (1986). Measurement scales and statistics: A clash of paradigms. *Psychological Bulletin, 100*, 398–407.
Michell, J. (1990). *An introduction to the logic of psychological measurement*. Hillsdale, NJ: Erlbaum.
National Mathematics Advisory Panel. (2008). *Foundations for success: Final report*. Washington, DC: U.S. Department of Education.
Programme for International Student Assessment. (2006). *PISA technical report*. Washington, DC: Organization for Economic Cooperation and Development.
Rasch, G. (1960). *Studies in mathematical psychology: I. Probabilistic models for some intelligence and attainment tests*. Oxford, UK: Nielsen & Lydiche.
Reckase, M. D. (2009). *Multidimensional item response theory*. New York: Springer.
Reckase, M. D., & McKinley, R. L. (1991). The discriminating power of items that measure more than one dimension. *Applied Psychological Measurement, 15*, 361–373.
Spelke, R. (2005). Sex differences in intrinsic aptitude for mathematics and science. *American Psychologist, 60*(9), 950–958.
Stevens, S. S. (1946). On the theory of scales of measurement. *Science, 103*, 667–680.
Torgerson, W. S. (1958). *Theory and methods of scaling*. New York: Wiley.
Tourangeau, R. (2000). Remembering what happened: Memory errors and survey reports. In A. A. Stone, J. S. Turkkan, C A. Bachrach, J. B. Jobe, H. S. Kurtzman, & V. S. Cain (Eds.), *The science of self-report: Implications for research and practice* (pp. 29–48). Mahwah, NJ: Erlbaum.
U.S. Department of Education. (2001). *The longitudinal evaluation of school change and performance (LESCP) in Title I schools: Vol. 1. Executive summary* (Document No. 2001-20). Washington, DC: Office of the Deputy Secretary.
U.S. Department of Education. (2009). *The nation's report card: Mathematics highlights 2000* (NCES Publication No. 2001-518). Washington, DC: National Center for Education Statistics, Office of Educational Research and Improvement.
van der Linden, W., & Hambleton, R. (1997). *Handbook of modern item response theory*. New York: Springer-Verlag.

CHAPTER 7

Investigating Factorial Invariance in Longitudinal Data

ROGER E. MILLSAP
HEINING CHAM

In the study of development and change, longitudinal studies collect data on individuals over repeated occasions. These data often consist of psychological self-report or rater-report measures in a variety of areas: cognition, personality, emotions, attitudes, and behaviors. When the longitudinal study includes individuals experiencing relatively rapid change (e.g., children) or when the study spans many years (e.g., lifespan development), questions about the continued validity of these measures may be important. A given measure may have been designed to measure a particular psychological construct. Does the measure relate to this construct in the same way at age 8 and at age 18? For example, substance abuse as an indicator of externalizing problems may relate differently to externalizing problems at age 8 and at age 18. The relationship of cognitive test scores to the dimensions underlying the test items may change with age, depending on the age range. In these examples, the same measures are being used at each occasion, but their relationships to the constructs or latent variables may be changing. These changes may jeopardize the interpretations of change based on the analyses of the measured variables.

The problem of changing relations between measures and the latent variables underlying those measures is a special case of the general problem of measurement invariance (Meredith, 1993). Psychologists are most familiar with this concept in the form of factorial invariance, which has been a topic of study since the early 20th century (Ahmavaara, 1954; Meredith, 1964; Thomson & Lederman, 1939; Thurstone, 1947). Factorial invariance holds when certain features of the factor structure remain the same across multiple populations or multiple time points. Confirmatory factor analysis is the most widely used method at present in studies of factorial invariance (Jöreskog, 1971). Longitudinal factor analysis has received less attention than the multiple population case, but a literature exists on this topic (Bieber & Meredith, 1986; Chan, 1998; Corballis & Traub, 1970; Jöreskog, 1970; Marsh & Grayson, 1994; Meredith & Horn, 2001; Molenaar, 1985; Tisak & Meredith, 1989; Tisak & Tisak, 2000; Widaman, Ferrer, & Conger, 2010).

This chapter describes the use of confirmatory factor analysis in the investigation of factorial invariance in longitudinal data. We begin with a general description of measurement invariance, along with some assumptions that underlie what follows. The longitudinal factor analysis model is then described. We next describe the sequence of steps that can be followed in determining whether invariance holds and in what form it might hold. A real example in a longitudinal study of coping is then given. The final section considers issues in conducting and interpreting studies of factorial invariance in the longitudinal context.

Central Issues

We begin by supposing that $\mathbf{X}_t$ is a $p \times 1$ vector of measured random variables on occasion t, $t = 1, 2, \ldots, T$. These measures might be test scores, questionnaire scores, or item scores, but they are regarded as continuous in scale. We define $\mathbf{W}_t$ as an $r \times 1$ vector of latent variables on occasion t, representing the constructs that the variables in $\mathbf{W}_t$ are intended to measure. The complete set of measures and latent variables can be grouped by occasion as

$$(\mathbf{X}_1, \mathbf{W}_1), (\mathbf{X}_2, \mathbf{W}_2), \ldots, (\mathbf{X}_T, \mathbf{W}_T). \tag{7.1}$$

We assume that a common group of N individuals is measured on $\mathbf{X}_t$ on each of the T occasions. Problems of missing data or attrition are common in longitudinal studies, but we do not address that issue here. We do make one important assumption about relations among the measured and latent variables that applies throughout the chapter. We assume that the measures $\mathbf{X}_t$ are conditionally independent of the latent variables at earlier occasions, given the latent variables at the present occasion t. The assumption means that we do not have to model any lagged direct effects of earlier latent variables on the present measures. Instead, the effects of earlier latent variables on $\mathbf{X}_t$ are strictly mediated by the present latent variables underlying $\mathbf{X}_t$. This assumption may be violated in some applications, but its use greatly simplifies the investigation of measurement invariance.

We can now define longitudinal measurement invariance. This definition parallels definitions for the independent population case (Mellenbergh, 1989; Meredith & Millsap, 1992; Lord, 1980). We will say that longitudinal measurement invariance holds in relation to occasions $t = 1, 2, \ldots, T$ if and only if for $\mathbf{W}_t = \mathbf{W}_{t+k}$,

$$F(\mathbf{X}_t|\mathbf{W}_t) = \mathrm{F}(\mathbf{X}_{t+k}|\mathbf{W}_{t+k}) \tag{7.2}$$

where $F(\mathbf{X}_t|\mathbf{W}_t)$ is the conditional distribution function for $\mathbf{T}_t$ given $\mathbf{W}_t$, or $P(\mathbf{X}_t \leq \mathbf{x}_t|\mathbf{W}_t)$, for any given fixed value $\mathbf{x}_t$ of $\mathbf{X}_t$. Equation 7.2 is defined for all t, k such that $t + k \leq T$. This definition says that for the same latent variable scores at two different occasions, we expect the conditional distributions of the measured variables to also be the same. In other words, systematic changes in the probability of achieving any given score on $\mathbf{X}_t$ come about only through changes in $\mathbf{W}_t$ and do not arise from other influences. The definition assumes that there are r latent variables at each occasion, with no changes in the number of latent variables. Changes in the number of latent variables would constitute violations of measurement invariance. The point of the preceding definition of measurement invariance is that a given score on the latent variable should correspond to the same distribution of scores on the measured variable, regardless of which occasion of measurement we are considering. If the measured variables meet this condition for measurement invariance, it does not preclude change on the measured variables over time. Equation 7.2 implies that any systematic changes in the measured variables are due to changes in the latent variables.

Conceptual Principles and Statistical Assumptions

The preceding definition of measurement invariance can accommodate many different types of latent variable models. The focus here is the common factor model. Factorial invariance is a weaker condition than measurement invariance as defined earlier because the factor analytic approach does not generally consider the entire distribution $F(\mathbf{X}_t|\mathbf{W}_t)$, and instead considers just the conditional mean and variance of $\mathbf{X}_t$ (Millsap, 2011). We turn now to this factor model.

The Longitudinal Factor Model

We now consider the case of a common factor vector $\mathbf{W}_t$ for r common factors at time t. Under the common factor model, we can express $\mathbf{X}_t$ as

$$\mathbf{X}_t = \boldsymbol{\tau}_t + \boldsymbol{\Lambda}_t\mathbf{W}_t + \mathbf{u}_t. \tag{7.3}$$

Here $\boldsymbol{\tau}_t$ is a $p \times 1$ vector of measurement intercept parameters at time t, $\boldsymbol{\Lambda}_t$ is a $p \times r$ factor loading matrix, and $\mathbf{u}_t$ is a $p \times 1$ vector of unique factor scores. We assume that the following holds for $\mathbf{W}_t$ and $\mathbf{u}_t$:

$$E(\mathbf{W}_t) = \boldsymbol{\kappa}_t \qquad E(\mathbf{u}_t) = 0 \tag{7.4}$$

$$\text{Cov}(\mathbf{W}_t) = \boldsymbol{\Phi}_t \qquad \text{Cov}(\mathbf{u}_t) = \boldsymbol{\Theta}_t \qquad \text{Cov}(\mathbf{W}_t, \mathbf{u}_t) = 0 \tag{7.5}$$

Here the $p \times p$ covariance matrix $\boldsymbol{\Theta}_t$ is assumed to be diagonal. Lagged covariances between the elements of $\mathbf{u}_t$, $\mathbf{u}_{t+k}$ are permitted, confined initially to covariances between the same variables measured at the two time points. These covariances are assembled in a $p \times p$ lagged covariance matrix:

$$\text{Cov}(\mathbf{u}_t, \mathbf{u}_{t+k}) = \boldsymbol{\Theta}_{t,t+k} \tag{7.6}$$

This lagged covariance matrix is assumed to be diagonal, with each diagonal element being the covariance between the unique factor for the same measured variable on two occasions. Under this structure, a unique factor may correlate with itself across time but not with other unique factors. In contrast, the common factors may freely correlate across time:

$$\text{Cov}(\mathbf{W}_t, \mathbf{W}_{t+k}) = \boldsymbol{\Phi}_{t,t+k} \tag{7.7}$$

Each of these lagged covariance matrices is a submatrix within a larger $s \times s$ supermatrix, where $s = rT$. This supermatrix contains the covariances among the common factors at every pair of occasions:

$$\Phi = \begin{vmatrix} \Phi_{11} & \Phi_{12} & \cdots & \Phi_{1T} \\ \Phi_{21} & \Phi_{22} & \cdots & \Phi_{2T} \\ \vdots & \vdots & \ddots & \vdots \\ \Phi_{T1} & \Phi_{T2} & \cdots & \Phi_{TT} \end{vmatrix} \tag{7.8}$$

We can also construct a factor-loading supermatrix that is $q \times s$, with $q = pT$. This superloading matrix has the block structure

$$\Lambda = \begin{vmatrix} \Lambda_1 & 0 & \cdots & 0 \\ 0 & \Lambda_2 & \cdots & 0 \\ \vdots & \vdots & \ddots & \vdots \\ 0 & 0 & \cdots & \Lambda_T \end{vmatrix} \tag{7.9}$$

We can define the supervectors for the measured variables, common, and unique factor scores as

$$\mathbf{X} = \begin{vmatrix} \mathbf{X}_1 \\ \mathbf{X}_2 \\ \vdots \\ \mathbf{X}_T \end{vmatrix} \qquad \mathbf{W} = \begin{vmatrix} \mathbf{W}_1 \\ \mathbf{W}_2 \\ \vdots \\ \mathbf{W}_T \end{vmatrix} \qquad \mathbf{u} = \begin{vmatrix} \mathbf{u}_1 \\ \mathbf{u}_2 \\ \vdots \\ \mathbf{u}_T \end{vmatrix} \tag{7.10}$$

Here $\mathbf{X}$ and $\mathbf{u}$ are each $q \times 1$, and $\mathbf{W}$ is $s \times 1$. We can also define a $q \times 1$ measurement intercept supervector as

$$\tau = \begin{vmatrix} \tau_1 \\ \tau_2 \\ \vdots \\ \tau_T \end{vmatrix} \tag{7.11}$$

Finally, the supermatrix $\mathbf{\Theta}$ will contain all of the submatrices $\mathbf{\Theta}_{t,t+k}$ in a band-diagonal structure (i.e., each submatrix is itself a diagonal matrix)

$$\Theta = \begin{vmatrix} \Theta_{11} & \Theta_{12} & \cdots & \Theta_{1T} \\ \Theta_{21} & \Theta_{22} & \cdots & \Theta_{2T} \\ \vdots & \vdots & \ddots & \vdots \\ \Theta_{T1} & \Theta_{T2} & \cdots & \Theta_{TT} \end{vmatrix} \tag{7.12}$$

This supermatrix is a $q \times q$ matrix.

Putting all of these elements together, the factor model for **X** across all occasions is

$$\mathbf{X} = \boldsymbol{\tau} + \boldsymbol{\Lambda}\mathbf{W} + \mathbf{u} \tag{7.13}$$

Under the earlier assumptions, the $q \times q$ covariance matrix for **X** is

$$\boldsymbol{\Sigma} = \boldsymbol{\Lambda}\boldsymbol{\Phi}\boldsymbol{\Lambda}' + \boldsymbol{\Theta} \tag{7.14}$$

The covariance structure for the measured variables is similar to the usual factor representation, aside from the special structuring of the loading and unique covariance matrices. To define the mean structure across occasions, we define the $s \times 1$ factor mean supervector and the $q \times 1$ mean supervector for the measured variables as

$$\boldsymbol{\kappa} = \begin{vmatrix} \boldsymbol{\kappa}_1 \\ \boldsymbol{\kappa}_2 \\ \vdots \\ \boldsymbol{\kappa}_T \end{vmatrix} \qquad \boldsymbol{\mu} = \begin{vmatrix} \boldsymbol{\mu}_1 \\ \boldsymbol{\mu}_2 \\ \vdots \\ \boldsymbol{\mu}_T \end{vmatrix} \tag{7.15}$$

Then the measured variable means can be expressed in terms of the factor model across occasions as

$$\boldsymbol{\mu} = \boldsymbol{\tau} + \boldsymbol{\Lambda}\boldsymbol{\kappa} \tag{7.16}$$

Again, apart from the special structure in the loading matrix, this expression is identical to the model for the means in a single occasion.

Model Identification

The factor model just described is not identified without further constraints. A general treatment of identification in factor analysis is beyond our scope, and so we confine discussion to models with two features. First, we assume that each common factor has a minimum of three indicators at each occasion. Second, we assume that each measured variable loads on only a single factor. Models with multiple factors per occasion are permitted, but each factor must have indicators that do not also load on other factors.

With these restrictions, the longitudinal factor model can be identified in several ways. First, some factor loadings and/or factor variances must be fixed to nonzero values. If the factor loadings are invariant across occasions, both the loadings and the factor covariance matrices can be identified by fixing all of the factor variances to 1.0 in one occasion (e.g., the first occasion). If no invariance constraints have been imposed on the factor loadings, identification can be achieved by fixing the loading for one chosen indicator per factor to 1.0 at each occasion. The chosen indicator is often denoted the "reference indicator" for the factor. For a given factor, one would choose the same reference indicator across occasions. Second, some measurement intercepts and/or factor means must be fixed to identify the mean structure. If the measurement intercepts are invariant across occasions, the intercepts and factor means can be identified by fixing the factor means to zero in one occasion (e.g., the first occasion). If no invariance constraints have been imposed on the measurement intercepts, identification is achieved by fixing the measurement intercept for one chosen indicator per factor to zero in each occasion. The chosen intercept is ordinarily for the reference indicator mentioned earlier.

Evaluating Invariance

A traditional framework for testing factorial invariance in multiple population studies (Meredith, 1993; Meredith & Millsap, 1992; Widaman & Reise, 1997) can be applied to the longitudinal context with some modifications. The framework consists of a nested series of increasingly constrained models that incorporate invariance restrictions on model parameters. These restrictions are introduced in a particular order to help locate the source of any violation of invariance, if invariance is rejected. In longitudinal studies, the restrictions are equality constraints that are placed on elements of the parameter supermatrices described earlier.

The Baseline Model

A longitudinal invariance investigation begins with the factor model described earlier, with no invariance constraints introduced. This baseline model says that r common factors exist in each occasion and that the factors in any occasion have the same pattern of fixed and free loadings. This baseline model is often denoted the *configural invariance* model (Thurstone, 1947). The configural model may not fit the data. The number of factors may not remain constant across occasions, or the pattern of nonzero loadings may change. Rejection of the configural model will undermine further tests of invariance, unless an alternative configural model is available. All further models beyond the configural model will include additional constraints and will not show better fit to the data. The baseline configural model should represent a good fit to the data.

A poor fit for the configural model will lead some investigators to modify the model by either adding factors, altering the loading pattern, or permitting unique factors to covary. Adding factors changes the definition of what is being measured by the measured variables. In this case the invariance study might be premature, given that a clear understanding of what is being measured is still evolving. Alterations to the loading pattern will often permit variables to load on more than one factor, assuming that no additional factors are used. We do not consider such loading structures here, but there is no barrier to using such structures in invariance studies if they are interpretable. As a third alternative, some investigators will choose to permit nonzero covariances among the unique factors. In the model described in equations 7.3–7.16, some of these covariances are already permitted between occasions but not within occasions. There may be plausible explanations for further nonzero covariances. One common example concerns items whose wording is quite similar, inducing a larger correlation between that pair of items. As more of these covariances are permitted, however, we move farther away from the idea of the common factor as the basis for explaining the correlations among the measures.

Metric Invariance

The next step places equality constraints on the elements of the factor-loading supermatrix Λ so that the loading for a given variable on a factor is the same across occasions:

$$\Lambda_1 = \Lambda_2 = \ldots = \Lambda_T \tag{7.17}$$

This set of constraints represents the *metric invariance* model (Horn & McArdle, 1992; Thurstone, 1947). Metric invariance applies within each variable separately across time. If metric invariance is rejected, it suggests that the loadings for one or more variables are changing over time. A logical next step is to locate which loadings are varying. We address that type of search later.

Metric invariance is important and fundamental, but this level of invariance is not sufficient to permit clear interpretations of change scores. Comparisons of means across time are still ambiguous under metric invariance because the measurement intercepts are varying, and these influence the means directly. A large mean change on the measured variables could instead be due to lack of invariance in the measurement intercepts. The reverse situation is also possible: Lack of invariance in intercepts could mask real change.

Strong Invariance

If metric invariance holds for the loadings across occasions, the next step is to introduce invariance constraints on the intercepts. The combination of metric invariance with invariant intercepts is known as *strong factorial invariance* (Meredith, 1993) or *scalar invariance* (Steenkamp & Baumgartner, 1998). In addition to the constraints in equation 7.17, we require that

$$\tau_1 = \tau_2 = \ldots = \tau_T \tag{7.18}$$

The measurement intercept for each measured variable is the same across all occasions. Under strong factorial invariance, systematic changes in the mean structure on **X** are due to changes in the common factors. If strong invariance holds, we can study mean trends in the measured variables over time without questioning whether the trends are due to influences apart from the common factors. If strong factorial invariance fails to hold, we can conclude that one or more of the measurement intercepts are varying over occasions.

Strict Invariance

Assuming that the strong factorial invariance model has been evaluated, the final stage will evaluate invariance constraints on the unique factor variances and also possibly on any nonzero covariances between unique factors at different occasions. Under *strict factorial invariance* (Meredith, 1993), strong factorial invariance holds, and the unique factor variances are also invariant over occasions:

$$\Theta_{11} = \Theta_{22} = \ldots = \Theta_{TT} \tag{7.19}$$

Strict factorial invariance implies that changes over time in the means and variances of the measured variables are due to changes in the common factors. DeShon (2004) points out that violations of strict invariance for a given measure could be explained by the actions of unmodeled influences on the measure that would alter its interpretation. A portion of the unique factor variance is also measurement error variance, and so another explanation for changing unique variance lies in changes in the amount of measurement error. Although we feel that strict factorial invariance is useful and should be investigated, the review reported in Vandenberg and Lance (2000) noted that investigators often stop with strong invariance and do not test strict invariance.

Before presenting an example of the full sequence of model evaluations, it is useful to state the model fit criteria we use to determine when to retain or reject models. Our fit criteria include three global fit indices: the chi-square fit statistic, the root mean square error of approximation (RMSEA), and the standardized root mean square residual (SRMR). For the baseline configural model, we want our model to have an RMSEA estimate less than .08, with a 90% confidence interval that includes .05. We also want the SRMR estimate to be less than .08. Ideally, the chi-square statistic is not significant at the .05 alpha level, but this standard is seldom achieved in practice. For all subsequent nested models, we want the change in the chi-square statistic to be nonsignificant at the .05 alpha level. We also want the change in the RMSEA statistic to be less than or equal to .001. Considerable disagreement exists concerning the appropriate cut points for these global fit indices when the chi-square statistic itself is statistically significant (Beauducel & Wittmann, 2005; Fan & Sivo, 2005; Marsh, Hau, & Wen, 2004; Yuan, 2005). Global fit indices should also be supplemented with scrutiny of local fit indices, such as residuals, expected parameter change statistics, and modification indices (Saris, Satorra, & van der Veld, 2009). Patterns in local misfit can suggest the likely source of misspecification in a model.

Illustration

The data for this example come from a randomized field trial of an intervention designed to help bereaved children cope with the death of a parent (Sandler et al., 2003). Children's ages ranged from 8 to 16 (mean = 11.39, SD = 2.43) at the time of recruitment. Sandler and colleagues (2003) describe the recruitment and randomization for the sample. Four waves of measurement were completed and are used here, with the first wave completed at pretest and the next three waves following treatment (3 months, 11 months, 6 years). Our analyses are confined to the control condition (N = 109), which involved a self-study program.

The measures to be analyzed are from the active coping dimension of the Children's Coping Strategies Checklist (CCSC; Ayers, Sandler, West, & Roosa, 1996). The active coping dimension measures how often the child adopts coping strategies of focusing on the stressful event either to change the situation or to think about it more positively. The analyses use four out of the six subscales of the active coping dimension in the CCSC: Cognitive Decision Making, Direct Problem Solving, Control, and Optimism. Analyses are conducted at the subscale level, making $p = 4$ in all four occasions. The Mplus (Muthén & Muthén, 1998–2010) software program was used in all factor analyses. Missing data were handled using the full information maximum likelihood (FIML) option in Mplus.

Table 7.1 presents the means, standard deviations, and correlations for the four coping variables at each of the four waves of measurement. All statistics in Table 7.1 are adjusted for missing data using the FIML option. Each subscale is created as an average of the items in that subscale, and so the scale range for the subscales is identical to that of the items. Scores range from 1 to 4, with high scores meaning higher use of the coping strategy. The means on each of the four subscales in Table 7.1 are fairly stable over time. For each of the subscales, the correlations between waves appear in a simplex pattern, with lower

TABLE 7.1. Correlations, Means, and Standard Deviations for the Measured Variables

		CDM				DPS				CNT				OPT			
		T1	T2	T3	T4	T1	T2	T3	T4	T1	T2	T3	T4	T1	T2	T3	T4
CDM	T1	1															
	T2	.360	1														
	T3	.244	.448	1													
	T4	–.008	.151	.280	1												
DPS	T1	.553	.399	.283	–.021	1											
	T2	.245	.737	.397	.195	.337	1										
	T3	.337	.498	.734	.199	.229	.501	1									
	T4	.059	.138	.277	.726	.092	.222	.236	1								
CNT	T1	.473	.208	.176	.121	.570	.255	.276	.219	1							
	T2	.204	.553	.273	.145	.307	.694	.348	.194	.303	1						
	T3	.247	.417	.685	.142	.247	.466	.676	.289	.283	.378	1					
	T4	.025	.101	.194	.618	.090	.247	.150	.629	.226	.304	.333	1				
OPT	T1	.560	.201	.197	.072	.541	.226	.308	.116	.555	.247	.381	.280	1			
	T2	.215	.507	.267	.032	.299	.609	.354	.212	.203	.565	.418	.156	.426	1		
	T3	.229	.423	.652	.185	.209	.380	.559	.225	.102	.259	.752	.247	.384	.439	1	
	T4	.053	.057	.216	.514	.062	.255	.238	.616	.033	.169	.288	.641	.255	.234	.203	1
Mean		2.621	2.535	2.596	2.625	2.661	2.651	2.601	2.715	2.546	2.569	2.602	2.737	2.810	2.684	2.644	2.676
SD		0.588	0.635	0.649	0.606	0.620	0.674	0.589	0.617	0.654	0.686	0.662	0.631	0.774	0.726	0.726	0.672

Note. CDM, cognitive decision making; DPS, direct problem solving; CNT, control; OPT, optimism. FIML estimated descriptive statistics; $N = 109$.

correlations at greater lags. The Optimism scale departs from this pattern to some degree. Also, the correlations within each wave among the four subscales are substantial, supporting the idea of a common factor.

Table 7.2 reports the fit statistics for all of the models tested. Our initial model M1 uses the baseline configural model described earlier, except that no covariances between unique factors are permitted. The intent of this model is to evaluate a simple model that ignores any unique factor covariances. The fit results for M1 are not indicative of a good fit by our standards. As a result, we create model M2, which adds covariances for unique factors across time within each of the four variables, as in equation 7.12. M2 fits much better than M1, and M2 meets our criteria for an acceptable baseline configural model. The need for covariances across time in the unique factors suggests that these factors contain more than pure measurement error. We retained M2 as the baseline model and moved to evaluate further invariance constraints.

Model M3 imposes metric invariance, requiring the factor loadings for each measured variable to be invariant across time. In Table 7.2, M3 shows some loss of fit in comparison with M2, with a significant change in chi-square and a change in RMSEA larger than .001. After examining residuals and modification indices, we remove the invariance constraint on Direct Problem Solving in wave 3. The resulting model, M4, is an example of "partial" metric invariance (Byrne, Shavelson, & Muthén, 1989) in which some, but not all, loadings are invariant. M4 shows improved fit in comparison with M3 and is acceptable in relation to M2. The residuals and modification indices in M4 do not clearly show further loadings to

TABLE 7.2. Fit Statistics for the Invariance Models

Model	Chi-square	*df*	*p*-value	RMSEA (90% interval)	SRMR
M1 Configural No covar. Unique	201.360	98	< .0001	.098 (.079, .118)	.059
M2 Configural	111.509	74	.0032	.068 (.040, .093)	.057
M3 Metric	130.310	83	.0007	.072 (.047, .095)	.080
M4 Part metric	119.377	82	.0045	.065 (.037, .089)	.065
M5 Part strong	140.819	90	.0005	.072 (.048, .094)	.068
M6 Part strong II	130.889	89	.0026	.066 (.040, .089)	.071
M7 Part strict	148.150	101	.0016	.065 (.041, .087)	.074

Note. RMSEA, root mean square error of approximation; SRMR, standardized root mean square residual.

free. The loading for Direct Problem Solving at wave 3 is smaller than at the other waves. We retain M4 as a model representing partial metric invariance.

Next we add invariance constraints on all measurement intercepts except the intercept for Direct Problem Solving in wave 3. The loading for this variable was permitted to vary, and so the measurement intercept must also be allowed to vary. The intercept constraints worsen the fit for M5 in comparison with M4. Residuals and modification indices suggest that the intercept for Optimism at wave 1 should be allowed to vary. We relax the invariance constraint on this variable, creating model M6. M6 improves the fit considerably in comparison with M5 and is closer to M4 in fit. Residuals and modification indices do not suggest further removal of the invariance constraints on the intercepts. The final model adds invariance constraints on the unique factor variances in model M6, resulting in model M7. No invariance constraints are added on the covariances among the unique factors. The change in fit from M6 to M7 is small and meets our standards, supporting the plausibility of the invariance constraints. Model M7 represents partial strict invariance due to the single loading at wave 3 and the intercepts at waves 1 and 3, which all depart from invariance.

Table 7.3 presents the parameter estimates from model M7, the partially strict model. Among the factor loadings, the only change is at wave 3 for DPS. The intercept difference was also permitted for this variable at wave 3, but as shown in Table 7.3, the difference in

TABLE 7.3. Parameter Estimates from Model 7

	Wave 1	Wave 2	Wave 3	Wave 4
Factor loadings				
CDG	.460	.460	.460	.460
DPS	.532	.532	.411	.532
CNT	.480	.480	.480	.480
OPT	.492	.492	.492	.492
Measurement intercepts				
CDG	2.591	2.591	2.591	2.591
DPS	2.657	2.657	2.607	2.657
CNT	2.596	2.596	2.596	2.596
OPT	2.803	2.648	2.648	2.648
Factor correlations and means				
Wave 1	1.0			
Wave 2	.438	1.0		
Wave 3	.383	.604	1.0	
Wave 4	.144	.285	.307	1.0
Means	0[a]	–.039	.007	.146

[a]Fixed for identification.

the intercept at this wave is very small. In our judgment, the loading and intercept differences here are too small to cause concern. In the measurement intercept estimates, the only other violation of invariance occurs at wave 1 for Optimism. To judge the size of this intercept difference, we can compare the Optimism mean at wave 1 to its mean at wave 2. From Table 7.1, that mean difference is .126. The difference in intercepts at the two waves is .155. All of the difference in means is accounted for by the change in intercept, suggesting that the observed change in the mean on this variable from wave 1 to wave 2 is due to influences apart from the common factor. In absolute terms, the change in the means here is only about one-sixth of a standard deviation on the measured scale, and so this is not a large change. The factor correlations show the simplex pattern that is commonly found in longitudinal studies. None of the factor means is significantly different from zero, suggesting no mean change at the latent level. Overall, the results suggest that the partial invariance in the loadings and intercepts is good enough to warrant comparisons of means on the measured variables across time, as in growth modeling, for example. Invariance in the unique factor variances imply that increases in the variances of the measured variables over time in Table 7.1 are due to increasing variability on the common factor.

Future Directions

We describe here some general issues that should be considered when conducting an investigation of factorial invariance in longitudinal data. Some issues concern data conditions that can affect the outcome of the investigation. Others address points of strategy in conducting the analyses, or issues of interpretation. In some cases, the optimal strategies are unclear, and future directions for research are described.

Partial Invariance

If the metric invariance model is rejected, the next step is usually to determine which factor loadings are invariant and which are not. Similarly, if strong invariance is rejected, we conduct further analyses to determine which intercepts are invariant. In both cases, the likely outcome is a model representing partial invariance, as illustrated in the example. How should the search for variables that violate invariance be conducted? This question is part of a more general problem in structural equation modeling: How should a model that does not fit the data be altered or respecified to improve fit (Kaplan, 1988; MacCallum, 1986; MacCallum, Roznowski, & Necowitz, 1992)? Although there are no simple answers to this question in general, the invariance application has some simplifying features. The number of alternative models is limited and relatively small. One could examine all possible models in a brute force approach, but it is more helpful to apply any theory that might suggest which variables are likely to be violators of invariance. Past research with similar variables may help.

Is it better to start with a fully constrained model, gradually releasing constraints, or should we start with no invariance constraints and then add them? The two strategies may not lead to the same final model. In both cases, many tests are conducted, and Type I errors are likely to multiply. False discovery rate procedures (Benjamini & Hochberg, 1995) control the expected number of Type I errors in a series of tests and are often more powerful than traditional multiple comparison procedures. If we expect that few violations of invariance are present, it may be better to start with the fully constrained model so that fewer fit evaluations are needed. Yoon and Millsap (2007) illustrate the use of this approach for the multiple group case. The search problem is magnified when many variables or occasions are included in the model. The available power studies (Meade & Bauer, 2007; Meade & Lautenschlager, 2004; Yoon & Millsap, 2007) suggest that specification searches are more successful when few violations of invariance are present, the violations that are present are moderate or large in size, and the variable communalities (i.e., proportions of variance accounted for by the common factors) are high (e.g., > .60).

An additional search complication lies in the need to constrain some parameters for identification purposes. For example, if some loadings must be fixed to unit values across time for identification purposes, those loadings cannot be evaluated for invariance. If these parameters violate invariance and go undiscovered, distortions in the other parameter estimates may follow (Johnson, Meade, & DuVernet, 2009; Yoon & Millsap, 2007). This problem has been studied in the multiple population case, with some reasonable procedures being proposed (Rensvold & Cheung, 2001; Woods, 2009; Yoon & Millsap, 2007). Rensvold and Cheung (2001) systematically vary the placement of the identification constraints to judge which placement is best. Woods (2009) selects the measures to be used for identification using item-level bias test statistic values ranked high to low, with the selected measures having the lowest values. Yoon and Millsap (2007) use modification indices to relax invariance constraints within a metric invariance model. This topic deserves more study in the longitudinal case.

When is the level of partial invariance too "partial" to be acceptable? How many factor loadings, for example, can be different across time before the resulting measures become useless for longitudinal inference? Here we must distinguish two different domains of inference. The first domain is that of the measured variables. Historically, factorial invariance was studied to determine whether the measures themselves could be used in further analyses without worrying that their properties are changing over time. In contrast to this domain, advances in modeling have made it possible to work at the latent variable level within complex structural models, as in longitudinal latent path models. These structural models shift the focus from the measured variables to the latent variables and their relations across time.

Applied to the first domain, the question of when invariance is too partial is amenable to study. What distortions in the conclusions from the analyses of the measured variables would follow from partial invariance? By "distortion" we mean that the conclusion about change based on the measured variables would differ from the conclusion we would reach if we had the latent variable scores. In multiple group studies of invariance there have been efforts to look at the impact of partial invariance on conclusions drawn from measured variables (Millsap & Kwok, 2004; Stark, Chernyshenko, & Drasgow, 2004). Stark and colleagues (2004) examined the impact of item-level bias on conclusions from total scale scores. Millsap and Kwok (2004) examined the impact of total score bias on accuracy of selection decisions when the score is used to select people for jobs, treatment programs, or other interventions.

In the second latent domain, fewer answers are available. Suppose that we have a simple autoregressive path model among the latent variables underlying our measures, but we have only partial metric invariance over time. How many loadings must be different across time before our inferences about the latent autoregressions are compromised? There is no necessary mathematical relation between a latent autoregression coefficient and the factor loadings. Hence it is not at all clear how one should answer the preceding question. Intuitively, we might argue that large changes in loadings could indicate that the same latent variables are no longer being measured and hence that the latent autoregressions are no longer "autoregressions" but are rather regressions involving different latent variables. On the other hand, metric invariance itself is no guarantee that the same latent processes are operating at each occasion (see Widaman, Little, Geary, & Cormier, 1992, for a counterexample). At present, the best approach in this second domain may be to ask: Are the violations of invariance extensive enough to indicate that the same latent variables are not being measured across occasions?

Data Conditions

Some issues to consider when evaluating invariance concern data conditions that can affect the results of the analyses. In some cases, changes in the method of analysis can surmount these challenges, whereas others may preclude a conventional analysis.

Discrete Measures

The longitudinal factor model described earlier is formulated for continuous measured variables, but in practice the measured variables may be discrete in scale. For example, the measured variables may be item scores that are binary or Likert-type with few categories. In such cases, the use of the continuous factor model can lead to biases in parameter estimates (Carroll, 1945, 1983; McDonald & Ahlawat, 1974). An alternative approach is to use a factor model designed for discrete or ordered categorical measures (Bartholomew, 1983; Browne & Arminger, 1995; Christoffersson, 1975; Jöreskog, 1993; Maydeu-Olivares, 2005; Mislevy, 1986; Muthén, 1984; Wirth & Edwards, 2007). This model is not yet widely used in invariance studies (but see Millsap & Tein, 2004). The sequence of model evaluations under this form of factor analysis is similar to that described earlier, but depending on software, the measurement intercepts are replaced by threshold parameters. The factor model for ordered categorical measures has potentially more parameters than the continuous model, with larger sample size demands. New estimation methods help reduce these demands (Flora & Curran, 2004).

A different alternative in the discrete case is to use models from item response theory (IRT) (de Ayala, 2009; Embretson & Reise, 2000; Fischer & Molenaar, 1995; Lord, 1980; van der Linden & Hambleton, 1997). These models are designed for item-level measures, and they offer a wide variety of model types. Invariance studies using these models are common in the multiple population case, with fewer applications in the longitudinal case. The factor model for discrete measures is actually equivalent to an IRT model (Lord & Novick, 1968; Takane & de Leeuw, 1987). IRT can be viewed as a more general modeling framework for invariance modeling, but one that is still less familiar to psychologists than the factor model. Millsap (2011) provides a general introduction to the use of IRT in invariance modeling in the multiple population case.

Changing Measures

In some longitudinal studies, the measured variables are not identical across occasions, unlike what was assumed in the earlier description of the factor model. Particularly in studies spanning long time intervals, different measures may be introduced that are more age appropriate. In other cases, changes in standardized measures are introduced to reflect new normative data or new item content. These changes disrupt the modeling approach described earlier because we do not expect actual invariance longitudinally when different measures are used.

What can be done in this situation? In test theory, the traditional approach to this problem has been to develop equating procedures that would transform scores on different measures to a common scale that could then be used in place of the original scales (Kolen & Brennan, 2010). A fundamental assumption in such equating studies, however, is that the same latent variable underlies the different measures. In longitudinal studies, that assumption may be more or less plausible. Invariance studies can help address this question, but we cannot do a traditional invariance study when measures vary across occasions.

If longitudinal data are available with different measures at each occasion, and it is hypothesized that these measures are all measuring a common factor, this hypothesis is easily investigated. The supervector **X** in equation 7.10 would now consist of different measures at different occasions. A single factor model can be fit to **X** with no restrictions of invariance on model parameters. It may be necessary to account for occasion effects by permitting some covariances between unique factors within occasions. If a single factor model fits the data, support for the original hypothesis is found, and some form of equating may be possible.

A very different approach to longitudinal invariance modeling is represented in recent work by Nesselroade and colleagues (Nesselroade, Gerstorf, Hardy, & Ram, 2007). This approach eliminates the invariance restrictions described earlier (metric, strong, strict) and instead operates with configural invariance combined with invariance restrictions on the factor covariance matrices Φ_t. The focus in this approach is strictly on the latent domain, the argument being that invariance in relations among the latent variables is an indication that the same latent variables are measured at each occasion. Factor loadings are not required to be invariant. In the absence of traditional forms of invariance, the question is whether invariance in the factor covariance matrices Φ_t is convincing evidence that the same latent variables are being measured across time. The answer is not clear generally, but there may well be applications in which a plausible case can be made.

To conclude, the investigation of longitudinal factorial invariance is useful whenever it is suspected that the relations between the measured variables and their hypothesized factors are changing over time. If undetected, these changing relations can lead to erroneous conclusions about growth and development. We have described the use of confirmatory factor analysis in such investigations. Widely available software makes it possible to efficiently implement the method across a variety of data conditions. Longitudinal factor analysis also has limitations, but the largest barrier to wider use of the method is a general lack of awareness among investigators regarding its use. We hope that this chapter will help remove this barrier.

References

Ahmavaara, Y. (1954). The mathematical theory of factorial invariance under selection. *Psychometrika, 19,* 27–38.

Ayers, T. S., Sandler, I. N., West, S. G., & Roosa, M. W. (1996). A dispositional and situational assessment of children's coping: Testing alternative models of coping. *Journal of Personality, 64*, 923–958.

Bartholomew, D. J. (1983). Latent variable models for ordered-categorical data. *Journal of Econometrics, 22*, 229–243.

Beauducel, A., & Wittmann, W. (2005). Simulation study on fit indices in confirmatory factor analysis based on data with slightly distorted simple structure. *Structural Equation Modeling, 12*(1), 41–75.

Benjamini, Y., & Hochberg, Y. (1995). Controlling the false discovery rate: A practical and powerful approach to multiple testing. *Journal of the Royal Statistical Society: Series B, 57*, 289–300.

Bieber, S. L., & Meredith, W. (1986). Transformation to achieve a longitudinally stationary factor pattern matrix. *Psychometrika, 51*, 535–547.

Browne, M. W., & Arminger, G. (1995). Specification and estimation of mean and covariance structure models. In G. Arminger, C. C. Clogg, & M. E. Sobel (Eds.), *Handbook of statistical modeling for the social and behavioral sciences* (pp. 185–249). New York: Plenum Press.

Byrne, B. M., Shavelson, R. J., & Muthén, B. (1989). Testing for equivalence of factor covariance and mean structures: The issue of partial measurement invariance. *Psychological Bulletin, 105*, 456–466.

Carroll, J. B. (1945). The effect of difficulty and chance success on correlations between items and between tests. *Psychometrika, 26*, 347–372.

Carroll, J. B. (1983). The difficulty of a test and its factor composition revisited. In H. Wainer & S. Messick (Eds.), *Principles of modern psychological measurement* (pp. 257–283). Hillsdale, NJ: Erlbaum.

Chan, D. (1998). The conceptualization and analysis of change over time: An integrative approach incorporating longitudinal mean and covariance structures (LMACS) and multiple indicator latent growth modeling (MLGM). *Organizational Research Methods, 1*, 421–483.

Christoffersson, A. (1975). Factor analysis of dichotomized variables. *Psychometrika, 40*, 5–32.

Corballis, M. C., & Traub, R. E. (1970). Longitudinal factor analysis. *Psychometrika, 35*, 79–95.

de Ayala, R. J. (2009). *The theory and practice of item response theory*. New York: Guilford Press.

DeShon, R. P. (2004). Measures are not invariant across groups without error variance homogeneity. *Psychology Science, 46*, 137–149.

Embretson, S. E., & Reise, S. P. (2000). *Item response theory for psychologists*. Mahwah, NJ: Erlbaum.

Fan, X., & Sivo, S. A. (2005). Sensitivity of fit indices to misspecified structural or measurement model components: Rationale of the two-index strategy revisited. *Structural Equation Modeling, 12*(3), 343–367.

Fischer, G. H., & Molenaar, I. W. (Eds.). (1995). *Rasch models: Foundations, recent developments, and applications*. New York: Springer-Verlag.

Flora, D. B., & Curran, P. J. (2004). An empirical evaluation of alternative methods of estimation for confirmatory factor analysis with ordinal data. *Psychological Methods, 9*, 466–491.

Horn, J. L., & McArdle, J. J. (1992). A practical guide to measurement invariance in research on aging. *Experimental Aging Research, 18*, 117–144.

Johnson, E. C., Meade, A. W., & DuVernet, A. M. (2009). The role of referent indicators in tests of measurement invariance. *Structural Equation Modeling, 16*, 642–657.

Jöreskog, K. G. (1970). Factoring the multitest–multioccasion correlation matrix. In C. E. Lunneborg (Ed.), *Current problems and techniques in multivariate psychology* (pp. 68–100). Seattle: University of Washington Press.

Jöreskog, K. G. (1971). Simultaneous factor analysis in several populations. *Psychometrika, 36*, 409–426.

Jöreskog, K. G. (1993). Latent variable modeling with ordinal variables. In K. Haagen, D. J. Bartholomew, & M. Deistler (Eds.), *Statistical modeling and latent variables* (pp. 163–171). Amsterdam: North-Holland.

Kaplan, D. (1988). The impact of specification error on the estimation, testing, and improvement of structural equation models. *Multivariate Behavioral Research, 23*, 69–86.

Kolen, M. J., & Brennan, R. L. (2010). *Test equating, scaling and linking: Methods and practices* (2nd ed.). New York: Springer.

Lord, F. M. (1980). *Applications of item response theory to practical testing problems*. Hillsdale, NJ: Erlbaum.

Lord, F. M., & Novick, M. E. (1968). *Statistical theories of mental test scores*. Reading, MA: Addison-Wesley.

MacCallum, R. C. (1986). Specification searches in covariance structure modeling. *Psychological Bulletin, 100*, 107–120.

MacCallum, R. C., Roznowski, M., & Necowitz, L. B. (1992). Model modifications in covariance structure analysis: The problem of capitalization on chance. *Psychological Bulletin, 111*, 490–504.

Marsh, H. W., & Grayson, D. (1994). Longitudinal confirmatory factor analysis: Common, time-specific, item-specific, and residual-error components of variance. *Structural Equation Modeling, 1*, 116–145.

Marsh, H. W., Hau, K.-T., & Wen, Z. (2004). In search of Golden Rules: Comment on hypothesis-testing approaches to setting cutoff values for fit indexes and dangers in overgeneralizing Hu and Bentler's (1999) findings. *Structural Equation Modeling, 11*(3), 320–341.

Maydeu-Olivares, A. (2005). Linear item response theory, nonlinear item response theory, and factor analysis: A unified framework. In A. Maydeu-Olivares & J. J. McArdle (Eds.), *Contemporary psychometrics* (pp. 73–100). Mahwah, NJ: Erlbaum.

McDonald, R. P., & Ahlawat, K. S. (1974). Difficulty factors in binary data. *British Journal of Mathematical and Statistical Psychology, 27*, 82–99.

Meade, A. W., & Bauer, D. J. (2007). Power and precision in confirmatory factor analytic tests of measurement invariance. *Structural Equation Modeling, 14*, 611–635.

Meade, A. W., & Lautenschlager, G. J. (2004). A Monte Carlo study of confirmatory factor analytic tests of measurement invariance. *Structural Equation Modeling, 11*, 60–72.

Mellenbergh, G. J. (1989). Item bias and item response theory. *International Journal of Educational Research, 13*, 127–143.

Meredith, W. (1964). Notes on factorial invariance. *Psychometrika, 29*, 177–185.

Meredith, W. (1993). Measurement invariance, factor analysis, and factorial invariance. *Psychometrika, 58*, 525–543.

Meredith, W., & Horn, J. (2001). The role of factorial invariance in modeling growth and change. In L. M. Collins & A. G. Sayer (Eds.), *New methods for the analysis of change* (pp. 203–240). Washington, DC: American Psychological Association.

Meredith, W., & Millsap, R. E. (1992). On the misuse of manifest variables in the detection of measurement bias. *Psychometrika, 57*, 289–311.

Millsap, R. E. (2011). *Statistical approaches to measurement invariance*. New York: Routledge.

Millsap, R. E., & Kwok, O.-M. (2004). Evaluating the impact of partial factorial invariance on selection in two populations. *Psychological Methods, 9*, 93–115.

Millsap, R. E., & Tein, J. Y. (2004). Assessing factorial invariance in ordered-categorical measures. *Multivariate Behavioral Research, 39*, 479–515.

Mislevy, R. J. (1986). Recent developments in the factor analysis of categorical variables. *Journal of Educational Statistics, 11*, 3–31.

Molenaar, P. C. M. (1985). A dynamic factor model for the analysis of multivariate time-series. *Psychometrika, 50*, 181–202.

Muthén, B. O. (1984). A general structural equation model with dichotomous, ordered categorical and continuous latent variable indicators. *Psychometrika, 49*, 115–132.

Muthén, L., & Muthén, B. O. (1998–2010). *Mplus user's guide* (6th ed.). Los Angeles: Authors.

Nesselroade, J. R., Gerstorf, D., Hardy, S. A., & Ram, N. (2007). Idiographic filters for psychological constructs. *Measurement, 5,* 217–235.

Rensvold, R. B., & Cheung, G. W. (2001). Testing for metric invariance using structural equation models: Solving the standardization problem. In C. A. Schriesheim & L. L. Neider (Eds.), *Research in management* (Vol. 1, pp. 25–50). Greenwich, CT: Information Age.

Sandler, I. N., Ayers, T. S., Wolchik, S. A., Tein, J. Y., Kwok, O., Haine, R. A., et al. (2003). The Family Bereavement Program: Efficacy evaluation of a theory-based program for parentally bereaved children and adolescents. *Journal of Consulting and Clinical Psychology, 70,* 587–600.

Saris, W. E., Satorra, A., & van der Veld, W. M. (2009). Testing structural equation models or detection of misspecifications? *Structural Equation Modeling, 16,* 561–582.

Stark, S., Chernyshenko, O. S., & Drasgow, F. (2004). Examining the effects of differential item (functioning and differential) test functioning on selection decisions: When are statistically significant effects practically important? *Journal of Applied Psychology, 89,* 497–508.

Steenkamp, J. E. M., & Baumgartner, H. (1998). Assessing measurement invariance in cross-national consumer research. *Journal of Consumer Research, 25,* 78–90.

Takane, Y., & de Leeuw, J. (1987). On the relationship between item response theory and factor analysis of discretized variables. *Psychometrika, 52,* 393–408.

Thomson, G. H., & Lederman, W. (1939). The influence of multivariate selection on the factorial analysis of ability. *British Journal of Psychology, 29,* 288–305.

Thurstone, L. L. (1947). *Multiple factor analysis.* Chicago: University of Chicago Press.

Tisak, J., & Meredith, W. (1989). Exploratory longitudinal factor analysis in multiple populations. *Psychometrika, 54,* 261–281.

Tisak, J., & Tisak, M. S. (2000). Permanency and ephemerality of psychological measures with application to organizational commitment. *Psychological Methods, 5,* 175–198.

Vandenberg, R. J., & Lance, C. E. (2000). A review and synthesis of the measurement invariance literature: Suggestions, practices, and recommendations for organizational research. *Organizational Research Methods, 3,* 4–70.

van der Linden, W. J., & Hambleton, R. K. (Eds.). (1997). *Handbook of modern item response theory.* New York: Springer.

Widaman, K. F., Ferrer, E., & Conger, R. D. (2010). Factorial invariance within longitudinal structural equation models: Measuring the same construct across time. *Child Development Perspectives, 4,* 10–18.

Widaman, K. F., Little, T. D., Geary, D. C., & Cormier, P. (1992). Individual differences in the development of skill in mental addition: Internal and external validations of chronometric models. *Learning and Individual Differences, 4,* 167–213.

Widaman, K. F., & Reise, S. P. (1997). Exploring the measurement invariance of psychological instruments: Applications in the substance abuse domain. In K. J. Bryant (Ed.), *Alcohol and substance use research* (pp. 281–324). Washington, DC: American Psychological Association.

Wirth, R. J., & Edwards, M. C. (2007). Item factor analysis: Current approaches and future directions. *Psychological Methods, 12,* 58–79.

Woods, C. M. (2009). Empirical selection of anchors for tests of differential item functioning. *Applied Psychological Measurement, 33,* 42–57.

Yoon, M., & Millsap, R. E. (2007). Detecting violations of factorial invariance using data-based specification searches: A Monte Carlo study. *Structural Equation Modeling, 14,* 435–463.

Yuan, K. H. (2005). Fit indices versus test statistics. *Multivariate Behavioral Research, 40,* 115–148.

PART II

Approaches to Data Collection

CHAPTER 8

Foundational Issues in Longitudinal Data Collection

LEA PULKKINEN
KATJA KOKKO

Pioneering longitudinal studies demonstrated the value of a longitudinal research strategy to understanding individual development and the factors affecting it, and consequently this approach became common in developmental psychology. There are special challenges in the study of the same individuals over time, but guidelines for planning and conducting a longitudinal study are difficult to find. The present chapter discusses basic issues and practical problems, such as the researchers' motivation and commitment to the study, timing of data collection, sample attrition, and validity of data, that should be considered before launching a longitudinal study. Much can be learned from previous studies. We start with conceptual definitions and a brief history of early longitudinal studies.

A Brief History of Early Longitudinal Data Collections

Longitudinal Research Strategy and the Concept of Development

A longitudinal study refers to a research method that studies an individual across time with measurements at periodic intervals. For the study of individual development, it is necessary to collect data on a given characteristic (e.g., intelligence) of the same individual at different times (i.e., longitudinally). The term *longitudinal study* does not specify the duration of the study, which may vary from a few days to tens of years, nor the intervals of data collection, which may also vary from days to years, nor the frequency of data collection points. Rather, a linkage of time points provides longitudinal data; at least two time points are needed, as in Robins's (1966) pioneering follow-up study of children attending a child guidance clinic. As noted by Rutter (1994), not all longitudinal data are prospective or real time. Data may also be "followed back" register data or "linked" register data, ethics permitting.

A cross-sectional method refers to data collected at a given point in time from a sample of participants making up different age groups. Cross-sectional data are valuable for the description of the characteristics of each age group. Cross-sectional data do not, however, reveal whether differences between groups are due to developmental changes in the individuals or to some other factors, such as schooling, that may have affected the studied characteristic differently in different age groups.

Early longitudinal studies were focused on childhood, along with the contemporaneous concept of development. Childhood has been seen as the start of physical and psychological processes in, for instance, perceptual and motor behavior, language, thinking, intelligence, and adaptation to society. Gesell (1928) was especially concerned with physical maturation and developed observational tools and techniques for assessing it. Collecting descriptive data about individual children at different ages has been necessary to better understand development. The question of whether the origin of human behavior and development is in inherent biological factors or external environmental factors has been debated by researchers since the earliest developmental studies. Advances in behavior genetics and molecular genetics have reactivated this discussion. Additive genetic factors explain only part of the variation of a studied characteristic or capacity in the population, leaving an important role for environmental factors. As noted by Rutter (2006), an outcome is the sum of the effects of genes, the effects of the environment, and the effects of the "co-action of genes and environment through gene–environment correlations and interactions" (p. 211).

It is difficult to make inferences regarding causes and effects in development, but the timing of events observed in longitudinal studies warrants some conclusions. Rutter (1994) discussed several possibilities for testing cause-and-effect relationships with longitudinal data. One of them is a "natural experiment" that was successfully conducted by Elder (1974) in his study of the effects of economic depression on children and adolescents. Another possibility is to test competing hypotheses by combining cross-sectional and longitudinal data, as in the study of the effects of parent–child separation on children. Advanced statistical methods also enable a researcher to make some inferences from the relations between studied variables in respect to the direction of effects between them.

"The concept of development is fundamentally biological," argued Harris (1967, p. 3). Development was seen to be associated with the organization of living structure and life processes over time toward the complexity of organization and large units or "wholes." Rapid biological maturation in infants allows almost all changes to be interpreted as development, but when maturation slows, the interpretation of development becomes more complex. Much discussed has been the endpoint or telos of development. A kind of identity crisis among researchers in the field of developmental psychology arising from the lack of a commonly accepted concept of development was documented in a series of conceptual articles in the 1970s reviewed by Montada and Schmitt (1982). There was no consensus about the areas of content in developmental theory and research or about the appropriate methods to use to study them. Experimental child psychology was a dominant trend in developmental psychology, but its contribution to understanding human development was limited. Questions also arose as to whether the main target of developmental psychology was the study of age-related processes of change or, rather, the analysis of interacting antecedents of change and methods of interventions.

The crisis prompted the rise of the lifespan orientation to development from a psychological perspective (reviewed by Baltes, Lindenberger, & Staudinger, 1998) and the rise of a life-course orientation from a sociological perspective (reviewed by Elder, 1998).

Lifespan theory and research is concerned with interindividual regularities and differences, intraindividual plasticity in development, and three major influence systems on lifespan development: age graded, history graded, and non-normative. A basic assumption is that various adaptive processes are involved from conception to old age. "Life course" refers to a sequence of socially defined events and roles in people's lives in association with four paradigms: location in time and place, linked lives, human agency, and timing of events. Furthermore, the rise of psychological gerontology (Birren & Schaie, 1977) clarified the scope and goals of developmental psychology.

In the 1920s and 1930s, Charlotte Bühler presented the view that development is not limited to childhood but encompasses the whole lifespan (Keller, 2000). It took several decades, however, before adult development and aging were accepted into the core of developmental psychology; even today developmental psychological research tends to be oriented to childhood. The extension of the concept of development to the years after childhood and adolescence is partly a result of longitudinal studies that continued from childhood into adulthood. Consequently, changes in the concept of development pushed research to become more longitudinal, and longitudinal studies altered the concept of development.

The Beginning and Expansion of Longitudinal Studies

We present a brief history of early longitudinal studies that involved psychological research, that studied participants from childhood onward for a period of at least 15 years, and that were initiated by the end of the 1960s (Pulkkinen, 1993; Schneider & Edelstein, 1990; Verdonik & Sherrod, 1984; Young, Savola, & Phelps, 1991) to demonstrate the origins and expansion of the longitudinal research method. Early longitudinal studies were generally multidisciplinary, most often involving medicine (pediatrics), psychology, education, and/or sociology. Other disciplines, such as anthropology, psychiatry, epidemiology, criminology, economics, and genetics, entered as partners in later studies.

Some of the first large-scale longitudinal studies were conducted in California in the United States. The United Kingdom and Sweden also led in early longitudinal studies. The first large-scale longitudinal study was initiated in California in 1921. It was called Genetic Studies of Genius, later renamed the Gifted Children Study. It was aimed at investigating the maintenance of children's and adolescents' intellectual superiority. Other early California longitudinal studies include the Berkeley Growth Study on mental, motor, and physical growth from birth onward, initiated in 1928; the Berkeley Guidance Study on the effects of parental counseling on personality development, initiated in 1928; and the Oakland Growth Study on physical, physiological, social, and biological factors in personality development, initiated in 1931. One of the motivations of the longitudinal studies initiated in the late 1920s and early 1930s was to investigate the effects of the Great Depression on child development. Longitudinal research programs were also established outside California. One of them was the Fels Longitudinal Study, initiated in 1929 in Ohio, where the Fels Research Institute was established with the goal of studying development from birth to adulthood—a novel idea at the time. Another novel idea was to study the impact of the juvenile justice system and developmental background on delinquency in the One Thousand Juvenile Delinquents Study and the Cambridge–Somerville Youth Study, initiated on the East Coast of the United States in the 1920s and 1930s.

Longitudinal studies begun in the 1930s and 1940s include the Scottish Mental Surveys, in which IQ-type test scores were collected in schools in 1932 and 1947, testing tens of thousands of children born in 1921 and 1936, respectively, and the British National Survey of Health and Development, concerning the age cohort born in 1946. The Malmö Study on the influence of schooling on intelligence, talent, and career opportunities was initiated in Sweden in 1938, and the Lundby study, a survey of the mental health of a Swedish population, was commenced in 1947.

The boom of longitudinal studies began in the 1950s. Among several studies initiated was a new British cohort study, the National Child Development Study on education, health, family, employment, and housing, started in 1958. In the United States, the Patterns of Child Rearing Study was initiated in 1951; the Kauai Longitudinal Study on resilient children and youth in relation to developmental stress in 1954; the Longitudinal Study of Moral Development in 1955; the Louisville Twin Study on the contributions of genetic and environmental factors to physical growth and mental development in 1959; and the Columbia County Longitudinal Study on child aggression in 1959.

In the 1960s, many studies were initiated that continue to be productive. In the United States, these include the National Longitudinal Surveys, in which representative samples of older and younger women and men were followed biennially. In Europe, the Cambridge Study in Delinquent Development was initiated in the United Kingdom in 1961; the study From Year to Year on abilities, education, and labor markets was initiated in the Netherlands in 1965; and three longitudinal studies were launched in Sweden: the Individual Statistics Project, the Project Metropolitan, and the Individual Development and Adjustment study in 1961, 1964, and 1965, respectively. Two longitudinal studies were started in Finland: the Healthy Child Study in 1963 and the Jyväskylä Longitudinal Study of Personality and Social Development (JYLS) in 1968.

Since the 1960s, the number of longitudinal studies has increased, and the longitudinal approach to development has become a recognized research method. In Finland alone, the number of longitudinal studies in psychology and related disciplines begun in the 1970s, 1980s, and 1990s number up to 125 (Sihvo & Pulkkinen, 2002). Numerous reviews and handbooks have been written about developmental processes based on the outcomes of longitudinal studies. Furthermore, the statistical analysis of longitudinal data has received considerable attention, as reviewed by Collins (2006). Guidelines for planning and conducting a longitudinal study are more difficult to find. Among a few guidebooks are those edited by Nesselroade and Baltes (1979), Magnusson and Bergman (1990), and Giele and Elder (1998).

Characteristics of the First Longitudinal Studies

To illustrate the characteristics of longitudinal studies, a few well-known longitudinal studies are described here in regard to both productive and critical aspects. It is clear that historical conditions frame theory and methods, which may limit later research options. Earlier longitudinal studies are often used as models for new ones. Mishaps can be avoided through an awareness of critical issues.

Early longitudinal studies were often motivated by educational goals: the possibility of advancing or steering child development. This was the case with the Gifted Children Study that was begun by Lewis Terman in 1921 (Terman & Oden, 1959). Terman thought that by identifying gifted children and giving them a good education, society would gain talented individuals in leadership positions. The intelligence of children and adolescents ages 3–19 years was tested in urban areas of California, and 857 boys and 671 girls with IQs above

135 were selected for the study. Terman initially planned to follow the participants for 10 years, but the study transitioned into a long-term longitudinal study. Terman died in 1956, but the Gifted Children Study has been continued by Stanford University. By the 1990s, 13 data waves had been collected, generally two in each decade (from 1922 to 1992). The Gifted Children Study started with an emphasis on children's intelligence and their homes and schools, but many aspects of human life, including education and marriage, military experience, work and achievements, and aging and retirement became study objectives as the participants grew older (Elder & Pellerin, 1998). The results showed that a stereotypic conception that giftedness is accompanied by deficiencies in other areas (i.e., physical or social weakness) was incorrect. Generally positive outcomes were associated with superior intellectual ability.

The two Oakland studies, the Guidance Study initiated by Macfarlane (1938) and the Oakland Growth Study initiated by Jones in 1938, featured more representative samples. The sample of the Guidance Study consisted of the families of every third baby born in Berkeley over an 18-month period, totaling 248 infants and their families. They were allocated to either a "guidance" condition or a "control" condition with matched socioeconomic status. The sample of the Oakland Growth Study consisted of 212 fifth-grade children from five elementary schools. The data from these two studies were later merged and archived at the Institute of Human Development, University of California, Berkeley. In 1957–1958, funding was obtained for the study of all available participants from the samples of both studies.

A specific feature of these longitudinal studies is that extensive and well-documented data have been fruitfully utilized in many secondary analyses. *A secondary analysis* refers to the process whereby a researcher recodes data for his or her specific research purposes and poses questions not originally presented, perhaps even decades after the data collection. The duration of time required to study continuity and change in behavior and early precursors of later behavior may be beyond the reach of individual researchers (Brooks-Gunn, Phelps, & Elder, 1991). Researchers age with their study participants and encounter other real-life demands.

Archival data from the Guidance Study and the Oakland Growth Study (for 84 males and 87 females) were utilized by Block (1971) in his research on personality development. Clinical psychologists judged the participants at several points in time on the basis of interview documents using the 100-item California-Q-Set that Block devised for this purpose. Data were collected during junior and senior high school and in adulthood. Block analyzed personality development with a person-oriented approach by searching for patterns of behavior, studying their continuity across the age stages, and analyzing life conditions associated with each personality type. Archival data from the Guidance Study and the Oakland Growth Study were also used by Elder (1974) in his study of the effects of the Great Depression in the United States on the development of children (Guidance Study) and adolescents (Growth Study). By comparing the two age cohorts of the two longitudinal studies, Elder showed that cultural–historical change does not have a uniform impact on development; the age at which people experience change may be important. For instance, adolescent boys who found part-time jobs and emotional support outside their homes coped with economic hardship quite well, but among young boys who were more dependent on their families, the impact of economic strain was severe.

In the area of social and personality development, assessment methods lacked the degree of standardization that is typical of intelligence tests. As noted by Kagan and Moss

(1962), this fact limited the findings from the first longitudinal studies of social and personality development. Mainly anecdotal and biographical information was collected in the early studies on constancies in personality, and the samples were small (e.g., 6 or 15 children; see Kagan, 1964). A larger sample was followed at the Fels Research Institute. The original sample consisted of 89 children. Participants were followed up to adolescence and on into early adulthood (mean age 24 years). In the summary of their book, Kagan and Moss (1962) state: "The most dramatic and consistent finding of this study was that many of the behaviors exhibited by the child during the period of 6 to 10 years of age, and a few during the age period 3 to 6, were moderately good predictors of theoretically related behaviors during early adulthood" (p. 266).

Pioneering long-term longitudinal studies raised much enthusiasm, but their methodology has also been criticized by, for example, Block (1971) and Honzik (1965). These criticisms are also relevant in the evaluation of current longitudinal studies. One criticism concerned the lack of emphasis on theoretical ideas and specific hypotheses. The studies were focused on practical problems, such as how to educate talented individuals, how to support parenting, and what the effects of economic depression are on children. Block also criticized the timing of adult data collection in studies that were originally focused on children and youths and that transitioned into long-term longitudinal studies when data collection was continued in adulthood. He argued that data for adulthood should not be collected before age 30, for example at age 24, because the participants may not have settled down, and their personal style of adaptation may not have sufficiently developed before age 30. Furthermore, the samples of the first studies were relatively small, limiting data analysis, and some were highly selective, limiting generalizations. For instance, the social background of gifted children was good, and the effects of intelligence and home environment on outcomes could therefore not be separated. In the Fels Study, the 89 children in the sample were from only 63 different families; the participation of siblings biased statistical analyses.

Typically, the coverage of variables in the first longitudinal studies was large at the outset, then enlarged further when researchers became interested in additional aspects of the life paths of the studied participants as they became older. On the negative side, variables were poorly defined, and there were differences between childhood–adolescence and adult variables. Generally, a variety of measures were used for data collection, but only one rater may have been employed over many years, so the rater's framework may have affected the results. On the positive side, rich data collected in these longitudinal studies have been carefully documented, archived, and made available for other researchers. Consequently, secondary analyses are possible with new methodological inventions and theoretical ideas.

A Case Study on the Initiation of a Longitudinal Study

A theory-based longitudinal study is vulnerable to becoming outdated when ways of thinking change, because every study is planned and conducted in the prevailing intellectual climate of its time. Current research and theories, as well as measurement techniques and statistical tools, both inspire and set limits on new studies. A researcher who is planning a new study benefits from skepticism about current trends, careful observations of a phenomenon, theoretical thinking, a combining of recent trends in science, and some intuition about the implementation of these considerations into the hypotheses of a new study.

As a demonstration of how a long-term longitudinal study may be started from a doctoral dissertation, we describe the JYLS (Pitkänen, 1969; Pulkkinen, 2006, 2009), initiated by Lea Pulkkinen (formerly Pitkänen) in 1968 and conducted with her colleagues to the present day. Pulkkinen began her training at the University of Jyväskylä, Finland, in 1958, where she was introduced to the experimental study of personality, learning theories, child development, differential psychology, and advanced statistical methods such as factor analysis. She first worked as her mentor's research assistant but started to develop her own ideas when she became skeptical about the interpretation of aggression as a need or a personality trait. She was interested in the many facets of aggression. Learning theories, in particular the emergence of the social learning theory, guided her to understand aggression as a behavior that varied in type and strength within a child's behavioral repertoire depending on learning history. She developed a descriptive model of aggression and tested it with children in daycare (Pitkänen, 1969, p. 29).

After noticing that only a small proportion of children were frequently aggressive, Pulkkinen became interested in alternative behaviors to aggression in coping with conflict situations. She had an insight into the cognitive regulation of emotional behavior. Based on this idea, she developed a two-dimensional impulse control model for the description of different coping strategies (Pitkänen, 1969, p. 102). It was a novel idea, because in the 1960s emotions were generally understood as states; the study of emotion regulation became a focus of mainstream research only about 20 years later. Another novel idea was to conceptualize positive prosocial behaviors as alternatives to aggression in conflict situations. The opposite of aggression (nonaggression) was generally referred to as the "inhibition of aggression," which was negatively evaluated from a psychodynamic point of view, because it might result in personality pathology. Only a few studies on positive behaviors had been published up to that time. Pulkkinen tested her model in 1968 with 369 second-grade Finnish children at 8 years of age. Inspired by the book *Birth to Maturity* by Kagan and Moss (1962), Pulkkinen noted in the discussion section of her doctoral dissertation that "a longitudinal study would make it possible to examine the stability of the individual patterns of behaviour" (Pitkänen, 1969, p. 190). The sample was traced at age 14 and again for major data collections at ages 27, 36, 42, and 50.

There was pressure to use international personality inventories, recently standardized in Finland, for data collection when she tested her impulse control model with 8-year-old participants. Her previous observations while collecting inventory data on children and comparing them with teacher ratings had, however, made her skeptical about children's capacity to assess their personalities through inventories. Pulkkinen wanted to secure findings by using several measures. Besides inventories, she used teacher ratings, even though at the time such ratings had a bad reputation because a "halo" effect resulted from the correlation of teacher ratings with school achievements and home background. At that time, researchers expected that children's socioemotional behavior would be independent of background factors such as parenting; these relationships are now better understood. Pulkkinen additionally chose a peer nomination method (Walder, Abelson, Eron, Banta, & Laulicht, 1961). Fortunately, she chose some items that had been used by Walder and colleagues (1961), which made it possible for researchers in Finland and the United States to conduct comparative studies decades later, when both studies were continued into middle age (Dubow, Huesmann, Boxer, Pulkkinen, & Kokko, 2006; Kokko, Pulkkinen, Huesmann, Dubow, & Boxer, 2009). This similarity between the measures of the longitudinal studies is called the *harmonization of measures*. It means sharing and using the same measures with other researchers to increase comparability of research findings between different studies.

The two-dimensional model was confirmed (e.g., Pulkkinen, 2009), and most findings from the longitudinal study were based on teacher ratings and peer nominations; inventory data collected at age 8 have not had much use in the JYLS due to their low validity with rating data. The use of multiple measures for basic data collections was of particular importance. In a longitudinal study, poor data collected at a certain age cannot be remedied later.

Launching a New Longitudinal Study

Block (1971) highlights many problems in the method of longitudinal study. In fact, he says "the motivations for *not* initiating a longitudinal research program are many" (p. 3). Problems include locating and maintaining a proper subject sample, making fundamental procedural decisions for the future, receiving criticism for these decisions from researchers years later based on their retrospective wisdom, the fact that more immediate professional rewards can be obtained from quick and neat designs, and knowing that one's successors may harvest one's efforts, as the most interesting findings may not be available within one's own career span or lifetime. He notes, however, that "magnetically, psychologists are now increasingly drawn toward longitudinal studies for the ineluctable reason that there simply is no other way by which certain questions regarding development, cause and effect may be approached" (p. 3).

In making a decision about launching a longitudinal study, several issues, some of them applicable to any study, should be considered. First, a rationale and motivation for conducting a study are needed. Second, there are many choices to be made concerning the selection of an optimal design and the sampling of participants. These choices affect the quality of data and the generalizability of the results. Third, management and analysis of data demand expertise, as well as the capacity to store data for secondary research. These issues are discussed in the following sections, along with examples from previous studies. Our goal is to assist those who may be launching new longitudinal studies.

Rationale and Motivation for Launching a Longitudinal Study

An important question to be answered is whether a research problem requires a longitudinal study. There are two answers to this question as noted by Rose (2006). A longitudinal perspective is necessary if one is interested in, *first*, investigating consistency and change in the individual characteristics and, *second*, the developmental consequences of individual characteristics over time. Only by means of a longitudinal study is it possible to examine whether early individual differences in, for example, social behavior remain consistent over time and whether mechanisms, such as environmental mediating factors, promote continuity or change.

A related question is whether research problems are sustainable over the planned duration of the study. The researcher has to be aware of the historical context and prevailing intellectual climate, as these can play important roles in planning a study. A study that is to be sustained over many years presupposes that the researcher will anticipate the future of science in the area of study in question. Above all, a longitudinal study needs a principal researcher who has a long-standing interest in and motivation for the study. Motivation is needed, in particular, when research questions change as participants age. In order to pose developmentally relevant research questions and to use appropriate methods for answering them, the researcher has to become knowledgeable about each new developmental phase. The principal investigator also needs the motivation and capacity to organize collaborations with students and other researchers and the ability to cope with stress and the mess caused by hundreds or thousands of variables and overlapping processes for planning and collecting new data and analyzing and publishing previously collected data.

The researcher's commitment to the developmental understanding of the phenomenon in question affects his or her commitment to the length of the longitudinal study, which in turn is dependent on the availability of funding. Securing funding for a longitudinal study may be a problem, particularly if the duration of the study is longer than the normal funding period of an agency and if the researcher is young and not yet established in the scientific field. For instance, in the JYLS, the interviews of participants at ages 14 and 20 were made by unpaid university students. A lack of travel funding limited the number of participants who could be interviewed and even the number and quality of audio tapes that could be purchased for recording the interviews. In large national studies, funding can be guaranteed through institutional decisions, but for individual researchers and research groups funding has to be received through competition, often for each data collection wave. This may make it difficult to regulate the periodic intervals of data collection.

In large, multidisciplinary research groups, the principal investigator plays an important role in coordinating various research interests and in choosing and balancing theoretical and disciplinary orientations, as well as measures to be used. Researchers commonly prefer optimal measures for studying their particular areas, but participants cannot be loaded with a data collection that is too long and extensive. This means that in extensive, multidisciplinary longitudinal studies, it is necessary to make compromises concerning the number and length of measures but at the same time to use measures that are as reliable and valid as possible. In a smaller scale study, the principal investigator is more independent in the choice of measures, but human capital and other resources for the study may be more limited. Furthermore, the principal investigator has to train or coordinate the training of the research staff. The goal of training a team of investigators to collect the data is to reduce the "researcher effects" on the results.

Practical Considerations

Permissions and Respect of Participants

Various permissions are needed before a research project can go ahead. Universities and research institutes have organized committees to review research applications from ethical points of view. In a longitudinal study, specific concerns may include the treatment of participants, the planned duration of the study, multiple measures to be used, permission to use and save documentary data, saving data in data archives, and the users of the data. Specific permission is also needed to conduct the study in a school or other relevant context and to obtain documentary data or addresses of the participants; the researcher has to sort out all permissions required, each with the correct provider. In addition, an informed consent has to be obtained from each participant (and the parents of participating children) separately for each data collection stage and for each part of the study.

Research methods used in a longitudinal study easily grow in number, because the same methods used in previous data collection waves have to be repeated in order to secure the comparability of findings across ages and because there is a pressure to add, with careful consideration, measures that are age relevant and relevant to successive developmental phases. For instance, in the study of middle-aged participants, retirement and aging should be anticipated. The load on participants must be evaluated. Often abbreviated measures are used to reduce the load.

During the course of a longitudinal study, there are various ways in which researchers can maintain contact with participants with the aim of encouraging them to remain in the study. Birthday cards have been sent in some studies; these also serve the function of keeping track of addresses. Researchers must respect all reasons for declining to participate but be persistent with those who need flexibility regarding data collection arrangements. Sometimes measures have to be tailored to specific requirements; for example, a telephone interview may be conducted instead of a face-to-face interview. Confidentiality of the participants has to be respected and the anonymity of the stored data secured. The attractiveness of measures encourages participants to respond to them, and receiving feedback about research is an important incentive for participation.

Timing of Data Collection

In addition to the duration of the study, the researcher has to consider the timing and frequency of the data collection waves. One has to decide whether data can be collected at regular intervals or coinciding with expected developmental transitions and/or life events (e.g., starting or finishing school) that trigger developmental changes. A further question to be considered is whether to collect data intensively at close intervals, or at longer intervals over a lengthy period of time, or to undertake a data collection that is somewhere between these two approaches (Collins, 2006). Process-oriented research questions (e.g., daily mood fluctuations) require more intensive collections of data than do studies of the long-term stability of, or changes in, personality traits, for example. Furthermore, many developmental changes are more rapid in childhood than in adulthood, making it necessary to collect data on children with more frequency than on adults.

While making decisions about the frequency of data collection, it is important to consider the effect of repeated measurements on participants. Measurements repeated too often may be experienced as intrusive and could in turn affect the studied phenomenon. In a long-term longitudinal study in which participants are seen once in 6 or 8 years, repeated measures most likely do not affect behavior that is generally not easily modified, as known from intensive therapies, but long intervals may limit the possibilities for studying developmental processes.

Selection of a Sample

In longitudinal studies, several kinds of samples can be found, such as a birth cohort sample, a random sample, a selective sample, or a convenience sample. The birth cohort sample includes all individuals born during a certain period of time in certain areas. Examples from the United Kingdom are the National Survey of Health and Development (age cohort born in 1946), the National Child Development Study (1958), the British Cohort Study (1970), and the Millennium Cohort Study (2000; Elliott & Vaitilingam, 2008; Ferri, Bynner, & Wadsworth, 2003; Smith & Joshi, 2002); from the United States, the Kauai Longitudinal Study (1955 birth cohort; Werner & Smith, 2001); and from New Zealand, the Dunedin Multidisciplinary Health and Development Study (age cohort born between April 1, 1972, and March 31, 1973; Moffitt, Caspi, Rutter, & Silva, 2001). In regard to size, the sample in cohort studies may consist of thousands of participants.

A Finnish longitudinal study of twins is an example of the extension of the birth cohort study design. In the study (from ages 12 to 17), all twins born within 5 consecutive years (about 600 pairs of twins per year) were included in the sample in order to have a sufficient sample size for data analysis (Kaprio, 2006); thus, it was necessary to wait for 5 years before a certain wave of data was collected from the whole sample. Nested in this epidemiological population-based sample was a subsample composing about 40% of all twins, formed for the intensive assessment of twin families. Most (72%) of the subsample was selected at random, but this random sample was then enriched with twins assumed to be at elevated familial risk for alcoholism based on one or both parents' elevated scores on an alcoholism screening test. Enrichment increases the incidence of the studied phenomenon in the sample, and its effect can be controlled statistically.

A basic assumption beyond statistical inferences is that the researcher randomly selects a *representative* sample from the population for which research findings will be generalized (e.g., Coolican, 2009). Researchers often compromise this assumption, as remarked by Bergman and Magnusson (1990): "Considering the nonrandom nature of most samples that are studied, it is surprising to note the strong importance that sometimes is given to the results of significance tests for which the assumptions are not even remotely fulfilled" (p. 11). The goal of randomness can be achieved by selecting, for example, a simple or systematic random sample. The latter applies to cases in which demographic characteristics (e.g., ethnicity, education) are expected to be related to the psychological characteristic(s) of interest. It is then possible to make a random selection from the known subgroups (i.e., strata) to have a representation of each of them. A random sample can also be drawn from a certain geographical area, as was done in the JYLS, in which 12 second-grade school classes were randomly selected and all pupils ($N = 369$) in them were included in the sample. In adulthood, the studied sample has been compared with, in regard to demographic variables, the age cohort of the general population born in the same year by using information from Statistics Finland. It is important for conclusions to estimate how well the demographic characteristics of the sample correspond to the characteristics of the general population to which the results are to be generalized.

An example of using a selective sample (for gender, socioeconomic status [SES], and linguistic culture) is the Montreal Longitudinal and Experimental Study started in 1984, in which 6-year-old boys ($N = 1{,}037$) were selected from French-speaking, low-SES areas of Montreal, Canada (Tremblay, Vitaro, Nagin, Pagani, & Séguin, 2003). The study participants were followed up until young adulthood. There is also a British study, titled the Cambridge Study in Delinquent Development, in which a sample of 8-year-old boys ($N = 411$) was selected from a working-class urban area in Cambridge (West & Farrington, 1977). Their path of criminal activity has been followed through middle age. The use of selective samples, such as those representing a certain geographical area and certain SES background, has to be considered in the interpretation of the findings.

Practical reasons often limit the possibility of using a random sample. Furthermore, it is not always clear what the cost–benefit ratio of the randomness would be and whether answering the research problem requires a random sample. Many psychological processes are expected to be universal, which is a possible reason for the fact that psychological findings in experiments and other studies have often been obtained with convenience samples consisting of, particularly, university students. College students have also been followed up over a period of decades in well-known and productive longitudinal studies: Vaillant's (1977) longitudinal study was made up of Harvard male graduates ($N = 163$), and Helson's

(Helson & Srivastava, 2002) longitudinal study consisted of female Mills College graduates ($N = 120$).

In regard to sampling, a researcher needs to consider the power of the study, which is defined as the probability of correctly rejecting a false null hypothesis (i.e., there is no difference between studied groups) (Cohen, 1992). A researcher should estimate the sample size needed to produce enough statistical power to reveal the expected difference; previous studies can be utilized for estimating the size of the difference. A statistical term for the size of the difference is *effect size*. A way to calculate an effect size is to use *Cohen's d*, in which the mean of one population (e.g., a risk group) is subtracted from the mean of another population (e.g., a nonrisk group) and the resulting figure is divided by the standard deviation of the common population (Coolican, 2009, pp. 389–390). Cohen (1992) labels a *d* of 0.20 as small, 0.50 as medium, and 0.80 as large in effect size. They represent the 85, 67, and 53 percent overlaps of distribution, respectively. If the researcher expects that the difference is large, then the sample size can be smaller, but it cannot be too small, as there is a risk of not having enough statistical power to detect the difference. If the expected difference is small, a larger sample size is needed.

Because the power to evaluate an effect size is affected by the sample size, the use of a large sample size may result in producing statistically significant differences that have no real meaning and that obscure a weak study design (Coolican, 2009). It is also evident that the larger the sample, the more expensive and time-consuming the data collection. Thus the researcher needs to carefully consider the positive and negative aspects of a sample size when planning to start a new longitudinal study.

Sample Attrition

Attrition refers to the loss of participants from a study. Sample attrition is often a problem in a longitudinal study. A dropout at a particular measurement point may result in some characteristics of the participants being overrepresented. An individual's refusal to participate may have consequences. *First*, refusing participation in the beginning of the study may distort the representativeness of the original sample in comparison with the population because refusal may affect some subgroups more than others. *Second*, across the years the sample may become selective because of refusal by participants. However, a longitudinal study also offers possibilities to estimate effects of the attrition. Information is often available for a majority of the dropouts from earlier waves, and it can be used to compare those who drop out and those who do not (Bergman & Magnusson, 1990).

In a longitudinal study, the sample size and attrition (or the participants' retention in the study) can be described in many terms and figures. There is a great variety and inconsistency both in the terminology used and in the sample sizes reported in publications. We propose four types of samples that should be reported in a longitudinal study (see Figure 8.1). First, there is the size of the *intended sample*, based on the sampling design from a population and consisting of individuals who are approached for consent to participate in the study. Second, there is the *initial sample* that consists of those individuals in the intended sample who give their consent to the study and who participate in it at the outset. Third, when follow-up data are collected, there is the *eligible sample* that consists of those members of the initial sample who could be reached for the follow-up. The initial sample is often reduced in the eligible sample, because some participants may have died, may decline to continue in the study, or cannot be traced. When the study continues for a long time, the eligible sample generally becomes smaller. Fourth, there is the *effective sample* of each data wave, consisting of participants who have actually continued their participation in the data collection. If the data collection comprises several parts, such as an interview, inventories, medical examinations, and laboratory tests, the effective sample may vary. The maximum size of the effective sample is described by the number of individuals who participated in at least one part of the data collection during a certain wave.

The terms *initial sample* and *effective sample* were proposed by Bergman and Magnusson (1990), and the term *eligible sample* is commonly used in the literature (e.g., Moffitt et al., 2001). We have added the term *intended sample* to show how many individuals were reached in order to compose the initial sample. It may indicate the selectivity of the sample that should be considered in the interpretation of findings. There is still one more sample size to be given. In longitudinal studies, it has become common and recommended to use statistical methods to treat missing data, based on the available data for some participants whose data are lacking in certain measures at a certain study point. In this way, the representativeness of the sample may be secured and the power of the study increased. There is no consistent way in research reports to express the size of the imputed sample. We propose that it would be described alongside other sample sizes.

The following rates can be presented in the description of the participants' retention in the study: first, the *initial participation rate*, that is, the proportion of the initial sample of the intended sample at the beginning of the study; second, the *eligibility rate*, that is, the proportion of the eligible sample in a certain wave of the initial sample; and third, the *participation rate*, that is, the proportion of the effective sample in a certain wave of the eligible sample. Fourth, the proportion of the effective sample in a certain wave of the initial sample shows the *retention* rate in the study. It is to be noted that in a longitudinal study, there are individuals who temporarily decline to participate in a given wave of data collection for various reasons, such as health, work, and family matters, but who recommence participation at a later time. Thus the retention rate may fluctuate from wave to wave.

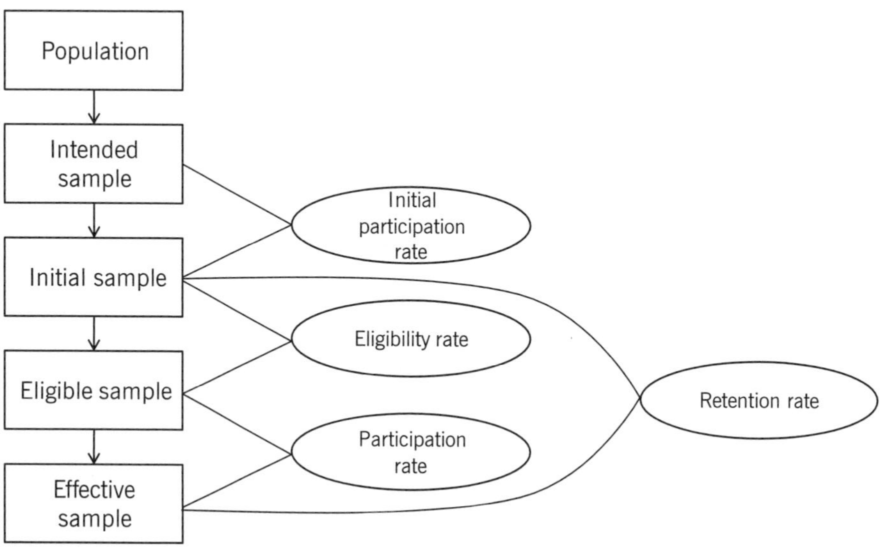

FIGURE 8.1. Sample size and attrition in a longitudinal study.

These rates can be illustrated by the New Zealand Dunedin Study, in which the initial participation rate was 100%, because perinatal data were obtained at delivery for every baby. The initial sample size was 1,661. In the first follow-up at age 3, the size of the eligible sample was one-third smaller, 1,139, and the size of the effective sample, or the sample seen (Moffitt et al., 2001), was 1,037. Thus the participation rate was 91% (1,037/1,139). As shown by Moffitt and colleagues (2001), the participation rate remained very high until young adulthood—97% at age 21. The size of the eligible sample also remained about the same until adulthood—1,020 at age 21. At age 32, the size of the eligible sample was 1,015, and the participation rate was 96% (972/1,015). Due to the attrition between data collected at birth and at age 3, the eligibility rate at age 3 (the eligible sample compared with the initial sample) was 69% (1,139/1,661), but thereafter, eligibility declined very slowly, to 61% (1,015/1,661) at age 32. The overall retention rate was also at this level when the effective sample was compared with the initial sample, because the number of participants seen was close to the eligible sample; at age 3, 1,037 participants were seen, and at age 32, 972 participants were seen out of 1,661 participants in the initial sample. Thus the retention rates were 62% (1,037/1,661) and 59% (972/1,661), respectively.

In the JYLS, the initial participation rate of 8-year-old schoolchildren (N = 369) was also 100%, because the permission of school authorities was sufficient for data collection at school in the 1960s. By age 50, the eligibility rate was 88% (323/369); the eligible sample had declined to 323, because 3.3% had died and 9.2% had declined entirely. The participation rate from the eligible sample (271/323) was 83.9%, and the retention rate from the initial sample (271/369) was 73%. In the Cambridge Study of Delinquent Development, great efforts have also been made to maximize the retention rate, because the most elusive males tended to be most antisocial, as noted by Farrington, Ttofi, and Coid (2009). In this study, the initial sample was 411 males. At age 48, 394 were still alive (eligibility rate 96%), and 365 of them participated in the study (participation rate 93%). The effective sample was 88.8% of the initial sample, showing a high retention rate.

Quality of Data

The quality of the data in a longitudinal study is largely associated with the validity of the data (Bergman & Magnusson, 1990). Deficient planning of data collection has long-term consequences, because problems with the data cannot be remedied later. Therefore, the researcher has to ascertain that his or her methods will permit a valid comparison of individuals. Data have to reflect the aspects of individual characteristics that they are expected to reflect. This presumes a theoretical construct analysis and the content analysis of measures; it may be necessary to extend the analysis to close or parallel constructs while choosing the measures. Pure operationalization is not sufficient; there should be a solid foundation of theory that connects the construct to be measured (e.g., intelligence) and its measure (content). The use of multiple measures to study complex constructs is recommended; this facilitates the formation of a latent construct to represent the studied construct.

Research methods must be adjusted to a new age group, and the comparability of measures must be maintained across ages. In a longitudinal study spanning from childhood to adulthood, it may be necessary to use different measures and informants for the same construct in different developmental phases. This makes it impossible to study absolute continuity in the construct (e.g., comparing the level of aggression in childhood and adulthood), but it may allow the study of differential continuity, that is, rank order stability (e.g., whether more aggressive children become more aggressive adults). Whenever possible, it is advisable to use the same measures, unmodified, for the different data waves. Likewise, reliable and well-validated research instruments should be used to make research findings comparable across different studies, whenever possible. A longitudinally studied sample is too valuable for ad hoc and nonvalidated measures. A new research instrument should be piloted with another sample and administered with the old instrument in at least one wave of data collection, or the longitudinal continuity of the construct will be lost.

For the comparability of research findings in different studies, attention has recently been given to the harmonization of measures between studies, that is, using the same measures and items in different studies. This practice is valuable to the field of psychological science because it increases the accumulation of knowledge and reduces the use of constructs and measures that are not comparable between studies.

Data quality is threatened by missing data, which cannot be avoided in a longitudinal study. One or more data collection waves may be missing participants, variables, and/or items. Missing data may reduce the validity of findings, affect the power of the study by reducing the number of participants, and bias the representativeness of the sample. Statistical tools have been developed for handling missing data; their use is recommended. There are also other means to avoid the flaws caused by missing data, such as calculating the means of scales instead of using sum scores and studying the same topic with different measures, such as by a questionnaire and an interview, which makes it possible to replace missing information. As another example, the use of a life history calendar on which certain events such as participants' education and employment are systematically recorded helps with filling in gaps in other measures and with the formation of valid variables on individuals' life experiences.

Data quality can be improved in a longitudinal study—compared with a cross-sectional study—by utilizing many sources of data for the formation of variables. For instance, work history, marriage status, and even the number of children are complex variables that are more validly assessed if data are collected from several sources at different times. The data files of participants collected over years are valuable for checking the coding of variables, understanding possible outliers in the data, and learning about the context of a participant's responses.

Data Archiving and Dissemination of Findings

Funding agencies may set recommendations for and demands on making data publicly available. Many extensive longitudinal data sets have already been archived, such as the Oakland Studies at the Institute of Human Development, University of California, Berkeley; the JYLS in the Finnish Social Science Data Archive; and the British birth cohort studies in the United Kingdom data archives. The archives are assumed to take care of the updating of digital records so that future scholars have access to them despite changes in formats and technologies. In many cases, such as in the JYLS, hard copies of data arranged in participants' files without identification data are also kept at least for some periods of time, which makes it possible to check details on individual life paths. According to Finnish legislation, institutes have to prepare descriptions of registers and archives and keep them publicly available. The participants' identification data are kept in a safe, separate from all other research materials. Access to identification data is restricted to only principal and co-principal investigators.

A decision to archive empirical data leads to many other decisions. One of them concerns the point at which data should be archived—whether after each data collection wave or later. Related decisions concern the time at which to open the data archive for the scientific community and the researchers' right to publish results analyzing prior data. Other decisions concern the types of data to be archived; these may vary from primary data (including all participants' responses at the variable level) to more advanced data (including cleaned variables and variables formed from the data set). For instance, the formation of a variable for the length of education, socioeconomic status, or identity status may require collecting information from different variables and measures, coding data, and calculating coding reliabilities. There are also variables, such as lifetime duration of unemployment, that can be created using information collected in several data waves. The labeling of variables and information provided about the coding of variables (e.g., reversed items and their coding) and the language in which to code all this information are also to be considered. In countries in which the native language is not English, the researcher has to supply resources for the translation of measures, variable labels, and coding systems, if the data archive is meant to be internationally available. In every instance, the anonymity of the participants has to be guaranteed.

A longitudinal study produces much information, but publishing research findings demands planning and a publication strategy. There are differences between longitudinal studies in their overall productivity and publishing outlets. Some longitudinal studies have been reported mainly in books, some in journal articles. In the case of several collaborators, it has to be decided who is involved in publication and how to avoid publishing overlaps. A related issue is the question of how long to wait before publishing the results of a longitudinal study. Data collection for the whole duration of the study may take years, so it may be necessary to publish results based on separate data collection phases before all phases are completed. In addition, researchers have to consider how to effectively communicate the findings to a general public, the media, and those who may apply results in practice.

Summary

The longitudinal design in the study of human development has established its position in science gradually during the past hundred years. The concept of development has affected the investigation of human development longitudinally, but longitudinal studies have also affected the concept of development. Earlier studies were focused on children and adolescents, but when the participants became older the studies were extended into adulthood. Consequently, longitudinal studies have increased understanding of developmental processes, not only in childhood and adolescence but also in adulthood and old age.

Studying individual development longitudinally is an attractive approach to research, but conducting a longitudinal study sets demands that should be critically considered in the planning stage of the study. Important considerations include, for example, a long-term commitment to the study, funding, sampling, estimating the duration and needed frequencies of data collection and the feasibility of tracing the sample over time, the availability of relevant measures across the studied ages, and the sustainable quality of the data. The first consideration, of course, is whether a longitudinal study is needed for solving the research problems in question. In general, longitudinal research is needed in psychology if the problem concerns consistency and change in individual characteristics and their developmental consequences over time.

Acknowledgments

The preparation of this chapter was supported by funding from the Academy of Finland to Lea Pulkkinen (Grant No. 127125) and Katja Kokko (Grant Nos. 118316 and 135347).

References

Baltes, P. B., Lindenberger, U., & Staudinger, U. M. (1998). Life-span theory in developmental psychology. In W. Damon (Series Ed.) & R. M. Lerner (Vol. Ed.), *Handbook of child psychology: Theoretical models of human development* (5th ed., pp. 1029–1143). New York: Wiley.

Bergman, L. R., & Magnusson, D. (1990). General issues about data quality in longitudinal research. In D. Magnusson & L. R. Bergman (Eds.), *Data quality in longitudinal research* (pp. 1–31). New York: Cambridge University Press.

Birren, J. E., & Schaie, K. W. (Eds.). (1977). *Handbook of the psychology of aging*. New York: Van Nostrand Reinhold.

Block, J. (1971). *Lives through time*. Berkeley, CA: Bancroft Books.

Brooks-Gunn, J., Phelps, E., & Elder, G. H., Jr. (1991). Studying lives through time: Secondary data analyses in developmental psychology. *Developmental Psychology, 27*, 899–910.

Cohen, J. (1992). A power primer. *Psychological Bulletin, 112*, 155–159.

Collins, L. M. (2006). Analysis of longitudinal data: The integration of theoretical model, temporal design, and statistical model. *Annual Review of Psychology, 57*, 505–528.

Coolican, H. (2009). *Research methods and statistics in psychology*. London: Hodder Education.

Dubow, E. F., Huesmann, L. R., Boxer, P., Pulkkinen, L., & Kokko, K. (2006). Middle childhood and adolescent contextual and personal predictors of adult educational and occupational outcomes: A mediational model in two countries. *Developmental Psychology, 42*, 937–949.

Elder, G. H., Jr. (1974). *Children of the Great Depression*. Chicago: University of Chicago Press.

Elder, G. H., Jr. (1998). Life course and human development. In W. Damon (Series Ed.) & R. M. Lerner (Vol. Ed.), *Handbook of child psychology: Theoretical models of human development* (5th ed., pp. 939–991). New York: Wiley.

Elder, G. H., Jr., & Pellerin, L. A. (1998). Linking history and human lives. In J. Z. Giele & G. H. Elder (Eds.), *Methods of life course research: Qualitative and quantitative approaches* (pp. 264–294). Thousand Oaks, CA: Sage.

Elliott, J., & Vaitilingam, R. (Eds.). (2008). *Now we are 50: Key findings from the National Child Development Study*. London: Centre for Longitudinal Studies.

Farrington, D. P., Ttofi, M. M., & Coid, J. W. (2009). Development of adolescence-limited, late-onset, and persistent offenders from age 8 to age 48. *Aggressive Behavior, 35*, 1350–1363.

Ferri, E., Bynner, J., & Wadsworth, M. (Eds.). (2003). *Changing Britain, changing lives: Three generations at the turn of the century*. London, UK: Bedford Way Papers.

Gesell, A. (1928). *Infancy and human growth*. New York: Macmillan.

Giele, J. Z., & Elder, G. H. Jr. (1998). Life course research: Development of a field. In J. Z. Giele & G. H. Elder, Jr. (Eds.), *Methods of life course research: Qualitative and quantitative approaches* (pp. 5–27). Thousand Oaks, CA: Sage.

Harris, D. B. (Eds.). (1967). *The concept of development: An issue in the study of human behavior*. Minneapolis, MN: Jones Press.

Helson, R., & Srivastava, S. (2002). Creativity and wisdom: Similarities, differences, and how they develop. *Personality and Social Psychology Bulletin, 28*, 1430–1440.

Honzik, M. (1965). Prediction of behavior from birth to maturity [Review of the book *Birth to maturity*]. *Merrill-Palmer Quarterly of Behavior and Development, 11*, 77–88.

Jones, H. E. (1938). The California Adolescent Growth Study. *Journal of Education Research, 31*, 561–567.

Kagan, J. (1964). American longitudinal research on psychological development. *Child Development, 35*, 1–32.

Kagan, J., & Moss, H. A. (1962). *Birth to maturity*. New York: Wiley.

Kaprio, J. (2006). Social behaviors and health in twins: The Finn Twin Studies. In L. Pulkkinen, J. Kaprio, & R. J. Rose (Eds.), *Socioemotional development and health from adolescence to adulthood* (pp. 76–91). New York: Cambridge University Press.

Keller, H. (2000). Developmental psychology: I. Prenatal to adolescence. In K. Pawlik & M. R. Rosenzweig (Eds.), *The international handbook of psychology* (pp. 235–260). London: Sage.

Kokko, K., Pulkkinen, L., Huesmann, L. R., Dubow, E. F., & Boxer, P. (2009). Intensity of aggression in childhood as a predictor of different forms of adult aggression: A two-country (Finland and United States) analysis. *Journal of Research on Adolescence, 19*, 9–34.

Macfarlane, J. W. (1938). Studies in child guidance: I. Methodology of data collection and organization. *Monographs of the Society for Research in Child Development, 3*(Whole No. 19).

Magnusson, D., & Bergman, L. R. (Eds.). (1990). *Data quality in longitudinal research*. New York: Cambridge University Press.

Moffitt, T. E., Caspi, A., Rutter, M., & Silva, P. A. (2001). *Sex differences in antisocial behaviour: Conduct disorder, delinquency, and violence in the Dunedin Longitudinal Study*. New York: Cambridge University Press.

Montada, L., & Schmitt, M. (1982). Issues in applied developmental psychology: A life-span perspective. In P. B. Baltes & O. B. Brim, Jr. (Eds.), *Life-span development and behavior* (Vol. 4, pp. 1–32). New York: Academic Press.

Nesselroade, J. R., & Baltes, P. B. (Eds.). (1979). *Longitudinal research in the study of behavior and development*. New York: Academic Press.

Pitkänen, L. (1969). *A descriptive model of aggression and nonaggression with applications to children's behaviour.* Jyväskylä, Finland: University of Jyväskylä.

Pulkkinen, L. (1993). Longitudinal approaches to adult lifestyles. In M. Vartiainen (Ed.), *European views in psychology: Keynote lectures* (pp. 13–37). Helsinki: Finnish Psychological Society.

Pulkkinen, L. (2006). The Jyväskylä longitudinal study of personality and social development. In L. Pulkkinen, J. Kaprio, & R. J. Rose (Eds.), *Socioemotional development and health from adolescence to adulthood* (pp. 29–55). New York: Cambridge University Press.

Pulkkinen, L. (2009). Personality: A resource or risk for successful development. *Scandinavian Journal of Psychology, 50*, 602–610.

Robins, L. (1966). *Deviant children grown up*. Baltimore: Williams & Wilkins.

Rose, R. J. (2006). Genetic and environmental influences on social behavior and health. In L. Pulkkinen, J. Kaprio, & R. J. Rose (Eds.), *Socioemotional development and health from adolescence to adulthood* (pp. 56–75). New York: Cambridge University Press.

Rutter, M. (1994). Beyond longitudinal data: Causes, consequences, changes, and continuity. *Journal of Consulting and Clinical Psychology, 62*, 928–940.

Rutter, M. (2006). *Genes and behavior: Nature–nurture interplay explained*. Oxford, UK: Blackwell.

Schneider, W., & Edelstein, W. (1990). *Inventory of European longitudinal studies in the behavioral and medical sciences*. Munich: European Science Foundation.

Sihvo, T., & Pulkkinen, L. (2002). *Suomalaisia pitkittäistutkimuksia psykologian alalta ja lähitieteistä* [Finnish longitudinal studies in the field of psychology and related disciplines]. Jyväskylä, Finland: University of Jyväskylä, Department of Psychology.

Smith, K., & Joshi, H. (2002). The Millennium Cohort Study. *Population Trends, 107*, 30–34.

Terman, L. M., & Oden, M. H. (1959). *Genetic studies of genius: V. The gifted group at mid-life*. Stanford, CA: Stanford University Press.

Tremblay, R. E., Vitaro, F., Nagin, D., Pagani, L., & Séguin, J. R. (2003). The Montreal Longitudinal and Experimental Study: Rediscovering the power of descriptions. In T. P. Thornberry & M. D. Krohn (Eds.), *Taking stock of delinquency: An overview of findings from contemporary longitudinal studies* (pp. 205–254). London: Kluwer Academic.

Vaillant, G. E. (1977). *Adaptation to life*. Boston: Little, Brown.

Verdonik, F., & Sherrod, L. R. (1984). *An inventory of longitudinal research on childhood and adolescence*. New York: Social Science Research Council.

Walder, L., Abelson, R., Eron, L., Banta, T., & Laulicht, J. (1961). Development of a peer-rating measure of aggression. *Psychological Reports, 9*, 497–556.

Werner, E., & Smith, R. S. (2001). *Journeys from childhood to midlife: Risk, resilience, and recovery*. Ithaca, NY: Cornell University Press.

West, D. J., & Farrington, D. P. (1977). *The delinquent way of life: Third report of the Cambridge Study in Delinquent Development*. London, UK: Heinemann Educational Books.

Young, C. H., Savola, K. L., & Phelps, E. (1991). *Inventory of longitudinal studies in the social sciences*. Newbury Park, CA: Sage.

CHAPTER 9

The Use of Large-Scale Data Sets for the Study of Developmental Science

PAMELA DAVIS-KEAN
JUSTIN JAGER

Central Issues

This chapter examines the use of large-scale data sets for examining research questions in the developmental sciences. The use of large-scale data sets in developmental science has been relatively rare and generally limited to sociologists and economists interested in examining children and families. In the past two decades, however, many large-scale data sets have been made available to the research community (through archiving institutions such as the Inter-University Consortium for Political and Social Research [ICPSR] and the Henry A. Murray Research Archive) that, in addition to focusing on children and their families, also include the process or explanatory variables that are of interest to disciplines such as psychology. These data sets have some important advantages in examining developmental questions, as well as limitations, and we discuss some of these issues in this chapter. First, however, we begin by defining large-scale data sets and discussing the most common types that are used in developmental science. Then we discuss the various advantages and disadvantages of these data sets for developmental science, helping the reader decide which type of data set is best suited for his or her own research questions. We then discuss some specific statistical issues in using large-scale longitudinal data sets and end with a section on how to apply the use of this method to developmental science questions.

What Is a Large-Scale Data Set?

The first issue that should be addressed is what is meant by the term *large-scale* data set. Basically, a large-scale data set is a data set that has broad or expansive research applications. These types of data sets need not be "large" in terms of sample size (i.e., a large N), but they do need to serve as a rich source of research, whether the source of the data is primary or secondary. Secondary data analyses are often represented by large national population studies. These data sets are collected for all researchers to use and thus are not the "primary" data of any single researcher or research team. Primary data sets, however, are often associated with community samples in which individual researchers have collected data based on their own theories or models. These data sets have generally been proprietary and not available to other researchers except those on the research team. Thus the distinguishing element between primary and secondary data is whether or not the researcher(s) collected the data themselves. However, both types of data are "large-scale" data sets provided that they can be used to answer a broad array of research questions.

Large-scale data sets typically fall into one of two categories: *population* or *process*. Population data sets can be thought of as national, representative data sets. These data sets are usually collected by research organizations that gather data across the country, and the sample is chosen by a specific sampling strategy to make sure that all racial/ethnic, gender, and economic groups are represented in the data set. They are generally collected to be used by the general research community and may not be based on any particular theory of development or family functioning. A prime example of a population data set is the National Longitudinal Study of Adolescent Health (Add Health). Add Health (Bearman, Jones, & Udry, 1997) is a longitudinal study of a nationally representative sample of 7th–12th graders in the United States in the 1994–1995 school year and includes measures on individual social, economic, psychological, and physical well-being, as well as contextual data on the family, neighborhood, school, friends, and romantic relationships. The Add Health cohort (N = 20,745) has been followed into young adulthood with four in-home interviews, the most recent being in 2008, when the sample was ages 24–32. Though full access to the data requires a contractual agreement with the Add Health administrators, a public-use data set is available through ICPSR (see Table 9.1). The public-use data set is limited to waves 1, 2, and 3 and a random subsample (N = 6,500) of the original sample, but it does include all the original measures.

In contrast to population data sets such as Add Health, process data sets are generally guided by the theory of the research group that is collecting the data and often are collected at the community level as opposed to the national level. These types of data sets often are representative of the community of focus, but they can also be based on convenience samples. Because process data sets are typically based on theory and guided by groups of researchers with expertise in the specific area of research being examined, these data sets often include abundant measures of constructs germane to the particular research area of focus and sparse measures on other research areas and topics. Often, process data sets are not initially available for use outside of the research teams but become available across time for use by other researchers. The National Institute of Child Health and Human Development (NICHD) Study of Early Child Care and Youth Development (SECCYD) is an example of a process data set (NICHD Early Child Care Research Network, 1994). This data set is a birth cohort longitudinal data set that was collected at 10 locations across the United States starting in 1991. Though the data set was collected from multiple sites, it was not designed to be nationally representative of children born in the United States in 1991. The data design is also censored such that mothers who (1) did not speak English fluently, (2) had an obvious disability, (3) were hospitalized more than 7 days postpartum, (4) were planning on moving out of the catchment area within 3 years, and (5) were younger than 18 years old

TABLE 9.1. Resources for Longitudinal Data

Resource	Website
Data Archives	
Murray Research Archives	*www.murray.harvard.edu*
Inter-University Consortium for Political and Social Research (ICPSR)	*www.icpsr.umich.edu/icpsrweb/ICPSR*
Population data sets	
Early Childhood Longitudinal Study—Birth Cohort (ECLS-B)	*nces.ed.gov/ecls/birth.asp*
Early Childhood Longitudinal Study—Kindergarten Cohort (ECLS-K)	*nces.ed.gov/ecls/kindergarten.asp*
Panel Study of Income Dynamics—Child Development Supplement (PSID-CDS)	*psidonline.isr.umich.edu/CDS*
The National Longitudinal Study of Adolescent Health (Add Health)	*www.cpc.unc.edu/projects/addhealth*
Process data sets	
NICHD Study of Early Child Care and Youth Development (SECCYD)	*www.icpsr.umich.edu/icpsrweb/ICPSR/series/00233*
Maryland Adolescent Development in Context Study (MADICS)	*dvn.iq.harvard.edu/dvn/dv/mra/faces/study/StudyPage.xhtml?globalId=hdl:1902.1/01066*
Child Development Project (CDP)	*www.cdp.auburn.edu*
Minnesota Longitudinal Study (MLS)	*www.cehd.umn.edu/icd/parent-child/default.html*
Michigan Longitudinal Study (MiLS)	*www.med.umich.edu/psych/sub/razprojects.htm*
Data collection institutes	
Survey Research Center (SRC/ISR)	*www.src.isr.umich.edu*
National Opinion Research Center (NORC)	*www.norc.uchicago.edu/homepage.htm*
Westat	*www.westat.com*
Research Triangle Institute (RTI)	*www.rti.org*
Statistical training	
Inter-University Consortium for Political and Social Research (ICPSR)	*www.icpsr.umich.edu/icpsrweb/ICPSR*
University of Kansas Quantitative Training	*www.quant.ku.edu*

when they gave birth were not included in the sample. Even with these sample limitations, the NICHD SECCYD provides a wealth of data related to child development that include measures on individual, social, economic, psychological, and physical well-being and development in multiple contexts that include child care, schooling, and out-of-school activities. These data are also collected with a variety of methods, including surveys, laboratory and field observations, multiple developmental and achievement assessments, and census information. The NICHD SECCYD cohort (1,364) has been followed from birth to adolescence across four waves of data collection (phase I: 0–3-year-olds; phase II: 54 months through first grade; phase III: 2nd–6th grade; phase IV: 14–15 years of age) and from years 1991 to 2008. During this period of time the sample size was reduced from the original 1,364 to 1,056 adolescents still being followed at 15 years of age. The data in this data set are restricted data and must be obtained from a contractual agreement through ICPSR (see Table 9.1). However, obtaining the data is a relatively easy process and should not deter you from the use of this rich data set. Throughout the remainder of this chapter we use Add Health and SECCYD as the exemplars of population and process data sets, respectively. When applicable, we ground our discussion of population and process data sets in real-world examples using Add Health and SECCYD.

It is important to note that there is a lot of overlap between secondary and primary data and between national and process data sets (i.e., secondary data are often national data sets, and vice versa). In general, if you are analyzing a data set that you did not personally design or collect (including data of a mentor or colleague), then you are performing a secondary data analysis. If you are analyzing a data set that you designed and collected, then you are performing primary data analysis. Data that are collected from experiments are almost always primary data, because the researcher has created an experiment that is specific to a series of questions. Correlational data can be either primary or secondary data depending on the specific goals of the research and, as noted previously, can be either process or population data sets. Thus, when deciding on which type of large-scale data set to use, one has many options among the types of data sets that are available, and often the decision is based on the researcher's need for depth in the process of behavior or desire to generalize behaviors to the population. There are a few data sets that will give you the ability to do both (e.g., the Early Childhood Longitudinal Studies—Birth Cohort and Kindergarten, which are national data sets rich in measurements of multiple constructs; see Table 9.1).

Process or Population: What Should I Use to Answer My Questions?

Why are there such differences in the ways that data are collected to study questions relevant to developmental science? The answers lie within the differences between the disciplines that study the development of children and families. Psychologists generally examine how aspects of the individual predict behavior, whereas sociologists and economists focus more on how aspects of society and demographic characteristics of the individual (e.g., race/ethnicity, gender, marriage status, etc.) influence behavior. Though these areas of focus at times overlap, they are distinct enough that these disciplines train their students in different methods, and these methods often dictate the data collection and research done by these disciplines. In the next sections we spend some time discussing these disciplinary differences and how they influence the methods used to understand behavior.

Examining Process

Often developmental researchers are interested in examining relations between different variables. Based on a theoretical model, researchers make specific predictions regarding the relations being examined. For example, a researcher may wish to study how early success in reading relates to later academic motivation and, in turn, academic achievement or how maternal depression prior to birth relates to mother–child attachment during early childhood. Opposed to being population-based, these types of questions are process-based. Process-based questions typically focus on how different factors, constructs, or variables relate to or influence one another. Unlike population-based studies, which focus on the incidence of a behavior, the goal of process-based studies is to uncover the origins or pathways to those behaviors.

Just as the research aims of population-based studies and process-based studies often vary, so too does the structure of the data used to explore those research aims. Data sets used to explore process-based research tend to be smaller in size (i.e., a smaller *N*), less diverse in terms of race/ethnicity and social class, and measure a narrower band of constructs. But those constructs that are measured are usually measured with greater depth and specificity. Some examples of these types of data sets are the Maryland Adolescent Development in Context Study (MADICS), the Child Development Project (CDP), the Minnesota Longitudinal Study (MLS), and the Michigan Longitudinal study (MiLS). None of these projects aims to make inferences about a particular population; instead, they aim to examine how different factors interplay to inform individual development. Generally speaking, these types of data sets are used more by developmental psychologists, who are more interested in models of behavior within individuals or groups than in the prevalence of behaviors at an aggregate level or among a population.

Generalizing to the Population

Unlike developmental scientists who are examining the process of individual development, there are those who want to examine how demographic, policy, or social categories may have important predictive power on behavior. These societally oriented variables can be elements of socioeconomic status (e.g., education, income, occupation), government policies (e.g., availability of quality child care, poverty policies, education policies), and even the influence of societal norms (e.g., collective vs. individualistic societies) on human behavior. These examples are not comprehensive of all the topics examined in these social sciences, but the point is that the mechanisms by which these various topics influence behavior is not necessarily as important for these scientists as whether or not they are prevalent across the population and whether these predictors are unbiased. Thus, compared with developmental scientists who study process, these scientists want to know how generalizable or inferential these predictors are across the population. In other words, can they create a model that predicts human behavior across the population?

The methods used primarily by sociologists and economists to study developmental science questions rely on population samples. Unlike process data sets, which as mentioned earlier focus on community samples, population data sets are collected to be representative of a well-defined population (e.g., country, region). The sample can be constructed in various ways, but the primary goal is to have a data set that can be used to represent the population of interest such that researchers can generalize from this sample to the full

TABLE 9.2. Decision Matrix for Using Population or Process Data Sets

	Does your research question entail or demand . . .				
	Population norms (functional forms, prevalence or incidence rates)	Generalizability	Mechanisms (mediation/ moderation)	Subgroup comparisons	Power to detect small effects
Process data sets	No	No	Yes	No[a]	No
Population data sets	Yes	Yes	No[a]	Yes	Yes
Process–population combination	Yes	Yes	Yes	Yes	Yes

[a]It is often possible to use these data sets for these goals, but they are not necessarily the best choice.

population. In many cases generalization is to the national population, but at other times it may be to a specific subgroup, such as families with autistic children or minority groups such as Latinos, African Americans, or Asian Americans. For population data sets, the size of the samples tends to be large, because often a large sample is needed to accurately represent the population of interest.

Though it may appear that population data sets would be a positive avenue for studying developmental science questions due to the sample size and generalizability advantage, what is lost is often the important process of why these variables are predicting behavior. Often the question of importance at the population level, such as employment of certain gender or racial groups, does not measure the process of the way employment may influence the mother when a child is born. Thus, deciding what type of data set to use is based primarily (as all research should be) on the question that the researcher is asking. In Table 9.2, we have provided a decision matrix to help in making choices regarding the type of data set that might be useful for answering questions across developmental science. Depending either on your disciplinary or theoretical background, you will make decisions based on the type of question you are interested in answering. This will lead to the type of data that you may want to collect or to find in social science data archives.

Conceptual Principles and Statistical Assumptions

After making the decision regarding what type of data (process or population) are most relevant to your research question, you will then need to address important conceptual principles and statistical assumptions inherent to large-scale developmental data sets.

Developmental Methods and Attrition

Longitudinal data are complex and often a challenge to analyze. The size and scope of large-scale longitudinal data sets, whether process based or population based, only increases that challenge. Most users need to be quite advanced in their statistical skills so that they can take advantage of the rich longitudinal data that both process-based and population-based data sets provide. Unfortunately, an introduction to advanced longitudinal methods is well beyond the scope of this chapter. However, no matter the statistical technique, chances are that there are online resources (e.g., *statmodel.com*, *semnet.com*) or statistical workshops (ICPSR and the University of Kansas, among others, offer a broad array of short yet effective statistical workshops; see Table 9.1) that fit your experience level. Readers looking for an introduction to contemporary methods for analyzing longitudinal data are encouraged to read Preacher, Wichman, MacCallum, and Briggs (2008) or Burchinal, Nelson, and Poe (2006).

When it comes to longitudinal research, the proper handling of missing data is also vital. Practically speaking, every longitudinal study has dropouts, though some more than others. The problem for researchers is that attrition (i.e., respondents dropping out of the study) is rarely random (Johnston, O'Malley, Bachman, & Schulenberg, 2008; Levin, Katzen, Klein, & Llabre, 2000; Siddiqui, Flay, & Hu, 1996). Instead, certain subgroups are more likely to drop out than others, such as those of lower socioeconomic status, those in poorer physical and mental health, and those who are members of a racial minority group (Johnston et al., 2008; Levin et al., 2000; Siddiqui et al., 1996). As a consequence of this differential attrition, over time the retained sample no longer represents the original sample, leading to biased estimates (Collins, Schafer, & Kam, 2001; Widaman, 2006). Unfortunately, this bias can rarely be eliminated; however, if properly applied, today's missing data techniques (i.e., multiple imputation [MI] or missing data algorithms such as full information maximum likelihood [FIML]) can reduce it substantially (Enders, 2010). In addition to introducing bias, attrition also results in a reduced sample size and subsequently a loss of statistical power (Collins et al., 2001). Readers interested in a more detailed account of attrition and useful methods for adjusting for it should consult Enders (2010).

Sample Weights and Complex Sample Designs

Population-based studies often include "sample weights" that, when applied to the data, result in parameter estimates (i.e., estimates of totals, proportions, and associations) that are representative of the national population from which the sample was collected. Although the purpose of a sample weight is simple enough, there are often multiple weights to choose from, and determining which weight is the right one for you can be tricky. For example, most longitudinal population-based studies also include weights that adjust for attrition. So instead of using the methods that adjust for attrition, mentioned briefly earlier (and in more detail by Enders, 2010), it is also possible (though less optimal) to adjust for attrition through reweighting. The conceptual distinction between a sample weight and an attrition weight is a tricky but important one. The purpose of a sample weight is to adjust sample estimates so that they "represent" a larger population (e.g., adjust sample estimates so that they represent all the families in the United States or all of the middle-school children in California). So, even if there is no attrition (i.e., no reduction in sample size across collection periods), a sample weight would still need to be applied to the data in order to attain estimates that represent the larger population. The purpose of an attrition weight is to adjust estimates of a sample reduced by attrition so that the estimates represent the original, full sample. Depending on the population data set used, the weights provided may be sample weights, attrition weights, or, more often than not, a combination of the two. For example, Add Health provides four separate sample weights from which to choose, one for each wave of data collection. The wave 1 weight (GSWGT1) is a sample weight only. The wave 2–wave

4 weights (GSWGT2–GSWGT4) are combination sample–attrition weights. For example, in addition to adjusting the estimates so that they are representative of the U.S. population, GSWGT4 also adjusts for attrition between waves 1 and 4. Which Add Health weight should you use? If you are not adjusting for attrition in some other manner (i.e., MI, FIML), then you should apply the sample–attrition combination weight for the most recent wave that you are using. If you are adjusting for attrition in some other manner, then you should apply the wave 1 sample weight (GSWGT1). More detailed information on the Add Health weights and their application is available in Chantala (2006). Most other population-based studies have similar reference articles or user guides. Researchers should consult these publications carefully when selecting the appropriate set of weights.

Most large national data sets take advantage of complex sampling procedures. On large populations, using simple random sampling is often extremely labor-intensive and not economically feasible. Instead, complex sampling designs are used, such as stratified sampling, which entails sampling units of existing clusters or groups (e.g., schools, families, neighborhoods, or classrooms). Although these sampling methods are certainly convenient, they do complicate the estimation of variances and standard errors. When compared with *N* randomly selected individuals, the individuals within a group or cluster of *N* individuals (say a family) are more likely to resemble each other in terms of attitudes, demographics, and so forth (Kish, 1957). Thus, naturally existing groups of individuals are more homogeneous than a similarly sized group put together based on random selection. From a technical standpoint, the greater degree of homogeneity within naturally existing groups violates the assumption of independence, an assumption that most of the statistical techniques used by social scientists make. From a practical standpoint, the greater degree of homogeneity within naturally existing groups results in an underestimation of variances (and, in turn, standard errors). This systematic bias leads to an increased likelihood of Type I errors. Depending on the degree of homogeneity within the clusters and the size of the clusters, the bias can be substantial (i.e., a 50–50 chance of a Type I error; Kish, 1957). The remedy is to use statistical software that is capable of properly analyzing data collected via a complex sampling design. In "designed-based" analyses such as these, a "stratification" variable and a "primary sampling unit" variable are incorporated into the analyses in order to adjust for the sampling design. By design, the primary sampling unit variable is nested within the stratification variable. Fortunately, many of the widely used statistical packages (e.g., SUDAAN, SAS, SPSS, STATA, and Mplus) are capable of such analyses. Using the Add Health stratification variable REGION (based on the Northeast, Midwest, South, and West regions of the United States) and cluster variable PSUSCID (based on school), Chantala (2006) provides syntax templates for SUDAAN, SAS, STATA, and Mplus. Even if you are using a data set other than Add Health, these syntax templates and the detailed explanations provided are a helpful starting point. The user guide for your favorite statistical software package is also a great resource, as most user guides contain program-specific instructions for the analysis of complex sample data.

In sum, when using a population data set, check to see whether (1) sampling weights are provided, (2) those weights are combination sample/attrition weights, and (3) data were collected via a complex sampling design. If sampling weights are provided, then they will need to be applied to obtain accurate point estimates. If the sampling weights are also attrition weights, then users should take care to select the weight that is most appropriate, which often depends on the combination of time points analyzed and whether other techniques were used to adjust for attrition. Finally, if data were collected via a complex sampling design, then analytical techniques that adjust for the sampling design will need to be used in order to obtain accurate variance estimates.

Causality and the "Third Variable"

Next we turn to conceptual principles relevant to the use of process data sets. The issue of causality in correlation research is an important topic and is well addressed in many publications (e.g., Bullock, Harlow, & Mulaik, 1994; Cohen & Cohen, 1983; Cook & Campbell, 1979; Foster, Chapter 2, this volume; Kline, 2011); thus, we do not reiterate these issues in the chapter but would like to highlight these issues in relation to large-scale longitudinal data sets. As is often stated in both statistics and methodology classes, "correlation is not causation," and we have to be quite careful not to forget this when using the power of large-scale longitudinal data sets. It is tempting to believe that, with all the variables that can be used in studying the human condition in the population or large community data sets/samples, we should be able to "control" for many of the differences between groups and thus be able to make causal statements such as that participation in a reading program or reading to your child "causes" differences between groups. All we can say is that they are related.

Many developmental scientists who are interested in process questions use structural equation modeling (SEM) to study their questions. SEM was often referred to as "causal modeling." Yet, when using a longitudinal data set, the closest we get to causality is often what is referred to as temporal precedence, or the fact that we know that data were collected prior to another variable of interest (Kline, 2011). Temporal precedence is a criterion for establishing causality, and depending on how you ask your developmental question, it is always available in longitudinal studies but is not the only criterion that must be met (Kline, 2011). Again, many variables may be related to the reason that a relation between two variables is found, including an unmeasured "third variable." This unmeasured third variable can be a particular problem when issues of selection may be an issue, such as in convenience samples.

Selection issues are of particular concern to those using convenience samples because of the lack of control in the way a community is sampled. This lack of control may lead, for example, to groups of people joining who may be doing so to earn money from the study, who are highly educated and interested in participating in studies, or who have family members who have the time and transportation available to participate, as well as many other possible factors that may not be measured yet are related to the results found in the study (Grimes & Schultz, 2002; Heckman, 1979). Because they are representative by design, population data sets are certainly better for dealing with issues of selection. Even so, they are still based primarily on correlational designs and thus are also limited, even in a highly controlled study, in making statements about causality other than temporal precedence.

Though not a substitute for the ability to test for causality, one avenue that can be used with both convenience and population samples is replication. Often the population samples and community samples have used either the same measurement or a very similar measurement to examine important developmental questions. When this situation arises, a researcher can test his or her questions using both types of data sets and the same types of variables in both analyses. This cross-validation can strengthen the claims by the researcher that his or her phenomena are important and replicable in multiple data sets. Developmental researchers often use replication in laboratory settings in order to show that their results are generalizable to other populations. Thus process-oriented developmental scientists can use a similar strategy in order to see whether their findings generalize across multiple types of studies. This strategy has been successfully used already in multiple studies in developmental science (Davis-Kean et al., 2008; Duncan et al., 2007). Thus, using this type of replication technique (discussed later in the chapter) provides another avenue for developmental scientists to use the strength of large-scale data sets to validate their theories and research.

Developmental Applications

So far we have reviewed the various issues regarding the use of large-scale data sets to study process and population questions in developmental science and some questions about why this may differ by social science disciplines and statistical issues that may be important in the use of these data sets. In this section we focus specifically on the benefits to developmental science in using large-scale data sets either at the national or community level. We have discussed or alluded to some of these issues earlier, but they are now specifically addressed.

Using Large-Scale Process Data Sets for Developmental Research

A defining feature of national data sets is breadth of measures; they typically cover a broad range of measures. In contrast, a defining feature of process data sets is the depth of measures. Though process data sets often lack the breadth of measures that typifies national data sets, those measures that are included in the data sets are often measured in far greater detail. With respect to research application, process data sets' focus on depth at the cost of breadth has its advantages as well as disadvantages. One important advantage is that process data sets and their detailed measures allow for a far more nuanced examination of how factors influence or are associated with other factors. More specifically, these sorts of data sets allow for the focused exploration of moderation (i.e., interactions) and mediation (i.e., indirect effects). Issues of mediation and moderation are ubiquitous in developmental research in general and psychological research in particular. Perhaps the best illustration of this, using our example of the NICHD SECCYD data set, is a recent publication by Brooks-Gunn, Han, and Waldfogel (2010) that examined the influence of a mother's returning to work (either full or part time) in the first year of a child's life. Using SEM, they were able to test for both moderator and mediator effects on child outcomes of a mother's returning to work in the first year of a child's life. Contrary to early work on this data set, this research found little influence of moderators (maternal occupation, gender, temperament) but found that any effects of mother's returning to work on child outcomes are mediated through aspects of the home environment and maternal sensitivity. Their conclusion is that a mother's return to work in a child's first year of life is related to both positive and negative outcomes in children but that they offset each other, producing a neutral influence. Thus this very careful analysis of process data was able to give a much more nuanced examination of the issue of maternal employment and child care.

One key disadvantage of process data sets is the lack of generalizability. Process data sets are often based on convenience samples. When they are not, they are based on community samples. Either way, these data sets are rarely representative of the general population and at best are representative of a particular community. As a result, it can be difficult to determine to whom the findings may generalize. Thus, the NICHD SECCYD example showed the power of examining process data, but the data set is not nationally representative, so the results apply only to those families living within the communities in which the data was collected and who agreed to participate in the study. This data set is also not representative of the socioeconomic distribution or race/ethnic distribution in the United States. Little can be said, then, about how the use of child care is related to various social class groups and races/ethnicities. Indeed, a rather large disadvantage of the NICHD SECCYD is the lack of racial/ethnic diversity in the data set.

Another disadvantage of process data sets is that often they do not contain all of the measures you wish to include in your study. The researchers and principal investigators responsible for these sorts of data sets created the data sets to address specific research questions related to their areas of focus, expertise, and theoretical perspective. The domains and measures that you find interesting or important may not be central to their original research aims. As a result, a particular process data set may not contain all of the measures you need to conduct your study properly. In the case of a community sample, we are often missing good information on socioeconomic status, neighborhood safety, wealth, multiple resources, multiple caregivers living in the home, and other demographic and descriptive data that are often found in the national data sets.

Also, as mentioned earlier, sample size may be an issue with the smaller scale community samples. The smaller sample size of many of these data sets prohibits the researcher from having the power needed to find effects—especially in psychological research, in which effect sizes may be small (r = .10–.20; Cohen & Cohen, 1983). Sample size is also important when investigators want to use more advanced multivariate analyses and SEMs, for which sample sizes less than 100 are not adequate (Tabachnick & Fidell, 2007). Thus, finding a process data set that fits your data needs can be a challenge.

Using Population Data Sets for Developmental Research

Population and national data sets give developmental researchers the ability to generalize their findings beyond the community and to study diverse populations. They also, in general, have the sample sizes that allow the researcher to find effects even when they are small. These characteristics of population-based data sets provide rather powerful and important reasons for developmental scientists who do not use these data sets or are not aware of them to spend time exploring them and taking advantage of what is available in them to study. A cursory glance through many psychological journals, for example, will show studies in which small and unrepresentative samples have been used, the authors of which make claims or allude to the idea that their findings are true for the more general population. These types of studies would be strengthened if the researchers could test their questions in a larger sample, perhaps already available in one of the developmental population studies. When using population data sets to replicate findings based on small, unrepresentative samples, it will not always be possible to find the exact measure or variables. Still, it is worth the effort to see whether they are available and can be studied in a larger population.

Another advantage is the breadth of measures available within these data sets. For example, in addition to socioemotional, physiological, and biological information on the child, Add Health also has information on parents, peers, siblings, and romantic partners, and on income, education, occupation, schools, and neighborhoods. The ability to examine how the environment of a child changes as the child changes is another important advantage of these large-scale population studies in developmental science. Because these studies are generally collecting contextual data at the same time that they are collecting child and family data, more complicated models can be tested on how children develop within changing contexts over time (Bronfenbrenner & Morris, 1998). Because population data sets aim to be representative, they are typically larger and more diverse in race/ethnicity, gender, and other categories that are important when examining the population at large (e.g., employed–not employed; high education–low education; married–not married). Thus the use of large-scale data sets has some distinct advantages for developmental science, especially for those researchers who are interested in the influence of context or for those seeking diversity in the samples that they study.

Population data sets also have their disadvantages. These data sets are often collected by large data collection groups such as Westat, the Survey Research Center (SRCLISR), the Research Triangle Institute (RTI), and the National Opinion Research Center (NORC) (see Table 9.1) and are expensive to undertake, and the surveys are often more general than specific. Thus what is gained in breadth of the sample is often detrimental to the depth of the types of questions being asked. This lack of depth can compromise the psychometrics of the scales or questions in the study such that scales that were developed and validated at certain lengths and content are now reduced and the comparability to the original scales is unknown. The ability of researchers to test the original theory underlying these scales (e.g., self-esteem, depression, anxiety) may also become compromised.

Another concern is that many of the studies relevant to developmental science are supplements to larger surveys that were not originally meant to study developmental questions concerning children and families (e.g., the Panel Study of Income Dynamics—Child Development Supplement and the National Longitudinal Study of Youth) and thus may not have as many of the measures of psychological constructs (e.g., depression, self-esteem, personality, anxiety) that might be found in the smaller scale process data sets. Hence, developmental researchers who may want to have the generalizability and statistical power of the population studies may find that they cannot answer their questions of interest because the key variables are often not well represented in these types of data sets.

Future Directions

We have discussed some of the advantages and disadvantages of using population and process data sets, but there are also methods that can take advantage of both types of data sets and lead to new insights in developmental science. Two possibilities that we discuss further are replicated analyses across a variety of data sets and integrative data analysis (IDA), by which multiple data sets with similar measurements can be combined (pooled) for analysis. Both of these analyses take advantage of the fact that different data sets often include some of the same measurements or latent constructs and that by either combining the data (i.e., IDA) or by using the same analytic technique (i.e., replicated studies) one can gain power and generalizability past what any single data set would allow. Both of these techniques may be useful in combining the positive aspects of process and population data sets to give developmental researchers more opportunities to tests their theories in varied populations.

Perhaps the best example of using multiple process and population data sets to answer developmental questions is a study conducted by Duncan and colleagues (2007) in which they used replicated analyses across six multinational longitudinal data sets. Their goal was to examine what predicted school readiness from a set of predictors that had been found in the literature to relate to entry to school. Prior to the Duncan and colleagues article, research had found that social skills and behavior problems were related to achievement outcomes. Duncan and colleagues examined this relation, as well as those with early math, reading, and attention skills. Each of the data sets identified each of these constructs in their data set, and then a set of replicated analyses was done for each data set. Finally, through meta-analysis techniques, they combined effect sizes across the studies to determine effect sizes for each construct. By using this type of replicated analyses, Duncan and colleagues found that early math, reading, and attention skills had the strongest predictive power on later achievement and that social skills and problem behaviors had close to zero effects. By using this method, these researchers were able to test and replicate their findings across multiple countries (United States, United Kingdom, and Canada), leading to new insights on how socioemotional and achievement skills are related to school readiness. The researchers used both population and process data sets in their replications and specifically used the process data sets due to the better measurement of the constructs of interest.

Clearly, this is a valuable way to examine developmental questions when data sets are available that have measured similar constructs around the same ages. One of the potential disadvantages is not having access to multiple data sets for the replicated analysis. As mentioned earlier, data sets that are important to answering developmental science questions are now accessible in data archives such as ICPSR and the Radcliffe Murray Center at Harvard.

Another technique that is valuable in combining information from multiple data sets is integrative data analysis (IDA). Unlike meta-analysis, which uses summary data from existing studies, IDA uses pooled data from original data sets (Curran & Hussong, 2009). This method can use data from multiple independent data sets with data that were collected at different time points using different methods and were sampled in different areas of the country or other countries. The major difference in this method is that the data are actually combined in a single data set in which characteristics of the samples can be used as predictors, as would be done in any analysis of a complete data set. There are multiple advantages to this technique, especially for process data sets: increased sample size and power, increased heterogeneity of the sample (and therefore greater generalizability), and potentially increased age coverage (i.e., together the data sets cover a larger age range than any of the individual data sets). As an example of this technique, consider multiple independent data sets that have measured alcohol use and have similar predictors but in different settings, such as hospitals, inpatient clinics, or community referral. These data sets on their own have fairly small samples but good measurement of their phenomena, and all are looking at similar issues. In this situation, IDA can pool the data and use the setting as a variable within the data set to account for variations of the setting (as well as other variations). This new pooled data set will have a larger sample size, which leads to more power to answer the central questions of the researchers. This technique is a powerful tool for developmental scientists to use as they consider the limitations of their studies and how those can be overcome by pooling data with other researchers examining similar topics.

Summary and Conclusion

The purpose of this chapter was to discuss the use of large-scale data sets in developmental science. We have reviewed the definition of a large-scale data set, discussed how data sets can be thought of in terms of studying questions of process or population generalizability, the advantages and disadvantages of these data sets, the importance of research questions, statistical issues, and some ways in which developmental science can be enhanced by using process and population data sets. Large-scale data sets provide a powerful tool for developmental researchers to use to study both the *breadth* and *depth* of child and family development. The process data sets often examine multiple mechanisms of development across time. The population data sets offer complexity in information on contexts and the ability to generalize to the population when appropriate weights are used. These characteristics of population-based data sets give developmental scientists some very strong tools to answer their questions of interest. This is not to say that collecting one's own data is not also valuable. As we have discussed, any one data set may not have all the variables or constructs that an individual researcher may want. Thus, new data must be collected in order to isolate a particular phenomenon of interest to the researchers. However, there are many constructs that are well measured and collected in the large-scale data sets, and being able to examine their depth (process) or breadth (population) in ways that cannot easily be done with new data collection is a strength of these types of data sets and, with the use of replication and pooled data techniques, can lead to new and exciting answers to developmental questions.

References

Bearman, P., Jones, J., & Udry, J. (1997). The National Longitudinal Study of Adolescent Health: Research design. Chapel Hill, NC: Carolina Population Center. Available at *www.cpc.unc.edu/projects/addhealth/design.html.*

Burchinal, M., Nelson, L., & Poe, M. (2006). IV. Growth curve analysis: An introduction to various methods for analyzing longitudinal data. *Monographs of the Society for Research in Child Development, 71*(3), 65–87.

Bronfenbrenner, U., & Morris, P. A. (1998). The ecology of developmental processes. In W. Damon & R. M. Lerner (Eds.), *Handbook of child psychology: Vol. 1. Theoretical models of human development* (pp. 993–1028). New York: Wiley.

Brooks-Gunn, J., Han, W.-J., & Waldfogel, J. (2010). First-year maternal employment and child development in the first 7 years. *Monographs of the Society for Research in Child Development, 75*(2), 1–147.

Bullock, H. E., Harlow, L. L., & Mulaik, S. A. (1994). Causation issues in structural equation modeling research. *Structural Equation Modeling: A Multidisciplinary Journal, 1*(3), 253–267.

Chantala, K. (2006). *Guidelines for analyzing Add Health data*. Chapel Hill, NC: Carolina Population Center. Available at *www.cpc.unc.edu/projects/addhealth/data/guides/wt-guidelines.pdf.*

Cohen, J., & Cohen, P. (1983). *Applied multiple regression/correlation analysis for the behavioral sciences* (2nd ed.). Hillsdale, NJ: Erlbaum.

Collins, L. M., Schafer, J. L., & Kam, C. (2001). A comparison of inclusive and restrictive strategies in modern missing data procedures. *Psychological Methods, 6*(4), 330–351.

Cook, T. D., & Campbell, D. T. (1979). *Quasi-experimentation: Design and analysis for field settings.* Chicago: Rand McNally.

Curran, P. J., & Hussong, A. M. (2009). Integrative data analysis: The simultaneous analysis of multiple data sets. *Psychological Methods, 14*(2), 81–100.

Davis-Kean, P. E., Huesmann, L. R., Jager, J., Collins, W. A., Bates, J. E., & Lansford, J. (2008). Changes in the relation of beliefs and behaviors during middle childhood. *Child Development, 79*(5), 1257–1269.

Duncan, G. J., Dowsett, C. J., Claessens, A., Magnuson, K., Huston, A. C., Klebanov, P., et al. (2007). School readiness and later achievement. *Developmental Psychology, 43*(6), 1428–1446.

Enders, C. K. (2010). *Applied missing data analysis*. New York: Guilford Press.

Grimes, D. A., & Schulz, K. F. (2002), Bias and causal associations in observational research. *Lancet, 359*, 248–252.

Heckman, J. J. (1979). Sample selection bias as a specification error. *Econometrica, 47*(1), 153–161.

Johnston, L. D., O'Malley, P. M., Bachman, J. D., & Schulenberg, J. E. (2008). *Monitoring the Future national survey results on drug use, 1975–2007: Vol. 2. College students and adults ages 19–45* (NIH Publication No. 08-6418B). Bethesda, MD: National Institute on Drug Abuse.

Kish, L. (1957). Confidence intervals for clustered samples. *American Sociological Review, 22*(2), 154–165.

Kline, R. B. (2011). *Principles and practice of structural equation modeling* (3rd ed.). New York: Guilford Press.

Levin, B. E., Katzen, H. L., Klein, B., & Llabre, M. L. (2000). Cognitive decline affects subject attrition in longitudinal research. *Journal of Clinical and Experimental Neuropsychology, 22*(5), 580–586.

NICHD Early Child Care Research Network. (1994). Child care and child development: The NICHD Study of Early Child Care. In S. L. Friedman & H. C. Haywood (Eds.), *Developmental follow-up: Concepts, domains, and methods* (pp. 377–396). New York: Academic Press.

Preacher, K. J., Wichman, A. L., MacCallum, R. C., & Briggs, N. E. (2008). *Latent growth curve modeling*. Thousand Oaks, CA: Sage.

Siddiqui, O., Flay, B. R., & Hu, F. B. (1996). Factors affecting attrition in a longitudinal smoking prevention study. *Preventive Medicine, 25*, 554–560.

Tabachnick, B. G., & Fidell, L. S. (2007). *Using multivariate statistics* (5th ed.). Boston: Allyn & Bacon.

Widaman, K. F. (2006). III. Missing data: What to do with or without them. *Monographs of the Society for Research in Child Development, 71*(3), 42–64.

CHAPTER 10

Telemetrics and Online Data Collection

Collecting Data at a Distance

JOSHUA WILT
DAVID M. CONDON
WILLIAM REVELLE

Central Issues

Throughout history, technological advances have paved the way for scientific discovery. One of the most famous examples of this phenomenon is Galileo's telescope. By improving the Dutch invention that allowed visual perception of distant objects as if they were nearby, Galileo laid the groundwork for modern astronomy. We call attention to the ability to observe data from afar, or *telemetrics* (derived from the Greek roots *tele* = "remote" and *metron* = "measure"). Telemetric technology is exemplified by online data collection via the Internet, though that is just one of the methods available for collecting data from afar. Additional examples—many of which are increasingly integrated with Internet technology—include data collection via mobile phones and more recently developed self-tracking devices. These tools represent some of the greatest technological advances over the past 20 years. Telemetric technologies facilitate research because they allow instantaneous communication, quick exchange of data, and a high degree of interconnection among people (Birnbaum, 2004; Duffy, 2000). Furthermore, by virtue of their user-friendly interfaces, these technologies have the potential to attract large numbers of participants and thus revolutionize research on developmental theories.

Web-based research is by far the most popular telemetric method (and it receives the most attention in this chapter as a result, though several other technologies are noted as well). A rapid increase in computer literacy over the past several years has been a primary factor contributing to the growth of Web-based research. The Internet is fast becoming the communication method of choice for the young and elderly alike (*Different people*, 2004). Whereas younger individuals gravitate toward social networking sites such as Facebook, MySpace, and Twitter to keep in touch with their friends, communities, and the world, older individuals are avid users of e-mail. Young and old alike use the Internet daily for a wide variety of tasks, including school and work-related projects, checking the news and weather, paying bills, playing games, and making travel plans. The growth in general Internet usage has been accompanied by a boom in online research (Birnbaum, 2004). Utilization of the Internet for conducting research will continue to increase in popularity due to low cost and increasing ease of use (Barchard & Williams, 2008). A plethora of websites are devoted to directing participants to online studies and websites that provide resources for those interested in designing their own Web-based studies, but it is difficult and time-consuming to browse each individual site. However, we believe that the three websites in Table 10.1 have done an exemplary job of compiling comprehensive lists of the websites we consider to be most helpful for those interested in designing their own Web-based studies.

Advantages over Traditional Methods and Potential Drawbacks

In the process of opening lines of communication on a global scale, the Internet has put researchers in contact with people from all parts of the world. Many Web-based studies take advantage of this increased participant pool and are designed to collect data from a large number of participants, and millions of people around the world have participated in online psychological research. It seems that any psychological topic may be studied online on a large scale, as evidenced by the broad array of surveys, tests, and experiments listed on Web pages devoted to advertising online psychological research. We can attest to the almost unfathomable ease in obtaining participants that the Internet provides, as, over the past 8 years, we have collected in excess of 250,000 participants through our own Web-based study. Prior to the advent of online research, this volume of participation was

TABLE 10.1. Exemplary Websites That Provide Guides to Online Studies and Resources for Online Researchers

Name	Website	Description
Psychological Research on the Net	*psych.hanover.edu/research/exponnet.html*	Links to online studies divided by area and links to resources for conducting online research, such as designing surveys, creating and hosting Web experiments, and managing data collected online
Social Psychology Network	*www.socialpsychology.org/expts.htm#services*	Online studies in social psychology and personality psychology, and links to "how-to" guides, online data collection services, and software to help researchers design online studies
Online Psychology Research UK	*www.onlinepsychresearch.co.uk*	Lists of online studies, resources for developing studies, information about Web hosting and programming, and marketing online studies

likely unthinkable. In contrast to studies aimed at obtaining extremely large sample sizes, research on a smaller scale may also be conducted on the Internet. This flexibility is especially evident and advantageous for studies of select groups or hard-to-reach populations. These populations include the very elderly, physically and/or mentally disabled individuals, and individuals residing in rural locations. In fact, the ability to study such populations at all is one of the more compelling benefits of online research. Researchers should be aware, however, that the increase in overall responses may come with a decrease in the response rates of individuals enrolled in online studies (Granello & Wheaton, 2004). Along with access to a wide variety of participants come increases in the potential generalizability of results (Birnbaum, 2004). Results from online research may be able to avoid the routine caveat that the findings may be generalizable only to a small subset of the population; however, this advantage must be considered, along with the possibility that Internet users may not make up a representative sample, depending on the nature of one's investigation (Granello & Wheaton, 2004). Researchers may also be more confident in the precision of their results due to the increased statistical power of using large samples. Estimates of population parameters and effect sizes can be incredibly precise when sampling from thousands of participants.

The advantages that online research affords to the *process* of conducting research are just as compelling as those related to sampling (Ahern, 2005; Duffy, 2002). In particular, the costs of online research can be substantially reduced relative to other methods. Participants in online studies are also routinely compensated with feedback about their responses to the study instead of monetary payments. Beyond a computer and website domain, there are few material costs in running online studies. Expenses associated with hiring staff are decreased as tasks typically done by human research assistants (recruiting, running studies, data entry) are automated. However, researchers must routinely check for potential technical difficulties that could hinder these processes (Granello & Wheaton, 2004).

Data collection and entry may be completed quickly with online methods. Advertising a study is often as easy as posting a link on a Web page or sending an e-mail—a method that can be used to reach many people in a short amount of time. After participants are made aware of the study, they often respond more quickly as well; for example, on average, participants respond to mail-based surveys within months, to phone-based surveys within weeks, but to Web-based surveys within days (Granello & Wheaton, 2004). Willingness to participate in online research is boosted by potential participants' perceptions of increased anonymity. Data typically are transmitted instantaneously and stored in a form that is easily transferable to statistical packages. The ability to stay in close contact with participants is another desirable feature of online research (Gosling, Vazire, Srivastava, & John, 2004). Web pages may contain links to more information about the study. Dynamic Web pages can be designed to give feedback to participants about their responses. Follow-up is easy and nearly instantaneous via e-mail. Researchers should be aware, however, that in contrast to the ease with which participants may be contacted, those same participants may just as easily refuse to respond and thus be lost to attrition.

It is important to note that the power of online research does not preclude the need for fundamentally sound research design. Due to the sheer magnitude of potential studies and the absence of face-to-face interaction, the ability to make valid comparisons across cultures may require researchers to focus more closely on issues related to the sampling of participants, the clarity of instructions given to participants from distinct cultures, and the design of research instruments. On a more general note, the benefits of online research do not come automatically with the use of technology; they require proper use of the tools employed and consideration of the possible impact that those tools may have (Hine, 2005).

Types of Telemetric Research

A wide and growing variety of telemetric tools are available for developmental research. Among these, the Internet has certainly had the most meaningful impact to date, as even the most traditional forms of "offline" research are often facilitated by electronic communications at some point. The Internet's central role in telemetry is also likely to continue as the number of Internet-enabled devices continues to grow. In fact, it is increasingly the case that the Internet is being used in conjunction with other technologies that are used to record or access data.

The most ubiquitous telemetric tool is the mobile phone. Although the penetration rates of mobile phones that are Internet enabled has increased dramatically over recent years (Federal Communications Commission [FCC], 2010), even less expensive mobile phones can be used in a research capacity via text messaging technology (Wilt, Funkhouser, & Revelle, 2011). A unique method of telemetric research comes from the use of "electronically activated recorders" (Mehl, Vazire, Holleran, & Clark, 2010; Mehl, Vazire, Ramirez-Esparza, Slatcher, & Pennebaker, 2007), also known as the "Big EAR." These devices are digital voice recorders capable of collecting short audio recordings. Researchers who use this technology can record the sounds and conversations of participants at various intervals throughout the day in order to measure characteristics of their interactions. As these technologies and many more like them expand in functionality over the coming years, the breadth of variables that *can* be measured telemetrically will continue to expand rapidly.

In the meantime, there is a more established set of methodologies employed by developmental scientists that are well suited for use on the Internet. The most common of these include self-reports, informant reports, open-response questionnaires, observational reports, ability tests, and experiments. Because each of these methods can be and has been adapted in various ways for use online, the remainder of this section is devoted to addressing the telemetric issues related to each.

Self-Report and Informant Report

Self-report involves, quite simply, asking participants to describe themselves by responding to items or questions. Self-reports were traditionally administered as paper-and-pencil measures and now likely constitute the most popular form of online research. It is relatively straightforward to transfer self-report methodology from paper to the Internet, as no specialized personnel or materials are required. Several free sites even eliminate the need to program forms to present, score, and store the items, as well as devise a method for error checking. Researchers must still consider common pitfalls such as missing data and duplicate responses.

Important considerations must be made before administering self-reports online. First, it is necessary to evaluate the goals of the research and to select scales for measuring the constructs of interest. Here it is essential to keep the questions and format of the items as simple as possible (Wood & Griffiths, 2007). Web pages should be easy to navigate, with instructions directing participants through each section of the self-report form. Although not commonly used, computer-assisted self-interviewing (CASI) techniques may be particularly well suited to guiding participants through an online self-report questionnaire efficiently (De Leeuw, Hox, & Kef, 2003).

In addition to self-reports, researchers may also benefit by collecting the perspectives of others through informant reports. These can be used either in conjunction with self-reports as a means of increasing validity or as a substitute for self-reports when it is impossible to evaluate the subject in question. From a developmental perspective, informant reports may be especially useful for children or elderly participants with cognitive deficits. Online research methods have made the previously difficult task of obtaining informant reports relatively easy (Vazire, 2006). Typically this is done by asking participants to provide contact information for peers or family members who may best be able to rate the participant on a variety of characteristics. E-mail makes contacting informants easy and also allows the researcher to include instructions about the study and even links to the study Web pages.

Open-Response Questionnaires

Open-response questionnaires—the online equivalent of face-to-face interviews—can save both time and expense over traditional methods. Participants may find online questionnaires more attractive and convenient, as well. Whether responding on Web pages or via e-mail, this method reduces the pressure to provide quick responses (Wood & Griffiths, 2007). Participants have time to reflect more about their answers and generate richer, more accurate data. Open-response questionnaires can also be particularly beneficial for studying sensitive issues. It is likely that participants feel more anonymous and less embarrassed when responding in this manner, thereby prompting disclosure of details they may not have chosen to reveal in a traditional interview setting (Tourangeau, 2004; Whittier, Seeley, & St. Lawrence, 2004). In contrast, e-mail and instant messaging may increase spontaneity, which may be desired if it is believed to indicate more truthful or less filtered responses. Asynchronous methods may change experiences of time and space and therefore have myriad substantive effects on the resultant data. Researchers aiming to simulate traditional interview settings may rely on instant messaging programs or software that allows video interviews (e.g., Skype). Video interviews also provide access to potentially valuable behavioral and emotional information, as facial and body movements and tone of voice may be coded to supplement the interview data.

Observational Research

Observing behavior as it occurs is sometimes referred to as the gold standard of psychological methods (Funder, 2001). Although it may at first seem as if this method is not transferrable to online research, it is indeed possible to observe many social phenomena or group behavior using telemetric methods. With proper permissions, video cameras may send live streaming feeds from school classrooms, business meetings, or social gatherings back to a computer that may store video and audio data. In addition to actual behavior being recorded, social phenomena such as group behavior that occurs online may also be studied (Bos, Olson, Gergle, Olson, & Wright, 2002; Bruckman, 1999). Additionally, Internet chat rooms and bulletin boards provide a rich sample of human behavior that can be mined for studies of communication. Adding to the flexibility of online methods, participants could be given expectations or goals regarding the interaction (McKenna & Bargh, 2000).

Ability Tests

Ability tests are designed to measure how well individuals can perform in a given domain based on their ability to solve problems related to that domain. Well-known examples include the SAT and the Wechsler Adult Intelligence Scale. Although there is considerable potential for increasing sample sizes and reducing the cost of administering ability tests telemetrically, several challenges make it difficult to ascertain the validity of online ability tests that lack supervised administration. The most formidable of these challenges relates to the fact that most ability tests include a "speed" component, either by limiting the amount of time available or by taking the time to completion into account during scoring. Concerns related to timing are exacerbated by the inability to control the extent to which participants are using outside resources, such as other people or websites, to solve test items. Researchers can partially compensate for these difficulties through careful test design and programming, but these options remain inferior to supervised test administration. Another formidable challenge comes from the need to control the dissemination of ability items, as failure to do so can compromise the validity of the item. However, with the advent of computer-generated test items of known difficulties and discriminations, it is possible to address this challenge by generating very large sets of unique items (Embretson, 2004).

In addition to following the guidelines used for designing self-report assessments, online ability tests may involve audio or visual presentation of items, and thus necessitate more careful attention to browser capabilities. It is also typical for ability tests to be administered using computerized adaptive testing (CAT), which is based on item response theory and allows for more efficient testing (Embretson & Reise, 2000). CAT presents items in a response-dependent fashion and therefore may require more advanced programming capabilities. Advanced programming also may be required for researchers interested in recording information other than item responses that may serve as valid measures of ability, such as response latency, problem-solving strategies, and so forth.

Experiments

Random assignment of participants to different conditions in order to conduct "true" experiments online is relatively straightforward, though these procedures are not necessarily pursued in most online assessments. In fact, most researchers using the previously described methods are looking for relationships between variables without manipulating aspects of the study between individuals. As with traditional research, correlational methods are most fruitful when combined with experimental methods (Revelle & Oehlberg, 2008), as randomization serves to break the correlation between experimentally manipulated *independent variables* (IVs) and nonobserved but potentially *confounding variables* (CVs). Transfer of computer-based lab experiments to the Internet generally involves relatively little difficulty, though more advanced experiments may benefit from the use of specialized software applications that allow advanced graphics and more sensitive timing.

Researchers must also be aware of special circumstances that could potentially bias experimental results from online studies. It is crucial to protect against repeated participation in experimental designs (recommended safeguards are discussed in the subsection "Data Quality") and to standardize procedures and Web pages as much as possible across participants. One may also record information about the computer and browser participants are using, as well as asking about the environment in which they are taking the experiment as a means of measuring potential confounds. Familiarity with computers and the Internet, as well as computer anxiety, may be especially relevant confounds for online experiments. Interestingly, researchers do not have to worry about the confounding effects of experimenter–participant interactions. However, this advantage comes with the limitation that participants are not able to ask for immediate clarification of instructions, unless the website is equipped with a "live help" button. Inclusion of such a function would necessitate that personnel be available at all times that the survey is active. A clear, simple, and thorough presentation of instructions and an easily accessible help function are therefore mandatory. Previously mentioned CASI techniques may prove useful here.

Designing an Internet Study

There are a plethora of programming tools to choose from when deciding how to design online studies. Presenting a comprehensive list of these options is beyond the scope of this chapter, but there are a number of articles (Barchard & Williams, 2008; Birnbaum, 2004; Cantrell & Lupinacci, 2007) and an excellent handbook (Gosling & Johnson, 2010) that contain detailed lists of resources and instructions for their proper usage.

Researchers can flexibly customize their Web pages to meet the specific aims of each study. Online studies may include both static pages, which present identical information to every participant, and active pages, which can differ depending on characteristics of the users, their computers, the time of day, and so forth (Cantrell & Lupinacci, 2007). Items may be presented in a variety of ways. They may be ordered one after another on a single page, with subsets of questions on separate pages, or even as one question per page. Items do not have to be presented in the same order to each participant. With the tremendous flexibility afforded by online methods, Web-based studies will likely differ from each other greatly in terms of formatting and design, yet there are a number of principles to which all studies should adhere (Granello & Wheaton, 2004). All pages should use clearly delineated buttons and easy-to-read font; plain Web pages without color are recommended. Forms can present special problems for persons with visual impairments, especially those using screen readers; thus, all documents should be accessible to persons with disabilities (see the website *www.w3.org/WAI* for detailed instructions). Participants should also receive acknowledgment that they have finished the study shortly after completion.

Before putting the site into production, there are many steps that one should take to ensure that everything runs smoothly. Some ways to do this include (1) submitting multiple entries of the data, filling in every field on the survey; (2) downloading the data frequently to make sure it appears in the correct format; (3) trying to find errors by purposely making the system fail; and (4) observing a pilot group as they complete the study (Wyatt, 2000). Each of these steps decreases the chances that users will discover programming bugs after the study is active. As no study is perfect, it is likely that system maintenance will be necessary; if so, it is advised that researchers be careful when taking down active studies, as it is bad form to interrupt participants while they are still in the process of completing the study.

Once the study is operational, it is time to recruit participants. Researchers can allow open access to the study or restrict participation to participants who meet certain criteria—either through the use of screening questions or by sending invitations to members of the targeted population (Nosek, Banaji, & Greenwald, 2002). Deciding where and how to advertise should be guided by the goal of obtaining a sample that accurately reflects the characteristics of the desired population. One may wish to post on websites likely to be frequented by members of the population or send out e-mails to mailing lists likely to contain individuals who meet the inclusion criteria. The existence of online communities (specialized or generalized) may also help one find individuals who fit each study's specific needs (Couper, 2000). Various commercial resources may be used to identify and select samples or to post surveys to a nationally representative panel. Advertisements should include a short summary of the research proposal, outline how the results will be used, and provide details about how individuals can participate or obtain more information about the study.

Feedback

When giving participants feedback about their scores, it is important to use neutral and descriptive rather than evaluative language, as people may be sensitive to negative feedback about their abilities. As in any research study, it is a good idea to write a detailed and clear debriefing in order to decrease the chances that participants misinterpret their feedback. Researchers must also be careful not to provide feedback or advice that is beyond their professional knowledge, as they have no chance to clarify such feedback.

Conceptual Principles and Statistical Assumptions

Is Online Research Valid?

All of the advantages conferred by online research would be rendered null if it were shown that these methods had low validity. Indeed, there are still a number of potential hindrances to validity that merit consideration. Self-selection may present a large problem; for example, online intelligence tests may attract relatively intelligent individuals, and the ones who finish the test without dropping out may be even more intelligent than the average test taker (Preckel & Thiemann, 2003). Internet users in any particular study may be rather homogeneous in terms of their computer skills, their computer anxiety, and their motivation to do well. The problem of self-selection may be compounded by the tendency for individuals to drop out of online studies at a higher rate than for those conducted in the laboratory (Birnbaum, 2004). Lack of control over the environment may also hinder the validity of online research, especially for online experiments. Individuals can participate from nearly any location, whether from a quiet library on a desktop computer or a crowded party on an Internet-enabled mobile phone. They may also consult with other people and other online resources, regardless of instructions not to do so. Additionally, members of a defined population may not have equal access to the technology needed to complete the online study (Granello & Wheaton, 2004), resulting in further stratification of the obtained sample. In contrast to these potential deficits, online methods may be more valid than traditional methods in terms of obtaining representative samples and therefore more generalizable results. With its nearly unlimited reach, online research offers a way to recruit a highly diverse sample in terms of age, ethnicity, socioeconomic status, and various other demographic variables. Although the sample will likely not be as similar to the target population as it would be if representative sampling were used, it probably will be more representative than commonly used introductory psychology course and high school samples.

Empirical research on the validity of online research has been accumulating steadily. In a review of nine studies, Krantz, Dalal, and Birnbaum (2000) found that results from traditional methods and online methods show a high degree of convergence. Research on the effects of computer-based testing (CBT) and CAT showing similar results to paper-and-pencil tests also support the conversion of personality and ability tests to online versions (Clariana & Wallace, 2002). A recent study examined potential differences between Web-based and paper-and-pencil assessments when completed in freely chosen contexts (Hardre, Crowson, & Xie, 2010). Web-based studies showed a slightly higher percentage of data loss and lower overall time to complete relative to paper-and-pencil studies, whereas paper-and-pencil studies produced higher overall mean scores across measures, greater variability in responses, and higher positive affect for responding. Administration methods showed no difference on internal consistency, positive-response bias, or strength of interscale correlations. A comprehensive examination of the validity of online research was conducted by Gosling and colleagues (2004). Online samples were found to be more diverse demographically than traditional samples. Internal consistency of measures and indicators of psychological adjustment were similar to those obtained using traditional samples and similar across different online presentation formats (e.g., radio button vs. dropdown menus). It is clear that much more research is needed on the topic of validity; however, the results to this point are promising for online research.

Data Quality

Validity depends in large part on the quality of data that studies are able to obtain. Data quality is maximized when participants are able to understand items and thus provide meaningful answers. Steps that increase the probability of collecting high-quality data include the use of clear instructions, formats that are standardized and accessible to all participants (Nosek et al., 2002), and, if possible, Web pages that are designed to guide participants through the study (De Leeuw et al., 2003). Even if most participants provide meaningful data, some will answer randomly or answer all questions with the same (or only slightly different) responses. Others may withhold effort, submit duplicate forms, or lie. All of these introduce noise into the data. Researchers may take steps to reduce the chances that their data will be compromised in the face of these insidious threats. Researchers must pursue means of detecting random and duplicate data. Studies may include duplicate questions with definitive answers (e.g., When is your birthday?) to catch users who are not paying attention to the study. Detecting lies about age, location, and other demographic characteristics can be difficult, though there are options for offsetting these hazards where necessary (such as requiring participants to register through an online service that can verify their information). Researchers should also consider strategies aimed at reducing multiple entries from the same participant, such as (1) simply asking participants whether they have previously completed the study, (2) disabling "back" or "reload" buttons, and/or (3) using "cookies" when allowable. Those concerned with the time that participants are taking on each part of the study may set timers on different parts of the test, record a time stamp, or forward participants through the survey after a predetermined time (Nosek et al., 2002).

Is Online Research Ethical?

For any study, ethical research practices include protecting human subjects from physical and emotional risks, minimizing coercive features of the study, delivering adequate informed consent and debriefing, and ensuring confidentiality of data obtained from participants

(Barchard & Williams, 2008). Online research involves little or no physical risk. Emotional risks, just as with traditional research, depend on the content of each individual study. However, there are vital differences between traditional and online methods that carry significant ethical implications.

An obvious difference is that researchers are unable to be physically present during the study. The absence of a researcher may decrease social pressure to participate or remain in a study when a participant is feeling discomfort. Therefore, online studies inherently carry less risk of coercion. Lack of researcher presence may also have the beneficial effect of increasing anonymity. Indeed, researchers may ensure participant anonymity by deciding not to collect identifying information.

In contrast to the benefits previously discussed, unless the website is equipped with a "live help" button, it is difficult—if not impossible—to capture verbal and nonverbal cues from participants or to promptly answer their questions. These deficits may result in participants not receiving adequate informed consent or debriefing procedures. An additional threat to receiving adequate debriefing is that participants may decide to exit the study early. These problems should further motivate researchers to be especially careful in designing the statements of consent and debriefing. Including a "quit" button that directs participants to a debriefing page is thus recommended.

Because researchers cannot visually verify that participants are of the appropriate age to participate, they may want to institute safeguards that decrease the probability of the participation of minors: asking for participant age, advertising on sites that minors are not likely to visit, modifying the advertisement to appeal to adults, or having participants register through a service that can verify their age (Nosek et al., 2002). As no safeguard is 100% effective, researchers should also consider the potential implications should a breach of confidentiality occur for participants outside of the defined age range for the study (Barchard & Williams, 2008). As with any ethical dilemma in a research study, one should weigh the possibility and consequences of such a breach against the benefits of conducting the research.

With the new and evolving risks that online technology presents to privacy in general, it should be no surprise that risks to participant confidentiality are relatively complicated. There are at least three differences between traditional and online methods with regard to privacy that merit careful consideration. First, the line between public and private behavior is blurred on the Internet (Kraut et al., 2008). Researchers should thus be sure to inform participants of the following issues on the statement of consent: (1) whether their responses will be identifiable or anonymous, (2) which parts of the information that they provide are being stored (as well as how data will be stored), and (3) which parts of their responses will be made public or remain private. Second, data are transmitted across servers and thus may be intercepted. Some researchers may decide against collecting identifying information because programs may be able to intercept confidential information (Social Security numbers, credit card numbers, etc.) in transit (Kraut et al., 2008). It is important to note here that one may even elect not to record Internet protocol addresses because, although they do not directly identify the participant, they give location, as well as machine information (Nosek et al., 2002). If it is necessary to collect identifying information, researchers may choose to separate the times at which they obtain participant responses and identifying information. If one collects identifying information at the same time as participant responses, encryption may be used as a means to separate content from identifying information (Nosek et al., 2002). Third, because data are stored electronically, respondents should be made aware of the risks and benefits of electronic records. The risks that hackers pose make it advisable to store data offline whenever possible, as no online database can be made completely secure (Koocher, 2007). It is worth emphasizing finally that the increased risks to confidentiality necessitate that extra care be taken when researching sensitive issues (Nosek et al., 2002). Researchers interested in meeting Health Insurance Portability and Accountability Act compliance levels may purchase RedCAP and RedCAP Survey software.

Developmental Applications

The ease of communication provided by telemetric techniques facilitates tasks crucial to developmental research, such as participant recruitment (Birnbaum, 2004) and informational interactions. Online tools allow more effective and efficient interactions, which in turn allow researchers to attract participants more precisely, whether in terms of specific attributes or representativeness to the general population. With regard to data collection itself, there are some telemetric issues that are particularly relevant to developmental research, several of which are discussed next.

Collecting Data in the Natural Environment

The ability to measure variables at a distance is of considerable benefit in that it allows participants to remain in their natural environments. There are a variety of circumstances in which this flexibility is valuable. Especially in cases involving infants and young children, the ability to gather data outside of a laboratory can make participation significantly less intrusive in that it allows measurements to be taken in environments more comfortable for children and parents alike. This simultaneously reduces error and increases the flexibility to gather data at times that are conducive to the child's natural schedule. Certainly, the nature of the technology being used to gather data affects the degree to which remote data collection will be successful. In cases in which strict controls and/or specialized training are required to collect accurate measurements (as may be the case with imaging technologies, for example), it may not be feasible to collect accurate data in the natural environment without supervision by a trained researcher. But in cases in which the quality of data collection does not depend on specialized skills, such as with self-reports and open-response questionnaires, remote data collection can be an attractive alternative.

Longitudinal Research

The appeal of remote data collection is perhaps most evident with longitudinal research due to the inherent need for multiple interactions between researcher and participant. Maintaining contact with participants over time has traditionally been one of the most challenging and resource-demanding aspects of longitudinal research. By collecting some or all of the data remotely, researchers can reduce many of the costs associated with repeated measurements while simultaneously reducing the inconveniences imposed on participants. Thus it may be possible to include participants who would not otherwise be able or willing to participate due to physical or geographical constraints imposed by the need to visit the lab on a fixed schedule. A number of longitudinal studies employ online research methods to great effect, including the Study of Mathematically Precocious Youth (Lubinski & Benbow, 2006) and the Dunedin longitudinal study (Moffitt & Caspi, 2001; Moffitt, Caspi, Rutter, & Silva, 2001; Robins, Caspi, & Moffitt, 2002).

This flexibility also provides longitudinal researchers the freedom to increase the reliability and frequency of assessment. Brief longitudinal studies, such as those designed to measure diurnal effects or developmental changes over critical periods, often require participants to provide information on a specific schedule. Before the advent of remote data collection technology, researchers using time-sensitive longitudinal data were dependent on participants' honest compliance. Using more recent technologies, researchers can prompt participants to provide information automatically according to a fixed or random schedule and verify the time that the data were collected with an electronic time stamp. As discussed earlier, technologies such as the Big EAR even make it possible for researchers to collect information remotely without the participants' involvement (Mehl et al., 2007; Mehl et al., 2010).

Longitudinal studies for which the time sensitivity of data collection is less relevant, such as with longevity and life outcome studies, can still benefit from remote data collection. One of the biggest challenges to long-term longitudinal research relates to the amount of time required to produce meaningful findings (Costa & McCrae, 1992). Researchers who conduct studies spanning several years or decades invest substantial time and funding and are therefore increasingly motivated to retain participants as the study progresses. As a result, the need to minimize attrition has been a strategic factor in the organization of many prominent longitudinal studies.

Illustration

Among the many examples of online data collection in psychological research, one that is particularly illustrative of the benefits and challenges is the ongoing Synthetic Aperture Personality Assessment (SAPA) study. This procedure, which takes its name from the analogous procedure of synthetic aperture measurement in radio astronomy, allows researchers to capitalize on the large sample sizes achieved by administering surveys on the Internet. Several aspects of the SAPA design make it flexible enough for use in studying a wide variety of psychological constructs, including many germane to developmental researchers. A thorough description of SAPA can be found in Revelle, Wilt, and Rosenthal (2010). For the purposes of this illustration, discussion is focused on the origin of the items presented, the method by which the survey is constructed, and the technology used to analyze the results.

Selecting Items to Be Assessed

Although the ability to collect data from more (and more diverse) participants is a considerable benefit of online data collection, it does not sidestep the constraint that each individual participant is willing and able to respond to only a limited number of items. The SAPA procedure is designed to address this constraint, which is particularly relevant when a single construct can be measured in multiple ways (i.e., by distinct survey items or ability measures). For example, a greater number of survey items have been proposed to measure the five-factor personality model than could be reasonably administered to a single participant. Each SAPA participant is given a subset of the items related to the construct(s) being measured. One possibility might include multi-item scales aimed at measuring extraversion in conjunction with both adult and adolescent attachment measures, with age-appropriate measures of attachment being administered based on the age at which participants enter the survey. Through random rotation of the items across many participants, each possible pairing of items will be presented. In our example, the covariance matrix of several hundred items measuring extraversion and attachment can be synthetically formed even though each participant is responding only to approximately 60 items. Statistical analysis of the resulting synthetic matrix allows for evaluation of the relationship between each pair of items, as well as the higher level structure of multiple constructs (as if they were measured simultaneously). Note that the missing data in these sets due to the random rotation of items (rather than the age-dependent assignment of attachment items) are missing completely at random (MCAR), allowing for use of the same analytic techniques as would be used if the data set were complete.

Perhaps the most challenging aspect of measuring a given construct is the process of selecting the tools by which to measure it. For many of the personality constructs assessed by SAPA, this obstacle was substantially overcome by the independent development of the International Personality Item Pool (IPIP) by Lewis R. Goldberg (Goldberg et al., 2006). This pool is a repository of public-domain items designed to assess a growing array of constructs. Though the pool currently contains more than 3,100 unique items, SAPA also provides researchers the flexibility to develop and validate items of their own design.

Survey Development

Aside from selecting the appropriate measures, there are a number of important strategic considerations, including the recruitment of participants, the design of the user interface, and the logistics for data handling. For Internet-based surveys, it is generally necessary to provide some motivation in order to attract participants. In the case of SAPA, participants are motivated by the prospect of receiving a dynamically generated report describing their personalities in terms of the Big Five dimensions. The scoring for this report is based on an algorithm that compares their item responses against those of other participants of approximately the same age and gender. In addition to their scores and confidence intervals, participants are given brief textual descriptions of their placement on each dimension, which are largely adapted from prior work by John Johnson (2005). Of course, it is difficult to overstate the importance of these reports, as they represent a tacit agreement with the participant that the time spent filling out the survey will be worth his or her while. Participants are encouraged to share their results and/or a link to the survey, and their willingness to do so is, to some extent, dictated by the accuracy and utility of their score reports.

The user experience also plays an important role in the success of the survey. To that end, frequent improvements have been made to SAPA since its inception, including recent updates to improve aesthetics and increase the specificity of demographic data collected from participants. In order to maintain participant confidentiality, none of the demographic data requested can be used for identification purposes, and database access is password protected. The databases themselves, which include item responses, demographic information, and participant feedback, are regularly backed up offline.

Data Analysis

As is implied by the structure of SAPA, none of the participants provides responses to the full set of items, and, in most cases, large samples are needed in order to evaluate the stable structure of constructs based on pairwise correlations. Although these specific aspects of data collected through SAPA may be somewhat unique, it is often the case that data collected online requires powerful and flexible software for statistical analysis. The R computing environment is an excellent resource in that it offers more than 3,000 specialized statistical packages and can be downloaded for free from the Comprehensive R Archive Network (CRAN) website (R Development Core Team, 2010). The *psych* package in R is of particular relevance for researchers who are interested in analyzing synthetic correlation matrices such as those used with SAPA, as well as a variety of other psychometric functions (Revelle, 2011).

Current and Future Directions

Though well established in some respects, the adoption—and development—of online data collection techniques is still evolving rapidly. In particular, the increasing functionality and penetration of wireless technologies have led to a proliferation of portable tools capable of gathering data at the participant level and then transmitting back to the researcher via the Internet. The best and most ubiquitous example of such a tool is the mobile phone.

Mobile phones themselves are not a new technology; however, their increasing functionality for the transmission of data has affected the ways in which users interact. In 2008, for example, voice usage among mobile phone users in the United States decreased from the prior year while the rate of data usage increased dramatically, with the bulk of the growth related to text messaging (FCC, 2010). Particularly among younger populations, penetration rates for text messaging are now quite high (FCC, 2010), and a growing number of researchers have begun adapting their methods to take advantage of this technology.

Of course, there are several ways in which text messaging studies are distinct from "computer-based" research. Prior to the recent introduction of "smartphones" (which offer computer-like functionality in a mobile handheld device), text messaging studies were distinguished by being more portable than studies that required a computer and an Internet connection. Smartphone adoption has been rapid in recent years (FCC, 2010), but studies that are dependent on such technology are more subject to sample biases because smartphones are more expensive than traditional mobile phones with text messaging capability.

Text messaging studies also differ in terms of user experience. Text messages are limited in length to 160 characters, and, on phones without full keyboards, multiple button taps are required in order to input each letter. These limitations require researchers to develop questions and tasks that can be communicated briefly and answered with short responses. Likert-type items and multiple-choice items are ideal. One recent example of text messaging–based research (Wilt et al., 2011) relied on the distribution of items to participants in advance. In this particular case, each participant was given a preprinted card with items intended to measure experiences in real time at fixed intervals (every 3 hours) by asking about moods and current activities. Researchers interacted with participants largely through the use of automated e-mails received by participants as text messages. In this way, initial instructions and automatically generated reminders could be sent out at the precisely designated intervals. Participants sent their responses via text message to an e-mail inbox for later data analysis (Wilt et al., 2011). These data collection strategies allowed participants to quickly and discreetly respond to the questionnaires in a way that was minimally disruptive to their current activities.

Text messaging offers several advantages over more traditional methods for measuring experiential data. Relative to paper-and-pencil diaries, text messaging is both more accurate and more efficient. Researchers can be assured that responses are given at the designated time, and the responses can be logged with considerably less effort for both the researcher and the participant. Relative to the use of personal digital assistants (PDAs) and/or other specialized technologies, text messaging is more familiar and generally less expensive (Steeh, Buskirk, & Callegaro, 2007; Wilt et al., 2011). Unless face-to-face interaction between the researcher and participants is required, text messaging studies also provide an effective means of interacting with participants from diverse locations. Among the challenges to consider before embarking on a text messaging study, researchers must evaluate whether the technology is appropriate for the targeted population and how they plan to recruit cooperative participants.

Beyond text messaging, there are a variety of emergent technologies with potential for widespread use among researchers, including several related to the nascent field of personal informatics. This field, also known as self-tracking, is fueled by individuals who collect—and in many cases analyze—important information about their own lives for a wide variety of purposes. Though the specific rationale for self-tracking varies from one person to the next, it is typically motivated by the desire to improve or maintain aspects of one's health, finances, productivity, or interpersonal relations (Li, Dey, & Forlizzi, 2010). Broadly interpreted, this includes the widespread use of social networking services (such as Facebook and Twitter) on which individuals can broadcast their feelings, thoughts, activities, and desires in unlimited detail.

Personal informatics also includes the more precise ways in which individuals are taking measure of their own lives. Owing in large part to the decreasing size and increasing sophistication of electronic circuitry, practically all types of "everyday" accessories (including shoes, jewelry, eyeglasses, and even clothing) are now being transformed into wearable wireless measurement tools (Goodwin, Velicer, & Intille, 2008). In biological terms, the list of commonly self-tracked measures already includes caloric intake, body weight, the dosage and side effects of medications, and time spent sleeping (Li et al., 2010). As it becomes more cost effective to collect and remotely transmit more involved biological measures (such as the presence of exogenous and endogenous substances in the skin or bloodstream), these factors will be added to the list. In terms of behavior, a number of extant tools and services facilitate the tracking of an individual's movements (through global positioning system [GPS] trackers and accelerometers in mobile phones) (Goodwin et al., 2008), spending habits (via electronic bank statements and financial software) (Li et al., 2010), personal correspondence (by e-mail and phone records), and productivity (through the use of specialized computer software programs). Each of these tools offers the potential to measure individuals with an amazing degree of precision. Although few people are motivated to analyze their own lives in such detail, the technology for doing so already exists. To the extent that people are comfortable with the complicated issue of sharing this information, the personal informatics field offers tremendous research opportunities.

More generally, the future of online data collection is likely to bring continued expansion across a broad variety of technologies. As the number and type of electronic devices connected to the Internet increase, the distinction between data collected online and offline will decrease. Although traditional paper-and-pencil measures are not yet near extinction, the need for such measures will dwindle as new technologies such as touch-screen computers facilitate their migration online. However, increased connectivity will not eliminate the primary obstacles to good research, nor will the resultant efficiency and affordability substitute for fundamentally sound research designs. To the contrary, the likelihood that researchers will soon be capable of collecting staggeringly large amounts of data makes ethical conduct among the research community all the more imperative. It also highlights the need for ongoing development of data analytic skills and tools capable of organizing and interpreting enormous data sets. The future of online data collection techniques is limited only by the innovations of those who employ them.

References

Ahern, N. R. (2005). Using the Internet to conduct research. *Nurse Researcher, 13*(2), 55.

Barchard, K. A., & Williams, J. (2008). Practical advice for conducting ethical online experiments and questionnaires for United States psychologists. *Behavior Research Methods, 40*(4), 1111–1128.

Birnbaum, M. H. (2004). Human research and data collection via the Internet. *Annual Review of Psychology, 55*, 803–832.

Bos, N., Olson, J., Gergle, D., Olson, G., & Wright, Z. (2002). Effects of four computer-mediated communications channels on trust development. In *Sigchi Conference on Human Factors in Computing Systems: Changing our world, changing ourselves* (p. 140). Minneapolis, MN: Association for Computing Machinery.

Bruckman, A. (1999). The day after net day: Approaches to educational use of the Internet. *Convergence, 5*(1), 24.

Cantrell, M. A., & Lupinacci, P. (2007). Methodological issues in online data collection. *Journal of Advanced Nursing, 60*(5), 544–549.

Clariana, R., & Wallace, P. (2002). Paper-based versus computer-based assessment: Key factors associated with the test mode effect. *British Journal of Educational Technology, 33*(5), 593–602.

Costa, P., & McCrae, R. R. (1992). Multiple uses for longitudinal personality data. *European Journal of Personality, 6*(2), 85–102.

Couper, M. P. (2000). Review: Web surveys: A review of issues and approaches. *Public Opinion Quarterly, 64*(4), 464.

De Leeuw, E., Hox, J., & Kef, S. (2003). Computer-assisted self-interviewing tailored for special populations and topics. *Field Methods, 15*(3), 223–251.

Different people use the Internet in different ways. (2004). Available at *www.infoplease.com/ipa/A0931238.html*.

Duffy, M. (2000). Web-based research: An innovative method for nursing research. *Journal of Canadian Oncology Nursing, 10*(2), 45.

Duffy, M. E. (2002). Methodological issues in Web-based research. *Journal of Nursing Scholarship, 34*(1), 83–88.

Embretson, S. E. (2004). The second century of ability testing: Some predictions and speculations. *Measurement: Interdisciplinary Research and Perspective, 2*(1), 1–32.

Embretson, S. E., & Reise, S. P. (2000). *Item response theory for psychologists*. Mahwah, NJ: Erlbaum.

Federal Communications Commission. (2010). Fourteenth annual report on mobile wireless competition (Technical Report). Washington, DC: Author. Available from *www.fcc.gov/14report.pdf*.

Funder, D. C. (2001). Personality. *Annual Review of Psychology, 52*, 197–221.

Goldberg, L. R., Johnson, J. A., Eber, H. W., Hogan, R., Ashton, M. C., Cloninger, C. R., et al. (2006). The international personality item pool and the future of public-domain personality measures. *Journal of Research in Personality, 40*(1), 84–96.

Goodwin, M. S., Velicer, W. F., & Intille, S. S. (2008). Telemetric monitoring in the behavior sciences. *Behavior Research Methods, 40*(1), 328–341.

Gosling, S. D., & Johnson, J. A. (Eds.). (2010). *Advanced methods for conducting online behavioral research*. Washington, DC: American Psychological Association.

Gosling, S. D., Vazire, S., Srivastava, S., & John, O. P. (2004). Should we trust Web-based studies? A comparative analysis of six preconceptions about Internet questionnaires. *American Psychologist, 59*(2), 93–104.

Granello, D. H., & Wheaton, J. E. (2004). Online data collection: Strategies for research. *Journal of Counseling and Development, 82*(4), 387–393.

Hardre, P. L., Crowson, H. M., & Xie, K. (2010). Differential effects of Web-based and paper-based administration of questionnaire research instruments in authentic contexts-of-use. *Journal of Educational Computing Research, 42*(1), 103–133.

Hine, C. (2005). *Virtual methods: Issues in social research on the Internet*. Oxford, UK: Berg.

Johnson, J. A. (2005). Ascertaining the validity of individual protocols from Web-based personality inventories. *Journal of Research in Personality, 39*(1), 103–129.

Koocher, G. P. (2007). Twenty-first century ethical challenges for psychology. *American Psychologist, 62*(5), 375–384.

Krantz, J. H., Dalal, R., & Birnbaum, M. H. (2000). Validity of Web-based psychological research. In M. H. Birnbaum (Ed.), *Psychological experiments on the Internet* (pp. 35–60). San Diego, CA: Academic Press.

Kraut, R., Olson, J., Banaji, M., Bruckman, A., Cohen, J., Couper, M., et al. (2008). Psychological research online: Report of Board of Scientific Affairs' advisory group on the conduct of research on the internet. In D. N. Bersoff (Ed.), *Ethical conflicts in psychology* (4th ed., pp. 426–433). Washington, DC: American Psychological Association.

Li, I., Dey, A., & Forlizzi, J. (2010). A stage-based model of personal informatics systems. *Chi 2010*, pp. 557–566.

Lubinski, D., & Benbow, C. P. (2006). Study of mathematically precocious youth after 35 years: Uncovering antecedents for the development of math–science expertise. *Perspectives on Psychological Science, 1*(4), 316–345.

McKenna, K. Y. A., & Bargh, J. A. (2000). Plan 9 from cyberspace: The implications of the Internet for personality and social psychology. *Personality and Social Psychology Review, 4*(1), 57–75.

Mehl, M. R., Vazire, S., Holleran, S. E., & Clark, C. S. (2010). Eavesdropping on happiness. *Psychological Science, 21*(4), 539–541.

Mehl, M. R., Vazire, S., Ramirez-Esparza, N., Slatcher, R. B., & Pennebaker, J. W. (2007). Are women really more talkative than men? *Science, 317*, 82.

Moffitt, T. E., & Caspi, A. (2001). Childhood predictors differentiate life-course persistent and adolescence-limited antisocial pathways among males and females. *Development and Psychopathology, 13*(02), 355–375.

Moffitt, T. E., Caspi, A., Rutter, M., & Silva, P. A. (2001). *Sex differences in antisocial behavior: Conduct disorder, delinquency, and violence in the Dunedin longitudinal study*. Cambridge, UK: Cambridge University Press.

Nosek, B. A., Banaji, M. R., & Greenwald, A. G. (2002). E-research: Ethics, security, design, and control in psychological research on the Internet. *Journal of Social Issues, 58*(1), 161–176.

Preckel, F., & Thiemann, H. (2003). Online- versus paper–pencil version of a high potential intelligence test. *Swiss Journal of Psychology, 62*(2), 131–138.

R Development Core Team. (2010). *R: A language and environment for statistical computing* [Computer software manual]. Vienna, Austria: Author.

Revelle, W. (2011). *Procedures for psychological, psychometric, and personality research* [Computer software manual]. Available at *personality-project.org/r/psych.manual.pdf* (R package version 1.1.09).

Revelle, W., & Oehlberg, K. (2008). Integrating experimental and observational personality research: The contributions of Hans Eysenck. *Journal of Personality, 76*(6), 1387–1414.

Revelle, W., Wilt, J., & Rosenthal, A. (2010). Individual differences in cognition: New methods for examining the personality–cognition link. In A. Gruszka, G. Matthews, & B. Szymura (Eds.), *Handbook of individual differences in cognition: Attention, memory and executive control* (pp. 27–49). New York: Springer.

Robins, R. W., Caspi, A., & Moffitt, T. E. (2002). It's not just who you're with, it's who you are: Personality and relationship experiences across multiple relationships. *Journal of Personality, 70*(6), 925–964.

Steeh, C., Buskirk, T. D., & Callegaro, M. (2007). Using text messages in U.S. mobile phone surveys. *Field Methods, 19*(1), 59–75.

Tourangeau, R. (2004). Survey research and societal change. *Annual Review of Psychology, 55*, 775–801.

Vazire, S. (2006). Informant reports: A cheap, fast, and easy method for personality assessment. *Journal of Research in Personality, 40*(5), 472–481.

Whittier, D. K., Seeley, S., & St. Lawrence, J. S. (2004). A comparison of Web- with paper-based surveys of gay and bisexual men who vacationed in a gay resort community. *AIDS Education and Prevention, 16*(5), 476–485.

Wilt, J., Funkhouser, K., & Revelle, W. (2011). The dynamic relationships of affective synchrony to perceptions of situations and personality states. *Journal of Research in Personality, 45*(3), 309–321.

Wood, R. T. A., & Griffiths, M. D. (2007). Online data collection from gamblers: Methodological issues. *International Journal of Mental Health and Addiction, 5*(2), 151–163.

Wyatt, J. C. (2000). When to use Web-based surveys. *Journal of the American Medical Informatics Association, 7*(4), 426.

CHAPTER 11

Collecting and Analyzing Longitudinal Diary Data

BERNHARD SCHMITZ
JULIA KLUG
SILKE HERTEL

Developmental scientists aim to describe and explain, as well as predict, the effects and interference of, intraindividual variations in the behavior and experience of humans and interindividual differences within these variations. The focus on ontogenetic development over the lifespan, as well as the aim to learn more about changes over time, requires systematic longitudinal data collection. This promotes the use of diaries that deliver time series data for data collection. Diaries are a flexible instrument; they can be used to collect data on a broad set of variables. Observations can be accomplished by the subject of him- or herself (self-observation) or, in research focusing on infants and young children, by close others, mostly parents, participating in the situation (participant observation).

Diaries as an approach to data collection have a long tradition in developmental research. Very famous are the diary records of Wilhelm Preyer (1882), Jean Piaget (1936), Stern and Stern (1907), and Stern (1914) who observed and documented their own children's development. Many of those early approaches to the collection of data on lifespan developmental processes are still important today. Already at that time, it was recognized that cross-sectional data were not sufficient to investigate developmental processes. The choice of the diary as a method of data collection promoted longitudinal approaches.

Building on early approaches to diary-based data collection, process research allows systematic investigation of development. Early diary data collection was not systematic in terms of time lags between observations and was not standardized in terms of what was observed, how the data were collected (e.g., written notes), or who the observers were (e.g., parents and close relatives introduce observation bias). Observations were not embedded in a theoretical framework of children's development. Finally, most of the observations were single case studies that did not allow for generalization. Nowadays, diary data collection in research settings must be conducted to allow statistical analyses of the data. Diaries should be standardized in terms of the aspects that are observed, the time lags between the observations, and the way the data are collected.

Conceptual Principles and Statistical Assumptions

Standardized diaries provide us with time series data that are amenable to sophisticated designs and statistical analyses. Schmitz (1989, p. 1) defines a time series as a sequence of measurements of one or more variables in consecutive points of time. Shadish et al. (2002) recommend 100 measurement points, but in special cases with specific research questions, results from a shorter period of time are sufficient. A big advantage of diary data is that they are gathered in real-life situations, so they have high external validity (Hertel, Klug, & Schmitz, 2010).

Diary research must be planned thoroughly. First, there needs to be a theoretical background, which leads to the central questions addressed in the diary. Second, the target group needs to be specified. The investigator must determine whether the target shall work on his or her own diary or whether the work on the diary will be done by a participant observant (e.g., a parent). Third, the time period within which the diary shall be completed and the frequency of entry need to be fixed. Fourth, the format must be selected. Options include using an open format in which participants reflect on what they have done or a standardized or partly standardized format in which questions and answers are provided. The advantage of structured diaries with forced-choice questions and answers lies in their ease of analysis and interpretation. If a standardized version is chosen, the items need to be formulated as states because trait measures are assumed to be stable. Finally, a study design needs to be chosen, which leads to different ways of analyzing the gathered process data. In the following section, we address some statistical assumptions before we give examples of developmental applications and ways of analyzing time series data gathered from diaries.

Statistical Assumptions

Different measures of data quality can be computed for time series data. It is of importance that quality measures, which are normally calculated for samples, are calculated for individuals. Consider this example of diary measures for positive affect. One needs data from different observers to assess objectivity. In the case of positive affect, diary data are collected about a couple for a period of 50 days. Each day, a man and a woman living together work on the Positive and Negative Affect Scale (PANAS; Watson, Clark, & Tellegen, 1988). The man evaluates his own positive affect, and the woman rates the positive affect of the man. Correlating these measures gives an indicator of objectivity for the individual. On the basis of the man's positive affect diary data, one could calculate Cronbach's alpha for this individual's internal consistency. Regarding individual retest reliability, one could correlate the positive affect measure for odd days with that on even days for this individual. Similarly, one could divide the observation period into two equal parts, days 1–25 and days 26–50, and correlate positive affect on the 1st, 2nd, and 3rd days with the related measures on the 26th, 27th, and 28th days, and so on.

If one is interested in the validity of the measurement of this man's positive affect, one could ask him to work on the PANAS and another daily measure of positive affect, for example, a graphical analog scale with extreme labels reaching from 1, "no positive affect," to 100, "very high positive affect." Daily PANAS values can be correlated with graphical analog values. Based on the daily PANAS, individual factor analyses can also be conducted (Cattell, 1951).

In a sample of individuals, the quality indicators can be calculated for each individual separately. For instance, one could compute Cronbach's alpha for each individual and look at the distribution of these characteristics. If some individual alphas are low, these individuals could be eliminated from further analyses. This is a powerful method to control the quality of the data for the whole sample. In addition to evaluating the distribution of the individual quality criteria, one could aggregate these values by certain kinds of averaging (e.g., weighted mean). One important way to aggregate time series data is accomplished by the chain technique following Cattell (1951).

The analysis of individuals' courses is an advantage of time series data gathered with diaries. Especially in the study of development, single cases are often of interest. Schmitz (2006), discussing nomothetical and idiographic approaches, points out that it is not possible to draw conclusions about an individual from a sample. He illustrates the problem of aggregation for a bivariate process with a vivid numeric example that shows the difference between cross-sectional (interindividual) and process (intraindividual) relations between two variables.

Consider Table 11.1. In column 1, the data of two variables (positive affect and understanding) provided by four individuals on one occasion are presented. Computing the

TABLE 11.1 Hypothetical Example Regarding the Relation between Intra- and Interindividual Correlation for Positive Affect and Understanding

		Occasions					
Subject	Variables	1	2	3	4	Mean across time	Intraindividual correlation
1	Positive affect	120	120	101	99	110	–1.0
	Understanding	101	99	120	120	110	
2	Positive affect	120	120	99	101	110	–1.0
	Understanding	99	101	120	120	110	
3	Positive affect	80	80	99	101	90	–1.0
	Understanding	99	101	80	80	90	
4	Positive affect	80	80	101	99	90	–1.0
	Understanding	101	99	80	80	90	
	Correlations of means (aggregated across time) +1.0						
Aggregated across individuals							
	Positive affect	100	100	100	100		
	Understanding	100	100	100	100		
One-occasion cross-sectional correlation		.00	.00	.00	.00	.00[a]	

[a]Mean of one-occasion cross-sectional correlation.

correlation between the two variables yields a coefficient of .0. This is the cross-sectional correlation for occasion 1. The cross-sectional correlation for occasion 2 is computed similarly to occasion 1 and also yields a coefficient of .0, as do the cross-sectional correlations of occasions 3 and 4. Obviously, the cross-sectional correlation for the four occasions is identical (.0). From a process (intraindividual) perspective, in row 1 the data for two variables (positive affect and understanding) are displayed for subject 1 over four occasions. Computing the correlation for this individual over time yields a coefficient of –1.0. The same procedure for subjects 2, 3, and 4 leads to a process (intraindividual) correlation of –1.0. Again, all correlations are equal (–1.0). This example shows that all interindividual correlations are the same, all intraindividual correlations are the same, but inter- and intraindividual correlations differ strongly. Hence, these two kinds of correlations are conceptually different, refer to different ways of collecting data, and can have completely different numerical values.

Nevertheless, by using diary data, the course of individual development can be examined without loss of meaningfulness. Developmental processes can be described more precisely due to the great number of measurements, even in individual cases, and even inferential statistics can be calculated for individual cases (Schmitz, 1990). What information can we get out of an individual's trajectory? Schmitz (2006) describes several questions that can be answered by analyzing an individual's course: Is the development continuous or discontinuous? If it is discontinuous, are there one or more jumps? Are there plateaus or drawbacks? Does development follow a linear, quadratic, or cubic trend? Is development characterized by high or low variability? Are there phases of different quality in development? Does the course show regularity or rhythm (e.g., daily, weekly, yearly)? All of these questions can be answered by looking at the trajectory of a single individual. Furthermore, the relation between the courses of two or more variables in an individual can be analyzed. Using autocorrelations, correlations, and cross-correlations can tell us if there are synchronous or lagged relations in or between variables. Equally, the relation between the courses of two or more variables can be analyzed.

Developmental Applications

The deficits of cross-sectional designs in studying development are commonly known. Human development can be conceptualized as a process, which can be approximated best by process analyses (e.g., time series analysis). Diaries are best suited to measure changes that occur over a relatively short period of time, given that the diary is completed regularly. Diaries can be applied in every age group, to cover the whole lifespan.

It is possible to measure cognitive and emotional development, as well as the development of morals or the development of language, with the help of diaries. A child can work on a diary, or parents can reflect on their observations of the child in a diary. The time courses of the observed variables can then be analyzed using such methods as trend analysis and spectral analysis. With the help of trend analyses, the presence of a linear trend can be tested. A simple linear regression is estimated whereby the points of measurement serve as predictors. A linear trend can be positive or negative. In addition to linear trends, the data can be tested for the presence of polynomial trends such as quadratic or cubic ones. There could be a weekly rhythm (e.g., for tiredness), which is always at its peak on weekends. In the plot of spectral analysis, you might find this peak on day 7.

As Shapiro and Cole (1999) point out in their overview article, "self monitoring is viewed as both an assessment tool and an intervention technique" (p. 448). Using diaries not only helps to measure developmental processes and to gather time series data, but it also fosters specific desired behavior. Working on diaries is a form of self-monitoring that can lead to a reactivity effect (Korotitsch & Nelson-Gray, 1999). Reactivity effects can be desirable, but they can also introduce bias such that the original behavior cannot be measured properly. It is important to consider the possibility of reactivity effects when collecting data with diaries.

Children are not the only targets of diary research. Sliwinski, Almeida, Smyth, and Stawski (2009), for example, examined intraindividual change and variability in the within-person coupling of daily stress and negative affect using diary data from adults. They examined the bivariate relations between variables over time using multiple regression analysis. In this case, cross-correlations and multivariate autoregressive integrated moving average (ARIMA) models would also have been a suitable method of analysis. ARIMA models are fitted to time series data to better understand the data or to predict future points in the series (forecasting). If the data show nonstationarity at the beginning, a differentiating step is needed, in which linear trends are detected and eliminated. This is the integration step. The residuals can be further analyzed for autoregressive processes. Using means of values of earlier points in time, the values of later points in time can be predicted. Additionally, a time series may be checked for moving average processes. The latter usually includes a linear regression of the current value of the series against previous (unobserved) white noise error terms or random shocks.

Multivariate time series analyses address two or more variables for which process data are available. Similarities in the courses of the two variables can be studied. For example, Valiente, Fabes, Eisenberg, and Spinrad (2004) examined the relations between parents' expression of emotion and children's daily stress, measured with diaries.

Multivariate time series analyses can also be conducted with two intraindividual variables. It is well known that correlations do not allow causal interpretation. Applied to time series, cross-correlation refers to a relation between two time courses (Schmitz, Klug, & Schmidt, 2011). By using cross-correlations, it is possible to detect dynamic interactions and thereby discover references to the direction of causality. The assumption is that what happens earlier in time can have an effect on what happens later. Lagged cross-correlations can be used to provide references of causality due to temporal sequence. To illustrate a dynamic interaction, consider the example of the intraindividual relation between a child's ability to cope with stress and his or her ability to concentrate on tasks. Figure 11.1 shows the possible cause–effect relations schematically.

If the ability to cope with stress at time t predicts the ability to concentrate at time t + 1, a temporal sequence is demonstrated, and it seems plausible that coping causally contributes to concentration. Although the causal interpretation of time-lagged relations is often correct, time lag does not necessarily prove causality. Schmitz (1989) discussed the issue of time-lagged relations and causality in detail.

The ϕ coefficients in Figure 11.1 represent the time-lagged path coefficients of the bivariate process. The phi coefficient is a measure of association of two binary variables. It is similar to the Pearson correlation coefficient in its interpretation, but it does not range from –1 to +1. Its maximum value is determined by the distribution of the two variables. By estimating the ϕ parameters, the investigator can describe how the dynamic system works (Schmitz, 2006).

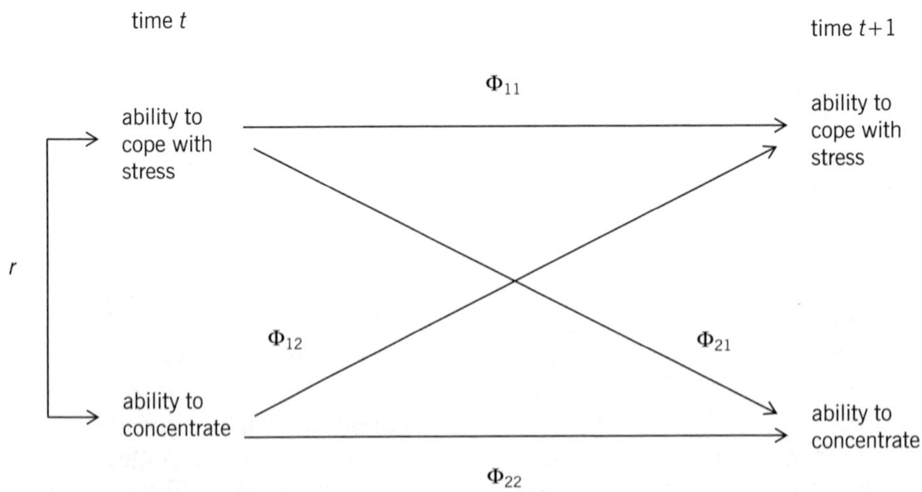

FIGURE 11.1. Schematic diagram of the dynamic interaction between a child's ability to cope with stress and his or her ability to concentrate on tasks.

Figure 11.2 shows the possible resulting ϕ matrices, which can be interpreted as follows. The parameters ϕ_{11} and ϕ_{22} give information about the autocorrelations in a single time series. For example, if ϕ_{11} was significantly positive, then earlier ability to cope with stress would influence the ability to cope with stress later. The parameters ϕ_{12} and ϕ_{21} give information about the time-lagged dynamic interactions of the two time series. ϕ_{12} shows the effect of the ability to concentrate on the ability to cope with stress, whereas ϕ_{21} denotes the effect of the ability to cope with stress on the ability to concentrate. The synchronous correlation *r* does not provide information about the cause–effect relation. For further information on ARIMA models, see Schmitz (1987).

Most diary studies are, by definition, longitudinal designs. Another aspect to consider is whether one is interested in changes in the original course due to maturation or changes fostered by an intervention. Most analytical methods apply to both cases. One exception is

$$\begin{bmatrix} 0 & 0 \\ 0 & 0 \end{bmatrix}$$

white noise

$$\begin{bmatrix} \phi_{11} & 0 \\ 0 & \phi_{22} \end{bmatrix}$$

just autocorrelations

$$\begin{bmatrix} \cdots & \phi_{12} \\ 0 & \cdots \end{bmatrix}$$

causal relation 2→1

$$\begin{bmatrix} \cdots & 0 \\ \phi_{21} & \cdots \end{bmatrix}$$

causal relation 1→2

$$\begin{bmatrix} \cdots & \phi_{12} \\ \phi_{21} & \cdots \end{bmatrix}$$

feedback

FIGURE 11.2. Phi matrices.

the interrupted time series analysis, which is unique to intervention studies. The "interrupted time-series design is one of the most effective and powerful of all quasi-experimental designs . . . it is a particularly strong quasi-experimental alternative to randomized designs" (Shadish, Cook, & Campbell, 2002). The interrupted time series design can assess treatment effects. At the point in time at which an intervention takes place, the time series should show an interruption. That means that there should be a break in the former course of measured values, for example, an abrupt rise after an intervention. This interruption can appear in different forms, permanence and immediacy.

Two exemplary interrupted time series designs are (1) the simple interrupted time series design and (2) the time series design with a no-treatment control group. A simple interrupted time series design consists of a number of consecutive measurements within one group before and after an intervention takes place. O_1 to O_5 represent the measurements before the intervention, X stands for the intervention, and O_6 to O_{10} represent the measurements after the intervention took place.

Baseline measurements					Intervention	Post measurements				
O_1	O_2	O_3	O_4	O_5	X	O_6	O_7	O_8	O_9	O_{10}

Imagine a group of children who have learning difficulties studying at home. Using a learning diary, their daily study routines are measured (baseline measurements). After several weeks they take part in a training program for students, which is designed to foster self-regulated learning. The contents of the training might include structuring homework, organizing the study environment, using adequate learning strategies, and monitoring the learning process. These variables represent the intervention. After the training, daily routines continue to be measured with the learning diary for several weeks (post measurements). Daily learning routines should change in a positive way after taking part in the training, with an increase in positive learning routines in the post measurement period in contrast to the baseline measurement period.

Meanwhile, events that cannot be controlled pose a threat to the internal validity of simple interrupted time series designs. When this happens, a change in the measurement phase is due not to the intervention but to other things that happened in the meantime (e.g., maturation). Other sources of internal validity threats are the systematic loss of participants, a change in the instruments used, and a reactivity effect due to working with the same instruments over a period of time (Shadish et al., 2002).

Adding a no-treatment control group to the interrupted time series design helps to avoid some of these threats. Hence, data from the experimental group, which received the treatment, can be compared with data from the control group, which did not receive the treatment. In each group, baseline data and post intervention data are collected.

	Baseline measurements					Intervention	Post measurements				
EG	O_1	O_2	O_3	O_4	O_5	X	O_6	O_7	O_8	O_9	O_{10}
CG	O_1	O_2	O_3	O_4	O_5	—	O_6	O_7	O_8	O_9	O_{10}

EG stands for the experimental group, whereas CG stands for the control group.

To continue with the former example, another group of children with learning difficulties is added. This new group also works on a learning diary for the whole time, but with one difference: They do not participate in the training on self-regulated learning. Their improvement can then be compared with the improvement of the training group. The interrupted time series design with control group is one of the most valid quasi-experimental designs.

What information do we get from interrupted time series studies? Interrupted time series analysis provides answers to questions about *whether* an intervention works and *how* an intervention works (see Yaffee & McGee, 2000). Intervention effects can be examined either for an individual or for an aggregated sample. If the intervention is effective, the values of the dependent variable show a change in the designated direction. Interventions can lead to such effects as (1) a change in level or intercept; (2) a change in drift, trend, or slope; (3) continuous or discontinuous effects, which describe whether the effect persists over time; and (4) immediate or delayed effects (Shadish, Cook, & Campbell, 2002).

In the following section, we take a more detailed look at two studies that used diaries and time series analysis in developmental research. Some of the presented methods are applied in interrupted time series designs.

Illustration

The following examples are drawn from a series of studies dealing with self-regulated learning. Self-regulated learning is central to lifelong learning (Bolhuis, 2003). The overall development of self-regulation is conceptualized as a linear trend. Among the most important theoretical topics discussed with respect to self-regulated learning are the questions of whether and how it can be enhanced effectively by interventions and whether and how the components of self-regulated learning are interrelated. Examples presented here integrate two perspectives. One is designed to give answers to theoretical questions, and the other is designed to demonstrate applications of powerful methods of analyses based on diary data. There are three detailed research questions. First, is it possible to enhance special components of self-regulated learning for students by step-by-step training of these single components? Second, is training for students with respect to a group of components of self-regulated learning able to change overall self-regulation? The third question deals with the dynamic relations between important components of self-regulation: Are there time-lagged relations between components?

The diaries all have a similar outline and were adapted with respect to the age of the students. As an example, we describe one standardized diary for students in grade 5. The diary for fifth graders is a short version of a longer form given to eighth graders (Perels, Gürtler, & Schmitz, 2005). For a similar version for university students, see Schmitz and Wiese (2006). The diary was applied in an intervention study in which training was presented to parents and fifth-grade children to enhance the child's self-regulated learning and problem solving. The evaluation of the training was performed by an experimental–control group pre–post comparison. We also conducted a process evaluation based on time series analyses of diary data, which we focus on here.

The diary has origins in our process model of self-regulation (Schmitz & Wiese, 2006). Details on the diary are provided in Appendix 11.1. The diary addresses student homework. Students completed the diary before doing homework and after finishing homework. The diary functions as a data collection technique. In some studies it can also function as a kind of self-monitoring instrument, which means that the questions in the diary could stimulate self-reflection processes that can change behavior. In the prehomework part of the diary, students were asked for the current time and day and to list a goal for the week. In addition, the diary asked for actions to be taken to reach that goal. If there is no homework to be done that day, the diary asks for a reason. Affect before learning is measured with items for positive and negative affect. The next questions concern the subjects for which homework has to be done. These are followed by questions about the phase before learning with respect to planning, fun in learning, and self-efficacy.

Next, the student has time to do the homework without being interrupted by questions. Students who interrupt their homework are asked for the reason and for what would motivate resumed learning. When finished, the student is asked about which subjects he or she did homework for, how much time was needed, and how much of that time involved concentration. Then the student reports about the strategies applied. After homework is finished, the diary asks whether the student applied the following strategies during learning: volition, motivation, effort, self-monitoring, concentration, and help seeking. Regarding behavior after learning, the following topics were measured: reaching the goal, approximating the weekly goal, whether learning was fun, and satisfaction with the learning result. Positive and negative affect were measured in the same way as before the learning. Finally, an open-ended question addresses the actions intended to be done the next day.

Is it possible to enhance special components of self-regulated learning for students by step-by-step training of these single components? Data stem from a study by Schmidt, Perels, and Schmitz (2010), which contains more details. In this study a training to enhance self-regulated learning is presented. Participants were 84 fifth-grade students in a German secondary school (Gymnasium). There were three different training groups: a control group that received no training ($N = 40$), a group in which only the students received training ($N = 22$), and a group in which both students and parents were trained ($N = 22$). The students worked with the diaries for a period of 70 days. Data were excluded if fewer than three items were answered, if no reasons were given for not answering the main part of questions, or if diaries were not returned at all. In sum, 729 (22.2%) diaries had to be excluded, and 2,351 diaries could be analyzed. The training was presented in weekly sessions. The training dealt with important aspects of self-regulated learning. In the learning diary of the students, the overall scale Self-Regulation (7 items) measures the components planning, motivation, volition (3 items), and self-monitoring (2 items). The internal reliability of the overall Self-Regulation scale was satisfactory ($\alpha = .78$). Split-half reliability (odd–even coefficient) was high ($r = .91, p < .00$). By means of the diary data, we were able to conduct a process evaluation with the help of time series analyses. Trend analyses were computed. Figure 11.3 shows the significant linear trend for the overall Self-Regulation scale for students ($b_0 = 3.18$, $b_1 = .005$, $p < .00$). In the course of the training sessions, the students' self-regulated learning increased steadily.

In a similar study (Schmitz & Wiese, 2006), we instructed university students in self-regulated learning in a series of weekly sessions. The topics included avoiding procrastination as an important part of volitional strategies. Students in the intervention group also worked with standardized diaries. It was intended to test the effect of the single training session dealing with procrastination (presented on day 14) by comparing the procrastination variable measured in the diary before the intervention (baseline) and after the intervention. The results of the interrupted time series analysis showed that training on the topic of procrastination had significant effects (see Figure 11.4): Procrastination decreased by .40 after the training session was introduced. In a similar way, the effects of other training contents

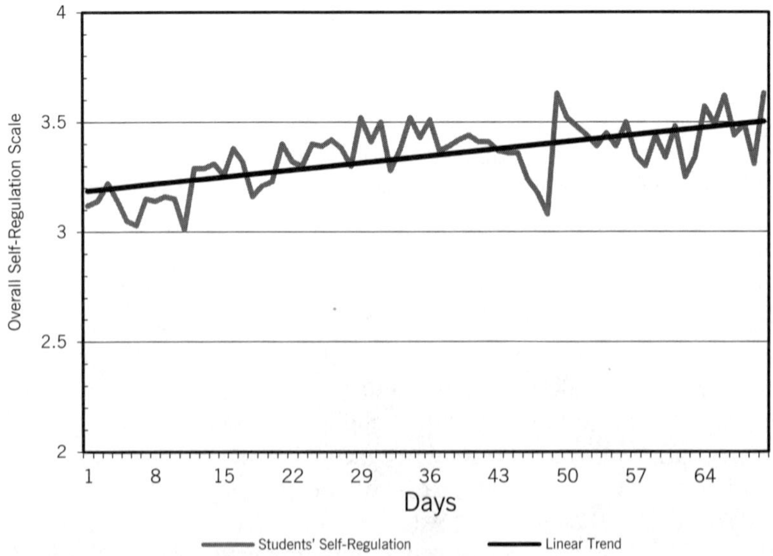

FIGURE 11.3. Linear trend of students' overall self-regulation.

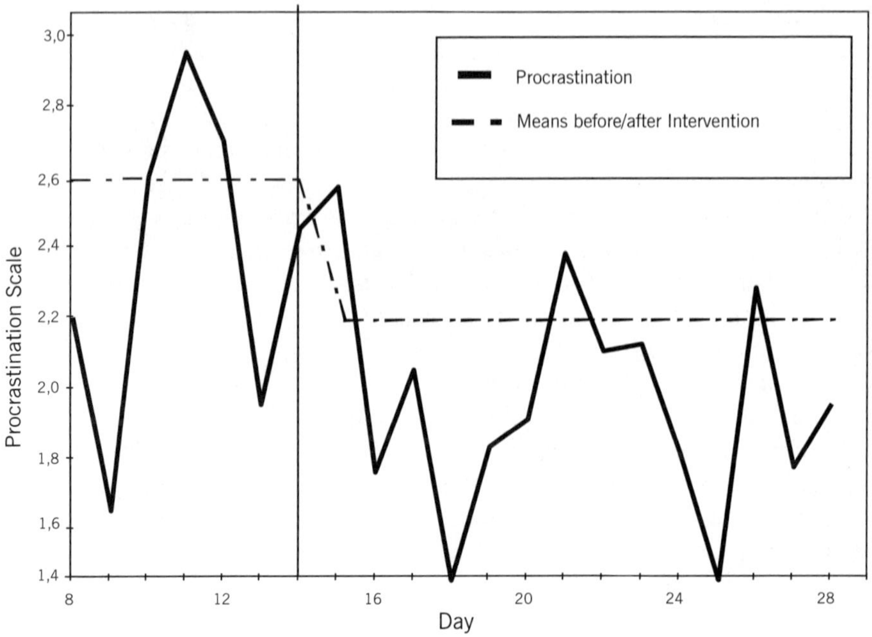

FIGURE 11.4. Interrupted time series analysis for the procrastination scale.

can be evaluated. In sum, this kind of evaluation does not give a conclusion about whether the training program as a whole was effective but instead allows detailed analyses of which components of the training program worked well.

One important application of time series analyses is the analysis of time-lagged relations. For this question we take data from Schmitz (2006). The diary used is similar to the one in the appendix but more elaborate. Regarding the model of self-regulated learning, we consider three important variables: self-efficacy, effort, and goal attainment. The results of multivariate time series analyses for two individuals are presented in Table 11.2, which on one hand contains the causal (time-lagged) relations given by the phi matrix and on the other hand the synchronous relations of the variables. As mentioned earlier, the phi matrix contains the lagged relations between the variables and has to be interpreted as the column variables having a time-lagged effect on the row variables. Student A shows the following time-lagged relations: In addition to the univariate autoregressive effect of self-efficacy, self-efficacy is raised one time unit after goal attainment is enhanced, and goal attainment changes one time unit after self-efficacy is enhanced. In contrast, student B does not show any time-lagged relations because the phi matrix is not significant for any element. Table 11.2 also contains the pattern of synchronous correlations of these variables.

Future Directions

The chapter shows how human development processes can be measured and analyzed in a systematic way by process analyses. Diaries are an appropriate method for measuring human processes and can be applied to every age group, covering the whole lifespan and different contents, such as relationships, stress, self-regulation, learning, clinical issues, and training content. A challenge lies in the implementation of time series designs, which are more time-consuming and expensive than cross-sectional studies. We want to motivate researchers to make this additional effort and to use methods of time series analysis to get deeper insight into human development processes into different age groups and with varying content.

Some limitations of diary data are due to the fact that they depend on self-reports (see Veenman, Van Hout-Wolters, & Afflerbach, 2006). Furthermore, a high level of compliance

TABLE 11.2. Results of Intraindividual Time Series Analyses: Phi Matrices and Residual Correlations for Two Individuals

		Phi matrix			Synchronous correlations		
Student	Variables	Self-efficacy	Effort	Goal attainment	Self-efficacy	Effort	Goal attainment
Student A	Self-efficacy	.34*	–.16	.32*	1.	.40*	.24
	Effort	.01	.19	.24	.40*	1.	.41*
	Goal attainment	.30*	.04	.04	.24	.41*	1.
Student B	Self-efficacy	.01	–.11	.01	1.	.68*	.53*
	Effort	.13	–.14	.01	.68*	1.	.76*
	Goal attainment	.24	.02	–.09	.53*	.76*	1.

*$p < .05$.

by the participants is needed. A lack of compliance could result in a high dropout rate, which can reduce external validity of the data. In addition to that, it is necessary to consider the reactivity effect. Although a change due to diary completion is desirable from an intervention perspective, reaction effects confound measurement and intervention effects (Schmitz, 2006). A further limitation of diaries (Spörer & Brunstein, 2006) is that their validity depends on motivation (i.e., the quality of the reported data will be higher in cases of motivated participants) and on writing skills (i.e., incompetence in writing can undermine the quality of the diary data). The use of standardized diary format can reduce problems arising from the latter.

To compensate for these limitations in diaries, researchers can include further forms of data, such as observational measures, archival measures, or physiological measures. Fahrenberg, Myrtek, Pawlik, and Perrez (2007) argue in their position paper for the use of computer-assisted methodology in measuring daily activities in order to enhance ecological validity. There is an ongoing discussion about the advantages and disadvantages of paper–pencil or Web-based diaries. One central issue is the question of participants' compliance in filling in diaries. Broderick and Stone (2006) described some issues with paper–pencil diaries. Green, Rafaeli, Bolger, Shrout, and Reis (2006) compared electronic with paper-and-pencil diaries and found only minor differences between methods.

Although the limitations are important, the advantages of the use of diaries far exceed their disadvantages. A diary is a flexible instrument, which can be used to measure processes. Diaries allow the investigation of psychological variables in daily life situations. By means of diaries, it is possible to collect and analyze data with a high level of ecological validity. Furthermore, diaries can capture and analyze developmental process data with a variety of sophisticated statistical methods. Clearly, diaries hold great promise for studying developmental processes in the future.

References

Bolhuis, S. (2003). Towards process-oriented teaching for self-directed lifelong learning: A multidimensional perspective. *Learning and Instruction, 13*, 327–347.

Broderick, J. E., & Stone, A. A. (2006). Paper and electronic diaries: Too early for conclusions on compliance rates and their effects: Comment on Green, Rafaeli, Bolger, Shrout, and Reis (2006). *Psychological Methods, 11*(1), 106–111.

Cattell, R. B. (1951). P- technique: A new method for analyzing the structure of personal motivation. *Transactions of the New York Academy of Sciences: Series 2, 14*, 29–34.

Fahrenberg, J., Myrtek, M., Pawlik, K., & Perrez, M. (2007). Ambulatory assessment: Monitoring behavior in daily life settings: A behavioral-scientific challenge for psychology. *European Journal of Psychological Assessment, 23*(4), 206–213.

Green, A. S., Rafaeli, E., Bolger, N., Shrout, P. E., & Reis, H. T. (2006). Paper or plastic? Data equivalence in paper and electronic diaries. *Psychological Methods, 11*, 87–105.

Hertel, S., Klug, J., & Schmitz, B. (2010). Quasi-experimentelle Versuchspläne [Quasi-experimental designs]. In H. Holling & B. Schmitz (Eds.), *Handwörterbuch der Psychologie: Methoden und Evaluation* [Psychological dictionary: Methods and evaluation] (pp. 49–62). Göttingen, Germany: Hogrefe.

Korotitsch, W., & Nelson-Gray, R. O. (1999). An overview of self-monitoring research in assessment. *Psychological Assessment, 11*(4), 415–425.

Perels, F., Gürtler, T., & Schmitz, B. (2005). Training of self-regulatory and problem-solving competence. *Learning and Instruction, 15*, 123–139.

Piaget, J. (1952). *La naissance de l'intelligence chez l'enfant* [The origins of intelligence in children]. London: Routledge & Kegan Paul.
Piaget, J. (1980). *Adaptation and intelligence: Organic selection and phenocopy*. Chicago: University of Chicago Press.
Preyer, W. (1882). *Die Seele des Kindes* [The soul of a child]. Leipzig, Germany: Grieben.
Schmidt, M., Perels, F., & Schmitz, B. (2010). How to perform idiographic and a combination of idiographic and nomothetic approaches: Comparison of time-series analyses and hierarchichal linear modelling. *Journal of Psychology, 218*, 166–174.
Schmitz, B. (1987). *Zeitreihenanalyse in der Psychologie: Verfahren zur Veränderungsmessung und Prozessdiagnostik* [Time-series analysis in psychology: Methods for measuring changes and for diagnosing processes]. Weinheim, Germany: Beltz.
Schmitz, B. (1989). *Einführung in die Zeitreihenanalyse* [Introduction to time-series analysis]. Bern, Germany: Huber.
Schmitz, B. (1990). Univariate and multivariate time-series models: The analysis of intraindividual variability and intraindividual relations. In A. v. Eye (Ed.), *Statistical methods in longitudinal research: Vol. 2. Time series and categorical longitudinal data* (pp. 351–368). New York: Academic Press.
Schmitz, B. (2006). Advantages of studying processes in educational research. *Learning and Instruction, 16*, 433–449.
Schmitz, B., Klug, J., & Schmidt, M. (2011). Assessing self-regulated learning using diary measures with university students. In B. Zimmerman & D. Schunk (Eds.), *Handbook of self-regulation of learning and performance* (pp. 251–266). New York: Routledge.
Schmitz, B., & Wiese, B. (2006). New perspectives for the evaluation of training sessions in self-regulated learning: Time-series analyses of diary data. *Contemporary Educational Psychology, 31*, 64–96.
Shadish, W. R., Cook, T. D., & Campbell, D. T. (2002). *Experimental and quasi-experimental designs for generalized causal inference*. Boston: Houghton Mifflin.
Shapiro, E. S., & Cole, C. L. (1999). Self-monitoring in assessing children's problems. *Psychological Assessment, 11*(4), 448–457.
Sliwinski, M. J., Almeida, D. M., Smyth, J., & Stawski, R. S. (2009). Intraindividual change and variability in daily stress processes: Findings from two measurement-burst diary studies. *Psychology and Aging, 24*(4), 828–840.
Spörer, N., & Brunstein, J. C. (2006). *Erfassung selbstregulierten Lernens mit Selbstberichtsverfahren: Ein Überblick zum Stand der Forschung* [Assessing self-regulated learning with self-report measurements: A state-of-the-art review]. *Zeitschrift für Pädagogische Psychologie, 20*(3), 147–160.
Stern, C., & Stern, W. (1907). *Die Kindersprache: Eine psychologische und sprachtheoretische Untersuchung* [Children's language: A psychological and language-theoretical investigation]. Leipzig, Germany: Barth.
Stern, W. (1914). *Psychologie der frühen Kindheit* [Psychology of early childhood]. Leipzig, Germany: Quelle & Meyer.
Valiente, C., Fabes, R. A., Eisenberg, N., & Spinrad, T. L. (2004). The relations of parental expressivity and support to childrens's coping with daily stress. *Journal of Family Psychology, 18*(1), 97–106.
Veenman, M. V. J., Van Hout-Wolters, B. H. A. M., & Afflerbach, P. (2006). Metacognition and learning: Conceptual and methodological considerations. *Metacognition and Learning, 1*, 3–14.
Watson, D., Clark, L. A., & Tellegen, A. (1988). Development and validation of brief measures of positive and negative affect. The PANAS scales. *Journal of Personality and Social Psychology, 54*, 1063–1070.
Yaffee, R. A., & McGee, M. (2000). *Introduction to time series analyses and forecasting. With applications of SAS and SPSS*. San Diego, CA: Academic Press.

APPENDIX 11.1. Excerpt of a Diary for Fifth-Grade Students

Please always fill out the grey-colored fields even if you don't do any homework or studying.

☐☐ . ☐☐ . ☐☐ ☐☐ : ☐☐

date time

For the next week I set myself, related to math, the following goal:

____

To attain my goal I will

____

If you don't do any homework or studying today, please say why

____

At the moment I feel . . .

	Totally Disagree	Partially Disagree	Partially Agree	Totally Agree
active	☐	☐	☐	☐
interested	☐	☐	☐	☐
annoyed	☐	☐	☐	☐
distressed	☐	☐	☐	☐

Only fill out the following if you have homework to do or you are studying!

How much time do you schedule for it? ☐☐ minutes

Refer the following statements to your math exercise. If you don't have exercises for math today, please choose <u>one</u> other subject and write it down:________

	Totally Disagree	Partially Disagree	Partially Agree	Totally Agree
I consider exactly how I will proceed.				
I really feel like studying today.				
I am sure that I will finish what I have planned to do.				

Please do your homework now!

Only fill out this section, if you pause doing your homework or studying!

Why did you interrupt your homework or studying?

☐ Right now I am not in the mood to keep on.
☐ I've been distracted.
☐ Something has cropped up.

I will do the following to go on working.

☐ I will split the remaining tasks (schedule breaks).
☐ Concentration exercises.
☐ Disable distractors (close my room door, don't talk on telephone with friends).

Continue here if you have finished your homework!!!

How long did it take to do your tasks today? __________ minutes.
How many minutes did you work while concentrating? __________ minutes.

	Totally Disagree	Partially Disagree	Partially Agree	Totally Agree
I didn't let myself get distracted from studying.	☐	☐	☐	☐
Although I was not in the mood, I continued learning.	☐	☐	☐	☐
Today I put much effort into my work.	☐	☐	☐	☐
While learning, I thought about my procedure.	☐	☐	☐	☐
While learning, I paid attention to my concentration.	☐	☐	☐	☐
If I didn't understand a task I asked for help. From whom?	☐	☐	☐	☐
Today I achieved everything that I had planned.	☐	☐	☐	☐
Today I made a step towards my week's goal.	☐	☐	☐	☐
Homework/studying was fun today.	☐	☐	☐	☐
Today I am satisfied with my learning results.	☐	☐	☐	☐

For tomorrow I intend to do the following (think of your week's goal)

____

CHAPTER 12

Retrospective Methods in Developmental Science

ANDREA FOLLMER GREENHOOT

Central Issues

How accurately can individuals report their own or others' past characteristics, feelings, behaviors, and experiences? Retrospective methods for measuring these types of variables are not unusual in the empirical literature, and they may present a particularly attractive solution to some of the design challenges inherent in developmental science. Developmental investigations are often designed to examine patterns of change and stability in individuals over time, but it is expensive and time-consuming to wait for development to happen, and prospective longitudinal methods may be especially impractical for investigating the antecedents or origins of infrequent and atypical developmental outcomes. Methods that rely on participants' recall of traits, behaviors, internal states, or experiences at earlier ages permit researchers to circumvent the complexities of assessing individuals at two or more time points often separated by years. Nevertheless, it is well established that human remembering is imperfect and that we are prone to forgetting, distortions, and illusions, particularly as the delay between an event and its later recollection increases. Therefore, the goals of this chapter are (1) to review the common uses of retrospective methods in developmental science and (2) to evaluate the reliability of these methods for addressing developmental questions from the perspective of the literatures on memory and memory development.

Conceptual Principles

Self-, parent, and other (e.g., teacher) report methods are quite common in the literature on human development and are used to assess all sorts of constructs. The limitations of such methods, particularly the tendency to respond to researchers' questions in socially desirable ways and the influence of demand characteristics, have been studied extensively (e.g.,

Crowne & Marlowe, 1964). In spite of these limitations, self-report methods are quite well accepted in the psychological research literature, particularly if they are combined with other methods that provide convergent measurement. But new sources of error and bias are introduced when the reports are retrospective in nature. Retrospective report methods ask participants to reflect, recall, and report on traits, behaviors, internal states, experiences, and other variables of interest after some delay. Technically, even reports of past states, behaviors, or experiences after very short delays (i.e., days or weeks rather than years) involve memory, but the role of memory processes in what is reported becomes increasingly important with the passage of time. By definition, then, memory is central to retrospective methodology and is the single feature that discriminates retrospective report methods from basic self-report methods. Thus, any evaluation of the validity of data collected with retrospective methods requires an analysis of research on memory and memory development, with a special emphasis on the factors that are likely to influence the reliability of reports of past traits, behaviors, internal states, and experiences from previous periods of development. The analysis provided here begins with an overview of basic memory principles, followed by a treatment of the memory research relevant to the most common applications of retrospective methods in developmental science.

Basic Principles of Remembering

In order to provide an accurate retrospective report, an individual has to encode information about the phenomenon of interest (i.e., the behavior, experience, or characteristic), preserve the resulting memory representation over a delay, and eventually retrieve and report it. According to the memory literature, however, maintaining the accuracy of these processing steps is not a simple and straightforward matter. Indeed, since Bartlett's seminal research (1932), psychologists have known that human remembering is not a simple reproductive process that stores memories in a verbatim or photographic form but rather is an active, constructive process that is vulnerable to errors and knowledge-driven distortions. Memory encoding is thought of as a process of construction, as individuals use background knowledge, attitudes, and beliefs to interpret and elaborate on to-be-remembered information. The resulting memory representations are conceptualized by current models as dynamic patterns of features that are activated and bound together during the encoding process (e.g., Conway & Pleydell-Pearce, 2000; Schacter, Norman, & Koustaal, 1998).

Memory retrieval is seen as a similar process of reconstruction that involves the reactivation of component features and pattern completion, again guided by current knowledge, attitudes, and beliefs. Expectations that are provided by knowledge about familiar events, people, or objects may be translated into retrieval cues, resulting in superior recall of knowledge-relevant, as opposed to knowledge-irrelevant, information (Brewer & Nakamura, 1984). But a critical feature of this reconstructive retrieval process is that the "memory" that gets retrieved and reported can be dramatically influenced, changed, and reorganized by a number of factors, including the simple passage of time; relevant knowledge, attitudes, and beliefs; exposure to intervening experiences; and the social and physical context of remembering. For instance, individuals may incorrectly activate features that are consistent with knowledge but are not a part of the to-be-remembered event, resulting in errors in recall (Greenhoot, 2000; Ornstein et al., 1998). Furthermore, it is well established that events that occur during the delay interval between an event and its later recall, such as related experiences or exposure to another person's account, may be confused with a target event during retrieval, leading to recall distortions (Bruck & Ceci, 1999; Johnson, Hashtroudi, & Lindsay, 1993). Memory errors, moreover, are more likely to occur as the delay interval between initial encoding and retrieval increases, as memory representations decay and become more difficult to reconstruct over time (Myles-Worsley, Cromer, & Dodd, 1986; Ornstein et al., 1998). Finally, characteristics of the retrieval context are known to affect remembering. Remembering is generally enhanced by recall conditions (e.g., one's physical surroundings or mental state) that resemble those that were in place when an event occurred (Godden & Baddeley, 1975; Tulving & Thompson, 1973), and the social context can also alter the likelihood of retrieving and reporting information (e.g., Davis & Bottoms, 2002; McCloskey & Zaragoza, 1985; Roediger, Meade, & Bergman, 2001).

Most retrospective reporting is likely to rely on a particular form of memory called *autobiographical* memory, which consists of our memories for our own personal histories, including personally experienced events and general "facts" and knowledge about ourselves. Theories of autobiographical memory argue that it serves several functions besides memory per se (e.g., Conway & Pleydell-Pearce, 2000; Nelson & Fivush, 2004). Specifically, autobiographical memory contributes to our self-concepts, our relationships and sense of shared history with others, and emotion regulation processes and affective experience. It turns out, however, that these autobiographical memory functions can also shape and bias the recall of personal memories in some systematic ways; some recall distortions serve to enhance views and presentations of the present self, and others cause people to perceive the experiences of their lives as more pleasant than unpleasant (e.g., Ross, 1989; Walker, Skowronski, & Thompson, 2003; Wilson, Gunn, & Ross, 2009; Wilson & Ross, 2003).

In sum, basic principles from the theoretical and empirical literatures on memory suggest that recall is fallible and that previous states, traits, and behaviors can be forgotten and altered in memory via a range of factors, particularly as the delay interval between the to-be-remembered event and the report of it increases. The types and severity of errors and distortions depend on a number of variables, including the characteristics of the individual doing the reporting; the identity of the individual being reported on (self versus other); individual and developmental differences in relevant knowledge, attitudes, and beliefs; and the context of the reporting.

Developmental Applications

The most common applications of retrospective methods in developmental science fall into three broad categories: (1) adults' (e.g., parents' and teachers') reports of children's past states, traits, behaviors, and experiences; (2) adults' reports on their own pasts; and (3) children's reports of their own pasts. The sections that follow provide a treatment of the research relevant to evaluating the validity each of these three developmental applications.

Adult Reports on Children's Pasts

Adult retrospective reports have been used in the recent developmental literature to gather information about children's early life circumstances, personality and physical characteristics, and achievement of developmental milestones (Germo, Goldberg, & Keller, 2009; Roizen et al., 2007). One of the most common uses of this method is to identify the antecedents or origins of atypical, infrequent developmental patterns that emerge during childhood, such as a diagnosis of a childhood disorder, delinquent or violent behavior, or peer rejection (e.g., Herrenkohl, Huang, Tajima, & Whitney, 2003; Pierce, Vinokur, & Buck, 1998; Rork & Morris, 2009; Sandstrom & Coie, 1999) or to measure antecedent variables prior to an unexpected event such as a parent's military deployment (O'Connor, Bredenkamp, & Rutter, 1999). Because the population of interest is defined by an uncommon or unexpected outcome, prospective longitudinal work would require tracking a large enough sample so as to include enough positive cases for predictive analyses. Such work tends to be time-consuming, costly, and impractical, and researchers who lack sufficient resources sometimes turn to retrospective reports from parents of children in the population of interest (or from other adults in the child's life) to gather information about their previous behaviors and experiences.

Although there are many practical reasons for the adoption of these methods, parent retrospective reports have raised concern since the 1960s, when a flurry of studies cast doubt on their accuracy (e.g., Brekstad, 1966; Haggard, Brekstad, & Skard, 1960; Wenar & Coulter, 1962; Yarrow, Campbell, & Burton, 1970). In the most comprehensive of these studies, Yarrow and colleagues (1970) compared parents' retrospective reports with baseline measures of their children's characteristics collected 3–30 years previously and found only very small (albeit significant) correlations between parents' retrospective reports and the baseline data. However, the overlap between the two types of measures tended to be higher when there were shorter delays between the baseline and the retrospective report (Yarrow et al., 1970) and when the reports focused on physical traits, such as height and weight, rather than behavioral and personality characteristics, such as manageability (Burton, 1970).

None of these findings is all that surprising when one considers basic, well-established principles of remembering. First and foremost, as is the case with any parent or teacher report measure, parents can accurately report on only those behaviors and experiences that were encoded and stored in memory in the first place. But even those phenomena that are encoded may be forgotten or misremembered after a delay or in response to intervening events. For example, parents may misattribute events that happen during the delay interval, including changes in children's behaviors and characteristics, to the target time period. Research on memory dating shows that adults are often inaccurate in estimating the timing of previous events (e.g., Thompson, Skowronski, Larsen, & Betz, 1996), and an extensive literature on source monitoring demonstrates that confusion about the sources of information can lead to recall distortions, particularly after long delays (e.g., Johnson et al., 1993).

An additional source of error in parents' reports of their child's past attributes is their current "knowledge," including attitudes and beliefs, about the child. Not only does current knowledge guide the way people retrieve memories, but also individuals may reinterpret, add, or omit information such that what is eventually recalled is consistent with current understandings (Anderson & Pitchert, 1978; Ross, 1989; Snyder & Uranowtiz, 1978; Spiro, 1977; Wilson & Ross, 2003). Investigations of the accuracy of parent retrospective reports have found that many reporting errors appear to be biased in the direction of desirability, precocity, and fewer difficulties; in other words, parents generally remember their children's attributes more positively than originally reported in the baseline documentation, especially when the delay interval is quite long (e.g., Yarrow et al., 1970). Furthermore, there is evidence that when adults' impressions of another person change over time, they modify their recall of that person's behaviors and characteristics in ways that are consistent with newly acquired views (Snyder & Uranowitz, 1978; Spiro, 1977). All the same, sometimes our knowledge may bias us to perceive and report *changes* rather than consistency over time, through the operation of implicit theories of personal change. Such implicit theories include general beliefs about development and the conditions that produce stability and change in personal characteristics (e.g., "Adolescents are far more idealistic than adults"), as well as more specific personal beliefs about oneself (e.g., "I was much less confident when I was 15 than I am now"), and such beliefs can bias the way previous attributes are recalled. For instance, when people possess theories of improvement, they systematically distort their memories of the past by exaggerating the inferiority of their past attributes (e.g., Ross, 1989). Although research on implicit theories has focused on theories of the self, a logical extension is that adults' intuitive theories about children's development may similarly influence the way they retrospectively report their children's characteristics.

In sum, the memory literature highlights the potential hazards of relying on parents' retrospective reports of their children's attributes or experiences as objective measures of the constructs they are intended to measure. Nevertheless, most retrospective reports are at least minimally associated with baseline measurements, and the methodology may be most appropriately used in contexts that involve short delays and that ask parents to report on phenomena that are unlikely to evoke strong beliefs, attitudes, or implicit theories about their children's developmental trajectories.

Adult Reports on Their Own Pasts

Researchers sometimes ask adults to report on their own past states, traits, behaviors, and experiences to gather information about past parenting behaviors and other family variables. For example, 7–17 months following 9/11, Mowder, Guttman, Rubinson, and Sossin (2006) asked parents who worked near Ground Zero to recollect their parenting behaviors and beliefs prior to and immediately after 9/11. Their reports suggested that there had been shifts in their parenting perceptions immediately after 9/11, but they returned to baseline over time. Adult reports of their own childhoods, like adult reports of their children's behaviors, are often used to investigate the predictors of relatively uncommon outcomes, such as violent behavior, incarceration, substance abuse, disease, and psychopathology in adulthood (e.g., Henry, Moffitt, Caspi, Langley, & Silva, 1994; Manuzza, Klein, Klein, Bressler, & Shrout, 2002; Sudman & Bradburn, 1973; Widom, Weiler, & Cottler, 1999). In fact, some adult diagnoses, such as adult attention-deficit/hyperactivity disorder (ADHD), actually require a positive retrospective diagnosis of childhood ADHD (American Psychiatric Association, 2000).

Many of the memory principles that apply to the previous category of retrospective reports also apply to this category, but there are also some important dissimilarities. First, it is well established that memory is more accurate and complete for phenomena that are directly experienced than for those that are only witnessed (e.g., Engelkamp & Dehn, 2000; Greenhoot, McCloskey, & Glisky, 2005), and for this reason adults could be more accurate in reporting on their own past states, traits, and behaviors than on those of their children. Nevertheless, the mnemonic benefits of direct experience may be dwarfed by the impact of the dramatic cognitive changes that take place across childhood and adolescence. As mentioned previously, there is ample empirical evidence that we retrieve, reinterpret, and reorganize old memories in light of our current knowledge and perspectives (e.g., Anderson & Pitchert, 1978; Greenhoot, 2000; Ross, 1989; Snyder & Uranowtiz, 1978; Spiro, 1977;

Wilson & Ross, 2003), and these findings raise questions about how an adult trying to remember the distant past can escape from his or her current state of knowledge. What's more, our knowledge about the self often includes intuitive theories about how we used to be and how we have come to be our current selves, and these beliefs also have implications for what is remembered (Ross, 1989). For example, Conway and Ross (1984) found that participants in a study skills program overestimated their improvement (and, consequently, the effectiveness of the program) by exaggerating how poor their skills had been prior to the program. Moreover, 6 months later, when asked to recall the grades they had received just after the program, participants reported better grades than they had actually obtained. In fact, the program did not significantly affect the participants' grades at all.

Reports of one's own past may also be affected by autobiographical memory biases related to self-enhancement and emotion regulation functions. Many intuitive theories, for instance, serve to maintain or enhance positive views of the self. In this regard, Wilson and Ross (2003) have shown that people tend to evaluate their past selves more negatively than their current selves, particularly when the attribute in question is important to them, although these patterns may be moderated by factors such as self-esteem and depression. Furthermore, the literatures on memory for unpleasant events and on coping and emotion regulation suggest that adults' recall of past experiences may be altered by their attempts to regulate emotion (e.g., Compas, Connor-Smith, Staltzman, Harding Thomsen, & Wadsworth, 2001; John & Gross, 2004; Walker, Skowronski, & Thompson, 2003). Coping strategies such as cognitive restructuring and reappraisal involve transforming one's view of an event; if this processing is carried out after an event has unfolded, it by definition involves restructuring a recollection so as to reduce distress.

Consistent with this litany of potential retrospective biases, research on the validity of adults' reports of their childhood histories suggests that the accuracy of such reports is questionable. Some evidence comes from a study by Widom, Weiler, and Cottler (1999) on the relation between adult substance abuse and prospective and retrospective measures of childhood victimization. Analyses using retrospective reports replicated the findings of previous retrospective studies that abused individuals are at increased risk for substance abuse, whereas analyses using prospective reports found no increase in risk associated with victimization. One explanation for the robust findings with retrospective measures is that current involvement in problem behavior influences participants' ability and willingness to recollect difficult childhood experiences; in other words, accurate retrospective reporting of childhood victimization may well differ for individuals with and without current substance abuse problems.

Research on adult ADHD provides additional evidence for retrospective biases in childhood reports. Manuzza and colleagues (2002) compared prospective and retrospective reports of childhood ADHD symptoms in a sample of adults with and without a positive history; almost all of the adults with a childhood diagnosis were identified by their retrospective reports, yet only 27% of those "diagnosed" through retrospective reports actually had childhood ADHD. This pattern suggests that participants' reports of their childhood behaviors and characteristics may have been guided (and distorted) by general beliefs about childhood and development. Additionally, adults have been shown to "bring forward in memory" the temporal distance of the age of onset of childhood and adolescent behaviors such as smoking and substance use; in other words, people tend to report the onset of such behaviors as taking place at older ages than those at which they actually occurred (e.g., Sudman & Bradburn, 1973). Thus, although retrospective reports may provide important information about adults' perspectives on their past, these measures do not appear to be objective measures of past states, traits, and behaviors.

Children's Reports on Their Own Pasts

Retrospective reports by children and adolescents about their own pasts are less common than parent or adult reports, but they have been used in the recent literature to collect data on a wide range of variables, including children's past interactions with parents (e.g., Calam, Waller, Cox, & Slade, 1997), experiences with abuse (Herrenkohl et al., 2003), peer relationships (e.g., Sandstrom & Coie, 1999; Vernberg, Greenhoot, & Biggs, 2006), the onset of deviant behavior or substance use (Nurco, Blatchley, Hanlon, & O'Grady, 1999), and pretrauma experiences and characteristics (Pfefferbaum et al., 1999). For example, in an evaluation of middle and high school students exposed to the Oklahoma City bombing 7 weeks after the event, Pfefferbaum and colleagues (1999) found that retrospective reports of their initial responses to the explosion predicted their posttraumatic stress levels at 7 weeks.

For obvious reasons, the delays involved in this category of retrospective reports are shorter than the delays involved when adults report on childhood, but because the reporters are necessarily younger at the time of retrieval, some of the errors and difficulties observed with adult retrospective self-reports are magnified in children's and adolescents' retrospective self-reports. The literature on memory development has yielded substantial evidence of age-related improvements in children's abilities to encode, maintain, and retrieve memories (e.g., Baker-Ward, Ornstein, Gordon, Larus, & Clubb, 1993; Brainerd, Kingma, & Howe, 1985); the younger the child, the weaker the memory representation, and the more vulnerable the memory will be to forgetting and to influences from knowledge and intervening events.

The few studies that have examined the validity of children's or adolescents' retrospective reports suggest that they are prone to errors. For instance, Capaldi (1996) compared adolescent boys' recall of their first sexual intercourse with prospective measures marking the same event. Although the boys were highly consistent over time in reporting whether or not they had had intercourse, they were quite inaccurate in reporting the date or age of the experience. Yarrow and colleagues' (1970) study of children's recollections of their physical and behavioral characteristics as preschoolers found that their reports were more similar to their mothers' retrospective reports (described earlier) than they were to the baseline records. Thus, the children's recollections may have been influenced by factors such as discussions and family stories that were shaped by the mothers over the delay interval.

Nonetheless, it should also be pointed out that there are some adult memory biases that are unlikely to afflict children. Emotion regulation functions, for instance, are still developing across childhood (Brenner & Salovey, 1997; Compas et al., 2001). Furthermore, because the development of identity and a coherent life story is only just beginning in the teen years (e.g., McAdams, Diamond, de St. Aubin, & Mansfield, 1997), children and to some extent adolescents are unlikely to exhibit recall biases driven by implicit theories of the self or motivation for self-enhancement. Thus, children's and possibly adolescents' retrospective memory errors may be more random than systematic.

In sum, there are numerous applications of retrospective methods in developmental science, and each of these suffers from some significant shortcomings that are linked to the fallibility of memory. The memory literature suggests that the histories we recall are our subjective impressions of how we used to be, often reflecting intervening experiences and current beliefs about how we have changed. The next section presents data from one of my own investigations (Greenhoot et al., 2005) to provide a comprehensive illustration of the use and pitfalls of retrospective methods in developmental studies.

Illustration: Children's and Mothers' Reports of Family Violence

This illustration of retrospective methods draws on data from Greenhoot and colleagues (2005) to compare mothers' and children's accounts of family violence and control events with baseline data collected 6 years previously. This investigation was carried out in the context of a prospective longitudinal study of women and children exposed to family violence, directed by Laura McCloskey (see McCloskey, Figueredo, & Koss, 1995, for further details). The study was originally designed to examine the impact of domestic violence and abuse on women's and children's mental health, but our follow-up assessments on this sample have provided a rich and unique opportunity to examine the children's and mothers' memories and retrospective reports. In the first year of the study, McCloskey and colleagues (1995) recruited 363 battered and nonbattered women and one of their children between the ages of 6 and 12 years to participate in a study on families. The children and mothers participated in separate interviews, during which an abbreviated version of the Conflict Tactics Scale (Straus, 1979) was used to question mothers and children about the frequency of the mother's partner's use of specific forms of aggression (e.g., hitting with an object) against the mother (e.g., being pushed, beaten, or kicked) or child (i.e., being pushed, kicked, or burned) in the previous year. Children whose year 1 reports were not sufficiently corroborated by their mothers were excluded from this analysis along with their mothers, as were dyads that did not participate in the follow-up interview at year 6. A final sample contained 234 dyads; 81 of these (the control group) reported no year 1 exposure to mother- or child-directed family violence, and 153 (the exposed group) reported some form of family aggression in year 1. Several nonabusive control events (e.g., grandparent dying, changing schools, losing a friend, moving to a new home) and family and life circumstances (e.g., name of teacher, location of home, names of others living in home) were also documented at the baseline assessment.

Six years later, when the children were 12–18 years of age, mothers and youths participated in separate 3-hour interviews that included questions about family relationships, social adjustment, psychopathology, and criminal behavior. In this interview, they were asked open-ended questions about their year 1 life circumstances and a series of open-ended and yes-or-no questions about the occurrence of specific forms of family aggression in year 1 and the control events. The exposed youths reported slightly more than half of the child-directed acts that they had disclosed 6 years earlier and less than half of the previously disclosed mother-directed acts. In contrast, their rates of correct "no" responses to questions about acts that had not occurred were quite high. Thirty-four percent of the teens exposed to spousal violence did not report any spousal violence at all, and 21% of those exposed to child-directed aggression failed to recall or report it altogether. Finally, the data in the bottom half of Table 12.1 show that youths in the control group very rarely reported family violence in their retrospective reports of year 1. Together, these patterns

TABLE 12.1. Proportions of Year 1 Family Violence Acts Reported and Correctly Rejected at Year 6 in Exposed and Control Groups

	Reporter	
Variable	Youth	Mother
Exposed group		
Child-directed aggression		
% reported (correct recall)	.56 (.38)	.58 (.44)
% correctly rejected	.87 (.26)	.62 (.37)
Mother-directed aggression		
% reported (correct recall)	.44 (.41)	.63 (.53)
% correctly rejected	.75 (.73)	.69 (.40)
Control group		
Child-directed aggression		
% reported (false alarms)	.06 (.14)	.07 (.21)
% correctly rejected	.86 (.29)	.56 (.41)
Mother-directed aggression		
% reported (false alarms)	.01 (.05)	0.0 (0)
% correctly rejected	.96 (.19)	.83 (.41)

Note. "Correct recall" refers to the proportion of violent acts disclosed at year 1 that were correctly reported at year 6 by the exposed group; "false alarms" refer to the proportion of violent acts that did not occur in the control group, reported at year 6; "correct rejections" refer to the proportion of acts that did not occur at year 1 that were correctly denied or rejected at year 6, either group.

suggest that the adolescents tended to retrospectively underreport their childhood exposure to year 1 violence, particularly when they were not the victims. Indeed, on the basis of their retrospective reports, about one-third would not have been identified as exposed to spousal abuse, and one-fifth would not have been classified as exposed to physical punishment or abuse. There are numerous explanations for these retrospective reporting errors. One possibility is that some participants chose not to disclose past family violence to the interviewer. Indeed, Femina and her colleagues (Femina, Yeager, & Lewis, 1990) reported that when asked about their failures to recollect adolescent experiences of physical abuse, young adults often admitted to deliberate nondisclosures to protect their parents, to avoid embarrassment, or to attempt to forget the experiences. Nonetheless, we found that measures of participants' willingness to disclose other personal information in the interviews were unrelated to memory for family aggression, suggesting that nondisclosure cannot completely account for the retrospective errors we observed. Additional analyses on the child data showed that, consistent with the basic memory principles outlined at the beginning of this chapter, retrospective errors were least likely to occur when the children were older at year 1, when their attitudes about mothers' partners were more in line with aggressive and abusive behavior, and when their recent experiences (e.g., exposure to recent family violence) were more similar to those at year 1.

The data in the right column of Table 12.1 suggest that mothers in the exposed group showed less underreporting of year 1 family violence than their children. Interestingly, the mothers reported a similar percentage of the child-directed acts from year 1 to that reported by their children and a higher percentage of year 1 mother-directed aggression. At the same time, exposed mothers' rates of correct rejections were quite low, suggesting that they were confused about the specific details of their family violence histories from year 1. On the basis of the retrospective reports, 47% of the mothers would have been misclassified as nonexposed to mother-directed aggression, and 30% of the children would have been misidentified as nonexposed to child-directed aggression. As shown in the bottom half of Table 12.1, mothers in the control group were quite accurate in reporting their exposure (or lack therefore) to spousal violence in year 1, yet they did make some errors of commission (i.e., false alarms) on child-directed aggression. Such errors may reflect normative beliefs and attitudes about physical punishment in this sample, as corporal punishment (e.g., pushing, spanking) was quite common in both the exposed and control groups (McCloskey et al., 1995). Thus, these errors could reflect confusion between specific forms of corporal punishment at the time of recall.

Finally, in response to the questions about major nonabusive life events (e.g., changing schools, moving to a new home) from year 1, the teens correctly reported only 38% of the events, and the mothers recalled about 20% (see Table 12.2), rates that are even lower than those observed for reports of family violence events. Both mothers and teens correctly remembered about 75% of their year 1 life circumstances (e.g., name of teacher) during that same year. Thus, adults' and youths' retrospective reporting of specific life events appears to be more prone to error than reporting of more enduring life circumstances.

Taken together, these data suggest that youths' and mothers' retrospective reports of events and circumstances after a 6-year delay underestimated their previous exposure to family violence, as well as the occurrence of nonabusive control events. Furthermore, nonexposed mothers and youths whose baseline documentation classified them as nonexposed rarely retrospectively reported any family violence in year 1, with the exception of mothers' reports of child-directed punishment and abuse. Thus, the most common retrospective errors in this data set were errors of omission rather than commission. The few errors of commission may well reflect widely held beliefs about childrearing.

TABLE 12.2. Proportions of Year 1 Control Events Reported and Correctly Rejected at Year 6, Collapsed across Exposed and Control Groups

	Reporter	
Variable	Youth	Mother
% correct recall	.38 (.35)	.20 (.19)
% correct rejections	.83 (.19)	.35 (.21)

Note. "Correct recall" refers to the proportion of control events disclosed at year 1 that were correctly reported at year 6; "correct rejections" refers to the proportion of acts that did not occur at year 1 that were correctly denied or rejected at year 6.

Future Directions

In sum, current memory theory and research suggest that retrospective report methods may not always accurately measure the constructs that they are intended to measure. The fact that retrospective methods have a number of shortcomings is not a new insight. Myrtle McGraw questioned the wisdom of memory as a source of objective data seven decades ago (McGraw & Molloy, 1941). The contemporary literature on memory and memory development provides information about when and why reports might be biased and in doing so sheds light on the conditions that lead to their optimal application. Memory-based reporting errors may be minimized by conditions that involve shorter delays and older rememberers, and that evaluate directly observable phenomena that do not activate strongly held beliefs about child or self-development.

In spite of these cautions, some researchers have argued that retrospective methods have an important place in developmental science. In contrast to Widom and colleagues' (1999) findings, several studies have revealed similar predictive values for some variables whether they are measured retrospectively or prospectively (e.g., Herrenkohl et al. 2003; Sandstrom & Coie, 1999; Schwebel, Brezausek, Ramey, & Ramey, 2004; Shaffer, Huston, & Egeland, 2008). Furthermore, others have pointed out that retrospective methods for identifying child maltreatment may identify those for whom there were ongoing cases of abuse during the original, prospective measurement (Kendall-Tackett & Becker-Blease, 2004), although the findings of Greenhoot and colleagues (2005) provide little support for this argument. Nevertheless, sometimes researchers are interested in the subjective representation of childhood itself rather than an objective measure of reality, and in these situations retrospective reports are highly appropriate. For example, the Adult Attachment Interview, another very common tool involving retrospective reports, was designed for just such a purpose (George, Kaplan, & Main, 1985).

What are some alternatives for surmounting the design challenges that so often prompt retrospective methodology? One option that could be employed in studies of atypical or infrequent developmental outcomes is to conduct focused prospective studies that begin with identification of a vulnerable sample (e.g., Rogers, 2009). For instance, if it is known that individuals in particular subgroups have an increased likelihood of a particular developmental pattern, one might choose to track outcomes in an "at risk" sample over time. Another option is to collect convergent data so that retrospection from a single individual is not the only measure on each participant (Shaffer et al., 2008).

Conclusions

In sum, a reliance on retrospective reports should be discouraged in developmental research if at all possible, but there are several principles to keep in mind should this methodology be the only option for data collection in a developmental investigation. First and foremost, a consideration of the age at which the reported items occurred is critical. Individuals are unlikely to retain memories of information and events that occurred during the period of infantile amnesia (roughly 0–5 years), and even after that period there are age-related increases in the ability to encode and maintain memories over the long term. Similarly, caution should be used in interpreting retrospective reports of past events, behaviors, or attributes after extensive delays, especially if there has been exposure during the delay interval to intervening events or misinformation. Thus, retrospective reports may be most defensible and valid under the following conditions:

- The reporters were adults or adolescents at the time of the events, behaviors, or attributes being reported.
- The delay interval between the target events, behaviors, and attributes and the time of reporting is short.
- Exposure to related intervening events or potential sources of misinformation has been minimal.
- The reporter is unlikely to have strongly held beliefs about the domain being reported on.
- The researchers are interested in the participants' subjective representations of the past rather than an objective measure of reality.

References

American Psychiatric Association. (2000). *Diagnostic and statistical manual of mental disorders* (4th ed., text rev.). Washington, DC: Author.

Anderson, R. C., & Pitchert, J. W. (1978). Recall of previously unrecallable information following a shift in perspective. *Journal of Verbal Learning and Verbal Behavior, 17*, 1–12.

Baker-Ward, L., Ornstein, P. A., Gordon, B. N., Larus, D., & Clubb, P. A. (1993). Young children's long-term retention of a pediatric examination. *Child Development, 64*, 1519–1533.

Bartlett, F. C. (1932). *Remembering: A study in experimental and social psychology*. New York: Cambridge University Press.

Brainerd, C. J., Kingma, J., & Howe, M. L. (1985). On the development of forgetting. *Child Development, 56*, 1103–1119.

Brekstad, A. (1966). Factors influencing the reliability of anamnestic recall. *Child Development, 37*, 603–612.

Brenner, E., & Salovey, P. (1997). Emotion regulation during childhood: Developmental, interpersonal, and individual considerations. In P. Salovey & D. Sluyter (Eds.), *Emotional literacy and emotional development* (pp. 168–192). New York: Basic Books.

Brewer, W. F., & Nakamura, G. V. (1984). The nature and function of schemas. In R. S. Wyer & T. K. Srull (Eds.), *Handbook of social cognition* (Vol. 1, pp. 119–160). Hillsdale, NJ: Erlbaum.

Bruck, M., & Ceci, S. J. (1999). The suggestibility of children's memory. *Annual Review of Psychology, 50*, 419–439.

Burton, R. V. (1970). Validity of retrospective reports assessed by the multitrait–multimethod analysis. *Developmental Psychology Monograph, 3*(No. 3, Part 2), 1–15.

Calam, R., Waller, G., Cox, A., & Slade, P. (1997). Eating attitudes in young teenage girls: Parental management of "fussy" eating. *Eating Disorders: The Journal of Treatment and Prevention, 5*, 29–40.

Capaldi, D. M. (1996). The reliability of retrospective report for timing first sexual intercourse for adolescent males. *Journal of Adolescent Research, 11*, 375–387.

Compas, B. E., Connor-Smith, J. K., Saltzman, H., Harding Thomsen, A., & Wadsworth, M. E. (2001). Coping with stress during childhood and adolescence: Problems, progress, and potential in theory and research. *Psychological Bulletin, 127*(1), 87–127.

Conway, M. A., & Pleydell-Pearce, C. W. (2000). The construction of autobiographical memories in the self-memory system. *Psychological Review, 107*(2), 261–288.

Conway, M., & Ross, M. (1984). Getting what you want by revising what you had. *Journal of Personality and Social Psychology, 47*, 738–748.

Crowne, D. P., & Marlowe, D. (1964). *The approval motive: Studies in evaluative dependence*. New York: Wiley.

Davis, S. L., & Bottoms, B. L. (2002). Effects of social support on children's eyewitness reports: A test of the underlying mechanism. *Law and Human Behavior, 26*(2), 185–215.

Engelkamp, J., & Dehn, D. M. (2000). Item and order information in subject-performed tasks and experimenter-performed tasks. *Journal of Experimental Psychology: Learning, Memory, and Cognition, 26*, 671–682.

Femina, D. D., Yeager, C. A., & Lewis, D. O. (1990). Child abuse: Adolescent records vs. adult recall. *Child Abuse and Neglect, 14*, 227–231.

George, C., Kaplan, M., & Main, M. (1985). *Adult Attachment Interview*. Unpublished manuscript, University of California, Berkeley.

Germo, G. R., Goldberg, W. A., & Keller, M. A. (2009). Learning to sleep through the night: Solution or strain for mothers and young children? *Infant Mental Health Journal, 30*(3), 223–244.

Godden, D. R., & Baddeley, A. D. (1975). Context-dependent memory in two natural environments: On land and underwater. *British Journal of Psychology, 66*, 325–331.

Greenhoot, A. F. (2000). Remembering and understanding: The effects of changes in underlying knowledge on children's recollections. *Child Development, 71*, 1309–1328.

Greenhoot, A. F., McCloskey, L., & Glisky, E. (2005). A longitudinal study of adolescents' recollections of family violence. *Applied Cognitive Psychology, 19*(6), 719–743.

Haggard, E. A., Brekstad, A., & Skard, A. G. (1960). On the reliability of the anamnestic interview. *Journal of Abnormal and Social Psychology, 61*, 311–318.

Henry, B., Moffitt, T., Caspi, A., Langley, J., & Silva, P. A. (1994). On the "remembrance of things past": A longitudinal evaluation of the retrospective method. *Psychological Assessment, 6*(2), 92–101.

Herrenkohl, T. L., Huang, B., Tajima, E. A., & Whitney, S. D. (2003). Examining the link between child abuse and youth violence: An analysis of mediating mechanisms. *Journal of Interpersonal Violence, 18*, 1189–1208.

John, O. P., & Gross, J. J. (2004). Healthy and unhealthy emotion regulation: Personality processes, individual differences, and life span development. *Journal of Personality, 72*(6), 1301–1333.

Johnson, M. K., Hashtroudi, S., & Lindsay, D. S. (1993). Source monitoring. *Psychological Bulletin, 114*(1), 3–28.

Kendall-Tackett, K., & Becker-Blease, K. (2004). The importance of retrospective findings in child maltreatment research. *Child Abuse and Neglect, 28*(7), 723–727.

Manuzza, S., Klein, R. G., Klein, D. F., Bressler, A., & Shrout, P. (2002). Accuracy of adult recall of childhood attention deficit disorder. *American Journal of Psychiatry, 159*, 1882–1888.

McAdams, D. P., Diamond, A., de St. Aubin, E., & Mansfield, E. (1997). Stories of commitment: The psychosocial construction of generative lives. *Journal of Personality and Social Psychology, 72*, 678–694.

McCloskey, L. A., Figueredo, A. J., & Koss, M. P. (1995). The impact of systemic family violence on children's mental health. *Child Development, 66*, 1239–1261.

McCloskey, M., & Zaragoza, M. (1985). Misleading postevent information and memory for events: Arguments and evidence against the memory impairment hypotheses. *Journal of Experimental Psychology: General, 114*, 3–18.

McGraw, M., & Molloy, L. B. (1941). The pediatric anamnesis: Inaccuracies in eliciting developmental data. *Child Development, 12*, 255–265.

Mowder, B. A., Guttman, M., Rubinson, F., & Sossin, K. M. (2006). Parents, children, and trauma: Parent role perceptions and behaviors related to the 9/11 tragedy. *Journal of Child and Family Studies, 15*(6), 733–743.

Myles-Worsley, M., Cromer, C., & Dodd, D. (1986). Children's preschool script reconstruction: Reliance on general knowledge as memory fades. *Developmental Psychology, 22*, 22–30.
Nelson, K., & Fivush, R. (2004). The emergence of autobiographical memory: A social cultural developmental theory. *Psychological Review, 111*, 486–511.
Nurco, D. N., Blatchley, R. J., Hanlon, T. E., & O'Grady, K. E. (1999). Early deviance and related risk factors in the children of narcotic addicts. *American Journal of Drug and Alcohol Abuse, 25*(1), 25–45.
O'Connor, T. G., Bredenkamp, D., & Rutter, M. (1999). Attachment disturbances and disorders in children exposed to early severe deprivation. *Infant Mental Health Journal, 20*, 10–29.
Ornstein, P. A., Merritt, K. A., Baker-Ward, L., Gordon, B. N., Principe, G. F., & Furtado, E. (1998). Children's knowledge, expectation, and long-term retention. *Applied Cognitive Psychology, 12*, 387–405.
Pfefferbaum, B., Nixon, S. J., Tucker, P. M., Tivis, R. D., Moore, V. L., Gurwitch, R. H., et al. (1999). Posttraumatic stress responses in bereaved children after the Oklahoma City bombing. *Journal of the American Academy of Child and Adolescent Psychiatry, 38*(11), 1372–1379.
Pierce, P. F., Vinokur, A. D., & Buck, C. L. (1998). Effects of war-induced maternal separation on children's adjustment during the Gulf War and two years later. *Journal of Applied Social Psychology, 28*, 1286–1311.
Roediger, H. S., Meade, M. L., & Bergman, E. T. (2001). Social contagion of memory. *Psychonomic Bulletin and Review, 8*(2), 365–371.
Rogers, S. J. (2009). What are infant siblings teaching us about autism in infancy? *Autism Research, 2*, 125–137.
Roizen, N. J., Antshel, K. M., Fremont, W., AbdulSabur, N., Higgins, A. M., Shprintzen, R. J., et al. (2007). 22q11.2DS deletion syndrome: Developmental milestones in infants and toddlers. *Journal of Developmental and Behavioral Pediatrics, 28*(2), 119–124.
Rork, K. E., & Morris, T. L. (2009). Influence of parenting factors on childhood social anxiety: Direct observation of parental warmth and control. *Child and Family Behavior Therapy, 31*(3), 220–235.
Ross, M. (1989). Relation of implicit theories to the construction of personal histories. *Psychological Review, 96*, 341–357.
Sandstrom, M. J., & Coie, J. D. (1999). A developmental perspective on peer rejection: Mechanisms of stability and change. *Child Development, 70*(4), 955–966.
Schacter, D., Norman, K. A., & Koustaal, W. (1998). The cognitive neuroscience of constructive memory. *Annual Review of Psychology, 49*, 289–318.
Schwebel, D. C., Brezausek, C. M., Ramey, S. L., & Ramey, C. T. (2004). Interactions between child behavior patterns and parenting: Implications for children's unintentional injury risk. *Journal of Pediatric Psychology, 29*, 93–104.
Shaffer, A., Huston, L., & Egeland, B. (2008). Identification of child maltreatment using prospective and self-report methodologies: A comparison of maltreatment incidence and relation to later psychopathology. *Child Abuse and Neglect, 32*, 682–692.
Snyder, M., & Uranowitz, S. W. (1978). Reconstructing the past: Some cognitive consequences of person perception. *Journal of Personality and Social Psychology, 36*, 941–950.
Spiro, R. (1977). Remembering information from text: The "state of the schema" approach. In R. C. Anderson, R. J. Spiro, & W. E. Montague (Eds.), *Schooling and the acquisition of knowledge* (pp. 137–165). Hillsdale, NJ: Erlbaum.
Straus, M. A. (1979). Measuring intrafamily conflict and violence: The Conflict Tactics (CT) Scales. *Journal of Marriage and the Family, 41*(1), 75–88.
Sudman, S., & Bradburn, N. M. (1973). Effects of time and memory factors on response in surveys. *Journal of the American Statistical Association, 63*, 805–815.
Thompson, C. P., Skowronski, J. J., Larsen, S. F., & Betz, A. (1996). *Autobiographical memory: Remembering what and remembering when*. Hillsdale, NJ: Erlbaum.

Tulving, E., & Thompson, D. M. (1973). Encoding specificity and retrieval processes in episodic memory. *Psychological Review, 80,* 352–373.

Vernberg, E., Greenhoot, A. F., & Biggs, B. K. (2006). Intercommunity relocation and adolescent friendships: Who struggles and why. *Journal of Consulting and Clinical Psychology, 74*, 511–523.

Walker, W. R., Skowronski, J. J., & Thompson, C. P. (2003). Life is pleasant—and memory helps keep it that way! *Review of General Psychology, 7,* 203–210.

Wenar, C., & Coulter, J. B. (1962). A reliability study of developmental histories. *Child Development, 33,* 453–462.

Widom, C. S., Weiler, B. L., & Cottler, L. B. (1999). Childhood victimization and drug abuse: A comparison of prospective and retrospective findings. *Journal of Consulting and Clinical Psychology, 67*(6), 867–880.

Wilson, A. E., Gunn, G. R., & Ross, M. (2009). The role of subjective time in identity regulation. *Applied Cognitive Psychology, 23,* 1164–1178.

Wilson, A. E., & Ross, M. (2003). The identity function of autobiographical memory: Time is on our side. *Memory, 11*(2), 137–149.

Yarrow, M. R., Campbell, J. D., & Burton, R. V. (1970). Recollections of childhood. *Monographs of the Society for Research in Child Development, 35,* 1–83.

CHAPTER 13

Peer Ratings

WILLIAM M. BUKOWSKI
ANTONIUS H. N. CILLESSEN
ANA MARIA VELÁSQUEZ

For at least 80 years, measures derived from various forms of peer ratings have been used extensively to assess multiple aspects of children's and adolescents' experiences with their age-mates, including individual differences in fundamental aspects of social behavior, social and individual competence, and patterns of liking and disliking. The word *peer* in the expression *peer ratings* has two distinct but interrelated meanings. It is used to refer to both a *source* of information that is used to create a set of measures and the *phenomena* that these measures are intended to index. To put it succinctly, the expression *peer ratings* refers to measures based on peer reports that tell us about what goes on in children's and adolescents' experiences within the peer group. Most studies of peer relations use peer ratings in one form or another. Their pervasive and indispensable role in peer research justifies the inclusion of a chapter on peer ratings in handbooks of developmental methods (e.g., Thompson, 1960).

Central Issues

By absolute and comparative standards, there is much to recommend peer ratings. As a particular form of measurement they are efficient, rich, and direct. Peer ratings are relatively easy to collect, code, and score. One can collect a lot of information inexpensively. They are also highly amenable to multiple forms of statistical analysis. The relative simplicity of their administration in conjunction with the power and depth of the measures they create has led to their use in a wide range of contexts (e.g., school classrooms and summer camp groups in at least 40 countries.)

Compared with measures that rely on other sources of information, such as parents and teachers, peer ratings provide breadth, depth, reliability, and validity. The first advantage of peer ratings derives from the broad array of contexts in which peers observe each other. Peers see each other in multiple contexts, including the school classroom, the lunch room, the playground and neighborhood, the school hallways, and even the washrooms. They also have access to the verbal and cyber-based peer grapevine about who did what with whom and in what circumstances. Teachers have access to some of these observational contexts, especially the classroom and the school hallways, but their knowledge of what children are like in other contexts, including some school-based contexts (e.g., the locker room and schoolyard) is, at best, meager. Parents' observations are limited also. Although they can observe their own children in several contexts (e.g., in the home, in the immediate neighborhood, and at some school-related events), their sense of base rate may be tenuous because they have few opportunities to observe other children. The access that peers have to such a broad set of observational contexts not only gives them an extensive database about the characteristics of each of their age-mates but also helps them develop a fuller recognition of the frequencies and base rates for a wide range of characteristics.

A second advantage of peer ratings is that they are derived from multiple assessors. By using multiple assessors, peer-based measures take advantage of the collective knowledge of the group. This practice increases reliability and decreases the biases (or invalidity) inherent in procedures that use a single source of information. It has been known for more than a century (Galton, 1907) that the collective voice of the people can be more accurate than the voice of any particular person (Surowiecki, 2004). The advantage of having multiple assessments gives peer ratings a clear edge over self-ratings or ratings obtained from teachers and parents.

The third advantage of peer ratings concerns perspective. Direct insider information can be critical for some forms of measurement. Measures of liking, for instance, are likely to be most valid when the information is provided by the liker him- or herself rather than by an outsider who, at best, has seen indications of liking without having experienced it directly. Although there are some circumstances in which an outsider's views may be as useful as those of an insider, these cases are likely to be relatively rare.

Put simply, to conduct or understand research on peer relations requires familiarity with the conceptual, methodological, and statistical issues related to the use of peer ratings. This chapter is aimed at describing these issues.

What Kind of Peer Ratings Are Used?

Traditionally, peer ratings have been used in three measurement domains: peer assessment, sociometry, and group structure. In our discussion we focus on the first two. Peer assessments and sociometric methods share two basic characteristics that serve very different functions, namely the use of peer ratings and the utility for making measures of phenomena related to functioning in the peer domain. If there has been a fundamental terminological weakness in peer research, it is probably the all too frequent confusion about the distinction between peer assessment techniques and sociometry. Peer assessment techniques, such as the revised class play (Masten, Morison, & Pellegrini, 1985), are used to collect information about the characteristics of individual children. Sociometric techniques are used to measure the social forces that exist between individuals. Although these methods are often used together, they serve different purposes and produce different types of information.

In a peer assessment procedure, each child in a group indicates, using either a nomination or rating scale system, whether or not each of his or her peers presents particular characteristics (e.g., "someone who helps others"). Data from peer assessments are used to create measures for each child on multiple dimensions of functioning, such as aggression, social withdrawal, and sociability. The social forces that are measured by sociometric measures can be positive (i.e., attraction) or negative (i.e., repulsion). Sociometric methods collect information about the extent to which each child in a group likes or dislikes each of the other children in the group. These forms of information provided by individual children about which peers they like and which they dislike are used to compute measures of acceptance (i.e., how a much a child is liked) and rejection (i.e., how much a child is disliked) for every child in the group. A simple sentence captures the distinction between them: *Peer assessment techniques assess what a child is like; sociometric techniques assess whether a child is liked*. The intricacies of peer assessments and sociometric measures are described in the following sections.

Conceptual Principles and Statistical Assumptions

Peer Assessment Techniques

If there is a particular project that brought the use of peer assessments into a modern format, it is probably Mitchell's (1956) study of the use of a "guess who?" technique with a group of fourth graders. Prior to this study, "guess who?" or "who are they?" techniques had been used by Hartshorne, May, and Maller (1929), Raths (1943), and Havighurst and colleagues (1952). These early uses of peer assessments were typically focused on measuring a particular construct of interest (e.g., moral behavior). Their procedures asked children to match characteristics to the individuals in the group. Raths (1943), for example, used the following item:

> Do we have any boys or girls in our room who lose their temper, who get mad very quickly, who become angry and excited when things go wrong? Then when they do lose their tempers, they often do things or say things that are very rude and very impolite. Who are the children who do this?

Children who took part in Raths's procedure simply identified which of their peers fit this description. The number of times that each child was chosen for an item was used as an index of the extent to which each child manifested the characteristic described in the item. Mitchell's description of how these nominations are used to create scores for individual children remains true more than 50 years later. He wrote:

> The number of nominations received by each child for each description is computed and this score constitutes the child's score for this item. The score for this item is then added to the scores for other descriptive items that are supposed to measure . . . this same form of behavior. This total score [summed across these items] is regarded as an index of the extent to which a particular child shows this more general form of behavior. (Mitchell, 1956, p. 379)

This succinct description explains the basic premise of the meaning ascribed to the frequency measures derived from peer assessments.

The use of "guess who?" or "who are they?" techniques flourished in the 1950s. Two aspects of this flourishing are particularly notable. One feature concerns the content of the assessments and the conceptual structure used to organize the observed scores. Although the initial use of peer assessment techniques had been focused either on particular forms of behavior (e.g., self control; Hartshorne et al., 1929) or on broad dimensions of behavior (e.g., "good adjustment" and "bad adjustment"; Raths, 1943; Tuddenham, 1952), Mitchell (1956) recognized their potential to provide a comprehensive assessment of a child's or adolescent's social and personal functioning. He expanded the scope of these techniques with the use of a large and heterogeneous set of items indicating different features of social behavior in conjunction with a factor analysis of the observed scores on the 19 items. With his sample of fourth graders, he observed three large factors: *Leadership Ability* (sample item: "Who are the boys and girls who make good plans?"), *Aggressive Maladjustment* (sample item: "Who are the ones who break rules, rules of the school and rules of games?"), and *Withdrawn Maladjustment* (sample item: "Who are the boys and girls who stay out of games? They don't like to play hard."). Three smaller factors were identified: *Practical Intelligence, Friendship*, and *Negative Friendship*.

The most important advance in Mitchell's project was the presentation of an empirically supported structure for organizing the peer assessment items into conceptually meaningful factors that were useful for multiple research strategies. This same three-factor structure has been seen in most of the better known techniques that came after it, including Bower's (1957) class play, the Peer Nomination Inventory (Wiggins & Winder, 1961; Winder & Wiggins, 1964), the Peer Evaluation Inventory (Pekarik, Prinz, Liebert, Weintraub, & Neale, 1976), and the revised class play (Masten et al., 1985). This use of the same three factors is not surprising, as they roughly fit the three fundamental dimensions of social behavior: moving toward others (i.e., sociability), moving away from others (i.e., withdrawal), and moving against others (i.e., aggression).

A second aspect of the flourishing of peer assessment in the 1950s was the recognition by Bower (1957, 1960) and others (Wiggins & Winder, 1961; Winder & Wiggins, 1964) that peer assessment techniques could be used to identify high-risk children. They saw that the rich database possessed by the peer group could be used to target the children with problematic social functioning. A likely reason for the frequent use of peer assessment measures is their utility for assessing individual differences in basic forms of social behaviors across a broadly defined distribution that would include normal and at-risk children. Although the procedures used by Bower and by Winder and Wiggins to identify at-risk children were largely similar in their essential features to those of Mitchell (1956), they had to include a new set of procedures so that the normal children could be distinguished from those at risk. These new procedures included the creation of a reasoned cutoff score to distinguish typical from atypical and the establishment of a common frame of reference across groups in spite of differences in their size.

The strategy they chose was to standardize the observed scores. By transforming the observed scores into standardized scores, using the mean and standard deviation for each group, variations between groups were eliminated. This process controlled for variations in group size and created a comparable metric across groups. Although a distinction was typically made between scores based on same-sex and other-sex nominations, the standardized scores from these two parts of the peer group were usually added together to create a single index for each item. The combined same-sex plus other-sex scores for items that represented the same domain were simply added together to create a dimensional index. These aggregated scores were then standardized again to create an apparently tidy index whose mean and standard deviation were invariant across groups.

This invariance across groups was perceived to form a common framework for assigning children to extreme groups based on deviations expressed in standard deviation units (e.g., using a cutoff score of + or –1.65 as a 95% threshold). This standardize-and-then-add-them-up approach became a nearly universal procedure in peer assessment. This computational simplicity in conjunction with the simplicity of the data collection itself and the ability to set cutoffs based on a statistical criterion helped make peer assessment a widely used technique to measure individual differences in aggression, sociability, and withdrawal in the peer group.

In spite of these apparent advantages, however, there were reasons to be concerned about the conceptual validity of these general procedures. One problem concerns the homogeneity of the content of the items included in the broad scales of aggression, withdrawal, and sociability. Beginning in the late 1980s several researchers raised concerns about whether the items within these scales were indexing the same thing. They decided to create more finely articulated indices of these broad dimensions. Rubin and Mills (1988), for example, showed that the items used to measure withdrawal were not indices of the same phenomenon but were indices of at least two constructs, one representing the tendency to prefer to be alone (i.e., "active withdrawal") and the other representing the experience of being isolated or excluded from the group (i.e., "passive withdrawal"). The value of this distinction was confirmed in subsequent studies (Bowker, Bukowski, Zargarpour, & Hoza, 1998; Younger & Daniels, 1992).

At least four independent projects discovered more specific factors within the revised class play's Sociability/Leadership factor. Using an exploratory factor analysis with a sample of low-SES urban children, Luthar and McMahon (1996) found two factors: One was labeled Responsible Leader, and the other was called Popular. Similar factors (Leadership and Social Etiquette) were identified by Realmuto, August, Sieler, and Pessoa-Brandao (1997) and by Casiglia, LoCoco, and Zappulla (1998). More recently, Zeller, Vannatta, Schafer, and Noll (2003) discovered two slightly different factors (Popular-Leadership and Prosocial) in which aspects of leadership were more strongly associated with prosocial skills than with popularity.

There have also been several efforts to expand the range and the specificity of peer assessments. These include Coie and Dodge's (1987) proposal that aggression should not be measured as a unitary or single phenomenon but instead that it can be assessed according to whether it is reactive or proactive, as well as other proposals that peer assessments of aggression need to differentiate between social/relational aggression forms and physical/direct forms (Bjorkqvist, Lagerspetz, & Kaukiainen, 1992; Crick & Grotpeter, 1995; Galen & Underwood, 1997). Taken together, these reassessments indicate that persons who use peer assessment as a method of measurement need to be wary of the broadband three-factor approach and instead should focus on more specific forms of social action. It is a strength of the peer assessment method that it has the flexibility to be applied to many forms of content, including aspects of affect (Bukowski, Laursen, & Hoza, 2010), illness and physical stature (Noll, Bukowski, LeRoy, Rogosch, & Kulkarni, 1991; Sandberg, Bukowski, Fung, & Noll, 2004), social prominence (Newcomb & Bukowski, 1983), and self-distortions (Bukowski, Schwartzman, Santo, Bagwell, & Adam, 2009).

A second reason for concern is the use of unit weights to aggregate item scores to create scale scores. An inherent assumption of the just-add-them-together approach is that each item has the same value as an index of the latent construct. Although this practice is completely consistent with the concept of parallel scores taken from classical test theory, it is inconsistent with evidence taken from techniques such as factor analysis. Consider, for example, the factor loadings reported by Masten and colleagues (1985) for the items in the Aggressive Disruptiveness factor. Although the weight for the item "picks on other kids" is substantially larger (.85) than the weight for the item "interrupts when other children are speaking" (.62), these items are given equal weight when the items are combined to form a composite index. This practice compromises the accuracy and the validity of the scale.

A third implicit assumption concerns the practice of asking each participating peer to nominate just one same-sex peer and one other-sex peer for each item included in the assessment. This practice appears to be based on the rather dubious assumption that only one same-sex peer and only one other-sex peer (no more and no fewer) in each group fits each characteristic. Surely there must be some groups (if not all groups) for which this assumption is untrue. Ironically, earlier techniques, such as Mitchell's (1956), collected multiple nominees per item. In this way, recent techniques were a step backward rather than a step forward. The use of multiple nominations instead of just one is likely to create more accurate and valid measures.

A fourth reason for concern is the use of standardization practices. Although transforming raw scores into standardized scores solves one problem (i.e., eliminating potential biases in scores due to variations in group size), in doing so it creates others. The resulting appearance of uniformity across groups is more illusory than real unless from the outset there are no differences between groups in their means and variability. Given that this circumstance is highly unlikely, standardization distorts the nature of the actual differences between groups. This distortion makes it difficult, if not impossible, to examine differences between some aspects of group functioning. Accordingly, although standardization is useful for solving some problems, it is otherwise a conceptually misguided and empirically flawed strategy.

Sociometric Methods

Sociometric methods include a large class of methods that assess the positive and negative links (i.e., the attractions and repulsions) that occur between persons within a group. The basic principle of the sociometric method is that every group member has the capacity to evaluate every other group member on one or more criteria in a round-robin design. In this section, the basic procedure and basic elements of a sociometric procedure, as well as the methodological variations within each of the building blocks of the procedure, are discussed.

The Basic Procedure

Coie, Dodge, and Coppotelli (1982) and Newcomb and Bukowski (1983, 1984) presented a sociometric method that has served as the standard since the 1980s. In the Coie and colleagues (1982) procedure, children are asked to name three classroom peers they like most (acceptance) and three they like least (rejection). Nominations received for both questions are counted for each child and standardized within classrooms to control for differences in classroom size. A continuous score for social preference is created by taking the difference between the standardized acceptance and rejection scores and again standardizing the resulting scores within classrooms. A continuous score for social impact is created by summing the standardized acceptance and rejection scores and restandardizing the results. Finally, using detailed decision rules (see Coie et al., 1982), each child is assigned to one of five sociometric status types: popular (liked by many, disliked by few), rejected (disliked by many, liked by few), neglected (neither liked nor disliked), controversial (liked by some and disliked by others), and average (around the means of acceptance and rejection). In Coie and

Dodge (1987), the average group is simply everyone who does not meet the criteria for the first four groups. Assignment to the extreme groups was based on whether a child's score on the critical variable was common or rare. Cutoffs based on standardized scores were used for this purpose.

Newcomb and Bukowski (1983, 1984) recommended a modified approach. They measured acceptance with three "best friend" nominations rather than "liked most," and they proposed a probability-based criterion to identify whether a child's level of acceptance and rejection was common or rare and to control for differences in classroom size. As a consequence, the criteria for the assignment of children to the five sociometric status groups changed as well. Terry and Coie (1991) demonstrated that there is a high concordance of sociometric status assignments between the Coie and colleagues (1982) and Newcomb and Bukowski (1983) methods.

Basic Elements of the Sociometric Procedure

Sociometric procedures consist of the following basic components: reference group, voter population, nominee population, sociometric criteria, data collection method, quantification method, method of standardization, sociometric dimensions, and classification method. The *reference group* is the collection of persons (group or social network) within which status is determined. In most applications, the reference group is the classroom or grade, but other possibilities are sports teams, hobby clubs, or children in an after-school program. It is important to realize that peer status is relative to the reference group in which it is assessed. Decisions about the proper reference group for a study should be driven by considerations of ecological validity. In North America, the reference group for kindergarten and elementary school children is typically the classroom; for early adolescents in middle school, it is all peers in their grade; and for adolescents in high school, it is also the entire grade level or even all peers in school across grades. In other cultures with a different structure of secondary education, the proper reference group may continue to be the classroom beyond elementary school.

The *voter population* consists of the children or adolescents who participate as evaluators in a sociometric test. The *nominee population* includes the children or adolescents who are being evaluated. Ideally, all members of the reference group (e.g., classroom or grade) participate as both voters and those voted on. It is recommended that once the reference group is chosen, no restrictions are imposed on the list of voters or nominees. In practice, restrictions of the voter population are almost impossible to avoid due to absenteeism on the day of testing or lack of permission to participate. However, acceptable sociometric scores can still be obtained when the voter population is incomplete. With limited nominations, a minimum participation rate of 70% is required (Crick & Ladd, 1989). With unlimited nominations, stable constructs are still obtained with a 60% participation rate (Wargo Aikins & Cillessen, 2007). Restrictions of the nominee population are avoidable, although some researchers intentionally ask participants to evaluate only same-sex peers, peers of one ethnicity, or randomized subsets of all peers in the reference group. Restrictions of the nominee population can potentially have serious consequences. If they are large and not random, it changes the nature of the reference group and hence the validity of status obtained relative to the reference group that was originally intended. In most studies, the voter and nominee populations are subgroups of the reference group, and the former is smaller than the latter, making the voter-by-nominee matrix rectangular rather than the ideal square.

Three methods of *data collection* are commonly distinguished: peer nominations, ratings, and paired comparisons. Peer nominations are the most common. Technically, the peer nomination method is a method of partial rank ordering. For any given criterion, the voter ranks nominees at the top of the distribution of the variable and leaves the remainder of the peer group (those who are not nominated) unranked. Peer ratings continue to be used, although they are not as common as peer nominations. Maassen, van der Linden, Goossens, and Bokhorst (2000) demonstrated that ratings have certain statistical advantages over nominations, but the impracticality of collecting peer ratings in large reference groups (such as entire grades) often prevents researchers from using them. In the method of paired comparisons, children are presented with all possible pairs of peers in the nominee population or a random subset. For each dyad, they are asked to indicate which member best fits the criterion. This method yields highly reliable scores but is also exceptionally time-consuming. It is an excellent method for collecting sociometric data in small groups of very young children (kindergarten or preschool groups).

An issue of some importance when using peer nominations is whether to collect limited or unlimited nominations. In the first sociometric studies with children in the 1940s and 1950s, both fixed and free nominations were used. Fixed nominations were more common but not always limited to three. Because Coie and colleagues (1982) and Newcomb and Bukowski (1983) solicited three nominations, this practice was followed in many studies. There are two reasons why some researchers decided to revisit this issue. First, during sociometric data collection it is not uncommon for participants to indicate that they want to name fewer or more peers for certain questions. In those cases, letting the number of nominations be free rather than restricting them to a fixed number seems more ecologically valid. Second, researchers increasingly collect sociometric data in large reference groups, such as middle and high school grades. In those contexts, nominations fixed to a small number are problematic for participants. Based on these considerations, the use of unlimited nominations has increased.

The *quantification method* refers to the way scores are computed for each participant in a sociometric study. For peer nominations, one first computes the total number of nominations that each child received for each sociometric criterion. For peer ratings, it is average ratings received. For the method of paired comparisons, it is the number of times participants were chosen across all dyads in which they appeared.

An important issue in the quantification of peer nominations was raised in the discussion of peer assessments. This issue is that the number of votes received is positively correlated with the size of the voter population. Thus raw scores are not comparable between groups, classrooms, or grades that differ in size. The *standardization method* refers to the method of controlling for these differences. There are three methods: standard scores, probability scores, and proportion scores. The standard score method (Coie et al., 1982) is the most common method and the easiest to use. In this method, raw nominations received are standardized to z scores within the nominee population. Thus this method is closely linked to the idea that status is relative to the group in which it is assessed. The probability score method was first proposed by Bronfenbrenner (1945) and refined by Newcomb and Bukowski (1983). This method was originally intended for limited nominations. Using the binomial distribution, the probability of occurrence of each raw number of votes received is calculated based on the number of voters, the number of nominees, and the number of nominations requested. Ten Brink (1985) extended this method to unlimited nominations using the generalized binomial distribution. The proportion score method entails dividing the number of nominations received by the number of nominators, creating scores that express the proportion of all possible voters who chose the participant for each question (e.g., Hodges & Perry, 1999).

Two basic and two derivative measures can be created with the nominations collected in sociometric measures. The two basic measures are *acceptance* (i.e., the number of "liked most" choices a child receives) and *rejection* (i.e., the number of "liked least" nominations a child receives). Acceptance is an index of attractions, whereas rejection is an index of repulsions. The two derivative measures are known as *social preference* and *social impact*. Social preference is the difference between the standardized measures of acceptance and rejection; it serves as a measure of relative likableness. Social impact is the sum of the standardized measures of acceptance and rejection; it is a measure of notoriety in the peer group.

These scores have been used by themselves as indices of a child's experiences with peers, and they have been used together in classification systems that assign children to sociometric groups. Sociometric classification is a time-honored component of peer relations research. Starting in the 1940s, peer researchers used the basic and the derivative sociometric measures to create groups whose members showed similar patterns of acceptance, rejection, preference, and impact. The *popular* group was high in preference, acceptance, and impact and low in rejection; the *rejected* group was low in preference and acceptance and high in impact and rejection; the *average* group showed moderate scores on preference and impact; the *neglected* group was low in impact and moderate in preference; and the *controversial* group was average in preference and very high in impact. In spite of their wide use for several decades, especially during the 1980s, these groupings are now rarely used because statistical techniques that rely on dimensional measures have become more available and more powerful. A meta-analysis conducted in the early 1990s provides a summary of the findings from studies that used sociometric classification (Newcomb, Bukowski, & Pattee, 1993). Beyond providing a comprehensive report of research on differences between children in sociometric groups, this review served as a eulogy for the group-based approach to understanding peer relations.

Developmental Applications

Three developmental issues are related to the use of peer assessments: (1) whether age differences appear in the use of peer assessments and sociometric measures, (2) whether age differences in aspects of social behavior and experience with peers can be detected with peer assessment and sociometric measures, and (3) whether associations between peer assessment measures and sociometric measures vary as a function of age.

Age differences in the use of peer assessments and sociometric measures have been discussed before (Bukowski & Hoza, 1989; Wasik, 1987) and deserve little elaboration. The bottom line can be stated succinctly. Basic forms of sociometric methods have been used in reliable and valid ways with children as young as 4 or 5 years of age (e.g., children in preschool or kindergarten classrooms). By adapting procedures to account for their inability to read (e.g., by using pictures in one-on-one interviews instead of using written lists of names as part of a group administration), it is possible to collect information from young children about whom they see as their friends and whom they dislike or tend to stay away from. The use of peer assessments is a bit more challenging, not because of procedural issues but because of limitations in the complexity of young children's schemas for social behaviors. The best demonstration of this point comes from the work of Younger, Schwartzman, and Ledingham (1985, 1986), who showed that early school-age children had more difficulty than older children distinguishing between negative forms of adaptation (i.e., aggression and withdrawal). For this reason, the use of peer assessments with young children can probably be relied on to produce reasonably valid measures of very broad aspects of sociability, but it cannot produce differentiated indices of specific aspects of maladjustment.

Peer assessment and sociometric measures have been used to assess age differences. The use of peer assessment techniques to study age differences in social behavior is rare. One reason for this infrequent use of peer assessments to assess developmental differences may be related to the extensive use of limited nomination procedures that may lead to very restricted differences in mean values across groups. In at least one case, however, peer assessments were used to assess age differences in two forms of social behavior. Crick and Grotpeter (1995) did not observe age differences in a measure of aggression used with a school-age sample, but they did observe an age-related decrease in a peer-based measure of social isolation for girls. In regard to age differences in measures taken from sociometric measures, there is evidence from sociometric data (Maccoby, 1988) that levels of liking for same-sex peers, relative to that of other-sex peers, increases from early childhood through much of the school-age period. A fundamental assumption of these analyses is that the phenomenon that is indexed by the measures does not vary with age.

A final developmental issue concerns age-related variations in measures derived from peer ratings. Perhaps the best known examples of this approach can be seen in recent reports that measures of aggression and social status are typically negative during the school-age years but become positive during early adolescence (Cillessen & Mayeux, 2004). These findings point to the utility of peer assessment measures for studying age effects in associations between constructs.

Challenges and Illustrations

The use of peer ratings is not without challenges. In this section we discuss three matters related to the use of peer ratings. One concerns differences in group size, one concerns the level of analysis, and the third concerns the use of limited and unlimited nomination procedures.

Adjusting for Differences in Group Size

A well-recognized challenge to the use of peer nominations is the fact that they can be affected by the size of the peer group. Higher scores are more likely to be observed in larger classes than in smaller classes. A goal for researchers who use nomination-based measures has been to find a way to eliminate the variations in the size of observed scores that arise from differences in group size. This presumed inflation of scores from larger groups is believed to be due to the larger number of opportunities to be chosen in these groups. One can assume that when the number of nominators increases, the likelihood that a particular child would be chosen also will increase. Although it is generally believed that nomination-based scores are positively associated with class size, there is reason to expect that this association may be negative. Indeed, as the number of potential nominees increases, the likelihood that a particular child would be chosen by any other child is likely to decrease. If a nominator can choose from a larger pool of peers, the likelihood that she or he will choose any particular peer will be smaller than when there are fewer peers in the pool.

The typical technique for dealing with the potential biases that may result from differences in group size is to standardize the observed raw scores. This widely used strategy has several advantages. It is easy to implement, it appears to get the job done, and it produces scores that are in a metric that is widely understood. Nevertheless, standardization may cause more problems than it solves. Perhaps the biggest problem that standardization creates is that it does its job too well: It completely eliminates the differences between groups in their means and their variances. When between-group differences are artificially eliminated, groups take on the appearance (illusion?) of being more similar than they really are.

Recently two of us proposed a new way to deal with the problems associated with variations in group size. We (Velásquez, Bukowski, & Saldarriaga, 2011) propose a regression-based technique designed to make content-free estimates of the linear and curvilinear effects that group size has on the size of observed scores. These estimates are then used to adjust observed scores according to the expected level of inflation or deflation due to deviations in group size relative to the size of a target median group. This technique has several advantages, including (1) ease of application, (2) keeping the scores in their original metric, and (3) maintaining the real differences between groups in their means and variances.

This technique makes use of regression analysis to empirically estimate and remove the effect of group size on peer nomination scores. First, the linear and quadratic effects of group size (i.e., number of nominators minus one) are used as predictors of the average number of nominations received by individuals within the group across the items of a questionnaire (e.g., peer assessment). These effects provide information about how much the nomination scores are likely to increase as a function of a one-person increase in the group size. Next, a group reference size is chosen, and raw nomination scores for each individual in each item are adjusted according to the deviation of each individual's group size from the reference size. In this way, for each unit increase in group size, scores are decreased based on the coefficients. Similarly, for each unit decrease in group size, scores are increased.

Distinguishing between Levels of Analysis

At the outset of this chapter we extolled the virtues of methods that capitalize on the collective knowledge of the group. The basic premise regarding the value of measures derived from peer ratings is that the use of multiple assessors increases validity and accuracy. Another apparent strength of scores derived from peer ratings is the practical advantage of having a single indicator for each person on each dimension of interest. For much of the past 80 years following the initial use of peer ratings in the 1920s, this tidy practice of having a single indicator for each child on each variable of interest matched the demands of the available statistical procedures, such as correlational techniques. It was a match made in the methodological heaven of the 1920s to the 1990s.

Currently, however, the availability of hierarchical forms of analysis that can estimate and distinguish between effects from different levels of analysis, such as the individual and the group, has given us the chance to step back and think about how peer ratings are used in peer research. Perhaps the most basic way to begin this reconsideration is to remind ourselves that the correlation between two peer assessment measures is essentially a correlation between two totals. The correlation between two peer assessment scores tells us the extent to which high totals on one measure covary with high (or low) totals on the other. It is important to keep in mind that these observed totals are aggregates from across the entire nominating group. It may be that such correlations are reflections of a process that takes place at the level of the individual, but a correlation between two group measures cannot tell us directly about an individual-level process.

Consider the following example. There is evidence that in early adolescence the correlation between a measure of aggression and a measure of social status is positive and of a moderate size. For example, in a sample of 334 early adolescent boys and girls, the correlation between a measure of aggression and a measure of status within the group was observed to be .35 (Bukowski et al., 2011). In a more recent set of analyses, we (Bukowski, Vitaro, Velásquez, & Bagwell, 2011) investigated whether the association between the total number of times that a child was chosen for items indicating aggression and the total number of times the child was chosen for roles indicating status was present at the level of the individual nominator. The analysis showed that the frequency of instances in which a child chose the same peers for items indicating aggression and those indicating status was low (less than 6% of the potential number).

This finding suggests that the correlation between aggression and popularity is not due to processes of perception at the level of the individual but that it reflects dynamics across the peer group. This evidence of a difference between associations at the level of the individual and at the level of the group could be due to several factors (e.g., within- and between-clique variations in how peers are perceived on positive and negative dimensions). At a larger level, this finding illustrates the opportunity to use peer ratings in ways that differ from their typical use in the past nine decades. Perhaps it is time to leave this wonderful legacy behind us and to adapt peer measures to currently available statistical techniques that allow us to understand peer processes and dynamics at multiple levels of social complexity.

Limited and Unlimited Nominations

One issue of some importance related to the use of peer nomination methods in developmental research is whether nominations are to be limited or unlimited. The standards set for sociometric studies in the 1980s (Coie et al., 1982; Newcomb & Bukowski, 1983) asked for limited or fixed numbers of nominations. In the 1990s, Terry (2000) began recommending the use of unlimited nominations, a practice that has been followed in a number of other studies, especially when grade is the reference group (e.g., Cillessen & Mayeux, 2004). However, other studies have continued the practice of requesting three or fewer nominations. There are also studies that use hybrid forms, including unlimited nominations capped at a maximum or limited nominations for some questions and unlimited nominations for others. Given the variety of practices in sociometric research, the relative advantages of both methods should be reviewed and investigated further.

Using Limited or Unlimited Nominations

When limited nominations are used, students to name up to a particular number of peers (e.g., three) for each question on the sociometric instrument. The use of limited nomination was frequent from the earliest days of sociometry. Its use can still be seen in some prominent research groups today, typically in studies of elementary school children. When unlimited nominations are used, students are asked to name as many or as few peers as they wish for each sociometric question. This practice was initiated in the 1980s, usually in research conducted in middle and high schools with grade as the reference group, or in the upper grades of elementary schools in which students were allowed to choose peers from parallel classrooms of their own grade level in their school. In some studies students are allowed to name peers across all four grade levels of their high school (e.g., Franzoi, Davis, & Vasquez-Suson, 1994).

Hybrid Forms

There are several hybrid forms of the unlimited-nominations procedures. One common method allows students to name as many or as few peers as they wish for each question in the instructions but cap the number of total nominations on the data collection forms (e.g., Bellmore, Jiang, & Juvonen, 2010; Bukowski et al., 2010; Peters, Cillessen, Riksen-Walraven, & Haselager, 2010). An example of another hybrid form is a study by Cillessen, de Bruyn, and LaFontana (2009) of early adolescents in the second year of secondary school. For all behavioral reputation questions, early adolescents were asked to name two peers from their classroom who engaged in each behavior the most. For all peer status and affiliation questions (liking, popularity, friendship), participants could name as many or as few peers as they wanted from all classrooms of their grade level.

Critical Issues

When we compare results on similar themes (e.g., the behavioral correlates of acceptance, rejection, and popularity) across studies using these different methods, consistent findings emerge (e.g., Newcomb et al., 1993). From this perspective, methodological choices such as the use of limited or unlimited nominations may seem trivial, and in the broad perspective of building a database of essential knowledge about social relationships with peers that serves theoretical and practical knowledge, this issue may be of little importance. Accordingly, some researchers may conclude that the choice of method should depend primarily on practical considerations of the classrooms or schools in which sociometric data are collected, the testing time available, the cognitive level of the participants, or what is simply most convenient given the research circumstances.

However, it is important to strive for the greatest level of precision and accuracy in sociometric research. For that reason, the issue of limited versus unlimited nominations deserves additional attention as it is related to ecological validity, reference group size, the quantification and standardization of sociometric scores and stability. We turn to each of these issues separately.

Ecological Validity

The main reason to consider unlimited nominations is ecological validity (Terry, 2000). In sociometric research in middle schools, students would often indicate that they wished to name more than three peers for certain questions (e.g., Who do you like? Who cooperates and shares?), whereas they sometimes had trouble coming up with three names for questions about constructs such as aggression and (extreme) withdrawal or shyness. An important motivation behind considering unlimited nominations was to make the nomination process as ecologically valid as possible for the participants.

Reference Group Size

An advantage of limited nominations is that they are less likely to be influenced by reference group size. If one is asked to name one's top three choices for a certain criterion, the meaning of this process is expected to be the same regardless of the size of the reference group (given a certain minimum required for the sociometric process to be valid). However, this creates a double-bind situation, as the previous criterion of ecological validity dictates that students in large grades often wish to name more peers than the usual fixed number of three. Leaving the total number free means that nominations received become less exclusive compared with circumstances in which all participants are required to name exactly three peers.

The issue of reference group size is most critical in the comparison of elementary school classrooms with middle or high school grades. In middle or high school, it is often untenable to limit students to three nominations per question. Elementary classrooms range in size from around 25 to 30 across continents and countries, so the choice of method seems to be less critical. When the classroom is the reference group, the number of nominations spontaneously given centers around three anyway (somewhat larger for positive questions such as most liked, and somewhat smaller for negative questions such as least liked). In middle and high school grades, the criterion of ecological validity seems to dictate letting the number of nominations go free, at the cost of control over exclusivity.

Quantification

A solution to this problem can be found in the quantification and standardization of sociometric scores. Quantification of sociometric scores begins with a simple count of the number of nominations received for a question. In older sociometric studies, nominations received were sometimes weighted by their order, but this practice was abandoned because weighted and unweighted scores correlated highly. The issue has returned in discussions about the quantification of unlimited nominations.

In sociometric research, standardization refers to controlling for reference group size. There are three common methods of standardization: standard scores, probability scores, and proportion scores (Cillessen, 2009). Neither the standard score nor the proportion score is influenced by the nomination method (limited vs. unlimited) or the size of the reference group (classrooms and grades of different sizes), except that with unlimited nominations and in larger reference groups, the resulting distributions of standardized scores have more possible values and are therefore better estimates of the population distribution (although not necessarily normal).

The probability score method goes back to work by Bronfenbrenner (1943, 1944) and was reintroduced by Newcomb and Bukowski (1983, 1984). In this method, the probability associated with raw scores received is determined according to whether the score can be classified as rare (e.g., probability of occurrences less than 5%). With fixed nominations, these probabilities are based on the binomial distribution. With unlimited nominations, these probabilities are based on the generalized binomial distribution (ten Brink, 1985). Because this method of standardization adjusts to the number of nominations given, it is more advanced than the previous two methods. When the generalized binomial distribution is applied to unlimited nominations, a vote from a student who names more peers counts for less than a vote from a student who is exclusive in her or his nominations.

This principle is also built into the most sophisticated method to quantify and standardize unlimited nominations, a procedure developed by Terry (2000) that used the item response theory (IRT; Thissen & Steinberg, 1986) framework. In this approach, the nominees in the reference group are seen as equivalent to items on a test; each has his or her own individual distribution of the likelihood of being named. The distribution is taken into account, as well as individual differences between the voters in their own voting tendencies. This approach provides the most sophisticated way of scoring sociometric data, whether collected with limited or unlimited nominations, irrespective of the size of the reference group. Unfortunately, because this method requires special software and is labor-intensive, it has not been used frequently in the sociometric literature so far (but see Coie et al., 1999; DeRosier & Thomas, 2003).

Stability

An early observation in studies using unlimited nominations is that they seem to yield higher correlations of sociometric scores over time (Terry, 2000, based on an unpublished study). Jiang and Cillessen (2005) conducted a meta-analysis of stability coefficients of continuous sociometric scores. Stability coefficients from longitudinal studies using unlimited nominations were at the high end of the distributions. Direct comparisons of the stability of limited and unlimited nominations are scarce. In addition to Terry's (2000) unpublished study, Gommans and Cillessen (2010) recently conducted a comparison in fifth- and sixth-grade classrooms that confirmed higher over-time correlations for constructs assessed with unlimited nominations. However, it should be noted that the stability coefficients obtained for limited nominations found that sociometric dimensions of acceptance, rejection, preference, and popularity are comparable to coefficients for the most stable constructs in social and personality development research (e.g., aggression and extraversion).

Summary

Peer assessments and sociometric measures are powerful and enduring methods that have become indispensable in research on peer relations. They are relatively easy to apply, and the measures they produce are amenable for use in many forms of statistical analysis. In spite of their general utility, these techniques are not without their challenges and limitations. One set of challenges derives from what would appear to be one of their strengths, specifically the continuity of their application. In some respects peer assessments and sociometric measures may have outlived the statistical and historical circumstances in which they were developed and in which they flourished. Current advances in methodology (e.g., multilevel modeling) provide new avenues for the use of peer ratings in research on the features and effects of children's experiences with their age-mates.

Acknowledgment

William M. Bukowski's work on this chapter was supported by the Social Sciences and Humanities Research Council of Canada and by a Concordia University Research Chair.

References

Bellmore, A., Jiang, X. L., & Juvonen, J. (2010). Utilizing peer nominations in middle school: A longitudinal comparison between complete classroom-based and random list methods. *Journal of Research on Adolescence, 20*, 538–550.

Bjorkqvist, K., Lagerspetz, K. M. J., & Kaukiainen, A. (1992). Do girls manipulate and boys fight? Developmental trends in regard to direct and indirect aggression. *Aggressive Behavior, 18*, 117–127.

Bower, E. M. (1957). A process for identifying disturbed children. *Children, 4*, 143–147.

Bower, E. M. (1960). *Early identification of emotionally handicapped children in school*. Springfield, IL: Charles C. Thomas.

Bowker, A., Bukowski, W. M., Zargarpour, S., & Hoza, B. (1998). A structural and functional analysis of a two dimensional model of social isolation. *Merrill-Palmer Quarterly, 44*, 447–463.

Bronfenbrenner, U. (1943). A constant frame of reference for sociometric research: Part I. Theory and technique. *Sociometry, 6*, 363–397.

Bronfenbrenner, U. (1944). A constant frame of reference for sociometric research: Part II. Experiment and inference. *Sociometry, 7*, 40–75.

Bronfenbrenner, U. (1945). The measurement of sociometric status, structure and development. (*Sociometry Monographs*, no. 6). New York: Beacon House.

Bukowski, W. M., & Hoza, B. (1989). Popularity and friendship: Issues in theory, measurement, and outcome. In T. J. Berndt & G. W. Ladd (Eds.), *Peer relations in child development* (pp. 15–45). New York: Wiley.

Bukowski, W. M., Laursen, B., & Hoza, B. (2010). The snowball effect: Friendship moderates overtime escalations in depressed affect among avoidant and excluded children. *Development and Psychopathology, 22*, 751–759.

Bukowski, W. M., Lisboa, C., Bagwell, C., Velásquez, A. M., Saldarriaga, L. M., & Cillessen, A. H. N. (2011). *Status and aggression: Using a person centred approach to reconsider issues of risk and age-related trajectories*. Manuscript in preparation.

Bukowski, W. M., Schwartzman, A. E., Santo, J. B., Bagwell, C., & Adam, R. (2009). Reactivity and distortions in the self: Narcissism, types of aggression, and the functioning of the HPA axis during early adolescence. *Development and Psychopathology 21*, 1249–1262.

Bukowski, W. M., Vitaro, F., Velasquez, A. M., & Bagwell, C. (2011). *Aggression and status: Different levels, different findings*. Manuscript in preparation.

Casiglia, A. C., LoCoco, A., & Zappulla, C. (1998). Aspects of social reputation and peer relationships in Italian children. *Developmental Psychology, 34*, 723–730.

Cillessen, A. H. N. (2009). Sociometric methods. In K. H. Rubin, W. M. Bukowski, & B. Laursen (Eds.), *Handbook of peer interactions, relationships, and groups* (pp. 82–99). New York: Guilford Press.

Cillessen, A. H. N., de Bruyn, E. H., & LaFontana, K. M. (2009, April). *Behavioral effects of prioritizing popularity*. Paper presented at the biennial meeting of the Society for Research in Child Development, Denver, CO.

Cillessen, A. H. N., & Mayeux, L. (2004). From censure to reinforcement: Developmental changes in the association between aggression and social status. *Child Development, 75*, 147–163.

Coie, J. D., Cillessen, A. H. N., Dodge, K. A., Hubbard, J. A., Schwartz, D., Lemerise, E. D., et al. (1999). It takes two to fight: A test of relational factors and a method for assessing aggressive dyads. *Developmental Psychology, 35*, 1179–1188.

Coie, J. D., & Dodge, K. A. (1987). Continuities and changes in children's social status: A five-year longitudinal study. *Merrill-Palmer Quarterly, 29*, 261–281.

Coie, J. D., Dodge, K. A., & Coppotelli, H. (1982). Dimensions and types of social status: A cross-age perspective. *Developmental Psychology, 18*, 557–571.

Crick, N. R., & Grotpeter, J. K. (1995). Relational aggression, gender, and social-psychological adjustment. *Child Development, 66*, 710–722.

Crick, N. R., & Ladd, G. W. (1989). Nominator attrition: Does it affect the accuracy of children's sociometric classifications? *Merrill-Palmer Quarterly, 35*, 197–207.

DeRosier, M. E., & Thomas, J. M. (2003). Strengthening sociometric prediction: Scientific advances in the assessment of children's peer relations. *Child Development, 74*, 1379–1392.

Franzoi, S. L., Davis, M. H., & Vasquez-Suson, K. A. (1994). Two social worlds: Social correlates and stability of adolescent status groups. *Journal of Personality and Social Psychology, 67*, 462–473.

Galen, B. R., & Underwood, M. (1997). A developmental investigation of social aggression among girls. *Developmental Psychology, 33*, 589–600.

Galton, F. (1907). Vox populi. *Nature, 75*, 450–451.

Gommans, R., & Cillessen, A. H. N. (2010). *A comparison of limited and unlimited peer nomination methods*. Unpublished manuscript, Radboud University Nijmegen, Behavioural Science Institute.

Hartshorne, H., May, M., & Maller, J. (1929). *Studies in service and self-control*. New York: Macmillan.

Havighurst, R. J., DeHaan, R. E., Dieterich, W. J., Hackamack, H., Johnson, L., & King, R. D. (1952). A community youth development program. *Supplementary Educational Monographs, 75*.

Hodges, E., & Perry, D. (1999). Personal and interpersonal antecedents and consequences of victimization by peers. *Journal of Personality and Social Psychology, 76*, 677–685.

Jiang, X. L., & Cillessen, A. H. N. (2005). Stability of continuous measures of sociometric status: A meta-analysis. *Developmental Review, 25*, 1–25.

Luthar, S. S., & McMahon, T. J. (1996). Peer reputation among inner-city adolescents: Structure and correlates. *Journal of Research on Adolescence, 6*, 581–603.

Maassen, G. H., van der Linden, J. L., Goossens, F. A., & Bokhorst, J. J. (2000). A ratings-based approach to two-dimensional sociometric status determination. In A. N. Cillessen & W. M. Bukowski (Eds.), *Recent advances in the measurement of acceptance and rejection in the peer system* (pp. 55–73). San Francisco: Jossey-Bass.

Maccoby, E. E. (1988). Gender as a social category. *Developmental Psychology, 24*, 755–765.

Masten, A. S., Morison, P., & Pellegrini, D. S. (1985). A revised class play method of peer assessment. *Developmental Psychology, 21*, 523–533.

Mitchell, J. V. (1956). The factor analysis of a "guess who" questionnaire designed to identify significant behavior patterns in children. *Journal of Personality, 24*, 376–386.

Newcomb, A. F., & Bukowski, W. M. (1983). Social impact and social preference as determinants of children's peer group status. *Developmental Psychology, 19*, 856–867.

Newcomb, A. F., & Bukowski, W. M. (1984). A longitudinal study of the utility of social preference and social impact sociometric classification schemes. *Child Development, 55*, 1434–1447.

Newcomb, A. F., Bukowski, W. M., & Pattee, L. (1993). Children's peer relations: A meta-analytic review of popular, rejected, neglected, controversial, and average sociometric status. *Psychological Bulletin, 113*, 99–128.

Noll, R. B., Bukowski, W. M., LeRoy, S. S., Rogosch, F. A., & Kulkarni, R. (1991). Peer relationships and adjustment of children with cancer. *Journal of Pediatric Psychology, 16*, 307–326.

Pekarik, E. C., Prinz, R. J., Liebert, D. E., Weintraub, S., & Neale, J. M. (1976). The Pupil Evaluation Inventory: A sociometric technique for assessing children's social behavior. *Journal of Abnormal Child Psychology, 4*, 83–97.

Peters, E., Cillessen, A. H. N., Riksen-Walraven, J. M., & Haselager, G. J. T. (2010). Best friends' preference and popularity: Associations with aggression and prosocial behavior. *International Journal of Behavioral Development, 34*, 398–405.

Raths, L. (1943). The development of a "guess who" type of test. *Educational Research Bulletin, 22*, 70–72.

Realmuto, G. M., August, G. J., Sieler, J. D., & Pessoa-Brandao, L. (1997). Peer assessment of social reputation in community samples of disruptive and nondisruptive children: Utility of the revised class play method. *Journal of Clinical Child Psychology, 26*, 67–76.

Rubin, K. H., & Mills, R. S. L. (1988). The many faces of social isolation in childhood. *Journal of Consulting and Clinical Psychology, 6*, 916–924.

Sandberg, D., Bukowski, W. M., Fung, C., & Noll, R. (2004). Height and social adjustment: Are extremes a cause for concern and action? *Pediatrics, 114*, 744–750.

Surowiecki, J. (2004). *The wisdom of crowds: Why the many are smarter than the few and how collective wisdom shapes business, economies, societies, and nations*. New York: Doubleday.

ten Brink, P. W. M. (1985). *The generalized binomial distribution as an alternative for the computation of sociometric status according to the probability model*. Unpublished master's thesis, Radboud Universiteit Nijmegen, Department of Psychology.

Terry, R. (2000). Recent advances in measurement theory and the use of sociometric techniques. In A. H. N. Cillessen & W. M. Bukowski (Eds.), Recent advances in the measurement of acceptance and rejection in the peer system. *New Directions for Child Development, 88* (pp. 27–53). San Francisco: Jossey-Bass.

Terry, R., & Coie, J. D. (1991). A comparison of methods for defining sociometric status among children. *Developmental Psychology, 27*, 867–880.

Thissen, D., & Steinberg, L. (1988). Data analysis using item response theory. *Psychological Bulletin, 104*, 385–395.

Thompson, G. G. (1960). Children's groups. In P. H. Mussen (Ed.), *Handbook of research methods in child development* (pp. 821–853). New York: Wiley.

Tuddenham, R. D. (1952). Studies in reputation: I. Sex and grade differences in school children's evaluations of their peers. II. The diagnosis of social adjustment. *Psychological Monographs, 66*(1, Whole No. 333).

Velásquez, A. M., Bukowski, W. M., & Saldarriaga, L. (2011). *Adjusting for group size effects in peer nomination data*. Manuscript submitted for publication.

Wargo Aikins, J., & Cillessen, A. H. N. (2007). *Stability and correlates of sociometric status in early adolescence*. Unpublished manuscript, University of Connecticut, Department of Psychology.

Wasik, B. H. (1987). Sociometric measures and peer descriptors of kindergarten children: A study of reliability and validity. *Journal of Clinical Child and Adolescent Psychology, 16*, 218–224.

Wiggins, J. S., & Winder, C. L. (1961). The Peer Nomination Inventory: An empirically derived sociometric measure of adjustment in preadolescent boys. *Psychological Reports, 9*, 643–677.

Winder, C., & Wiggins, J. (1964). Social reputation and social behavior: A further validation of the peer nomination inventory. *Journal of Abnormal and Social Psychology, 68*, 681–684.

Younger, A., & Daniels, T. (1992). Children's reasons for nominating their peers as withdrawn: Withdrawal vs. active isolation. *Developmental Psychology, 28*, 955–960.

Younger, A., Schwartzman, A. E., & Ledingham, J. (1985). Age-related changes in children's perceptions of aggression and withdrawal in their peers. *Developmental Psychology, 21*, 70–75.

Younger, A., Schwartzman, A. E., & Ledingham, J. (1986). Age-related differences in children's perceptions of social deviance: Changes in behaviour or perspective? *Developmental Psychology, 22*, 531–542.

Zeller, M., Vannatta, K., Schafer, J., & Noll, R. B. (2003). Behavioral reputation: A cross-age perspective, *Developmental Psychology, 39*, 129–139.

PART III

Interindividual Longitudinal Analysis

CHAPTER 14

Foundational Issues in Investigating Development as Interindividual Variation

JARI-ERIK NURMI

One of my colleagues and a scholar in developmental science, Lars Bergman, once made a statement that all researchers in the field need to take seriously. He suggested that "in order to understand development, you need to investigate development." Although this sounds like a truism, it crystallizes two crucial issues. First, if we are interested in investigating development, we need to have longitudinal data over appropriate time points that allow us to investigate the developmental mechanisms that we are interested in. Second, we have to use statistical tools that allow us to model properly these developmental mechanisms.

There are many statistical frameworks that can be used to examine development and its mechanisms. The concept "development as interindividual differences" refers to investigating development by comparing the development of one individual with the development of other individuals. In other words, development is examined by determining an individual's score on some variable against other individuals' scores on the same variable and comparing that score against other individuals' scores on that variable. In turn, the concept "development as intraindividual differences" refers to examining how the values of an individual on a certain variable predict the subsequent values for the same individual on the same or different variables later on. This means, in fact, that development is modeled across time by using data on only one individual, as is the case in time series analysis (see Molenaar & Lo, Chapter 20, in this volume). Some statistical analyses, such as latent growth modeling, combine these two frameworks and examine interindividual differences in intraindividual patterns of variation across time (see Selig & Little, Chapter 16, this volume). The vast majority of developmental research has used and still uses a framework that focuses on investigating development from the point of interindividual differences. This is also the topic of this chapter.

The analysis of the relations between variables becomes not only interesting but also challenging when it is combined with the analysis of developmental changes, associations, and changing patterns of characteristics over time. In their efforts to better understand the key mechanisms of development, scholars have formulated many kinds of questions. Examples of such questions include: To what extent do children's academic skills develop when they move from preschool to kindergarten and further to elementary school? Does children's learning motivation predict their subsequent skill development, or is it rather academic skills that predict learning motivation later on? What are the best predictors of learning to read from kindergarten to elementary school? How does the speed of learning to read predict subsequent academic achievement in secondary school?

The statistical methods that are currently used to analyze interindividual differences were introduced more than a century ago. For example, Yule introduced multiple correlation and Galton regression and correlation coefficients, in the late 19th century (Cudeck, 2007). A few years later, in the early 20th century, several researchers became interested in the structure of mental abilities. In this work, Spearman was one of the pioneers of factor analysis. During the next decades, many researchers joined in developing various forms of this method, for example Thurstone, Cattel, and Burt (Jöreskog, 2007). In the early 1920s Wright introduced path analysis for analyzing the predictive associations between independent and dependent variables. Although exploratory factor analysis was for a long time the major statistical method used for investigating interindividual differences, in the 1960s several researchers, including Jöreskog, introduced a new way to combine variables into broader constructs, namely confirmatory factor analysis (Jöreskog, 2007). Whereas explorative factor analysis is a data-driven approach, confirmatory factor analysis is a theory-driven framework that draws on ideas about the constructs underlying the individual variables. A decade later, influenced by path analysis as employed in sociology and some related methods used in econometrics, structural equation modeling (SEM) was introduced. SEM aimed at not only modeling the factor structure but also investigating the associations between the factors/constructs over time (Jöreskog, 2007). Thus the foundation for investigating development as interindividual differences was laid.

In this chapter, I first discuss some of the key issues in investigating development as interindividual differences. Then I illustrate how such issues are typically handled in the framework of SEM. Next, I discuss some new developments in investigating development that extend the traditional framework with its reliance on solely interindividual differences. I conclude the chapter with a discussion of some possible future approaches to the investigation of human development.

Central Issues

The investigation of individual development is based on several conceptual principles that provide the guidelines for any empirical research effort. These include (1) how to conceptualize and operationalize the phenomenon of interest over its development, (2) how to investigate the causality involved in development, (3) how to investigate the complex associations between variables (mediation and moderation) so that they best describe the developmental mechanisms under study, (4) how to decide about the appropriate timing of the measurements, and (5) how to handle the fact that the cases under study are not independent but have a nested structure. These topics are briefly discussed next.

Definition of Constructs and Variables

One important step before starting any research is the definition of the key constructs under study and the formulation of the model to be tested. The formulation of constructs and models is typically based, on one hand, on previous theories and cumulative evidence and, on the other hand, on previous observations (either prestudy or current data). In many cases the models and the constructs are simply revisions of those used previously, and therefore the definition of the constructs and how they should be operationalized are already available. For example, if a theory focuses on age changes in children's coping, previous research typically provides guidance about how coping should be defined and measured. In some cases, scholars may have developed a new theoretical model that requires additional construct development, as well as operationalization concerning how the constructs should be measured. If the theory introduces new constructs, scientific traditions in the field (language communities) provide guidelines on how to define and measure these new constructs. New observations or data (from either prestudy, previous studies, or current studies) are typically needed to make sure that the constructs and variables are formulated in a reliable and valid manner.

Construct Similarity across Time

Whether we are interested in examining changes in the mean of some construct across time, the interindividual stability of the construct, or the cross-lagged associations between constructs, it is important to measure the same phenomenon at each time point. Although construct similarity is an ideal situation, from the practical point of view measuring constructs identically across time is often challenging and sometimes even impossible. In particular, in longitudinal studies extending over several years, even decades, measuring identical constructs over time is difficult. A good example is the measurement of children's academic skills from kindergarten through secondary school.

There are four possibilities in respect to construct similarity over time. In the first and most straightforward situation, we have measured the same construct with identical items at different measurement points. Then the invariance of the measurement models (e.g., across time t, time $t + 1$, and time $t + 2$) can be tested by confirmatory factor analysis. The second and less favorable situation is that, although we have measured the constructs by identical items, some parts of the model cannot be estimated to be identical over time (i.e., some parts of the measurement model are not invariant). For example, factor loadings may turn out to be different at different time points. This is problematic, as the meaning of the construct also changes across the measurements, and this needs to be taken into account at least when interpreting the findings of the study. If the structure of the construct changes across time, the interpretation of the associations over time, and particularly any mean changes, becomes difficult, if not impossible.

In the third situation, we have measured the same construct at different time points but by using different items. In this case, of course, it is impossible to test whether the construct measures the same phenomenon at the different time points. This is not an unusual case in developmental research, but it substantially restricts the conclusions that can be drawn from the study. For example, low stability of the construct across time may be due either to low stability of the phenomenon or to the change in the measurement model. Also, the changes in the mean across time become uninterpretable.

In the fourth case, we test the invariance of a latent construct with nominal variables using a latent class model (Kaplan, 2008). Latent classes are nominal factors arising from the patterns of response frequencies to categorical items. These response frequencies are similar to the correlation matrix in factor analysis. Under an a priori assumption of a latent nominal variable (with a certain number of classes), the model is then fitted to the observed nominal data.

Causality

One of the key research topics in developmental science is identifying mechanisms that direct individual development. By definition, these mechanisms imply causality, such as to what extent a certain method of teaching reading leads to improved reading performance in the future or to what extent a certain kind of parenting decreases problem behavior among children. In order to conclude that X is a cause of Y, the following assumptions need to be fulfilled: (1) X has taken place before Y, that is, X has been measured at time t and Y at time $t + 1$; (2) Y at time $t + 1$ should be a function of X at time t: $Y_{t+1} = fX_t$; (3) Y at time t should not vary as a function of X at time t or, alternatively, Y at time $t + 1$ should be a function of X at t, after controlling for Y at time t; and (4) there should not be any "third variable" that explains the function $Y_{t+1} = fX_t$.

Experimental and Intervention Studies

The classical way to test causality in science is to conduct an experiment. In a typical experiment, a sample, A, is chosen from a population. Sample A is then randomized into subsamples A_1, A_2, . . . and A_c. This randomization is the key principle in any experiment, and its key rationale is to create groups that do not differ in respect to any other variables ("third variable"; Hoyle & Smith, 1994). In practice, to succeed in randomization, one needs an original sample containing hundreds rather than tens of participants. Next, Y is measured at time t and time $t + 2$. Then, groups A_1 and A_2 are subjected to different manipulations (X_1, X_2) at time $t + 1$, and group Ac is used as a control group. Finally, conclusions about the causal impact of manipulation (X) on Y can be drawn on the basis of the change in Y from time t to time $t + 2$ in groups A_1, A_2, and A_c.

The use of experiments in developmental science is difficult for several reasons. First, developmental processes take a relatively long time to occur, and therefore experimental manipulations are practically impossible to carry out. Second, short experimental manipulations carried out in laboratory settings lack ecological validity. In other words, it is not credible that such manipulations would cause changes in individuals' behavior. Third, the exposure of individuals to some circumstances that might be assumed to influence their later development (e.g., poor teaching practices at school) is unethical and cannot be done.

Causality can also be examined by conducting an intervention study. The logic and the procedure of an intervention study follow that of an experiment. A sample, A, that might be assumed to benefit from the intervention is first selected. Sample A is then randomized into subsamples A_1 and A_c. Group A_1 is then exposed to the intervention, and A_c is used as a control group. By comparing the changes in Y between time t and time $t + 2$, we can conclude whether intervention was effective or not.

Intervention studies can be very important in examining causality, because evidence-based interventions also enable understanding of the possible mechanisms that are responsible for the changes in the phenomenon under study (Piantadosi, 1997). Moreover, they may avoid some of the ethical problems found in experimental studies. The typical ethical problem associated with an intervention occurs when the control group is not provided with the possibility to participate in the intervention. This is usually handled by using a waiting list, so that the control group is given an opportunity to receive the intervention after the original study is finished.

A quasi-experiment is similar to an experiment (Rutter, 1994). In this procedure, researchers typically have been following a sample of individuals that later on can be divided into "experimental" (who have experienced the event) and "control" (who have not experienced the event) groups on the basis of some event happening to them. An example of such an event might be a natural catastrophe, such as an earthquake. By comparing the groups, researchers can obtain important information about the consequences of the event. Another example might be a large-scale longitudinal study in which researchers are able to differentiate between groups that do not differ in age but differ in whether they have attended kindergarten or not during the past year. The key limitation of a quasi-experimental study is that randomization cannot be assured.

Cross-Lagged Longitudinal Study

Cross-lagged longitudinal studies in developmental science provide another design for the investigation of causality, although in a restricted sense (Hoyle & Smith, 1994). In such studies, the same variables are measured across different time points. The causality between X and Y can be inferred in the following case: (1) X at time t predicts Y at time $t + 1$, after controlling for Y at time t. This prediction should hold after controlling for any third variables that might explain the association between X and Y.

Inference of causality from cross-lagged longitudinal studies has some limitations. The chief limitation is that because, unlike an experiment, the procedure is not based on randomization, it is possible that some third variable exists that explains the association between X and Y. In other words, if such an unknown third variable had been identified and controlled for in the model, it might have explained the cross-lagged association found between X and Y. Examples of such a third variable include intelligence, when predicting children's skill development from their parents' SES, or shared genes among parents and their children when predicting how parental divorce predicts children's subsequent problem behavior.

There are at least two ways in which this problem of a third variable can be tackled in cross-lagged longitudinal studies. First, researchers may make an effort to define, on the basis of theory and previous research, what the most likely third variables might be and then measure them. These third variables can be entered in the statistical analyses as control variables. Second, researchers may use a cross-lagged longitudinal procedure in which the measurements are spaced over relatively short time periods, for example every month, every second month, or every half year. In a research design of this kind, one can assume that at least some third variables, such as shared genes or personality traits, should not influence the cross-lagged associations between the variables, because such third variables are unlikely to change within such a short time span.

Correlational Longitudinal Studies

In the case of longitudinal studies, only a minority include a fully cross-lagged longitudinal procedure, whereas most can be described as correlational longitudinal studies. In such studies, even those in which individuals are followed several times across their development, the measured constructs will vary from one measurement to another. If previous levels of the dependent variable (Y at time t) cannot be controlled for when predicting Y at time $t + 1$ by X at time t, then the design and related statistical analyses do not allow causality to be addressed. Such research may, of course, inform researchers about other important aspects of development, such as the previous correlates of subsequent development.

Developmental Mechanisms

In addition to causality, scholars in developmental science are typically interested in the mechanisms via which, and conditions under which, a construct X influences another construct Y (see Fritz & MacKinnon, Chapter 18, this volume). These mechanisms have been described in terms of two concepts: mediation and moderation.

Mediation

Once we have found that X predicts Y, it is important to determine via which mechanism this association is actualized (Baron & Kenny, 1986; Cohen & Cohen, 1983; Fritz & MacKinnon, Chapter 18, this volume). One way to examine such a mechanism is to identify a mediator (Z) at time $t + 1$ that mediates the impact of X at time t on Y at time $t + 2$. To infer that Z is a mediator between X and Y, the following should hold: (1) X at time t predicts Y at time $t + 2$, (2) X at time t predicts Z at time $t + 1$, (3) Z at time $t + 1$ predicts Y at time $t + 2$, and (4) after entering Z at time $t + 1$ to predict Y at time $t + 2$, X at time t should no longer predict Y at time $t + 2$ (full mediation), or the prediction of X on Y should decrease substantially (partial mediation, McKinnon, 2008).

Moderation

When the associations between the variables X and Y vary under different conditions depending on the values of some third variable Q, the variable Q is described as a moderator. To infer that Q is a moderator of the association between variables X and Y, the following should hold: X at time t predicts Y at time $t + 1$ differently depending on the values of Q. A typical way to investigate whether Q is a moderator between X and Y is first to predict Y by X and Q and then add into the equation the product of X and Q (Cohen & Cohen, 1983). If the product of X and Q adds to the impact of X and Q, then Q serves as a moderator between X and Y. This is then typically investigated by categorizing variable Q and then calculating the association between variables X and Y separately for each category of Q.

Reliability and Validity

We can test a theory or model only if we have been able to create reliable and valid constructs and variables. Reliable measurement means that the measurement of the construct does not include (too much) measurement error and that, if the measurement is repeated soon after, the two measurements yield similar results. The most common way to measure reliability is to calculate the internal consistency of the items involved (e.g., Cronbach's alpha). This internal consistency reliability is, however, sometimes problematic in estimating the reliability of an evolving phenomenon (e.g., academic performance). The reason for this is that when measuring such a construct, different items on the scale typically tap different parts of the distribution: Some items differentiate between individuals at the lower end of the distribution, whereas others differentiate between individuals at the higher end of the distribution. In such cases, other reliability measures, such as split-half reliability and the stability coefficient of the construct over time, are better choices for estimating reliability than internal consistency.

In addition to reliability, the validity of the construct is important for appropriate testing of a theory or model. Validity means that the construct measures what it is supposed to measure. This is not always self-evident. For example, a paper-and-pencil measure of reading skills may not measure reading skills alone but also motor skills. Similarly, self-rating items on self-esteem may also reflect, along with self-esteem, a person's tendency to give a positive view of him- or herself. The validity of a measurement can be tested in several ways, such as estimating whether the structure of the subcomponents of the construct is congruent with the theory (structural validity) or whether the construct is associated with other constructs that measure the same phenomenon (criteria validity).

Timing of Measurement

One important issue for scholars interested in developmental mechanisms is to define the appropriate timing of measurements (Little, Bovaird, & Slegers, 2006); in other words, the timing of measures of the construct under study should in some way reflect what is previously known about the nature of the phenomenon. Let us assume, for example, that a researcher is interested in the development of personality traits, such as the Big Five. As previous research has shown that such traits are relatively stable across time, there is no need to measure them every month. By contrast, if someone is interested in evolving emotions in social interactions, then, because emotions are known to fluctuate across time, there is a need to plan a study in which emotions and social interactions are measured several times a day.

Careful consideration of the nature of the phenomenon under study with respect to timing is important, because if it is not taken into account, the findings from the study may not give an appropriate view of the developmental mechanisms involved. For example, if personality traits and interpersonal relations are measured weekly, it is unlikely that any cross-lagged impacts with other variables will be found. Similarly, investigation of emotions once a year is unlikely to tap the key developmental mechanisms in affective reactions and social interactions in an ecologically valid way.

Many psychological mechanisms show both interindividual and mean-level stability most of the time. Given that scholars are interested in change, one possibility is to investigate the phenomenon during transition periods, when substantial changes in environmental contexts take place. Examples of such critical transitions include moving from kindergarten to primary school, the transition from primary to secondary school, becoming a parent, or retirement. The key assumption of this critical transition framework is that the contextual changes also lead to changes in many psychological mechanisms, because individuals need to deal with new environmental challenges and demands by adapting their thinking and emotions accordingly. It is, of course, possible that after a period of critical transition the developing system returns to the original set point. This is, however, an important research question, as it marks a step toward understanding the nature of developing systems.

Nested Data

In many cases, participants in a longitudinal study are not independent of each other but rather form a nested structure (Hox, 2002; Raudenbush & Bryk, 2002). Examples of such nested structures include students who are nested within classrooms, parents or siblings nested within families, and families nested in their living environments (e.g., neighborhoods). If individuals are investigated in respect to the same behaviors or attitudes in different situations, for example across different life domains (school, peer groups, and family), the behaviors could be conceptualized as being nested within individuals.

Identifying whether longitudinal data have a nested structure is important for two reasons. First, failure to account for a nested structure may lead to biased estimates (Heck & Thomas, 2009). A nested data structure increases the likelihood of biased estimates of effects, because the effect of interest is then compared with an underestimated error estimate. Second, nested data raise important research questions in their own right. Examples of such questions include: Are parents in the same family similar in respect to their parenting styles? What family-level variable might explain this similarity? Are students in the same classrooms similar to each other? What classroom-level variables might explain this similarity?

Illustrations of Investigating Development as Interindividual Differences by SEM

During the past decades SEM has become one of the major statistical tools in developmental science. In this section, I illustrate some of the theoretical principles discussed previously in more general terms in the context of SEM. There are good reasons for selecting the SEM approach (Hoyle & Smith, 1994): SEM provides tools to build measurement models of constructs, to test their similarity across time, to investigate their reliability and validity, to test cross-lagged associations between constructs over time, and to determine mediation and moderation. For example, the relations between variables and constructs, which were previously done by exploratory factor analysis (measurement model), and the association between constructs that was traditionally done by regression analysis (structural model) can be simultaneously analyzed by SEM models (Figure 14.1).

Building Constructs and Models across Time

Once a researcher has decided on the constructs to be studied in the model, SEM can be used to test whether the construct measures the same phenomenon across time (i.e., invariance). This can be tested by: (1) setting the loading of each item (e.g., x_{11}, x_{12}, and x_{13}) to be identical across measurement points, (2) allowing the error terms of the same items to be associated across time, and (3) allowing the constructs to be associated between different time points (Hoyle & Smith, 1994; McArdle, 2007; Millsap & Meredith, 2007). In addition, changes in the stability and in the mean of the constructs across consecutive time points can be estimated.

Besides construct invariance, SEM also provides a possibility of estimating the reliability of the construct (Hoyle & Smith, 1994). Construct reliability can be tested as item and scale reliability, as well as retest reliability across time. A particular application of SEM,

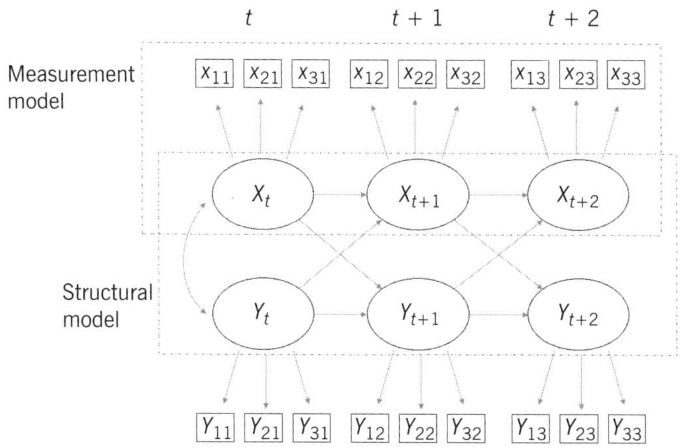

FIGURE 14.1. Schematic presentation of structural equation modeling.

the simplex model, is able to estimate the reliability of constructs that consist of only one item, given that the item is measured over several time points (Jöreskog, 2007). In validity estimation, SEM is an excellent tool for estimating structural, criteria, and predictive validities.

Investigating Causality, Mediator Effects, and Moderator Effects

SEM models are widely used in investigating causality. An example of such a model is given in Figure 14.1. If construct X at time t predicts Y at time $t + 1$ and construct X at time $t + 1$ predicts Y at time $t + 2$, after controlling for Y at time t and time $t + 1$, we can conclude that X is a cause of Y. Moreover, possible candidates for third variables can be controlled in SEM to investigate whether the inclusion of such third variables will decrease the cross-lagged paths from X to Y (Hoyle & Smith, 1994).

Investigation of mediator effects is straightforward in SEM (see Fritz & MacKinnon, Chapter 18, this volume). First, the association between X at time t and Y at time $t + 2$ is examined. If an association is found, then a mediator, Z, at time $t + 1$ is added to the model. If, after entering Z into the model, the influence of X at time t to Y at time $t + 2$ becomes nonsignificant, then it can be concluded that Z mediates the cross-lagged association between X and Y (Figure 14.2). In SEM, the statistical significance of the indirect impact from X at time t to Y at time $t + 2$ via Z at time $t + 1$ can also be tested (Hoyle & Smith, 1994).

Furthermore, the investigation of a moderator effect is straightforward in the SEM framework (see Selig & Little, Chapter 16, this volume). If Q is a nominal variable, the cross-lagged model is conducted using a "multisample procedure" (Jöreskog & Sörbom, 1993). This procedure estimates whether the same model fits to the data given different values of Q. If the same model does not fit to the different subsamples, it can be concluded that Q is a moderator variable between X and Y (Farrell, 1994). If Q is a continuous variable, a product of X and Q can be entered into a cross-lagged model to test whether the impact of this moderator effect is statistically significant. To illustrate the moderator effect, Q is categorized, and the procedure described previously is repeated.

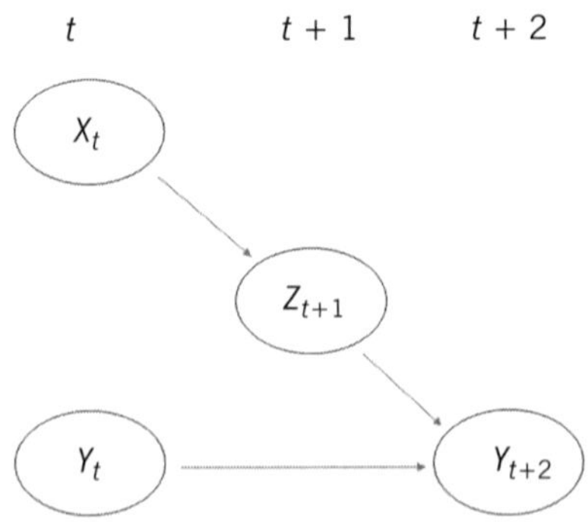

FIGURE 14.2. Schematic presentation of testing a mediation effect.

Although the traditional SEM discussed here is an excellent tool for analyzing many developmental issues, it also has one important limitation: It can be used only when the variables/constructs under study are continuous, dummy coded, or in ordinal scale. However, currently, in some applications of SEM—for example, the Mplus program—it is also possible to include nominal variables in the analysis.

New Developments

Although the investigation of development as interindividual differences provides a basis for understanding many important developmental phenomena, this framework also has its limitations. First, the SEM framework does not provide a tool to differentiate groups of individuals who show different trajectories of development. Second, it does not allow researchers to investigate whether the developmental mechanisms of interest vary across individuals. Finally, traditional SEM does not allow, as such, examination of developmental mechanisms simultaneously at different levels of data (nested data). Next, I briefly introduce some new tools that overcome these limitations of SEM.

Differentiating Interindividual and Intraindividual Differences across Time

As compared with the traditional SEM approach, growth curve modeling provides a tool to examine interindividual differences in intraindividual patterns of change across time. On one hand, growth curve modeling identifies various growth components that describe intraindividual variation over time. On the other hand, it investigates interindividual differences in various components of intraindividual change (e.g., level, linear growth, and quadratic growth) and how such components of interindividual variation are associated.

Whereas SEM focuses on the constructs and their associations within and across time, in growth curve modeling the mean of the various growth components—such as level (intercept), linear growth (slope), and quadratic growth—and variation across these means are determined over several time points (Bryk & Raudenbush, 1987; Muthén, 2008). This requires the variables to be measured identically over time. In addition to level, linear, and quadratic growth, different "parts" of the growth components can be modeled by using piecewise growth curve modeling (Li, Duncan, Duncan, & Hops, 2001). For example, if reading performance has been measured twice a year from kindergarten up to the second grade, the researcher can create separate growth components for the development that has taken place in kindergarten and for that which occurred during the first 2 school years.

One important feature of growth curve modeling is that it provides a tool to examine developmental dynamics between various growth components. For example, in the case of a single construct, a positive association between level and linear growth suggests that the construct under study shows an accelerating developmental pattern over time: High starting values predict accelerating development, whereas low starting values predict decelerating development. By contrast, a negative association between level and growth suggests that the construct under study shows decreasing individual variation over time and that high starting values predict decelerating development, whereas low starting values predict accelerating development. Even this kind of single construct analysis may increase our understanding of the developmental dynamics of a particular phenomenon (Leppänen, Niemi, Aunola, & Nurmi, 2004). Growth curve modeling also provides a possibility of examining the associations between the growth components of two or more constructs. Similarly, growth components can be predicted by some antecedents, and they can be used to predict some outcomes.

There are two major ways to conduct growth curve modeling (Chou, Bentler, & Pentz, 1998). One is latent growth modeling (LGM), in which growth components are defined as constructs (similar to the way construct is defined in SEM). The major strength of this approach is that it provides a tool to estimate constructs that are based on measurement models. Another possibility is to use hierarchical linear modeling (HLM; Bryk & Raudenbush, 1987). In this approach measurements across time are dealt with as measurements nested within individuals. The benefit of this hierarchical approach is that the measurement points across which the growth components are estimated can vary according to the number of measurements.

Mixture Modeling

An important alternative for investigating development as interindividual variation is to use a person-oriented approach (Bergman, Magnusson, & El-Khouri, 2003). Here, the aim is to identify groups of individuals who differ in the pattern of values they exhibit on different variables. One way to carry out such a person-oriented approach is to use mixture modeling, described also as "model-based clustering" (Muthén & Muthén, 2000). In its basic form, mixture modeling is conducted on a set of variables measured at a certain time point.

From the standpoint of this chapter, a particularly noteworthy application of this approach is latent mixture modeling. Whereas latent growth modeling investigates interindividual differences in intraindividual variation, latent mixture modeling complements it by a person-oriented approach. In fact, the starting point for latent mixture modeling is latent growth modeling. When the different growth components have been identified, they are used as criterion variables to identify different subgroups of the sample that follow homogeneous developmental trajectories over time. In identifying subgroups that display different trajectories, different criteria can be used. Subgroup identification can be based on the means of the trajectories, the pattern of variation and covariation across mean, or both. Latent mixture modeling can be carried out with one variable over time or alternatively with many variables. After different groups showing different developmental trajectories have been identified, the grouping can be predicted by certain antecedents, and the groups can be used to predict some outcomes.

Latent mixture modeling expands the results of latent growth modeling by identifying different groups of individuals showing different trajectories of development. Identification of such groups may serve three functions. First, it provides examples of how growth patterns come into being in the case of concrete individuals. It also provides a basis for identifying qualitatively different trajectories of development. Second, in the case in which the growth components of several constructs have been studied, latent mixture modeling may identify some crucial interactions between the different growth components. Third, latent mixture modeling also provides information on how big a proportion of the sample follows each of the different developmental trajectories.

Regression Mixture Modeling

Researchers have, for a long time, been interested in moderation effects, that is, whether the impact of X on Y varies as a function of some other variable Q. A new tool for analyzing a somewhat similar problem has recently been developed. Regression mixture modeling (RMM; van Horn et al., 2009) can be used to investigate whether different groups of individuals can be identified on the basis of how and to what extent X predicts Y (Figure 14.3). In RMM, besides the mean, variances, and covariances of the outcomes (Y), the effects of predictors (X) on the outcome (Y) are also allowed to vary between latent classes (van Horn et al., 2009). In other words, RMM aims to identify subgroups of individuals who show different impacts from X to Y. After identifying the best latent class solution, the researcher typically interprets that solution. Next, membership of each latent group can be predicted by certain antecedents, and the resulting latent group memberships can be used to predict various outcomes. As is evident, RMM is a very data-driven method.

Multilevel Modeling of Nested Data

Many developmental studies have a nested data structure. For example, students are nested within classrooms, siblings and parents are nested within families, and behaviors and attitudes are nested within individuals. When analyzing developmental phenomena, a nested data structure may be a problem, but it may also provide an option for examining research questions that increase understanding of the nature of the target phenomenon.

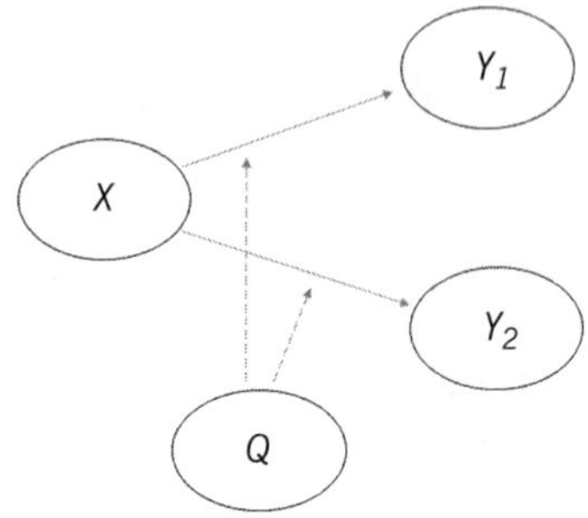

FIGURE 14.3. Schematic presentation of a regression mixture model.

The key idea of the multilevel modeling of nested data is that the variance of a variable or a construct is divided into several parts that refer to different hierarchical levels of the data (Duncan et al., 1997; Hox, 2002; Raudenbush & Bryk, 2002). In the case of two-level data, the first part of the variance, which is explained by the clustering variable and which also refers to the differences between the clusters, is typically described as between-level variation or level 2 variation. The rest of the variation is described as within-level variation or level 1 variation, and it refers to variation concerning individuals within the clusters. These kinds of analyses often provide important information on developmental mechanisms. For example, if classroom members share similar developmental patterns, we have good reason to assume that there is some classroom-related factor that can explain these differences. Similarly, if siblings share similar developmental trajectories, we can try to identify some family-related factors that may explain these similarities. In principle, most of the statistical tools, such as regression analysis, factor analysis, path analyses, SEM, and LGM, can be extended to multilevel models.

However, multilevel modeling also provides more sophisticated ways to investigate individual development. It is possible, for example, to estimate cross-level interaction, that is, whether the prediction from X to Y at the within level varies at the between level (i.e., between the clusters). If this is the case, then we can try to predict the variation in this prediction at the between level by using some between-level predictors. For instance, if we have found that the impact of teaching practice on children's skill development varies across classrooms, we can then examine whether some classroom-level predictors, such as classroom size or teacher's experience, predict the extent to which teaching practices contribute to the development of children's academic skills.

Which Method for Which Purpose?

In this chapter I have introduced some key issues on investigating development as interindividual differences and illustrated how they can be investigated by using SEM. In addition, I have discussed how this framework can be expanded to examine development as intraindividual differences, individual trajectories, and development in nested contexts. As many statistical tools were introduced, it is not always obvious which methods should be used to investigate which kinds of research questions. In this section I give some advice on suiting methods to purposes (see also Table 14.1).

SEM is particularly useful for the examination of causal relations between different constructs across specific time points. No other statistical tool is as useful for this purpose. SEM is also well suited for investigating mediator effects (although there are other methods as well; see Fritz & MacKinnon, Chapter 18, this volume) and moderator effects. Moderator effects can also be examined by using RMM and multilevel SEM in cases in which the moderator functions at the between level (Table 14.1).

If the researcher is interested in examining developmental processes spanning several measurement points or trends in these processes or associations between these trends, LGM is a good choice. LGM (or growth modeling with time as nested within individuals) is also a valuable tool for investigating the acceleration and deceleration of constructs across time (Table 14.1). If the researcher is interested in identifying the kinds of developmental trajectories individuals show across time, and if individuals show qualitatively different kinds of trajectories, latent mixture modeling is the preferred choice. When researchers

TABLE 14.1. Which Method for Which Purpose?

	Purpose					
Method	Causality over time	Mediation	Moderation	Developmental trends and processes over time	Developmental trajectories	Variation in relations between individuals
Structural equation modeling (SEM)	X	X	X			
Latent growth modeling (LGM)				X		
Latent mixture modeling				X	X	
Regression mixture modeling (RMM)			X			X
Multilevel SEM	X		X			X

assume that some mechanisms operate differently among different individuals (i.e., the associations between constructs vary), regression mixture modeling and multilevel SEM (in the case of nested data) will be valuable tools for investigating such individually varying processes.

Future Perspectives

Most research on developmental mechanisms has relied on investigating interindividual differences within and across different time points. Although some basic statistics have been available for more than 100 years, about 50 years ago new and more sophisticated methods began to be devised to investigate developmental mechanisms by using longitudinal data. One important method was SEM. More recent developments in the field have included many new tools, such as methods of analyzing nested data, methods of examining intraindividual variation and methods focusing on identifying groups of individuals who show different developmental trajectories or different associations between the key constructs. Progress, in fact, has been so fast that keeping track of novel methods has become challenging for scholars who lack expertise in statistics and mathematics.

Other methods are available that are likely to change how scholars think about development and how it can be investigated. For example, SEM has been expanded to include models that can deal with nominal variables, such as latent class models (Muthén, 2002) and a generalized linear latent framework (Moustaki, 2007). One limitation of many previous methods in investigating interindividual differences has been that associations have been assumed to be linear. This is no longer the case, as SEM has been extended to include nonlinear modeling (Wall & Amemiya, 2007). Although time series data and analyses have been used for decades in econometrics, investigating the developmental mechanisms of individual cases across time has been rare in the behavioral sciences (for exceptions, see Molenaar, 1985; Sang, Schmitz, & Tasche, 1993; see also Molenaar & Lo, Chapter 20, this volume). Time series analysis is one approach that is likely to become more popular during the next few years among scholars interested in increasing their understanding of the mechanisms of evolving individuals.

Acknowledgments

The preparation of this chapter was made possible by a fund from the Academy of Finland (Grant Nos. 213486 and 126043). I would like to thank Kaisa Aunola, Noona Kiuru, Asko Tolvanen, and Minna Torppa for valuable feedback on this chapter.

References

Baron, R. M., & Kenny, D. A. (1986). The moderator–mediation variable distinction in social psychological research: Conceptual, strategic, and statistical considerations. *Journal of Personality and Social Psychology, 51*, 1173–1182.

Bergman, L. R., Magnusson, D., & El-Khouri, B. M. (2003). *Studying individual development: A person-oriented approach* (Vol. 4). Mahwah, NJ: Erlbaum.

Bryk, A. S., & Raudenbush, S. W. (1987). Application of hierarchical linear models to assessing change. *Psychological Bulletin, 101*(1), 147–158.

Chou, C.-P., Bentler, P. M., & Pentz, M. A. (1998). Comparisons of two statistical approaches to study growth curves: The multilevel model and the latent curve analysis. *Structural Equation Modeling, 5*(3), 247–266.

Cohen, J., & Cohen, P. (1983). *Applied multiple regression/correlation analysis for the behavioral sciences*. Hillsdale, NJ: Erlbaum.

Cudeck, R. (2007). Factor analysis in the year 2004: Still spry at 100. In R. Cudeck & R. C. MacCallum (Eds.), *Factor analysis at 100: Historical developments and future directions* (pp. 1–7). Mahwah, NJ: Erlbaum.

Dorman, C. (2001). Modeling third variables in longitudinal studies. *Structural Equation Modeling, 8*, 575–598.

Duncan, T. E., Duncan, S. C., Alpert, A., Hops, H., Stoolmiller, M., & Muthén, B. (1997). Latent variable modeling of longitudinal and multilevel substance use data. *Multivariate Behavioral Research, 32*(3), 275–318.

Farrell, A. D. (1994). Structural equation modeling with longitudinal data: Strategies for examining group differences and reciprocal relationships. *Journal on Consulting and Clinical Psychology, 62*(3), 477–487.

Heck, R. H., & Thomas, S. L. (2009). *An introduction to multilevel modeling techniques*. London: Routledge.

Hox, J. (2002). *Multilevel analysis: Techniques and applications*. Mahwah, NJ: Erlbaum.

Hoyle, R. H., & Smith, G. T. (1994). Formulating clinical research hypotheses as structural equation models: A conceptual overview. *Journal of Consulting and Clinical Psychology, 62*(3), 429–440.

Jöreskog, K. R. (2007). Factor analysis and its extensions. In R. Cudeck & R. C. MacCallum (Eds.), *Factor analysis at 100: Historical developments and future directions*. Mahwah, NJ: Erlbaum.

Jöreskog, K., & Sörbom, D. (1993). *LISREL 8: Structural equation modeling with the SIMPLIS command language*. Hillsdale, NJ: Erlbaum.

Kaplan, D. (2008). An overview of Markov chain methods for the study of stage-sequential developmental processes. *Developmental Psychology, 44*(2), 457–467.

Leppänen, U., Niemi, P., Aunola, K., & Nurmi, J.-E. (2004). Development of reading skills among preschool and primary school pupils. *Reading Research Quarterly, 39*, 72–93.

Li, F., Duncan, T. E., Duncan, S. C., & Hops, H. (2001). Piecewise growth mixture modeling of adolescent alcohol use data. *Structural Equation Modeling, 8*, 175–202.

Little, T. D., Bovaird, J. A., & Slegers, D. W. (2006). Methods for the analysis of change. In D. K. Mroczek & T. D. Little (Eds.), *Handbook of personality development* (pp. 181–211). Mahwah, NJ: Erlbaum.

McArdle, J. J. (2007). Five steps in the structural factor analysis of longitudinal data. In R. Cudeck & R. C. MacCallum (Eds.), *Factor analysis at 100: Historical developments and future directions* (pp. 99–130). Mahwah, NJ: Erlbaum.

McKinnon, D. P. (2008). *Introduction to statistical mediation analysis*. New York: Erlbaum.

Millsap, R. E., & Meredith, W. (2007). Factors invariance: Historical perspectives and new problems. In R. Cudeck & R. C. MacCallum (Eds.), *Factor analysis at 100: Historical developments and future directions* (pp. 131–152). Mahwah, NJ: Erlbaum.

Molenaar, P. (1985). A dynamic factor model for the analysis of multivariate time series. *Psykometrika, 50*, 181–202.

Moustaki, I. (2007). Factor analysis and latent structure of categorical and metric data. In R. Cudeck & R. C. MacCallum (Eds.), *Factor analysis at 100: Historical developments and future directions* (pp. 293–314). Mahwah, NJ: Erlbaum.

Muthén, B. (2002). Beyond SEM: General latent variable modeling. *Behaviormetrika, 29*(1), 81–117.

Muthén, B. (2008). Overview of old and new models. In R. Gregory, K. Handcock, & M. Samuelsen (Eds.), *Advances in latent variable mixture models*. Los Angeles: University of California, Los Angeles.

Muthén, B., & Muthén, L. K. (2000). Integrating person-centered and variable-centered analyses: Growth mixture modeling with latent trajectory classes. *Alcoholism: Clinical and Experimental Research, 24*(6), 882–891.

Piantadosi, S. (1997). *Clinical trials: A methodological perspective*. New York: Wiley.

Raudenbush, S. W., & Bryk, A. S. (2002). *Hierarchical linear models: Applications and data analysis methods*. Thousand Oaks, CA: Sage.

Rutter, M. (1994). Beyond longitudinal data: Causes, consequences, changes, and continuity. *Journal of Consulting and Clinical Psychology, 62*(5), 928–940.

Sang, F., Schmitz, B., & Tasche, K. (1993). Developmental trends in television coviewing of parent–child dyads. *Journal of Youth and Adolescence, 22*(5), 531–542.

van Horn, M. L., Jaki, T., Masyn, K., Landesman Ramey, S., Smith, J. A., & Antaramian, S. (2009). Assessing differential effects: Applying regression mixture models to identify variations in the influence of family resources on academic achievement. *Developmental Psychology, 45*(5), 1298–1313.

Wall, M. M., & Amemiya, Y. (2007). A review of nonlinear factor analysis and nonlinear structural equation modeling. In R. Cudeck & R. C. MacCallum (Eds.), *Factor analysis at 100: Historical developments and future directions* (pp. 337–361). Mahwah, NJ: Erlbaum.

CHAPTER 15

Analysis of Experimental and Quasi-Experimental Data

Pinpointing Explanations

RICHARD GONZALEZ
TIANYI YU
BRENDA VOLLING

A major function of data analysis is to facilitate inferences about psychological and behavioral processes. Analytical tools help us learn about underlying processes. But textbooks typically do not highlight this key function of data analysis, instead focusing on the multitude of problems one must address when analyzing data, such as correcting the p-value for multiple tests or using the right error term in an F-test or discussing what goodness-of-fit measures to report in a paper. Textbooks tend to ignore the nonstatistical issues that can interfere with making solid inferences from data, even when one computes a p-value correctly.

In this chapter we present data analysis in a different light. We highlight the role of data analysis in making solid inferences about psychological, behavioral, and developmental processes from experimental and quasi-experimental designs. As researchers, we conduct studies because we want to learn something we did not already know (though sometimes studies are conducted for other reasons, such as gathering information to make predictions). The goal is to ensure that the design and data analytical procedures we use do not interfere with our ability to learn about underlying developmental processes. The chapter highlights how design decisions and data analytical procedures work together in service of illuminating our understanding of development, which sometimes goes beyond the practice of computing p-values in a test of significance.

The classic monographs by Campbell and Stanley (1963), Cook and Campbell (1979), and Shadish, Cook, and Campbell (2002) are consistent with this general view. These influential works list problems that can interfere with a researcher's ability to make solid inferences from data. Their lists can be characterized as "top pitfalls to avoid in psychological research." Random assignment into treatment conditions bypasses many of these pitfalls, but often research settings in developmental psychology do not allow randomizing units into conditions. One cannot randomize participants into levels of gender (male or female) or randomize participants into having or not having an older sibling. The list of pitfalls, or threats to internal and external validity as Cook and Campbell called them, has played an important role in strengthening developmental research by bringing to mind a standard set of alternative explanations.

Several generations of psychologists have been influenced by this work. Our focus in the present chapter is more on what needs to be done in developmental research rather than what needs to be avoided (we do discuss what to avoid as well). To make a nonresearch analogy: A novice chef will not get very far when learning how to make a soufflé if she or he is provided with a list of what not to do in the kitchen; she or he also needs a set of instructions about what to do in order to make a successful soufflé. This analogy holds in data analysis as well: Researchers need a set of instructions for conducting successful developmental research.

This chapter takes a contemporary perspective on a few of the points raised by Campbell and his colleagues, presents them in a constructive manner, and highlights a few of the newer analytical tools. This chapter serves as an introduction to the topic and, we hope, will motivate readers to pursue the more detailed, book-length treatment in Shadish and colleagues (2002).

Design for the Research Question

Allen Edwards, an early methodologist in psychology, pointed out that the real concern in psychological research should be not in finding the significance of hypotheses but rather in finding significant hypotheses to test. All too often researchers become focused on concerns of significance testing, such as whether there is sufficient statistical power to detect differences or in using a fancy new statistical procedure, but they do not give sufficient attention to developing research hypotheses that are worth testing. We suggest spending time finding good research questions. Several researchers have written advice pieces about how to generate research ideas (McGuire, 1973; Wicker, 1985).

Once you have the research question and have decided that it is an empirical question (i.e., a question that data, in principle, can answer), the next step is to conceive of a research design that can test that research question. You need to consider a design that can answer the research question in a manner that is as clean as possible from alternative explanations. The design should be able to test the research question. If the research question is to test two competing predictions, then the design should be one that can produce data to adjudicate between the two theories. What tasks will you give the research participants? How will you recruit them into the study? Who are the appropriate participants for the research question? What will you measure or observe? What will you manipulate or control or counterbalance? Will you be able to make sense of other patterns in the data besides the one that you predict may emerge from the study? This last question can salvage a study because, if it is considered in advance, you may be able to include the appropriate measure or control that will permit conclusions from an alternative data pattern.

The selection of research design turns out to be critically connected to the research question. Typically, one cannot choose from among a set of ready-made research designs but must tailor the research design to fit the research question. It takes much effort, which is the reason that having an important or "significant" research hypothesis from the beginning is so important. The research question has to be worth the effort.

We include this point about selecting the research design in a chapter on data analysis because often the best data analysis advice is to think through one's design from the beginning so analyses can be straightforward and simple. Too often, complicated and fancy statistical techniques are necessary because there were problems with the research design. Had those problems been addressed up front, perhaps there would be no need for heroic, lifesaving, complicated data analytical procedures. Our own bias is that simple data analysis, when warranted, is best, and careful planning in the early stages of the research process can sometimes lead to simpler analytical procedures. Of course, sometimes the research question entails using more complicated statistical methods.

Attributing Explanations to Data Patterns: Experiments

Some methodologists and researchers have treated the lab experiment as the gold standard in psychological research. The experiment is characterized by (1) a manipulation of some sort by which some participants are placed in one condition and other participants are placed in different conditions, such as a control group; and (2) random assignment to those different conditions. In the case of two conditions, both conditions should be identical in all respects except for the key component that is manipulated. The comparison of these two groups allows us to assess the role of the key component because the two intervention groups are treated in an identical manner except for the key component. Any difference between the two groups on the outcome measures can be attributable to the key component. For example, in a developmental study on emotion regulation, the manipulation, say, could be whether the mother is present or absent in the testing situation. The presence of the mother would be the key component that distinguishes the two conditions; the conditions are identical in all other respects.

If the two intervention, treatment, or manipulation groups differed on more features, then it would be difficult to attribute the reason for the outcome differences to the key component (unless the components are arranged in a factorial design that permits teasing apart their separate influences). If the researcher selected, say, left-handed children to receive one intervention and right-handed children to receive the other, the assignment would be based on handedness. This would introduce a confound, the potential for an alternative explanation, because the two groups of children could differ on the measured variable because of their handedness rather than because of the difference between the treatments they received. Thus the ability to attribute the difference between group averages to the key component would be compromised—the observed difference could be due to the key component, could be due to handedness, or could be due to some combination of handedness and the key component. Random assignment to conditions helps reduce such attributional ambiguity in explaining differences between groups.

Furthermore, the researcher needs to check that only the intended component was manipulated. The experimenter may intend both emotion regulation conditions to be identical in all respects except for the presence or absence of the mother, but in practice it may not turn out that way. For example, the research assistant may interact more with the child in the mother-absent condition, making it difficult to pinpoint the explanation for the difference observed on the dependent variable. Is the difference between conditions attributable to the mother's absence, attributable to a change in the quality of the interaction between child and research assistant, or a combination of both? Differences between conditions can exist for many reasons, not only the intended manipulation, and sometimes those differences are not readily apparent to the researcher.

It is best to tackle these issues before the data collection phase. For example, children can be assigned to intervention groups through a random process. Under traditional statistical theory, random assignment to conditions allows one to rule out many alternative explanations when comparing differences across levels of a manipulation, such as two types of treatments, in which children who receive a new kind of instruction are compared with children who receive a traditional type of instruction. The experiment provides a level of control that permits clean explanations of data patterns.

However, in no way is random assignment sufficient for such inferences. Other details could cloud the ability to explain the findings, or "to make causal inferences," as some like to say. For example, an invalid measure for the outcome variable could damage an otherwise well-designed study that used random assignment, or the manipulation may involve more features than the researcher intended (such as in the emotion regulation example mentioned earlier in which the research assistant interacted differently with the participants in the different conditions). Random assignment is not sufficient, but it goes a long way toward eliminating many alternative explanations. Random assignment can eliminate alternative explanations involving comparison of different conditions, but it doesn't help much with other problems, such as issues with measurement.

There is an important lesson here. Sometimes a study is made stronger by careful thought and decision making before data are ever collected; this can sometimes make subsequent data analysis relatively easy. Too many researchers rely on complicated data analytical procedures to fix problems that sometimes could be addressed through relatively simple design decisions.

Attributing Explanations to Data Patterns: Quasi-Experiments

Random assignment to intervention, condition, or treatment group is not always possible. For example, a researcher studying the effect of divorce on children's academic performance cannot randomly assign families to the divorced or not divorced conditions. The researcher could, however, compare children whose parents divorced to children whose parents did not divorce. There is value in such a comparison, but the researcher must exercise care in interpreting group differences because the two conditions (divorced and nondivorced families) may differ on other attributes in addition to divorce status (e.g., Stewart, Copeland, Chester, Malley, & Barenbaum, 1997). Other variables commonly used in developmental research that cannot be subject to random assignment include gender and age.

Many research questions involve comparisons of naturally occurring groups. The researcher can compare boys with girls, divorced with nondivorced families, 3-year-olds with 5-year-olds, late adolescents with adults with older adults, and children who start first grade early with those children who delay first grade for 1 year. In these cases there is a natural "comparison" across levels, even though random assignment is not possible. But the researcher needs to deal with alternative explanations that are present in making such comparisons of naturally occurring groups. There are ways of dealing with such confounds, which gave rise to quasi-experimental designs. These types of designs provide useful ways of minimizing alternative explanations, mostly through careful construction of comparison groups but sometimes through careful data analysis.

The validity of a research paradigm can be characterized on two major features: *internal validity* and *external validity*. Internal validity is the ability to make solid inferences about the process. Does the study design allow one to attribute an explanation to the correct key component without contamination from alternative explanations? External validity is the ability to generalize the findings to other subject populations, other types of research settings (e.g., from lab to classroom), or other types of stimulus materials (e.g., from printed page to computer screen or from a paradigm that uses stuffed animals with children to one that uses real pets). Methodologists have tended to view these two types of validity as a zero-sum game (you can have one only at the expense of the other). If you want to optimize internal validity, the common wisdom instructs, then you need well-controlled studies with clear manipulations and random assignment in order to attribute findings to relatively unambiguous explanations. If you want to optimize external validity, then you sacrifice internal validity in favor of generalizability, not only in terms of subject population but also in other senses, such as the robustness of findings across different settings (e.g., when classrooms naturally vary on many dimensions). We do not discuss other types of validity that have been studied in the literature (e.g., construct validity, predictive validity, face validity, discriminant validity).

New designs can be developed that yield both high internal validity and high external validity. There is a sense in which the Cook and Campbell tradition attempted to do this by focusing on quasi-experiments with their list of pitfalls, but there was still an element of sacrificing internal validity with the modifier *quasi* in front of the term *experimental*. There is room for much more innovation and creativity in developing new research designs that yield both high internal validity and high external validity. Shadish and colleagues (2002) offer some preliminary solutions using multiple methods across studies.

There has been an interesting counterproposal in the recent methodology literature that challenges the gold standard status of the experiment—that is, a challenge to the standard belief that internal validity has a higher priority than external validity. This gold standard status has not typically been given to the experiment in other social sciences such as economics and sociology. Indeed, some, such as the Nobel laureate econometrician James Heckman (2005a, 2005b), have argued that social science researchers should make the field experiment the gold standard because it maximizes external validity and because one can do a decent job at achieving internal validity if appropriate statistical techniques are used. A theme of the general argument is that sometimes threats to internal validity can be addressed through statistical means much easier than can threats to external validity. (An example is provided later in the chapter.) So, to paraphrase, his recommendation is to design studies to maximize external validity (which involves design decisions made before data are collected) and let statistical techniques deal with issues of internal validity (Heckman, 2005a, 2005b). It is still too early to tell whether this approach will be fruitful for developmental researchers, but it is worthwhile at least to think about the rarely challenged assumption in developmental psychology that the true experiment should be the gold standard. At minimum, we should give more attention to the general concerns of external validity in our research and to the creation of new designs that permit solid causal inferences when random assignment is not possible.

The Right Comparison Group: Matching and Propensity Scores

The implicit assumption in experiments and quasi-experiments is that there are two or more groups that can be compared on the key components. Regardless of whether the study is an experiment or a quasi-experiment, the researcher should construct good comparison groups. Returning to the example of the effect of parental divorce on a child's academic performance, we could compare children whose parents have divorced with children whose parents have not divorced. But then we would need to be careful about equating all other differences. We could match families on demographic variables, such as age of parents and children, number of siblings, socioeconomic status, parents' race and ethnicity, parents' immigration status, parents' education, whether other family members such as grandparents live at home, and so forth. Hopefully, we could find pairs of families that are similar on all those dimensions, attributes, and variables except that one set of parents is divorced and the other is not. In effect, this is trying to mimic the result from a randomized experiment in which groups vary on key components and not much else. Such matching would be difficult to implement in practice, but it provides one option for creating natural comparison groups (see Shadish et al., 2002, for a nice review of matching). One example of a research paper using matching in the context of divorce is by Lansford and colleagues (2006), who used data analytical procedures that allowed sophisticated matching.

A new house on the methodological block is a set of techniques based on propensity scores. The logic of propensity scores is relatively simple (for more details, see Rubin, 1997, or the book-length treatment by Gao & Fraser, 2009). One takes a two-step approach to the data analysis problem. The first step is to use the available covariates to model the propensity to be in the treatment group. For example, although families cannot be randomly assigned to be divorced or not divorced or to have a second child or not to have one, it is possible to model the propensity for a family to be divorced or to have a second child. Thus a propensity to be divorced can be predicted from covariates such as the parents' employment and level of education, the length of the marriage, and so on. This first step resembles risk models seen in epidemiology and biostatistics in which the dependent variable, say, is a binary outcome (such as divorced–not divorced), and a set of covariates, or predictors, provides a basis for a logistic regression. The predicted scores from the logistic regression can be transformed into probabilities, and they become propensity scores.

With propensity scores in hand, the analyst can proceed to step 2. The analyst can create a subset of the data with suitable matches on propensity scores (e.g., two families with the same propensity score, with one divorced and the other not). There are several ways of accomplishing this matching on propensity (see Gao & Fraser, 2009). Another way to perform step 2 is to stratify the sample on the propensity score. For example, create five groups having propensity scores between 0 and 20%, 21 and 40%, 41 and 60%, 61 and 80%, and 81 and 100% (e.g., Rubin, 1997). Then, within each propensity group, compute mean differences between those families who are divorced and those who are not and perform tests within each propensity group. This general procedure works well and provides a diagnostic in that if there is an interaction between the five strata of propensity scores and the divorce status (say, in the context of a two-way ANOVA with treatment and propensity group as the two factors), then the first step may have been misspecified because there still is a relation between propensity and "treatment" (e.g., maybe the first step missed important predictors, or more complicated nonlinear or interaction terms are needed in the logistic regression in step 1). This approach also provides another diagnostic: It can identify whether there are a sufficient number of participants in each group to make an appropriate comparison. For instance, if there are no participants in one group (e.g., at the lowest propensity level there are no divorced families), then one cannot estimate a treatment effect for that propensity subgroup.

The propensity score approach is one way to model self-selection into treatment conditions. This becomes important when modeling the primary dependent variable of interest, which could lead to biased results if propensity or self-selection effects are not properly controlled. This is one example of the kind of "statistical fix" to improve internal validity that Heckman had in mind when arguing for the field study as the gold standard, though Heckman's own techniques to deal with self-selection are different from propensity score techniques. Heckman (2005b) makes the important point that sometimes the theory that one is testing suggests different ways of handling covariates that may not be the same as that suggested by a general purpose statistical technique such as propensity scores.

A less desirable approach at step 2 would be to run an analysis of covariance (ANCOVA) using the propensity score as a covariate; this approach imposes strict assumptions on the relation of the propensity score and the "treatment" effect. ANCOVA is commonly used in developmental research for dealing with the problem of "equating" different groups when random assignment cannot be done. It adjusts statistical parameters by removing the linear and additive role of the confounding variables. In practice, most researchers merely enter the covariate as a linear predictor without also checking whether nonlinear or interaction terms are necessary. If the data suggest a nonlinear relation of the covariate but the analysis merely includes a linear term, then the analysis does not completely remove all variance associated with the covariate. Another problem with the ANCOVA approach to dealing with confounds is that one cannot easily assess whether the groups overlap on values of the covariate, which is an important condition for the logic of ANCOVA to apply. In general, ANCOVA methods depend on many assumptions, and the newer propensity score approaches may be preferred. ANCOVA is still a useful alternative to difference scores when modeling change, but that is a different use from the one we are describing here.

Indeed, much of the modern literature in statistics has not been kind to ANCOVA approaches to correcting for covariates and adjusting models. Psychologists have mostly ignored the important new developments in other social sciences, statistics, and computer science that have provided new methods for making causal inferences (e.g., Pearl, 2000), with propensity scores and selection models being two examples. Some psychologists have argued that ANCOVA tends to work relatively well in most cases and perhaps not much worse than the newer methods (e.g., Steiner, Cook, Shadish, & Clark, 2008). Still, it will be useful for developmental researchers to be aware of alternatives to ANCOVA, such as propensity scores.

The propensity score method provides one way of equating groups, because it can equate along multiple dimensions simultaneously. This is seen as a strength by some, given that many dimensions and attributes are addressed in the matching process, but it could be criticized by others as not being clear on the manner in which the units are matched. To illustrate, consider the many different ways a developmentalist could construct comparison groups to examine the effect of divorce on academic performance. One could compare single-parent homes of, say, widows and widowers to single-parent homes of divorced parents. In this case, the single-parent status is held constant but what varies is the reason for the single-parent status (divorce or death of parent). However, the death of a parent obviously has its own psychological consequences that may be different from the effects of a divorce, so this comparison could be criticized as not being a fair comparison, even when holding all other aspects constant except divorce status. Another logical comparison could be to compare divorced couples who share equal custody of children with married couples who live in different cities due to work and whose children spend equal time in both households. The process of switching households is similar in the two types of families, but one family is divorced and the other family is not. Is this a fair comparison? It may be a good comparison if the goal is to equate the process of having children move around different households, but this may not be a fair comparison with which to examine the effects of divorce. Maybe couples who work in different cities have different financial struggles, so any difference between the two sets of families could be due to divorce status or could be due to differences in, say, financial difficulties.

Overall, researchers should take seriously the problem of comparison and how to handle situations in which random assignment is not possible. Careful thought about design and construction of comparison groups (including matching, propensity score methodology, and ANCOVA approaches) will facilitate clear inferences from one's research.

Comparisons over Time versus Comparisons over Groups

There are other ways of addressing the comparison problem. Rather than focus on two different groups, it is possible to focus on change over time for a single group. For example, the researcher could collect data on the child's academic performance before and after the divorce. This is a different line of attack on the problem of addressing the role of divorce on academic performance. It compares the same child with him- or herself by examining the child before and after the divorce or by following the child multiple time periods after the divorce to estimate trajectories. The analyses of such data can be handled by repeated-measures and latent growth curve approaches.

This design approach, however, is not free from inferential problems. How far back in time before the divorce should the researcher go in the school records to collect data on academic performance? Maybe family life was affected by predivorce events that eventually led to the divorce, and those events may have affected the child's academic performance. Comparing predivorce to postdivorce academic performance may provide a biased estimate of the effect of divorce given that the predivorce academic performance score could have been influenced by emerging family dynamics. How far back in time does one go to assess the "pre"? How far into the future should the research collect "post" data? Does the process act relatively quickly within the same school year, or are the effects more distal, taking several years to show marked effects? Does the time course vary by individual?

There are clever hybrid designs that combine two types of comparison techniques—the comparison over two or more times and the comparison of two or more groups. For example, the researcher could compare families who have divorced to those families who have not in the context of a predivorce versus postdivorce temporal comparison. So, academic achievement could be tracked, say, 2 years prior to the divorce (e.g., by retrospective data collection) and 2 years after the divorce, and data could be collected over the same time frame for matched families who did not divorce. This type of comparison will allow, for instance, an examination of whether there were initial retrospective differences predivorce between the two types of families. It will also permit comparison of the trajectories, that is, changes over time, of these two types of families. If the children of divorced couples show a change in academic performance patterns over time that differs from those of the nondivorced couples, especially if the two groups of students were relatively similar 2 years before the divorce, then we can be more confident about divorce as an explanation for the performance effect (e.g., Lansford et al., 2006). The analysis of such designs can proceed with repeated-measures or latent growth curve models, with the inclusion of a grouping variable to address the between-subjects comparison. The matching of divorced and nondivorced families provides an inferential boost when interpreting the effect of divorce on the academic performance trajectories.

Time: A Fundamental Developmental Variable

Developmental psychology is concerned with development, and development occurs over time. The issue of how best to capture the unfolding change over time in a research project turns out not to be as straightforward as one might think. Two simple research designs that may occur to the reader are to compare two groups that differ in age, such as comparing 3-year-olds with 5-year-olds, and to compare a single group of participants as they develop, such as observing a group of children at age 3 and then again 2 years later when they are 5 years old. The former design, making use of two groups of different ages, is called a *cross-sectional* design; the latter design, making use of a single group of participants over time, is called a *longitudinal* design. The analysis of these two basic designs is relatively simple. The independent sample *t*-test serves as a basis for the cross-sectional design (comparing two means from different groups of participants), and the paired *t*-test (comparing two means from the same group of participants) serves as a basis for the longitudinal design. When cross-sectional designs have more than two groups, then between-subjects analysis of variance (ANOVA) can be used to analyze data; when longitudinal designs include more than two testing times, then repeated-measures ANOVA can be used. Both types of ANOVA can be generalized to include covariates (though consider our previous discussion of ANCOVA with respect to covariates), to include more complicated random effects and error structures, especially in the case of longitudinal designs and latent growth curve models, and to include other types of dependent variables such as binary data. Both cross-sectional designs and longitudinal designs have their pros and cons, as we saw in the previous section with the example on divorce.

Consider a developmental question about emotion regulation. The researcher believes that there is a key developmental process that occurs roughly at age 3 or 4, so decides that the key comparison to make in a study is between children of age 2 and children of age 5. The researcher designs a laboratory task with behavioral observation to test the question and carefully administers the task to both age groups to avoid floor or ceiling effects (i.e., not using a task that is too difficult for the 2-year-olds or too easy for the 5-year-olds). There still is a choice to make between a cross-sectional and a longitudinal design. Should the researcher compare a group of 2-year-olds with a group of 5-year-olds (i.e., compare two different groups of participants) or measure a group of 2-year-olds, then wait 3 years until they are 5 years old to test them again (i.e., compare the same participants with themselves at different ages)? The answer rests mostly on whether one wants to study age differences or age changes, in addition to practical considerations such as whether waiting for the longitudinal data is feasible in the time frame of a dissertation, funding considerations, and so forth.

If the researcher hopes to collect data the same year, say 2012, then the cross-sectional design could be useful. Cross-sectional designs allow estimation of age differences. This design also has drawbacks. Development is not directly assessed because the comparison is between different groups of participants, or cohorts. Maybe the two cohorts had different exposure to television shows (e.g., a new public television show for toddlers targeting emotion regulation aired in late 2011, such that many of the 2-year-olds were exposed to a type of information that was not available to the 5-year-olds when they were 2). Maybe the social interaction with the experimenter differed (the 5-year-olds interacted with the research assistant in a different way than the 2-year-olds), which may have affected the performance on the experimental task. In this case, the difference between the two age groups may not be attributable to the development of the emotion regulation construct but to, say, social interaction, so comparing the mean difference between groups of 2- and 5-year-olds may not lead to solid inferences. The researcher needs to be careful about making comparisons between different groups of participants when participants were not randomly assigned to those groups. Techniques such as matching and propensity scores may control for some alternative explanations, but a cross-sectional design is silent about age change.

One way to view a cross-sectional design is that it has many missing data—2-year-olds are not observed at age 5, and the 5-year-olds were not observed at age 2. These missing data preclude direct examination of change over time and require additional assumptions in order to justify the usual comparison of means between a group of 2-year-olds and a group of 5-year-olds (e.g., Maris, 1998). It is difficult to make claims about individual growth or change patterns (*intra*individual comparisons) when one does not observe change directly but must infer change from cross-sectional data (*inter*individual comparison). If the goal is to make claims about a difference between two time points for a particular person but the researcher has cross-sectional data, then he or she can compare the means of two or more groups. This requires making assumptions, such as the similarity of change processes over the set of individuals, that justify the computation of a group mean. Such assumptions should be evaluated for plausibility.

The longitudinal version of this research design—observing a group of toddlers at age 2 and the same children again when they are 5 years old—more directly addresses change over time by focusing on comparisons within the same participants. This design offers a more direct assessment of development, the estimation of age changes, because data can be analyzed by comparing scores at age 2 and at age 5 for each child, something that cannot be done in the cross-sectional design. Although longitudinal designs have advantages, they also present interesting challenges, such as dealing with practice effects that can confound estimation of age change (Greenwald, 1976).

Obviously, for this longitudinal example data collection cannot happen completely in 2012. The researcher using a longitudinal design can collect data in 2012 when the toddlers are 2 years old and then again in 2015 when they are 5 years old. There may be practice or learning effects on repeated observation. For example, if a laboratory task is administered both at age 2 and at age 5, the 5-year-olds may remember aspects of the task, so that differences in performance may not be due solely to maturation but to other processes, such as memory, as well. There are also similar problems to those with cross-sectional designs. Events and experiences may have happened between observations, not all related to the particular maturation process under study, that may add confounds when attributing explanations to observed differences on the dependent variable.

Methodologists have offered hybrid designs that optimize the advantages of both cross-sectional and longitudinal designs. One such design begins with a cross-sectional design, such as collecting data in 2012 from a group of 2-year-olds and a group of 5-year-olds. Then the researcher assesses the same children in 2013 and again in 2014, so there is a longitudinal design for a group of 2-year-olds that started in 2012 and a separate longitudinal design for a group of 5-year-olds that also started in 2012. This type of dual cross-sectional and longitudinal design, called cross-sequential design, permits the kinds of comparisons that characterize each of their component designs (Baltes, Reese, & Nesselroade, 1988). For example, within the same design one can compare age differences in 2012 by testing whether the mean on the dependent variable of interest differs between the 2-year-old group and the 5-year-old group. One can also examine longitudinal questions within the same design by comparing means on the same children over time (such as the group of 2-year-olds in 2012, then again in 2013 and in 2014). These hybrid designs also permit additional comparisons not possible with cross-sectional-only or longitudinal-only designs. For example, one can compare data from the 5-year-olds collected in 2012 with data from the 5-year-olds collected in 2015 to test whether 5-year-olds in 2012 differ from 5-year-olds in 2015. For a recent example of a quasi-experimental longitudinal design examining the effect of a school-based life skills intervention on alcohol use, see Spaeth, Weichold, Silbereisen, and Wiesner (2010).

The analysis of such hybrid designs turns out to be somewhat difficult. It appears on the surface that there are three factors: age of child, cohort, and time of measurement (see Masche & van Dulmen, 2004; Schaie, 1970). But it turns out that these three variables are related to each other. As Baltes (1968) showed, if you know two of the variables (such as age of child and cohort), you automatically know the third variable (time of measurement). One can conduct two-way ANOVA analyses on such designs (e.g., treating age of child as a within-subjects factor and cohort as a between-subjects factor). There are alternative analyses that permit comparisons of all three variables in a reduced design (e.g., sacrificing some of the higher-order interactions). These analyses allow the simultaneous study of age–cohort–period relations by making some simplifying assumptions, such as an equality assumption that two adjacent ages have the same effect (e.g., Mason, Mason, Winsborough, & Poole, 1973). Sometimes such simplifying assumptions may be reasonable (such as setting a constraint that the effect for 8-year-olds is the same as the effect for 10-year-olds in the context of a study that also includes 5-year-olds and 20-year-olds, given that 8- and 10-year-olds may not differ much on the dependent variable). But one must be careful that such equality constraints do not mask important data patterns (e.g., one may not want to set the effect for 3-year-olds to be the same as for 5-year-olds if one believes that relevant developmental processes have occurred during that period). Some advances have also been made in merging the analysis of longitudinal and cross-sectional data in the context of structural equation modeling (e.g., McArdle, Hamagami, Elias, & Robbins, 1991).

Describe What You Observed and What You Didn't

Data analysts spend much time on the details of the statistical test—choosing the model, checking its assumptions, fitting the model, learning the computer program, evaluating the fit, and reporting tests of significance. These are indeed important aspects of data analysis. Unfortunately, too little time is spent communicating the results in terms of what was observed. Too often researchers report the statistical model and its significance without also reporting the corresponding descriptive statistics that give substantive meaning to the results section. How often have we read sentences such as "A two-way ANOVA supported the predicted interaction; no main effects were observed" with little else to inform the reader about the observed data pattern? Report and discuss the descriptive statistics such as means, correlations, regression slopes, and relevant variance differences.

As with most use of descriptive language, one needs to be mindful that the words match the conclusions that are possible from the design. For example, in a cross-sectional study, one could correctly report means and standard errors, but it would be incorrect to discuss patterns in the means across cohorts as "age change" because change was not directly observed. Use the phrase "age difference" when discussing differences between means in a cross-sectional design, and use the phrase "age change" when discussing patterns of means in a longitudinal design.

Good descriptive reporting can include a table of measures of central tendency such as means and their corresponding standard errors. Or a table of correlations or regression slopes, along with their respective standard errors, can be reported if the association between variables represents the key measure. We support the recent trend to report confidence intervals for the key parameter estimates (e.g., Cumming & Finch, 2005). The combination of reporting parameter estimates and their confidence intervals highlights both the effect (such as differences between parameters) and its uncertainty (the confidence interval). A statistical test could have a p-value of 0.04 because the differences in parameters are small but the confidence interval is also small, or the same p-value of 0.04 could arise because the differences in parameters are relatively large but the confidence intervals are wide. But as statistical models become more complicated and dozens of parameters emerge, such as in a latent growth curve model, structural equation model, or mixture model (e.g., indicators of latent variables, error variances, covariances between factors and between errors, different parameter values for different latent classes, random effect variances, etc.), the suggestion of reporting parameters and confidence intervals can get unwieldy. Methodologists need to develop better visualization methods, especially for the case of multivariate longitudinal data that communicate the parameters, their variability, and the model fit.

We should also be mindful of dealing with what we did not observe. This is the point in the chapter at which we discuss the elephant in the developmental living room—missing data. Much of developmental research, especially in longitudinal studies, suffers from missing data. There could be many reasons, such as that the participant no longer wants to participate, or he or she can no longer be contacted, or the parent had to leave the session early so that the child could not finish the battery of tests, and so forth. It is important to report "missingness," such as percentages of missing data across conditions or data collection waves, much as any other descriptive statistic is reported. The handling of missing data is a major topic in data analysis and can get somewhat complicated if the missing data are related to variables or processes. Just because a statistical technique advertises that it can "handle" missing data does not mean that the user can proceed mindlessly with the analysis. The analyst should be mindful that proper inferences from such analytical tools depend on a set of important assumptions being satisfied and that those assumptions cannot always be checked. We refer the reader to the book-length treatment on missing data by Little and Rubin (2002). Learning how to handle missing data appropriately can go a long way to improve the inferential quality of the observations one has in hand.

Model the Statistical Process in Developmentally Meaningful Ways

We now turn to the important role of statistical models in data analysis. Even the simplest parameters or descriptive measures are computed in the context of a statistical model. When we compare the difference between the mean of 3-year-old boys and the mean of

3-year-old girls, we are making many assumptions. We are assuming that the mean is a good representation of the data. Does that single number for the boys provide an adequate summary of the observations? In order to attach a *p*-value to the difference between two means, we need to make assumptions about the nature of the variance (e.g., in the classical statistical test, that the population variance for the boys is assumed equal to the population variance for the girls). Maybe that is an unrealistic assumption for the particular data set. Maybe there are developmental or cohort reasons that the variances could differ across the two groups. In many classical statistical tests, the emphasis is on testing particular parameters such as means, with other parameters such as the variance playing supporting roles. There is no a priori reason that that should be the case. Maybe the difference in variance is the key research question that needs to be tested; then, rather than using a remedial measure such as transforming the data to eliminate the variance differences, one could test the variances themselves and let them serve as the key hypothesis test. We encourage developmental researchers to focus on parameters that are developmentally relevant and to consider statistical models that directly estimate and test those developmentally relevant parameters.

Variances also can play a more critical role in complicated models. In latent class models that are becoming popular in developmental psychology, it is common to make an equal variance assumption across classes. The typical assumption of equal variances across classes could be questioned. Why should variances be equal across classes? Of course, sometimes an equal variance assumption is necessary to identify the model, but this is an area to which methodologists should give much more attention. How can the equal variance assumption be relaxed in a way that minimizes convergence problems? How can substantive hypotheses about different variances across clusters or changes in variance across time be tested appropriately? General latent class and mixture models that relax many of the restrictive assumptions can be estimated using modern Bayesian statistical methods and their associated Monte Carlo sampling techniques. Psychologists have lagged behind other social scientists in the adoption of modern Bayesian statistical methods, which can sometimes solve problems that appear intractable or quite complicated from the perspective of the usual frequentist statistical theory that characterizes much of the statistics used in developmental psychology. For an introduction to Bayesian methods as applied to general regression methods, see Gelman and Hill (2006).

Heterogeneity: Random Effect Models and Latent Class Models

Developmental psychologists realize that the heterogeneity present in developmental studies can illuminate key developmental processes. For some research questions, capturing the heterogeneity present in a population is critical, whereas for other research questions one strives to minimize the heterogeneity present in the sample under investigation. The former is usually a concern in quasi-experimental designs and the latter in experimental designs. Capturing heterogeneity can be viewed as one step toward external validity (capturing the variability present in the population), whereas reducing heterogeneity can be viewed as one step toward internal validity (controlling the variability present in the population). Sometimes, though, heterogeneity can be modeled directly and can provide meaningful process information in both experimental and quasi-experimental designs.

The main point about heterogeneity is that every research participant can respond differently, and this variability can be quantified within a statistical model as a parameter of interest. This is easiest to see in longitudinal designs, which produce trajectories over time for each participant. Suppose the researcher is testing the developmental trajectory of violent behavior in adolescent boys and assesses boys at ages 12, 14, 16, and 18 on a battery of aggressive measures. The researcher could compute the mean for each of the four times and draw a single curve that represents the average research participant. Does that average curve represent the majority of the data? Does it misrepresent important alternative data patterns? The mean curve may be fitted well by a line, meaning that a slope and intercept provide convenient summaries of the growth pattern, but there may be variability in the slopes and intercepts. Given the longitudinal nature of the design, in principle, it is possible to estimate separate regressions for each boy, thus computing a slope and intercept for each boy. If the study had 100 boys each measured four times, there would be 100 slopes and 100 intercepts. The slopes represent the linear (constant) change over time, and time can be scaled so that, for example, the intercept represents the starting level of aggression at age 12. We can conduct analyses to test which variables predict those boys who started relatively high versus relatively low (intercept differences) and which variables predict those boys who stayed relatively flat over time compared with those who increased (positive slope) or decreased (negative slope) over time. We can conduct analyses comparing different demographic groups, or different groups of boys, for different patterns in slope or intercept.

It turns out that we do not actually run separate regressions for each participant because that is inefficient and can introduce bias in some cases, such as in the presence of missing data. Instead, we use modern statistical models that estimate the regressions simultaneously. These models are referred to by many names, including random effect models, multilevel models, and latent growth models, but they are all essentially the same underlying model. The key idea is that there is variability around the slope and intercept. It is not the case that a researcher can simply estimate a single slope and intercept for the entire data set; these models estimate separate slopes and intercepts for each participant within a single, simultaneous regression model (these models also include "fixed effect" terms that capture the average patterns in the data). It does not matter whether we say that the slope is a random effect (a parameter with a distribution), that the slope is a dependent variable at a higher level of analysis (hierarchical modeling), or that there is a latent slope of which each participant represents an observation (growth curve modeling). In all those cases, we are allowing the slope to vary by person; the models lead to identical results given comparable identification constraints. The single, simultaneous model can also take into account differences in variance. For example, some participants may exhibit more variability, or volatility, than others—two participants may have the same slope and intercept but one person's data points are close to the regression line, whereas the other person's data points are more variable around the regression line. These models can also handle some types of missing data.

The standard repeated-measures ANOVA is a special case of the more general random effect model. The traditional repeated-measures ANOVA is a "random intercept model" in the sense that participants are treated as a random effect; it imposes a relatively restrictive set of assumptions on the covariances between the time points. More general latent growth models allow for more complicated random effects, such as both a random intercept and a random slope, as well as more general covariance patterns across time. One of the benefits of all this is that we can summarize individual subject trajectories to maintain the heterogeneity present in the data. We can then study those trajectories, such as figuring out what predicts the slopes and intercepts or what the slopes and intercepts predict on the outcome variable. If age change trajectories are important in developmental psychology, then knowing what predicts them and what they predict could be valuable in both theory development and theory testing. The new technology of random effect terms allows us to maintain the heterogeneity in both our analyses and our theories.

We can see that the model specifics become important. For example, the model fitting linear regressions for each boy assumes that a straight line (slope and intercept) represents each boy's pattern well. What about the boy who exhibited low levels of aggression at ages 12 and 18 but high levels at ages 14 and 16? A straight line would not do justice to that boy's data pattern. We may need more complicated regression models to account for nonlinearities. In that case, the data are more complicated than mere slopes and intercepts. Blindly assuming linear relations in data may hold back theoretical advances if those linear relations are not present in the data. We believe developmental theory will progress more rapidly by tackling nonlinearity directly, finding ways to estimate it so that nonlinearity can be predicted, assessed, understood, and used to predict other variables.

We should not equate nonlinearity with polynomial regression (linear, quadratic, etc.). Nonlinearity is a more general concept, with polynomials as a special case. Sometimes it is possible to express nonlinear parameters directly in relation to theoretical parameters of interest. For example, in a study of adolescent drinking behavior, perhaps key parameters of interest are the age at which the adolescent begins to drink alcohol and, once the adolescent begins to drink, how quickly he or she accelerates his or her drinking behavior (if at all). Such processes can be modeled directly using nonlinear regression techniques by which a parameter can be assigned to the "liftoff," that is, the point at which the curve moves away from no drinking, and a second parameter assesses the degree of curvature (e.g., assessing the rate of increase). This type of direct assignment of a statistical parameter to a psychological parameter cannot always be accomplished in the context of polynomial regression, which is why more general nonlinear approaches are sometimes needed (Gonzalez, 2009b). The heterogeneity we discussed related to estimating separate parameters for each participant can be extended to nonlinear models as well.

An alternative method for dealing with heterogeneity is to define subsets of participants with similar parameters (i.e., similar trajectories). This latter method treats each subset as an equivalence class—participants in the same subset or equivalence class are treated as indistinguishable, but the subsets can be different from each other. There has been much progress in the past two decades on these kinds of models, which are also known by different names, such as latent class analysis and mixture models. Once the clusters are identified, then new research questions emerge about what predicts cluster membership (e.g., are there risk factors that can predict those boys who start low but increase their aggression over time, or are there any buffering processes that help maintain a low level of aggression in the group of boys who start low in aggression and remain low) or about what these clusters predict (e.g., does cluster membership predict future aggression, performance in school, or impulsivity?).

The general approach offered by latent growth mixture models holds promise in its usefulness for testing developmental theory. The ability to model trajectories for each participant, the ability to model hetereogeneity, and the ability to deal with missing data will likely lead to major new advances in testing developmental theory. It can also lead to new theory development as researchers ponder the developmental processes that yield heterogeneity.

Measurement Error

Developmental studies have the usual issue of measurement error that is typical in many psychological studies. This issue can be addressed through classic psychometric theory, modern structural equation models, or item response theory. Measurement error can have two key effects on the statistical analyses: It can reduce statistical power to detect differences, and it can introduce bias. The former effect is relatively innocuous and can be addressed by increasing the number of participants, reducing extraneous noise in one's procedure, or using statistical methods to create latent variables. The latter effect of measurement error, however, is more serious, especially in the context of multiple regression models. Measurement error in predictor variables can bias the coefficients (the "betas") of other variables in the model. The bias can be in either direction and can even change the sign of a regression coefficient. For instance, the population regression coefficient for a variable could actually be positive, but in a sample regression, the estimated coefficient could be negative due to measurement error on a different variable that is included in the model. The role of measurement error has mostly been underappreciated by developmental psychology, except in the context of estimating difference scores and change. But measurement error in predictor variables also needs attention and careful modeling.

The role of measurement error becomes important for developmental psychology in the context of change scores. At first blush, change seems so simple to estimate and describe—for example, take the difference of two time points and, *voila*, you have an estimate of change. Such a simple measure of change is at the heart of the standard paired *t*-test, which is typically used in a before–after design when one wants to compare the means between two time points. There is nothing wrong with the use of such difference scores as long as they are used appropriately (Rogosa, Brandt, & Zimowski, 1982). The paired *t*-test and the repeated-measures ANOVA, which can be conceptualized as using weighted difference scores in the form of contrasts over time (e.g., Gonzalez, 2009a; Maxwell & Delaney, 2004), tend to be legitimate uses of difference scores. Problems arise when one wants to use the difference score in other ways, for instance, as a measure of discrepancy (see Griffin, Murray, & Gonzalez, 1999). One needs to be careful about measurement error when interpreting difference scores directly or using them as predictors of other variables. For example, if one wants to use change in parental depression as a predictor of a child's behavior problems, then change is a measured variable with error. There are exciting new approaches that model change as a latent variable and that thus can take advantage of standard ways latent variables deal with measurement error (McArdle, 2009). These newer models still require more development and understanding (e.g., identification issues), but they hold promise for testing theory in developmental psychology.

Future Directions and Conclusions

Throughout this chapter, we viewed the problem of data analysis in experimental and quasi-experimental designs as one of reducing the number of alternative explanations and confounds to observed differences on the dependent variable. For us, the primary problem of data analysis is setting up a design and using analytical tools that facilitate clean inferences about explanatory mechanisms.

This chapter highlighted opportunities for innovation in methodology as related to developmental research. These include new designs that provide strength in both internal and external validity, as well as new statistical procedures for the measurement and modeling of change. Other open problems are currently receiving attention from methodologically minded researchers. For example, it is not always possible to use the same dependent variable across time or with different age groups (e.g., there may be floor or ceiling effects). This problem also arises when pooling multiple studies that used different measures. The change in dependent variable introduces a confound, making it difficult to explain differences in age groups or changes over time. Some interesting attempts to tackle this problem have recently been studied (e.g., Curran & Hussong, 2009; McArdle, Grimm, Hamagami, Bowles, & Meredith, 2009). We hope that methodologists and developmental psychologists continue working together to create new tools that facilitate the testing of developmental theory and advance our understanding of developmental processes.

The punch line of this chapter is that there is no substitute for good design. Statistics cannot salvage a poorly designed study. It is possible for a well-designed study to provide useful information when the data analysis is simple or even weak. Researchers should strive for research that is based on solid design principles. Good data analysis is necessary but not sufficient for making solid inferences from one's data. This is one of the major lessons we have learned from scholarship in quasi-experimental designs.

Acknowledgments

We thank Lindsay Bell, Jonathan Lane, and Julie Maslowsky for helpful suggestions on earlier versions of this chapter.

References

Baltes, P. (1968). Longitudinal and cross-sectional sequences in the study of age and generation effects. *Human Development, 11*, 145–171.

Baltes, P., Reese, H., & Nesselroade, J. (1988). *Life-span developmental psychology: Introduction to research methods*. Hillsdale, NJ: Erlbaum.

Campbell, D., & Stanley, J. (1963). *Experimental and quasi-experimental designs for research*. Boston: Houghton Mifflin.

Collins, L., & Horn, J. (1991). *Best methods for the analysis of change*. Washington, DC: American Psychological Association.

Cook, T., & Campbell, D. (1979). *Quasi-experimentation: Design and analysis issues for field settings*. Boston: Houghton Mifflin.

Cumming, G., & Finch, S. (2005). Inference by eye: Confidence intervals, and how to read pictures of data. *American Psychologist, 60*, 170–180.

Curran, P., & Hussong, A. (2009). Integrative data analysis: The simultaneous analysis of multiple data sets. *Psychological Methods, 14*, 81–100.

Gao, S., & Fraser, M. (2009). *Propensity score analysis: Statistical methods and applications*. Thousand Oaks, CA: Sage.

Gelman, A., & Hill, J. (2006). *Data analysis using regression and multilevel/hierarchical models*. New York: Cambridge University Press.

Gonzalez, R. (2009a). *Data analysis for experimental design*. New York: Guilford Press.

Gonzalez, R. (2009b). Transactions and statistical modeling: Developmental theory wagging the statistical tail. In A. Sameroff (Ed.), *Transactional processes in development: How children and contexts shape each other* (pp. 223–245). Washington, DC: American Psychological Association.

Greenwald, A. (1976). Within-subjects designs: To use or not to use? *Psychological Bulletin, 83*, 314–320.

Griffin, D., Murray, S., & Gonzalez, R. (1999). Difference score correlations in relationship research: A conceptual primer. *Personal Relationships, 6*, 505–518.

Heckman, J. (2005a). Rejoinder: Response to Sobel. *Sociological Methodology, 35*, 135–162.

Heckman, J. (2005b). The scientific model of causality. *Sociological Methodology, 35*, 1–97.

Lansford, J., Malone, P., Castellino, D., Dodge, K., Pettit, G., & Bates, J. (2006). Trajectories of internalizing, externalizing, and grades for children who have and have not experienced their parents' divorce or separation. *Journal of Family Psychology, 20*, 292–301.

Little, R., & Rubin, D. (2002). *Statistical analysis with missing data* (2nd ed.). Hoboken, NJ: Wiley.

Maris, E. (1998). Covariance adjustment versus gain scores: Revisited. *Psychological Methods, 3*, 309–327.

Masche, J., & van Dulmen, M. (2004). Advances in disentangling age, cohort, and time effects: No quadrature of the circle, but a help. *Developmental Review, 24*, 322–332.

Mason, K., Mason, W., Winsborough, H., & Poole, W. (1973). Some methodological issues in cohort analysis of archival data. *American Sociological Review, 38*, 242–258.

Maxwell, S., & Delaney, H. (2004). *Designing experiments and analyzing data* (2nd ed.). Mahwah, NJ: Erlbaum.

McArdle, J. (2009). Latent variable modeling of differences and changes with longitudinal data. *Annual Review of Psychology, 60*, 577–605.

McArdle, J., Grimm, K., Hamagami, F., Bowles, R., & Meredith, W. (2009). Modeling life-span growth curves of cognition using longitudinal data with multiple samples and changing scales of measurement. *Psychological Measurement, 14*, 126–149.

McArdle, J., Hamagami, F., Elias, M., & Robbins, M. (1991). Structural modeling of mixed longitudinal and cross-sectional data. *Experimental Aging Research, 17*, 29–52.

McGuire, W. (1973). The yin and yang of progress in social psychology: Seven koan. *Journal of Personality and Social Psychology, 26*, 446–456.

Pearl, J. (2000). *Causality: Models, reasoning and inference*. Cambridge, UK: Cambridge University Press.

Rogosa, D., Brandt, D., & Zimowski, M. (1982). A growth curve approach to the measurement of change. *Psychological Bulletin, 92*, 726–748.

Rubin, D. (1997). Estimating causal effects from large data sets using propensity scores. *Annals of Internal Medicine, 127*, 757–763.

Schaie, K. W. (1970). A reinterpretation of age related changes in cognitive structure and functioning. In L. R. Goulet & P. B. Baltes (Eds.), *Life-span developmental psychology: Research and theory* (pp. 485–507). New York: Academic Press.

Shadish, W., Cook, T., & Campbell, D. (2002). *Experimental and quasi-experimental designs for generalized causal inference*. Boston: Houghton Mifflin.

Spaeth, M., Weichold, K., Silbereisen, R., & Wiesner, M. (2010). Examining the differential effectiveness of a life skills program (IPSY) on alcohol use trajectories in early adolescence. *Journal of Consulting and Clinical Psychology, 78*, 334–348.

Steiner, P., Cook, T., Shadish, W., & Clark, M. (2008). The importance of covariate selection in controlling for selection bias in observational studies. Available at *www.northwestern.edu/ipr/events/workshops/QEPPTs/CovariateSelection08.pdf*.

Stewart, A., Copeland, A. P., Chester, N. L., Malley, J. E., & Barenbaum, N. B. (1997). *Separating together: How divorce transforms families*. New York: Guilford Press.

Wicker, A. (1985). Getting out of our conceptual ruts: Strategies for expanding conceptual frameworks. *American Psychologist, 40*, 1094–1103.

CHAPTER 16

Autoregressive and Cross-Lagged Panel Analysis for Longitudinal Data

JAMES P. SELIG
TODD D. LITTLE

The type of models we discuss in this chapter fall under the larger heading of structural equation models (SEMs) for longitudinal data. Many different names have been used for these models, including causal models (Bentler, 1980; Kenny, 1979), cross-lagged panel models (Mayer, 1986), linear panel models (Greenberg & Kessler, 1982), and autoregressive cross-lagged models (Bollen & Curran, 2006). These models are also related to the autoregressive model and the simplex model. For simplicity, we refer to these models as panel models. What all these hold in common is that they are used to examine the structural relations of repeatedly measured constructs. Recently, several authors have critiqued the frequent use of panel models. We believe that, although many of the criticisms are justified, the panel model remains a useful tool for developmental scientists.

Figure 16.1 shows a path diagram for a two-wave, two-variable panel model. Here two latent variables, X and Y, are measured on two occasions. For convenience, only the structural portion of the model is displayed, and the underlying measurement model with multiple indicators is omitted. See Little (in press) and Little, Preacher, Selig, and Card (2007) for a thorough treatment of measurement models for longitudinal data. This model can be described with the two following equations:

$$X_2 = \beta_1 X_1 + \beta_2 Y_1 + \zeta_X$$
$$Y_2 = \beta_3 Y_1 + \beta_4 X_1 + \zeta_Y$$

Here, X and Y are two different constructs measured at two time points (denoted with a subscript 1 for time 1 and 2 for time 2). The linear regression coefficients β_1 and β_3 describe the autoregressive effects, or the effect of a construct on itself measured at a later time. The autoregressive effects describe the stability of the constructs from one occasion to the next.

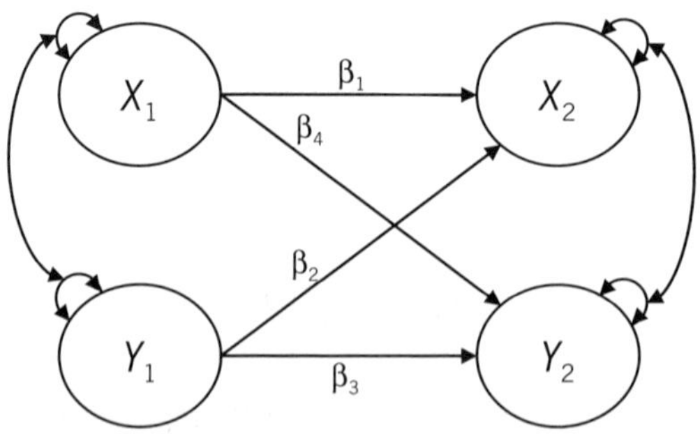

FIGURE 16.1. Path diagram for a two-wave, two-variable panel model.

More precisely, the autoregressive effects describe the stability of individual differences from one occasion to the next. A small or zero autoregressive coefficient means that there has been a substantial reshuffling of the individuals' standings on the construct over time. In contrast, a sizable autoregressive coefficient means that individuals' relative standings on the construct has changed very little over time.

The regression coefficients β_2 and β_4 represent cross-lagged effects, or the effect of a construct on another measured at a later occasion. Here again, these effects depend on individual differences on the constructs. Thus if individuals' standings on X at time 1 are related to their standings on Y at time 2, there will be a significant cross-lagged effect. A feature of the model is that the cross-lagged effects, for example of X_1 predicting Y_2, are estimated controlling for the prior level of the construct being predicted. The inclusion of the autoregressive effects means that the variance in Y_2 that can be predicted by X_1 is residual variance controlling for previous levels of Y_1 (i.e., the stable portion). This statistical feature is the reason this model is sometimes referred to as a residual change model. The fact that prior levels of the outcome construct are controlled for allows one to rule out the possibility that a cross-lagged effect is due simply to the fact that X and Y were correlated at time 1. Gollob and Reichardt (1987) and Cole and Maxwell (2003) make compelling arguments for the need to include autoregressive effects in order to minimize bias in the estimation of cross-lagged effects. The preceding model can be extended to more than two occasions and more than two constructs. The autoregressive and cross-lagged effects retain the same meaning.

Conceptual Principles and Statistical Assumptions

In the next sections, we review some of the fundamental issues in the use of panel models in developmental research. We consider critical views of the use of the panel model, in addition to the strengths of the model. As with any statistical model, panel models have numerous assumptions that must be met and various threats to validity that must be addressed.

Theory of Change

Collins (2006), in her comprehensive review of longitudinal modeling, argues that any analysis of longitudinal data must be preceded by considering "the nature of the change phenomenon that is to be observed" (p. 507). Aspects of the theoretical model of change can entail, among many other factors, the expected pattern or trajectory of change for a variable; whether change in the variable is monotonic (i.e., changing only in one direction); and what other variables will predict change. Collins's description of the theoretical model of change focuses primarily on how one variable will change over time, but it certainly encompasses how one variable is expected to induce change in another.

A potential limitation of the panel model is that it lacks an explicit theory of change, or at least that the model's theory of change may not align with the researcher's implicit theory of change. Though it is possible, using SEM, to include the mean structure in panel models, most applications of the panel model ignore information about variable means and change in means over time. Thus the way that X and Y are changing over time is not emphasized in the typical panel application (but means can be included if one has a theory of mean-level changes).

Hertzog and Nesselroade (1987) address just this issue in critiquing autoregressive models. The problem with autoregressive effects is that they describe stability in individual differences but do not describe within-person stability for the measured variable. For example, a large autoregressive coefficient for Y can mean any of the following: (1) individuals do not change on Y over time, (2) individuals uniformly increase or decrease in their levels of Y over time, or (3) individuals systematically increase and decrease over time such that one's initial level determines the direction and degree of change over time (i.e., displaying a fan-spread pattern of change over time).

A similar state of affairs exists for cross-lagged effects in the panel model. A relatively weak or nonspecific model of change for a cross-lagged effect could specify that increases in X, or the presence of X, should lead to decreasing levels of Y. For example, a researcher may believe that cognitive behavioral therapy (CBT) at time 1 will lead to a decrease in depressive symptoms at time 2. A panel model based on measures of the number of CBT sessions attended and levels of depressive symptoms for two occasions could examine whether individuals who attended more sessions also had lower scores on depressive symptoms.

Interindividual versus Intraindividual Change

Many of the potential limitations of the panel model stem from the fact that panel models focus on individual differences (interindividual variability) whereas some theories of change pertain to within-individual change (intraindividual variability). Given the previous discussion of autoregressive effects, it should be clear that although the parameters of the panel model are affected by intraindividual change (e.g., the magnitude of the autoregressive coefficient is affected by individual-level change), the parameters of the panel model are not sensitive to the type of individual-level change. The panel model could then be viewed as a potentially useful model with the limitations that it cannot easily incorporate a theory of intraindividual change and that the autoregressive and cross-lagged effects are not specific to the type of individual level-change observed over time.

Panel Models in Developmental Research

To examine the place of panel models in developmental research, we briefly review critiques of the model and then highlight its potential for use in developmental research. Critics of panel models, such as Rogosa (1987), argue that path models, such as the panel model, should be avoided because they do not begin with an explicit statement of the expected change process. Rogosa offers latent growth curve models (LGCMs) as an alternative that begins by specifying how individuals are expected to change and proceeds to identify correlates of within-person change. On the other hand, LGCMs can be viewed as models of mean structure change that are not sensitive to covariation patterns across time among the variables. For those situations in which there is neither strong theory for the change process nor a strong expectation for the trajectory of change over time or in which the research question is about the pattern of influence (and not direction of change), the panel model can be useful to explore the relations between variables over time. In this light, the results of the panel model can provide a piece of the puzzle regarding the examined association.

Reciprocal Effects

In spite of the limitations of the panel model, much of its appeal derives from the fact that it provides a means of examining relations that stem directly from theory. For example, there is a great deal of interest in the developmental sciences in reciprocal relations. Systems theory (Sameroff, 1983) places a heavy emphasis on such reciprocal relations such as those that exist between the parent and child or between the individual and his or her environment or context. Panel models make it easy to examine such reciprocal relations in that for a simple bivariate model the existence of cross-lagged effects can describe reciprocal relations. Results from a panel analysis can be used to determine whether cross-lagged effects occur in both directions (i.e., whether X_1 predicts Y_2 and Y_1 predicts X_2) and to assess the relative strength of the cross-lagged effects. For example, data based on the observation of a parent–child dyad could be analyzed to see whether a parent's behavior affects the child's subsequent behavior or the child's behavior affects the parent's subsequent behavior and even to see which of the two cross-lagged effects is stronger.

Mediation

Cole and Maxwell (2003) describe how the panel model can be used to examine mediation. A mediator is a variable that in part explains the association between two other variables. For example, Maxwell and Cole (2007) examine a hypothetical model in which the relation between parental depression and child depression is explained by problematic parenting. Panel models are useful for mediation in that the direct and indirect effects allow a statistical evaluation of mediation and are easy to estimate in the context of a panel model. The longitudinal nature of the data from the panel design provides an advantage over mediation models estimated using cross-sectional data (Cole & Maxwell, 2003; Maxwell & Cole, 2007). See MacKinnon (2008, Chapter 8) and Selig and Preacher (2009) for more information on the use of mediation models with longitudinal data.

Moderation

Panel models also make it relatively easy to examine moderation, or statistical interactions (Aiken & West, 1991). Moderation occurs when the magnitude of the relation between two variables depends on a third variable. When using measured variables, moderation can be tested by using the multiplicative product of two variables as a predictor. The effect of this product term then indicates whether moderation exists. When using latent variables, introducing a moderator is more of a challenge (but see Little, Slegers, and Card, 2006, for an approach to moderation with latent variables). Recent changes to SEM software such as Mplus (Muthén & Muthén, 2009) also make it easier to include a moderator in a latent variable model.

To sum up this section on the use of the panel model in developmental research, we acknowledge that panel models have limitations and should not be thought of as the default model for longitudinal data analysis. However, we do believe there is a place for the use of the panel model in developmental research. Results from a panel model may lead to better understanding of the longitudinal relations between variables. The results could suggest future analyses (e.g., looking for reciprocal effects, mediation, or moderation) that would shed further light on these relations. The results may also provide information on the within-person processes that correspond to the panel analyses and lead to the analysis of intraindividual data to test those ideas. In common with many statistical results, the results from a panel model will rarely be a final destination but instead will be an invitation to further investigation.

Reliability of Measurement

The ability to arrive at unbiased parameter estimates relies on the assumption that the variables are measured without error. Measurement error can be addressed using latent variables with multiple indicators (Brown, 2006). In this situation, there are two important parts of the panel model. The structural model will look much the same whether latent or measured variables are used; however, the latent variable model will have an underlying measurement model in which the specific relations between the observed measured variables and the unobserved latent variables will be specified. Use of latent variables is often desirable because, in addition to correcting for measurement error, the use of the latent variable model requires the researcher to be more explicit in stating the way the constructs in the model are defined, and a confirmatory factor analysis can be used to evaluate the success of the measurement model.

Factorial Invariance

Factorial invariance is another key assumption of longitudinal panel models. That is, is the instrument measuring the same construct at different time points? Factorial invariance is also referred to as measurement equivalence or measurement invariance (all these terms are synonymous; see Meredith, 1993). Factorial invariance does not mean that the constructs are unchanging. It addresses only the equivalence of measurement of the construct to ensure that the differences in the constructs are true differences and not confounded with problems such as changes in the discrimination (loading information) or changes in the sensitivity (mean-level information) of one or more of the indicators of a construct. The basic idea of factorial invariance is that if the construct changes over time, then this change is conveyed as changes in all the indicators in the same direction and the same amount. If one or more indicators changes differently from what was expected, then this item is no longer invariant. Factorial invariance and differential item functioning (DIF) are the same concept, with factorial invariance the method for testing indicators that are roughly continuous and DIF being the method of testing indicators that are dichotomous or polytomous in nature (Reise, Widaman, & Pugh, 1993).

Factorial invariance is assumed in any model with multiple time points or multiple groups. When only observed, or manifest, variables are used in a panel model, factorial invariance is an untestable assumption. By using latent variables with multiple indicators, however, this assumption can be tested. The procedures for testing factorial invariance are spelled out in detail in sources such as Little, Card, Slegers, and Ledford (2007).

Sample Selectivity and Selective Attrition

Two related threats to validity cover the researcher's ability to generalize results to the target population. *Sample selectivity* occurs when the sample is a nonrepresentative sample from the population. This threat to validity for panel studies (and any developmental study, for that matter) is often ignored in most research reports. Sample selectivity can be related to a poor sampling framework on the part of the experimenter or to selective participation. To the degree that population characteristics are known, one can compare the sample characteristics with the population characteristics to determine the nature of the selectivity. Reweighting the sample to adjust the sample characteristics to follow more closely the population can help reduce any bias due to sample selectivity. *Selective attrition* occurs when participants drop out of a study in a predictable way (e.g., low-socioeconomic-status [SES] participants may be more likely to drop out than higher SES participants). To the degree that characteristics of the dropout process are measured and represented on the data set, the missing data mechanism would be classified as missing at random (MAR). When missing data are due to the MAR mechanism, the information lost can be recovered with modern techniques for handling missing data.

Retest Effects

Another threat to the validity of conclusions from panel models involves retest effects. Retest effects arise from the fact that construct-irrelevant variance is often introduced when participants are measured repeatedly with the same instrument. These effects can occur when respondents remember presented material, react to repeated questioning, or lose interest in the study, to list a few examples. Such effects are mostly ignored and rarely estimated, even though powerful designs exist that allow for the control of retest effects. With the advancement of modern methods for handling missing data, planned missing-data-collection designs can also be used both to control for retest effects and to estimate the size and direction of retest effects (see discussion of planned missing designs later in the chapter and in Enders, 2010).

Model Specification

Another assumption is that the panel model is properly specified. The broad issue of specification incorporates separate assumptions. For example, all the relations examined using a panel model are assumed to be linear, or at least linear in the parameters. Model specification also entails properly structuring the associations among the variables. For example, omitting an important cross-lagged effect in an estimated model can bias the other parameter estimates. This issue is often less relevant for panel models with a smaller number of variables, but when there are many variables and many occasions, analysts will often omit paths in the pursuit of model parsimony. Therefore, care in parameter pruning is warranted.

Correct model specification also entails the assumption that all the important predictors are included in a model. For example, given the two-variable, two-wave model previously described, the cross-lagged effect of X on Y may be biased if in fact the relation between X and Y can be completely explained by their mutual dependence on some third variable Z. This assumption is arguably one of the most difficult to satisfy because there are often dozens, if not hundreds, of possible determinants of human behavior. It is difficult to argue that a bivariate model includes all relevant variables, although logic, prior research, and plausibility arguments can help narrow the field in terms of potential confounds to a study's findings.

Panel Models and Causal Claims

In the past, it was common to refer to panel models as causal models (Bentler, 1980; Kenny, 1979). Their introduction into many fields created great optimism that panel models could determine causal relations between variables in a manner similar to the way an experiment with random assignment can lend support to a causal effect. This optimism may have stemmed from the fact that panel models are in alignment with two fundamental aspects of causal inference. First, by measuring putative causes prior to the effects, temporal precedence of the cause is supported, and second, by simultaneously modeling the unique effect of several causes, it may be possible to support a causal explanation of one variable over another.

However, we view it as a positive result that panel models are no longer commonly referred to as causal models. No statistical model can determine causal relations apart from strong theory and solid research design. Furthermore, causal claims are especially difficult to make in developmental research, as a great many potential causes cannot be manipulated due to either practical or ethical limitations (Baltes, Reese, & Nesselroade, 1977).

The possible exception to the rule that results from a panel analysis provide weak support for making causal claims is the case in which the data come from an experimental design. In this case, it is the fact that the putative cause is manipulable through the random assignment of individuals to receive different levels of the causal variable, and not any property of the model itself, that supports causal inference.

There are several reasons to use caution when attempting to draw causal inference based on panel model results. For example, the putative causes often cannot be manipulated or cannot be manipulated independently from other variables in the model. In addition, proper causal inference rests on model assumptions such as including all relevant predictors. As noted earlier, this assumption can be difficult to establish.

Although it can be difficult to support causal claims using results from a panel model, we believe the panel model can be an important tool in building an argument for a causal effect of one variable on another. This support for a causal argument is especially true when the evidence from the panel model is a component in a much broader examination of the effect.

Role of Time in Panel Models

Though it is possible to use panel models with cross-sectional data, there are many advantages to using longitudinal data instead. Using longitudinal data allows the investigator to more precisely specify the hypothesized direction of effects. The temporal precedence of one variable before another can lend support to a causal claim. Finally, it allows the investigator to focus on change over time rather than static relations.

One of the fundamental choices for the use of a panel model is when to measure participants. In other words, at what developmental epoch would we expect the see the hypothesized cross-lagged and autoregressive effects? Here it is assumed that, just as the level of a variable can change as individuals develop, so too can the relation between two or more variables.

The choice of time between observations for a panel model is often not given sufficient attention. Whenever associations between variables change over time, any autoregressive or cross-lagged effect from the model is specific to the chosen lag. Thus the analyst assumes that a reasonable lag was used, meaning that it was not too long or too short and the time was appropriate to see the effect emerge. An interesting implication arises from this assumption. Most panel designs measure all variables on a fixed lag schedule. The fact that all variables are measured at the same time implicitly assumes that the time for the cross-lagged effect of X on Y and Y on X is the same. It is not difficult, however, to imagine a scenario in which the two cross-lagged effects emerge on different schedules.

When choosing time lags for a panel design, the designer must choose a lag that will provide sufficient time for the effect to occur but not so much time that the effect will have disappeared. The analyst using a panel model must assume that an appropriate lag was chosen to detect the hypothesized effect. It cannot be assumed that the appropriate lag for each relation will be the same.

Developmental Applications

Belsky, Fearon, and Bell (2007) used a panel model to examine the longitudinal relations among three constructs: parental sensitivity, child attentional control, and child externalizing behavior. Each construct was assessed on four occasions. The hypothesized relation among these constructs was that the child's attentional control would mediate the relation between quality of parenting and problem behavior. Thus the change suggested by the model was that sensitive parenting would support the child in developing attentional control, and this in turn would serve to reduce problem behaviors. In this analysis, Belsky and colleagues are capitalizing on many of the strengths of panel models. First, they examine longitudinal effects (e.g., the effect of sensitive parenting at time 1 on attentional processes at time 2), which gives them the ability to rule out possible effects (e.g., time 2 variables cannot affect time 1 variables) and the ability to explicitly test for relations in the opposite direction of those specified by theory. For example, the authors directly test for relations, such as earlier attentional processes, that predict later sensitive parenting. The panel model approach can be especially useful in testing for such reciprocal effects. Finally, the analyses of Belsky and colleagues highlight the utility of panel models for testing indirect, or mediated, effects. The authors are also careful to state that "it is risky to embrace causal conclusions without direct experimental manipulation, even with longitudinal data" (Belsky et al., 2007, p. 1239).

Illustration

Children of depressed mothers are often at risk for several negative outcomes (Downey & Coyne, 1990). In particular, children of depressed mothers are themselves at risk for experiencing issues related to depression and anxiety. Several authors, such as Downey and Coyne (1990) and Cummings and Davies (1994) describe models for family functioning in which there are reciprocal parent–child effects such that maternal depression may affect the functioning of the child and the functioning of the child may have an impact on the mother's depressive symptoms. In the following example, we examine the longitudinal association between a mother's level of depressive symptoms and her child's level of internalizing symptoms. The model presented is simplified to illustrate the key elements of the autoregressive cross-lagged model and the information that can and cannot be gained from such a model. This model is incomplete, as many other important constructs are omitted. For example, the quality of the mother–child relationship may act as a mediator between maternal depressive symptoms and the child's internalizing symptoms, or a contextual factor such as family financial strain may moderate the association between these constructs. However, the model does describe the relation between two constructs and highlights the potential reciprocity between these constructs.

The data for this example are from the NICHD Study of Early Childcare (*secc.rti.org*). Mothers and children were assessed once when the focal child was approximately 24 months of age and again when the child was approximately 36 months of age. Maternal depressive symptoms were measured using the Center for Epidemiological Studies—Depression scale (CES-D; Radloff, 1977). The 21 items of the CES-D are often reported as a single score representing depressive symptoms. To create multiple indicators for a maternal depressive symptoms construct, we created three parcels (Little, Cunningham, Shahar, & Widaman, 2002). Here the item parcels are averages of three items. Children's internalizing symptoms were assessed using the Child Behavior Checklist (CBCL; Achenbach, 1992). We used three subscales from the CBCL as indicators of an internalizing symptoms latent variable: Anxious/Depressed, Withdrawn, and Somatic Symptoms.

All analyses were conducted using Mplus 5.21. Full information maximum likelihood estimation was employed to make use of all available data. Of the original mother–child dyads, 130 were missing data for all variables and therefore excluded from the analyses, leaving a total sample size of 1,234 dyads. Latent variables were identified by setting the latent variance to 1.0, and the scale for the mean structure was set by fixing the latent means to 0. When factor loadings were equated (e.g., to test the weak invariance model), latent variances at the second occasion were freely estimated, and when intercepts were equated across occasions (e.g., to test the strong invariance model), latent means at the second occasion were freely estimated.

Prior to estimating the structural model for the longitudinal associations between maternal depressive symptoms and child internalizing symptoms, we conducted tests for longitudinal factorial invariance. Model fit indices for the configural, weak, and strong invariance models, in addition to the formal model comparisons using the nested model chi-square test, are presented in Table 16.1. Based solely on the nested model chi-square comparisons, the weak invariance constraints (i.e., equating factor loadings across occasions) significantly diminished model fit as compared with the configural invariance model ($p = .02$). However, by the change in CFI standards of either Cheung and Rensvold (2002) or Meade, Johnson, and Brady (2008), the weak invariance model is supported. The strong invariance constraints (i.e., equating indicator intercepts across occasions) did not result in a significant decrease in model fit as compared with the weak invariance model ($p = .38$) and are thus supported by any standard.

Table 16.2 shows the results for the two-wave, two-variable model. All autoregressive and cross-lagged effects are statistically significant ($p < .001$). The autoregressive

TABLE 16.1. Model Fit Indices for the Configural, Weak, and Strong Invariance Models

Model	χ^2	*df*	CFI	RMSEA (90% CI)	$\Delta\chi^2$	Δdf	*p*
Configural	81.80	42	0.995	0.028 (0.019–0.037)	—	—	—
Weak	93.19	46	0.994	0.029 (0.020–0.037)	11.39	4	.02
Strong	98.67	50	0.994	0.028 (0.020–0.036)	5.48	4	.24

coefficients for maternal depressive symptoms and child internalizing behavior show that individual differences in both constructs are relatively stable over the 12-month lag between occasions of measurement. The cross-lagged effect of maternal depressive symptoms on child internalizing behavior confirms previous findings that mothers with higher levels of depressive symptoms tend to have children with higher levels of internalizing symptoms, even when controlling for the child's previous levels of internalizing symptoms. There is also evidence of mother–child reciprocity because children with higher levels of internalizing symptoms tend to have mothers with higher levels of depressive symptoms, even when controlling for the mother's prior level of depressive symptoms.

The model accounts for over a third of the variance in maternal depressive symptoms at 36 months ($R^2 = .37$) with lagged maternal depressive symptoms accounting for 25% of the variance and child internalizing behavior accounting for just over 4%. More of the variance for child internalizing behavior at 36 months is accounted for by the model ($R^2 = .59$), with prior levels of child internalizing behavior accounting for 51% of the variance and prior levels of maternal depressive symptoms accounting for just over 1%.

TABLE 16.2. Structural Model Parameter Estimates, Standard Errors, and Standardized Estimates

Effect	Coefficient	*SE*	Standardized
Maternal depressive symptoms$_1 \rightarrow$ Maternal depressive symptoms$_2$	.48	.03	.50
Child internalizing behavior$_1 \rightarrow$ Child internalizing behavior$_2$	.75	.03	.71
Maternal depressive symptoms$_1 \rightarrow$ Child internalizing behavior$_2$	.13	.03	.12
Child internalizing behavior$_1 \rightarrow$ Maternal depressive symptoms$_2$	.20	.03	.20
Maternal depressive symptoms $_1 \leftrightarrow$ Child internalizing behavior$_1$	.39	.03	.39
Maternal depressive symptoms $_2 \leftrightarrow$ Child internalizing behavior$_2$	.09	.02	.18

Consistent with our previous discussion of the use of panel models for causal inference, we do not see these results as support for a causal effect of maternal depressive symptoms on child internalizing behavior or of child internalizing behavior on maternal depressive symptoms. The present analyses identify an interesting association that warrants further research, but with only two variables in the model and given the impossibility of manipulating either maternal depressive symptoms or child internalizing behavior, the results should not be used to bolster a causal claim without further supporting evidence.

Future Directions

Variable-Lag Models

Time plays a role in panel models in that associations are structured by time and variables are measured on multiple occasions. The role that time plays in panel models is characteristically different compared with the role of time in other models for longitudinal data that explicitly include time (e.g., LGCMs). In a panel model the autoregressive or cross-lagged effects are specific to the chosen lag between observations, but traditional panel models do not consider whether, or how, the autoregressive or cross-lagged effects may have differed if a different lag had been chosen. The use of fixed lags also complicates cross-study comparisons of similar effects. We have recently been exploring variations on the panel model in which time lags are included as predictors and the magnitude of autoregressive and cross-lagged effects can be moderated by lag (Selig, 2009; Selig, Preacher, & Little, 2009). This lag as moderator approach relies on a variable-lag design in which the lag between measurements is intentionally varied across participants (cf. McArdle & Woodcock, 1997, who used a variable lag design in conjunction with a latent growth model). We see these models as useful in that they allow one to examine how an effect changes with lag and may lead to a deeper understanding of the relations examined with panel models and a greater ability to make cross-study comparisons of effects.

Continuous Time Models

In line with our earlier comments about the role of time in panel models, we note that panel models use time in a discrete rather than a continuous fashion. A cross-lagged effect occurs across a discrete time lag. The effect is represented as static even though intuition may suggest that an effect of this sort unfolds over time. Models that use time in a continuous rather than a discrete fashion are not new. Coleman (1968) proposed continuous time models. Continuous time models would diminish the importance of choosing an appropriate lag and ease cross-study comparison of effects. Recent work by Oud (2002) demonstrates the use of continuous time models using data from a traditional panel design.

Random Effects Models

Traditional panel models treat all autoregressive and cross-lagged effects as fixed, meaning that the same regression weight is expected to apply to all members of the population. Random effects models, in contrast, hold that effects can vary across persons. Thus a particular cross-lagged effect, such as the previously described effect of maternal depressive symptoms on child internalizing symptoms, could vary across parent–child dyads. Such random effects models usually involve a time series or pooled cross-sectional design, and therefore issues of stationarity can arise (Rovine & Walls, 2006). However, the random effects approach to panel models hold great promise for examining how effects vary across persons and what person-level predictors may explain variation in these effects.

Planned Missing Designs

As mentioned earlier, many planned missing data designs exist that would be particularly useful for increasing the validity of inferences based on panel model data. For example, the three-forms questionnaire approach can reduce the fatigue associated with large protocols by randomly assigning participants to a questionnaire form. Each form would have approximately one-third of the item content randomly missing (the proportion missing is flexible). Because the random nature of the planned missing data is controlled by the experimenter, the missing data mechanism is missing completely at random and readily recoverable with modern missing data treatments (Enders, 2010; Graham, Taylor, Olchowski, & Cumsille, 2006). For controlling and estimating retest effects, participants can be randomly assigned to measurement occasion. The key here is, again, random assignment at the beginning of the study. By virtue of experimental (and statistical) control, the participants who were measured at the first assessment occasion are no different from those who did not experience the first occasion. At the second measurement occasion, any differences in the response patterns between first-time respondents and second-time respondents would be the amount and nature of the retest effects (see Graham, Olchowski, & Gilreath, 2007).

Conclusion

In summary, the panel model is especially useful for identifying the relations between variables across time. Such models are useful for initial research into the effect of one variable on another and also when the researcher seeks to elaborate on how or for whom the effect occurs (e.g., mediation or moderation). Panel models are a poor choice when the goal is to show the functional form of systematic (mean-level) change in a variable over time or if the theoretical emphasis is on intraindividual change.

In common with many statistical models, the utility of panel model results for making causal claims is much more a consideration of the data and research design than of any particular quality of the statistical model. Results from panel models using quasi-experimental or observational data should not be used as the sole support for a causal claim. However, such results could be used in conjunction with theory and other empirical results as one element in a larger argument in favor of a causal relationship. Although we acknowledge critiques of the use of the panel model for longitudinal data, we believe it has the potential to shed light on longitudinal associations between variables that can further our understanding of developmental processes.

References

Achenbach, T. M. (1992). *Manual for the Child Behavior Checklist 2–3 and 1992 Profile*. Burlington: University of Vermont, Department of Psychiatry.

Aiken, L. S., & West, S. G. (1991). *Multiple regression: Testing and interpreting interactions*. Newbury Park, CA: Sage.

Baltes, P. B., Reese, H. W., & Nesselroade, J. R. (1977). *Life-span developmental psychology: Introduction to research methods*. Monterey, CA: Brooks/Cole.

Belsky, J., Fearon, R. M. P., & Bell, B. (2007). Parenting, attention and externalizing problems: Testing mediation longitudinally, repeatedly and reciprocally. *Journal of Child Psychology and Psychiatry, 48*, 1233–1242.

Bentler, P. M. (1980). Multivariate analysis with latent variables: Causal modeling. *Annual Review of Psychology, 31*, 419–456.

Bollen, K. A., & Curran, P. J. (2006). *Latent curve models: A structural equation approach*. Hoboken, NJ: Wiley.

Brown, T. A. (2006). *Confirmatory factor analysis for applied research*. New York: Guilford Press.

Cheung, G. W., & Rensvold, R. B. (2002). Evaluating goodness-of-fit indexes for testing measurement invariance. *Structural Equation Modeling, 9*, 233–255.

Cole, D. A., & Maxwell, S. E. (2003). Testing mediational models with longitudinal data: Questions and tips in the use of structural equation modeling. *Journal of Abnormal Psychology, 112*, 558–577.

Coleman, J. S. (1968). The mathematical study of change. In H. M. Blalock & A. B. Blalock (Eds.), *Methodology in social research* (pp. 428–478). New York: McGraw-Hill.

Collins, L. M. (2006). Analysis of longitudinal data: The integration of theoretical model, temporal design, and statistical model. *Annual Review of Psychology, 57*, 505–528.

Cummings, E. M., & Davies, P. T. (1994). Maternal depression and child development. *Journal of Clinical Psychology and Psychiatry, 35*, 73–112.

Downey, G., & Coyne, J. C. (1990). Children of depressed parents: An integrative review. *Psychological Bulletin, 108*, 50–76.

Enders, C. K. (2010). *Applied missing data analysis*. New York: Guilford Press.

Gollob, H. F., & Reichardt, C. S. (1987). Taking account of time lags in causal models. *Child Development, 58*, 80–92.

Graham, J. W., Olchowski, A. E., & Gilreath, T. D. (2007). How many imputations are really needed?: Some practical clarifications of multiple imputation theory. *Prevention Science, 8*, 206–213.

Graham, J. W., Taylor, B. J., Olchowski, A. E., & Cumsille, P. E. (2006). Planned missing data designs in psychological research. *Psychological Methods, 11*, 323–343.

Greenberg, D. F., & Kessler, R. C. (1982). Equilibrium and identification in linear panel models. *Sociological Methods and Research, 10*, 435–451.

Hertzog, C., & Nesselroade, J. R. (1987). Beyond autoregressive models: Some implications of the trait–state distinction for the structural modeling of developmental change. *Child Development, 58*, 93–109.

Kenny, D. A. (1979). *Correlation and causality*. New York: Wiley-Interscience.

Little, T. D. (in press). *Longitudinal SEM*. New York: Guilford Press.

Little, T. D., Card, N. A., Slegers, D. W., & Ledford, E. C. (2007). Representing contextual effects in multiple-group MACS models. In T. D. Little, J. A., Bovaird, & N. A. Card (Eds.), *Modeling contextual effects in longitudinal studies* (pp. 121–147). Mahwah, NJ: Erlbaum.

Little, T. D., Cunningham, W. A., Shahar, G., & Widaman, K. F. (2002). To parcel or not to parcel: Exploring the question and weighing the merits. *Structural Equation Modeling, 9*, 151–173.

Little, T. D., Preacher, K. J., Selig, J. P., & Card, N. A. (2007). New developments in latent variable panel analysis of longitudinal data. *International Journal of Behavioral Development, 31*, 357–365.

Little, T. D., Slegers, D. W., & Card, N. A. (2006). A non-arbitrary method of identifying and scaling latent variables in SEM and MACS models. *Structural Equation Modeling, 13*, 59–72.

MacKinnon, D. P. (2008). *Introduction to statistical mediation analysis*. Mahwah, NJ: Erlbaum.

Maxwell, S. E., & Cole, D. A. (2007). Bias in cross-sectional analyses of longitudinal mediation. *Psychological Methods, 12*, 23–44.

Mayer, L. S. (1986). On cross-lagged panel models with serially correlated errors. *Journal of Business and Economic Statistics, 4*, 347–357.

McArdle, J. J., & Woodcock, R. W. (1997). Expanding test–retest designs to include developmental time-lag components. *Psychological Methods, 2*, 403–435.

Meade, A. W., Johnson, E. C., & Brady, P. W. (2008). Power and sensitivity of alternative fit indices in tests of measurement invariance. *Journal of Applied Psychology, 93*, 568–592.

Meredith, W. (1993). Measurement invariance, factor analysis and factorial invariance. *Psychometrika, 58*, 525–543.

Muthén, L. K., & Muthén, B. O. (2009). *Mplus user's guide* (5th ed.). Los Angeles: Authors.

Oud, J. H. L. (2002). Continuous time modeling of the cross-lagged panel design. *Kwantitatieve Methoden, 69*, 1–26.

Radloff, L. S. (1977). The CES-D scale: A self-report depression scale for research in the general population. *Applied Psychological Measurement, 1*, 385–401.

Reise, S. P., Widaman, K. F., & Pugh, R. H. (1993). Confirmatory factor analysis and item response theory: Two approaches for exploring measurement invariance. *Psychological Bulletin, 114*, 552–566.

Rogosa, D. (1987). Causal models do not support scientific conclusions: A comment in support of Freedman. *Journal of Educational Statistics, 12*, 185–195.

Rovine, M. J., & Walls, T. A. (2006). A multilevel autoregressive model to describe interindividual differences in the stability of a process. In J. L. Schafer & T. A. Walls (Eds.), *Models for intensive longitudinal data* (pp. 124–147). New York: Oxford University Press.

Sameroff, A. J. (1983). Developmental systems: Contexts and evolution. In W. Kessen (Ed.), *Handbook of child psychology: Vol. 1. History, theory, and methods* (pp. 237–294). New York: Wiley.

Selig, J. P. (2009). *Where has the time gone?: The role of time lags in models for longitudinal data*. Unpublished doctoral dissertation, University of Kansas.

Selig, J. P., & Preacher, K. J. (2009). Mediation models for longitudinal data in developmental research. *Research in Human Development, 6*, 144–164.

Selig, J. P., Preacher, K. J., & Little, T. D. (2009). Lag as moderator models for longitudinal data [Abstract]. *Multivariate Behavioral Research, 44*, 853.

CHAPTER 17

Analyzing Change between Two or More Groups

Analysis of Variance versus Analysis of Covariance

KAMALA LONDON
DANIEL B. WRIGHT

A critical question in much developmental research is whether different groups change in the same way. One of the most common methods used in developmental science is to test a particular measure in different groups of participants for the same event at two time points. We compare the two most popular statistical approaches in the situation: analysis of variance (ANOVA) on change scores and analysis of covariance (ANCOVA) partialing out initial scores. Although these techniques address related research questions, they can lead to different conclusions, what is known as *Lord's paradox*. We use recent data on children's memory to illustrate that these approaches can lead to opposite conclusions and discuss the analytical choices. The analytical choice depends on the specific research questions and assumptions, but we conclude that for most developmental research the ANCOVA is preferred to the ANOVA.

Central Issues

The very nature of development implies changes over time. Developmental scientists seek to elucidate how humans' (and other animals') physical, social, and cognitive attributes and abilities change with time and experience. Developmental research also addresses how development in one domain (e.g., hippocampal development) affects another domain (e.g., autobiographical memory). From a policy and practice perspective, clinicians are interested in identifying factors that promote and hinder optimal development in order to guide prevention and treatment efforts. Many questions regarding human development, then, require measuring some behavior at two or more points in time.

Developmental researchers often compare change between different groups. Sometimes participants can be randomly allocated into groups (e.g., treatment or no treatment), or the groups can be matched on initial scores on some variable (e.g., matching an intellectually disabled group with chronological or mental age-matched peers). Such designs allow researchers to assume that groups' initial scores are approximately the same, and this simplifies analytical choices. However, developmental researchers often seek to examine naturally occurring groups in cases in which random allocation is not feasible. For example, researchers interested in the effects of child abuse might compare some developmental outcome among abused versus nonabused children. Age is another predictor variable that is fundamental to developmental science in cases in which random allocation (to age groups) is not possible. This is often the case in developmental psychology, in which the groups correspond to different ages. Because differences that correspond with age are fundamental to developmental psychology, we present an example in this chapter looking at cognitive differences and changes across age.

The example we consider has a group of children, ages 4 to 9 years, who experienced a staged event, a magic show (London, Bruck, & Melnyk, 2009, Experiment 2). They were questioned about the event soon afterward and then again 10 months later. The number of pieces of information recalled by each child at these two points in time was recorded. London et al.'s question was about the relationship between forgetting and age. Two common analytical approaches are (1) running classic repeated-measures analyses such as the *t*-test or ANOVA and (2) running an ANCOVA on final scores, partialing out initial scores (related to doing an ANOVA on the residuals). With the ANOVA, or difference-score, approach, we subtract the amount recalled at the second test from the initial amount recalled and compare these difference scores with age. These are the alternatives considered in a famous statistical paradox.

Conceptual Principles and Statistical Assumptions

Lord's Paradox

Lord (1967) described a fictitious example in which two statisticians, faced with the same data set and the same basic research question, come to different answers. The research question was whether two groups differed on some measure at time 2 after taking into account values at time 1. The approaches the statisticians took were an ANOVA on the differences between the scores (i.e., time 2 – time 1, the classic repeated-measures *t*-test/ANOVA approach) and an ANCOVA partialing out time 1 scores. These two most popular analytical approaches continue to be used in this situation by psychologists and other scientists. Because both of these approaches appear to address very similar substantive questions and yet can produce different conclusions, this phenomenon has become known as *Lord's paradox*.

Discussion of Lord's paradox has been active within the statistics literature (e.g., Holland & Rubin, 1983; Maris, 1998; Senn, 2006; Wainer, 1991), with examples provided from either fictitious (e.g., Lord, 1967; Wright, 2006b) or relatively large-scale data sets (e.g., Wainer & Brown, 2004). The data presented here provide a particularly good example of Lord's paradox for several reasons. First, the sample is of a size similar to many developmental psychology studies ($n = 51$). Second, both approaches match onto theoretical and applied questions in developmental psychology. Third, the effect sizes for these two different approaches are large and in opposite directions. This example shows that Lord's paradox is not simply something that occurs with large or made-up data sets but that it must always be considered when comparing some measure by groups that differ on baseline scores.

Comparing Response Variables between Two Time Points by Age

Developmental researchers often investigate how some characteristic changes between two time periods and whether these changes are the same for different groups. This situation can lead to Lord's paradox. The groups in this example are children of different ages, and the interest is whether the time trajectory is the same for participants of different ages. When measurements are taken at many different time points, similar conceptual issues arise (see Singer & Willett, 2003). Here we concentrate on the situation with just two time points. Singer and Willett's (2003) textbook covers, in elegant detail, longitudinal designs with several time points.

The example used comes from London and colleagues (2009; Experiment 2). They examined 4- to 9-year-old children's long-term memories of a staged event 2 weeks after the event and again at a final interview after a 10-month delay. The particular measure of interest for the present chapter was the number of free recall utterances at the initial interview and at the final interview; the authors examined the amount of forgetting across the two time periods as a function of age. The researchers sought to explore developmental trends in event memory and also developmental trends in forgetting and remembering with delay.

Hand (1994) explained that Lord's paradox is paradoxical only because researchers do not precisely stipulate their hypotheses. Thus, if London and colleagues' (2009) hypothesis was simply that the change in the amount recalled at the two testing periods varied by age, then the appropriate analysis would involve subtracting the amount recalled at the initial interview from the amount recalled at the final interview (i.e., "change") and seeing whether this difference is associated with the children's age. The method of analysis implied is an ANOVA on these change scores, which was the method advocated by one of Lord's (1967) hypothetical statisticians.

Lord's other hypothetical statistician suggested using an ANCOVA with the scores from the initial interview partialed out. This method would be appropriate if London and colleagues' hypothesis involved predicting final scores. Formal comparison of the ANOVA on the change scores and the ANCOVA have led many statisticians to argue that if you are interested in whether the grouping variable is causing a difference in the response variable at time 2, then the ANCOVA approach is usually, but not always, preferred (Maris, 1998; Wainer, 1991; Wright, 2006b). What causation is and how to infer it are complex questions that philosophers have addressed since the beginnings of science and philosophy. We discuss in detail one recent approach that has become popular in statistics and medicine and that is gaining favor in psychology. Furthermore, ANCOVA is usually more statistically powerful than the ANOVA (Maxwell & Delaney, 2004; Oakes & Feldman, 2001).

A Brief Primer on Regression

Having some understanding of regression, up to the level covered in most introductory statistics courses, is useful for the following section. Because many readers will not have had a statistics course recently, in this section we present a very brief guide to basic univariate regression (see any introductory textbook for more details). Regression involves predicting one variable (called the dependent, outcome, or response variable) from one or more predictor (or independent) variables.

Using the data from the London and colleagues (2009) memory study example, to predict the number of items recalled at time 2 from the number of items recalled at time 1 the following equation could be used: time $2_i = \beta_0 + \beta_1$ time $1_i + e_i$. The subscripts tell the reader that each individual person can have a different value for these variables. The Greek letter β (beta) is used to stand for the numbers that regressions are used to estimate. β_0 is called the intercept and is the predicted number of items recalled at time 2 if no items were recalled at time 1. β_1 is called the slope. It shows how the number of items recalled at time 1 is related to the number of items recalled at time 2. The expectation is that this should be positive; if Michelle recalls more items than Obama at time 1, you would expect that she should also recall more at time 2. The e_i at the end is called the error or residual term. This tells us that the predictions will not be exactly right. The regression procedures try to find values of β_0 and β_1 that make the e_i values small. In particular, one common approach is to find the values of β_0 and β_1 that produce the smallest possible value for the sum of the squared residuals. This is called ordinary least squares regression and is the basis of the regressions discussed in this chapter (and is also used in ANOVAs).

Developmental Applications

How the grouping variable, age, is expressed can have important consequences for the results. In London et al. (2009) it could be a quantitative/metrical variable (measured in months or in years), or it could be categorical (e.g., three age groups). We use the acronyms ANOVA and ANCOVA regardless of whether the predictor variable is categorical or not, helping to reinforce that these are all linear models (Cohen, 1968). An extreme case of categorizing is dichotomizing the variable into just two groups: a *young* group and an *old* group. Although dichotomizing has been frowned upon for several decades (Cohen, 1983; MacCallum, Zhang, Preacher, & Rucker, 2002), it still needs to be considered, because it continues to be used in some branches of psychology. We present three different strategies for dealing with the age variable: dichotomizing, using years, and using months (the data and code for analyses/graphs using the freeware statistical program R and screenshots for SPSS are available at *www2.fiu.edu/~dwright/lord/Comparing.htm*). For purposes of exposition, we assume that the slopes for the regression lines are independent of the age variable and that age is a linear predictor. The six basic types of analysis are shown in Table 17.1.

The regression equations of the two approaches in Table 17.1 make clear that in one respect the only difference between the ANOVA and the ANCOVA approaches is that in the ANOVA approach it is assumed that the β_2 from the ANCOVA approach is 1, whereas for the ANCOVA this value is estimated. For both models, the predictor variable is the number of correct utterances recalled at the 10-month delayed posttest. With ANOVA, the dependent variable is the change in recall from the time 1 test to the time 2 test. For the ANCOVA model, the dependent variable is amount recalled at time 2; the covariate is amount recalled at the time 1 test. With the ANCOVA model, then, the dependent variable is the amount recalled at time 2, while holding constant the amount recalled at time 1.

The values for the β_1 parameter in Table 17.1 are those of most interest because they measure how much the amount recalled differs by age. The exact values should not be

TABLE 17.1. Estimates for the Two Approaches Described by Lord's Paradox, Using Data from London et al. (2009)

	Approach	
How age is treated	ANOVA on difference $\text{Final}_i = \text{Initial}_i + \beta_1 \text{Age}_i + \beta_0 + e_i$	ANCOVA $\text{Final}_i = \beta_2 \text{Initial}_i + \beta_1 \text{Age}_i + \beta_0 + e_i$
Dichotomize 4–6 versus 7–9	$\beta_0 = -2.17$ (0.80) $\beta_1 = -4.06$ (1.10) $H_0: \beta_1 = 0: t(49) = -3.68$	$\beta_0 = 1.21$ (0.51) $\beta_1 = 0.78$ (0.71) $\beta_2 = 0.17$ (0.07) $H_0: \beta_1 = 0: t(48) = 1.10$
In years	$\beta_0 = -2.59$ (2.38) $\beta_1 = -1.03$ (0.34) $H_0: \beta_1 = 0: t(49) = -2.99$	$\beta_0 = -1.53$ (1.17) $\beta_1 = 0.53$ (0.20) $\beta_2 = 0.11$ (0.07) $H_0: \beta_1 = 0: t(48) = 2.63$
In months	$\beta_0 = -3.06$ (2.44) $\beta_1 = -0.09$ (0.03) $H_0: \beta_1 = 0: t(49) = -3.11$	$\beta_0 = -1.73$ (1.22) $\beta_1 = 0.04$ (0.02) $\beta_2 = 0.11$ (0.07) $H_0: \beta_1 = 0: t(48) = 2.70$

Note. Standard errors are in parentheses.

compared because the scales differ, but their signs and their values divided by their standard errors (i.e., their t values) can be compared. We begin by comparing how the variable age is treated. In the first column (ANOVA), the magnitude of t is largest when dichotomizing the age variable. Given that having a larger t value is sometimes thought of as a desirable outcome in psychology (Meehl, 1967), this suggests that in this example at least, dichotomizing might be a good thing. However, a better interpretation of the data is that the association is nonlinear. Figure 17.1a shows a number of things. First, most of the points are below the difference = 0 dashed line. The data points above the dashed line are children who recalled more after the delay; the data points below the dashed line show that most of the children recalled less after the delay than initially. See Wright and London (2009a) for a tutorial on graphing the association among three variables.

Second, the difference appears related to age. The difference in recall at the two time points remains fairly stable at about two fewer utterances recalled at the 10-month interview than at the 2-week interview until about 70–80 months (~6–7 years; the first vertical dashed line is at 77 months), and then it declines until the difference again stabilizes at about 100 months (~8½ years), at which there are about seven fewer utterances (the second vertical dashed line is at 100 months). The point at which the dichotomization happens to occur is where the amount is changing the most, and therefore this happens to approximate this curve well. However, without justification for choosing this point of inflection or hypothesizing a possible mechanism for this sudden shift, there is no reason to believe that the dichotomized model is an accurate reflection of the underlying processes, and it is less likely to generalize to other situations than are models that more accurately account for the underlying processes. That the later two methods have similar t values, coupled with visual inspection of Figure 17.1a, suggests that little information is lost by collapsing the month data into years for examining the association between age and the difference in the amount recalled.

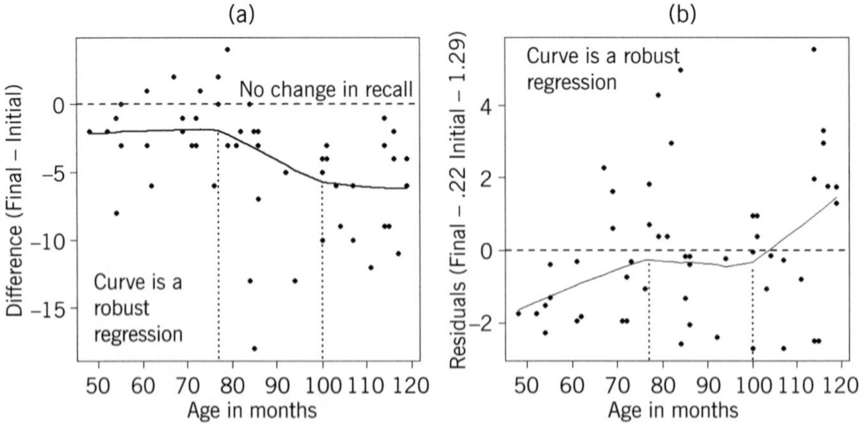

FIGURE 17.1. The relationship between the difference in amount recalled (final interview at 10 months minus initial exit interview at 2 weeks) with age in months (Figure 17.1a, *left panel*) and between the residuals of the model of final scores regressed on initial scores with age in months (Figure 17.1b, *right panel*). The vertical dashed lines correspond to 77 and 100 months of age.

Turning to the ANCOVA approach, the *t* value when age is dichotomized is smaller than it is when age is expressed in years or in months. Figure 17.1b shows the scatterplot of the residuals of the best-fitting least squares model, $e_i = \text{Final}_i - 1.29 - 0.22\ \text{Initial}_i$, as a function of age. The more precise methods of measuring age (i.e., in months and years) produce better fits. In terms of how to treat age in developmental science, we suggest researchers use months if information is lost by using the broader age grouping. With age over several years, usually little information is lost, so using years is fine. If the researcher has only a couple of years' worth of children, then months is probably preferable. Also, if you have sharp discontinuities at age points (e.g., alcohol statistics and 21st birthday) or expected cyclical patterns, then months should be used.

We now compare the ANOVA and ANCOVA approaches using these quantitative variables. For the ANOVA approach the age parameter is negative; the average decrease in the amount reported is larger for older than for younger children (the curve goes down in Figure 17.1a). In other words, according to this approach the older children *forget* more. With the ANCOVA approach, the values of β_1 are positive. In other words, controlling for initial scores, the older children have higher predicted final scores than do the younger children (the curve goes up in Figure 17.1b). In words, the older children are predicted to remember *more*.

ANOVA: older children *forget* more than younger children

ANCOVA: older children *remember* more than younger children

To summarize, Lord's paradox can occur any time a developmental researcher is examining change scores among different groups. Using two different statistical methods can yield different results, with apparently opposite interpretations. The method one chooses, then, goes beyond affecting statistical power and instead can affect the entire conclusions. How should the researcher proceed?

Illustration

The possible implications of these different models for use in the developmental arena are now illustrated with two scenarios. Suppose there were two eyewitnesses to a crime: a 5-year-old and a 9-year-old. For the first scenario, suppose that due to limited resources only one child can be interviewed soon after the crime and that the other child can be interviewed only after a 10-month delay. Which child should be interviewed first?

Denote the 5-year-old's initial interview score with I5, for Initial 5-year-old, and the 9-year-old's with I9, for Initial 9-year-old. If the 5-year-old is interviewed first, then the total amount that child recalls is I5. If the 9-year-old is interviewed second, then assuming that the regression equation in Table 17.1 applies (in column 1 with age in years), the total predicted number of utterances for this child would be (I9 – 2.59 – 9•1.03), which is I9 – 11.86. The total amount from the two children would be: I5 + I9 – 11.86. If the 9-year-old is interviewed first and the 5-year-old second, then the predicted total would be: I9 + (I5 – 2.59 – 5•1.03) = I5 + I9 – 7.74. Therefore, if the 9-year-old were interviewed first, then we would expect about four more utterances than if the 5-year-old were interviewed first. The older group remembers more. If the principal interest is whether the differences in amount recalled between the two time periods vary by age, then the ANOVA approach is appropriate. According to this analysis, the younger children on average show less decline in their free recall reports compared with the older children (i.e., they forget less). This accurate description of the data *suggests* that *younger* children's recall is less affected by the passage of time. But, as we will see, this apparently sound causal conclusion is based on a dubious assumption.

For the second scenario, suppose that the two children recalled the same amount at the initial interview (denote this value I); that 10 months later, at trial, only one of the children can be called to testify, and that it is best to choose the child who is likely to recall the most. Which child should be called? Assuming that the equation in column 2 of Table 17.1 with age in years applies, then the predicted number of utterances after a 10-month delay for the younger child is .11 I – 1.53 + 5•0.53 = .11 I + 1.12, and the comparable number for the older child is .11 I – 1.53 + 9•0.53 = .11 I + 3.24. Therefore, according to this scenario, the 9-year-old, who is predicted to recall two more utterances than the 5-year-old, should be selected. This accurate description of the data *suggests* that *older* children's recall is less affected by the passage of time. It will be argued that the assumption required to draw this causal conclusion is more reasonable than the one required for the previous inference.

We believe that the best interpretation of the data is that the younger children recalled very little at time 1 and that there was little room for their performance to drop. The older children recalled much more than the younger groups at time 1. However, although their absolute difference scores of time 2 minus time 1 were greater, the older group still recalled more than the younger group at time 2. The ANOVA approach would lead to the conclusion that the older group simply forgets more; the ANCOVA approach depicts the more complex story that the older children outperformed the younger children at both time points and that their memory scores had much more room to fall.

These data provide a striking example of Lord's paradox by showing how the choice of a statistical procedure may lead to opposing conclusions. The ANOVA approach shows that the decrease in the amount recalled increases with age, whereas the ANCOVA approach shows that, controlling for the initial amounts recalled, the older children recall more at the final interview. The causal conclusions suggested by these approaches are opposite, and each is large. The correlation between the difference in the amounts recalled and age in years was *negative* .39 (the ANOVA approach), and the correlation between the final test and age in years, partialing out initial recall, was *positive* .36 (the ANCOVA approach). Thus the choice of which approach is more appropriate determines the conclusions.

Although Lord (1967) did not say which approach was generally preferred, Rubin's model of causal inference (Holland & Rubin, 1983; Rubin, 1974, 1977; Wainer, 1991) has shown when each of these approaches is more likely to be valid for causal inference. For a recent discussion of Rubin's model with reference to psychology and in comparison with the Cook and Campbell (1979) approach to causation, see Maxwell (2010). Rubin's model is usually described in relation to experimental groups and causation, but it can also be used for quasi-experimental groups, in which interest is in an association rather than a cause (Wainer, 1991; Wright, 2006a). Age is different from most quasi-experimental variables because, as time progresses, people move from one group to another. Usually the effects are gradual, but sometimes there are more abrupt shifts, and some patterns are complex, such as the emergence between ages 2½ and 3 years of children's use of symbols to guide their searches of a large-scale space (see DeLoache, 2002, for a review).

The key to Rubin's model is that to make causal inference, one must make assumptions about two unobserved conditions. Suppose in a traditionally designed experiment there is a control group, G1, and an experimental group, G2. Both groups are assessed on the same variable at time 1 (label these measurements as G1T1 and G2T1) and then later at time 2, after G1 has experienced the control condition and G2 has experienced the experimental condition. Label these Control(G1T2) and Exper(G2T2). Because the interest is in any effects of the manipulation, ideally you would want to measure the same people in both the control and experimental conditions. The effects for G1 and G2, denoted Effect(G1) and Effect(G2), can be estimated by:

$$\text{Effect(G1)} = \textit{Exper(G1T2)} - \text{Control(G1T2)}$$

and

$$\text{Effect(G2)} = \text{Exper(G2T2)} - \textit{Control(G2T2)}$$

It is often assumed that these effects are the same and therefore an estimate of the effect for the population from which these samples were drawn can be calculated by averaging the group effects or by using either one. The problem is that the variables in *italics* have not been measured and therefore need to be estimated. If the groups had been determined randomly, we would expect that they would not differ greatly when placed in the same conditions, and therefore the expected value for *Control(G2T2)* would be Control(G1T2), and the expected value for *Exper(G1T2)* would be Exper(G2T2). If random assignment were used, a valid (though likely not the most statistically powerful) test of the difference between the control and experimental conditions would simply compare the time 2 measurements, often with an ANOVA (or, because there are only 2 groups here, a *t*-test). An ANOVA on the change scores and an ANCOVA would both be valid because the random assignment allows us to assume that before manipulation the groups do not differ systematically (G1T1 would be approximately the same as G2T1, and because these are measured this assumption can be tested). This situation presents no particular problems. As Cook and Campbell (1979, p. 5) put it, "random assignment is the great *ceteris paribus*—that is, other things being equal—of causal inference." In many situations it is either not possible or not practical to employ random assignment, as in the case of age. Children of different ages can be randomly assigned to different treatment conditions, but children cannot be randomly assigned to different age groups (or diagnoses). Therefore, the researcher must take into account varying baseline scores for such variables.

The difficulty is how to estimate the unmeasured variables when random assignment has not been used, as is the case with London and colleagues' (2009) quasi-experimental design in which the grouping variable is age. Group differences at the initial interview may exist, and in these data they do. According to Rubin's model, in order to conduct an ANOVA on change scores, it must be assumed that, in the absence of manipulation, the initial scores are good estimates of future scores (Wainer, 1991). Thus the assumption is: G2T1 is a good estimate for *Control(G2T2)*. Because *Control(G2T2)* is unmeasured, we cannot test this directly; but, because in almost all relevant research, memory levels decline with delay, this assumption appears unreasonable. For the ANCOVA approach, the assumption is that *Control(G2T2)* can be estimated by a linear predictor of G2T2 with time. Because this is a more general assumption, it is more likely to be met, or at least more likely to be an adequate approximation. Wainer (1991) and others stress that these assumptions only suggest which approach is better for inference and that both approaches offer valid descriptions of the data. Because the ANCOVA model is more flexible than the ANOVA model, with its one extra parameter estimated, it is easier to justify empirically. Research does show that linear decay is only a rough approximation of the forgetting function; alternatives that do not assume linear decay are discussed later in this chapter.

Returning to the London et al. (2009) example, the effect of interest is whether the transition from the initial interview to the final interview is similar for participants of different ages. In this example, the assumption for causal inference for the ANOVA with change scores is that, as time progresses, the children continue to recall approximately the same number of utterances. This assumption is not valid here; the participants of all ages tended to recall less at the final interview than at the initial interview and, with few exceptions, memory research shows that the amounts people recall decline with time. The assumption for the ANCOVA method is that the recall at time 2 is a linear predictor of that at time 1. This is a more realistic assumption, and therefore the ANCOVA approach is preferred here for causal inference and in most research in which the interest is in age differences.

ANOVA on change scores and ANCOVA are just two of an infinite number of possible ways to address these data, but they are the two most popular and, in terms of parameters estimated, two of the simplest. Other hypothesized relationships between the time 1 and time 2 variables, such as their ratio, can be used, and other methods, such as matching participants between groups, can be used (Rubin, 2006). A very general approach is to fit to the data an additive model with a curved line for the relationship between the initial interview and the final interview. Additive models (Hastie & Tibshirani, 1990) are now available in many of the main statistical packages.

Future Directions

The goal for any researcher should be to describe the data accurately, telling a story in a way that the reader can comprehend. As such, researchers need to be equipped with a variety of statistical methods in their toolboxes, because different data and different questions call for different tools. There are several extensions that can be made to the basic ANOVA and ANCOVA models. In this section, we summarize some extensions of the ANOVA and ANCOVA approaches described previously.

Check for Interactions!

First, the traditional ANCOVA approaches assume that there is no interaction between age and the effect as measured by the differences between groups (i.e., the assumption that Effect(G1) = Effect(G2)). This can be dealt with by including an interaction term in the models. An interaction term between, for example, age and initial recall is the product of these two variables. If you are using SPSS, you would create a new variable by multiplying these together and then add this variable to the model via the regression procedure. If the fit is significantly improved, the interaction is statistically significant. If the interaction is significant, it means that the effect of one of the variables depends on the value of the other variable. For the current example, a significant interaction would mean that the relationship between time 1 and time 2 scores depended on the age of the participants. Interactions can be conceptually difficult, particularly if it is among several variables. For the data in London and colleagues (2009), the interaction terms (i.e., the parameter for the product of age and initial recall) were small and nonsignificant. This means that we cannot reject the hypothesis that the slope of the relationship between time 1 and time 2 scores is the same for all age groups. The parallel slope assumption should be examined when conducting ANCOVAs (Rutherford, 2000; for examples using SPSS, see Field, 2009, Chapter 14).

Allowing the Data to Suggest a Nonlinear Relationship

Second, although only linear models were reported for the London et al. (2009) data, there are other options. Notably, there are many models that can be used to fit a smooth curve through the data. These models relax the assumption of linearity between age and variables of interest. The approach we describe is allowing what is called a spline to be fit to the data (see Wright & London, 2009b, Chapter 7, for an introduction). Additive models involve piecing together different curves, which are called splines, to map out the relationship between each predictor variable and the response variable. These are very flexible models and are most valuable either when graphically exploring data or when not wanting to make many assumptions about one predictor variable while looking at more specific models with another predictor variable.

Having Many Data Points

London et al. (2009) tested children at only two points in time. This is the simplest schedule for a longitudinal design. Researchers often test children at several times, and multilevel modeling approaches allow the times tested to be different (Pinheiro & Bates, 2000; Singer & Willett, 2003; Wright & London, 2009c). These are more complex situations, but the same issues apply as with the simpler design: how to use previous measurements within the models. The ANOVA approach would involve measuring change at each point, whereas the ANCOVA would involve regressing previous scores. The methods for this can be complex and are covered in Singer and Willett (2003) at a level appropriate for psychology graduate students. Because researchers usually assume that scores change over time, the norm is to decide on a covariance structure that is more akin to the ANCOVA approach.

Summary

This chapter has compared two statistical procedures that are commonly used in developmental science: ANOVA and ANCOVA. The principles in this chapter apply to many developmental studies in which people are measured at two points in time and measurements from the first time are used as a baseline measure. With ANOVA, the analysis is run on the difference scores (i.e., time 2 scores minus time 1 scores), whereas with ANCOVA we examine the time 2 scores while partialing out the initial scores.

In a classic 1954 paper, Lord described a paradox, referred to as Lord's paradox, and demonstrated that the use of ANOVA versus ANCOVA on repeated-measures data can yield different and sometimes contradictory findings. Hence the researchers' choice of ANOVA versus ANCOVA will depend upon the research question. In the example used in this chapter, we saw that ANOVA showed that older children forgot more than younger children after a 10-month delay. However, the results from the ANCOVA showed different results: Controlling for the initial amount recalled, the older children in fact still remembered more at the 10-month delay compared with the younger children. The ANOVA results were driven by the fact that, when compared with the younger children, the older children had much better memories at the initial recall. They still were recalling more at the posttest—it was just that their memories had much further to fall with delay given their superior baseline performance.

ANCOVA is a very useful approach when true random assignment cannot be used. For example, children cannot be randomly assigned to age groups. ANCOVA can partial out baseline differences attributable to age. The purpose of this chapter was not to say that the ANCOVA approach is always better but that researchers should consider several approaches and that, of these two, *usually* the ANCOVA approach will be preferred for making causal inference in situations in which two or more groups are compared at two time points.

References

Cohen, J. (1968). Multiple regression as a general data-analytic system. *Psychological Bulletin, 70,* 426–443.

Cohen, J. (1983). The cost of dichotomization. *Applied Psychological Measurement, 7,* 249–253.

Cook, T. D., & Campbell, D. T. (1979). *Quasi-experimentation: Design and analysis issues for field settings*. Boston: Houghton Mifflin.

DeLoache, J. S. (2002). The symbol-mindedness of young children. In W. W. Hartup & R. A. Weinberg (Eds.), *Child psychology in retrospect and prospect: The Minnesota Symposia on Child Psychology* (Vol. 32, pp. 73–101). Mahwah, NJ: Erlbaum.

Field, A. (2009). *Discovering statistics using SPSS* (3rd ed.). London: Sage.

Hand, D. J. (1994). Deconstructing statistical questions. *Journal of the Royal Statistical Society: A, 157,* 317–356.

Hastie, T., & Tibshirani, R. (1990). *Generalized additive models*. Boca Raton, FL: Chapman & Hall.

Holland, P. W., & Rubin, D. B. (1983). On Lord's paradox. In H. Wainer & S. Messick (Eds.), *Principles of modern psychological measurement* (pp. 3–35). Hillsdale, NJ: Erlbaum.

London, K., Bruck, M., & Melnyk, L. (2009). Post-event information affects children's autobiographical memory after one year. *Law and Human Behavior, 33,* 344–355.

Lord, F. M. (1967). A paradox in the interpretation of group comparisons. *Psychological Bulletin, 72,* 304–305.

MacCallum, R. C., Zhang, S., Preacher, K. J., & Rucker, D. D. (2002). On the practice of dichotomization of quantitative variables. *Psychological Methods, 7,* 19–40.

Maris, E. (1998). Covariance adjustment versus gain scores—revisited. *Psychological Methods, 3,* 309–327.

Maxwell, S. E. (2010). Introduction to the special section on Campbell's and Rubin's conceptualizations of causality. *Psychological Methods, 15,* 1–2.

Maxwell, S. E., & Delaney, H. D. (2004). *Designing experiments and analyzing data: A model comparison perspective* (2nd ed.). Mahwah, NJ: Erlbaum.

Meehl, P. (1967). Theory-testing in psychology and physics: A methodological paradox. *Philosophy of Science, 34,* 103–115.

Oakes, J. M., & Feldman, H. A. (2001). Statistical power for non-equivalent pretest–posttest designs: The impact of change-score versus ANCOVA models. *Evaluation Review, 25,* 3–28.

Pinheiro, J. C., & Bates, D. M. (2000). *Mixed-effects models in S and S-PLUS.* New York: Springer.

Rubin, D. B. (1974). Estimating causal effects of treatments in randomized and nonrandomized studies. *Journal of Educational Psychology, 66,* 688–701.

Rubin, D. B. (1977). Assignment to a treatment group on the basis of a covariate. *Journal of Educational Statistics, 2,* 1–26.

Rubin, D. B. (2006). *Matched sampling for causal effects.* Cambridge, UK: Cambridge University Press.

Rutherford, A. (2000). *Introducing ANOVA and ANCOVA: A GLM approach.* London: Sage.

Senn, S. L. (2006). Change from baseline and analysis of covariance revisited. *Statistics in Medicine, 25,* 4334–4344.

Singer, J. D., & Willett, J. B. (2003). *Applied longitudinal data analysis: Modeling change and event occurrence.* New York: Oxford University Press.

Wainer, H. (1991). Adjusting for differential base rates: Lord's paradox again. *Psychological Bulletin, 109,* 147–151.

Wainer, H., & Brown, L. M. (2004). Two statistical paradoxes in the interpretation of group differences: Illustrated with medical school admission and licensing data. *American Statistician, 58,* 117–123.

Wright, D. B. (2006a). Causal and associative hypotheses in psychology: Examples from eyewitness testimony research. *Psychology, Public Policy, and Law, 12,* 190–213.

Wright, D. B. (2006b). Comparing groups in a before–after design: When *t*-test and ANCOVA produce different results. *British Journal of Educational Psychology, 76,* 663–675.

Wright, D. B., & London, K. (2009a). *First steps in statistics* (2nd ed.). London: Sage.

Wright, D. B., & London, K. (2009b). *Modern regression techniques using R: A practical guide for students and researchers.* London: Sage.

Wright, D. B., & London, K. (2009c). Multilevel modelling: Beyond the basic applications. *British Journal of Mathematical and Statistical Psychology, 62,* 439–456.

CHAPTER 18

Mediation Models for Developmental Data

MATTHEW S. FRITZ
DAVID P. MACKINNON

Central Issues

The study of development is the study of change, regardless of whether the researcher is primarily interested in the ultimate outcome of the change or in the process that leads to the ultimate outcome. Mediation analyses are conducted in order to better understand the mechanisms by which one variable causes change in a second variable by examining the role of intermediary variables in this change. The parity in the goals of the study of development and mediation analysis—to better understand change—explains why mediation models are widely used in developmental research to test mechanisms of change in the development of a variety of different behaviors, attitudes, cognitive functions, physical characteristics, and psychological problems across the entire range of the human lifespan. For example, Kim and Cicchetti (2004) found a mediating role of self-esteem and social competence in the association between mother–child relationship quality and the children's development of maladjustment in a longitudinal sample of school-age children. And Salthouse (1996) describes how the effect of age on declines in memory is mediated by the individual's cognitive processing speed in a sample of adults ranging in age from 18 to 93 years old. These two examples are only a tiny subset of the developmental studies that have used mediation models, but they illustrate how researchers interested in developmental change in all age ranges and a variety of topics are using mediation models.

Conceptual Principles and Statistical Assumptions

Definition of Mediation

Mediation refers to any model in which the effect of an independent variable on a dependent variable is transmitted through a third intervening or mediating variable. That is, in order for a change in the independent variable to cause a change in the dependent variable, the change in the independent variable must first cause a change in the mediating variable, or mediator, and then the change in the mediator must cause a change in the dependent variable. A mediation model with a single mediator is illustrated in Figure 18.1, in which X is the independent variable, Y is the dependent variable, and M is the mediator. The effect of the independent variable on the dependent variable that is transmitted by the mediator is called the mediated or indirect effect because the independent variable indirectly affects the dependent variable through the mediator. Complete mediation occurs when the entire effect of the independent variable on the dependent variable passes through the mediator such that if the mediator was to be held constant, then a change in the independent variable would have no effect on the dependent variable. Partial mediation occurs when only part of the overall effect of the independent variable on the dependent variable is mediated. The piece of the overall effect of the independent variable on the dependent variable that is not mediated is called the direct effect. Partially mediated models exist on a continuum between completely mediated models and models with no mediation. Baron and Kenny (1986) note that partially mediated models are more likely to be encountered in the social sciences than completely mediated models because all of the shared variance between two variables is rarely accounted for by a single third variable.

Mediation models are distinct from another class of third variable models called moderation models. In a moderation model, an interaction exists between the independent variable and the third variable, called a moderator, such that the effect of the independent variable on the dependent variable is conditional on the values of the moderator. That is, the magnitude, and potentially the sign, of the effect of the independent variable on the dependent variable is different for different values of the moderator. Note that in a moderation

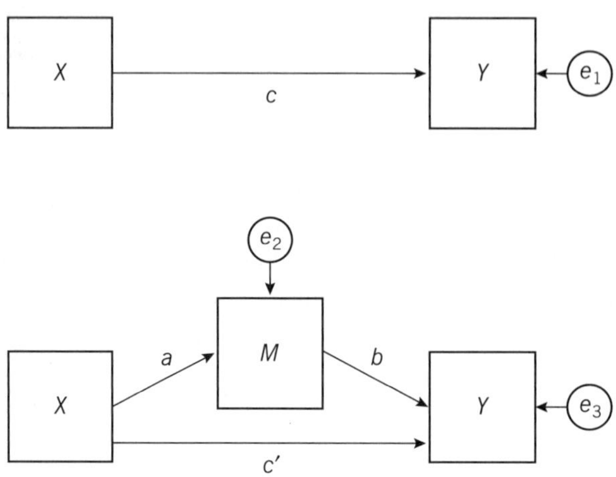

FIGURE 18.1. The single mediator model.

model, no assumptions of causality between the variables, especially between the independent variable and the moderator, are made. However, a mediation model is a causal chain that describes how the first link in the chain, the independent variable, affects the last link in the chain, the dependent variable, through all intermediary links, the mediators.

The Single Mediator Model

The single mediator model in Figure 18.1 can be represented using three ordinary least squares (OLS) regression equations:

$$Y_i = i_1 + cX_i + e_{1i} \tag{18.1}$$

$$M_i = i_2 + aX_i + e_{2i} \tag{18.2}$$

$$Y_i = i_3 + c'X_i + bM_i + e_{3i} \tag{18.3}$$

where c represents the total effect of X on Y, a is the effect of X on M, c' is the direct effect of X on Y after controlling for the mediator M, b is the effect of M on Y after controlling for X, i_1, i_2, and i_3 are intercepts, and e_{1i}, e_{2i}, and e_{3i} represent residual error terms for individual i. The mediated effect is equal to the product ab. In OLS regression, the overall effect of X on Y, c, is equal to the sum of the indirect and direct paths such that

$$\hat{c} = \hat{c}' + \hat{a}\hat{b} \tag{18.4}$$

where the hats indicate estimates of the population parameters.

Testing the Mediated Effect

Product-of-Coefficients Tests

Although MacKinnon, Lockwood, Hoffman, West, and Sheets (2002) describe three different categories of tests of mediation, including the causal-steps tests, the difference-in-coefficients tests, and the product-of-coefficients tests, only the product-of-coefficients tests will be described here because the other two categories of tests do not generalize well to longitudinal data. Product-of-coefficients tests assess mediation by testing the product of the estimates of the a and b paths, $\hat{a}\hat{b}$, for significance by dividing the product by the standard error of the product and comparing the resulting quantity with a normal distribution for significance. The primary distinction between the different product-of-coefficients tests described by MacKinnon and colleagues is the manner in which the standard error of the product is computed. The most commonly used estimate of the standard error of the product is the first-order standard error derived by Sobel (1982), which is equal to

$$\hat{\sigma}_{\hat{a}\hat{b}} = \sqrt{\hat{b}^2\hat{\sigma}^2_{\hat{a}} + \hat{a}^2\hat{\sigma}^2_{\hat{b}}} \tag{18.5}$$

MacKinnon (2008) describes several advantages the product-of-coefficients tests have over the causal-steps tests and the difference-in-coefficients tests, including equal or higher statistical power in most situations and the fact that an estimate of the mediated effect is produced. In addition, in multiple mediator models and mediation models for longitudinal data, the product-of-coefficients methods can test specific mediated effects for significance, as well as the overall mediated effect. This means that confidence intervals, effect sizes, and confidence intervals for the effect sizes may all be computed for each of these mediated effects.

Distribution of the Product Tests

The product-of-coefficients tests, as just described, have a fatal flaw in that the distribution of the product of two random variables, that is, *ab*, is not normally distributed in most cases and has a different shape depending on the values of *a, b*, and their standard errors (Springer & Thompson, 1966). This means that dividing $\hat{a}\hat{b}$ by the standard error in equation 18.5 and comparing this quantity to a normal distribution or using this standard error to create symmetric confidence intervals around $\hat{a}\hat{b}$ is incorrect in most situations. There are two methods for addressing the non-normality of *ab*. The first is to use the actual, non-normal distribution of *ab* for specific values of *a* and *b* in order to create asymmetric confidence intervals around $\hat{a}\hat{b}$. The second method is to use nonparametric tests that do not make the assumption that the distribution of *ab* is normally distributed.

MacKinnon, Fritz, Williams, and Lockwood (2007) developed a computer program called PRODCLIN that uses numerical integration to find the asymmetric critical values from the distribution of the product for specific values of *a* and *b*. These critical values are then used to create an asymmetric confidence interval around $\hat{a}\hat{b}$, allowing it to be tested for significance. In addition to being more accurate than standard symmetric confidence intervals, Fritz and MacKinnon (2007) found that the PRODCLIN test was more powerful than the first-order standard error test in all situations. Tofighi and MacKinnon (2010) have developed a new version of PRODCLIN for R (R Core Development Team, 2010) and have found that the PRODCLIN program also produced more accurate Type I error rates than the first-order standard error test.

Resampling Tests

Resampling tests, namely the bootstrap procedure, are a family of nonparametric tests that take samples from the original sample in order to create an empirical distribution of the underlying distribution of interest (Efron & Tibshirani, 1993). Resampling tests have been advocated as a method for testing indirect effects because these tests do not assume that the indirect effect is normally distributed (e.g., Bollen & Stine, 1990; Shrout & Bolger, 2002). Fritz and MacKinnon (2007) compared the percentile and bias-corrected bootstrap tests with the PRODCLIN test and found that the bias-corrected bootstrap test had more power than the percentile bootstrap or PRODCLIN tests, which had approximately equal power. However, Fritz, Taylor, and MacKinnon (2010) found that the bias-corrected bootstrap has elevated Type I error rates for small sample sizes, so this test should be used with caution.

Resampling tests currently have two advantages over the PRODCLIN test of mediation. First, resampling tests of mediation can be conducted in most general statistical software packages, such as SAS and R, and several software packages, such as Mplus (Muthén & Muthén, 2010), will compute bootstrap confidence intervals for any indirect effect. Second, at this time PRODCLIN is limited to two variables, meaning that for some longitudinal mediation models, PROCLIN cannot be used. Resampling tests of mediation can be used regardless of the number of paths in the indirect effect. For more information on bootstrap tests of mediation, as well as other resampling tests of mediation, see MacKinnon, Lockwood, and Williams (2004).

Assumptions of the Single Mediator Model

Several assumptions of the single mediator model must be met in order to correctly estimate the mediated effect. The first assumption is that the relationships between the variables are correctly specified. In equations 18.1, 18.2, and 18.3, the relationships between *X*, *M*, and *Y* are specified as linear and additive. If the form of the relationship is nonlinear or if an interaction occurs, then these equations can be adjusted to reflect this by including a higher order or interaction term. The second assumption requires that there be no omitted variables that cause the observed effects or influence these effects, such as a moderator. This assumption also implies that the causal ordering of *X* causing *M* causing *Y* is correct and, for example, *M* does not cause *X*. The third assumption requires that *X*, *M*, and *Y* are valid and reliable measures of the constructs of interest, because measurement error can lead to bias in the regression coefficients, especially for the *b* path (Hoyle & Kenny, 1999). The final assumption is that the residuals are uncorrelated with the predictors in their respective equations, are independent of the residuals in the other equations, and are homoscedastic. These four assumptions are common to all regression models, and violations of these assumptions can lead to bias in the parameter estimates or the standard errors. For more information on testing assumptions of regression models and the consequences of violating these assumptions see Cohen, Cohen, West, and Aiken (2003).

A second set of assumptions of the single mediator model concerns the inferences that may be made from the model (MacKinnon, 2008). The first assumption is that *X*, *M*, and *Y* are continuous, normally distributed variables. If any of the variable are continuous but not normally distributed, then transformations may be applied to the individual variables (Cohen et al., 2003). If *X* is categorical, then the tests of mediation described to this point are unaffected, provided *X* is coded correctly for a regression model. However, if either *M* or *Y* is a categorical variable, then ordinary least squares (OLS) regression is not suited for the analysis, and a different model must be chosen, such as a logistic regression model. The second assumption is that the distribution of the indirect effect is normally distributed, an assumption that, as described previously, is not met in a majority of mediation analyses, meaning that, in general, tests of the mediated effect, $\hat{a}\hat{b}$, that are based on normal theory should be avoided in favor of tests that do not assume normality, such as bootstrapping or PRODCLIN. A third assumption is that the estimates of *a* and *b* represent average causal effects. If individuals are randomly assigned to *X*, then in most circumstances $\hat{a}$ and $\hat{c}$ are considered causal effects, but because individuals are almost never randomly assigned to *M*, $\hat{b}$ and $\hat{c}'$ usually cannot be considered causal effects. When *a* and *b* are not average causal effects, then the inferences from the model are compromised and should be used with caution. For more information on causal inference in mediation, see MacKinnon (2008, pp. 347–367).

The fourth assumption involves identifying whether the mediation model in question is a macro-mediational model, meaning that the mediation model of interest is the whole causal chain, or a micro-mediational model, meaning that the mediation model of interest is a smaller piece of a larger model. For instance, Ranby and colleagues (2009) describe a model in which social norms mediated the effect of a program to develop a healthy body image and decrease the use of diet pills in high school female athletes on the outcome expectancy of taking diet pills. This model alone would be a macro-mediational model. However, outcome expectancies predicted intentions to use diet pills, which in turn predicted actual usage of diet pills, making the original model a micro-mediational piece of a larger macro-mediational model. A fifth assumption is that the mediation model being tested is a theoretical model, in which the constructs in the original theory are being tested, rather than an empirical model in which variables that have been found to be significantly related in previous research are being tested but may represent proxies of the constructs of interest (Kraemer, Wilson, Fairburn, & Agras, 2002). Both of these assumptions affect the generalizability and conclusions that can be reached from the mediation model. Two additional assumptions are temporal precedence of causes to effects and correct timing of measurements, which are discussed next.

Temporal Precedence and Longitudinal Data

Temporal Precedence

Temporal precedence is the idea that a cause must precede an effect in time, so that the effect one variable has on another variable requires some amount of time to occur, even if the amount of time required for the effect to occur is so short that the effect appears instantaneous. Temporal precedence is a fundamental assumption in mediation analysis, which is the reason that alternate names for X and Y in Figure 18.1 are the *antecedent* and the *consequent*, respectively, implying that a change in X must precede a change in Y. Temporal precedence presents a problem when a researcher tests a mediation model using cross-sectional data. Although it is usually not possible to measure multiple psychological variables at the exact same moment in time, for all intents and purposes the variables are measured at the same time in cross-sectional data. Measuring all of the variables at once does not take into account the time necessary for the antecedent to affect the mediator variable or the time necessary for the mediator variable to affect the consequent (Gollob & Reichardt, 1991). Thus, the use of cross-sectional data to investigate mediation violates temporal precedence and greatly decreases the validity of causal inference from the model. Instead, longitudinal data that measure variables at different points in time are needed.

Longitudinal Data

Kraemer, Yesavage, Taylor, and Kupfer (2000) question in their article, "How Can We Learn about Developmental Processes from Cross-Sectional Studies, or Can We?", whether the study of developmental processes should even be attempted with cross-sectional data. They conclude that drawing inferences about longitudinal relationships from cross-sectional studies is ill advised at best and often incorrect, although cross-sectional results may be used to plan longitudinal studies. These conclusions apply directly to mediation models. For example, Sliwinski and Hofer (1999) question the validity of mediation models in examining the relationship between age and memory loss due to the reliance on cross-sectional studies to make inferences about the relationship of two developmental variables that change with time. Maxwell and Cole (2007) support the conclusions of Kraemer and colleagues and Sliwinski and Hofer, noting that unless specific, but unlikely, assumptions are met, the results from a cross-sectional mediation analysis will be highly biased. Repeated measurements of variables have numerous other advantages as well, including the ability to study delayed effects, increased statistical power to find effects, and the ability to examine trends across time (Venter & Maxwell, 1999), as well as allowing for the study of within-unit and between-unit variation (MacKinnon, 2008). Also, cross-sectional data may make the interpretation of effect sizes difficult because there is no indication of the time interval to which the effect applies (Gollob & Reichardt, 1987).

Three characteristics of longitudinal relationships need to be considered when fitting mediation models to longitudinal data: stability, stationarity, and equilibrium (Kenny, 1979; see also Cole & Maxwell, 2003; Hertzog & Nesselroade, 1987; MacKinnon, 2008). Stability refers to the degree to which an individual's score on a variable changes over time relative to changes in other individuals' scores. Scores that do not change over time are more stable than those that do change over time. Kraemer and colleagues (2000) noted that researchers need to differentiate between trait variables and state variables in longitudinal studies. If a variable represents a trait, then instability is likely due to measurement error or a confounding variable, not actual changes in the trait, whereas instability in a state variable is more likely to represent actual changes in the individual's state across time. Stationarity is the degree to which relations among variables measured remain consistent across time. If the relation between two variables is constant across time, then the relationship is stationary. Nonstationarity could be caused by a change in the causal relationship across time (MacKinnon, 2008) or the presence of a time-varying moderator variable. Equilibrium refers to the consistency of within-wave (cross-sectional at each measurement occasion) covariances. Only after a model has reached equilibrium can the relations between the variables be accurately measured by cross-sectional data (James, Mulaik, & Brett, 1982; Maxwell & Cole, 2007). However, once a model has reached equilibrium, it may be of little interest to a researcher (Gollob & Reichardt, 1987). Although equilibrium is related to stability and stationarity, a model that is both stable and stationary is not necessarily at equilibrium, as illustrated by Cole and Maxwell (2003, pp. 560–561).

Timing Schema

How Many Waves of Data?

An important consideration when planning the measurement timing schema (i.e., the quantity and spacing of the measurements) for a longitudinal mediation model is how many times the variables must be measured. For mediation, a study with two waves of data is called a half-longitudinal design because when X, M, and Y are all measured on two occasions, then either the effect of X on M must occur instantaneously or the effect of M on Y must occur instantaneously in order to measure the mediated effect of X_1 on Y_2 using path tracing rules, where the subscript indicates the measurement occasion (Cole & Maxwell, 2003). As in the cross-sectional design, this means that there may not be sufficient time for X or M to exert its full effect. Also, specifying an instantaneous effect when time is needed for the effect to occur can greatly bias the results (Gollob & Reichardt, 1987). For this reason, rather than use an instantaneous effect in the estimate of the mediated effect, Cole and Maxwell recommend using the estimate of the effect of X_1 on M_2 and the effect of M_1 on Y_2 to form the estimate of the mediated effect because it will be less biased. However, this estimate of the mediated effect will not be unbiased unless the system has reached equilibrium such that the effect of M_1 on Y_2 is equal to the effect of M_2 on Y_3, which would require a third measurement to test. For more information on half-longitudinal designs, see MacKinnon (2008, pp. 199–201).

Due to potential problems with the half-longitudinal design, a fully longitudinal design in which the variables are measured at three or more points in time is preferred. Measuring the same variable three or more times allows a researcher to study many more aspects of a causal relationship. First, the more waves of data that are present, the better equipped a researcher is to investigate stability, stationarity, and equilibrium in the model, including delayed effects or decay in the effects. Second, the timing of measurement occasions should be based on theory, but there are numerous cases in which the time needed for a variable to have its full effect on another variable is unknown (James et al., 1982). When the exact period of time required for an effect to fully manifest is unknown, increasing the number of measurement occasions allows a researcher to better examine the proper time frame (Boker & Nesselroade, 2002; Cole & Maxwell, 2003; Collins & Graham, 2002). However, collecting more waves of data does not guarantee that enough time has passed for an effect to occur or that the effect has not already dissipated by the time the variables were measured.

Finally, variables can have effects on themselves at later time points, and these effects, known as autoregressive effects, may increase or decrease in magnitude over time (Gollob & Reichardt, 1991) or occur in cycles (Boker & Nesselroade, 2002). For instance, a child's externalizing behavior at one time point is likely to be highly related to the child's externalizing behavior at a future time point. Autoregressive effects are related to the stability of a variable across time and, as such, the effect of one variable on another variable can change as the time between the two measurements, known as a lag, increases. Continuing with the example of child externalizing behavior, the relationship between externalizing behavior at two consecutive time points (e.g., measurements 1 and 2) is likely to be stronger than the relationship between two nonconsecutive time points (e.g., measurements 1 and 3). Investigating effects over different time lags is a good method with which to examine the necessary time for a variable to exert its full effect and plan proper measurement occasions, as well as the equilibrium of a set of variables across time.

Fritz (2007) conducted a literature survey using the PsycINFO search engine to determine the number of waves of longitudinal data currently being used by researchers to analyze mediation models. The literature survey consisted of peer-reviewed journal articles published from 2000 to 2006 in American Psychological Association journals that contained the keywords *mediat** and *longitudinal*. The articles had to test at least one mediation hypothesis on a data set that contained two or more waves of data; studies in which only one wave of a multiwave data set was analyzed were not included, resulting in 69 articles. As illustrated in Table 18.1, the frequencies of studies using a particular number of waves decreased as the number of waves increased, with the largest percentage of studies using two waves of data, 47.89% ($n = 34$).

Variable Trajectories

A second important consideration when planning the measurement timing schema for a longitudinal mediation model is the shape of the trajectories of the individual variables across time. If the change in X, M, and Y across time is linear, then at least two measurement points are needed, and the spacing of the measurements is unimportant as the change is constant across time. However, if the trajectories of X, M, or Y are not linear but are instead

TABLE 18.1. Frequencies of the Number of Measurement Waves Used by Researchers in Longitudinal Mediation Models for Articles Appearing in American Psychological Association Journals Published between 2000 and 2006

Number of waves of data	Frequency	Percentage of studies
2	34	47.89
3	19	26.76
4	11	15.49
5	3	4.23
6	3	4.23
10	1	1.41

Note. Frequencies sum to 71 because two of the articles had two independent longitudinal data sets.

curvilinear, such as quadratic change; nonlinear, such as exponential decay; or discrete, such as a step function, then the timing schema is very important (see Blozis, Chapter 26, this volume). First, the number of measurements should meet or exceed the minimum number of points required to estimate a specific function. For example, quadratic change requires a minimum of three measurements to estimate, but more measurements give a better estimate of the quadratic function. Second, the spacing of the measurements needs to be planned to capture the parameters of the trajectory as accurately as possible. For curvilinear and nonlinear trajectories this means several closely spaced measurements around all inflection points and curves. If a variable decays exponentially across time, for example, then a measurement is required at the beginning of the process in order to estimate the initial value of the decay, a second measurement is required after most of the decay has occurred in order to estimate the value the decay asymptotes to, and several measurements are needed during the heart of the decay in order to estimate how quickly the variable decays from the initial value to the asymptote value. Determining when an inflection point or curve will occur can be problematic if individuals develop at different rates or X, M, and Y do not follow the same trajectories, but there is no requirement that the timing schema for each variable or each person must be the same.

Type of Longitudinal Effect

A third consideration when determining the measurement timing schema for a mediation model is the type of longitudinal effects that are theorized to occur. In cross-sectional data, each variable is measured only once at the same time point, which means that only a single effect between the two variables can be estimated. In longitudinal data, each variable is measured at multiple time points, allowing for a variety of different longitudinal effects to be present. The simplest longitudinal effect that can be estimated is a lag-independent constant effect. If the effect between two variables is a lag-independent constant, then the effect between the two variables is the same regardless of the elapsed time between the measurements. Consider X, M, and Y, each measured at the same four equally spaced points in time (i.e., $X_1 - X_4$, $M_1 - M_4$, and $Y_1 - Y_4$). If the effect of X on M is a lag-independent constant, then the effect of X_1 on M_2 would be the same as the effect of X_1 on M_3 or of X_3 on M_4.

A more realistic type of constant longitudinal effect for developmental theories is the lag-dependent constant effect. In a lag-dependent constant effect, the relationship between two variables is constant across time, but only for a specific elapsed time between the two measurements of the variables. When the elapsed time between the measurements of the two variables changes, then the magnitude, and possibly the sign, of the effect changes as well. Using the example of X, M, and Y measured at four equally spaced time points, if the effect of X on Y is a lag-dependent constant, then the effect of X on Y would be the same, regardless of which pair of measurements was considered, provided the elapsed time between the measurements was the same. Hence, the effect of X_1 on Y_2 and the effect of X_2 on Y_3 would be equal because the same amount of time elapsed between the measurements of X and Y. The effect of X_1 on Y_3 and the effect of X_2 on Y_4 would also be equal. However, the effect of X_1 on Y_2 would not be equal to the effect of X_1 on Y_3 because different amounts of time elapsed between the two sets of measurements. In most cases, as the elapsed time between measurements increases, the effect between the two variables decreases in magnitude, but it may increase.

In an extinguishing or diminishing effect, the magnitude of the effect between two variables decreases as a function of time. For example, the effect of M_1 on Y_2 is larger in magnitude than the effect of M_3 on Y_4. In an augmenting or intensifying effect, the magnitude of the effect between two variables increases as a function of time. For example, the effect of M_1 on Y_2 is smaller in magnitude than the effect of M_3 on Y_4. Neither the diminishing nor the augmenting effects are dependent on the elapsed time between measurements, only the time that has passed since the first measurement of the variables. Related to an augmented effect is a time-delayed effect in which a set amount of time must pass before the effect can be measured. For example, if the effect of X on M did not occur until between the third and fourth measurements, then the effect of X_3 on M_4 would represent the time-delayed effect of X on M, while the effect of X_1 on M_2 and of X_2 on M_3 would both be equal to zero.

Another type of longitudinal effect is a cumulative, or overall, effect. In a cumulative effect, not only the direct effect of one variable measured at a specific time on another variable measured at a specific later time must be considered but also the impact of the first variable on the second variable through all intermediated time points and variables. For example, in order to estimate the cumulative effect of X_1 on Y_4, a researcher cannot examine only the direct relationship between X_1 and Y_4 but must also take into account the indirect effect X_1 has on Y_4 through M_1–M_4 and Y_1–Y_3. Models in which a single measurement of a variable has direct effects on multiple measurements of another variable are called distributed lag models. Distributed lag models are frequently used in developmental research when a variable does not change across time but is expected to have a direct effect at every future measurement of the other variable, such as when X represents assignment to a treatment group or a control group.

Developmental Applications

Basic Regression Model

The simplest mediation model for longitudinal data would be to measure X only at the first time point, M only at the second time point, and Y only at a third time point in order to take into account temporal precedence. Equations 18.1–18.3 would then be fit to the data, and one of the product-of-coefficients tests described earlier could be used to estimate the mediated effect and test for significance. If a half-longitudinal design was used in which each variable was measured only once but the variables were measured only at two different occasions, then two of the variables must be measured at the same time point, necessitating a decision based on the underlying theory as to which two variables in the model should be measured at the same time, resulting in a potentially biased estimate of that effect. The basic regression mediation model is useful if there is no clustering present in the data and each of the variables is measured only once or additional measurements are ignored, which is not recommended.

ANCOVA and Change Score Models

Although measuring *X, M,* and *Y* once each at three different time points does address the temporal precedence assumption, this design does not control for values of these variables at previous time points. Therefore, a more practical design would be to measure all three variables at each time point. In equations 18.1–18.3, the previous measurement of the outcome variable could then be included as a predictor to create an analysis of covariance (ANCOVA) model. If a half-longitudinal design was used, a theory-based decision would need to be made as to which effect would have to be instantaneous. An alternative to the ANCOVA model for mediation is a difference or change score model (see London & Wright, Chapter 17, this volume). Change scores are computed by subtracting an individual's score on a variable at one time point from the individual's score on the same variable at the next time point. Mediation can be examined for change scores by substituting change scores for the corresponding variables in equations 18.1–18.3. ANCOVA and change score mediation models are useful if each variable is measured twice and is expected to have an effect on itself at a future time point or if the change between the two measurement occasions is of interest, provided no clustering is present in the data.

Autoregressive Models

ANCOVA models for mediation that include a previous measurement of the dependent variable as a predictor in equations 18.1–18.3 are a form of autoregressive mediation model because they include the effect of a variable on itself at a later time point. However, if *X, M,* and *Y* have all been measured at three different time points, then the ANCOVA model uses only five of the nine data points collected. Autoregressive models, as illustrated in Figure 18.2, use all of the available data and allow a researcher to investigate the stability, stationarity, and equilibrium of the variables in the model as described by Cole and Maxwell (2003). In addition, autoregressive models allow the researcher to investigate specific mediated effects (e.g., a_1b_2) for significance and to compare these specific effects with other specific effects (e.g., a_2b_3). The overall mediated effect may also be tested for significance. The overall mediated effect represents the effect of the first measurement of *X* on the last measurement of *Y* (i.e., the effect of X_1 on Y_4) and is equal to the sum of every indirect path between these two variables, including the autoregressive paths. In some cases, the overall mediated effect may be more interesting than specific mediated effects because, as noted by Cole and Maxwell, the overall mediated effect is an estimate of the extent to which *M* mediates the relationship between *X* and *Y* across the observed time period.

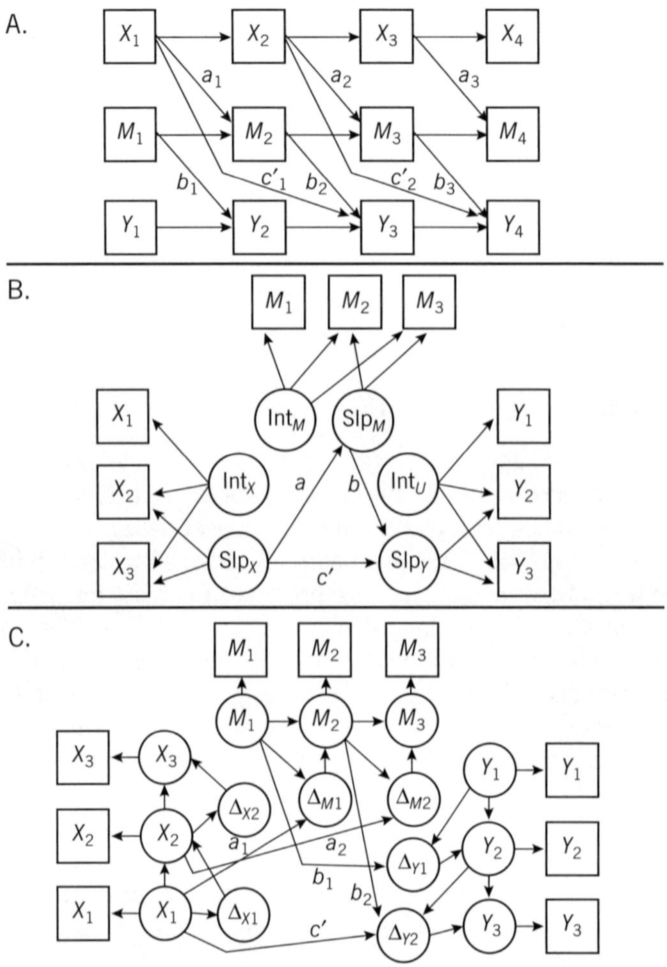

FIGURE 18.2. (A) An autoregressive mediation model. (B) A latent growth curve mediation model. (C) A latent change score mediation model. Disturbances have been removed in order to improve readability.

Several issues need to be considered when fitting an autoregressive mediation model, as described by MacKinnon (2008). The first issue is whether to keep variables within the same measurement wave (e.g., X_1, M_1, and Y_1) uncorrelated; to allow these variables to correlate, which requires the use of structural equation modeling (SEM) software; or to include contemporaneous causal effects between these variables. MacKinnon suggests that there are circumstances in which contemporaneous effects should be included but that these should be based on theory and not solely on a desire to improve model fit. The second issue is how different effects should be distributed across time. For instance, in the autoregressive model in Figure 18.2, should X also have a direct effect on Y at the next time point (e.g., X_1 on Y_2)? The distribution of the effects is a central issue in all longitudinal mediation models and must be based on the underlying theory being tested, as well as consideration of the elapsed time between measurements. A third issue is whether to include cross-lagged effects between *Y*, *M*, and *X* (e.g., Y_1 to X_2 or M_1 to X_2), which should be decided based on the underlying theory. Autoregressive mediation models are useful when each variable has been measured three or more times, when autoregressive effects are hypothesized to occur, and when the researcher is interested in the overall, as well as time specific, mediated effects. If an autoregressive mediation model is estimated using SEM software, then latent variables can also be incorporated into the model, as can clustering in the data if specific SEM software packages are used, such as Mplus.

Multilevel Models

Another category of models that can be used to test for mediation in longitudinal data are multilevel models. Krull and MacKinnon (1999, 2001; see also MacKinnon, 2008) discuss multilevel mediation models, with the primary issue being at which level the different variables are entered into the model. For instance, in a two-level model in which children are nested within classrooms, if *X*, *M*, and *Y* are all child variables, then *a* and *b* are level 1 effects, and if *X* and *M* are classroom variables, then *a* and *b* are level 2 effects. However, if *Y* and *M* are child variables and *X* is a classroom variable, then *a* is a level 2 effect and *b* is a level 1 effect. These models become more complex as the number of levels increases. Another level of complexity is added if either *a*, *b*, or both are allowed to be random, rather than fixed, effects. Preacher, Zyphur, and Zhang (2010) present a general framework for testing multilevel mediation models using SEM that allows the outcome variable to be at level 2. Multilevel mediation models are useful if there is clustering in the data and when the individual effects that make up the mediated effect are hypothesized to occur at different levels of the model.

Growth Curve Models

If *M* or *Y* has been measured three or more times, then multilevel models may also be used to fit a growth curve mediation model. In a multilevel growth model, level 1 represents repeated measures nested within an individual and time is a level 1 predictor. Rather than investigate the effect of one variable on another variable at a specific time point, growth models examine the effect a variable has on the change in the other variable across time. In mediation, this means that two models must be fit. The first model investigates the effect of *X* on the growth of *M* across time, where *X* is entered at level 1 if it is a time-varying variable such as depression and at level 2 if it is a time-invariant variable such as gender. The second model investigates the effect of *M* on the growth in *Y*, partialing out the effect of *X*, again selecting the correct level at which to include *M* and *X* depending on the nature of the variables.

A latent growth curve (LGC; see Grimm & Ram, Chapter 24, this volume) model for mediation was developed by Cheong, MacKinnon, and Khoo (2003). In an LGC mediation model, the intercept and slope for *X*, *M*, and *Y* are modeled as latent variables, called latent growth parameters, and the causal effects occur between these latent growth parameters. As illustrated in the LGC mediation model in Figure 18.2, a change in the linear slope of *X* across time causes a change in the linear slope of *M* across time, which in turn causes a change in the linear slope of *Y* across time. Additional causal paths can be added to LGC mediation models, including paths between intercepts and from intercepts to slopes, based on the underlying theory (MacKinnon, 2008). Additionally, researchers can specify curvilinear or nonlinear trajectories across time for *X, M,* and *Y* depending on the underlying theory (see Blozis, Chapter 26, this volume). Fritz (2007) developed an LGC mediation model in which both *M* and *Y* decayed exponentially across time.

If *X, M,* and *Y* are all measured on the same occasions, then the LGC model in Figure 18.2 is called a parallel process model because all three processes—that is, the change across time in *X, M,* and *Y*—are occurring during the same time period. The parallel process model does not meet the assumption of temporal precedence, making a sequential process model in which each process in the causal chain is measured after the preceding process more desirable but harder to estimate given the increased time frame over which *X, M,* and *Y* need to be measured. LGC mediation models are useful when a researcher hypothesizes that, rather than *X* affecting *M* at a specific time point that in turn affects *Y* at a specific time point, the change in *X* across time affects the change in *M* across time, which affects the change in *Y* across time.

Latent Change Score Models

A latent variable version of the change score mediation model has also been developed by MacKinnon (2008), based on work by McArdle (2001). In a latent change score (LCS) model, the change scores are latent variables that represent the error-free difference between the scores at two measurement occasions (Ferrer & McArdle, 2010). Several variations of LCS mediation models have been proposed, including a model in which the latent measurement of each variable affects the LCS between the same measurement occasion and the next measurement of the next variable in the mediation model, illustrated in Figure 18.2. LCS mediation models have not been widely utilized, but Selig and Preacher (2009) present an example in which LCS, LGC, and autoregressive mediation models are fitted to developmental data. LCS mediation models are useful when the variables have been measured three or more times and the researcher hypothesizes that the level of one variable at a specific time point or the change in that variable between two specific time points affects the change in another variable between two other specific time points. These models can also be extended to look at the effect of a variable on the change in the change (i.e., second-order change) of another variable.

Other Models

Several other longitudinal models could also be used to test for mediation in longitudinal data, although limited work has been done to date to test mediation with these models. One type is the autoregressive latent trajectory (ALT) model which combines an autoregressive model with an LGC model (Curran & Bollen, 2001). A second type is the survival model, which predicts time until an event (Singer & Willett, 2003; see also Keiley, Kirkland, Zaremba, & Jackson, Chapter 22, this volume). A third type is the latent transition model, which models how individuals change between latent classes (Collins & Lanza, 2010). Fritz (2007) examined the type of model used to test mediation in his literature survey, shown in Table 18.2. The most commonly used models were the SEM models with autoregressive effects (n = 17, 22.67% of the studies), then the SEM models without autoregressive effects (n = 13, 17.33% of the studies), and regression models without prior measurements as covariates (n = 13, 17.33% of the studies).

TABLE 18.2. Frequencies of the Longitudinal Mediation Models Used by Researchers for Articles Appearing in American Psychological Association Journals Published between 2000 and 2006

Method used	Frequency	Percentage of studies
Latent growth curve	6	8.00
Non-latent growth curve	4	5.33
Latent difference score	1	1.33
Non-latent difference score	9	12.00
SEM: Autoregressive	17	22.67
SEM: Nonautoregressive	13	17.33
Regression across waves (no ANCOVA)	13	17.33
ANCOVA	9	12.00
Cross-sectional analyses only	3	4.00

Note. Frequencies sum to 75 because two of the articles had two independent longitudinal data sets which models were tested for and four of the articles tested two non-nested models.

Illustration

In order to illustrate several of the concepts provided in the current chapter, we now present an empirical example using data from the Athletes Training and Learning to Avoid Steroids (ATLAS) program, which is a prevention program designed to decrease intentions to use anabolic steroids among high school football players (for more information, see MacKinnon et al., 2001). The data for the empirical example come from the first cohort of the ATLAS study ($N = 1{,}506$) and consist of four observations that were measured after completion of the ATLAS program. The mediated effect of interest is the effect of the ATLAS program on intentions to use steroids through the mediator perception of peers as an information source about steroids.

Although perception of peers and intentions to use steroids were originally modeled with linear trajectories (MacKinnon et al., 2001), theory suggests that a more likely trajectory across time is exponential decay, illustrated in equation 18.6:

$$Y(t) = \omega_0 + (\omega_1 - \omega_0) * Exp[\omega_2 * t] \qquad \textbf{(18.6)}$$

where ω_0, ω_1, and ω_2 are estimates of the asymptote value, initial value, and rate of decay of Y. Exponential decay was theorized because, if the program had an effect on these variables, it is likely that the effect would decay over time, but hopefully not back to the pretreatment levels. In order to test for mediation under the constraint that the trajectories of the mediator and outcome variables decay exponentially as a function of time, a nonlinear multilevel mediation growth model (Fritz, 2007) was fit to the data using SAS PROC NLMIXED. Two models were estimated, the first measuring the effect of group assignment, X (0 = control group, 1 = ATLAS group), on perceptions of peers, M, shown in equation 18.7, and the second measuring the effect of group assignment and perceptions of peers on intentions to use steroids, Y, shown in equation 18.8.

Model for M on X:

Level 1:

$$m_{it} = \omega_{m0i} + (\omega_{m1i} - \omega_{m0i}) * Exp[\omega_{m2i} * t] + e_{it}$$

Level 2:

$$\omega_{m0i} = \pi_{m00} + a_0 x_i + u_{m0i}$$
$$\omega_{m1i} = \pi_{m10} + a_1 x_i + u_{m1i} \qquad \textbf{(18.7)}$$
$$\omega_{m2i} = \pi_{m20} + a_2 x_i + u_{m2i}$$

where π_{m00}, π_{m10}, and π_{m20}, are estimates of the asymptote value, initial value, and rate of decay of M for the control group and a_0, a_1, and a_2 are the differences between the two groups such that $\pi_{m00} + a_0$, $\pi_{m10} + a_1$, and $\pi_{m20} + a_2$ are the asymptote value, initial value, and rate of decay of M for the ATLAS group, e_{it} is random error, and u_{m0i}, u_{m1i}, and u_{m2i} are random effects.

Model for Y on M and X:

Level 1:

$$y_{it} = \omega_{y0i} + (\omega_{y1i} - \omega_{y0i}) * Exp[\omega_{y2i} * t_t] + b_i m_{it} + e_{it},$$

Level 2:

$$\omega_{y0i} = \pi_{y00} + c'_0 x_i + u_{y0i} \qquad \textbf{(18.8)}$$
$$\omega_{y1i} = \pi_{y10} + c'_1 x_i + u_{y1i}$$
$$\omega_{y2i} = \pi_{y20} + c'_2 x_i + u_{y2i}$$
$$b_i = \pi_{y30}$$

where π_{y00}, π_{y10}, and π_{y20} are estimates of the asymptote value, initial value, and rate of decay of Y for the control, partialing out the effect of M, c'_0, c'_1, and c'_2 are the differences between the two groups in X partialing out the effect of M, such that $\pi_{y00} + a_0$, $\pi_{y10} + a_1$, and $\pi_{y20} + a_2$ are the asymptote value, initial value, and rate of decay of Y for the ATLAS group, b is the effect of M partialing out the effect of time (i.e., the natural exponential decay of Y) and the effect of X on the exponential decay of Y, e_{it} is random error, and u_{y0i}, u_{y1i}, and u_{y2i} are random effects.

In the model, group assignment had an effect on all three of the exponential decay parameters of the mediator, as shown in Table 18.3, such that individuals in the ATLAS program had higher perceptions of peers as sources of information at the initial measurement, as well as at the asymptote, and had a slower rate of decay than the control group. In addition, group assignment had an effect on all of the exponential decay parameters for the outcome, such that individuals in the ATLAS program had lower intentions to use steroids at the first measurement than the control group, slightly higher intentions at asymptote, and a faster rate of change, all partialing out the effect of the mediator. The $\hat{b}$ coefficient was significant as well, indicating that higher perception of peers as an information source at

TABLE 18.3. Parameter Estimates from the Empirical Example

Parameter	Estimate	Standard error	PRODCLIN (95% confidence intervals)
a_0	0.586	0.121	[–0.0708, –0.0294]
a_1	0.920	0.053	[–0.0899, –0.0671]
a_2	–0.017	0.005	[0.0006, 0.0023]
b	–0.085	0.004	
c'_0	1.072	0.065	
c'_1	–0.150	0.019	
c'_2	1.987	0.004	

Note. Each confidence interval was computed using PRODCLIN, the estimate of the b path, and the corresponding a path. All parameter estimates were significant at $p < .001$.

any time led to lower intentions to use steroids at that time. Confidence intervals computed using PRODCLIN are also presented in Table 18.3. The results then support the hypothesis that the ATLAS program affected intentions to use steroids through the mediating variable perception of peers as an information source.

Future Directions

Mediation models are widely used in the study of development to understand mechanisms of change across time, but researchers are in danger of focusing more on the significance of their chosen statistical model than on the actual longitudinal causal process that is being studied. Kenny, Kashy, and Bolger (1998) comment that in mediation "we must learn to model a process not just to analyze data" (p. 263). In order to model the process, rather than just analyze the data, Kraemer and colleagues (2000) recommend placing an increased emphasis on the specific developmental process being studied, the time scale of the process, the reliability of the measurements, and clarity in terminology. In practical terms, this means focusing on several key questions when planning a longitudinal mediation study. First, how exactly does the researcher wish to define the three variables in the mediation model, and what are the most reliable measures of these variables? Second, how is each of the three variables in the mediation model expected to change across time? Third, what types of longitudinal effects are expected to occur between each pair of variables in the mediation model? Fourth, in response to the second and third questions, how many repeated measurements are necessary for each variable, and what is the optimal spacing of these measurements to model the mediated effect? Finally, given the answers to these questions, which longitudinal mediation model best tests whether the hypothesized effects occurred or not? Methodologists continue to improve tests of mediation and create new mediation models to describe change. However, these new mediation models need a firm theoretical underpinning in order to be useful, which must come from developmental researchers focusing on the form and timing of the longitudinal processes that they study.

Acknowledgment

This research was supported by National Institute on Drug Abuse Grant No. DA009757.

References

Baron, R. M., & Kenny, D. A. (1986). The moderator–mediation variable distinction in social psychological research: Conceptual, strategic, and statistical considerations. *Journal of Personality and Social Psychology, 51*, 1173–1182.

Boker, S. M., & Nesselroade, J. R. (2002). A method for modeling the intrinsic dynamics of intraindividual variability: Recovering the parameters of simulated oscillators in multiwave panel data. *Multivariate Behavioral Research, 37*, 127–160.

Bollen, K. A., & Stine, R. A. (1990). Direct and indirect effects: Classical and bootstrap estimates of variability. *Sociological Methodology, 20*, 115–140.

Cheong, J., MacKinnon, D. P., & Khoo, S.-T. (2003). Investigation of mediational processes using parallel process latent growth curve modeling. *Structural Equation Modeling, 10*, 238–262.

Cohen, J., Cohen, P., West, S. G., & Aiken, L. S. (2003). *Applied multiple regression/correlation analysis for the behavioral sciences* (3rd ed.). Mahwah, NJ: Erlbaum.

Cole, D. A., & Maxwell, S. E. (2003). Testing mediational models with longitudinal data: Questions and tips in the use of structural equation modeling. *Journal of Abnormal Psychology, 112*, 558–577.

Collins, L. M., & Graham, J. W. (2002). The effect of the timing and spacing of observations in longitudinal studies of tobacco and other drug use: Temporal design considerations. *Drug and Alcohol Dependence, 68*, S85–S96.

Collins, L. M., & Lanza, S. T. (2010). *Latent class and latent transition analysis for applications in the social, behavioral, and health sciences*. Hoboken, NJ: Wiley Interscience.

Curran, P. J., & Bollen, K. A. (2001). The best of both worlds: Combining autoregressive and latent curve models. In L. M. Collins & A. G. Sayer (Eds.), *New methods for the analysis of change* (pp. 105–135). Washington, DC: American Psychological Association.

Efron, B., & Tibshirani, R. J. (1993). *An introduction to the bootstrap*. Boca Raton, FL: Chapman & Hall/CRC.

Ferrer, E., & McArdle, J. J. (2010). Longitudinal modeling of developmental changes in psychological research. *Current Directions in Psychological Science, 19*, 149–154.

Fritz, M. S. (2007). *An exponential decay model for mediation*. Unpublished doctoral dissertation, Arizona State University, Tempe.

Fritz, M. S., & MacKinnon, D. P. (2007). Required sample size to detect the mediated effect. *Psychological Science, 18*, 233–239.

Fritz, M. S., Taylor, A. B., & MacKinnon, D. P. (2010, June). *When does the bias-corrected bootstrap test of mediation produce elevated Type I error rates and why?* Poster presented at the annual meeting of the Society for Prevention Research, Denver, CO.

Gollob, H. F., & Reichardt, C. S. (1987). Taking account of time lags in causal models. *Child Development, 58*, 80–92.

Gollob, H. F., & Reichardt, C. S. (1991). Interpreting and estimating indirect effects assuming time lags really matter. In L. M. Collins & J. L. Horn (Eds.), *Best methods for the analysis of change* (pp. 243–263). Washington, DC: American Psychological Association.

Hertzog, C., & Nesselroade, J. R. (1987). Beyond autoregressive models: Some implications of the trait–state distinction for the structural modeling of developmental change. *Child Development, 58*, 93–109.

Hoyle, R. H., & Kenny, D. A. (1999). Sample size, reliability, and tests of statistical mediation. In R.

H. Hoyle (Ed.), *Statistical strategies for small sample research* (pp. 195–222). Thousand Oaks, CA: Sage.

James, L. R., Mulaik, S. A., & Brett, J. M. (1982). *Causal analysis: Assumptions, models, and data.* Beverly Hills, CA: Sage.

Kenny, D. A. (1979). *Correlation and causality*. New York: Wiley.

Kenny, D. A., Kashy, D. A., & Bolger, N. (1998). Data analysis in social psychology. In D. T. Gilbert, S. T. Fiske, & G. Lindzey (Eds.), *The handbook of social psychology* (4th ed., Vol. 1, pp. 233–265). New York: Oxford University Press.

Kim, J., & Cicchetti, D. (2004). A longitudinal study of child maltreatment, mother–child relationship quality, and maladjustment: The role of self-esteem and social competence. *Journal of Abnormal Child Psychology, 32*, 341–354.

Kraemer, H. C., Wilson, G. T., Fairburn, C. G., & Agras, W. S. (2002). Mediators and moderators of treatment effects in randomized clinical trials. *Archives of General Psychiatry, 59*, 877–883.

Kraemer, H. C., Yesavage, J. A., Taylor, J. L., & Kupfer, D. (2000). How can we learn about developmental processes from cross-sectional studies, or can we? *American Journal of Psychiatry, 157*, 163–171.

Krull, J. L., & MacKinnon, D. P. (1999). Multilevel mediation modeling in group-based intervention studies. *Evaluation Review, 23*, 418–444.

Krull, J. L., & MacKinnon, D. P. (2001). Multilevel modeling of individual and group level mediated effects. *Multivariate Behavioral Research, 36*, 249–277.

MacKinnon, D. P. (2008). *Introduction to statistical mediation analysis*. New York: Erlbaum.

MacKinnon, D. P., Fritz, M. S., Williams, J., & Lockwood, C. M. (2007). Distribution of the product confidence limits for the indirect effect: Program PRODCLIN. *Behavior Research Methods, 39*, 384–389.

MacKinnon, D. P., Goldberg, L., Clarke, G. N., Elliot, D. L., Cheong, J., Lapin, A., et al. (2001). Mediating mechanisms in a program to reduce intentions to use anabolic steroids and improve exercise self-efficacy and dietary behavior. *Prevention Science, 2*, 15–28.

MacKinnon, D. P., Lockwood, C. M., Hoffman, J. M., West, S. G., & Sheets, V. (2002). A comparison of methods to test mediation and other intervening variable effects. *Psychological Methods, 7*, 83–104.

MacKinnon, D. P., Lockwood, C. M., & Williams, J. (2004). Confidence limits for the indirect effect: Distribution of the product and resampling methods. *Multivariate Behavioral Research, 39*, 99–128.

Maxwell, S. E., & Cole, D. A. (2007). Bias in cross-sectional analyses of longitudinal mediation. *Psychological Methods, 12*, 23–44.

McArdle, J. J. (2001). A latent difference score approach to longitudinal dynamic structural analysis. In R. Cudeck, M. du Toit, & D. Sorbom (Eds.), *Structural equation modeling: Present and future* (pp. 341–380). Lincolnwood, IL: Scientific Software International.

Muthén, L. K., & Muthén, B. O. (2010). Mplus (Version 6.1) [Computer software]. Los Angeles: Authors.

Preacher, K. J., Zyphur, M. J., & Zhang, Z. (2010). A general multilevel SEM framework for assessing multilevel mediation. *Psychological Methods, 15*, 209–233.

R Core Development Team. (2010). R (Version 2.6.1) [Computer software]. Vienna, Austria: R Foundation for Statistical Computing.

Ranby, K. W., Aiken, L. S., MacKinnon, D. P., Elliot, D. L., Moe, E. L., McGinnis, W., et al. (2009). A mediation analysis of the ATHENA intervention for female athletes: Prevention of athletic-enhancing substance use and unhealthy weight loss behaviors. *Journal of Pediatric Psychology, 34*, 1069–1083.

Salthouse, T. A. (1996). General and specific speed mediation of adult age differences in memory. *Journal of Gerontology: Psychological Sciences, 51B*, P30–P42.

Selig, J. P., & Preacher, K. J. (2009). Mediation models for longitudinal data in developmental research. *Research in Human Development, 6*, 144–164.

Shrout, P. E., & Bolger, N. (2002). Mediation in experimental and nonexperimental studies: New procedures and recommendations. *Psychological Methods, 7*, 422–445.

Singer, J. D., & Willett, J. B. (2003). *Applied longitudinal data analysis: Modeling change and even occurrence*. Oxford, UK: Oxford University Press.

Sliwinski, M. J., & Hofer, S. M. (1999). How strong is the evidence for mediational hypotheses of age-related memory loss? *Gerontology, 45*, 351–354.

Sobel, M. E. (1982). Asymptotic confidence intervals for indirect effects in structural equation models. *Sociological Methodology, 13*, 290–312.

Springer, M. D., & Thompson, W. E. (1966). The distribution of products of independent random variables. *SIAM Journal on Applied Mathematics, 14*, 511–526.

Tofighi, D., & MacKinnon, D. P. (2010, June). *Distribution of the product of two normal random variables in R: Monte Carlo and QUADPACK*. Poster presented at the annual meeting of the Society for Prevention Research, Denver, CO.

Venter, A., & Maxwell, S. E. (1999). Maximizing power in randomized designs when *N* is small. In R. H. Hoyle (Ed.), *Statistical strategies for small sample research* (pp. 31–58). Thousand Oaks, CA: Sage.

PART IV

Intraindividual Longitudinal Analysis

CHAPTER 19

Foundational Issues in Intraindividual Longitudinal Analysis

MICHAEL J. ROVINE
LAWRENCE L. LO

Central Issues

Single-subject and person-specific approaches to the modeling of developmental processes are becoming more central in the description of complex and time-varying processes. These methods, which have a relatively long tradition in psychology (Kratochwill, 1978), have been labeled *idiographic* (Lamiell, 1981; Zevon & Tellegen, 1982) and have been used to describe intraindividual patterns of change (Nesselroade & Ford, 1985). The more general behavioral laws described through cross-sectional studies of a sample of individuals have been labeled *nomothetic*. Most researchers are aware of the problems inherent in interpreting results from cross-sectional data (Baltes, Reese, & Nesselroade, 1977). Many, however, are much less aware of the interpretive problems that arise when the data collected represent a few repeated occasions on a sample of individuals. Molenaar (2004) has described many of these problems and has indicated how these difficulties can often be resolved only with time series data. Although such data have long been collected in a number of different research areas (Jones & Nesselroade, 1990; Luborsky & Mintz, 1972), these data are often not available because of the difficulty and expense involved in collecting a large number of occasions. Fortunately, due to new technologies, time series data are becoming much easier and less expensive to collect, and methods for estimating many different models are being used more often (Walls & Schafer, 2006).

The availability of time series data (intensive data collected on each individual) through diaries, personal data assistants, and "smartphone" devices through measures of physiological characteristics (EKG, fMRI, heart rate, blood pressure, etc.); and by other means have brought time series approaches into the domain of the developmental sciences (Molenaar, 1994). Time series approaches, including Box–Jenkins type autoregressive integrated moving average (ARIMA) models (Box & Jenkins, 1970), multivariate vector autoregressive models (Luktepohl, 2005), P-technique factor models and dynamic factor models (Molenaar, 1985; Wood & Brown, 1994), and *state-space* models (Molenaar, 1994), among others, have been appearing more often in the developmental literature. Both time domain (Box & Jenkins, 1970) and frequency domain (Jenkins & Watts, 1968) approaches developed for engineering, econometric, and medical applications are now becoming important tools in the social sciences. As with the switch to any new set of methods, a certain amount of reluctance and misunderstanding exists. In this chapter we wish to discuss the following issues involved in these important approaches.

Person-Specific versus Group-Based Models

With separate models estimated for a set of individuals, it becomes possible to test whether a single model adequately describes the group. When only a single model is estimated based on the entire group's data, this becomes impossible. The assumption of such group-based models is that there is a common model that holds equally well for each member of the sample. By comparing separately estimated individual models with the group model using time series data, we can specifically test whether the individuals can be adequately described by a group model.

Because there is very often a fine line between a group-oriented approach and a person-specific approach, we review a number of different currently popular methods and describe the degree to which they are person specific. Because many models that generate measures of individual differences are based on parameters estimated on the group, we distinguish between these models (group based) and models in which parameters are estimated separately for each individual (person specific).

Time Series Analogues of Group-Based Models

Many different models for individual differences exist, some of which are person specific based on time series data and some of which provide individual descriptive statistics that are nevertheless based on group models. Two important modeling approaches that fall into the latter category are the lagged regression and path analytic approaches and the multilevel growth curve model and repeated-measures analysis of variance (ANOVA) approaches. Although these models generate descriptive statistics that can be used to describe individual differences, they are really group models that allow post hoc predictions of these individual differences. As a result, they provide limited person-specific information.

Single-Subject Models Based on Cattell's P-Technique Notion

Because the tradition of person-specific modeling comes, in part, from the assessment of interindividual differences in intraindividual change, we describe how the idea of the data box (Cattell, 1966) led to a family of approaches that come under the heading of *P-technique analysis*. By adding lagged variables to the P-technique data, we add a number of additional analytical possibilities, including longitudinal factor analysis, vector-autoregressive models, dynamic factor models, and state-space models.

What Constitutes a Sample

An important difference between group-based and person-specific analyses is the idea of a sample. In a group-based analysis, the parameters of the model are often used to generalize to a population of interest. If the sample is representative of the population, one can say something important about the population. In a person-specific analysis, the generalization is related to the individual model. Because time is essentially taking the place of number of participants, the generalization is made across the time dimension. Most typically, different models will arise for different individuals. Subgroups of individuals can be constructed by pooling those individuals whose models are identical. Nesselroade and Molenaar (1999) described methods for pooling (as opposed to sampling). As a simple example, P-technique factor analysis requires a multivariate time series collected on an individual. For more than one individual, the multiple P-technique analyses are akin to multiple group structural equation models (SEM). By constraining solutions equal across individuals we can test whether the same model holds for all.

Recursive Estimation and the State-Space Model

Estimation methods for many of these models fall into two general categories: complete data procedures that estimate parameters once all of the data have been collected and recursive estimation procedures in which parameters of the model are updated sequentially as each new observation appears. Once all of the data have arrived, the recursive and complete data estimates of the same statistical model typically result in the same parameter estimates. However, for certain types of problems, recursive estimation simplifies the computations. For problems in which the model changes as the data arrive, recursive procedures allow certain time-varying characteristics, including the possibility of estimating time-varying parameters in ways that would be difficult using the complete data approach. A very general model for describing recursive estimations is the *state-space model* (Harvey, 1989). We show a basic form of this model and suggest how it can be used to approach the solution to certain estimation problems.

Recursive estimation arguably began with Gauss and then disappeared until being rediscovered by Plackett (1950). It was generalized by Kalman as the famous *Kalman filter* (Kalman, 1960; Kalman & Bucy, 1961), which represented a general solution for estimating the state in the state-space model formulation. The filtering approach not only allowed the opportunity for estimation of time series parameters but also introduced the possibility of control; namely, having targets for certain variables in the model and changing other variables in the model to move toward the optimal target. Although the derivation of the filter by Kalman is based on a somewhat difficult area of mathematics, the filter can be described using regression concepts. To give a flavor of the recursive method of estimation, we show how regression models can be reconstituted in recursive form. The resulting regression equations have the form of a filter. Using the pieces that compose these equations, we can indicate the relationship between the recursive regression estimator and the Kalman filter.

P-Technique and Dynamic Factor Models

The Data Box

Cattell (1966) presented a schematic for describing data from a multivariate study. As shown in Figure 19.1, the data box has variables, individuals, and occasions, creating a three-dimensional structure. Each two-dimensional slice of the box represents a way of constructing an association matrix. The vertical axis indicates the dimension across persons. The horizontal planes contain axes that identify the dimension across variables (upper left to lower right) and the dimension across occasions (lower left to upper right). Each two-dimensional slice provides an association matrix for one dimension that pools across the other dimensional component. Cattell gave each two-dimensional facet a letter name. For example, the individuals-by-variables facet (pooled across individuals) was called *R*, and the factor analysis resulting from analyzing the *variable-by-variable* association matrix was call *R-technique*; this is the most common form of factor analysis. Although all facets were given names, some were more successful in generating interpretable research results than others. Important for studies of intraindividual differences was the *P* facet, which created an *occasion-by-variable* rectangular data set for a single subject (pooled across occasions). Factor analysis of this type of data set was referred to as *P-technique*. The R-technique (interindividual–vertical) and P-technique (intraindividual–horizontal) slices are represented in Figure 19.1.

P-Technique Factor Analysis

Research in which P-technique factor analysis has been used includes studies of stepchildren's emotional experiences (Corneal & Nesselroade, 1994), mood change (Bath, Daly, &

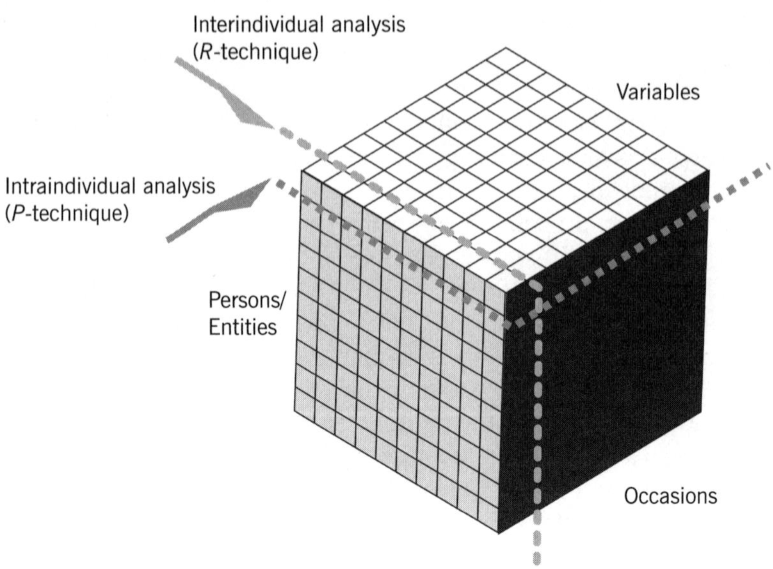

FIGURE 19.1. The data box, depicting the dimensions of persons, variables, and occasions.

Nesselroade, 1976), and attachment (Mitteness & Nesselroade, 1987). In P-technique factor analysis, occasions take the place of individuals in ordinary R-technique factor analysis. Aside from that, the analytic approach is the same. Although others had proposed similar approaches (e.g., Stone, 1947), factor analysis of multivariate time series became more generally accepted after Cattell's presentation.

The P-technique model is

$$y_t = \Lambda\eta_t + \varepsilon_t \qquad \textbf{(19.1)}$$

where y_t is a vector of observed variables at time t, Λ is a matrix of factor loading, η_t is a vector of latent variables at time t, and ε_t is a vector of residuals. The data set for the *P-technique* analysis is the horizontal rectangular data set highlighted in Figure 19.1. Pooling across occasions results in a *variable-by-variable* association matrix.

With multiple participants, we can estimate separate P-technique solutions. We can then compare the solutions to see whether the same model tends to describe different individuals. If that is the case, the separate data sets could be pooled to calculate a single group analysis. Most typically, that is not the case. As an example, in Table 19.1 we show two different P-technique factor analyses from a study of mood in which the Positive and Negative Affect Schedule (PANAS) was administered to stepchildren after an interaction with their stepparents (Rovine, Molenaar, & Corneal, 1999). The factor patterns show interesting and idiosyncratic patterns. Notice that factors include combinations of positive and negative items and that the factor correlations suggest that these factors are relatively independent. This contradicts the typical group results for the PANAS, which tends to produce positive and negative subscales. The interesting individual differences tend to be averaged out of such pooled analyses. In the event that certain subsets of the sample have structurally identical models, methods are available for pooling the results of the individual P-technique analyses (Nesselroade & Molenaar, 1999).

Although P-technique was relatively accepted as an important method for describing multivariate time series, a number of criticisms emerged (Anderson, 1963; Holtzman, 1962). Most notably, no lagged values of the variables appear in the data matrix. A lagged value or lagged relationship is the relationship between variables at two time points, where the degree of lag indicates the gap in time; for example, a lag 2 is the relationship between a variable at time t and the variable at time $t - 2$. For example, if we are measuring mood and satisfaction on a daily basis and today's mood predicts tomorrow's satisfaction, that is a lag 1 relationship. If today's mood predicts satisfaction 2 days later, that is a lag 2 relationship. If today's mood predicts today's satisfaction, that is a simultaneous relationship. P-technique models only simultaneous relationships among the data. Without the lags the timing of the components may be lost. Effects resulting from this omission were first presented by Anderson (1963). More recently Molenaar and Nesselroade (2009) demonstrated the relative robustness of the P-technique solution even in the presence of lagged relationships.

Going beyond P-technique, Molenaar (1985) presented a very general model, the dynamic factor model, that properly addressed the question of lags and the order of the lagged relationships. We can add lags to the P-technique data set by adding an offset version of each variable as an additional variable. In Figure 19.2 we add the first-order lags for each variable in the data set.

TABLE 19.1. P-Technique Factor Analyses for Stepsons A and B

Factor	Stepson A					Stepson B		
loadings	Interest	Anger	Anxiety	Affection	Closeness	Anger	Interest	Strength
Interest	.64						.77	
Excited	.67						.81	
Enthused	.72	–.38					.81	
Inspired	.42	–.36					.56	
Alert	.66		.34				.77	
Attentive	.74		.33				.58	
Satisfied	.62	–.59				–.58	.61	
Proud	.66	–.39				–.60		.65
Distressed		.85				.96		.92
Upset		.87		–.23			.92	
Strong	.51	.30	.23					.56
Hostile		.91		.29		.79		
Irritable		.88		–.32		.92		
Discouraged		.74	.33	.24		.82		
Accepting	.46	–.63					.65	
Notwant		.97				.74		
Deterred	.51	.34		.25				.75
Contented	.32	–.46				–.55	.57	
Scared			.71			.79		
Nervous			.92			.78		
Jittery		.45	.73	.27		.81		
Afraid			.98		–.13	.79		
Humiliated		.35		–.49		.57		
Loved				.43			.69	
Active	.43			.37				.81
Liking					.62		.72	
Ashamed			.49		–.41	.82		
Close					.73		.68	

Factor intercorrelations

	Interest	Anger	Anxiety	Affect	Closeness
Interest	1.00				
Anger	.36	1.00			
Anxiety	–.06	–.08	1.00		
Affection	.13	–.03	.11	1.00	
Closeness	.37	–.36	.14	.23	1.00

	Interest	Anger	Strength
Interest	1.00		
Anger	–.10	1.00	
Strength	.42	.65	1.00

Dynamic Factor Analysis

Molenaar's (1985) dynamic factor model represents a generalization of the P-technique model. Although particular versions of this model had been previously discussed by Priestley, Subba Rao, and Tong (1973), Brillinger (1975), and others, Molenaar provided a very general method that, among other things, translated nicely to the domain of structural equation modeling.

The dynamic factor model is

$$y_t = \sum_{u=0}^{s} \Lambda_u \eta_{t-u} + \varepsilon_t \qquad \textbf{(19.2)}$$

where Λ_u contains the factor loading for lag, u. With this model the researcher can determine the degree to which latent variables and residuals are correlated over time. The P-technique model is a special case of the dynamic factor model with $s = 0$ (i.e., only a contemporaneous factor loading matrix).

Because many find the model relatively complex, we think that it is helpful to consider a path diagram of a simple dynamic factor model. This helps to show how the addition of lags adds a set of required constraints to the model. In Figure 19.2 we show a dynamic factor for five observed variables with one factor and a lag order of 1 based on Wood and Brown (1994). The model includes variables at times t and $t - 1$. The model represents the fact that at any particular occasion, the observed variables are dependent on both a "today" factor and a "yesterday" factor (Wood & Brown, 1994). To also allow the $t - 1$ observed variables to be accounted for by a previous day, we also add a $t - 2$ latent variable. Notice that the observed variables are predicted by the concurrent and previous latent variables. No regression relationship is included between the lagged latent variables. Correlations among the residuals are included for the current and previous occasion variable pairs.

Although the model looks very similar to the more standard factor model, its inclusion of lags adds some additional technical complications to the estimation of the model. An ordinary covariance matrix is not the proper input matrix. The model requires a special type of input matrix (the block Toeplitz matrix) of simultaneous and lagged covariances. A routine for properly estimating the matrix can be found in Wood and Brown (1994).

The model requires the set of constraints indicated in Figure 19.2. Because of the redundancy of the model, fit indices for the model must be calculated by hand. These and other technical problems involved in estimating the model are discussed in Wood and Brown (1994).

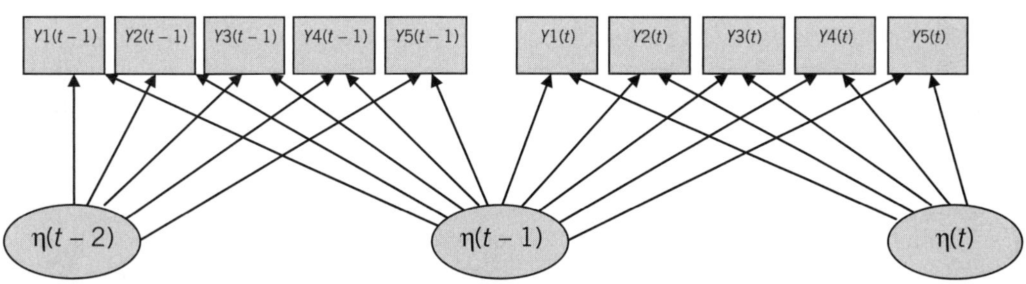

FIGURE 19.2. Dynamic factor model with lagged and concurrent factor loadings.

Molenaar, Sinclair, Rovine, Ram, and Corneal (2009) discuss situations in which the P-technique assumptions do not hold. Although the general dynamic factor model (Molenaar, 1985) would represent a proper alternative with sufficient data, that model requires a long time series to identify the proper order of the lagged relationship and to allow the computation of a stable model given the number of variables.

Person-Specific Individual Difference versus Group Models

A very subtle difference can exist between group-based models that generate statistics that describe differences in individuals and genuine person-specific models. The simplest way to make this distinction is to consider whether the parameters of a model are estimated based on the group or whether a separate model for each individual is used to generate the parameters. At the heart of the matter is what constitutes a subgroup. For the group-based models, a subgroup represents an a priori definition based on some known variable or, in the case of latent class or mixture models, a certain similarity based on group distributional characteristics. For the person-specific model, a subgroup represents a set of individuals who can be shown empirically to have identical or very similar model parameter values. Although both modeling approaches can provide useful information, the group-based model comes with one important assumption: namely, that the same model holds for all members of the sample.

The *ergodicity theorem* (Birkhoff, 1931) implies that for a result from a group-based model to properly apply to an individual, the group model has to be the appropriate model for each individual. In the absence of time series data, this is an untested assumption. Molenaar (2004) has shown dramatically how factor models derived from cross-sectional analysis on a group covariance matrix can have little to do with the models that best describe each individual. Using a data set provided by Borkenau and Ostendorf (1998), Molenaar has demonstrated the implications of violations of ergodicity for personality factors based on the Big Five; namely, for individuals, the Big Five seems to be a poor model. It is only when pooling across individuals that the five factors emerge. Rovine, Molenaar, and Corneal (1999; Molenaar, Rovine, & Corneal, 1999) showed a similar result based on time series assessments of mood, showing that the positive and negative factors of the PANAS may be an artifact of pooling.

The possible violation of the ergodicity assumption always lurks in the background in any study using either cross-sectional or short longitudinal data. Without either prior time series results validating the group model for individuals or concurrently collected time series data, this concern must at least be considered.

Other modeling approaches attempt to account for heterogeneity of intraindividual variation. Latent class growth analysis (Nagin, 1999) and growth mixture modeling (Muthén & Shedden, 1999) address group heterogeneity by extraction of subgroups that differ in structure. Although these methods allow heterogeneity, within an aggregate group they still assume homogeneity within subgroups (Sterba & Bauer, 2010). Consequently, these modeling approaches both make assumptions of *ergodicity*.

To show how the individual difference measures are generated from a group-based model, we will consider two commonly used models: the linear growth curve model (McArdle & Epstein, 1987) and the lagged regression or panel analysis model (Blalock, 2007; Little, Preacher, Selig, & Card, 2007).

A Linear Growth Curve Model

There are a number of equivalent ways to define the linear growth curve model (Bryk & Raudenbush, 1992; Goldstein, 1995; McArdle & Epstein, 1987; Rovine & Molenaar, 2005). One useful way is based on the linear mixed model (Laird & Ware, 1982). The linear mixed model can be written as

$$\vec{y}_i = X_i\vec{\beta} + Z_i\vec{\gamma}_i + \vec{\varepsilon}_i \quad \textbf{(19.3)}$$

where y_i is a vector of repeatedly measured dependent variable values; X_i is the design matrix (matrix of predictor variable values related to the fixed effects; $\vec{\beta}$ is the vector of fixed effect parameters; Z_i is the design matrix related to the random effects; $\vec{\gamma}_i$ is the vector of random effects parameters; and $\vec{\varepsilon}_i$ is the vector of residuals. Z_i, $\vec{\gamma}_i$, and $\vec{\varepsilon}_i$ can vary among individuals.

The linear growth curve model estimates a set of fixed effects parameters that define straight lines for the different groups. By including polynomial terms (powers, centered powers, or orthogonal polynomials), curves of any shape can be modeled. For two groups with four repeats, the fixed effects part of the model in matrix form becomes

$$\begin{bmatrix} y_{i1} \\ y_{i2} \\ y_{i3} \\ y_{i4} \end{bmatrix} = \begin{bmatrix} 1 & 0 & 0 & 0 \\ 1 & 1 & 0 & 0 \\ 1 & 2 & 0 & 0 \\ 1 & 3 & 0 & 0 \end{bmatrix} \begin{bmatrix} \beta_1 \\ \beta_2 \\ \beta_3 \\ \beta_4 \end{bmatrix} + \begin{bmatrix} 1 & 0 \\ 1 & 1 \\ 1 & 2 \\ 1 & 3 \end{bmatrix} \begin{bmatrix} \gamma_1 \\ \gamma_2 \\ \gamma_3 \\ \gamma_4 \end{bmatrix} + \begin{bmatrix} \varepsilon_{i1} \\ \varepsilon_{i2} \\ \varepsilon_{i3} \\ \varepsilon_{i4} \end{bmatrix} \quad \text{Group 1}$$

$$\begin{bmatrix} y_{i1} \\ y_{i2} \\ y_{i3} \\ y_{i4} \end{bmatrix} = \begin{bmatrix} 1 & 0 & 1 & 0 \\ 1 & 1 & 1 & 1 \\ 1 & 2 & 1 & 2 \\ 1 & 3 & 1 & 3 \end{bmatrix} \begin{bmatrix} \beta_1 \\ \beta_2 \\ \beta_3 \\ \beta_4 \end{bmatrix} + \begin{bmatrix} 1 & 0 \\ 1 & 1 \\ 1 & 2 \\ 1 & 3 \end{bmatrix} \begin{bmatrix} \gamma_1 \\ \gamma_2 \\ \gamma_3 \\ \gamma_4 \end{bmatrix} + \begin{bmatrix} \varepsilon_{i1} \\ \varepsilon_{i2} \\ \varepsilon_{i3} \\ \varepsilon_{i4} \end{bmatrix} \quad \text{Group 2} \quad \textbf{(19.4)}$$

where β_1 and β_2 are the respective intercept and slope for the first group and β_3 and β_4 are the respective differences in intercept and slope between the two groups. These parameters are fixed for the sample. γ_1 and γ_2 are the random effects (in this case random slopes and intercepts). These are predicted post hoc based on the group parameters. Given by Henderson (1975), the fixed and random effects are

$$\begin{bmatrix} \beta \\ u \end{bmatrix} = \begin{bmatrix} (X^TV^{-1}X)(X^TV^{-1}Y) \\ GZ^TV^{-1}(Y - X\beta) \end{bmatrix} \quad \textbf{(19.5)}$$

where $V = E[(Z_i\vec{\gamma}_i + \vec{\varepsilon}_i)(Z_i\vec{\gamma}_i + \vec{\varepsilon}_i)^T] = ZGZ^T + R$. G is the covariance matrix of the random effects under the assumption

$$\begin{pmatrix} \gamma_{1i} \\ \gamma_{2i} \end{pmatrix} \sim iid \begin{pmatrix} \begin{pmatrix} 0 \\ 0 \end{pmatrix}, \begin{pmatrix} \sigma^2_{\gamma 1} & \sigma_{\gamma 1 \gamma 2} \\ \sigma_{\gamma 2 \gamma 1} & \sigma^2_{\gamma 2} \end{pmatrix} \end{pmatrix}$$

Thus the random effects are group-based estimates. This is quite opposed to the metaphorical notion that each person's intercept and slope are estimated. They are post hoc predictions of the residuals based on the group model, not person-specific individual estimates.

The random effects typically described by investigators are measures of individual differences. These effects are basically regression residuals estimated under a specific set of assumptions for a particular regression model. In a growth curve setting, this becomes the requirement that each individual follow the same trajectory shape. Whereas the parameter values can differ from person to person, the parameterization of the curve typically does not. In situations in which the type of trajectory varies among individuals, the growth curve approach can misrepresent how individuals differ. In addition, the inference regarding the fixed effect parameters can be less than optimal when a single error model does not describe all individuals equally well (Liu, Rovine, & Molenaar, 2010).

The person-specific analogue to the growth curve model could require fitting a separate polynomial curve of an order to be empirically determined for each individual. With most typically designed studies, the number of occasions would be far too small to estimate parameters of this model with any precision. As a result, a growth curve along with its assumptions represents a necessary practical compromise.

Lagged Regression Models

Like the linear growth curve, the stability and lagged regression models are group-based models. The individual difference measures are actually *post hoc* predictions based on the group parameter estimates. Although this is perfectly acceptable for any question involving group differences, the question will always remain of whether the group model adequately describes any individual. Again, *ergodicity* remains an untested assumption.

Moving to a True Individual Difference Regression Model

To see how we can move to a true individual differences model, we can begin with a stability model for a variable, x, as described earlier. In Figure 19.3 we represent such a model for a single variable measured on five repeated occasions.

This figure represents a first-order autoregressive model (i.e., each occasion is regressed on only the prior occasion). To estimate the parameters of this model, we need a sample of individuals, n. The model is equivalent to estimating four separate regression equations with no restrictions on the parameters. We certainly could not estimate the model based on a single individual. However, with some modifications to that model, we

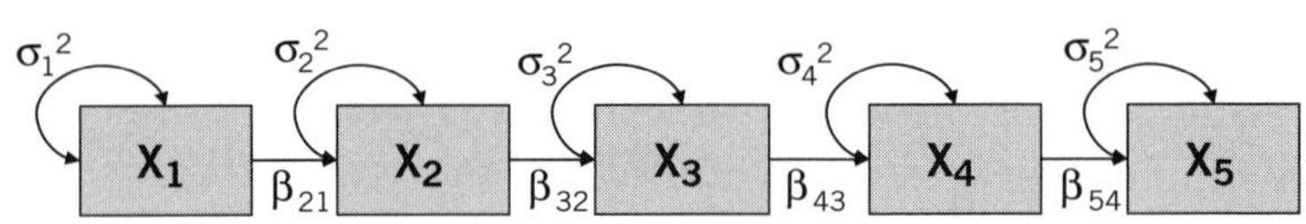

FIGURE 19.3. Stability model for a single variable measured on five occasions.

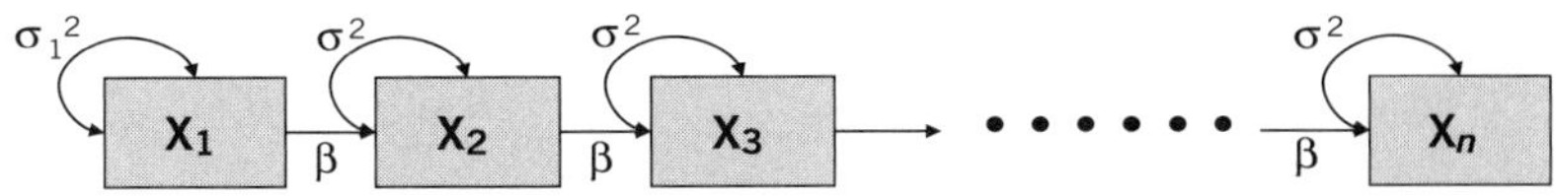

FIGURE 19.4. First-order autoregressive model for a single variable measured on n occasions.

can obtain parameter estimates for this model for a single subject. This alternative model is pictured in Figure 19.4. Here we extend the model from five occasions to n occasions. We constrain the parameters between each occasion to be equal. We also assume the variance of the residuals at each occasion (the innovations) to be equal. (The innovation is the difference between the observed value at time t and the predicted value based on prior information up to time t.) Because the regression coefficient for each pair of occasions is the same value, $\beta_{t,t-1}$, we can stack the data by lagging the variable, x, as described above. Regressing y_t onto y_{t-1} gives us the regression coefficient, $\beta_{t,t-1}$. This works because the regression of each occasion onto the previous occasion is the same value; so, wherever in the variable sequence one is, the prediction of the next occasion is always the same; hence the lagged variable. For a second-order autoregressive model, we would simply add y_{t-1} as a second predictor. Given this strategy we can easily extend this logic to any lagged or cross-lagged regression model. Consider the regression of y onto x for a single subject shown in Figure 19.5. Again, the assumption that the regression coefficient is identical across occasions requires the lagged variable as a predictor and allows the model to be estimated. This model can be expressed as the set of autoregression equations:

$$\begin{aligned} y_{t+1} &= \beta_{11} y_t + \beta_{12} x_t + \varepsilon_{1,t+1} \\ x_{t+1} &= \beta_{21} x_t + \varepsilon_{2,t+1} \end{aligned} \qquad \textbf{(19.6)}$$

where β_{11} is the stability coefficient for y and β_{12} is the lagged regression coefficient of y onto x.

Using the same logic we can define a cross-lagged regression model (see Figure 19.6) that is the time series analogue to the standard panel cross-lagged regression model. This model can be expressed as the set of autoregressive equations:

$$\begin{aligned} y_{t+1} &= \beta_{11} y_t + \beta_{12} x_t + \varepsilon_{1,t+1} \\ x_{t+1} &= \beta_{21} x_t + \beta_{22} y_t + \varepsilon_{2,t+1} \end{aligned} \qquad \textbf{(19.7)}$$

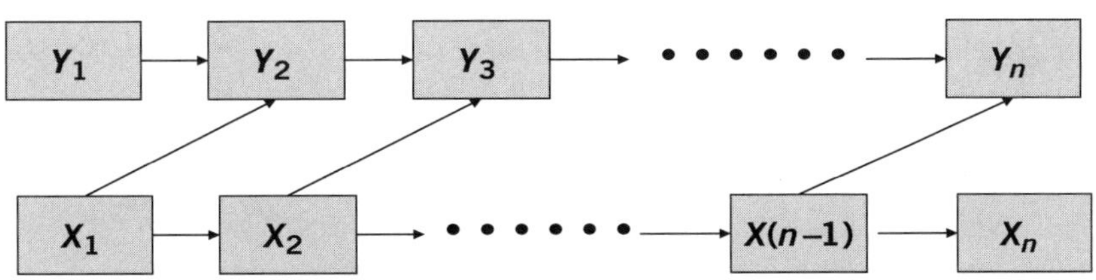

FIGURE 19.5. Lagged regression model for time series data.

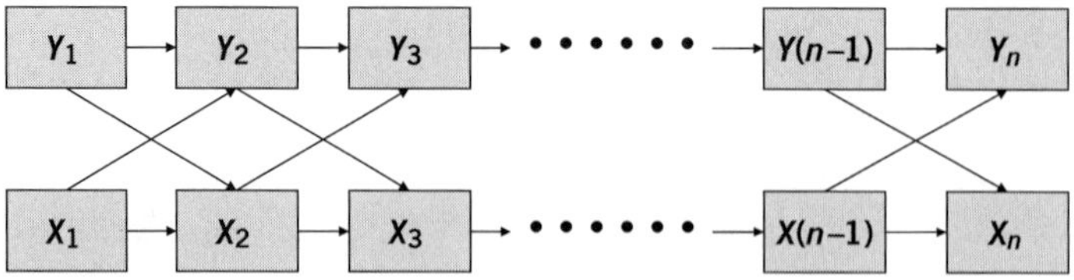

FIGURE 19.6. Cross-lagged regression model for time series data.

Autoregressive models have certain properties regarding error structure that make them suitable for analyzing developmental processes. Yule (1927) made the distinction between models that treat error as a superimposed component and as a process disturbance. The former perspective is characteristic of models such as the growth curve, in which error structures are added to a predefined trajectory that is a function of time. The latter perspective models error (or variance) as part of the dynamic process; error variance is conceptualized as a disturbance to the dynamic process that subsequently affects future values of the process. This second error structure perspective is characteristic of autoregressive models and more general dynamic models (e.g., state-space models).

The Vector Autoregression Model

Although it is perfectly permissible to write the lagged regression or the cross-lagged regression equations as shown previously, there are some major advantages to rewriting the set of equations as a single matrix equation. Most notably, in the matrix formulation, we can handle any number of variables and any degree of lagged relationships.

Consider the general situation, which we introduce as a cross-lagged regression between the two time series x and y. Rather than write the set of equations represented by this model, we write the single matrix equation. The first-order vector autoregressive equation can be written as

$$\vec{y}_{t+1} = B\vec{y}_t + \vec{\varepsilon}_{t+1} \tag{19.8}$$

For the model in Figure 19.5, this becomes

$$\begin{bmatrix} y_{t+1} \\ x_{t+1} \end{bmatrix} = \begin{bmatrix} \beta_{11} & \beta_{12} \\ \beta_{21} & \beta_{22} \end{bmatrix} \begin{bmatrix} y_t \\ x_t \end{bmatrix} + \begin{bmatrix} \varepsilon_{1t+1} \\ \varepsilon_{2t+1} \end{bmatrix} \tag{19.9}$$

where β_{11} and β_{22} are the stabilities and β_{12} and β_{21} are the cross lags.

Once we establish the individual models, we could determine whether there is variability in the stabilities and lags and whether the averaged values that we would obtain from a short time are reflective of the individuals. The matrix B represents the set of regression parameters that include both the stabilities and the cross-lagged regression coefficients. The vector autoregression (VAR) is equivalent to the equations in equation 19.9 for the cross-lagged regression model.

It is relatively simple to extend this model to any number of variables. The model can also be easily extended to higher order autoregressive models with any number of time series.

Moving to a True Individual Difference Curve Model from a Trend Model

As we mentioned before, the growth curve model (either latent or manifest) is a group-based model in which individual difference measures are predicted post hoc based on the common model and a set of relatively restrictive assumptions. Typically, all individuals are assumed to follow the same general shape with individual differences represented as best linear unbiased predictions (BLUPs) of the individual curves. With time series data, unique trends or curve shapes can be estimated separately for individuals.

In time series modeling, we know that in order to properly model the covariance relationships among the variables in the series, we require at least a weakly stationary series. The variance function must be a constant, the series must be detrended, and the covariance function among the different series must also be constant. A thorough discussion of ergodicity and the problems of making inferences about individual processes from group-level analysis is presented by Molenaar (2004). Regarding detrending, there are basically two approaches. If we are not interested in modeling the trend in the series, we can difference the series, where differencing simply means taking the difference score between each adjacent pair of measures and treating these differences as a new series. Differencing once removes linear trends, differencing twice removes quadratic trends, and so forth. If we are interested in modeling the trends, we can fit a trend model to each time series. A simple approach would involve fitting polynomials (linear, quadratic, cubic, etc.) to each series until the residuals of the resultant series have a constant mean function. We can then determine the order of the process for the residuals. With an overall linear trend and a first-order autoregressive process, the equation for this model would be

$$y_{t+1} = \beta_0 + \beta_1 t + \beta_2 y_t + \varepsilon_{t+1} \quad \textbf{(19.10)}$$

As in all person-specific approaches we can peruse individual models and determine which individuals can be pooled together.

Recursive Estimation and the State-Space Model

Typically in statistical analysis with cross-sectional or longitudinal data with relatively few occasions, we estimate the model using all of the data. Often the study is over, all of the data are collected, and the time for analysis is nigh. In a time series study, however, some subset of the data might be available, but a fair amount of time may pass before all of the data are in. There might be circumstances in which it is important to analyze whatever data are available (e.g., how effective a medical treatment is) and to update the results as each new data point arrives. Such problems suggest recursive estimation over a complete data analysis.

Recursive estimation simply means reestimating a statistic as each new data point arrives. For data that are received over time, a recursive estimator allows the estimator of the parameter to include all of the data that are currently available and to use them to provide a relatively simple formula to update the estimate as each new data point is encountered. Once all of the data are in, the parameter estimate derived recursively will be the same as that estimate using complete data. However, for many types of problems, including problems that unfold in real time, the recursive approach and, in particular, the Kalman filter has many advantages (Chow, Hamagami, & Nesselroade, 2007; Molenaar et al., 2009). We present a short introduction to recursive estimation and show how certain estimation equations can be rewritten recursively. Using this approach to regression, we provide a hopefully intuitive link to the Kalman filter.

Estimating a Mean Recursively

To estimate a mean recursively we consider the data set in Table 19.2. Given the formula for the mean

$$\overline{y_N} = \sum_{i=1}^{N} y_i \left(\frac{1}{N}\right) \tag{19.11}$$

we can rewrite this as

$$\begin{aligned}\overline{y_N} &= \sum_{i=1}^{N-1} y_i \left(\frac{1}{N}\right) + y_N \left(\frac{1}{N}\right) = \sum_{i=1}^{N-1} y_i \left(\frac{1}{N-1}\right)\left(\frac{N-1}{N}\right) + y_N \left(\frac{1}{N}\right) \\ &= \overline{y_{N-1}}\left(\frac{N-1}{N}\right) + \frac{y_N}{N}\end{aligned}$$

which gives the recursion relationship. Using the data in Table 19.2, we see that for line 6

$$\overline{y_6} = 3\left(\frac{5}{6}\right) + \frac{9}{6} = \frac{24}{6} = 4$$

which is the mean up to observation 6. As expected, once all of the data are in, the mean is identical to the mean of all observations. If we think of the sequence of numbers as a time series, with each new observation representing a new occasion, we could plot the means by occasion and observe how the mean develops over time.

To begin the recursion, we need to know the value of the mean at $N = 1$, which is trivially the value of the first observation. Note, however, that we could arbitrarily pick a

TABLE 19.2. Recursive Estimation of a Mean

N	y	$\bar{y}$
1	1	1
2	3	2
3	5	3
4	3	3
5	3	3
6	9	
7	4	
8	4	

number. If the sample were small, the effect of picking this number could be dramatic on the overall mean. As the sample gets larger, the effect of this initial selection would diminish.

Estimating a Simple Regression Recursively

The recursion for the mean is relatively simple. For a linear regression, the problem becomes slightly more complex. To show one way of developing the recursion, we begin with a simple linear regression model. To additionally simplify the model, we assume that the data have been centered, so the intercept of the model is 0.

The equation for the simple regression model is

$$y_i = X_i\beta_i + \varepsilon_i \qquad i = 1, \ldots, T \tag{19.12}$$

Given this equation, the regression weight is indexed by i to suggest that we are interested in estimating the regression for the first i observations.

Just using the first r observations, the regression coefficient is

$$\beta_r = \left(\sum_{i=1}^{r} x_i^2\right)^{-1} \left(\sum_{i=1}^{r} x_i y_i\right) \tag{19.13}$$

Using algebraic manipulations, this equation can be rewritten as

$$\beta_r = \beta_{r-1} + \left(\sum_{i=1}^{r} x_i^2\right)^{-1} x_r(y_r - \beta_{r-1}x_r) \tag{19.14}$$

The multiple regression model is a straightforward extension of the simple regression model (Brown, Durbin, & Evans, 1975; Plackett, 1950). As is very often the case, we can write the multivariate version of an equation by taking the univariate version and replacing the scalars in the model with the appropriate vectors and matrices. Taking equation 19.14, the recursive estimation formula for the simple regression, we can extend it to the multiple regression recursion

$$b_r = b_{r-1} + (X_r^T X_r)^{-1} x_r(y_r - x_r^T b_{r-1}) \tag{19.15}$$

The recursion typically includes a second recursion for the inverse of the sum of squares and cross-products (SSCP) matrix of the predictors, $(X_r^T X_r)^{-1}$. This recursion was originally presented by Plackett (1950).

The State-Space Model

The state-space model is a general recursion form that consists of two equations: the observation equation and the transition equation. Many variants of the basic model exist (Aoki, 1967; Durbin & Koopman, 2001; Harvey, 1989; Kim & Nelson, 1998; Simon, 2006), including continuous and discrete versions of the model. A good introduction to the concepts underlying the model and Kalman filter can be found in Maybeck (1979). Here we present a simple form of the discrete linear Gaussian state-space model. This can be expressed as two basic equations: the observation equation and the state or transition equation. A basic form of these equations (including no exogenous variables) includes the observation and state or transition equation.

$$y_t = Hx_t + \upsilon_t \quad \text{is the } \textit{observation equation} \tag{19.16}$$

Following conventions we name the state vector $x(t)$. Here y_t is a vector of observations. This equation has the form of a regression equation in which the parameter vector $x(t)$ can vary over time and $\upsilon(t)$ is a set of measurement errors. H is a design matrix that we will initially assume to be known.

$$x(t+1) = \Phi x_t + w_{t+1} \quad \text{is the } \textit{transition equation} \tag{19.17}$$

which is a first-order vector autoregressive model in which Φ represents a set of regression weights linking elements of the state at time t to the same elements at time $t + 1$. $w(t + 1)$ is the vector of *innovations* (differences between the predicted state and the actual state at time $t + 1$). The error term in the observation equation corresponds to the "superimposed" error, while the innovation term in the transition equation corresponds to the disturbance error that was characterized by Yule. In the most general model, all parameter matrices, including H and A, can be time varying.

To show a simple example of a state-space model, we can rewrite the second-order autoregressive model

$$y_{t+1} = \beta_{t+1,t}y_t + \beta_{t+1,t-1}y_{t-1} + \varepsilon_{t+1} \tag{19.18}$$

as

$$y_t = (1 \quad 1 \quad 1)x(t)$$

$$\begin{pmatrix} y_{t+1} \\ y_t \\ y_{t-1} \end{pmatrix} = \begin{bmatrix} \beta_{t+1,t} & \beta_{t+1,t-1} & 0 \\ 1 & 0 & 0 \\ 0 & 1 & 0 \end{bmatrix} \begin{pmatrix} y_t \\ y_{t-1} \\ y_{t-2} \end{pmatrix} + \begin{pmatrix} \varepsilon_{t+1} \\ 0 \\ 0 \end{pmatrix} \tag{19.19}$$

Even though this would not be the typical working representation of the AR(2) model, we show this form for transparency.

The Kalman filter addresses the problem of trying to estimate the state of a discrete time process as described here. The parameters of any model that can be written in state-space form can be estimated using the Kalman filter.

The Kalman Filter

A very general and extremely useful recursion algorithm is the Kalman filter (Kalman, 1960; Kalman & Bucy, 1961). It goes beyond the regression algorithms shown previously by allowing, among other things, time-varying parameters. Following Pollock (2003), we simply rewrite the least squares equations and provide names for some of the terms. This ad hoc approach allows us to define the filter gain that represents the improvement of the estimate obtained by the updating algorithm. As we will see, all of the concepts we define represent simple combinations of the quantities we have already dealt with.

The covariance matrix of the regression parameters is $D(\beta) = \sigma_\varepsilon^2 (X^T X)^{-1}$. If we define $P_r = (X^T X)^{-1}$, then $D(\beta) = \sigma_\varepsilon^2 P$, and equation 19.14 becomes

$$b_r = b_{r-1} + P_r x_r (y_r - x_r^T b_{r-1}). \qquad \textbf{(19.20)}$$

Now we give some definitions:

$$h_r = y_r - x_r^T b_{r-1} \qquad \textit{prediction error}$$

$$\sigma_\varepsilon^2 f_r = \sigma_\varepsilon^2 (1 + x_r{}^T P_{r-1} x_r) \qquad \textit{dispersion error} \qquad \textbf{(19.21)}$$

$$\kappa_r = P_{r-1} x_t f_r^{-1} \qquad \textit{filter gain}$$

With these definitions we can express the recursion. For the parameter updating equation

$$b_r = b_{r-1} + \kappa_r h_r \qquad \textit{parameter recursion} \qquad \textbf{(19.22)}$$

the update is the prediction error multiplied by the filter gain, which can be thought of as a weight indicating the importance of the prediction error in determining the regression coefficient. For the dispersion updating equation, a similar equation can be derived:

$$P_r = (I - \kappa_r x_r{}^T) P_{r-1} \qquad \textit{dispersion recursion} \qquad \textbf{(19.23)}$$

These two equations come directly from regression.

In the simplest sense the Kalman filter is a generalization of the previous recursion equations. The broad utility and incredible flexibility of the filter make it one of the most important technological innovations of the 20th century.

Given a state-space model in which observations arrive one occasion at a time, we can consider three different types of statistical estimation of the state, x: *prediction,* $x(-)$ uses all of the data up to but not including x; *filtering,* $x(+)$ updates the prediction based on the newest observation; and *smoothing,* $x(s)$ uses all of the observations to essentially filter to the end of the data set and work back to the newest observation.

The filter consists of a set of equations that first make a prediction of the next observation to arrive. Once those new data arrive, the prediction is adjusted based on the discrepancy between the prediction and the actual data point. The degree of adjustment is determined by the Kalman gain. The next observation arrives, and then the process is repeated.

This updating observation by observation allows some important additions to ordinary regression estimation in time series. One of the most important of these is the ability to have all parameters in the model time varying. This allows for possibilities in time series modeling well beyond many of the more standard techniques. Very readable discussion applications and variants of the basic filter appear in Grewal and Andrews (2001) and Simon (2006).

Conclusion

In this chapter we reviewed some of the issues regarding the estimation of person-specific and single-subject models. The possibility of estimating truly person-specific models becomes available only with the collection of time series data. At this point we remind the reader of the hopefully obvious fact that even though many methods are not truly person specific, those methods can still provide extremely helpful and useful information. However, when the data can feasibly be collected, in order to allow the possibility of different models for different individuals, time series person-specific approaches are certainly important to consider.

References

Anderson, T. W. (1963). The use of factor analysis in the statistical analysis of multiple time series. *Psychometrika, 28*, 1–25.

Aoki, M. (1967). *Optimization of stochastic systems: Topics in discrete-time systems*. Boston: Academic Press.

Baltes, P., Reese, H., & Nesselroade, J. (1977). *Life-span development psychology: Introduction to research methods*. Monterey, CA: Brooks/Cole.

Bath, K. E., Daly, D. L., & Nesselroade, J. R. (1976). Replicability of factors derived from individual P-technique analyses. *Multivariate Behavioral Research, 11*, 147–156.

Birkhoff, G. (1931). Proof of the ergodic theorem. *Proceedings of the National Academy of Sciences of the USA, 17*, 656–660.

Blalock, H. M. (2007). *Causal modeling in experimental designs*. New York: Aldine.

Borkenau, P., & Ostendorf, F. (1998). The Big Five as states: How useful is the five-factor model to describe intraindividual variations over time? *Journal of Research in Personality, 32*, 202–221.

Box, G., & Jenkins, G. (1970). *Time series analysis: Forecasting and control*. San Francisco: Holden-Day.

Brown, R., Durbin, J., & Evans, J. (1975). Techniques for testing the constancy of regression relationships over time. *Journal of the Royal Statistical Society: Series B, 37*, 149–163.

Brillinger, D. R. (1975). *Time series: Data analysis and theory*. New York: Holt, Rinehart & Winston.

Bryk, A., & Raudenbush, S. (1992). *Hierarchical linear models: Applications and data analysis methods*. Newbury Park, CA: Sage.

Cattell, R. B. (1966). The data box: Its ordering of total resources in terms of possible relational systems. In R. B. Cattell (Ed.), *Handbook of multivariate experimental psychology* (pp. 67–128). Chicago: Rand McNally.

Chow, S.-M., Hamagami, F., & Nesselroade, J. R. (2007). Age differences in dynamical emotion-cognition linkages. *Psychology and Aging, 22*, 765–780.

Corneal, S. E., & Nesselroade, J. R. (1994). A stepchild's emotional experience across two households: An investigation of response patterns by P-technique factor analysis. *Multivariate Experimental Clinical Research, 10*, 167–180.

Durbin, J., & Koopman, S. J. (2001). *Time series analysis by state space methods*. New York: Oxford University Press.

Goldstein, H. (1995). *Multilevel statistical models*. London: Edward Arnold.

Grewal, M., & Andrews, A. (2001). *Kalman filtering: Theory and practice using MATLAB*. New York: Wiley.

Harvey, A. C. (1989). *Forecasting, structural time series models and the Kalman filter.* Cambridge, UK: Cambridge University Press.

Henderson, C. R. (1975). Best linear unbiased estimation and prediction under a selection model. *Biometrics, 31,* 423–447.

Holtzman, W. H. (1962). Methodological issues in P-technique. *Psychological Bulletin, 59,* 243–256.

Jenkins, G. M., & Watts, D. G. (1968). *Spectral analysis and its applications.* San Francisco: Holden-Day.

Jones, C. J., & Nesselroade, J. R. (1990). Multivariate, replicated, single-subject designs and P-technique factor analysis: A selective review of the literature. *Experimental Aging Research, 16,* 171–183.

Kalman, R. E. (1960). A new approach to linear filtering and prediction problems. *Journal of Basic Engineering, 82,* 35–45.

Kalman, R. E., & Bucy, R. S. (1961). New results in linear filtering and prediction theory. *Journal of Basic Engineering, 83,* 95–108.

Kim, C. J., & Nelson, C. R. (1998). *State–space models with regime switching: Classical and Gibbs-sampling approaches with applications.* Cambridge, MA: MIT Press.

Kratochwill, T. R. (1978). *Single-subject research: Strategies for evaluating change.* New York: Academic Press.

Laird, N. M., & Ware, J. H. (1982). Random-effects models for longitudinal data. *Biometrics, 38,* 963–974.

Lamiell, J. T. (1981). Toward an idiothetic psychology of personality. *American Psychologist, 36,* 276–289.

Little, T. D., Preacher, K. J., Selig, J. P., & Card, N. A. (2007). New developments in SEM panel analyses of longitudinal data. *International Journal of Behavioral Development, 31,* 357–365.

Liu, S., Rovine, M., & Molenaar, P. (2010). *Selecting a linear mixed model for longitudinal data: Repeated-measures ANOVA and growth curve approaches.* Unpublished manuscript, Pennsylvania State University.

Luborsky, L., & Mintz, J. (1972). The contribution of P-technique to personality, psychotherapy, and psychosomatic research. In R. M. Dreger (Ed.), *Multivariate personality research* (pp. 340–410). Baton Rouge, LA: Claitor.

Luktepohl, H. (2005). *New introduction to multiple time series analysis.* Berlin: Springer-Verlag.

Maybeck, P. S. (1979). *Stochastic models, estimation, and control.* Boston: Academic Press.

McArdle, J. J., & Epstein, D. (1987). Latent growth curves within developmental structural equation models. *Child Development, 58,* 110–133.

Mitteness, L. S., & Nesselroade, J. R. (1987). Attachment in adulthood: Longitudinal investigation of mother–daughter affective interdependencies by P-technique factor analysis. *Southern Psychologist, 3,* 37–44.

Molenaar, P. C. M. (1985). A dynamic factor model for the analysis of multivariate time series. *Psychometrika, 50,* 181–202.

Molenaar, P. C. M. (1994). Dynamic latent variable models in developmental psychology. In A. von Eye & C.C. Clogg (Eds.), *Analysis of latent variables in developmental research* (pp. 155–180). Newbury Park, CA: Sage.

Molenaar, P. C. M. (2004). A manifesto on psychology as idiographic science: Bringing the person back into scientific psychology, this time forever. *Measurement, 2,* 201–218.

Molenaar, P. C. M., & Nesselroade, J. R. (2009). The recoverability of P-technique factor analysis. *Multivariate Behavioral Research, 44,* 130–141.

Molenaar, P. C. M., Rovine, M. J., & Corneal, S. E. (1999). Dynamic factor analysis of emotional disposition of adolescent stepsons toward their stepfathers. In R. K. Silbereisen & A. von Eye (Eds.), *Growing up in times of social change* (pp. 287–318). Berlin: de Gruyter.

Molenaar, P. C. M., Sinclair, K. O., Rovine, M. J., Ram, N., & Corneal, S. E. (2009). Analyzing

developmental processes on an individual level using non-stationary time series modeling. *Developmental Psychology, 45*, 260–271.
Muthén, B., & Shedden, K. (1999). Finite mixture modeling with mixture outcomes using the EM algorithm. *Biometrics, 55*, 463–469.
Nagin, D. S. (1999). Analyzing developmental trajectories: A semiparametric group-based approach. *Psychological Methods, 4*, 139–157.
Nesselroade, J. R., & Ford, D. H. (1985). P-technique comes of age: Multivariate, replicated, single subject designs for research on older adults. *Research on Aging, 7*, 46–80.
Nesselroade, J. R., & Molenaar, P. C. M. (1999). Pooling lagged covariance structures based on short, multivariate time series for dynamic factor analysis. In R. H. Hoyle (Ed.), *Statistical strategies for small sample research* (pp. 223–250). Thousand Oaks, CA: Sage.
Plackett, R. L. (1950). Some theorems in least squares. *Biometrika, 37*, 149–157.
Pollock, D. S. (2003). Recursive estimation in econometrics. *Computational Statistics and Data Analysis, 44*(1), 37–75.
Priestley, M. B., Subba Rao, T., & Tong, H. (1973). Identification of the structure of multivariable stochastic systems. In P. R. Krishnaiah (Ed.), *Multivariate analysis* (Vol. 3, pp. 351–368). New York: Academic Press.
Rovine, M.J., & Molenaar, P.C.M. (2005). Relating factor models for longitudinal data to quasi-simplex and NARMA models. *Multivariate Behavioral Research, 40*(1), 83–115.
Rovine, M. J., Molenaar, P. C. M., & Corneal, S. E. (1999). Analysis of emotional response patterns for adolescent stepsons using P-technique factor analysis. In R. K. Silbereisen & A. von Eye (Eds.), *Growing up in times of social change* (pp. 261–285). Berlin: de Gruyter.
Simon, D. (2006). *Optimal state estimation: Kalman, H infinity, and nonlinear approaches*. Hoboken, NJ: Wiley-Interscience.
Sterba, S. K., & Bauer, D. J. (2010). Matching method with theory in person-oriented developmental psychopathology research. *Development and Psychopathology, 22*, 239–254.
Stone, R. (1947). On the interdependence of blocks of transactions. *Journal of the Royal Statistical Society B, 9*, 1–32.
Walls, T. A., & Schaefer, J. L. (Eds.). (2006). *Models for intensive longitudinal data*. New York: Oxford University Press.
Wood, P., & Brown, D. (1994). The study of intra-individual differences by means of dynamic factor models: Rationale, implementation, and interpretation. *Psychological Bulletin, 116*, 166–186.
Yule, G. U. (1927). On a method of investigating periodicities in disturbed series, with special reference to Wolfer's sunspot numbers. *Philosophical Transactions of the Royal Society of London, Series A, 226*, 267–298.
Zevon, M. A., & Tellegen, A. (1982). The structure of mood change: An idiographic/nomothetic analysis. *Journal of Personality and Social Psychology, 43*, 111–122.

CHAPTER 20

Dynamic Factor Analysis and Control of Developmental Processes

PETER C. M. MOLENAAR
LAWRENCE L. LO

Central Issues

From a methodological perspective, developmental psychology always has been somewhat special in comparison with the other psychological subdisciplines, such as experimental psychology and social psychology. This is evident in the work, for instance, of Jean Piaget, one of the founding fathers of developmental psychology. Piaget's stagewise developmental model of cognitive development was based on the *méthode clinique*, a special observational approach that gave rise to much discussion in the English-speaking scientific world. Brainerd's (1978) critique of Piaget's stagewise developmental model is well known and typical, classifying that model as being merely descriptive and proposing a Markovian learning model as an alternative. This long-standing discussion about the merits of Piaget's stagewise developmental theory was resolved by Molenaar (1986a, 1986b) and van der Maas and Molenaar (1992), who showed, using a mathematical nonlinear dynamics approach, that developmental systems generally will display sudden qualitative changes in their evolution (so-called catastrophes, phase transitions, or bifurcations) of the kind described by Piaget. Consecutively, the catastrophe theoretical approach vindicated essential aspects of Piaget's model both in empirical research (e.g., Jansen & van der Maas, 2001, 2002; Raijmakers & Molenaar, 2004) and in theoretical respects (Wagenmakers, Molenaar, Grasman, Hartelman, & van der Maas, 2005).

The importance of nonlinear dynamics approaches within psychology certainly is not confined to developmental psychology, but these approaches had an especially profound impact on developmental psychological methodology and theory, starting as early as the 1980s and lasting up to the present (cf. Spencer, Thomas, & McClelland, 2009). Similar remarks can be made with respect to another feature of developmental psychological methodology, namely its reservations about variation between participants (interindividual variation) as a valid source of information concerning developmental processes. This criticism had a fundamental impact on developmental psychological methodology and theory. For example, Wohlwill's monograph on the study of behavioral development (Wohlwill, 1973) emphasizes the use of individual developmental functions while criticizing individual difference approaches. Similar remarks apply to Gottlieb's treatise on individual development and the genesis of novel behavior (Gottlieb, 1992) and to Ford and Lerner's seminal text on developmental systems theory (Ford & Lerner, 1992). Again this criticism was not confined to developmental psychology, as witnessed by the long-standing critical discussion of the relationship between average and individual learning curves (cf. several references to the early literature from 1931 onward in Sidman, 1960). But its impact on developmental methodology and theory stands out in comparison with other psychological subdisciplines.

In what follows we provide a definitive answer to the issue of whether interindividual variation constitutes a valid source of information concerning developmental processes. The answer will be predominantly negative, implying that analysis of developmental processes should be based on intraindividual variation, that is, time series analysis. Then, in the main part of this chapter, we focus on factor analysis of multivariate time series as an important tool for studying developmental processes. A hierarchy of increasingly complex dynamic factor models is presented, and ways to fit these models are considered in some detail. In the closing part of this chapter we address what we consider an exciting new extension of dynamic factor modeling, namely optimal control or guidance of individual developmental processes.

Interindividual versus Intraindividual Variation

Analysis of interindividual variation is the dominant approach to data analysis in psychology. For instance, analysis of variance, regression analysis, factor analysis, latent growth curve modeling, mixture analysis, and so forth, are all focused on interindividual differences in (sub)populations of participants. A random sample of participants is drawn from a presumably homogeneous population of interest and, consecutively, the variation between these participants is employed to carry out statistical tests about the true state of affairs in the population (generalization from sample to population of participants). The focus may be on mean differences between (sub)populations (as in analysis of variance) or on a description of the structure of individual differences in a population (as in factor analysis). But it is always the state of affairs at the population level that is of prime interest in standard psychological data analysis, and the source of information for such states of affairs is interindividual variation. This information is obtained by pooling the data of sampled participants. Pooling across participants is the hallmark of analysis of interindividual variation.

Variation in itself, considered quite independently from issues of modeling and statistical analysis, exists in two different forms: interindividual variation and intraindividual variation. The latter form, intraindividual variation, will be understood as pertaining to time-dependent differences occurring along a single individual's life trajectory. Hence intraindividual variation is associated with single-subject time series and implies a dynamic process perspective. Until recently, analysis of intraindividual variation (time series analysis) did not constitute a prominent approach in psychology. There are no principled reasons for this neglect in psychology of one of the two forms of variation; it appears to be the circumstantial result of historic contingencies (cf. Danzinger, 1990; Lamiell, 2003). It was assumed without much further reflection that states of affairs at the level of a population of individuals would generalize to equivalent states of affairs at the level of a single individual's life trajectory if that individual belonged to the population concerned. That is, it was assumed that the structure of interindividual variation in a homogeneous population of participants is equivalent to the analogous structure of intraindividual variation at the level of each individual belonging to that population. Given these assumptions (homogeneity of participants and equivalence of the structure of variation at the population and individual levels), it would seem to follow that it is sufficient to focus on the structure of interindividual variation and to generalize the results thus obtained to the level of intraindividual variation characterizing individual participants. For instance, if interindividual differences in personality obey a five-factor structure at the population level and the population is homogeneous (i.e., participants are exchangeable), then the structure of intraindividual variation characterizing each individual participant also would seem to have to obey the same five-factor structure.

Ergodicity

As we explain shortly, the assumption about the equivalence of a structure of interindividual variation at the population level and the analogous structure of intraindividual variation at the individual level is referred to as the *ergodic* assumption. It is reiterated that the ergodic assumption underlies all standard statistical analysis techniques in psychology. These techniques use only information provided by pooling across interindividual variation. As soon as results thus obtained are generalized to the level of the individual (e.g., in individual assessment or prediction), it is assumed that the ergodic assumption holds. Almost always the ergodic assumption is not stated or tested explicitly, but that does not mean that it is not required to make generalizations from states of affairs obtaining at the population level to the level of single participants.

The denotation *ergodic* is inspired by the so-called classical ergodic theorems (cf. Krengel, 1985). These theorems, in particular Birkhoff's individual ergodic theorem (Birkhoff, 1931), imply general mathematical conditions that have to be met by any measurable dynamic process in order to guarantee that the population structure of interindividual variation can be validly generalized to the level of intraindividual variation and vice versa. To ease the presentation, attention in this section is restricted to Gaussian (normally distributed) dynamic processes. Any ergodic Gaussian process has to obey the following two conditions (Molenaar, 2004):

- C_a: The Gaussian process has to be *stationary*. This implies (1) that the mean of the process has to be constant in time, (2) that the variance of the process has to be constant in time, and (3) that the sequential dependencies characterizing the process depend only upon the relative distance (lag) between time points.
- C_b: The Gaussian process also has to be *invariant across participants*. This implies that each participant in the population has to obey the same dynamic model.

Please notice that the two conditions are independent of each other. That is, a process may obey C_a without obeying C_b, or vice versa. In both of these cases the process is nonergodic, as it has to obey both conditions in order to be ergodic.

The requirement that ergodic processes have to be stationary (condition C_a) immediately rules out most developmental processes from being ergodic. Almost by definition, developmental processes have time-varying means and/or time-varying sequential dependencies and therefore are nonergodic. This implies that for most developmental processes the structure of interindividual variation at the population level is not equivalent to the structure of intraindividual variation at the level of individual participants. Consequently, the proper level required to obtain valid information about developmental processes violating condition C_a is the level of intraindividual variation within single participants. The latter conclusion—that the proper level at which to investigate development is not the population level (interindividual variation) but the level of individuals (intraindividual variation)—corroborates the old insight within developmental theory referred to previously.

The second ergodicity condition is C_b. This condition stipulates that all participants in the population have to obey exactly the same statistical model. In standard analysis of interindividual variation, this criterion is called the *homogeneity assumption*: populations (or, in mixture modeling, the subpopulations) have to be homogeneous in that each participant obeys exactly the same statistical model with the same numerical values for the fixed model parameters. It is the homogeneity assumption that underlies pooling the data of sampled participants, typical of analyses of interindividual variation. In particular, the homogeneity assumption is critical for the derivation of estimators for the parameters in statistical models. These estimators (e.g., maximum likelihood estimators) are derived on the explicit assumption that the population of participants is homogeneous. Consequently, if this assumption is violated—that is, if the population is heterogeneous—one would expect that this gives rise to bad model fits. It may come as a surprise that this is not at all the case.

In a series of simulation studies (e.g., Molenaar, 1997, 1999; Molenaar, Huizenga, & Nesselroade, 2003), heterogeneous data were generated according to several versions of factor models (including longitudinal and genetic factor models), in which each " participant" had its own factor model. That is, the values of factor loadings, measurement error variances, and so forth were subject specific. This constitutes a severe violation of the homogeneity assumption, which stipulates that these model parameters should be invariant across participants. Notwithstanding these violations of the homogeneity assumption, standard factor analysis of the simulated heterogeneous data yielded excellently fitting models. Hence it turns out that standard factor analysis is insensitive to violations of the homogeneity assumption. Or, stated otherwise, factor analysis of interindividual variation is insensitive to the presence of large-scale heterogeneity in the population. A formal proof of this result is presented in Kelderman & Molenaar (2007).

There exist theoretical reasons that human populations should be expected to be heterogeneous (i.e., violate the second ergodicity condition, C_b). Of particular importance from a theoretical perspective are the neural networks associated with cognitive and behavioral psychological processes. The growth of neural networks is governed by nonlinear epigenetic processes (e.g., McLachlan, 1999). The mathematical–biological models explaining these epigenetic processes create endogenous variation that is due neither to genetic nor to environmental influences but is caused by the nonlinear growth process itself (Molenaar, Boomsma, & Dolan, 1993). In mathematical biology a class of very successful models has been developed: the class of nonlinear reaction-diffusion models of biological pattern formation (e.g., Meinhardt, 1982). The key characteristic of nonlinear reaction-diffusion models is self-organization. The self-organizing nonlinear epigenetic processes represented by reaction-diffusion models of biological pattern formation also underlie the growth of neural networks (cf. Molenaar, 2007). Hence it can be expected that at the micro level human brain architecture will be quite heterogeneous. Insofar as human behavior and information processing are dependent on neural models or networks, this heterogeneity will be reflected in psychological measurements, thus causing violations of condition C_b. This conclusion has been corroborated in simulation studies of neural network growth (Kan, Ploeger, Kaijmakers, Dolan, & van der Maas, 2010; Molenaar & Raijmakers, 1999).

Conceptual Principles and Statistical Assumptions

In this section we present a review of statistical models for the analysis of intraindividual variation that is stationary in time. That is, it is assumed that the developmental processes under scrutiny obey the ergodic stationarity criterion C_a but possibly violate the ergodic homogeneity condition C_b. Hence the statistical models presented in this section can be used to test whether a developmental process is characterized by subject-specific dynamics (population heterogeneity). The focus is on factor models because these provide maximum generality in that all linear dynamic models can be reformulated as special instances of dynamic factor models (cf. Hannan & Deistler, 1987).

Dynamic Factor Analysis of Stationary Multivariate Time Series

Dynamic factor analysis is factor analysis of single-subject multivariate time series. It constitutes a generalization of Cattell's (1952) P-technique in that it takes account of lead-lag patterns in the dynamic relationships between latent factor series and observed series. In contrast, P-technique involves straightforward application of standard factor analysis to multivariate time series without accommodation of lead-lag sequential dependencies; the reader is referred to Molenaar and Nesselroade (2009) for further discussion of the domain of application of P-technique.

In what follows, boldface lowercase letters denote vectors; boldface uppercase letters denote matrices; an apostrophe (') attached to vectors or matrices denotes transposition. Let $\mathbf{y}(t) = [y_1(t), y_2(t), \ldots, y_p(t)]'$ be a p-variate time series, $p \geq 1$, observed at equidistant time points $t = 1,2, \ldots, T$. The mean of $\mathbf{y}(t)$ at each time point t is $E[\mathbf{y}(t)] = \mu(t)$. Considered as a function of t, $\mu(t)$ denotes the p-variate mean function (trend) of $\mathbf{y}(t)$. If $\mu(t) = \mu$, that is, if the mean function is constant in time, then $\mathbf{y}(t)$ has a stationary mean function. The sequential covariance of $\mathbf{y}(t)$ between a given pair of time points t_1 and t_2 is defined as $\Sigma(t_1, t_2) = \text{cov}[\mathbf{y}(t_1), \mathbf{y}(t_2)']$. Considered as a function of two-dimensional time, $\Sigma(t_1, t_2)$ denotes the (p,p)-variate covariance function of $\mathbf{y}(t)$. If $\Sigma(t_1, t_2)$ depends only on the relative time difference $t_1 - t_2 = u$, that is, $\Sigma(t_1, t_2) = \Sigma(t_1 - t_2) = \Sigma(u)$, $u = 0, \pm 1, \ldots, \pm T - 1$, then $\mathbf{y}(t)$ has stationary covariance function depending only on lag u. If both the mean function and covariance function of $\mathbf{y}(t)$ are stationary, then $\mathbf{y}(t)$ is called a weakly stationary p-variate time series.

In the first publication on dynamic factor analysis in psychology, the following model for weakly stationary multivariate Gaussian series was considered (Molenaar, 1985):

$$\mathbf{y}(t) = \mu + \Lambda(0)\eta(t) + \Lambda(1)\eta(t-1) + \ldots + \Lambda(s)\eta(t-s) + \varepsilon(t) \qquad \textbf{(20.1a)}$$

where $\mathbf{y}(t)$ is an observed p-variate time series, $\eta(t)$ is a latent q-variate factor series, and $\varepsilon(t)$ is a p-variate measurement error series. Because our main interest is not in the constant mean function μ, it is conveniently assumed that $\mu = 0$. Then all time series in equation 20.1a, $\mathbf{y}(t)$, $\eta(t)$ and, $\varepsilon(t)$, are zero mean weakly stationary.

The $\Lambda(u)$, $u = 0, 1, \ldots, s$, are (p,q)-dimensional matrices of lagged factor loadings, where $s \geq 0$ is the maximum lag. These lagged factor loadings allow for the possibility that the realization of the latent factor series $\eta(t)$ at each time t not only has an instantaneous effect on $\mathbf{y}(t)$ but also may have delayed effects at later time points $t + 1, \ldots, t + s$. The linear combination $\Lambda(0)\eta(t) + \Lambda(1)\eta(t-1) + \ldots + \Lambda(s)\eta(t-s)$ is called a convolution.

For later reference the limiting case of equation 20.1a is considered in which $s = 0$, that is, the case in which there are no lagged factor loadings:

$$\mathbf{y}(t) = \Lambda(0)\eta(t) + \varepsilon(t) \qquad \textbf{(20.1b)}$$

Equation 20.1b is a special instance of equation 20.1a. It has been assigned several labels, including state-space model (e.g., Molenaar, 1985) and process factor model (e.g., Browne & Nesselroade, 2005). In what follows, equation 20.1b is referred to as a state-space model. As we explain shortly, equation 20.1b has a special property not shared by equation 20.1a.

The dynamic factor model (equation 20.1a) was inspired by Brillinger's (1975) principal component analysis of multivariate weakly stationary time series. It differs from Brillinger's approach in a number of respects, perhaps the most important of which is that in equation 20.1a the convolution of lagged factor loadings and latent factor series is finite and depends at each time point t only on earlier realizations $\eta(t), \ldots, \eta(t-s)$ of the latent factor series, whereas in Brillinger's model this convolution is infinite and also depends on future realizations $\eta(t + 1), \eta(t + 2), \ldots$. Another important difference relates to the statistical characteristics of the measurement error series in each of the two models.

To complete the definition of the dynamic factor model under consideration, the covariance functions of the time series occurring in equations 20.1a and 20.1b have to be specified. Let diag-A denote a square diagonal matrix A (all off-diagonal elements being zero). Then the covariance functions associated with the right-hand side of equation 20.1a are:

$$\begin{aligned} \text{cov}[\varepsilon(t), \varepsilon(t-u)'] &= \text{diag-}\Theta(u);\ u = 0, \pm 1, \ldots \\ \text{cov}[\eta(t), \eta(t-u)'] &= \Psi(u),\ u = 0, \pm 1, \ldots \end{aligned} \qquad \textbf{(20.1c)}$$

The first equation in 20.1c defines the covariance function of the measurement error process. The univariate measurement error process $\varepsilon_k(t)$ associated with the k-th observed univariate series $y_k(t)$, $k \in \{1, \ldots, p\}$ is allowed to have nonzero sequential covariance: possibly $\text{cov}[\varepsilon_k(t), \varepsilon_k(t-u)] \neq 0\ \forall u$. However, measurement error processes $\varepsilon_k(t)$ and $\varepsilon_m(t)$ associated with different observed univariate series $y_k(t)$ and $y_m(t)$, $k \neq m \in \{1, \ldots, p]$ are assumed to be uncorrelated at all lags u: $\text{cov}[\varepsilon_k(t), \varepsilon_m(t-u)] = 0\ \forall u$. The second equation in 20.1c defines the covariance function of the latent factor series.

Some Intricacies Associated with Equation 20.1

It was proven in Molenaar (1985) that under certain conditions the covariance function of the latent factor series defined in equation 20.1c is not identifiable. That means that under certain conditions the variances and sequential covariances in $\Psi(u)$, $u = 0, \pm 1, \ldots$, cannot be estimated but have to be fixed a priori. The conditions concerned are twofold. First, the maximum lag s of the matrices of factor loadings $\Lambda(u)$, $u = 0, 1, \ldots, s$, has to be larger than zero: $s > 0$. Second, all factor loadings in $\Lambda(u)$, $u = 0, 1, \ldots, s$, should be free parameters. That is, the dynamic factor model should be exploratory, having no a priori pattern of fixed factor loadings.

If both these conditions obtain, then the covariance function of the latent factor series has to be fixed a priori. $\Psi(u)$, $u = 0, \pm 1, \ldots$, then can be fixed at any possible covariance function without affecting the goodness of fit of the model. In Molenaar (1985) the simplest covariance function for $\eta(t)$ was chosen: $\text{cov}[\eta(t), \eta(t-u)] = \delta(u)\mathbf{I}_q$, where $\delta(u)$ is the Kronecker delta ($\delta(u) = 1$ if $u = 0$; $\delta(u) = 0$ if $u \neq 0$), and $\mathbf{I}_q$ is the (q,q)-dimensional identity matrix. This particular choice implies that the latent factor series lacks instantaneous as well as sequential dependencies. Accordingly, $\eta(t)$ can be conceived of as a sequence of random shocks, often referred to in the engineering literature as a white noise sequence. But quite other choices are possible (cf. Molenaar & Nesselroade, 2001).

If the dynamic factor model is confirmatory—that is, if an a priori pattern of fixed factor loadings has been specified in $\Lambda(u)$, $u = 0, 1, \ldots, s$, then the covariance function of the latent factor series is identifiable. Also if $s = 0$, that is, if the state-space model equation 20.1b applies, then the covariance function of the latent factor series is identifiable. In these cases $\Psi(u)$, $u = 0, \pm 1, \ldots$, can be freely estimated or, alternatively, a parametric time series model for $\eta(t)$ (and hence for its covariance function) can be considered. For instance, the latent factor series $\eta(t)$ can be represented by a vector autoregression: $\eta(t) = B\eta(t-1) + \zeta(t)$, where B is a (q,q)-dimensional matrix of autoregression coefficients and $\zeta(t)$ is a q-variate white noise sequence lacking any sequential dependencies.

Given that for the state-space model equation 20.1b the covariance function (or a parametric time series model) of the latent factor series is always identifiable, it would seem rational to restrict attention to this type of model. At least for exploratory dynamic factor analyses, this would preclude the need to have to arbitrarily fix $\Psi(u)$, $u = 0, \pm 1, \ldots$, which is necessary in such applications of equation 20.1a. However, it can be shown that for certain types of psychological time series the state-space model is too restrictive. In particular, when the effect of $\eta(t)$ on $\mathbf{y}(t)$ is delayed, the state-space model will be inappropriate. For these time series one needs the general dynamic factor model equation 20.1a, in which $s > 0$. Such delays occur, for instance, in multilead electroencephalograph (EEG) registrations of electrocortical brain fields caused by a finite set of underlying neural sources. The activity of the neural sources is represented by the latent factor series $\eta(t)$ and the EEG registrations by the manifest series $\mathbf{y}(t)$. The effects of each neural source travel with finite speed along long-range axons to the target regions. Because target regions are located at different distances from a given neural source and the effects of a volley of action potentials of a neural source on the ongoing activity of target areas take time to dissipate, the relationships between $\eta(t)$ and $\mathbf{y}(t)$ will show complex patterns of delays.

Alternative Ways to Fit Equation 20.1

Analysis of stationary multivariate Gaussian time series based on the dynamic factor model equation 20.1 can proceed in various ways:

1. Based on the sequential covariance function, arranged in a so-called block-Toeplitz matrix (see Molenaar, 1985, for a detailed description). This can be carried out by means of commercially available structural equation modeling software. An important alternative implementation of the block-Toeplitz approach is the DyFa program by Browne and Zhang (2005). The DyFa program can be downloaded from *faculty.psy.ohio-state.edu/browne/software.php*.

2. Based on expectation–maximization (EM) of the raw data likelihood associated with state-space models (equation 20.1b), where the latent factor series is estimated by means of the recursive Kalman filter (expectation step) and the parameters are estimated by means of multivariate regression (maximization step). See Hamaker, Dolan, and Molenaar (2005) and Hamaker, Nesselroade, and Molenaar (2007) for explanations and applications. A similar approach uses maximum likelihood (ML) procedures, in which multiple filter recursions are executed for each free parameter to obtain analytical gradients (Harvey, 1989). These gradients are obtained iteratively within a quasi-Newton optimization routine for ML estimates. The software used in these applications can be obtained from *users.fmg.uva.nl/cdolan*.

3. In the frequency domain, after discrete Fourier transformation. This yields a set of frequency-dependent complex-valued factor models that can subjected to standard ML factor analysis (Molenaar, 1987). The software for dynamic factor analysis in the frequency domain can be obtained from the authors. Special nonlinearly constrained variants of this approach have been developed for the purpose of neural source estimation in brain imaging (Grasman, Huizenga, Waldorp, Böcker, & Molenaar, 2005). The software concerned can be obtained from *users.fmg.uva.nl/rgrasman*.

4. Rewriting the model as a state-space model, with the extended state containing not only the latent factor series but also the unknown parameters. This results in a nonlinear state-space model for which the extended Kalman filter is used to estimate the extended state, including the parameters. This is discussed further in the next section.

Dynamic Factor Analysis of Nonstationary Multivariate Time Series

Now we turn to a consideration of stationarity; that is, condition C_a for ergodicity. Although there exist statistical tests for nonstationarity (e.g., Priestley, 1988; Weber, Molenaar, & van der Molen, 1992), there is a lack of adequate statistical dynamic models for nonstationary psychological processes. What we have in mind are suitable generalizations of dynamic factor models having arbitrarily time-varying parameters (e.g., changing factor loadings, measurement error variances). To the best of our knowledge the only example of such a dynamic factor model for nonstationary time series was presented in Molenaar (1994) under the assumption that the factor loadings change according to polynomial functions of time. Recently (Molenaar, Sinclair, Rovine, Ram, & Corneal, 2009) this dynamic factor model was generalized to accommodate arbitrarily time-varying parameters, using a new statistical method to fit the model to the data. The latter model is described in some detail later and applied to an illustrative simulated data set. In closing this section we present a general interpretation of the model, linking the arbitrarily time-varying parameters to different time scales. According to this interpretation, the dynamic factor model with arbitrarily time-varying parameters provides a theoretical model integrating short-term and long-term developmental processes.

Consider the following state-space model with arbitrarily time-varying (nonstationary) parameters:

$$\begin{aligned} \mathbf{y}(t) &= \Lambda[\theta(t)]\eta(t) + \varepsilon(t) \\ \eta(t+1) &= \mathrm{B}[\theta(t)]\eta(t) + \zeta(t+1) \\ \theta(t+1) &= \theta(t) + \xi(t+1) \end{aligned} \qquad \textbf{(20.2a)}$$

In equation 20.2a, $\mathbf{y}(t)$ denotes the observed p-variate time series; $\eta(t)$ the q-variate latent factor series (state process). The first equation of (20.2a) shows that factor loadings in $\Lambda[\theta(t)]$ depend on a time-varying parameter-vector $\theta(t)$. The second equation describes the time evolution of the state process $\eta(t)$; the autoregressive weights in $\mathrm{B}[\theta(t)]$ depend on $\theta(t)$ and therefore can be arbitrarily time varying. The third equation in (20.2a) describes the time-dependent variation of the unknown parameters. The r-variate parameter vector process $\theta(t)$ obeys a random walk with Gaussian innovations $\xi(t)$.

The covariance functions associated with the innovation processes in equation 20.2a are given in 20.2b (remember that $\delta(u)$ is the Kronecker delta: $\delta(u) = 1$ if $u = 0$; $\delta(u) = 0$ if $u \neq 0$).

$$\begin{aligned} \mathrm{cov}[\varepsilon(t), \varepsilon(t-u)'] &= \delta(u)\mathrm{diag}\text{-}\Theta \\ \mathrm{cov}[\zeta(t), \zeta(t-u)'] &= \delta(u)\mathrm{diag}\text{-}\Psi \\ \mathrm{cov}[\xi(t), \xi(t-u)'] &= \delta(u)\mathrm{diag}\text{-}\boldsymbol{\Phi} \end{aligned} \qquad \textbf{(20.2b)}$$

To fit the state-space model with time-varying parameters to an observed multivariate time series, use is made of a combination of the second and fourth estimation techniques mentioned in the section "Alternative Ways to Fit"—that is, a combination of the EM algorithm and the extended Kalman filter/smoother. First, an extended state process is defined. The extended state process consists of the original latent factor series and the time-varying parameter process: $\mathbf{x}(t)' = [\eta(t)', \theta(t)']$. Then, using the extended state process $\mathbf{x}(t)$, equation 20.2a is rewritten as the following nonlinear state-space model:

$$\begin{aligned} \mathbf{y}(t) &= \mathbf{h}[\mathbf{x}(t), t] + \mathbf{v}(t) \\ \mathbf{x}(t+1) &= \mathbf{f}[\mathbf{x}(t), t] + \mathbf{w}(t) \end{aligned} \qquad \textbf{(20.3)}$$

The vector-valued nonlinear functions $\mathbf{h}[\mathbf{x}(t), t]$ and $\mathbf{f}[\mathbf{x}(t), t]$ consist of products of the entries of $\mathbf{x}(t)$. The $(q + r)$-dimensional innovations process $\mathbf{w}(t)$ is defined as the composition of the innovation processes $\zeta(t)$ and $\xi(t)$: $\mathbf{w}(t)' = [\zeta(t)', \xi(t)']$.

The extended state $\mathbf{x}(t)$ in the nonlinear state-space model (3) is estimated by means of the extended Kalman filter (EKF), of which the following schematic representation can be given:

$$\mathbf{x}(t+1|t+1) = \mathrm{EKF}[\mathbf{x}(t|t), \mathbf{y}(t+1), \mathbf{P}(t|t), \mathbf{f}_x, \mathbf{F}_{xx}, \mathbf{h}_x, \mathbf{H}_{xx}] \qquad \textbf{(20.4)}$$

where $\mathbf{x}(t|t)$ is the expected state at time t given information up to time t; $\mathbf{P}(t|t)$ is the covariance matrix of $\mathbf{x}(t|t)$; $\mathbf{h}_x$, $\mathbf{f}_x$ are Jacobians of $\mathbf{h}[\mathbf{x}(t), t]$ and $\mathbf{f}[\mathbf{x}(t), t]$; and $\mathbf{H}_{xx}$, $\mathbf{F}_{xx}$ are Hessians of $\mathbf{h}[\mathbf{x}(t), t]$ and $\mathbf{f}[\mathbf{x}(t), t]$.

The extended EKF depends on Taylor expansions of the vector-valued nonlinear functions in the nonlinear state model up to second order about the estimated state. The actual Kalman filter/smoother used in applications is much more complex. It is embedded in an EM algorithm and involves robust transformations of the recursions (extended Kalman filter and smoother; EKFIS). The EKFIS yields an estimate of the extended state at each time point. Because the state includes the time-varying parameters, one thus obtains for each estimated parameter a time series, or trajectory, spanning the whole observation interval.

There are several advantages of using the EKFIS. First, the EKFIS is exact for the linear state-space model with time-varying parameters because it keeps Taylor expansion terms up to second order. Also, the EKFIS uses covariance resetting to make the recursive estimation more robust. Another advantage is that the EKFIS applies not only filtering or recursive estimation of the state process forward in time but also smoothing or recursive filtering backward in time. In this way the information in the observed time series is used optimally. Additionally, EKFIS includes an iteration-within-recursion option, but we do not apply this option because in applications to the linear state-space model with time-varying parameters, the second-order linearization of the EKFIS is exact. Finally, EKFIS estimates the innovation variances in random walk for parameters by means of an EM algorithm, as is demonstrated next.

The equation used to embed EKFIS in the EM algorithm to estimate innovation variances in random walk for time-varying parameters is, according to equations 20.2a and 20.2b:

$$\theta(t+1) = \theta(t) + \xi(t+1)$$
$$\text{cov}[\xi(t), \xi(t-u)] = \delta(u)\text{diag-}\mathbf{\Phi}$$

where diag-$\mathbf{\Phi}$ is estimated in EM loop. When EKFIS is embedded in the expectation–maximization algorithm, two steps are performed within each iteration of this algorithm. First, the EKFIS yields a filtered estimate of the trajectory of the extended state process across the entire observation interval. Second, this filtered estimate of the extended state process is entered in the complete data likelihood, which is maximized in order to obtain an improved estimate of $\mathbf{\Phi}$, the variance of the process noise in the random walk model of the time-varying parameters. This model certainly is not the only one available to analyze nonstationary developmental processes. Several chapters in the volume edited by Molenaar and Newell (2010) present alternative approaches (see also Hamaker, Zhang, & van der Maas, 2009).

Developmental Applications

Potential applications of dynamic factor analysis are as widespread as current applications of standard factor analysis. This methodological framework can be used to analyze any psychological phenomenon involving a time series. The primary advantage of this method over other methods of longitudinal data analysis (e.g., standard longitudinal factor models) is the ability to answer questions regarding the dynamic structure(s) of the psychological construct(s) of interest; thus this method may be of interest to researchers interested in dynamic processes. Likewise, because this method focuses on an individual time series, it may be of interest to researchers interested in idiosyncratic psychological processes. As argued earlier, however, most developmental processes are likely both dynamic and idiosyncratic to some degree. In this section, we present several applications of dynamic factor analysis in several developmental domains.

Cognitive development has been a primary area for application of dynamic modeling. Several studies on Piaget's cognitive development theories were discussed earlier in this chapter. Another example of dynamic factor analysis within cognitive development is the study by Chow, Hamagami, and Nesselroade (2008) on the dynamic relationship between cognitive and affective processes. Dynamic factor analyses were implemented on individual time series and pooled to compare dynamic functioning between age groups. The authors found dynamic relationships between positive affect, negative affect, and cognitive ability that differed for younger and older adults. Older adults had stable affect that was unaffected by cognitive performance, whereas younger adults' affect was related to previous cognitive performance.

Dynamic processes of emotion and affect have also been studied via dynamic factor models outside of cognitive performance research. Ferrer and Nesselroade (2003) implemented dynamic factor analyses separately on a husband and wife, then investigated dyadic relationships by dynamic relationship between the two individuals' factor structures. They found that the husband and wife differed in terms of their factorial configuration and temporal organization. In the following dyadic analyses, they found a unidirectional relationship in which the husband's negative affect had a lagged relationship with the wife's subsequent negative affect. Molenaar and colleagues (2009) investigated the dynamics of children's emotional responses after interacting with their fathers. We take an in-depth look at this study in the following section in order to demonstrate the application of nonstationary time series modeling. Other excellent recent discussions and illustrations of dynamic factor analysis of psychological time series can be found in Browne and Nesselroade (2005), Browne and Zhang (2007), Ferrer (2006), Hamaker et al. (2005), Kim, Zhu, Chang, Bentler, and Ernst (2007), Mumma (2004), Nesselroade, McArdle, Aggen, and Meyers (2002), Sbarra and Ferrer (2006), Shifren, Hooker, Wood, and Nesselroade (1997), and Wood and Brown (1994).

Illustration

Molenaar and colleagues (2009) implemented intraindividual time series models for emotional responses of 16 boys after interactions with their fathers. The boys filled out a battery consisting of items measuring positive and negative affect after each of 80 interactions with their fathers. Detailed descriptions of the design and measures are given in Rovine, Molenaar, and Corneal (1999). The authors first conducted P-technique factor analyses on each of the individuals and found heterogeneity in factor structures for individuals. In this section we focus on the emotional dynamics of one of the boys studied.

The P-technique factor analysis for this individual yielded a three-factor solution consisting of Involvement, Anger, and Anxiety; this was based on the types of items that loaded on the factors (there was only one other boy who shared this factor structure).

The observed time series was converted to a lower dimensional factor time series corresponding to the number of factors using the regression factor score estimator derived from the P-technique analysis; this estimator has been shown to have the same precision as the Kalman filter recursive estimator (Molenaar & Nesselroade, 2009). This method is useful for splitting estimation problems in a sequence of two steps: The first step involves fitting the measurement model, and the second step fits the dynamic structure model.

The nonstationary model depicted in equation 20.2a was fit to the time series by the EFKIS method described in the section "Conceptual Principles and Statistical Assumptions." In this case, however, $y(t) = h(t)$ because the observed series has already been converted to a factor series. This particular model involved nine time-varying parameters, including three autoregressions and six cross-lagged regressions: Involvement(t + 1) from Involvement(t), Involvement(t + 1) from Anger(t), Involvement(t + 1) from Anxiety(t), Anger(t + 1) from Involvement(t), Anger(t + 1) from Anger(t), Anger(t + 1) from Anxiety(t), Anxiety(t + 1) from Involvement(t), Anxiety(t + 1) from Anger(t), and Anxiety(t + 1) from Anxiety(t). A graphical depiction of the EKFIS fit of the time-varying parameters is represented in Figure 20.1. For further technical details on implementation of the EFKIS in this analysis, refer to Molenaar and colleagues (2009).

The authors found several interesting features of the boy's dynamic process. The top panel of the figure indicates a change in polarity of the dynamic relationship between Involvement and Anxiety. The time-varying lagged-regression parameter of Involvement(t + 1) from Anxiety(t) changes from –0.19 at time 1 to 0.12 at time 80. Therefore, high Anxiety initially produces a decrease in the predicted value of Involvement at the next time point; however, this changes to an increase in the predicted value of Involvement at the next time point. This suggests a substantive change in the dynamics of the boy's emotional response to his father. Another noteworthy finding is seen in the dynamic relationship between Anxiety and Anger. As seen in the bottom panel of the figure, the time-varying cross-lagged regression of Anxiety(t + 1) from Anger(t) changes from 0.08 at time 1 to 0.39 at time 80. In this situation, Anger becomes a stronger predictor of subsequent Anxiety across time, even surpassing the Anxiety(t + 1) from Anxiety(t) autoregression.

As illustrated in this study, nonstationary time series analysis allows investigation of dynamic processes underlying psychological phenomena. This illustration demonstrates different ways that the relationship between psychological variables can change across time. Time-varying relationships of these variables can change in polarity, indicating a change in qualitative manner. They can also change in magnitude, indicating a change in quantitative degree. Such substantive findings are one of the primary benefits of nonstationary time series analysis.

Future Directions

General mathematical theorems in ergodic theory appear to have profound implications for the relationships between results obtained in analyses of interindividual variation and intraindividual variation (Molenaar, 2004). Development pertains to processes of change within individuals; thus the intraindividual perspective is fundamental (cf. Wohlwill, 1973). Consequently, standard analyses of interindividual variation will yield valid information about developmental processes only if lawful relationships exist between results thus obtained and results that would have been obtained in analogous analyses of intraindividual variation. Such lawful relationships exist, however, only if the developmental processes under scrutiny are ergodic. A Gaussian process is ergodic only if it obeys two strict conditions: the process has to be stationary, and different participants in the population have to

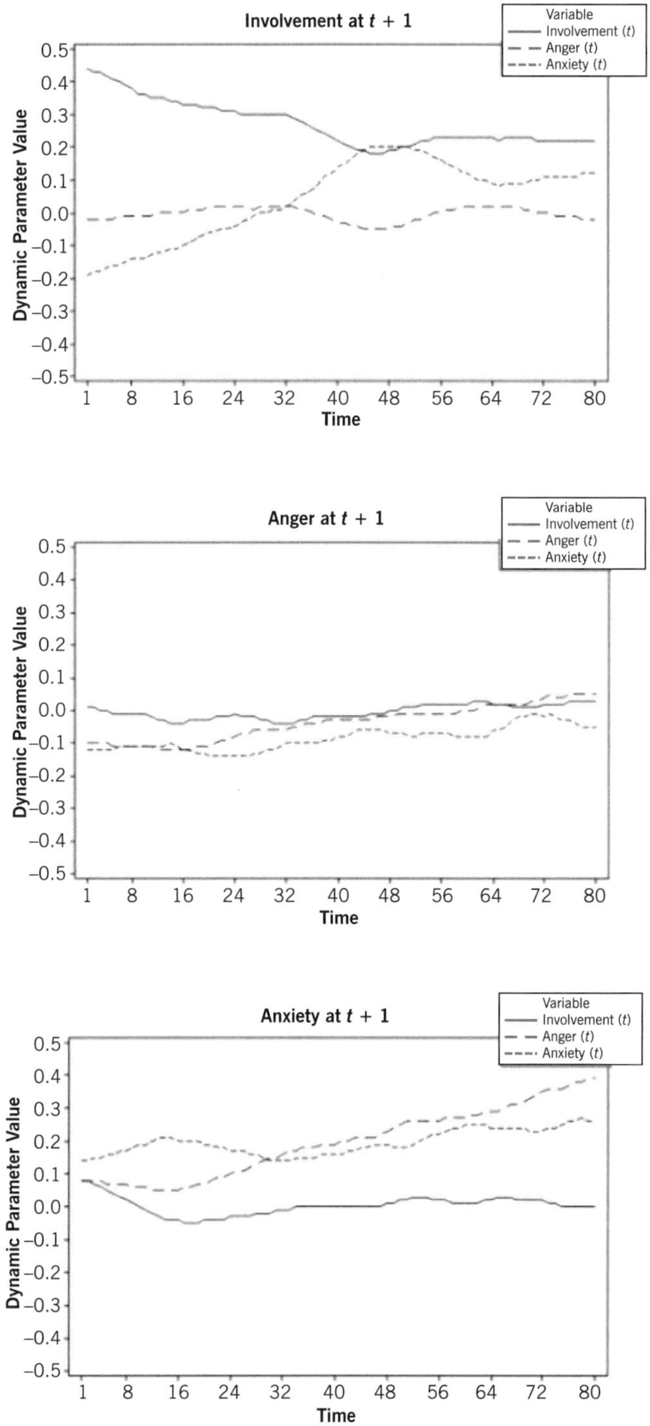

FIGURE 20.1. Graphic representation of the changing dynamic system characterizing the son's emotional reactions to interactions with his father. Lines indicate how the dynamic parameters change over time. The top panel depicts the time-varying contributions of Involvement, Anger, and Anxiety at time (t) to Involvement at time ($t + 1$). The middle panel depicts the contributions of the same to Anger at ($t + 1$), and the bottom panel depicts the contributions to Anxiety at ($t + 1$).

obey exactly the same dynamic model describing the process. Developmental processes generally are not stationary and hence are not ergodic. This implies that in order to obtain valid information about developmental processes, their analysis has to be based on intraindividual variation.

We are also conducting research on an exciting and powerful extension of dynamic factor modeling of intraindividual variation, namely computational optimal control. This extension has great potential for applied and theoretical work, in which it can be used to steer developmental processes in desired directions. It also involves a strong test of causality in that manipulating a time-varying covariate process will be effective only if it has a causal relationship with the state process under consideration. At present the combination of dynamic factor analysis of nonstationary processes and computational optimal control is successfully applied to patient-specific treatment in real time of diabetes type 1 (Zhou et al., 2010).

Since the first publication on dynamic factor analysis 25 years ago (Molenaar, 1985), progress has been slow but steady. Dynamic factor analysis of intraindividual variation has recently been recognized as the most complete methodology compatible with person-oriented approaches to developmental process analysis (Molenaar, 2010; Sterba & Bauer, 2010). This recognition will further induce progress in dynamic factor analysis, especially in the field of developmental psychopathology. In addition, importantly, the implications of ergodic theory will provide an enduring boost to this progress in that it stipulates that for the analysis of nonergodic processes such as developmental processes only intraindividual variation provides a valid source of information. This does not imply that the final goal of psychological science—to obtain nomothetic laws about psychological processes—has been left behind. It implies only that for nonergodic processes this goal has to be reached in a different methodological way, starting with dedicated analysis of intraindividual variation and then pooling in appropriate ways across results obtained in replicated time series designs. For nonergodic processes such as developmental processes, this will yield nomothetic laws about intraindividual variation and change.

References

Birkhoff, G. (1931). Proof of the ergodic theorem. *Proceedings of the National Academy of Sciences of the USA, 17,* 656–660.

Brainerd, C. J. (1978). The stage question in cognitive developmental theory. *Behavioral and Brain Sciences, 2,* 173–213.

Brillinger, D. R. (1975). *Time series: Data analysis and theory.* San Francisco: Holden-Day.

Browne, M. W., & Nesselroade, J. R. (2005). Representing psychological processes with dynamic factor models: Some promising uses and extensions of ARMA time series models. In A. Maydeu-Olivares & J. J. McArdle (Eds.), *Modern psychometrics: A festschrift to Roderick P. McDonald* (pp. 409–447). Mahwah, NJ: Erlbaum.

Browne, M. W., & Zhang, G. (2005). User's guide: DyFa: Dynamic factor analysis of lagged correlation matrices, version 2.03. Available at *quantrm2.psy.ohio-state.edu/browne/.*

Browne, M. W., & Zhang, G. (2007). Developments in the factor analysis of individual time series. In R. Cudeck & R. C. MacCallum (Eds.), *Factor analysis at 100: Historical developments and future directions* (pp. 265–292). Mahwah, NJ: Erlbaum.

Cattell, R. B. (1952). The three basic factor-analytic designs: Their interrelations and derivatives. *Psychological Bulletin, 49,* 499–520.

Chow, S.-M., Hamagami, F., & Nesselroade, J. R. (2008). Age differences in dynamical emotion–cognition linkages. *Psychology and Aging, 22*(4), 765–780.

Danziger, K. (1990). *Constructing the subject: Historical origins of psychological research*. Cambridge, UK: Cambridge University Press.

Ferrer, E. (2006). Application of dynamic factor analysis to affective processes in dyads. In A. Ong & M. van Dulmen (Eds.), *Handbook of methods in positive psychology* (pp. 41–58). Oxford, UK: Oxford University Press.

Ferrer, E., & Nesselroade, J. R. (2003). Modeling affective processes in dyadic relations via dynamic factor analysis. *Emotion, 3*, 344–360.

Ford, D. H., & Lerner, R. M. (1992). *Developmental systems theory: An integrative approach*. Thousand Oaks, CA: Sage.

Gottlieb, G. (1992). *Individual development and evolution: The genesis of novel behavior*. New York: Oxford University Press.

Grasman, R. P. P., Huizenga, H. M., Waldorp, L. J., Böcker, K. B. E., & Molenaar, P. C. M. (2005). Stochastic maximum likelihood mean and cross-spectrum modeling in neuron–magnetic source estimation. *Digital Signal Processing, 15*, 56–72.

Hamaker, E. J., Dolan, C. V., & Molenaar, P. C. M. (2005). Statistical modeling of the individual: Rationale and application of multivariate stationary time series analysis. *Multivariate Behavioral Research, 40*, 207–233.

Hamaker, E. J., Nesselroade, J. R., & Molenaar, P. C. M. (2007). The integrated state-space model. *Journal of Research in Personality, 41*, 295–315.

Hamaker, E. J., Zhang, Z., & van der Maas, H. L. J. (2009). Using threshold autoregressive models to study dyadic interactions. *Psychometrika, 74*, 727–745.

Hannan, E. J., & Deistler, M. (1987). *The statistical theory of linear systems*. New York: Wiley.

Harvey, A. C. (1989). *Forecasting, structural time series models and the Kalman filter*. Cambridge, UK: Cambridge University Press.

Jansen, B. R. J., & van der Maas, H. L. J. (2001). Evidence for the phase transition from rule I to rule II on the balance scale task. *Developmental Review, 21*, 450–494.

Jansen, B. R. J., & van der Maas, H. L. J. (2002). The development of children's rule use on the balance scale task. *Journal of Experimental Child Psychology, 81*, 383–416.

Kan, K. J., Ploeger, A., Raijmakers, M. E., Dolan, C. V., & van der Maas, H. L. (2010). Nonlinear epigenetic variance: Review and simulations. *Developmental Science, 13*, 11–27.

Kelderman, H., & Molenaar, P. C. M. (2007). The effect of individual differences in factor loadings on the standard factor model. *Multivariate Behavioral Research, 42*, 435–456.

Kim, J., Zhu, W., Chang, L., Bentler, P. M., & Ernst, T. (2007). Unified structural equation modeling approach for the analysis of multisubject, multivariate functional MRI data. *Human Brain Mapping, 28*, 85–93.

Krengel, U. (1985). *Ergodic theorems*. Berlin: de Gruyter.

Lamiell, J. T. (2003). *Beyond individual and group differences: Human individuality, scientific psychology, and William Stern's critical personalism*. Thousand Oaks, CA: Sage.

McLachlan, J. C. (1999). Developmental morphologies not directly specified by the genome of the individual. In M. A. J. Chaplain, G. D. Singh, & J. C. McLachlan (Eds.), *On growth and form: Spatio-temporal pattern formation in biology* (pp. 157–172). Chichester, UK: Wiley.

Meinhardt, H. (1982). *Models of biological pattern formation*. London: Academic Press.

Molenaar, P. C. M. (1985). A dynamic factor model for the analysis of multivariate time series. *Psychometrika, 50*, 181–202.

Molenaar, P. C. M. (1986a). Issues with a rule-sampling theory of conservation learning from a structuralist point of view. *Human Development, 29*, 137–144.

Molenaar, P. C. M. (1986b). On the impossibility of acquiring more powerful structures: A neglected alternative. *Human Development, 29*, 245–251.

Molenaar, P. C. M. (1987). Dynamic factor analysis in the frequency domain: Causal modeling of multivariate psychophysiological time series. *Multivariate Behavioral Research, 22*, 329–353.

Molenaar, P. C. M. (1994). Dynamic latent variable models in developmental psychology. In A. von Eye & C. C. Clogg (Eds.), *Analysis of latent variables in developmental research* (pp. 155–180). Newbury Park, CA: Sage.

Molenaar, P. C. M. (1997). Time series analysis and its relationship with longitudinal analysis. *International Journal of Sports Medicine, 18*, 232–237.

Molenaar, P. C. M. (1999). Longitudinal analysis. In H. J. Ader & G. J. Mellenbergh (Eds.), *Research methodology in the social, behavioral and life sciences* (pp. 143–167). London: Sage.

Molenaar, P. C. M. (2004). A manifesto on psychology as idiographic science: Bringing the person back into scientific psychology, this time forever. *Measurement, 2*, 201–218.

Molenaar, P. C. M. (2007). On the implications of the classical ergodic theorems: Analysis of developmental processes has to focus on intra-individual variation. *Developmental Psychobiology, 50*, 60–69.

Molenaar, P. C. M. (2010). Testing all six person-oriented principles in dynamic factor analysis. *Development and Psychopathology, 22*, 255–259.

Molenaar, P. C. M., Boomsma, D. I., & Dolan, C. V. (1993). A third source of developmental differences. *Behavior Genetics, 23*, 519–524.

Molenaar, P. C. M., Huizenga, H. M., & Nesselroade, J. R. (2003). The relationship between the structure of interindividual and intraindividual variation: A theoretical and empirical vindication of developmental systems theory. In U. M. Staudinger & U. Lindenberger (Eds.), *Understanding human development: Dialogues with lifespan psychology* (pp. 339–360). Dordrecht, The Netherlands: Kluwer Academic.

Molenaar, P. C. M., & Nesselroade, J. R. (2001). Rotation in the dynamic factor modeling of multivariate stationary time series. *Psychometrika, 66*, 99–107.

Molenaar, P. C. M., & Nesselroade, J. R. (2009). The recoverability of P-technique factor analysis. *Multivariate Behavioral Research, 44*, 130–141.

Molenaar, P. C. M., & Newell, K. M. (2010). *Individual pathways of change: Statistical models for analyzing learning and development*. Washington, DC: American Psychological Association.

Molenaar, P. C. M., & Raijmakers, M. E. J. (1999). Additional aspects of third source variation for the genetic analysis of human development and behavior: A commentary on Eaves et al. *Twin Research, 2*, 49–52.

Molenaar, P. C. M., Sinclair, K. O., Rovine, M. J., Ram, N., & Corneal, S. E. (2009). Analyzing developmental processes on an individual level using non-stationary time series modeling. *Developmental Psychology, 45*, 260–271.

Mumma, G. H. (2004). Validation of idiosyncratic cognitive schema in cognitive case formulations: An intraindividual idiographic approach. *Psychological Assessment, 16*, 211–230.

Nesselroade, J. R., McArdle, J. J., Aggen, S. H., & Meyers, J. M. (2002). Dynamic factor analysis models for representing process in multivariate time series. In D. S. Moskowitz & S. L. Hershberger (Eds.), *Modeling intraindividual variability with repeated measures data: Methods and applications* (pp. 235–265). Mahwah, NJ: Erlbaum.

Priestley, M. B. (1988). *Nonlinear and nonstationary time series analysis*. New York: Academic Press.

Raijmakers, M. E. J., & Molenaar, P. C. M. (2004). Modeling developmental transitions in adaptive resonance theory. *Developmental Science, 7*, 149–157.

Rovine, M. J., Molenaar, P. C. M., & Corneal, S. E. (1999). Analysis of emotional response patterns for adolescent stepsons using P-technique factor analysis. In R. K. Silbereisen & A. von Eye (Eds.), *Growing up in times of social change* (pp. 261–285). Berlin: de Gruyter.

Sbarra, D. A., & Ferrer, E. (2006). The structure and process of emotional experience following nonmarital relationship dissolution: Dynamic factor analysis of love, anger, and sadness. *Emotion, 6*, 224–238.

Shifren, K., Hooker, K., Wood, P., & Nesselroade, J. R. (1997). Structure and variation of mood in individuals with Parkinson's disease: A dynamic factor analysis. *Psychology and Aging, 12*, 328–339.

Sidman, M. (1960). *Tactics of scientific research: Evaluating experimental data in psychology*. New York: Basic Books.

Spencer, J. P., Thomas, M. S. C., & McClelland, J. L. (Eds.). (2009). *Toward a unified theory of development: Connectionism and dynamic systems theory reconsidered*. Oxford, UK: Oxford University Press.

Sterba, S. K., & Bauer, D. J. (2010). Matching method with theory in person-oriented developmental psychopathology research. *Development and Psychopathology, 22*, 239–254.

van der Maas, H. L. J., & Molenaar, P. C. M. (1992). Stagewise cognitive development: An application of catastrophe theory. *Psychological Review, 99*, 395–417.

Wagenmakers, E. J., Molenaar, P. C. M., Grasman, R. P. P., Hartelman, P. A. I., & van der Maas, H. L. J. (2005). Transformation invariant stochastic catastrophe theory. *Physica D: Nonlinear Phenomena, 211*, 263–276.

Weber, E. J. M., Molenaar, P. C. M., & van der Molen, M. W. (1992). A nonstationarity test for the spectral analysis of heart rate variability with an application to respiratory sinus arrhythmia. *Psychophysiology, 29*, 55–65.

Wohlwill, J. F. (1973). *The study of behavioral development*. New York: Academic Press.

Wood, P., & Brown, D. (1994). The study of intra-individual differences by means of dynamic factor models: Rationale, implementation, and interpretation. *Psychological Bulletin, 116*, 166–186.

Zhou, J., Wang, Q., Molenaar, P. C. M., Ulbrecht, J., Gold, C., & Rovine, M. J. (2010, June–July). *Closed-loop control of type 1 diabetic patients based on a data-driven state-space model*. Paper presented at the American Control Conference, Baltimore.

CHAPTER 21

P-Technique Factor Analysis

IHNO A. LEE
TODD D. LITTLE

Central Issues

People are complex. Our attitudes and behaviors are inconsistent, varying from one situation to the next; they collide with one another and are expressed depending on our immediate context (Corey, 1937; Wicker, 1969). Internal and external forces, such as personality, perceived control, the social environment, subjective norms, and the like, influence our attitudes and behaviors and how they change on a moment-to-moment basis (Ajzen, 1991; Shoda, Mischel, & Wright, 1994). At the individual level, within-person (i.e., intraindividual) variability is an index of how consistent (or inconsistent) an individual is when measured repeatedly and intensively (e.g., > 20 occasions) over time. How to best analyze and model such intraindividual change processes is the focus of this chapter.

Nesselroade and Ram (2004) suggest a taxonomy of intraindividual change that is differentiated by the extent to which change effects are fixed versus reversible or malleable—that is, those that may or may not be reversible (e.g., development, learning) and those that are more transient states (e.g., mood). Regardless of the nature of change, research across multiple domains (e.g., mood and emotion, personality, cognitive performance) has shown that reliable, systematic patterns of variability exist within an individual (Hooker, 1991; Siegler, 1994; Zevon & Tellegen, 1982).

The study of intraindividual variability is represented as one dimension of Cattell's (1952) data box, a three-dimensional depiction of the person, variable, and occasion characteristics of data samples. Analyses of intraindividual variability are based on relationships across time (variables by occasions) for one person, which is represented by a horizontal "P," or person, slice of the box. As such, P-technique factor analysis (Cattell, 1963; Cattell, Cattell, & Rhymer, 1947) is the corresponding multivariate method that targets these within-person change processes. By measuring an individual repeatedly, we can construct a more complete picture of his or her behavior with reference to previous life experiences (temporal context), environment and surrounding circumstances (spatial context), and interactions with others (person context).

Other occasion-specific analyses utilize vertical "S" and "T" slices, incorporating both person and occasion dimensions but from different perspectives. S-technique focuses on person clustering based on growth patterns (persons by occasions), whereas T-technique focuses on time-dependent clusters based on larger samples (occasions by persons). The standard method of factor analysis, formally R-technique, assesses cross-sectional data (variables by persons), represented by the vertical "R" slice.

The study of intraindividual change targets the behavior of a given individual. Like time-series analysis, P-technique utilizes repeated observations of a participant to make inferences about the relations among a set of variables. In other words, this method allows for large-sample, multivariate inferential tools to be utilized on the repeated observations provided by an individual, a small set of individuals, or even a larger sample (with all individuals intensively measured). P-technique can be contrasted with growth curve modeling, which is the study of interindividual differences in intraindividual change. Growth curve modeling requires larger samples (e.g., > 80 participants) and typically uses only a smallish set of observations (e.g., 3–7) per individual. Whereas large-sample methods are based on the combination of within-person and between-person change, P-technique targets the number of within-person observations to make inferences about the person.

Conceptual Principles and Statistical Assumptions

In the following section, we discuss the issues and assumptions that underlie the class of procedures used to analyze P-technique data. Some of these issues are specific to a particular analysis technique, whereas most are applicable to the class of techniques used for such data.

Single-Subject Designs

Cross-sectional studies are not suited to studying change, because they can capture processes only at a single point in time. Results are representative of only one occasion and under a specific set of circumstances. Whereas cross-sectional designs treat each individual as a "case" or unit of study, single-subject designs treat each time point within an individual as a single unit. For instance, these designs can address whether an individual's observed fluctuations in stress over a long period (e.g., 90 days) are representative of his or her general change patterns. Precise knowledge about individual processes, which is sacrificed in group designs, can be obtained.

Obtaining this person-level precision requires a trade-off in generalizability. Results gathered are specific to the individual; they may not generalize to others or represent the average tendencies of a larger group. Within a typical single-subject design, we cannot examine the individual in a broader context; that is, we cannot address the extent to which an individual is similar to or different from others.

This individual-versus-group trade-off, however, may be circumvented in some situations. One solution is to examine a small representative sample of individuals and, by conducting a multiple group analysis (in which each individual is treated as a "group"), evaluate the extent to which each person's change pattern is different from another's. However, this multiple group instantiation assumes that the set of individuals represents the entire population of interest (or a fixed set of the population). Alternatively, in using the capabilities of multilevel structural equation modeling (SEM), the set of individuals can represent a random sample from a larger pool to which we can generalize.

Another approach is chained P-technique, which utilizes a larger data set consisting of observations pooled across many individuals. Data from each of i individuals are stacked or "chained" to create a larger data set with a sample size of N (i*o_i; where i is the number of individuals and o_i is the number of observations on each individual). This pooling of data allows one to examine intraindividual processes within a group context—modeling the average intraindividual change, as well as how these trends differ from person to person. For example, studies have shown that mood fluctuation is entrained to the weekly calendar; individuals report lower levels of positive mood on Mondays and higher levels on weekends (Larsen & Kasimatis, 1990). By stacking data from many individuals, we can draw nomothetic conclusions about the average intraindividual change in day-to-day mood. This approach assumes that the change process is shared by all individuals.

Classical P-Technique

After many decades, classical P-technique factor analysis is still a viable method, under certain circumstances, for analyzing multivariate time series data. Its appeal may be due to its simplicity, as well as the commonsense notion that any process is best evaluated via intensive repeated measurements of multiple indicators (Molenaar & Nesselroade, 2009). As Bereiter (1963) stated, P-technique analysis is "the logical way to study change." This analysis is essentially a longitudinal factor analysis, applying the common factor model to the variance–covariance matrix of an individual's multivariate time series data. P-technique models examine the "correlation of occasions" (Cattell et al., 1947, p. 267), or how strongly an individual's standing on X is related to his or her standing on Y across many consecutive occasions. For example, during occasions on which a person is very anxious (i.e., has high anxiety scores), he or she could also be experiencing more stress (i.e., having concurrently high stress scores).

The distinctive feature of classical P-technique is acquiring an individual's scores from multiple items of a single construct across many time points. Many other time series procedures are not multivariate (in the sense that the underlying latent constructs are measured using multiple indicators), whereas P-technique is explicitly a latent variable approach to modeling time series data. For example, scores from three positive items (e.g., happy, cheerful, great) and three negative items (e.g., sad, down, unhappy) are collected over a span of 365 days. The resulting data structure will be a matrix of 365 rows (with day as the unit of measurement) by 6 columns, with each row corresponding to one measurement occasion and each column representing one item. The data set to be analyzed has repeated measurements of positive and negative items nested within a single person. From this data matrix, a 2-factor model of positive and negative affect can be fit (see Figure 21.1).

The classical P-technique factor model has two serious limitations. First, the application of the common factor model to time series data does not explicitly account for the time-dependent nature of the factors. The P-technique model assumes that the construct at time t influences the observed variables only at time t; in other words, it does not allow for any lagged or carryover effects in which prior factor levels can influence current observed scores. This limitation is a serious obstacle to modeling change processes. In studying mood fluctuation, for example, we would expect that yesterday's negative affect levels would carry over and exert some influence on today's affect.

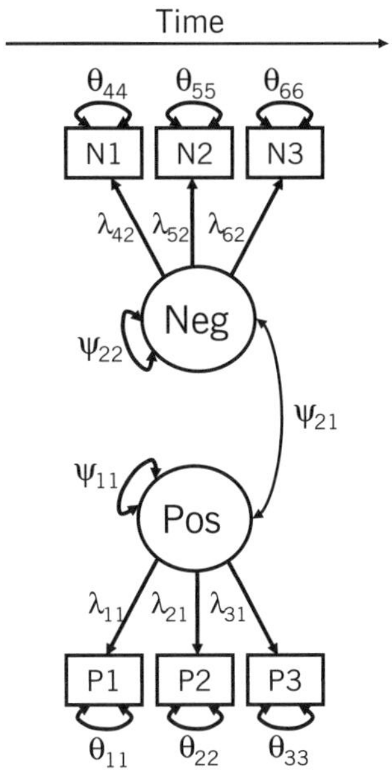

FIGURE 21.1. Classical P-technique factor analysis model of positive and negative affect.

A recent simulation study by Molenaar and Nesselroade (2009), however, demonstrated that classical P-technique analyses can recover parameters of dynamic processes (i.e., loadings and residuals of a construct's indicators) quite closely when these processes are restricted to the latent space. They advocated the utility of P-technique analyses as a way of quickly approximating the outcomes to be obtained from more complex, time-consuming methods (e.g., state-space models).

Second, classical P-technique models implicitly specify that the nature of the construct remains constant by assuming that factor loadings are invariant across time. The factor is assumed to influence the observed variables in the same way and to the same degree at all times, from day 1 through day 100 of a study. This assumption may not be reasonable if the factor structures are changing over time.

Dynamic Models

In addition to modeling concurrent relationships, dynamic models can examine the (lagged) relationships between variables that are separated in time. The same variable, measured on multiple occasions, will likely correlate with itself at a later time point. One's current standing may be predicted by yesterday's standing and, in turn, will reliably predict tomorrow's standing. Given this temporal sequence, we can make stronger claims about causality; logically, scores at a given time point (t) can influence only subsequent scores (time $t + 1$ or $t + 2$).

Lagging variables allows us to model these time-dependent structures. Creating lagged variables is accomplished by incorporating lags, or time-lapsed intervals, into the original data set; that is, values from a subsequent time point ($t + 1$) are inserted into the same row as those from the initial standing (time t). Variables measured at time t now represent lag

TABLE 21.1. Data Matrix with Lagged *X* and *Y* Variables

Time	X_t	X_{t+1}	Y_t	Y_{t+1}
.	—	x_{t1}	—	y_{t1}
1	x_{t1}	x_{t2}	y_{t1}	y_{t2}
2	x_{t2}	x_{t3}	y_{t2}	y_{t3}
3	x_{t3}	x_{t4}	y_{t3}	y_{t4}
...	...	...	...	...
99	x_{t99}	x_{t100}	y_{t99}	y_{t100}
100	x_{t100}	—	y_{t100}	—

0, whereas those measured at time $t + 1$ represent lag 1. The resulting data set has a wide-format structure, and the correlation between a variable X at adjacent time points, time t and time $t + 1$, can be calculated. See Table 21.1 for an example of a lagged data matrix for variables X and Y.

These lagged associations are summarized in a block-Toeplitz variance–covariance matrix, which includes the variances and covariances within and across lags. Figure 21.2 depicts a lagged covariance matrix of nine variables (with three variables indicating each of three constructs) at their initial standing (lag 0) and at two subsequent time points (lags 1 and 2). The within-lag relationships for lags 0, 1, and 2 are found within symmetric triangles (C) in the top left corner, middle portion, and bottom right corner of the matrix;

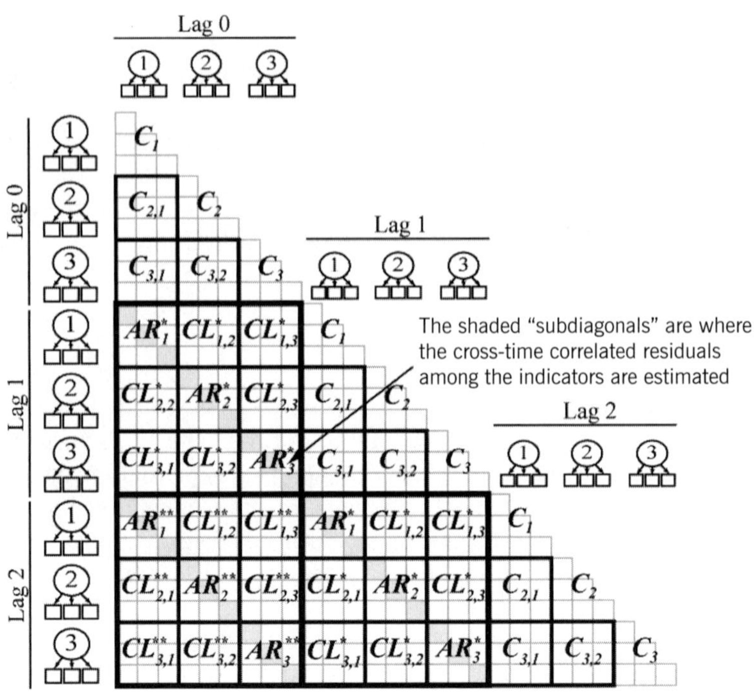

FIGURE 21.2. Block–Toeplitz matrix of variances and covariances (from nine variables, indicating three constructs) within and across two lags.

these values also appear in a regular variance–covariance matrix. The asymmetric, square portions of the matrix that cross lag 0 with lag 1 and lag 1 with lag 2 include the cross-lagged (CL) and autoregressive (AR) relationships; these square regions carry the same information because they represent one lag of separation. The CL relationships, depicted on the off-diagonals, show the association between different variables from one time point to another (e.g., scores on X at lag 0 with scores on Y at lag 1). Autoregressive correlations (i.e., covariances) are on the diagonal, which represents the association between scores (on the same variable) adjacent in time. The bottom left square of this matrix represents the two-lag interval between lag 0 and lag 2.

Dynamic factor analysis models explicitly represent these lags in the relations between the factors and manifest variables. Lags can be modeled directly or indirectly, so that their influence is exerted on the observed scores or on the factors themselves. The white noise factor score model (Molenaar, 1985) and the direct autoregressive factor score model (McArdle, 1982) are two well-established models that represent these autoregressive relationships; however, the mechanisms by which the factors influence the variables are quite different.

Direct Autoregressive Factor Score Model

The direct autoregressive factor score (DAFS) model was first used as an SEM and fit to psychological data by McArdle (1982). This model defines the mechanism of change at the latent level, where lagged influences travel via latent factors and affect observed scores indirectly. As in classical P-technique models, factors influence their corresponding items concurrently and in the same manner; in other words, the factor loading structure is invariant across time.

Lagged effects, or the amount of influence from prior factor levels, are transmitted through the autocorrelation of factors. The effect of previous levels of factor Y (at time $t-1$) on observed variables Y_1 and Y_2 is mediated by current levels of factor Y (at time t), as well as the amount of time elapsed (or number of lags). In other words, current Y_1 and Y_2 scores are affected by previous levels of factor Y to the extent that that current factor's (Y) scores are affected. Given a steady change process (i.e., simplex structure), the effect will be transmitted at a constant rate from one occasion to the next. If the amount of influence (or regression weight) is 0.5, for instance, the effect of Y at time $t-1$ would be diminished by 0.5; in turn, the effect of Y at time t would decrease further by 0.5 over the next interval. The effects of Y over two lags would be represented by a weighting of 0.25 (i.e., 0.5×0.5). Though it is possible for factor Y to directly influence factor scores at time $t+2$ (bypassing one interval), lagged effects that skip one or more time points are not very common. This model is easily expanded to include multivariate outcomes, in which previous levels of factor X can influence subsequent observed scores in Y, via factor Y. Figure 21.3a depicts the DAFS model.

In addition to the autocorrelation of factors, DAFS models specify an autocorrelation between an item's residual variances across all occasions. Because the same item appears at time 1, time 2, through time t, there is also a shared component that is due to the item itself and not to the latent factor. Regardless of the amount of time elapsed, this item-specific component will be consistent throughout the duration of study; thus all residual covariances can be constrained to equality when they are separated by the same time interval (e.g., residual correlations between lag 0 and lag 1 would be equal to their corresponding correlations between lag 1 and lag 2).

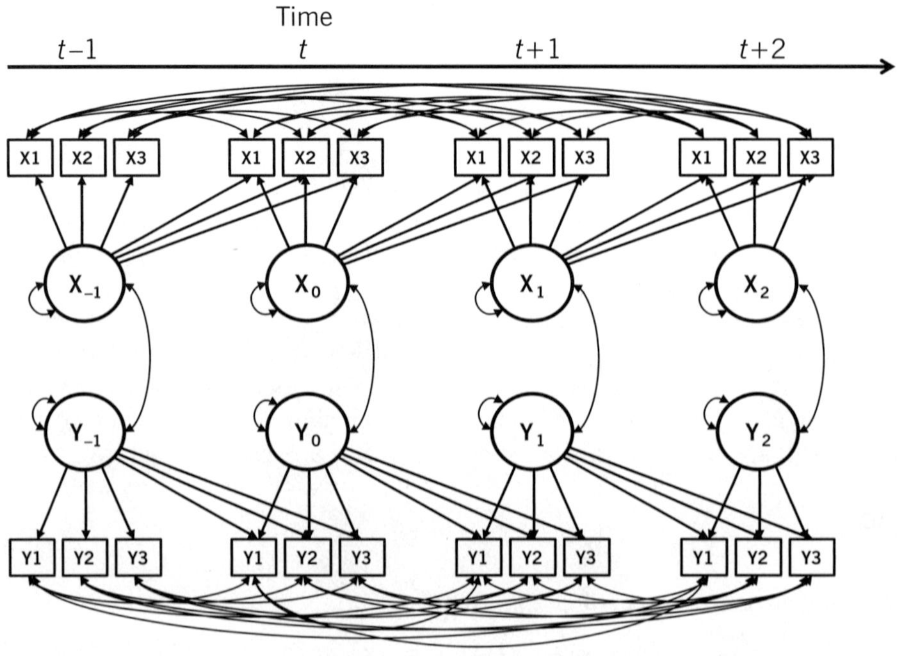

FIGURE 21.3a. Direct autoregressive factor score (DAFS) model. This figure depicts only one lag, though if given sufficient justification, two or more lags may be included.

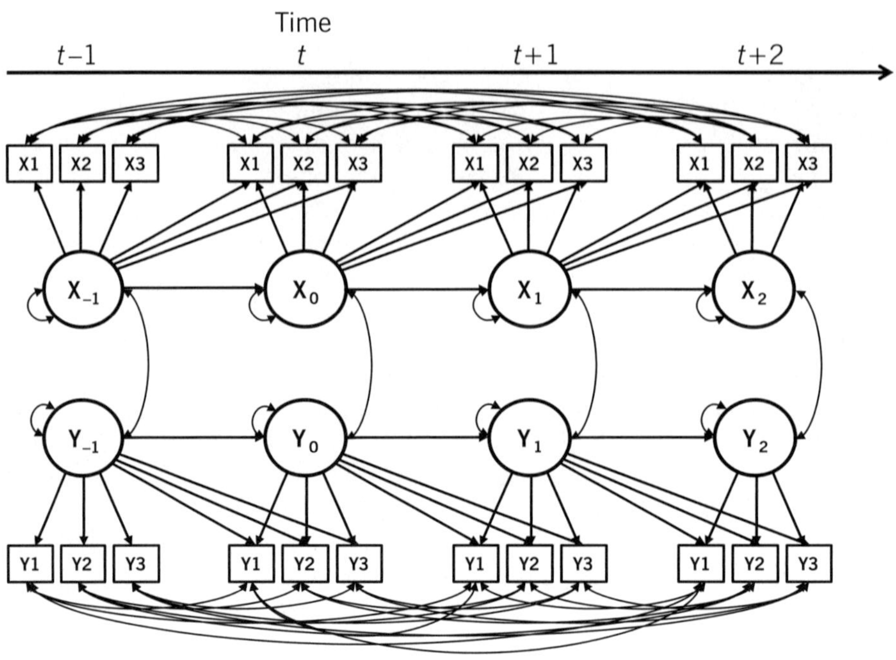

FIGURE 21.3b. White noise factor score (WNFS) model. This figure depicts only one lag, though, if given sufficient justification, two or more lags may be included.

White Noise Factor Score Model

Molenaar (1985) proposed an alternative dynamic factor model in which change is modeled from uncorrelated day-to-day factor scores. Renamed the white noise factor score (WNFS) model by Nesselroade, McArdle, Aggen, and Meyers (2002), this model specifies that all day-to-day blips or shocks that drive the system are determined independently from one another, or behave as a "white noise" series. As shown in Figure 21.3b, observed scores are directly influenced by three sources: current factor scores, previous factor scores, and current residual variances.

The influence of prior factor scores is transmitted via lagged factor loadings, the magnitude of which differs as a function of time; for instance, the effect of Y at $t-3$ on current Y_1 and Y_2 observed scores is likely to be weaker (i.e., represented by smaller factor loadings) than the effect of Y at $t-1$. As in the DAFS model, all within-lag factor scores, as well as an item's residual variance across time, are correlated. Correlated residuals of each observed variable are constrained to equality when separated by the same time interval.

Although both DAFS and WNFS models represent a dynamic process over time, the mechanisms driving each model are quite different in terms of how the factors relate to and influence the observed variables. The differences between the two models are illustrated in the following example, in which distress is the underlying latent factor that influences two indicators, cortisol level (a stress-related hormone) and self-reported stress level, measured over a period of hours. According to the DAFS model, cortisol and self-reported stress levels directly depend on an individual's current distress. Similarly, cortisol and self-reported stress measured 3 hours ago were directly dependent on the state of distress at that time, and in the same manner in which current levels relate to the current distress. In contrast, the WNFS model specifies that current cortisol levels and self-reported stress directly depend on the current state of distress, as well as previous distress (from 1 hour ago).

Suppose that the individual exercised 30 minutes ago and was able to alleviate some stress; as a result, the relationship between previous and current distress is attenuated. The WNFS model specification allows for previous distress to have some lingering influence on cortisol level, self-reported stress, or both. If, after exercising, cortisol and self-reported stress levels return to baseline at different rates, then this difference in recovery can be captured by the WNFS model. In contrast, the DAFS model is more restricted in that previous distress can influence cortisol and self-reported stress only in tandem, in an amount inversely proportional to the amount of attenuation.

To reiterate, given an event that disturbs the steady change process, the WNFS model can represent lagged effects with more specificity; this model can differentiate which variables are affected and to what extent by sacrificing a few degrees of freedom. However, if the disruption occurs at the construct level, the flexibility of the WNFS is not as advantageous; the DAFS model is a more parsimonious and preferred representation of the change process. Because factorial invariance is a tested assumption of the DAFS model, one can evaluate the nature of any disruptions to determine statistically which model would be appropriate.

Chained P-Technique

Chained P-technique (Cattell & Scheier, 1961) is a reduced form of the classical and dynamic P-technique data structure. Data from each of i individuals are stacked or "chained" to create a larger data set with a sample size of N (i*o_i; where i is the number of individuals and

o_i is the number of observations on each individual). By pooling individual data, chained P-technique analyses can borrow information from a larger subset and examine the individual within a broader group context. Furthermore, interindividual differences in intraindividual change, or how much within-person processes (e.g., mood fluctuation) vary from person to person, can be addressed with modern (multilevel) analysis approaches.

This pooling of data across individuals requires an assumption of structural equivalency (Molenaar, 2004). We must assume that all temporal relationships, the association between *X* at time 1 and *X* at time 2 (or any lagged relationships), are the same for all individuals. If this assumption is upheld, the aggregation of individual data will not distort the intraindividual relationships. In other words, the sample is ergodic; average relationships across the sample are representative of all relationships at the individual level. Conversely, the relationships within each individual also generalize to the larger group. We expect, however, that individuals may change in different ways and at different rates from one another. If this is the case, the sample is nonergodic. Pooling data from individuals with qualitatively different structures will distort relationships and should be avoided.

Intraindividual patterns of variability should be tested for similarity (i.e., "poolability") before data are aggregated. Various methods exist in testing for homogeneity of individual covariance matrices. One method utilizes a multiple group approach, in which each person is considered a "group." In brief, an omnibus test of homogeneity is conducted to verify whether one or more variance–covariance matrices differ across the sample. If this initial test is significant, follow-up tests should be implemented to identify which groups (i.e., individuals) differ in structure. Individuals with different patterns of variability should be removed from the sample until a homogeneous subgroup remains. The omnibus test is efficient in verifying homogeneity across the sample. If homogeneity is not met, however, the process of identifying deviant individuals can be somewhat tedious, particularly in larger samples.

A similar method, described by Nesselroade and Molenaar (1999), involves a two-step process to assess the poolability of individual data. First, a lagged covariance matrix for each person is retrieved to examine variability at the individual level. Second, a pooling algorithm compares the lagged relationships across individuals and returns a test statistic, *c*, to evaluate lack of equality. Finally, a test statistic is estimated to examine whether one or more lagged covariance matrices are not equivalent. When matrices are not equivalent, Nesselroade and Molenaar (1999) advocate the use of an elimination algorithm to identify the deviant individual(s). This algorithm eliminates each individual in turn, recalculating an intermediate value of *M* at each iteration, and retains the subsample giving the smallest value of *M*. This process repeats until all deviant individuals are removed and the sample is ergodic. When testing homogeneity among larger samples, this method is preferable to the multiple group approach. See Nesselroade and Molenaar for technical details of the elimination algorithm.

This assumption of homogeneity should not be taken lightly and may be difficult to meet, particularly with regard to intraindividual processes. A study of cognitive performance showed that only 10 of 31 individual data structures met the test of ergodicity (Nesselroade & Molenaar, 1999).

Developmental Applications

Development can be defined as the progression from one state to the next. Within psychology, this progression is viewed in terms of growth or maturation from an earlier stage to a more advanced stage. From a developmental perspective, these changes are characterized by transitions throughout the lifespan, such as moving from childhood to adolescence, or are indicated by milestone events (e.g., getting married). Recent studies have focused on changes occurring later in the lifespan. Hooker (1991) examined the intraindividual variability and stability in self-concept in four adults during the transition to retirement. Analyses of daily self-concept ratings over a 120-day period (prior to and following retirement) identified reliable dimensions of intraindividual change in self-concept (i.e., mental well-being, relation of self to others, competence/mastery) that challenged existing notions of self-concept as a stable construct. P-technique analyses were also used to examine the variability in daily exercise, monitoring of nutrition, and other health-seeking behaviors in older women (Quinn, Johnson, & Martin, 1996), as well as how therapeutic recreation activities positively influence the experiences of older adults residing in nursing homes (Voelkl & Mathieu, 1995).

P-technique models are often utilized in the domain of psychotherapy, in which the focus is on moment-to-moment behaviors, emotions, and experiences of clients (and in some cases therapists) while in therapy. The first P-technique analysis in psychotherapy was conducted by Luborsky (1953), in which biological variables (e.g., glucose levels, blood cell counts), physiological variables (e.g., stomach pains, amount of sleep), and various self-report measures from one client were obtained over 54 sessions. Results from a classical P-technique analysis showed that nine factors (e.g., Submissiveness, Surgency, Emotionality, Fatigue, Cyclothymia) yielded an accurate client profile.

More recently, Russell, Jones, and Miller (2007) reviewed a multitude of P-technique studies to identify the core components of psychotherapeutic processes. These studies examined over 400 clients being treated by 93 therapists across periods ranging from 1 month to 4 years. An utterance, or a full client or therapist statement, was the most frequently used unit of measurement, with an average of 700 utterances collected. Classical and dynamic P-technique analyses of individual utterances within therapy sessions identified several core client and therapist process areas (e.g., client affect, relationships, help seeking, therapist support, and disclosure) that contribute to a positive therapeutic outcome (Asay & Lambert, 1999; Bergin & Garfield, 1994; Essig & Russell, 1990).

Other applications of P-technique extend to cardiovascular activity (Friedman & Santucci, 2003), perceptions of control (Roberts & Nesselroade, 1986), and, in particular, mood fluctuation (Nesselroade & Ford, 1985).

Illustration

Lee and Little (2011) conducted a diary study using experience sampling methods (ESM) to examine systematic patterns of daily mood fluctuation, as well as predictors of this change, over 95 days. Eleven participants responded to questions regarding their moods, current states, and activities several times per day on a Palm Pilot device. To reduce participant burden, a planned missingness design was employed in which participants adhered to a fixed schedule and responded to questions only 4 or 5 days per week.

For this illustration, we fit a dynamic P-technique SEM to one participant's data (selected randomly) to examine the day-to-day effects of anxiety. The anxiety factor was specified using three indicators (e.g., "I feel nervous," "I feel anxious," "I feel worried") from the Inventory of Felt Emotion and Energy in Life (IFEEL) scale (Little, Wanner, & Ryan, 1997). Two lags were incorporated into the data structure to examine any carryover effects—that is, how anxiety on one day could influence anxiety levels over the next 2 days.

Because these data are nested within one individual, equality constraints of corresponding factor loadings and residual variances (i.e., strict factorial invariance) were enforced. Residual variances were correlated across lags.

Results showed that current anxiety reliably predicts tomorrow's anxiety with a standardized regression weight of 0.48, which in turn predicts anxiety levels on the 3rd day (see Figure 21.4). Anxiety exhibited an autoregressive simplex structure; in other words, this individual experienced a steady decrease in anxiety over a 2-day period. A direct relationship between anxiety levels on day 1 and day 3 was tested; however, results showed that anxiety is transmitted at a constant rate from day to day and does not directly predict subsequent levels 2 (or more) days in the future. Model fit was excellent ($\chi^2_{(32, N=95)} = 34.64$; RMSEA = $.027_{(.000; .083)}$; NNFI = .990; CFI = .991).

Future Directions

P-technique factor analysis remains an effective method of modeling intraindividual change. This method is best utilized when modeling stable constructs that are qualitatively consistent over time (e.g., positive affect, reading comprehension) and exhibit a steady change process. DAFS models are most appropriate when these change processes occur entirely in the latent space. Alternatively, WNFS models are more flexible and can represent lagged influences that are exerted directly on manifest variables.

The P-technique models described thus far assume that the factor loadings and covariances are constant across time. By implication, the definition of the construct is fixed, and all observed changes influence the magnitude of factor levels and not the nature of the factor itself. Development, by definition, is dynamic and nonstationary (i.e., exhibiting nonconstant mean and variance properties). Parameters (e.g., regression coefficients) are likely to vary across occasions; for instance, the autoregressive relationship of X at time 1 and time 2 may differ from that of X at time 9 and time 10. These nonstationary processes may be represented more effectively within other modeling frameworks.

Rausch (2009) introduced the time-varying factor structure (TIFS) model an extension of P-technique, as a way of representing nonstationary processes. The TIFS model utilizes a two-stage approach, in which classical P-technique models are initially fit to a series of smaller intervals (i.e., windows) of time; fitting a sequence of models generates

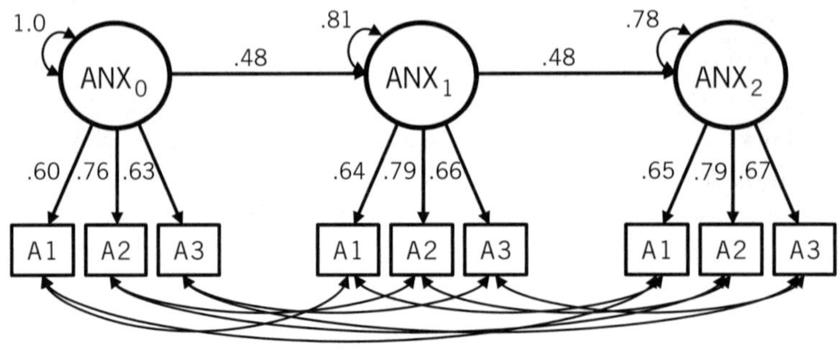

FIGURE 21.4. Dynamic P-technique model of anxiety with two lags. Residual variance estimates are not displayed.

multiple estimates, which may vary across intervals. Then latent growth curve models (with a polynomial trajectory) are fit to these windowed estimates to capture the variability across time. By allowing the factor loadings and covariances to change, this model allows for shifts (or development) in the nature of the construct. In an applied example, Rausch (2009) showed how the relationship between mood factors changes over time. The negative correlation between positive and negative affect increased from –.10 to approximately –1.0 over 40 windows (or 160 measurement occasions); this change in correlation is substantial (i.e., with a significant –.91 slope parameter; see Rausch, 2009). Note that factor scores (representing the within-person values of the construct) are not comparable across constructs with time-varying factor loadings due to the change in definition of the construct.

Advanced modeling techniques appropriate for nonstationary time series processes are still being explored. A recent study by Molenaar, Sinclair, Rovine, Ram, and Corneal (2009) elaborated on multivariate state-space techniques and introduced the extended Kalman filter with iteration and smoothing (EKFIS) as a method of estimating time-varying parameters. An application of the EKFIS technique was demonstrated, in which the emotional reactions (e.g., anger, involvement, anxiety) of two father-and-son pairs were estimated over a period of 6–8 weeks. The strength and direction of some factor relationships were found to differ according to the time of observation. Results from one father–son pair showed that the once-strong relationship between anger and involvement decreased toward the end of the observation period. Results from the second father–son pair showed a directional change in the association between involvement and anxiety, in which the regression coefficients changed from –.19 to .12 across the observation period.

These techniques may be applied to other research areas as well. A related study by Molenaar (2010) applied similar techniques to the modeling of phenotypic data from monozygotic and dizygotic twin pairs. The standard longitudinal genetic factor model (ACE) was transformed and adapted to the individual, with a focus on capturing intraindividual variation. The resulting iFACE model, a combination of the idiographic filter (iF) and the standard genetic factor model (ACE), allows for nonstationary change processes (e.g., heterogeneity of variance) and was found to perform well when fit to simulated phenotypic data.

The models previously described can represent only rates of change, how quickly factor levels change from one occasion to the next. Continuous time models, another class of analyses appropriate for modeling intraindividual processes, can examine how rates of change may be changing (i.e., accelerating) in a given system (or set of connected variables). The damped linear oscillator is one such model that specifies, via differential equations, how changes in acceleration are influenced by a system's equilibrium and velocity (Boker & Nesselroade, 2002). Instead of modeling observed values for each individual, the damped oscillator uses measurements of displacement from a baseline state (i.e., equilibrium), as well as its first and second derivatives; thus this model retains a sense of history of how a system behaves, so that recent activity can inform current change processes. Applications of this model extend to the areas of self-regulation and mood, in which current levels and rates of change are used to inform and adjust future states.

Acknowledgments

We would like to express our gratitude for the feedback and comments of our colleagues in the Center for Research Methods and Data Analysis (Todd D. Little, Director) at the University of Kansas.

This research was supported in part by a National Institutes of Health grant to the University of Kansas through the Mental Retardation and Developmental Disabilities Research Center (No. 5 P30 HD002528) and by various grants associated with the Center for Research Methods and Data Analysis at the University of Kansas (*www.CRMDA.KU.EDU*).

References

Ajzen, I. (1991). The theory of planned behavior. *Organizational Behavior and Human Decision Processes, 50*, 179–211.

Asay, T. P., & Lambert, M. J. (1999). The empirical case for the common factors in therapy: Quantitative findings. In B. L. Duncan, M. A. Hubble, & S. D. Miller (Eds.), *The heart and soul of change* (pp. 23–55). Washington, DC: American Psychological Association.

Bereiter, C. (1963). Some persisting dilemmas in the measurement of change. In C. W. Harris (Ed.), *Problems in measuring change* (pp. 3–20). Madison: University of Wisconsin Press.

Bergin, A. E., & Garfield, S. L. (Eds.). (1994). *Handbook of psychotherapy and behavior change* (4th ed.). New York: Wiley.

Boker, S. M., & Nesselroade, J. R. (2002). A method for modeling the intrinsic dynamics of intraindividual variability: Recovering the parameters of simulated oscillators in multiwave panel data. *Multivariate Behavioral Research, 37*(1), 127–160.

Cattell, R. B. (1952). The three basic factor-analytic research designs: Their interrelations and derivatives. *Psychological Bulletin, 49*, 499–520.

Cattell, R. B. (1963). The structuring of change by P-technique and incremental R-technique. In C. W. Harris (Ed.), *Problems in measuring change* (pp. 167–198). Madison: University of Wisconsin Press.

Cattell, R. B., Cattell, A. K. S., & Rhymer, R. M. (1947). P-technique demonstrated in determining psychophysical source traits in a normal individual. *Psychometrika, 12*, 267–288.

Cattell, R. B., & Scheier, I. H. (1961). *The meaning and measurement of neuroticism and anxiety*. New York: Ronald Press.

Corey, S. M. (1937). Professed attitudes and actual behavior. *Journal of Educational Psychology, 28*(4), 271–280.

Essig, T., & Russell, R. L. (1990). Analyzing subjectivity in therapeutic discourse: Rogers, Perls, Ellis, and Gloria revisited. *Psychotherapy: Theory, Research, Practice, and Training, 27*, 271–281.

Friedman, B. H., & Santucci, A. K. (2003). Idiodynamic profiles of cardiovascular activity: A P-technique approach. *Integrative Physiological and Behavioral Science, 38*(4), 295–315.

Hooker, K. (1991). Change and stability in self during the transition to retirement: An intraindividual study using p-technique factor analysis. *International Journal of Behavior Development, 14*(2), 209–233.

Larsen, R. J., & Kasimatis, M. (1990). Individual differences in entrainment of mood to the weekly calendar. *Journal of Personality and Social Psychology, 58*(1), 164–171.

Lee, I. A., & Little, T. D. (2011). *Inter- and intra-individual variability in daily mood fluctuation*. Manuscript in preparation.

Little, T. D., Wanner, B., & Ryan, R. (1997). Development and initial validation of the Inventory of Felt Emotion and Energy in Life (IFEEL) (ACCD Technical Report No. 5). Berlin: Max Planck Institute for Human Development and Education.

Luborsky, L. (1953). Intra-individual repetitive measurements (P-technique) in understanding symptom structure and psychotherapeutic change. In O. H. Mowrer (Ed.), *Psychotherapy: Theory and research* (pp. 389–413). New York: Ronald Press.

McArdle, J. J. (1982). *Structural equation modeling of an individual system: Preliminary results from "A case study in episodic alcoholism."* Unpublished manuscript, Department of Psychology, University of Denver.

Molenaar, P. C. M. (1985). A dynamic factor model for the analysis of multivariate time series. *Psychometrika, 50*, 181–202.

Molenaar, P. C. M. (2004). A manifesto on psychology as idiographic science: Bringing the person back into scientific psychology, this time forever. *Measurement, 2*(4), 201–218.

Molenaar, P. C. M. (2010). On the limits of standard quantitative genetic modeling of inter-individual variation: Extensions, ergodic conditions and a new genetic factor model of intra-individual variation. In K. E. Hood, C. T. Halpern, G. Greenberg, & R. M. Lerner (Eds.), *Handbook of developmental science, behavior, and genetics* (pp. 626–648). Malden, MA: Blackwell.

Molenaar, P. C. M., & Nesselroade, J. R. (2009). The recoverability of P-technique factor analysis. *Multivariate Behavioral Research, 44*, 130–141.

Molenaar, P. C. M., Sinclair, K. O., Rovine, M. J., Ram, N., & Corneal, S. E. (2009). Analyzing developmental processes on an individual level using non-stationary time series modeling. *Developmental Psychology, 45*, 260–271.

Nesselroade, J. R., & Ford, D. H. (1985). P-technique comes of age: Multivariate, replicated, single subject designs for research on older adults. *Research on Aging, 7*, 46–80.

Nesselroade, J. R., McArdle, J. J., Aggen, S. H., & Meyers, J. M. (2002). Dynamic factor analysis models for representing process in multivariate time-series. In D. S. Moskowitz & S. L. Hershberger (Eds.), *Modeling intraindividual variability with repeated measures data: Methods and applications* (pp. 235–265). Mahwah, NJ: Erlbaum.

Nesselroade, J. R., & Molenaar, P. C. M. (1999). Pooling lagged covariance structures based on short, multivariate time series for dynamic factor analysis. In R. H. Hoyle (Ed.), *Statistical strategies for small sample research* (pp. 223–250). Thousand Oaks, CA: Sage.

Nesselroade, J. R., & Ram, N. (2004). Studying intraindividual variability: What we have learned that will help us understand lives in context. *Research in Human Development, 1*, 9–29.

Quinn, M. E., Johnson, M. A., & Martin, P. (1996). Intraindividual change and interindividual differences in factors influencing older women's health-seeking behavior. *Health Care for Women International, 17*(2), 187–196.

Rausch, J. R. (2009). Investigating change in intraindividual factor structure over time. *Applied Psychological Measurement, 33*, 266–284.

Roberts, M. L., & Nesselroade, J. R. (1986). Intraindividual variability in perceived locus of control in adults: P-technique factor analyses of short-term change. *Journal of Research in Personality, 20*, 529–545.

Russell, R. L., Jones, M. E., & Miller, S. A. (2007). Core process components in psychotherapy: A synthetic review of P-technique studies. *Psychotherapy Research, 17*, 273–291.

Shoda, Y., Mischel, W., & Wright, J. C. (1994). Intra-individual stability in the organization and patterning of behavior: Incorporating psychological situations into the idiographic analysis of personality. *Journal of Personality and Social Psychology, 67*, 674–687.

Siegler, R. S. (1994). Cognitive variability: A key to understanding cognitive development. *Current Directions in Psychological Science, 3*, 1–5.

Voelkl, J. E., & Mathieu, M. A. (1995). Intraindividual variation in the subjective experiences of older adults residing in a nursing home. *Therapeutic Recreation Journal, 29*(2), 114–123.

Wicker, A. W. (1969). Attitudes versus actions: The relationships of verbal and overt behavioral responses to attitude objects. *Journal of Social Issues, 25*, 41–78.

Zevon, M. A., & Tellegen, A. (1982). The structure of mood change: An idiographic/nomothetic analysis. *Journal of Personality and Social Psychology, 43*(1), 111–122.

CHAPTER 22

Hazard, Event History, and Survival Modeling

MARGARET K. KEILEY
CASSANDRA KIRKLAND
ALI ZAREMBA
ASHLEY ANDERS JACKSON

Central Issues

In this chapter, we describe and illustrate the methodology of hazard modeling, often equivalently called event history analysis or survival analysis. Evolving from the fields of medicine and biology, this method is used to answer questions about whether and when events are likely to occur and what predicts those occurrences. For example, economists might want to know the effect of specific bank programs on economic recovery (e.g., Flores & Nooruddin, 2009), interventionists might need to know when clients are most likely to relapse to drinking and/or violence after alcohol treatment (Mignone, Klostermann, & Chen, 2009), and social scientists might wonder when adolescents and adults are most likely to have sexual intercourse for the first time (Canino, 2005; Keiley, Martin, Canino, Singer, & Willett, 2007). In addition, these researchers might also be interested in what predicts that event occurrence. What programs predict economic recovery? Is relapse to drinking related to the type of treatment received? Does being male predict earlier risk for sexual initiation? These types of questions about whether and when events occur and what predicts those occurrences are best answered by using the methodology of hazard modeling.

Researchers often have addressed these questions of when events occur and what predicts occurrence using techniques with which they are familiar: multiple regression, analysis of variance, or structural equation modeling. The problem with using these methods is that, because of the nature of the actual question—for example, When do adolescents and adults first have sexual intercourse?—some respondents in the sample will not have an *event time*; that is, some of these adolescents may not have had first sexual intercourse prior to the end of the study. A most perplexing question for the researcher becomes, What to do with participants of a study who do not experience the event during data collection? These respondents have unknown event times; that is, we do not know when, *if at all*, they will experience the event once data collection ends.

Conceptual Issues and Statistical Assumptions

One of the most important and unique aspects of event history analysis is that it provides a method for dealing with such respondents. Respondents with this kind of unknown event time are called "censored" observations.

Censoring

Three major reasons exist for censored cases. No matter when data collection begins or ends, some respondents may never experience the target event. In the sexual initiation example, some of the respondents may go through their lives never having first sexual intercourse. Another possibility is that respondents may experience the event, but only after data collection ends. These individuals are referred to as "right censored" individuals because they experience the target event *after* data collection ends. Finally, some individuals do or do not experience the event, but they drop out of the study prior to the end of data collection. They are censored at the age at which they no longer provide information about experiencing the target event. All individuals who do not experience an event during the window of data collection are censored at their current ages.

Censored cases are commonplace in almost any study of event occurrence, especially when the event itself may be uncommon. One traditional strategy to deal with censoring has been to set aside the censored cases and analyze only those cases for which event times are known. This strategy necessarily ignores an important source of information—those who have not experienced the event. The characteristics of respondents who are least likely to have experienced the target event in the time period of data collection may provide a fuller understanding of the phenomenon under study. In addition, this method introduces *length bias* because, in setting aside censored cases, the estimated average time to event is shortened. A second strategy has been to impute an event time for every censored person (usually the end of data collection) and use standard regression analysis or analysis of variance (ANOVA) to analyze the full sample, all of whom are considered now to have experienced the event at some point during data collection. The disadvantage of this strategy is obvious, as all "nonevents," or censored cases, are changed into "events"; thus the nature of the research question, and hence the phenomenon under study, is changed. With this method, too, length bias is introduced: longer event times are included but at shorter event times than is accurate, thus biasing the estimation of average time to event.

Perhaps a potentially less troubling strategy is a third solution, whereby investigators dichotomize event times by separating the respondents into two groups distinguished by whether or not respondents have experienced an event during the course of data collection or by some other point in time. For example, in studying time to first intercourse, if data collection ended when the respondents were age 22, the researcher might divide respondents into two groups—those who experienced the event and those who did not by the end of data collection—and then use logistic regression, for example, to estimate the odds of engaging in first intercourse by age 22. Alternately, an investigator might dichotomize participants into those who experienced the event prior to age 13, as an indicator of puberty, for instance, and those who experienced the event after age 13. In both examples, this dichotomization strategy may allow investigators to determine *whether* an event occurs within a proscribed time period, but valuable information is lost about *when* that event actually is most likely to occur.

The great importance of incorporating data from individuals with censored and noncensored event times simultaneously into data analyses is that the censored individuals are *not* a random subgroup of the sample. They are the ones who are *least likely* to experience the event; the ones who are the "longest lived" participants in the sample. They provide considerable information about the potential rarity of target event occurrence. Any credible investigation of event occurrence requires a data-analytic method that deals evenhandedly with both the noncensored and the censored observations. Therefore *survival analysis, event history,* and *hazard modeling* have now become invaluable to social scientists because they provide a sound and reasonable statistical basis for exploring the "whether" and "when" of all kinds of interesting target events in the lives of participants. As such, event history analysis provides information not only about event occurrence but also about event nonoccurrence. Indeed, the treatment of censored cases represents one of the major advantages of event history analysis over previous strategies for analyzing event data.

Later in this chapter, we describe and illustrate this methodology by using data from a study in which we investigated the occurrence of sexual initiation. Specifically, we examined the following research question: When are adolescents most likely to have sexual intercourse for the first time and what predicts that event occurrence? We investigated several hypotheses in this study, three of which are the focus of this chapter: (1) When are respondents most at risk for first sexual intercourse? (2) Does the gender or race of the respondent predict that risk? and (3) Is the respondent's idea of the best age at which to have a child related to that risk? We introduce this example along with our continued discussion of the conceptual issues and statistical assumptions.

We utilized the Urban Poverty and Family Life Survey of Chicago (Wilson, 1987) that was conducted in 1987 via personal and telephone interviews by the National Opinion Research Center. A stratified probability sample of census tracts was used that consisted of individuals from impoverished areas in the city of Chicago. The analytic sample for this example was 2,251 respondents, of whom 771 (34%) were men and 1,480 (66%) were women ranging in age from 18 to 47 (M = 31.8, SD = 7.1). Minorities were oversampled; respondents were primarily African American (AA; n = 1,093; 49%), with the remainder European American (EA; n = 331; 15%) and Hispanic (n = 827; 37%). On average the respondents thought that the best age at which to have a child was 23 years (SD = 3.3).

Framework for Investigating Event Occurrence

In order to begin the investigation of event occurrence, a researcher must first define the particular event in which he or she is interested. That event must satisfy several conditions, including a clear specification of states that are mutually exclusive and exhaustive. For example, in our study, "time of first intercourse" is the identified target event, signifying when an individual makes the transition from being a virgin to not being one; this transition is from one state to another. In this case, individuals are either sexual virgins or they are not; they cannot be both. The "states" are mutually exclusive and exhaustive of all other possible states.

Another condition that must be met prior to investigating event occurrence is the determination of the "beginning of time," a moment during which everyone in the population occupies one and only one of the states under investigation. This precise beginning of time is the time before which no one in the study has experienced the target event; that is, when everyone is still "at risk" for the event to occur. At the beginning of time all respondents are in the risk set. "Event time" will then be determined as the difference between the beginning of time, when no one has experienced the event and all are at risk, and the time at which the event occurs (if it does occur) for each person, at which point the person drops out of the risk set. In our example, although we did not expect any respondents in our study to report sexual initiation prior to the early childhood years, in actuality, the beginning of time is birth. At birth, all individuals are at risk for sexual initiation and thus all are in the accompanying risk set at that time.

A metric for time also must be established in meeting the conditions for survival/event history analysis. Two types of event history analysis, discrete and continuous, are differentiated by the metric indicated for time. In discrete-time event history analysis, events occur (or can be remembered to have occurred, in the case of retrospective data) across discrete periods, or separable and often large units of time. For example, in our study of time of first intercourse, a retrospective study, most respondents did not remember the exact age in days or months at which they first had intercourse but they did remember how old they were in years. Thus, in our case, time was measured in discrete units defined as age in years; these are discrete units as we do not know the exact date on which they had first intercourse. By contrast, if the exact time the event happens is known, time can be used in its continuous form. For example, if the event of interest is the timing of the birth of a first child, event time could be measured in continuous time, defined as the number of days, months, or years from the mother's own birth until the birth of her first child; continuous-time event history analysis then could be used. No single metric of time is suitable for all studies, and, as might be obvious, the same event can be measured using more than one metric of time. As Singer and Willett (2003) suggest, time should be measured in the smallest units possible as appropriate for each event examined. Though this recommendation favors continuous time over discrete when possible, we focus on discrete-time event history analysis in this chapter, as this framework allows for a more straightforward and simple explanation of the method of event history analysis itself. For more information on continuous-time event history analysis, see Singer and Willett (2003) or Allison (1995).

Describing Discrete-Time Event History Data

In order to introduce other concepts central to event history analysis, we illustrate the construction of a life table, which summarizes the distribution of event occurrence in sample data. We present the life table for the data on sexual initiation in Table 22.1. The first column indicates the discrete time periods and associated metric that we used in this analysis, in this case, age in years. The second column includes the risk set, or those respondents eligible to experience the target event (first sexual intercourse) during each time period. The third column indicates those respondents who had first sexual intercourse during each

TABLE 22.1. Life Table Describing the Age at Which Respondents First Had Sexual Intercourse

	Number			Proportion	
Age in years	Respondents at the beginning of the age period who had not had first sexual intercourse (risk set)	Respondents who had first sexual intercourse during this age period	Censored at the end of the age period	Respondents at the beginning of the age period who did have first sexual intercourse during this year (hazard function)	All respondents who still had not had first sexual intercourse at the end of the age period (survival function)
8	2,251	—	—	—	1.0000
9	2,251	20	0	0.0089	0.9911
10	2,231	11	0	0.0049	0.9862
11	2,220	22	0	0.0099	0.9764
12	2,198	62	0	0.0282	0.9489
13	2,136	128	0	0.0599	0.8921
14	2,008	205	0	0.1021	0.8010
15	1,803	312	0	0.1731	0.6624
16	1,491	398	0	0.2669	0.4856
17	1,093	338	0	0.3092	0.3355
18	755	264	0	0.3497	0.2182
19	491	167	2	0.3401	0.1440
20	322	93	2	0.2888	0.1024
21	227	87	140	0.3833	0.0632

Note. $N = 2{,}251$.

age/time period (who experienced the target event during that age). The fourth column includes those respondents who were censored (who did not experience the event during data collection). As seen in the life table, of the 2,251 respondents in the data set, 2,107 had first sexual intercourse between the ages of 9 and 21 and 144 were censored (did not have first sexual intercourse before data collection ended).

Hazard Function

From the life table, we can determine the hazard function by identifying, in each discrete time period, the pool of people who still remain at risk of experiencing the event in that period—these are the individuals who have reached this particular time period without already experiencing sexual initiation or being censored. They are referred to as the risk set. We compute the proportion of this risk set that actually experiences the target event *in* the time period, thereby obtaining an estimate of the hazard probability for this particular discrete time period, as follows:

$$\hat{h}(t_j) = \left(\frac{\text{\# in sample risk set who experience the target event in } j\text{th time-period}}{\text{\# in sample risk set in } j\text{th time-period}} \right) \quad \textbf{(22.1)}$$

Anyone who experiences the event or is censored (drops out of the study during the *j*th time period) within the current period is removed from the risk set for the following time period and is therefore not included in the estimation of the hazard probability for that subsequent period. The hazard function is the *conditional probability* that a person will experience the target event under investigation during time period *j*, given that he or she did not experience that event in a previous time period.

The hazard function for our data is displayed in column 5 of Table 22.1. At age 18, 755 respondents were eligible to have first sexual intercourse (i.e., they had not had intercourse during any earlier time period under study and were therefore in the risk set for that time period). Of those, 264 actually had first sexual intercourse before they turned nineteen. The hazard function for age period 18 is thus 264/755, or .3497. The hazard function represents the proportion of each age period's risk set who experienced the event during that age period, given that they had not had initiation of sex prior to that age. Thus, in our example, 35% had sex for the first time at age 18, given that they had not had sex prior to that time. The greater the hazard, the greater is the risk of event occurrence during that age period, and vice versa. Examination of the discrete time hazard conditional probabilities tells us the time of greatest risk for event occurrence, or when the event is most likely to occur. In this case, the first time period during which individuals are most at risk for first sexual intercourse is age 18 (i.e., at this age, the hazard function is largest), but a second peak occurs at age 21. Because the hazard function displays the unique risk associated with each age/time period, one can also determine the shape of the hazard function. When plotted, one can visually inspect whether this hazard function, or risk, increases, decreases, or remains constant over time (or whether it contains a combination of these trends). This shape can also be inferred from the life table. In the hazard function column of Table 22.1, one can see that the risk of first sexual intercourse increases fairly rapidly until age 18, at which time it reaches a peak of 35% and then decreases slightly to 29% at age 20, increasing again at age 21 to another peak of 38%. Though often only one peak is evident in the hazard function, indicating a single period during which the risk for an event is the greatest, other target events, such as the one we investigate here, are actually nonmonotonic, with a peak, a plateau, and another slightly higher peak.

Survival Function

In addition to using hazard function to examine the conditional risk of event occurrence *in each discrete time period*, we can also accumulate the period-by-period risks of event occurrence to assess the probability that a randomly selected individual will survive, that is, not experience the event. In any given discrete time period, the survival probability represents the probability that individual *i* will survive past the time period *j*, given that that individual had not experienced the target event in the *j*th period or any earlier period.

We can obtain values of the survival probability easily. At the beginning of time, t_0, here age 8, no one has yet experienced the target event; thus the survival probability, $S(t_0)$, is 1.00, or 100%. In the first discrete time period in which target events can occur, then, the risk set contains all members. In the first discrete period, age 9, the hazard probability is

$h(t_1)$, and therefore $\{1 - h(t_1)\}$, the complement of the hazard probability, describes the proportion of the first-period risk set that does not experience the target event in that period; these survive through the first discrete time period. Therefore the survival probability for the first discrete time period, which we label $S(t_1)$, is simply equal to $\{1 - h(t_1)\}$ of 1.00, the original $S(t_0)$. Similarly, in the second discrete time period, age 10, the hazard probability becomes $h(t_2)$, indicating that a fraction $\{1 - h(t_2)\}$ will now survive the period. Hence, the survival probability for the second period must be $\{1 - h(t_2)\}$ of the proportion who survived the first period, and that proportion is $S(t_1)$, giving us $\{1 - h(t_2)\}*S(t_1)$. The same algorithm can be repeated in each discrete time period successively, such that the survival probability in any discrete time period is simply equal to the complement of the hazard probability in that period multiplied by the survival probability in the previous period. By definition, the survival function will decrease over time and will never increase. Once a respondent has experienced the event, he or she is eliminated from the risk set. In the population, this algorithm can be represented as follows:

$$S(t_j) = \{1 - h(t_j)\} * S(t_{j-1}) \tag{22.2}$$

As an example, in age period 16, the survival function is the estimated survival for age period 15 (0.66) multiplied by 1 minus the estimated hazard in age period 16 (1 – 0.27 = 0.73) or 0.66*0.73 = 0.48.This survival function indicates that through age 16, about half of the sample is still "surviving"; they have not yet had first sexual intercourse. Alternatively, through age 16, approximately 50% of the sample has already had sex for the first time. The discrete time survival function for our data is shown in column 6 of Table 22.1. At the beginning of time (age 8) all are "surviving," and the survival function is 1. Over time, as respondents initiate first sexual intercourse, the sample survival function drops. Because most adults do end up having sexual intercourse *at some time* in their lives, the curves do decline toward a lower asymptote of zero.

Median Lifetime

So we have answered the question of when respondents are most at risk of experiencing sex for the first time, but what about the question of, on "average," how long it takes before respondents have sexual intercourse for the first time? Because of the presence of censoring, we cannot merely estimate the average age, but we can estimate a *median lifetime* from the sample survivor function. The median lifetime is the length of time that must pass until the value of the survivor function reaches one-half, or .50. In other words, it is the time by which half of the individuals in the study have experienced the target event. In our example, at age 15 the survivor function is greater than .50 (.6624), but at age 16, it is below .50 (.4856). We can interpolate to estimate that these respondents have a median lifetime of 15 years and 11 months, indicating that, on average, respondents are 1 month shy of 16 before initiating sexual intercourse. The median lifetime can be thought of as the "average" time to target event.

For target events that are rare, median lifetimes often cannot be estimated. Median lifetimes (as well as hazard and survival functions) can be estimated, however, for subgroups within a sample and can provide useful information about these groups. For example, we could estimate median lifetimes for the subgroups denoted by our dichotomous gender predictor (i.e., males vs. females).

Fitting Basic Discrete Time Hazard Models

Estimating sample hazard and survivor functions is useful for exploring whether and when a group of individuals is likely to experience a target event during the window of observation. These descriptive statistics can also be used to explore questions about differences between groups. When are children most likely to receive mental health services for the first time, and are European American (*EA*) children more likely than African American (*AA*) children to experience this event (Erath et al., 2009)? When do adolescents and adults first initiate sexual intercourse, and is the event influenced by their gender, race, or beliefs about the best age to have children? Both of these examples implicitly frame selected individual characteristics—such as race, gender, and beliefs about childrearing—as predictors of the risk profile describing the occurrence of the target events—mental health service and sexual initiation, respectively. In fact, we could construct a table similar to the one in Table 22.1 in which we examine the two sample hazard functions for males and females for the question of the timing of sexual initiation. In doing so, we would be implicitly treating gender as a predictor of the risk profile of first sexual intercourse.

The descriptive comparisons that we have done thus far lack the credibility of formal statistical tests, making it difficult to account for the impact of sampling idiosyncrasy and to generalize back to the population. Consequently, as in most quantitative analysis, we specify a formal statistical model of the discrete time hazard probability and then fit that model to our data. First, however, we must create a "person–period data set"—a data set in which each person has one record for every time period in which he or she is at risk for event occurrence (see table at *www.crmda.ku.edu/Guilford/HDRM*). In this person–period data set, a separate variable for each age period in which the respondent was at risk for first sexual intercourse is created. For our example of sexual initiation, these age variables are time dummy variables that we label A9 to A21. Each time dummy variable is equal to 1 in the time period for which it stands and 0 in all other time periods. We also create an indicator to denote event occurrence. This variable, *EVENT*, will ultimately serve as the *outcome* variable in our discrete time survival analyses. *EVENT* is coded with the value 0 at each age in which the respondent did *not* experience the target event and 1 at the single age at which the event was experienced. For each participant, once the event indicator has been coded 1 (and the target event has therefore occurred), no additional records are included in the person–period data set for that individual. An individual who experiences the event of interest—in this case, first experience of sexual intercourse—is no longer at risk of subsequent initiation, by definition, and therefore drops out of the risk set for this event. In our example, a European American male, respondent #168, experienced first sexual intercourse at the age of 11; thus *EVENT* takes on the value 0 in each of the time periods prior to age 11 but switches to value 1 in the discrete time bin corresponding to age 11. Then, once person #168 has experienced the target event, he is no longer at risk of experiencing sexual intercourse for the first time ever again; thus he contributes no further records to the person–period data set. A Hispanic female, respondent #812, initiates sexual intercourse at age 21. By contrast, an African American female, respondent #332, had not experienced first sexual intercourse for the first time by age 21. For her, *EVENT* is coded 0 in all 13 discrete time periods in the data set, from ages 9 through 21, and its value never switches from 0 to 1, meaning that the study ended without her experiencing the target event. She is therefore censored at age 21.

After specifying the statistical model (see the following subsection) we use this set of time dummies (13 dichotomous variables representing ages 9–21) as initial predictors of the timing of event occurrence (*EVENT* variable) in discrete time hazard modeling. Survival analysis does not *require* that we specify the metric of time in this very general way as a set of dichotomous time dummies; nothing would prevent us from using participants' (linear) age or powers of age (age, age^2, age^3, etc.) as the initial time predictors of event occurrence. Thus, instead of entering 13 variables to represent time, we would only enter 2 (age, age^2), if the hazard profile in the life table appeared to be quadratic, or 3 (age, age^2, age^3), if it appeared to be cubic. For more on alternative specifications of time see Keiley and Martin (2005) or Singer and Willett (2003). The series of time dummies usually provides the most successful starting point by estimating the typically irregular nature of any risk profile with age. We also include the variables in this person–period data set that we would like to use as predictors: gender, race, and "best age for having children." After creating the person–period data set, we can then fit the hazard model to the person–period data set using the procedure of logistic regression. The first model fit is the baseline model with only the variables representing time, and then we add our predictors.

Model Specification

The hypothesized statistical model for an event history analysis must describe the shape of the entire discrete time hazard function over time, not just its value at any one period. In addition, because the hazard is a conditional probability, the value of the discrete time hazard must be between 0 and 1. In order to deal with this limitation on the hazard's upper and lower bounds of 0 and 1, a transformation of the hazard function is needed. The common transformations for modeling probabilities are the odds and log odds (logit) transformations (Cox, 1972). A logit transformation is commonly used, both because it prevents the possibility of implausible predicted values and because it makes comparable the distances between the hazard functions represented by different predictors. That is, if we assume that the function is the same over time in the population for all subgroups denoted by the predictors, a logit transformation ensures that the distance between the discrete time hazard functions for the different groups is comparable over time. The logit transformation of the population hazard probability in the jth discrete time can be represented as follows:

$$\text{logit}\, h(t_j) = \log_e\left(\frac{h(t_j)}{1 - h(t_j)}\right) \tag{22.3}$$

Notice that in the brackets on the right-hand side of this equation is a quotient of the hazard probability and its complement. This quotient is the ratio of the probability that an event *will* occur ($h(t_j)$) to the probability that it *will not* occur ($1 - h(t_j)$) in the jth discrete time period (given that it had not occurred in an earlier time period). In other words, this quotient is the conditional *odds* that the target event will occur in this time period. In our example, for instance, it is the *odds* that an adolescent or adult will experience sexual intercourse for the first time in the jth time period, given that he or she had not experienced it earlier. We then take the natural logarithm of the conditional odds of event occurrence to obtain the logit transform or *log odds* of hazard. This new quantity ranges between minus and plus infinity as hazard ranges between 0 and 1, and is therefore unbounded.

Assumptions

As in all statistical methods, assumptions underlie the discrete time hazard model. In fact, three assumptions about the population allow us to hypothesize discrete time hazard models, estimate parameters, and assess goodness of fit. The first of these assumptions is that, for every value of a predictor of event occurrence, a hypothesized logit hazard function exists. For example, in the sexual initiation data, this assumption must be met for our predictors of interest—gender, race, and the best age for childbirth. We coded gender as a dichotomous variable, *FEMALE*, whose categories denoted the two genders (female: *FEMALE* = 1; male: *FEMALE* = 0). Accordingly, we hypothesized that the population had two logit hazard functions, one for females and one for males. The second variable we considered was the best age to have a child (*BST_AKID*, a continuous variable). This variable denoted the age at which the respondent felt it was best to have a child ($M = 22.7$; $SD = 3.3$; range: 14–35). Because the best age to have a child was a continuous predictor, we postulated as many logit hazard functions as there were values of the predictor. In combination with gender, we hypothesized as many functions as there were *combinations* of these predictors. Similarly, we coded race as two dichotomous variables denoting European Americans (EA = 1; AA = 0), African Americans (EA = 0; AA = 1), and Hispanics (EA = 0; AA = 0), with similar hypotheses about combination of these variables with the other two variables. This assumption is similar to the assumption for linear regression in which we hypothesize that for each value of any predictor, a distribution of the outcome exists.

The second assumption is that each of these logit hazard functions has an identical shape. In other words, we constrain the shape of each function to be the same for all predictors. In our example, in examining the life table we noted that the shape of the sample hazard function of risk of first sexual intercourse increased to a peak at age 18 and then leveled off and increased once again at age 21. Following this second assumption, often called the *linear additivity assumption*, we assumed, then, that the shape of the estimated hazard function for males and females would have this same shape. In addition, we assumed that the shape of the estimated hazard function for different values of the best time to have a child would also share this shape (i.e., increasing to a peak at age 18, leveling off, and then increasing again). But, if we suspect that the effect of the best age to have a child is different for males and females, we can fit a model in which we include the main effects of gender and the best age to have a child along with an interaction term of those two substantive predictors. Conducting a difference in deviance statistical test (described later) allows us to determine whether this assumption is violated. If it is, then usually we relax this assumption. Discrete time survival analysis has assumptions, but for this one, and the following, no penalty exists for violating them. In fact, the simple solution to violation of this assumption is to include the interaction of selected variables, because the interaction effects are substantively interesting.

The third assumption is called the *proportionality assumption*, namely, the distance between each of the logit hazard functions for each value of the predictors is assumed to be identical within each time period. The gap between the logit hazard functions will not be larger in some periods and smaller in others. The effect of any one predictor on the log odds of event occurrence is postulated to be constant over time. For our data, we may hypothesize that the difference between the estimated hazard functions for males and females is equidistant across adolescence and early adulthood. If that is true, then the logit hazard function itself would simply be shifted lower or higher for this predictor or other predictors, depending on the values of the logit hazard estimates for those predictors. The levels of each of these predictors denote various subgroups in the population. For example, for the gender predictor, one of the groups (*FEMALE* = 0 or male) can represent the baseline group, and the other level of the predictor (*FEMALE* = 1, or female) merely shifts the level of those logit hazard functions higher or lower from the level for the baseline group.

In the present example, as in many event history analyses, the proportionality assumption is often violated. In fact, the violation of this assumption, as with the previous assumption, is often substantively very interesting and adds greatly to the understanding of the profile of risk across time. We believed that the effect of a particular predictor, gender, on the risk of sexual initiation varied across time. Therefore, we included interactions between that variable, *FEMALE*, and time in the fitted model and tested whether adding those effects to the model improved the prediction of the risk. Indeed, as will be seen later when we introduce the fitting of hazard models, gender does interact with time in the prediction of sexual initiation. Investigators are encouraged to test whether the predictors in their event history analysis interact with time. If they do, then relaxing the proportionality assumption is appropriate.

Illustration

Fitting the Discrete Time Survival Model

We can now specify the model to answer the question about the risk of sexual initiation as a function of adolescent–adult age and gender for individual *i* in discrete time period *j*, as follows:

$$\text{logit}\, h_i(t_j) = \left[\alpha_9 A9_j + \alpha_{10} A10_j + \cdots \alpha_{21} A21_j\right] + \left[\beta_1 FEMALE_i\right] \tag{22.4}$$

The first set of predictors on the right-hand side of the discrete time hazard model in equation 22.4 provide the *baseline logit hazard profile*. The slope parameters associated with each of the dichotomous time predictors ($\alpha_9, \alpha_{10}, \ldots, \alpha_{21}$) represent the population values of the outcome—now a logit-transformed hazard probability—in each discrete time period for the group of *males* (for whom *FEMALE* = 0). We use "A" here to denote our time dummies, because time, in our example, is age. Substituting this predictor value into the model *for adolescents and adults who are male* yields the following:

$$\text{logit}\, h_i(t_j \mid FEMALE_i = 0) = \left[\alpha_9 A9_j + \alpha_{10} A10_j + \cdots \alpha_{21} A21_j\right] \tag{22.5}$$

In equations 22.4 and 22.5 the α's multiplied by their respective time dummies ($A9, A10, \ldots, A21$) act as multiple intercepts, one for each time period. As a group, these parameters represent the baseline logit hazard function, the value of logit hazard when all predictors are 0; in this case, our lone predictor is *FEMALE*. Each intercept parameter, $\alpha_9, \alpha_{10}, \ldots, \alpha_{21}$, represents the value of logit hazard (the log odds of event occurrence) in that particular time period for individuals in the "baseline" group, one in which all of the predictors are 0, here males. In the second part of equation 22.4 the β_1 multiplied by its respective predictor represents the shift (either up or down) in the baseline logit hazard function corresponding to a unit difference in the associated predictor. In this case, our predictor is *FEMALE*, and a 1-unit difference from 0 (denoting males) is a 1 that denotes females. Hence this slope parameter, β_1, tells us about the effect on event occurrence of a 1-unit difference in that predictor. In this case, β_1 indicates the shift in the baseline logit hazard profile—the male profile—that represents the baseline logit hazard profile for females. In this way, we designate one logit hazard function (in this case the male function) as the baseline logit hazard and then quantify the size of the additive shift between this baseline and the other functions obtained with a 1-unit increment in the predictors, in other words, a resultant shift in the baseline, here, the predictor, *FEMALE*. As in regression, these unit differences are interpreted within the scale of the predictor. For dichotomous variables, a 1-unit difference is a "state" difference (e.g., the difference between male, female or *AA*, *EA*, and Hispanic). For continuous variables, a 1-unit difference is interpreted as a shift in the hazard function per a 1-unit difference within the scale of that predictor, in our case the age that is considered best for someone to have a child. Because the first part of equations 22.4 and 22.5 serve as a set of time-related intercepts, we do not estimate an additional intercept in the model. For example, during the first time period, *A*9 is equal to 1, and all other time dummy variables, *A*10 to *A*21, drop out. Thus the intercept parameter during the first time period, α_9, can be thought of as the conditional log odds of event occurrence in the first time period, just as the intercept parameter during the second time period, α_{10}, represents the conditional log odds of event occurrence in the second time period, and so on.

Fitting a Discrete Time Hazard Model to Data and Interpreting the Results

Once we have created our person–period data set with the time variables, the *EVENT* variable, and our predictors, model fitting and parameter estimation are conducted by using standard logistic regression analysis to regress the binary outcome, *EVENT*, on the time dummies and on the substantive predictors in the person–period data set (see Singer & Willett, 2003, for a more complete explanation and how to program these models). We illustrate this here by fitting five discrete time hazard models to our data on adolescent and adult sexual initiation. Each of the fitted discrete time hazard models are shown in a table at *www.crmda.ku.edu/Guilford/HDRM*. The key elements of model 5 are shown in Table 22.2 on page 377. The first model contains the age dummies; the second model contains the age dummies and the *FEMALE* dichotomous predictor; the third model adds the continuous predictor, *BST_AKID*, the adolescent–adult's determination of the best age at which to have a child; and the fourth model includes the variables that denote race, *AA* and *EA* (with Hispanic as the comparison group). We are also including a fifth model that tests whether the effect of *FEMALE* on the risk of sexual initiation differs across the ages 9–21. That is, is the risk profile different for males and females, controlling for race and the best age to have a child? To do this, we create the interaction terms of *FEMALE* with each of the age dummies; thus the final model can be represented as:

$$\text{logit}\, h_i(t_j) = [\alpha_9 A9_j + \alpha_{10} A10_j + \ldots \alpha_{21} A21_j] + [\beta_1 BST\_AKID_i + \beta_2 AA_i + \beta_3 EA + \beta_4 FEMALE_i * \alpha_9 A9_j + \ldots \beta_{16} FEMALE_i * \alpha_{21} A21_j] \quad \textbf{(22.6)}$$

Comparison of Models

In logistic regression, a deviance statistic (–2 log likelihood) that is small and has a nonsignificant *p*-value indicates "good model fit." With large sample sizes, however, the deviance statistic is often significant, and good fit can be difficult to ascertain. Because we are interested in answering our research question about whether the risk of sexual initiation is related to our substantive predictors, we focus on determining whether adding these predictors one at a time *improves* the fit of the model by using the change in deviance statistics to compare two nested models. The hypothesis tests for our change in deviance statistics determined that, separately, *FEMALE, BST_AKID*, and race (*AA, EA*) each predict the risk of first sexual intercourse. The change-in-deviance statistic comparing Model 2 indicates that gender is a significant predictor of sexual initiation (Δ Deviance = 148.71, $df = 1$, $p < .001$); Model 3 indicates that the age that respondents think is the best age for having a child is a significant predictor of sexual initiation, even controlling for gender (Δ Deviance = 4.14, $df = 1, p < .05$). Race is also a significant predictor of sexual initiation, controlling for gender and the best age to have a child (Δ Deviance = 245.91, $df = 2, p < .001$). Finally, in comparing Model 5 with Model 4, the interaction of the variable *FEMALE* with time is significant in predicting the risk of first sexual intercourse, controlling for all else (Δ Deviance = 83.80, $df = 12, p < .001$). From this series of tests, we determined (1) that Model 5 is the best fitting model because it has the lowest deviance statistic (10028.70) and (2) that each of our predictors, added one at a time, is a statistically significant predictor of time to first sexual initiation (as shown via the four deviance-based hypothesis tests).

Examining the Final Fitted Model

In the table at *www.crmda.ku.edu/Guilford/HDRM*, the parameter estimates of each time period dummy variable in each model, A9–A21, indicate the shape of the baseline logit hazard function and whether the risk of having first sexual intercourse increases, decreases, or remains the same over time for a baseline group in the population. For Model 5 (see Table 22.2), the baseline group is defined differently from the baseline group for the model with just *FEMALE* as a predictor. In this model, Hispanic ($AA = 0, EA = 0$) males (*FEMALE* = 0) who believe that no age is best for having children (*BST_AKID* = 0) are the baseline group, that is, the group that has zero values on all the predictors in the model. In our sample, the baseline group is nonexistent because the values for the predictor, *BST_AKID*, are never zero, but in the population a baseline group would exist. Note that for the baseline group all of the interactions of time with *FEMALE* (now zero) are also zero; therefore, they drop out of the fitted equation, and we are left with just the parameter estimates for the time dummies at each age (see equation 22.7).

$$\text{logit}\, h_i(t_j | FEMALE_i = 0; EA = 0, AA = 0; BST\_AKID = 0) = [\alpha_9 A9_j + \alpha_{10} A10_j + \ldots \alpha_{21} A21_j] \qquad \textbf{(22.7)}$$

Transforming the logit hazard into hazard by exponentiating the logit *at each age* using equation 22.8 will allow us to determine the percentage of Hispanic males who believe that the best age for children is "never" who will have sex during each age period, given that they had not prior to that age. For example, at age 9:

TABLE 22.2. Parameter Estimates and Asymptotic Standard Errors (in Parentheses) from the Final Discrete Time Hazard Model Representing the Risk of First Sexual Intercourse in Adolescence–Adulthood as a Function of Age, Gender, Race, and Self-Report of the Age at Which Respondents Felt It Was Best to Have a Child

Predictor	Model 5
A_9	–4.03 (0.32)
. . .	. . .
A_{21}	0.23 (0.36)
F^*T_9	–1.78 (0.52)
. . .	. . .
F^*T_{21}	–0.56 (0.35)
Best age to have child	–0.02 (0.01)
EA	0.13 (0.08)
AA	0.85 (0.06)
Deviance statistic	10028.70
n parameters	29
AIC	10086.70
H_0: All $\beta s_{\text{female*time}} = 0$ simultaneously	83.80*** (12)

Note. $N = 2{,}251$; N events = 2,107; *F*, female; *T*, time.
$^{***}p < .001$.

$$h(t_j) = 1/(1+e^{-[\alpha_9]}) \quad \textbf{(22.8)}$$

Similarly, to understand the risk of first sexual intercourse for other subgroups, we can examine the effects of the other predictors in this model. The estimates for the race variables denote the shift from the baseline (Hispanic) that occurs for European Americans and African Americans. The estimates in Model 5 indicate the size of the risk differential that exists between the Hispanic group and the two other subgroups, European-American ($\beta_{EA} = 0.13$) and African American ($\beta_{AA} = 0.85$). The positive signs of these estimates indicate that European Americans and African Americans are at more risk for sexual initiation at every age than are Hispanics. The effect sizes, given by the estimated odds ratios, $e^{\beta EA}$ and $e^{\beta AA}$, are 1.14 and 2.34, respectively, indicating that at every age, the estimated odds of having sex for the first time are only slightly higher than even odds for European Americans compared with Hispanics and almost two and a half times higher for African Americans compared with Hispanics.

Coefficients of continuous variables can be interpreted in a similar manner. A primary question, however, is whether a 1-unit difference on the continuous scale under consideration is meaningful. That is, one should consider whether it is useful to examine two subgroups only 1 unit apart on a scale for which 1 unit may represent only a very small difference. For the continuous predictor, *BST_AKID* in Model 5, we chose to examine the size of the vertical differential in logit hazard corresponding to a 1 *SD* unit above and below the mean of *BST_AKID* (22.7 ± 3.3), controlling for *FEMALE*, race, and the interaction of *FEMALE* and time. The parameter estimate of *BST_AKID* is –0.02, indicating that the risk of first sexual intercourse is greater among those who think that it is best to have a child at a younger age, controlling for all else in the model. The estimated odds ratio for a 6.6-unit difference (2 *SD* or 6.6) in *BST_AKID* are $e^{\beta Bst\_akid*6.6} = e^{-.02*6.6} = .88$. The estimated odds of the target event occurring relative to a 6.6-unit difference in *BST_AKID*, therefore, are .88 to 1. Because odds ratios that are less than 1 are often more difficult to understand than those greater than 1, we can divide this estimate into 1, reverse the interpretation, and say, in this case, that the estimated odds of experiencing sexual intercourse for the first time for a person who scores approximately two SD *lower* than another person on the *BST_AKID* scale are only a little over 1 to 1 (1/.88 = 1.14), controlling for all else in the model.

Fitted Hazard and Survival Functions

A more useful way to interpret the results of a fitted model is to present plots of the predicted values for the fitted hazard and survival functions for prototypical adolescents–adults. In answer to our question about whether gender, race, and age at which respondents feel it is best to have children are related to the risk of sexual initiation, we plotted the fitted survival and hazard values for the 12 subgroups of interest from the "final" fitted model (Model 5, Table 22.2). In other words, we are interested in 12 prototypical individuals: individuals who are male or female, Hispanic, *EA*, or *AA*, and who feel it is best to have children at age 19 or age 26. We plot the fitted hazard functions for these 12 prototypes by substituting prototypical values of *FEMALE, EA, AA*, and *BST_AKID* into the fitted equation denoted in Model 5. The choice of values to illustrate the effects of attachment is straightforward; we use 0 and 1 for *FEMALE*; 0 and 1 in the proper combinations for race (*EA* = 0, *AA* = 0: Hispanic; *EA* = 1, *AA* = 1: European American; *EA* = 0, *AA* = 1: African American). For the best age at which to have a child, we chose to use values that were 1 *SD* above and below the mean of *BST_AKID*. A person who is 1 *SD* below and above the mean would not be "atypical" but would still be seen as wanting a child when young (19) or older (26), respectively. We can construct these plots via a two-step process. First, for the hazard plot, we substitute particular values of the predictors into the fitted model and calculate the predicted values of logit hazard. In our case, we plot the fitted survival and hazard function for Model 5 (Table 22.2), in which we included the interaction of female and the time dummies as well as the main effects of gender, race, and the age at which it is best to have a child (see equation 22.6). We then transform these values into fitted hazard values:

$$\hat{h}(t_j) = 1 / (1 + e^{-(\text{logit}\,\hat{h}(t_j))}) \quad \textbf{(22.9)}$$

The most efficient way to obtain these values is to program a series of "do loops" in a statistical package, transform the fitted hazard values in those "do loops," and print them out to use them in a graphics program. Sample scripts using SAS (SAS Institute, 2001) are available at *www.crmda.ku.edu/Guilford/HDRM*.

The fitted hazard plot for Model 5 presented in Figure 22.1 provides a graphical summary of the estimates from this fitted model and a clear picture of the risk of sexual initiation across the two genders and three races for typical respondents who feel that the best age for having children is younger (19). The remaining 6 prototypical risk profiles for those believing that it is best to have children at an older age (26) are similar to the ones in Figure 22.1, but shifted downward, indicating lowered risk. As these plots indicate, age 19 is the first age at which females are most at risk for initiating sexual intercourse for the first time.

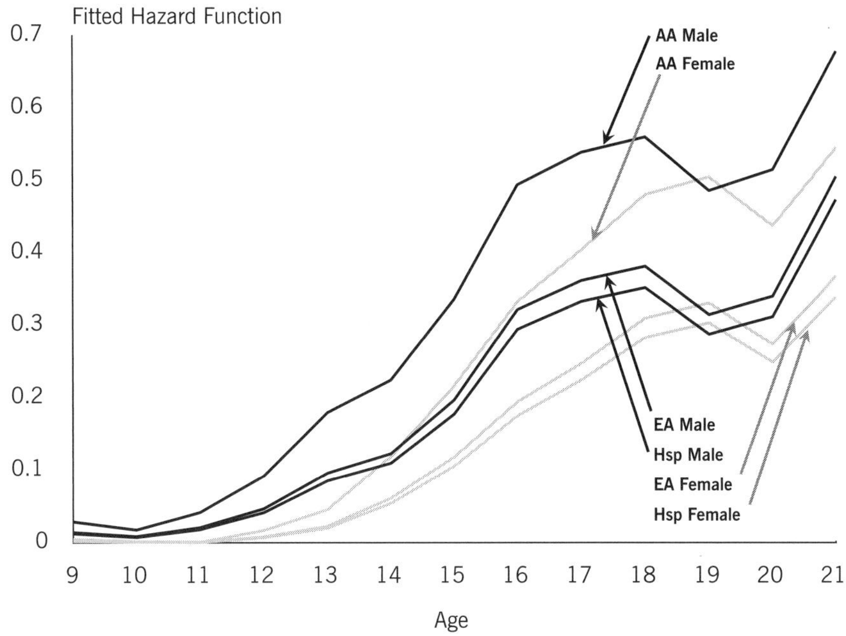

FIGURE 22.1. Prototypical profiles for the fitted hazard function for the age of first sexual intercourse from Model 5 that includes the effects of gender (male, female), race (AA, EA, Hispanic), and the interaction of gender with time. The best age to have children is included in this model, but we present only the prototypical profiles for those who feel the best age to have children is a younger age, 19. For those who feel the best age would be older, for example, age 26, all of the prototypical profiles would merely be shifted downward.

The risk then decreases at age 20, only to rise to a higher level at age 21. Males are most likely to have sex for the first time a year earlier than females, at age 18. They also have a decrease in risk 1 year later, at age 19, and then the risk increases rapidly to the greatest risk at age 21. This differential in times of greatest risk for males and females is the result of the interaction of the variable *FEMALE* with time. The risk profiles for the two genders are different across time. Fifty-six percent of African American males have sex for the first time at age 18, given that they had not prior to that time, but only 38% and 35% of European American and Hispanic males have sex for the first time at age 18, given that they had not had sex prior to that time. Fifty percent of African American females have sex for the first time at age 19, given that they had not had sex prior to that, whereas only 33% of European American and 30% of Hispanic females are initiating sex at that age. From age 14 onward, a greater percentage of African American females have first sex at the remaining ages, given that they had not had sex prior to that, than do all other females and European American and Hispanic males.

The fitted survival plots in Figure 22.2 indicate similar findings, but from the perspective of how long various prototypical individuals "survive" until age 21 without having first sexual intercourse. As can be seen, a median lifetime exists for each of the prototypical groups in which we are interested. Half of African American males have their first sexual intercourse shortly after they turn 14, and over half of other males and African American

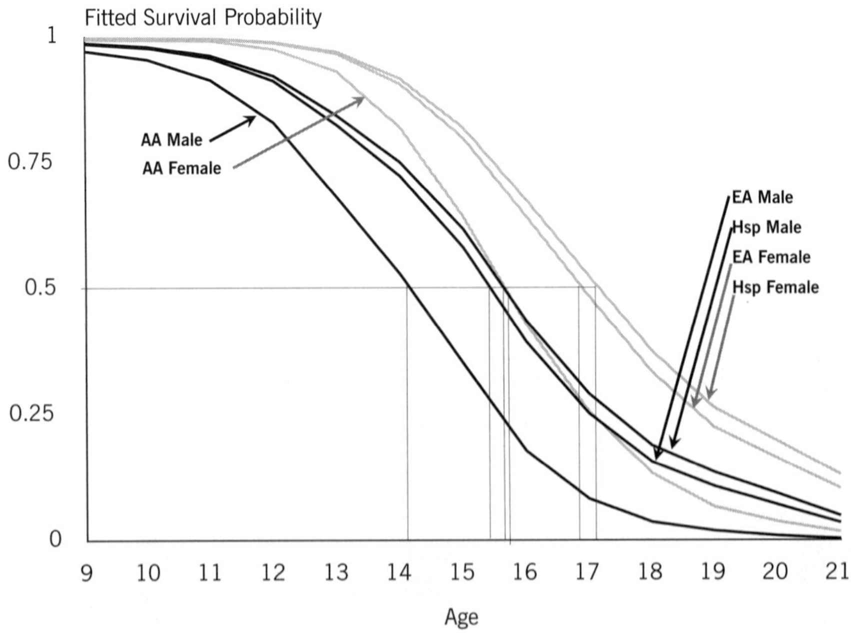

FIGURE 22.2. Fitted survival function for the age of first sexual intercourse from Model 5 that includes the effects of gender (male, female), race (AA, EA, Hispanic), and the interaction of gender with time. The best age to have children is included in this model, but we present only the prototypical profiles for those who feel the best age to have children is a younger age, 19. For those who feel the best age would be older, for example, age 26, all of the prototypical profiles would merely be shifted upward.

females have sex at about 15½ years old. Half of European American and Hispanic females have sex around 17 years of age. These latter individuals "survive" the longest without initiating sexual intercourse.

Two notes of caution regarding the interpretation of fitted prototypical plots such as these are worthy of mention. First, the apparent differences, as seen in the varying gap sizes between the fitted hazard functions for the different prototypical profiles, do not represent a time-varying effect of the predictors. Rather, this gap pattern is a function of the plotting scale. If we had plotted Model 5 in the metric of the logit hazard scale ($logit\ h(t_j)$) (equation 22.6) rather than exponentiating the hazard scale ($\hat{h}(t_j)$) (equation 22.9), the fitted lines for each of the subgroups would be parallel: No varying gap would be seen. We seldom plot on the logit hazard scale as the metric is difficult to interpret.

Second, the plots presented here represent fitted functions, *not* sample estimates from an analysis of subgroups of the sample. That is, we created the plots for various prototypical subgroups by using the parameter estimates from models fit to the *entire* sample, in which constraints were imposed on particular predictors' effects. We did not divide the sample into subgroups and conduct separate discrete time survival analyses. If we had done so, comparisons across the groups would have been less meaningful, because the models would have been fit to 12 different samples. This ability to generalize to the population is one of the strengths of fitting statistical models to sample data. Prototypical plots such as those presented here can be constructed in any analysis, regardless of the specific methodology used.

In sum, then, the event history analysis of our sexual initiation data yields several interesting findings. The age of greatest risk for sexual initiation for each of our prototypical groups is age 19 for females and 18 for males, controlling for race and the best age for having children. This finding illustrates that the effect of gender is different across time, as represented by the inclusion of the interaction of gender with time. Race has a pronounced effect on the timing of sexual initiation. African American individuals (male and female) have a greater risk, beginning at age 14, of having sex at every age, given that they had not before then. Interestingly, at age 19, the African American males and females are similarly likely to have sex, given that they had not prior to that; the risk for European American and Hispanic males and females to have sex at age 19 is also very similar, given that they had not had sex prior to that.

Developmental Applications

As noted at the beginning of this chapter, survival analysis has been used in several developmental areas to answer questions about the timing of events and what predicts that timing, but the utilization of this method has not yet reached its total potential. Researchers have used it to determine onset of behaviors, as we have in this chapter. For example, Dancy, Crittenden, and Ning (2010) investigated the time to first sexual intercourse for African American adolescent girls, and Trim, Schuckit, and Smith (2010) predict the onset of alcohol use in adolescents. In addition, researchers have examined when those in drug treatment relapse to drug use (Trujols et al., 2007) or terminate from therapy (Corning & Malofeeva, 2004). Many more applications of this methodology to other areas of developmental science await.

Conclusions

We have presented a discrete time event history analysis using a proportional odds model and discussed some of the relevant issues that arise in this type of analysis. Additional methods for modeling event history exist, however, and the reader is encouraged to explore these methods as well. For example, more than one type of event may be considered within the same analysis. In our example, one might be interested in whether individuals initiate their sexual experience by engaging in first sexual intercourse or by engaging in oral sex. A "competing risks" survival analysis could be conducted in which four mutually exclusive and exhaustive states include whether the respondent did not have any sexual experience, had only oral sex, had only first sexual intercourse, or had both oral sex and intercourse. In addition, if time is measured continuously rather than discretely, continuous-time survival analysis, in which proportional hazards models are commonly fit, can be explored (e.g., Allison, 1995; Singer & Willett, 2003). Clearly, event history analysis, or survival analysis, is a useful method for answering research questions related to the analysis of event times. Indeed, if researchers find themselves posed with the questions of *whether* and *when* certain events occur and what predicts those events, this methodology should almost always be the method of choice.

References

Allison, P. D. (1995). *Survival analysis using the SAS system: A practical guide*. Cary, NC: SAS Institute.

Canino, J. (2005). *Using survival analysis to explore the relationship among attachment theory, religiosity, and sexual initiation*. Unpublished doctoral dissertation, Purdue University.

Corning, A. F., & Malofeeva, E. V. (2004). The application of survival analysis to the study of psychotherapy termination. *Journal of Counseling Psychology, 51*, 354–367.

Cox, D. R. (1972). Regression models and life tables. *Journal of the Royal Statistical Society, B34*, 187–220.

Dancy, B. L., Crittenden, K. S., & Ning, H. (2010). African-American adolescent girls' initiation of sexual activity: Survival analysis. *Women's Health Issues, 20*, 146–155.

Erath, S., Keiley, M. K., Pettit, G., Lansford, J., Dodge, K., & Bates, J. (2009). Behavioral predictors of mental health service utilization in childhood through adolescence. *Journal of Developmental Behavioral Pediatrics, 30*, 481–488.

Flores, T. E., & Nooruddin, I. (2009). Financing the peace: Evaluating World Bank post-conflict assistance programs. *Review of International Organizations, 4*, 1–27.

Keiley, M. K., & Martin, N. C. (2005). Survival analysis in family research. *Journal of Family Psychology, 19*, 142–156.

Keiley, M. K., Martin, N. C., Canino, J., Singer, J., & Willett, J. (2007). *Discrete-time survival analysis: Predicting* whether, *and* if so when, *an event occurs*. In S. Menard (Ed.), *Handbook of longitudinal research: Design, measurement, and analysis* (pp. 441–463). Burlington, MA: Academic Press.

Mignone, T., Klostermann, K., & Chen, R. (2009). The relationship between relapse to alcohol and relapse to violence. *Journal of Family Violence, 24*, 497–505.

SAS Institute. (2001). Statistical analysis system. Cary, NC: Author. Available at *www.sas.com*.

Singer, J. D., & Willett, J. B. (2003). *Applied longitudinal data analysis: Modeling change and event occurrence*. New York: Oxford University Press.

Trim, R. S., Schuckit, M. A., & Smith, T. L. (2010). Predicting drinking onset with discrete-time survival analysis in offspring from the San Diego prospective study. *Drug and Alcohol Dependence, 107*, 215–220.

Trujols, J., Guardia, J., Pero, M., Freixa, M., Sinal, N., Tejero, A., et al. (2007). Multi-episode survival analysis: An application modeling readmission rates of heroin dependents at an inpatient detoxification unit. *Addictive Behaviors, 32*, 2391–2407.

Wilson, W. J. (1987). *The truly disadvantaged*. Chicago: University of Chicago Press.

PART V

Combining Interindividual and Intraindividual Longitudinal Analysis

CHAPTER 23

Foundational Issues in the Contemporary Modeling of Longitudinal Trajectories

JOHN J. McARDLE

Defining and Describing Trajectories Over Time

Figure 23.1 is a plot of longitudinal data from one of my favorite studies—the growth of verbal cognition in a set of children, originally carried out in a study described by Osborne and Suddick (1972). In this study, a special set of children ($N = 204$) were measured in school on the Wechsler Intelligence Scale for Children (WISC; Wechsler, 1970) on four separate occasions.

Figure 23.1a is a collection of dots and lines now commonly referred to as "longitudinal trajectories." The long history of this term is not widely known (see McArdle, 1988, 2001; McArdle & Nesselroade, 2003), but it is definitely popular (e.g., Raudenbush, 2001). One common definition is that "a trajectory is the path a moving object follows through space as a function of time" (*http://en.wikipedia.org/wiki/Trajectory*). In this case the people are thought of as moving through time (the X-axis), and the score they obtain on the WISC measure (Y-axis) is plotted as a dot; these dots are supposedly comparable over these ages. That is, we assume that the WISC score means the same thing at each time, so any score changes reflect changes in the people. Then the dots for the same person are connected by a straight line to form the individual trajectory. Of course, the scores could fluctuate in many ways between the dots (Wohlwill, 1973).

Figure 23.1b is a plot of the same WISC data, but here the information is presented in a scatterplot matrix. This shows the within-time univariate distributions on the diagonal and the time-to-time pairwise relationships among all persons on the off-diagonals. In this type of plot we can envisage data from all the people, and this even makes it easy to spot a few odd scores (the dots away from the main plot). There are many ways to plot longitudinal data (e.g., see Wainer & Spence, 2004), but it is hard to make the connections achieved by

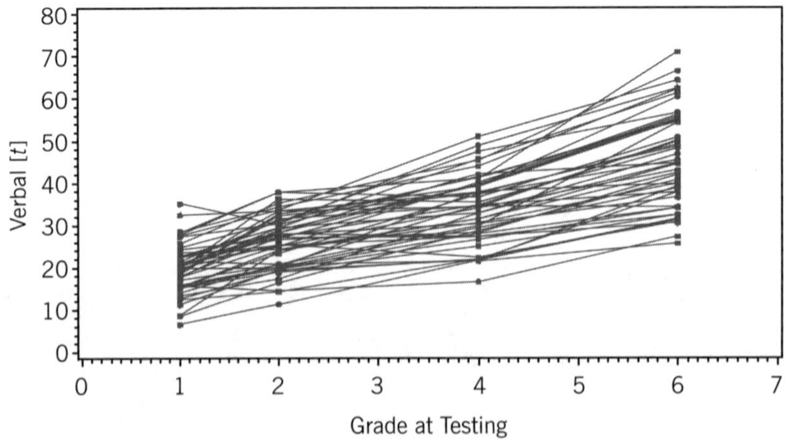

FIGURE 23.1a. Individual trajectories on the WISC Verbal scales ($N = 50$).

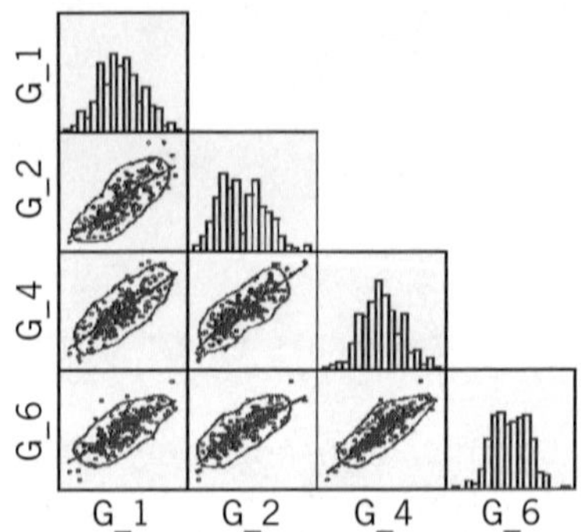

FIGURE 23.1b. A scatterplot matrix for four occasions of WISC data ($N = 204$). G, grade.

the simple lines and dots of Figure 23.1. In fact, it seems a bit easier to use Figure 23.1 to identify where a person has been and where he or she is going. Thus one advantage of the longitudinal trajectory plots is that they can help us tell a clear story about the person.

It has been my pleasure to deal with these longitudinal WISC data for about 20 years now, and I have tried many different kinds of analyses, including the beginnings of latent curve analysis (McArdle & Epstein, 1987), multivariate latent curve analysis (McArdle, 1988), multiple group factor analysis of latent curves (McArdle, 1989), autoregression versus latent curves (McArdle & Aber, 1990), multivariate analysis of variance (MANOVA) and the beginnings of latent change score analysis (McArdle & Nesselroade, 1994), and multivariate latent change score analysis (McArdle, 2001). I do not think I have found the best or most proper way to analyze these data, but I have certainly tried a lot of different forms of data analysis with these WISC data. I summarize my efforts here.

In a chapter on this topic Baltes and Nesselroade (1979) make a claim that, in studies of developing organisms, we often rely on some combination of information about (1) between-person differences, together with (2) within-person differences. In the prior literature on human development, these complex data collections are generally used for the study of intraindividual and interindividual differences. Instead of defining this in terms of algebraic relevance, they simply presented the five goals of longitudinal data analysis listed in Table 23.1.

What I am going to do now is use these five goals as my organization of our possible data analysis techniques and strategies. I am sure I will take some liberties with my reexpression of these earlier ideas, but I try to follow Baltes and Nesselroade (1979). Several decades ago longitudinal analyses were based largely on principles derived from linear growth models and formalized in terms of *analysis of variance* (ANOVA) techniques (e.g., Bock, 1975). In earlier work, these concepts were extended in the creation of randomized blocks and Latin squares (see Winer, 1962). Nowadays in research on human aging we often separate cross-sectional "age differences" from longitudinal "age changes" (see McArdle, 2009). Most of the newest analyses of developmental data analysis use information gathered from both cross-sectional and longitudinal selections in what are often termed "panel studies" (Hsiao, 2003).

The recent presentations on longitudinal data analysis are based on statistical procedures that combine these seemingly separate estimates. One way to do this is to create an "expected trajectory over time," in which the expected values are ***maximum likelihood estimates*** (MLE) and formal tests of hypotheses are encouraged (e.g., Hsiao, 2003; Miyazaki & Raudenbush, 2000; cf. McArdle & Bell, 2000). New computer programs for what are termed "latent curve" or "mixed effects" modeling allow model parameters to be estimated and used in making predictions and inferences. But this chapter is based on earlier work on longitudinal structural equation models (SEM; see McArdle, 2009). It is most important to recognize that we need to have some ways to understand these longitudinal data, and several theoretical statements have been formalized into "models" with useful statistical properties. These models allow us to consider alternative substantive ideas to fit these alternatives to our data and hopefully to make an informed choice about which alternatives are most useful. The great failure of any kind of analysis comes when a researcher reflexively applies any methods without thinking about what they mean and/or when the model predictions fail to look like the data.

I should state up front that, in my view, the current SEM approach is far less revolutionary than the past work. I think the new SEM techniques are not really much better than the old ones (cf. Raykov & Marcoulides, 2008). In my view, the classical techniques still form basic guideposts, and there are many worthwhile aspects of the older classical calculations. I mainly use SEM because it is convenient now.

TABLE 23.1. Five Objectives of Longitudinal Research

1. Direct identification of intraindividual changes.
2. Direct identification of interindividual differences in intraindividual changes.
3. Analysis of interrelationships in change.
4. Analysis of causes (determinants) of intraindividual change.
5. Analysis of causes (determinants) of interindividual differences in intraindividual change.

Note. Based on Baltes and Nesselroade (1979).

Issue 1: Studying Interindividual Changes with SEM

The very first issue we consider is how to organize information about the changes within a person. Baltes and Nesselroade (1979) used the term *intraindividual differences* but I now think it is better to state this as *within-person changes* (McArdle, 2009). There are two reasons for changing the prior terminology: (1) The term *within* is traditional ANOVA terminology to designate the separation of scores for the same person. This is in contrast to components that are "between persons." (2) The term *differences* rather than *changes* can then be reserved for models that imply the separation of different people.

A first important set of models for repeated-measures data has emerged from the "time-series" perspective and applied to panel data (see Andersen, 1971; Browne & Nesselroade, 2005). These models essentially suggest that the "future is predictable from the past" and that we should use this as a main feature of our analysis. The path diagrams of Figure 23.2 describe some options for these kinds of time series analyses of the WISC data. In general, a model is written in which the future deviation at time point [t] was predicted from deviation at the prior time point ([$t - 1$]) using a linear regression model with fixed parameters (b_0, b_1) and independent errors ($e[t]$). The utility of time series regression appeals to some researchers more than others (McArdle & Epstein, 1987).

The path diagrams of Figure 23.2 provide an exact translation of the necessary matrix formulation of these models (see McArdle, 1986, 1988), so none are provided. These path diagrams can be conceptually useful devices for understanding the basic modeling concepts. They are also practically useful because they can be used to represent the input and output of any computer program. In these path diagrams the observed variables are drawn as squares, and the unobserved variables are drawn as circles. Model parameters representing "fixed" or "group" coefficients are drawn as one-headed arrows, and "random" or "individual" characteristics are drawn as two-headed arrows. Here, the initial scores are random variables with no means but "random" variances ($\sigma_{[1]}{}^2$), and the effect of these scores on later scores is designated with regressions ($\beta[t]$). Standard deviations of the residual terms (Ψ_e) are also included (as in McArdle & Hamagami, 1991).

Figure 23.2a is a simple diagram in which everything in the past is used to produce (or predict) the future behaviors on the WISC. That is, the 1st-grade scores are used to produce the scores at the second grade, the fourth grade, and the sixth grade with unknown coefficients of proportionality ($\alpha[t]$). This implies that deviations from the mean for any person in the scores at later grades can be accounted for to some unknown degree by the early

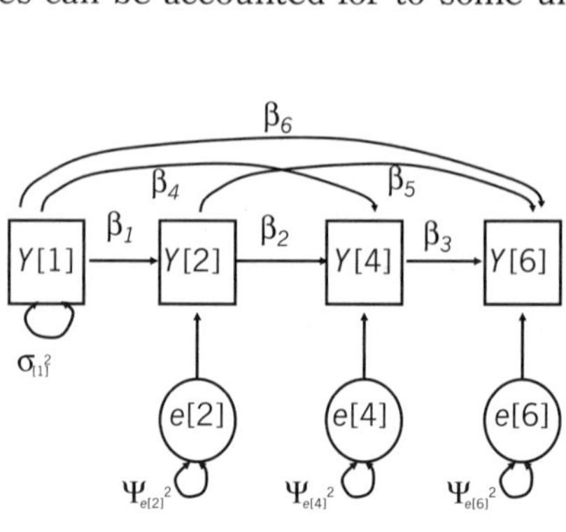

FIGURE 23.2a. A "fully recursive" Markov chain model with time-based effects.

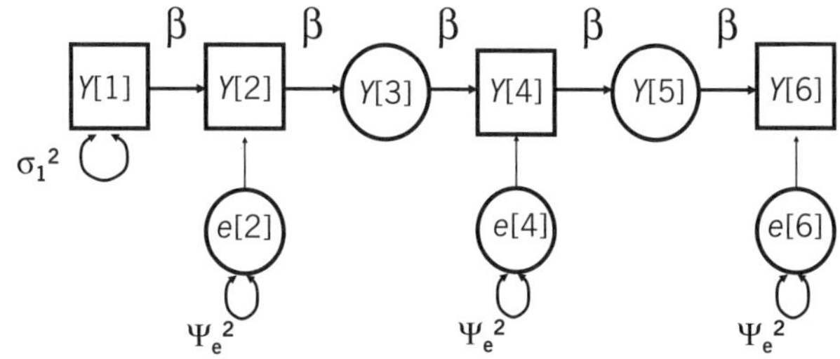

FIGURE 23.2b. An equal-time, equal-parameter "Markov simplex" model.

deviations from the mean. In a similar fashion, the second-grade scores are used to produce the fourth- and sixth-grade scores, and the fourth-grade scores are used to produce the sixth-grade scores. This kind of model is termed *fully recursive* because it requires as many parameters to be calculated as there are correlations observed in the data (Fig. 23.1b), so it is really not testing any major substantive idea here. To be clear, in this popular formulation, we are not really able to test whether or not the past predicts the future, or even vice versa, but we can use this approach to calculate the predicted values.

Figure 23.2a can have some important constraints. In a new version of this model, we can say that the only predictors needed for future scores are the ones in the immediate past. That is, the first affects the second, the second affects the fourth, and the fourth affects the sixth, and that is all that is needed to predict the future values. Because the time points are not equally spaced, we typically do not add further constraints to this model. This means we can eliminate three parameters from Figure 23.2a, and we can test this comparison of parameters as a formal hypothesis with three *degrees of freedom* (*df*). It is useful to restate that we are actually testing the importance of parameters that are not present, not the ones that are present. By fitting this alternative model, we can examine whether or not these simple time series restrictions seem reasonable for these WISC data.

We can add another important component to this model—a *latent variable* (LV), typically drawn as a circle with an arrow pointing directly to the square. This kind of LV is used because we want to assume that the time series process does not apply to the observed or *manifest variable* (MV), but the process applies to one key source of the variation in the MV—namely, the LV over time. Here we assume that there is one LV at each time, that the part of the MV that is not attributable to the LV is "unique," it may be partly "error of measurement," and it has the same variation at all times; this is exactly like a common factor model, but here the common factor has only one indicator, so it is not broad in any sense, nor is it tested in a rigorous way. But we should not underestimate the importance of this LV idea. One benefit of using LVs here is that we can estimate the process in the presence of random error (see Heise, 1975; Jöreskog & Sorbom, 1979). In this formulation, the time series for the LV is error-free, so we should find it to have predictions that are absent of error, and thus higher in accuracy. The model may fit the data better using this LV approach, but we do not have nor will we obtain estimated scores for the LVs. What we can examine is the effect of measurement error on our understanding of the process.

Figure 23.2b is an alternative and possibly simpler way to use LVs. Here we start with Figure 23.2a, but we then eliminate the parameters described earlier, and we add two LVs at the third and fifth grades to deal with the "unbalanced" data over time. In this conception, we assume that the children have verbal ability scores at each occasion, but we recognize that we did not measure them at these occasions. The main benefit of this type of LV model is that now we can consider a process that is measured over fairly equal units of time. That is, the interval of time between each LV is now 1 year, so we can constrain the parameter to be identical over time ($\beta[t] = \beta$). This simplifies the analysis because now we only have one parameter for any 1-year interval of time, and we have two additional *df*s to test the validity of this proportional prediction. Due to its simplicity, the prediction system is formally known as a "Markov simplex" model, but this seems to be misunderstood in the current literature (see Jöreskog & Sorbom, 1979; McArdle & Aber, 1990).

All of these time series models of Figure 23.2 were fitted to the WISC data, but they did not seem to fit very well; that is, the misfit index (χ^2) was large relative to the *df* (for details, see McArdle & Aber, 1990; McArdle & Epstein, 1987). The great success of time series models is that they allow us to make predictions about the future, and these predictions are fairly simple, but the failure to fit these models here means that these predictions were not very close to what had actually happened in the WISC scores. Part of this was the prior problem of "unbalanced" sequences (i.e., a 1-year gap, then a 2-year gap), but this seemed manageable (i.e., Figure 23.2b). But another part of the overall misfit of these models to the WISC data was clear—these time series models typically make an assumption of "stationarity"—that the variances (and covariances) remain the same over all times because the system has reached a "steady state of equilibrium" (see Heise, 1975). Equilibrium does not seem to be a reasonable assumption for verbal abilities in this young age range, and it is probably not a reasonable assumption for many other situations, either. Another assumption that was not tested is that the mean changes are not central to our understanding of the process. This problem does not create more of a misfit, but it can be a problem when the change for the whole group is a key part of the substantive questions.

To deal with some of these problems, a seemingly completely different set of models was also used. They are termed *latent curve models* (LCM), and they can be fitted by either approximate ANOVA methods or exact SEM methods (Meredith & Tisak, 1990; see McArdle, 1986, 1988; McArdle & Epstein, 1987; McArdle, Ferrer-Caja, Hamagami, & Woodcock, 2002). This LCM approach typically starts by assuming we have a *trajectory* equation for each occasion for each person formed as the sum of (1) unobserved or *latent scores* representing the individual's initial level (f_0), (2) unobserved or latent scores representing the individual *change over time* or *slope* (f_1), and (3) unobserved and independent unique features of measurements ($u[t]$). In this model the arrows from the latent slopes to observed variables are a set of group coefficients or *basis weights* that define the timing or *shape of the trajectory over time* (e.g., $\alpha[t] = t - 1$). We create this carefully selected set of basis weights (as $\alpha[t] = [0,1,3,5]$) so it takes care of the unbalanced time delay between occasions.

One version of this type of model is presented as a standard path diagram in Figure 23.3a. As before, the path diagrams of Figure 23.3 provide an exact translation of the necessary matrix formulation (see McArdle, 1986, 2007). In this case the initial level and slopes are often assumed to be random variables with "fixed" means (μ_0, μ_1) but "random" variances (σ_0^2, σ_1^2) and correlations (ρ_{01}). The standard deviations (σ_j) are drawn to permit the direct representation of the correlations (see McArdle & Hamagami, 1991). One new feature here is the use of a triangle to represent a measured variable that has no variation—that is, the unit constant. The key reason this new option is added to the path diagram is to allow us to make hypotheses about the group means. In LCM we want to make hypotheses

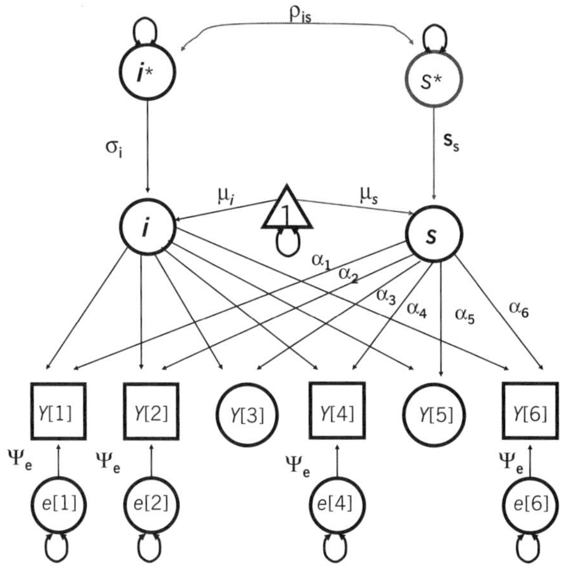

FIGURE 23.3a. A path diagram for a latent curve model with linear "slopes" based on weights $A[t]$.

about the group means and covariances that use the same parameters of proportionality (i.e., the basis $\alpha[t]$).

This LCM path diagram can also be interpreted as a two-common-factor model with means. The first latent factor score is an intercept or level score (labeled f_0), and the second latent factor score is a slope or change score (labeled f_1). The relationships between the latent levels f_0 and all observed scores $Y[t]$ are fixed at a value of 1. In contrast, the relationships between the latent slopes f_1 and all observed scores $Y[t]$ are assigned a value based on the time parameter $\alpha[t]$, which, depending on the application, may be fixed or estimated.

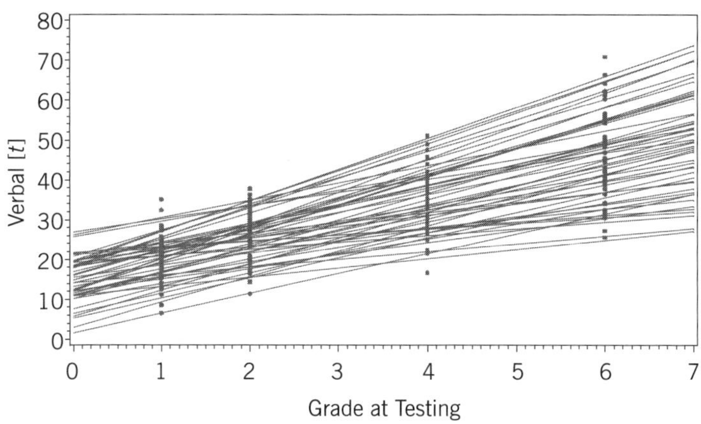

FIGURE 23.3b. Linear regression estimates of individual growth curves (n = 50).

For simplicity, the unique components ($u[t]$) are constant (Ψ_e) and uncorrelated with other components. In this longitudinal model the change score (f_1) is assumed to be constant *within* an individual, but it is not assumed to be the same *between* individuals. The latent variables are written in lower case (f_0, f_1) because they are similar to the predicted scores in a standard regression equation; that is, we do not use Greek notation because these scores do not need to be estimated (but see Figure 23.3b). Perhaps it is obvious, but this LCM is not the same as the prior time series model conception.

This simple linear LCM was fitted to the WISC data, and the results yielded a much better fit than found with other models (see McArdle & Aber, 1990). Several key issues can be seen in the simpler ordinary least squares (OLS) estimates of individual linear growth in Figure 23.3b. This plot is the result of extracting the longitudinal data for each individual and running a separate regression analysis for each person, whereas the WISC score was a simple linear function of time, and the plot included expected values. This yields estimates of linear equations with intercepts and slopes for each person, and this is a good way to see the key features of the LCM. First, the people vary at the first occasion, and this is a clear estimate of the intercept term in the LCM. In this figure it is clear that all persons are not alike—(1) we have an average intercept and a variation around this average; (2) we have a mean slope, a variation around this mean, and a possible covariance with the intercept score; and (3) we can see that the model does not fit all the data points (dots) in the plot. Thus we take the best parts of the LV approach, including the removal of independent unique variability, and the evaluation of systematic levels and slopes, and we add this to the individual and overall statistical indicators of goodness of fit.

Another interesting point is that the standard LCM is identical to the typical univariate repeated-measures ANOVA when the slopes are not allowed to vary (see McCall & Appelbaum, 1973). That is, the LCM approach offers a direct way to test the standard ANOVA as a simplified hypothesis (i.e., restricting the variance and covariance of the slopes to be zero results in "compound symmetry"). Although this standard ANOVA model may be reasonable in a number of circumstances, it is not reasonable with these WISC data because children do seem to vary in their slopes.

Although a linear scaling of the basis is very popular (see Singer & Willett, 2003), it is only one of many that could be used. For example, it is possible to add a lot of nonlinear complexity to the simple growth curve models for the study of within-person changes. For example, Wishart (1938) introduced a fundamental way to examine a nonlinear shape—the use of power polynomials to better fit the curvature apparent in growth data. The individual growth curve (consisting of $t = 1, T$ occasions) is summarized into a small set of linear orthogonal polynomial coefficients based on a fixed power series of time ($\alpha[t]$, $\frac{1}{2}\alpha[t]^2$, $\frac{1}{3}\alpha[t]^3, \cdots 1/p\ \alpha[t]^p$) describing the general nonlinear shape of the growth curve. A second-order (quadratic) polynomial growth model implies that the loadings of the second component are fixed to be a function of the first components (i.e., the derivative is linear with time).

The quadratic form of this basic model can be depicted as a path diagram as well (not included here). This can appear to be a bit complicated because it requires a third latent component with a basis that is related to the first one (i.e., $\frac{1}{2}\alpha[t]^2$), but all of this is done so that the implied change is linear with time (i.e., we add acceleration). Additional variance and covariance terms can be used to account for individual differences in these new LVs. In order to clarify these expressions, OLS quadratic regressions can be estimated for all the WISC scores on an individual basis (as in Figure 23.3b). Typically we find that introducing some curvature allows the model to approximate the data points more closely. Of course, a model of growth data might require this form of a second-order (quadratic), third-order (cubic), or even higher order polynomial model fitted to the data, and this family kind of nonlinear models are very popular (e.g., Bryk & Raudenbush, 1992).

One reason researchers like the LCM logic is that it permits many alternative extensions. A different alternative to the linear growth model was brought to light by Meredith and Tisak (1990)—the model proposed by Rao and Tucker in the form of summations of "latent curves." These innovative techniques were important because this made it possible to represent a wide range of alternative growth and change models by adding the benefits of the SEM techniques (McArdle, 1986, 1997; McArdle & Anderson, 1990; McArdle & Epstein, 1987; McArdle & Hamagami, 1991). Our use of this latent curve concept can be a minor adjustment to the LCM of Figure 23.3a: We allow the curve basis to take on a form based on the empirical data. In this example we simply write a model for the same person at multiple occasions in which the last two basis coefficients $a[3]$ and $a[4]$ are *free to be estimated* (the first two are still fixed at $a[1] = 0$ and $a[2] = 1$). The actual time of the measurement is known, but the basis parameters are allowed to be freely estimated so we can end up with different distances between time points—that is, an optimal shape for the whole curve. The estimated basis has been termed a "metameter" or "latent time" scale that can be plotted against the actual age curve for clearer interpretation (McArdle & Epstein, 1987). There are many ways to estimate these model parameters in an LCM framework, but this is very difficult to do with OLS, so these values are not estimated here.

The time series model and LCMs are only two approaches to the analysis of within-person changes that, while representing major modeling approaches, barely touch the surface of all other possibilities (e.g., see Walls & Schafer, 2006). These illustrations mainly show that any SEM, based on autoregressive (AR)-type models or LCMs, is used to make a prediction about the longitudinal trajectory based on a substantive issue. Thus both kinds of models have their place in the array of possible analytic frameworks, and choices between models are not often so easy. Some of these choices are simply defined by the data. For example, we might have a data set in which the individuals are measured repeatedly at more time points (e.g., $T = 100$). In this sense, this WISC collection of complete cases at a few time points ($T = 4$) is fairly easy to consider, even if the timing is unbalanced, and this allows us to go a bit further here.

Issue 2: Studying Interindividual Differences in Individual Changes with SEM

The second aspect of Baltes and Nesselroade's article (1979; see also Table 23.1) is the suggestion that we consider analyses focused on differences "between groups of persons in the way people change." In the WISC data we found that the original authors measured mothers' educational attainment levels before the children went to school at all; this showed a wide range across children, and we used this as the between-group variable (MOED). In one simple approach, we can just subdivide the WISC data into groups based on MOED and see whether or not the trajectories appear to differ.

At this time, we can consider four ways that the available SEM can be used to achieve these goals. We can (1) add measured variables (X) that define group differences into the previous expressions, (2) use the group variable to split the observed data into subsets for separate analyses, (3) define the grouping variable based on patterns of available data to deal with incomplete pieces, and/or (4) create latent groupings of people based on the pattern of available data. Of course, in any of these between-persons models the overall misfit can also be decomposed into individual components and outliers can be examined (e.g., McArdle, 1997).

Let us first add a measured variable (X = MOED) to characterize group differences directly into the previous linear expressions. Indeed, the most popular model used nowadays is the inclusion of the between-persons predictor in an LCM framework and having this static (one time of measurement) group variable account for systematic variation in the latent levels and slopes. As in any regression analysis, the coding and scaling of the between-person variable will lead to different estimates of effects. This type of SEM is depicted in Figure 23.4a and typically called by terms that are based on the history of its development with a substantive discipline: This model is termed an LCM in psychology (Meredith & Tisak, 1990), multilevel modeling in education (e.g., Bryk & Raudenbush, 1992), and a mixed-effects or random coefficients model in statistics (e.g., Longford, 1993). To be fair, there are advantages to considering these analyses within each discipline, but it is most important to note that variations of this analysis can be done using many computer programs, and the results are identical (see Ferrer, Hamagami & McArdle, 2004). In our prior WISC analyses, we have found that both the intercept and the slope were significantly higher for children whose mothers' educations were initially higher (see McArdle, 1989). Two of the limits of this popular approach quickly become evident: (1) We need to select an overall basis function for the entire group, and (2) the variance and covariance of the residuals of the latent variables must be the same over group.

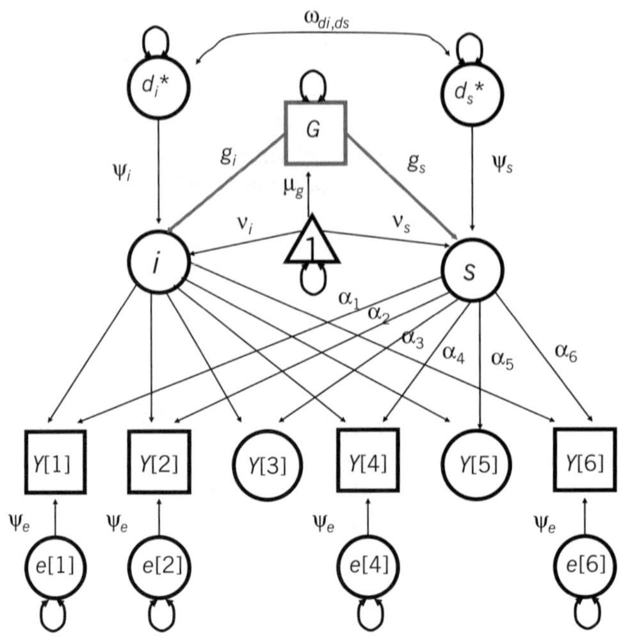

FIGURE 23.4a. A "multilevel" or "mixed-effects" model or LCM with an external G variable affecting both the latent levels and latent slopes.

A second analysis that does not require these constraints is to use the group variable to split the observed data into subsets for separate analyses. This is illustrated in the diagram of Figure 23.4b. This approach explicitly recognizes that separate models are allowed, so not all persons need to have the same within-person change model. In an SEM framework, checking whether or not the model and the model parameters are identical across independent groups is based on multiple group factor analysis (MGFA; Horn & McArdle, 1992; Sörbom, 1979).

Practical problems occur in any longitudinal study, including initial self-selection and dropout (or attrition). In prior work, a multiple-group SEM approach has been used (Jöreskog, 1971; McArdle & Hamagami, 1992) to deal with problems of "incomplete data" (see Cudeck, 2000; McArdle, 1994). In this situation, we can use the MGFA approach, defining the grouping variable based on patterns of available data to deal with incomplete pieces (with the incomplete data simply drawn as circles in the path diagram). We then assume that all parameters are invariant over all groups so that we mimic the assumptions of data missing at random (MAR; Little & Rubin, 1987; McArdle, 1994) and obtain tests of fit to represent MAR as a testable hypothesis.

In recent work much more complex models have been fitted using a raw data approach that does not require the data blocked into simple patterns (see Hamagami & McArdle, 2000; McArdle, Hamagami, Meredith, & Bradway, 2000; McArdle & Woodcock, 1997). Many of these can be seen from the perspective of multiple-group models with different numbers of data points on each person (McArdle & Hamagami, 1992). In this case, a model of "longitudinal convergence" (after Bell, 1954; McArdle & Bell, 2000) is a reasonable goal of many studies, but it is not always a hypothesis that can be tested with incomplete patterns (McArdle & Anderson, 1990). Instead, the MAR assumption is viewed as a convenient starting point, allowing us to use all the available information in one analysis, but it

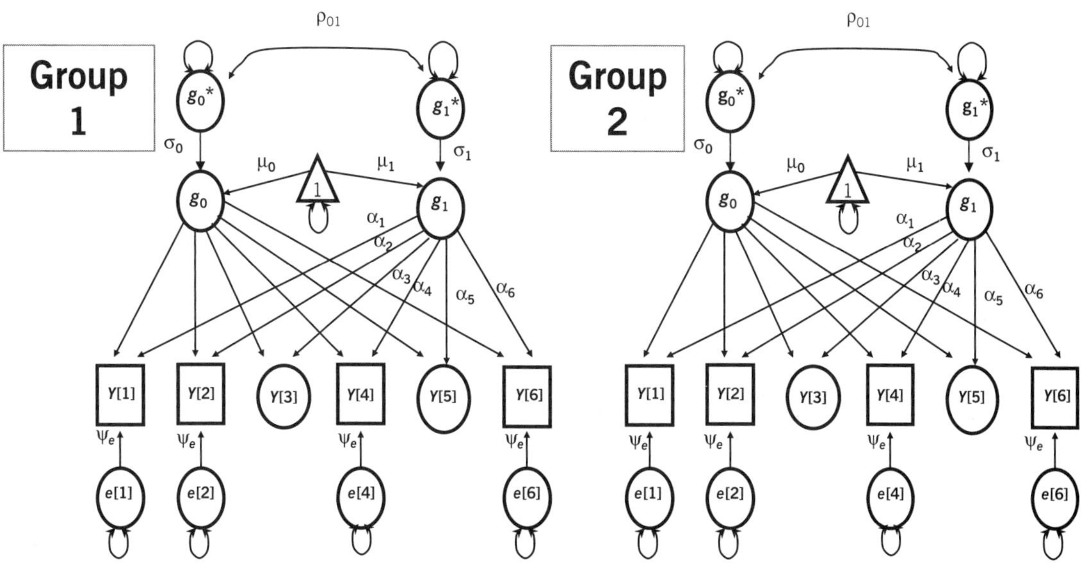

FIGURE 23.4b. Multiple-growth models for independent groups. The key question now is "Are any parameters not meaningfully the same (invariant) over groups?"

could be incorrect for a number of reasons (e.g., Cnaan, Laird, & Slasor, 1997; McArdle, 1994), but these key assumptions should be examined. Thus, instead of simply stating that MAR is a reasonable assumption, we should investigate methods for evaluating the failure of these assumptions. We can examine a model on the data that are already available, or we can gather extra information about the selection process (see Hedeker & Gibbons, 1997).

The benefits of considering incomplete group data are profound. For example, one of the corollary between-group issues is the potential for combining cross-sectional and longitudinal data. In one early resolution of these problems, Bell (1953) created a data collection he termed *accelerated* longitudinal data. To examine such ideas, Bell (1954) showed that by selecting data from a more time-consuming longitudinal study (i.e., by deletion of some of the existing data) he would get the same results. To ensure uniformity of the outcomes, Bell suggested a test of "convergence" of the cross-sectional and longitudinal data, created by joining together the shorter spans of data from people who were most similar at the endpoints. In contemporary work, this is now fitted with "invariance of the basis coefficients" (McArdle & Anderson, 1990). Bell (1954) demonstrated that estimates and inferences were basically the same, even though the data collection was accelerated, and we now do the same analysis using statistics for incomplete data (Hsiao, 2003; McArdle & Bell, 2000; Miyazaki & Raudenbush, 2000).

A fourth way of dealing with between-group differences is to create latent classes of different people based on the pattern of available data. It is always worth considering whether we have unmeasured subgroupings of people in our data set. It is now popular to explore these ideas with unobserved but heterogeneous subgroups, as in the SEM work on latent mixture models (LMM; Bauer & Curran, 2003; McLachan & Peel, 2000; Muthén, 2004, 2006). The defining feature of this model is that an SEM may be appropriate for each subgroup of persons, but there may be completely different SEMs for different unobserved subgroups; what we end up within the total group is a "mixture" of people. To better understand the class assignment of individuals, we can also write a prediction model (typically based on logistic regression) in which the probability of latent class membership is describable by other measured variables. The use of multiple parameters and a combined model is relatively new to this area, but it is potentially a reasonable and convenient way to deal with the problem of heterogeneity in a single-group data collection design. In the LCM context, this problem is often termed a "latent growth mixture model" (LGMM); this is essentially an effort to estimate the influences of LVs that are categorical, and this has an interesting history (see Bartholomew, 1987; Muthén & Shedden, 1999). This organization of information is the same as in Figure 23.4b, but, most important, the group membership is not known until the analysis is carried out. We have used LGMM with the WISC data and found this somewhat novel approach to be informative.

Issue 3: Studying Interrelationships in Individual Changes with SEM

The next question we face is what to do when we have multiple outcome variables. Figure 23.5a is a simple example of data from the WISC study. Here we plot both the longitudinal trajectory of the Verbal scales and the same for the Non-Verbal scales. The questions we ask begin with a surface look at the similarity of models across variables, but the deeper questions emerge about the time-dependent relationships of each variable to one another.

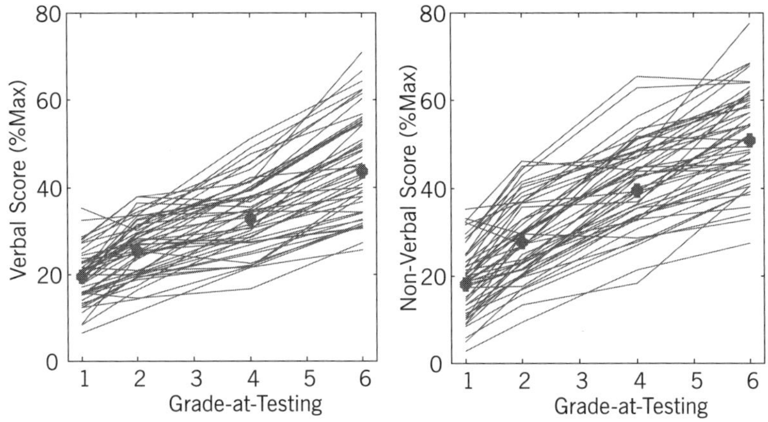

FIGURE 23.5a. Longitudinal WISC data on two variables (N = 204, plotted n = 50).

One natural model for multivariate longitudinal data is to examine the LCM of a common factor score. Basically, each MV is thought to be an indicator of one or more LVs, and it is this LV that carries the information over time. The key requirement here is that the factor pattern for the LV relationships is invariant over time (see McArdle, 1988, 2007). If invariance can be established, the LCM can then be applied to the LV[t] for examination of the common intercepts and slopes. In this model, the unique variance at the second level does not have any measurement error, so we have a clear indication of within-time variability that is not correlated over time (termed *state variance* by Cattell, 1959, as reported by McArdle & Woodcock, 1997). This model was termed a *curve of factor scores* (CUFFS; McArdle, 1988), and it still seems useful to some researchers (see Ferrer, Balluerka, & Widaman, 2008).

A different model for these same data is presented in Figure 23.5b. This model starts by fitting separate latent curves to each variable, and here we could establish any similarity of the curves—that is, we could first test the equality of the group slope parameters ($\alpha_1[t] = \alpha_2[t]$, etc.). Equality or invariance of this process is not required but can be studied. Most important, we can join these models at the individual level by correlating the latent intercepts and the slopes (see McArdle, 1989). That is, rather than correlating the variables at the same times, we correlated the components of the curves over time. The correlation of two or more latent slopes offers a broad single indication of whether one variable is changing in the same people as another variable. Testing the similarity of individual changes using the slope scores has proven to be a bit tricky, because the variances and covariances of the slopes need to be considered, and one is left wondering what to do about the intercept term. Basically, these are not separable concepts in most observational studies, because the intercepts and slopes are thought to occur at the same times. This SEM could be useful in the beginnings of an investigation into "correlated changes." If the correlation of components of change is our goal, we do not even need to measure the variables at exactly the same occasions or with exactly the same frequency.

One obvious extension of this logic is to examine common factors of the multiple intercepts and multiple slopes. One persistent problem with this model is the rather artificial separation of intercepts from slopes, because they are conceptually part of the same

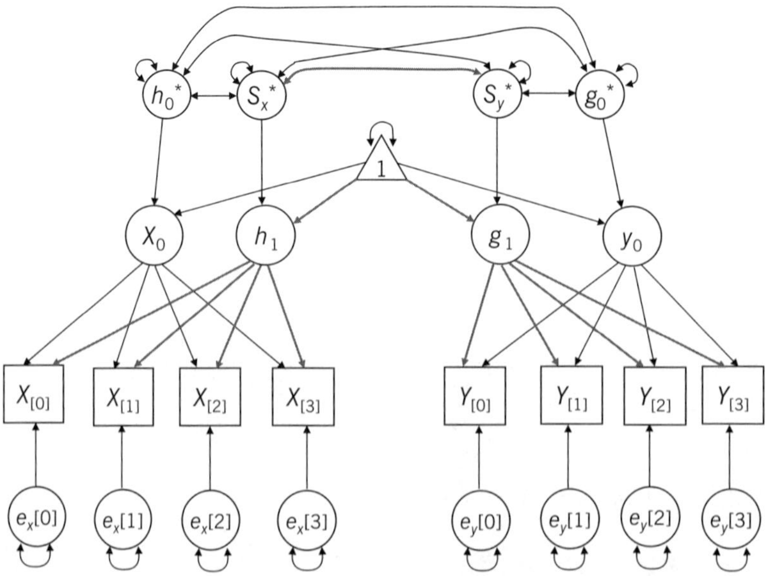

FIGURE 23.5b. A latent growth model for multiple variables. Based on McArdle (1988, 1989).

process. Nevertheless, such a model was initially termed a *factor of curves scores* (FOCUS; McArdle, 1988), and it is still considered useful by some researchers (see Duncan, Duncan, & Stryker, 2006).

No doubt there are many other models for multivariate longitudinal data that can be created to deal with this type of problem. However, most of these do not deal with specific timings, which was a direct focus of our autoregressive starting point. The bivariate and multivariate illustrations presented here dealt with the critical problem of interrelationships among different growth variables. In previous work, McArdle (1988, 1989, 1991) outlined some of these issues and fit a model in which the levels and slopes of one series was correlated with, or regressed upon, the levels and slopes of a different series. Similar multiple-variable latent variable modeling analyses have been used and reported by others (e.g., Raykov, 1997; Walker, Acock, Bowman, & Li, 1996). These kinds of analyses formalize an idea that the correlation among the slopes of two different variables may reflect the "common changes" (Griffiths & Sandland, 1984; McArdle & Nesselroade, 1994).

Issue 4: Studying Determinants (Causes) of Individual Changes with SEM

There are many alternative longitudinal models that can be fitted to these kinds of longitudinal data in Figure 23.5a (page 397), and some of these take into account the ordering of the responses. In these SEMs it is also important to recognize that models of *individual-differences relationships among dynamic variables do not necessarily reflect dynamic processes for the group*. The latter interpretation requires a focus on time-based parameters in the models and not on the time-independent correlation of the time-based scores (e.g., Gollob & Reichardt, 1987).

Following the previous work on common factor analysis and cross-lagged regression (Jöreskog & Sorbom, 1979) we can simply assume that, for the MV[*t*], the observed raw score measured can be decomposed into the sum of a common factor score and a unique score. This algebraic form is depicted in the path diagram of Figure 23.6a by having the latent variables and the error scores add to each other (i.e., with unit weights) to form the observed variables. Additional restrictive assumptions about random errors imply that the true scores include any common factors, as well as any specific factors.

Next we need to represent the changes within a person over time. We define a latent change score (LCS) between any two latent scores as the part of a later latent score at one time that is not part of it at the earlier time. We can simplify a lot of the required algebra by always assuming that the interval of time between LVs is the same. The simplifying assumption of equal latent intervals is not a testable feature of the model. In practice, it is not always possible and not always desirable to keep the MV intervals of time equal (see McArdle & Woodcock, 1997, 2000). We deal with this practical problem by making a clear definition of the patterns of complete and incomplete data (see Horn & McArdle, 2007; Jöreskog & Sorbom, 1979; McArdle, 1997; McArdle & Aber, 1990; McArdle & Bell, 2000; McArdle & Hamagami, 1991). In the path diagram of Figure 23.6a the LCS is drawn as a latent variable at each time, and the interpretation of this score as a change within a person is assured by the placement of the latent score at the first occasion and the LCSs (see McArdle & Nesselroade, 1994).

We can now create an SEM that allows for dynamic inferences and reinforces the key idea—we now have individual changes represented as LVs, and these are the key outcomes. What the researcher must now do is pose a model for the latent changes (see Ferrer & McArdle, 2010), and this can be difficult for a number of reasons. First, we are not used to

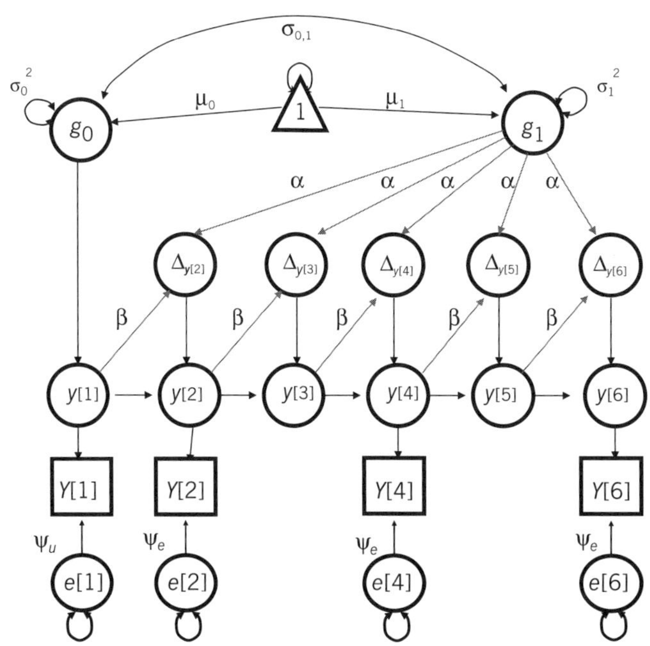

FIGURE 23.6a. The latent change score (LCS) model based on both LCM and AR(1).

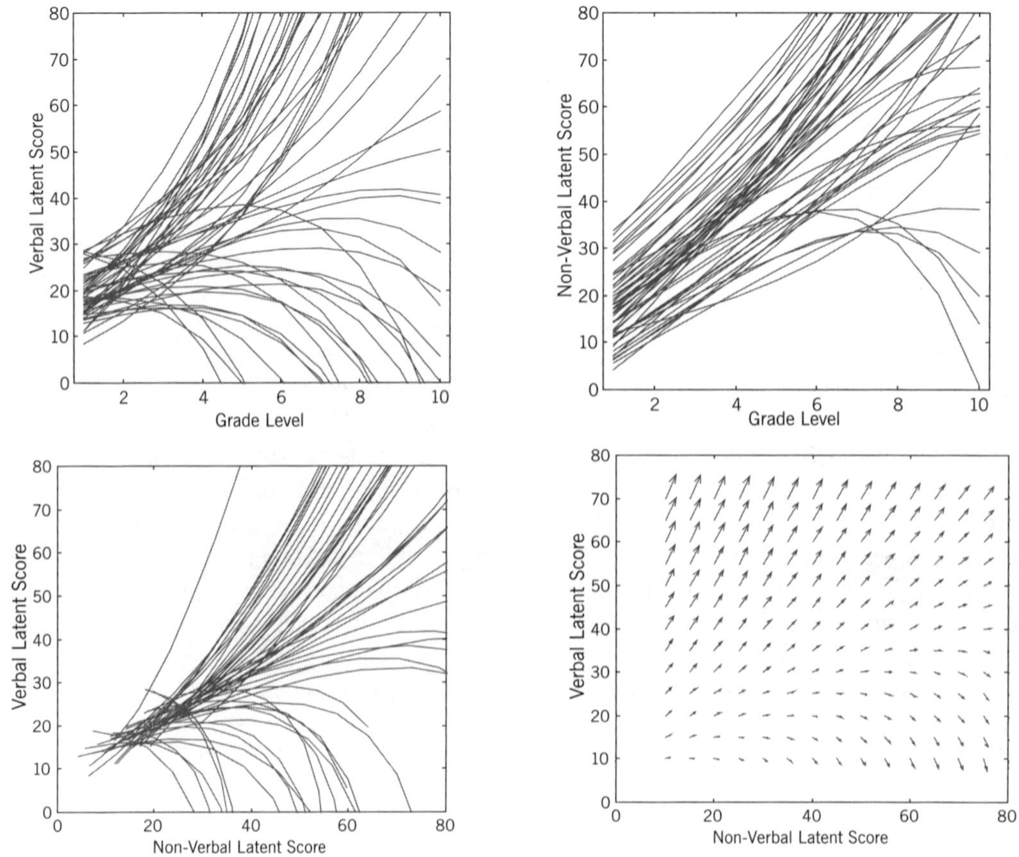

FIGURE 23.6b. Expected bivariate latent trajectories.

doing this kind of work on an a priori basis, but this is needed to create an expected set of trajectories. Second, we are typically willing to explore and try a lot of different models to see what looks like the best fit. In the SEM approach used here, we are not restrictive, and many models of change are possible.

These choices of dynamic models may be made on substantive or empirical considerations. In our initial examples, the model of latent change we used (Figure 23.6a) was based on a simple additive combination of the linear curve model and the autoregressive model (Figure 23.2, pages 388–389) and the linear latent curve model (Figure 23.3, page 391). This was written so time-based changes in the latent change score were allowed (1) to be constantly related to some alternative but fixed slope score ($\alpha[t]\, f_{1n}$), (2) to be proportional to the previous state ($\alpha[t]\ .\ y[t-1]_n$), and (3) to include an additive residual or disturbance term ($z[t]$). This dynamic SEM can be completed by adding several parameters for the multiple sets of latent variables. In all cases, we use fixed unit values to define the LCS, and we ensured the LCS were outcome variables. That is, the earlier LV in time is included as a predictor of the LCS, as is the common latent slope. All dynamic coefficients are repeatedly used for all occasions, but this is a hypothesis that should be tested. Due to our use of two additive change components, we termed this a *dual change score* model (DCS; McArdle,

2001; McArdle & Hamagami, 2001). This DCS model has some interesting properties, including its ability to bring together both the LCM and the AR–SEM as proper statistical subsets. We can assume that the latent trajectories are smooth deterministic curves or have uniform random residual properties by eliminating the variance of the residual ($z[t]$).

These kinds of univariate models were initially represented for the Verbal (V) and Non-Verbal (NV) scales of the WISC and were fitted using LISREL software. The results are presented graphically elsewhere (see McArdle, 2001). In each case (of V and NV) the models required at least as many parameters as were available in the DCS framework. That is, neither the autoregressive SEM nor the LCM fit these data very well, but the DCS was a great improvement. The resulting DCS equation for these trajectories for the overall group curve from the model parameters shows that the expected group mean will always increase both additively (by +2) and proportionally (by +0.09) per year. The simple substitution of specific time points (t = 0–10) into this equation results in the nearly straight average group curve. We note that trajectory estimates are made for grade 3 and grade 5, even though there were no group observations at this point, and also for $t > 6$ as a "forecast" of scores in future years. To better understand the meaning of the individual-differences parameters, individual latent curves were generated from the repeated application of the difference equation, and this yielded individual curves that follow the particular solution. The resulting individual latent curves (for $n = 50$) are presented elsewhere and show significantly more nonlinear curvature than the means (see McArdle, 2001). This collection of curves also shows increasing variance of a "fan spread" (Shadish, Cook, & Campbell, 2002).

These graphic illustrations from the WISC show only a sampling of the family of curves that can be generated from the few DCS model parameters. The results for the V model do not seem the same as the results for the NV; most obviously, one seems to grow up (V) and the other (NV) flattens out during this period of time. Tests for these kinds of bivariate models are well known in the SEM literature. A more challenging set of models is based on "time-varying covariates," or "systems models," and these are often not fully specified in SEM terms. However, let us now consider a bivariate model of change in which we write the prior difference equation for more than one dynamic variable.

If we want to identify the interplay of two variables that are changing over time, we can follow the previous SEM logic and write the LCS model in which the change in one latent variable is a function of both itself and another variable. The most important features of this bivariate change SEM include (1) the separation of individual scores from group parameters, (2) the assumption of a constant time interval, and (3) a separation of the true scores from the measurement error scores. Residual disturbances for each variable are included as well, but these will not be used. A path diagram of this bivariate dynamic model is presented in Figure 23.7a. As part of this SEM we include a representation of the change over time in the second LCS, including a constant change (α_x), a proportional effect (β_x) of the latent variable upon itself, and a "coupling effect" (γ_x) of the first variable. In this dynamic SEM it is clear that the predictors of one latent variable are embedded in the outcomes of the other variable and vice versa. In this bivariate form, model parameters may be simplified to deal with dynamic hypotheses about "coupling" or "lead-lag" relationships. Unlike all prior SEMs, these dynamic hypotheses may be considered in the presence of individual differences in constant growth and change. These alternatives can be examined in combination with restrictions on the univariate (μ and σ) parameters of change within each variable, and the results can be plotted as a statistical vector field (SVF; Boker & McArdle, 2005; McArdle & Hamagami, 2001).

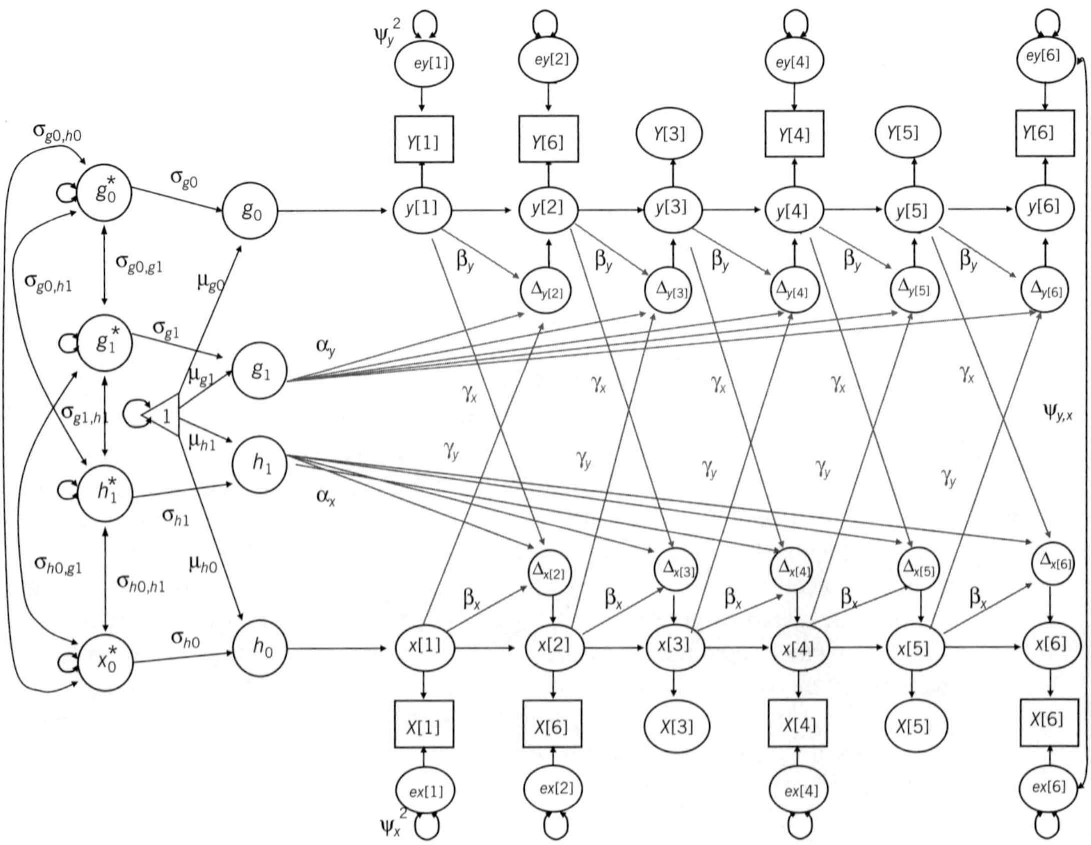

FIGURE 23.7a. A bivariate dual change score model.

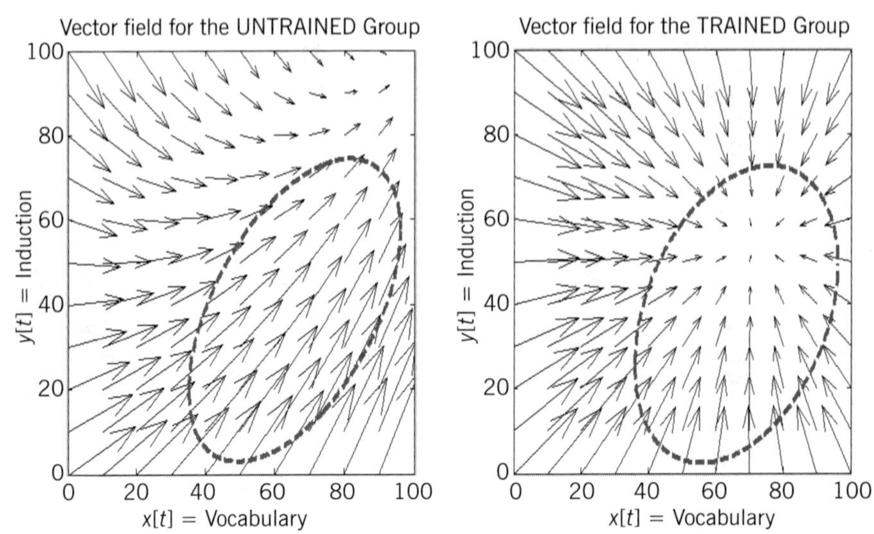

FIGURE 23.7b. Vector field plots for untrained and trained groups from the Berlin Aging Study of Training. Ellipse is 95% confidence around starting points.

The numerical results of fitting two bivariate DCS models to the four-occasion WISC V and NV scores (of Figure 23.5a, page 397) have been found using standard SEM programs, and some results are presented graphically in Figure 23.6b (page 400). In contrast to the univariate LCD results for V scores, here we obtained a large auto-proportion ($\alpha_y = +.5$), a small but negative mean slope ($\beta_{sy} = -1$), and a nontrivial coupling parameter from latent NV[t – 1] to LCS[V] ($\gamma_y = -.2$). In contrast, the model for NV scores includes a smaller autoproportion ($\gamma_x = -.0$), a smaller positive mean slope ($\mu_{sx} = 5$), and only a trivial coupling. These bivariate results were used to calculate the expected values for a longer time sequence ($t = 0$–10). The plot of the V latent scores now shows what appears to be a rapid fanning out at both the upper and lower portions of the initial scores, whereas the NV scores appear to have more steady increases. The bivariate equations lead to latent curves with downward trends for both variables, with a larger impact on the V than the NV curves.

The final two panels of Figure 23.6b represent a different kind of time-sequence plot because here, for each individual, we draw the V latent curve scores paired against the NV latent curve scores for the same occasions. This "state-space" pairing of latent growth curves seems to show that most individuals follow rapid increases in both variables with a few individuals dropping off toward lower V scores but higher NV scores. The initial levels and slopes are all positively correlated (e.g., $\rho_{sy,sx} = .8$), and these correlations are informative because they describe the location of the individual dynamic curves in the time-sequence plots. The final panel of Figure 23.6b is the SVF version of the same bivariate curves. Each arrow here shows the general direction of all curves within that specific region (equal-sized cells) of these curves. That is, for any pair of latent scores at a specific time (i.e., $x[t]$, $y[t]$), the small arrow points to where the pair of latent scores is expected to be at the next time ($x[t+1]$,$y[t+1]$). This final figure seems to emphasize the increases in the upper left-hand quadrant of the bivariate field.

A model with no effect of V on the NV changes was evaluated with a restriction that V[t – 1] did not affect LCS[NV], and this alternative fit the WISC data fairly well. In addition, a model with no effect of NV on the V changes was fit where the NV[t – 1] did not affect LCS[V], but this did not fit the data. The collection of bivariate latent change score results leads to a few substantive conclusions about this dynamic system: (1) The variables are growing, so the standard cross-lagged assumptions (i.e., no growth) are not a viable alternative for these WISC data; (2) there is no effect of the Verbal latent scores on the NV latent changes; and (3) the NV latent scores significantly and negatively affect the V latent changes. Thus *the NV scores are leading indicators of the growth in V scores, but not vice versa*. As it turns out, this result is consistent with aspects of some prior developmental theory in this area (see McArdle, Hamagami, Meredith, & Bradway, 2000). There are not many other SEMs that are used to establish time-ordered precedence (see Ferrer & McArdle, 2010; McArdle, 2009).

Issue 5: Studying Individual Differences in the Determinants of Individual Changes

Our final goal is to combine the concepts of the previous models but add separate group issues. One way to see this is as a multiple-group (MG) SEM, and this might start with the bivariate change model in Figure 23.7a. Without further detail, we should be able to see this path diagram for multiple groups (as in McArdle & Prindle, 2008). In any case, all forms of between-group analysis are of obvious importance in the study of dynamics: (1) MVs that are measured at one time (static) can be added into the dynamic model, and this could change the coupling parameters; (2) the MG–SEM approach allows all of these options, plus it allows the dynamic influences to be completely different across different manifest groups; (3) incomplete data modeling by MG–SEM or other approaches is fundamental in dynamic analysis (see Hamagami & McArdle, 2000); and (4) the determination of unobserved latent classes of persons who are following the same dynamic process is essential (see McArdle & Prindle, 2008). Variations on these MG–SEMs can be used to examine different combinations of variables or latent mixtures (Muthén & Muthén, 2005; Nagin, 1999).

The methods and results of research on group differences in dynamics have not been applied to these WISC data. But these kinds of SEMs are detailed in McArdle (2006) with data from the Berlin Age Training Study (with the permission of the authors, Baltes, Dittmann-Kohli, & Kliegl, 1986). The general purpose of this data collection was to evaluate theory of "cognitive plasticity," which suggested that older adults have untapped cognitive resources that can be stimulated by cognitive training. The study participants were randomly assigned to one of two groups: (1) one in which they were trained on one of two cognitive tasks (n = 161) or (2) a no-contact (not trained) control group (n = 87). The cognitive training program consisted of 10 consecutive sessions, and each dealt with training specifically focused on the improvement of aspects of "fluid intelligence" or "reasoning in novel situations" using training methods developed in earlier research. A cognitive measurement design included four rounds of repeated cognitive testing: (t = 0), a pretest measurement followed by 1 month of training or of no contact; (t = 1), a 1-week posttest measurement; (t = 2), a 1-month posttest measurement; (t = 3), and a 6-month posttest (t = 4) measurement. These time points were chosen because they were thought to represent critical junctures in the learning of these cognitive tasks. At each measurement session, a battery of cognitive tests was repeatedly administered, and two of these tests were used here: (1) Induction (IND), a "near-transfer" test expected to be directly affected by the specific training; and (2) Vocabulary (VOC), a "far-transfer" test not expected to be affected by this training.

Standard repeated-measures ANOVA models were used by Baltes and colleagues (1986), but these analyses were not intended to capture the possible within-persons changes, or individual transfer effects. Raykov (1997) reanalyzed one subset of these data using a model for multiple indicators of an Induction factor. The SEMs were based on factor analysis in multiple groups with correlated growth curves (McArdle, 1989). Raykov (p. 310) concluded, "the results indicate (a) group equivalence in the pattern of temporal development of ability variances, and (b) training effects in the experimental group that are stronger than the practice/experience effects in the control group, and both types of effects are maintained over the 6-month testing period." McArdle (2007) used the same data but asked the specific questions about group differences due to training as a dynamic system. The MG–SEM approach allows for differences in the latent means, slope variances, residual variance, and dynamic coupling of the respective trajectories. But the groups could have a different set of coupling parameters, implying a more fundamental impact of the experiment—*alterations in the dynamic system due to the treatment*.

These new results suggested that the Vocabulary scores exhibit proportionally more unique variance (and hence are less reliable, although the correlation among the latent levels is positive [+.5]). In terms of the group differences, one clear training impact is that the constant slopes are much higher in the trained group for both variables. This is interesting as the second variable (Vocabulary) is a "far-transfer" variable, and no real training differences were expected. This interpretation of mean changes for different variables is often characterized as a "transfer of training" (e.g., Baltes et al., 1986). The correlations among the latent slopes are high (+.8) in the control group and lower in the experimental group (+.5), but this is not what we expected as an impact when training is transferred. Further group differences include parameters with different signs, so their total impacts are hard to interpret directly or individually. In the control group, all parameters were accurately different from zero, so this was a *coupled system* of latent scores. In contrast, the results for the treated group suggested higher autoproportions and no accurate coupling parameters, so this was as an *uncoupled system* of latent scores.

The net result of the experimental training manipulation was that the treatment both raised and uncoupled the scores on the two variables. This result suggests no strong evidence of a transfer of training across these variables, This result could be due to the fact that training helped focus the persons on all tasks and especially focused on the Induction-like tasks (near transfer). At the same time the pattern of individual differences apparent here suggests that the specific training seems to have set the Induction variable farther away from the Vocabulary variable than it was before. The expected values from these parameters are those displayed as *vector field plots* for each group in Figure 23.7b (page 402). Both figures show an interesting dynamic property—*the change expectations of a dynamic model depend on the starting point*. Thus, the training seems to have isolated the abilities that were trained and possibly moved these scores toward other, unmeasured variables.

It may be clear that these kinds of dynamic differences due to training are not easy to see in the typical comparison of changes in the means, as in repeated-measures ANOVA. An updated version of this kind of MG–SEM dynamic analysis has also been carried out for a different set of randomized experimental data in McArdle and Prindle (2008) and for observational data in Grimm and McArdle (2007).

Discussion: Studying Longitudinal Data with Contemporary SEM

This analysis of longitudinal trajectories can be a great deal of fun for the eager analyst. One has an overwhelming sense that something useful, something special, could emerge from analyzing longitudinal data. After all, almost any longitudinal data collection takes a lot more time and effort than the more typical cross-sectional data collection. So, whether or not it is deserved, longitudinal analyses often take on a special importance. But, for very similar reasons, these analyses can be very difficult. Longitudinal analyses can be difficult to organize. It can be difficult to do something very simple and useful (such as plotting the data) and difficult to know when to stop with advanced analyses. To deal with these issues, I have placed SEM in the context of five goals suggested by Baltes and Nesselroade (1979). I suggest you consider what you or others have done within the context of the five steps outlined earlier; it is not necessary to carry them out in order, but it could be easier. Each step can build on the results from the previous steps.

There are many motivations to use contemporary SEM for longitudinal analyses, and SEM has both benefits and limitations. Among many benefits, we can see a required clarity of process definitions, easy programming of complex ideas, clear tests of parameter equivalence, and generally simple tests of otherwise complex ideas. A few of these SEM techniques even lead to novel ideas for data analysis, especially dealing with ordinal measurements. Perhaps SEM path diagrams provide a clearer way to think about longitudinal analyses. Unfortunately, among many SEM limitations, we need large and representative samples of persons for reasonable estimation, and we also need normal distribution of residuals (or uniquenesses) to create appropriate statistical tests. But, most important, we need to state what we want to examine about dynamic influences in advance of the data analysis. In this way any SEM requires the kind of clear thinking we have probably not yet achieved in behavioral sciences. In common practice, we get stuck using the SEM models in ways that are far simpler than is possible. That is, we seem to focus on issues 1, 2 and 3 and rarely reach issues 4 and 5.

Once again, the choice of a dynamic model is intimately tied to the substantive theory and the available data. The choice between using an autoregressive approach, a linear latent basis, or a polynomial or other nonlinear model can be substantively important. The initial idea from Wishart (1938) was that the basic shape of each individual curve could be captured with a small number of fixed parameters and random variance components. In some cases a fixed-basis polynomial model is more parsimonious than a free-basis model (see McArdle & Bell, 2000). But many recent textbooks overlook the latent-basis model (e.g., Duncan et al., 2006; Singer & Willett, 2003), and this option remains a most useful empirical choice.

One way to combine recent ideas about dynamics and retain the statistical and practical benefits of SEM is to use a model based on the LCS (Hamagami & McArdle, 2000; McArdle, 2001; McArdle & Hamagami, 2001). Indeed, the introduction of individual differences in change analyses has led to a great deal of statistical controversy in model fitting (e.g., Nesselroade & Cable, 1974; Sullivan, Rosenbloom, Lim, & Pfefferman, 2000). These kinds of "difference" or "gain" score calculations are relatively simple and theoretically meaningful, but the potential confounds due to the accumulation of random errors has been a key concern in previous studies using observed change scores or rate of change scores (e.g., Burr & Nesselroade, 1990; Rogosa & Willett, 1985; Willett, 1990). This recent SEM approach allows us to write expectations in terms of the first- or second- or higher order latent differences, and we can have the SEM program automatically generate the required nonlinear expectations of the scores.

Practical problems in the fitting of any statistical model with longitudinal data begin with scaling and metrics. These ideas can be examined at the item level by forming a scoring system for any construct; we used concepts from item response theory (IRT) (see McArdle, Grimm, Hamagami, Bowles, & Meredith, 2009; McArdle & Hamagami, 2004). Additional scaling issues deal with the exact timing of observations (e.g., Boker & McArdle, 2005) and, as usual, transformations can change the statistical patterns. Optimal measurement collections are a major challenge for new empirical research and worthy of much further discussion (McArdle, 2010).

The SEM analyses presented here make specific assumptions about latent changes in individuals and groups (as in McArdle & Prindle, 2008; Meredith & Tiask, 1990; Muthén & Curran, 1997). But the SEMs presented here were developed to be a reasonable match to the *goals of longitudinal data analysis* proposed by Baltes and Nesselroade (1979; Table 1). The representation of change processes can be accomplished using the variety of methods we have been referring to as latent curve, mixed effect, multilevel, or multiple-group modeling. With this in mind, we need to be careful not to forget the important lessons of the past. At the same time, we do need to invent new ways to collect the optimal sets of data needed for powerful tests of hypotheses about development. These are among the most important challenges for contemporary and future longitudinal research, and my hope is that some of the SEM ideas presented here can be useful in this work.

Acknowledgments

This work was supported by NIA Grant AG-7137-21 to John J. McArdle. I thank my colleagues John R. Nesselroade (University of Virginia), Kevin Grimm (University of California at Davis), John Prindle (University of Southern California), and Todd Little (University of Kansas) for their important contributions to an earlier version of this work.

References

Andersen, T. W. (1971). *The statistical analysis of time series*. New York: Wiley.

Baltes, P. B., Dittmann-Kohli, F., & Kliegl, R. (1986). Reserved capacity of the elderly in aging-sensitive tests of fluid intelligence: Replication and extension. *Psychology and Aging, 1*(2), 172–177.

Baltes, P. B., & Nesselroade, J. R. (1979). History and rationale of longitudinal research. In J. R. Nesselroade & P. B. Baltes (Eds.), *Longitudinal research in the study of behavior and development* (pp. 1–39). New York: Academic Press.

Bartholomew, D. J. (1987). *Latent variable models and factor analysis*. Gurnee, IL: Kenner Books.

Bauer, D. J., & Curran, P. J. (2003). Over-extracting latent trajectory classes: Much ado about nothing? *Psychological Methods, 8*, 384–393.

Bell, R. Q. (1953). Convergence: An accelerated longitudinal approach. *Child Development, 24*, 145–222.

Bell, R. Q. (1954). An experimental test of the accelerated longitudinal approach. *Child Development, 25*, 281–286.

Bock, R. D. (1975). *Multivariate statistical methods in behavioral research*. New York: McGraw-Hill.

Boker, S., & McArdle, J. J. (2005). Vector field plots. In P. Armitage & P. Colton (Eds.), *Encyclopedia of Biostatistics* (2nd ed., Vol. 8, pp. 5700–5704). Chichester, UK: Wiley.

Browne, M. W., & Nesselroade, J. R. (2005). Representing psychological processes with dynamic factor models: Some promising uses and extensions of ARMA time series models. In A. Maydeu-Olivares & J. J. McArdle (Eds.), *Advances in psychometrics: A festschrift to Roderick P. McDonald* (pp. 415–451). Mahwah, NJ: Erlbaum.

Bryk, A. S., & Raudenbush, S. W. (1992). *Hierarchical linear models in social and behavioral research: Applications and data analysis methods*. Newbury Park, CA: Sage.

Burr, J., & Nesselroade, J. R. (1990). Change measurement. In A. von Eye (Ed.), *Statistical methods in longitudinal research* (Vol. 1). New York: Academic Press.

Cnaan, A., Laird, N. M., & Slasor, P. (1997). Using the general linear mixed model to analyse unbalanced repeated measures and longitudinal data. *Statistics in Medicine, 16*, 2349–2380.

Cudeck, R. (2000). An estimate of the covariance between two variables which are not jointly observed. *Psychometrika, 65*, 539–546.

Duncan, T. E., Duncan, S. C., & Stryker, L. (2006). *An introduction to latent variable growth curve modeling* (2nd ed.). Mahwah, NJ: Erlbaum.

Ferrer, E., Balluerka, N., & Widaman, K. F. (2008). Factorial invariance and the specification of second-order latent growth models. *Methodology, 4*, 22–36.

Ferrer, E., Hamagami, F., & McArdle, J. J. (2004). Modeling latent growth curves with incomplete data using different types of structural equation modeling and multilevel software. *Structural Equation Modeling, 11*(3), 452–483.

Ferrer, E., & McArdle, J. J. (2010). Longitudinal modeling of developmental changes in psychological research. *Current Directions in Psychological Science, 19*(3), 149–154.

Ferrer-Caja, E., & McArdle, J. J. (2004). Alternative structural models for multivariate longitudinal data analysis. *Structural Equation Modeling, 10*(4), 493–524.

Gollob, H. F., & Reichardt, C. S. (1987). Taking account of time lags in causal models. *Child Development, 58*, 80–92.

Griffiths, D., & Sandland, R. (1984). Fitting generalized allometric models to multivariate growth data. *Biometrics, 40*, 139–150.

Grimm, K. J., & McArdle, J. J. (2007). A dynamic structural analysis of the potential impacts of major context shifts on lifespan cognitive development. In T. D. Little, J. A. Bovaird, & N. A. Card (Eds.), *Modeling contextual effects in longitudinal studies* (pp. 363–386). Mahwah, NJ: Erlbaum.

Hamagami, F., & McArdle, J. J. (2000). Advanced studies of individual differences linear dynamic models for longitudinal data analysis. In G. Marcoulides & R. Schumacker (Eds.), *New developments and techniques in structural equations modeling* (pp. 203–246). Mahwah, NJ: Erlbaum.

Hedeker, D., & Gibbons, R. D. (1997). Application of random-effects pattern-mixture models for missing data in longitudinal studies. *Psychological Methods, 2*, 64–78.

Heise, D. R. (1975). *Causal analysis*. New York: Wiley-Interscience.

Horn, J. L., & McArdle, J. J. (2007). Understanding human intelligence since Spearman. In R. Cudeck & R. MacCallum (Eds.), *Factor analysis at 100 years* (pp. 205–247). Mahwah, NJ: Erlbaum.

Hsiao, C. (2003). *Analysis of panel data*. New York: Cambridge University Press.

Jöreskog, K. G. (1971). Simultaneous factor analysis in several populations. *Psychometrika, 36*, 409–426.

Jöreskog, K. G., & Sorbom, D. (1979). *Advances in factor analysis and structural equation models*. Cambridge, MA: Abt Books.

Little, R. T. A., & Rubin, D. B. (1987). *Statistical analysis with missing data*. New York: Wiley.

Longford, N. T. (1993). *Random coefficient models*. London: Clarendon Press.

McArdle, J. J. (1986). Latent variable growth within behavior genetic models. *Behavior Genetics, 16*(1), 163–200.

McArdle, J. J. (1988). Dynamic but structural equation modeling of repeated measures data. In J. R. Nesselroade & R. B. Cattell (Eds.), *Handbook of multivariate experimental psychology* (2nd ed., pp. 561–614). New York: Plenum Press.

McArdle, J. J. (1989). Structural modeling experiments using multiple growth functions. In P. Ackerman, R. Kanfer, & R. Cudeck (Eds.), *Learning and individual differences: Abilities, motivation, and methodology* (pp. 71–117). Hillsdale, NJ: Erlbaum.

McArdle, J. J. (1991). Structural models of developmental theory in psychology. *Annals of Theoretical Psychology, 7*, 139–160.

McArdle, J. J. (1994). Structural factor analysis experiments with incomplete data. *Multivariate Behavioral Research, 29*(4), 409–454.

McArdle, J. J. (1997). Modeling longitudinal data by latent growth curve methods. In G. Marcoulides (Ed.), *Modern methods for business research* (pp. 359–406). Mahwah, NJ: Erlbaum.

McArdle, J. J. (2001). A latent difference score approach to longitudinal dynamic structural analysis. In R. Cudeck, S. du Toit, & D. Sorbom (Eds.), *Structural equation modeling: Present and future* (pp. 342–380). Lincolnwood, IL: Scientific Software International.

McArdle, J. J. (2006). Dynamic structural equation modeling in longitudinal experimental studies. In K. van Montfort, H. Oud, & A. Satorra (Eds.), *Longitudinal models in the behavioural and related sciences* (pp. 159–187). Mahwah, NJ: Erlbaum.

McArdle, J. J. (2007). Five steps in the structural factor analysis of longitudinal data. In R. Cudeck & R. MacCallum (Eds.), *Factor analysis at 100 years* (pp. 99–130). Mahwah, NJ: Erlbaum.

McArdle, J. J. (2009). Latent variable modeling of differences and changes with longitudinal data. *Annual Review of Psychology, 60*, 577–605.

McArdle, J. J. (2010). Contemporary challenges of longitudinal measurement using HRS data. In G.

Walford, E. Tucker, & M. Viswanathan (Eds.), *Sage handbook of measurement* (pp. 509–536). London: Sage.

McArdle, J. J., & Aber, M. S. (1990). Patterns of change within latent variable structural equation modeling. In A. von Eye (Ed.), *New statistical methods in developmental research* (pp. 151–224). New York: Academic Press.

McArdle, J. J., & Anderson, E. (1990). Latent variable growth models for research on aging. In J. E. Birren & K. W. Schaie (Eds.), *Handbook of the psychology of aging* (pp. 21–43). New York: Plenum Press.

McArdle, J. J., & Bell, R. Q. (2000). An introduction to latent growth curve models for developmental data analysis. In T. D. Little, K. U. Schnabel, & J. Baumert (Eds.), *Modeling longitudinal and multiple-group data: Practical issues, applied approaches, and scientific examples* (pp. 69–107). Mahwah, NJ: Erlbaum.

McArdle, J. J., & Epstein, D. B. (1987). Latent growth curves within developmental structural equation models. *Child Development, 58*(1), 110–133.

McArdle, J. J., Ferrer-Caja, E., Hamagami, F., & Woodcock, R. W. (2002). Comparative longitudinal multilevel structural analyses of the growth and decline of multiple intellectual abilities over the life-span. *Developmental Psychology, 38*(1), 115–142.

McArdle, J. J., Grimm, K., Hamagami, F., Bowles, R., & Meredith, W. (2009). Modeling life-span growth curves of cognition using longitudinal data with multiple samples and changing scales of measurement. *Psychological Methods, 14*(2), 126–149.

McArdle, J. J., & Hamagami, F. (1991). Modeling incomplete longitudinal and cross-sectional data using latent growth structural models. In L. Collins & J. L. Horn (Eds.), *Best methods for the analysis of change* (pp. 276–304). Washington, DC: American Psychiatric Association.

McArdle, J. J, & Hamagami, F. (2001). Linear dynamic analyses of incomplete longitudinal data. In L. M. Collins & A. G. Sayer (Eds.), *New methods for the analysis of change* (pp. 137–176). Washington, DC: American Psychological Association.

McArdle, J. J, & Hamagami, F. (2004). Methods for dynamic change hypotheses. In K. van Montfort, J. Oud, & A. Satorra (Eds.), *Recent developments in structural equation models* (pp. 295–336). London: Kluwer Academic.

McArdle, J. J., Hamagami, F., Meredith, W., & Bradway, K. P. (2000). Modeling the dynamic hypotheses of Gf–Gc theory using longitudinal life-span data. *Learning and Individual Differences, 12*(1), 53–79.

McArdle, J. J., & Nesselroade, J. R. (1994). Using multivariate data to structure developmental change. In S. H. Cohen & H. W. Reese (Eds.), *Life-span developmental psychology: Methodological innovations* (pp. 223–267). Hillsdale, NJ: Erlbaum.

McArdle, J. J., & Nesselroade, J. R. (2003). Growth curve analyses in contemporary psychological research. In J. Schinka & W. Velicer (Eds.), *Comprehensive handbook of psychology: Vol. 2. Research methods in psychology* (pp. 447–480). New York: Pergamon Press.

McArdle, J. J., & Prindle, J. J. (2008). A latent change score analysis of a randomized clinical trial in reasoning training. *Psychology and Aging, 23*(4), 702–719.

McArdle, J. J., & Woodcock, J. R. (1997). Expanding test-rest designs to include developmental time-lag components. *Psychological Methods, 2*(4), 403–435.

McCall, R. B., & Appelbaum, M. I. (1973). Bias in the analysis of repeated-measures designs: Some alternative approaches. *Child Development, 44*, 401–415.

McLachlan, G., & Peel, D. (2000). *Finite mixture models*. New York: Wiley.

Meredith, W., & Tisak, J. (1990). Latent curve analysis. *Psychometrika, 55*, 107–122.

Miyazaki, Y., & Raudenbush, S. W. (2000). Tests for linkage of multiple cohorts in an accelerated longitudinal design. *Psychological Methods, 5*(1), 24–63.

Muthén, B. (2004). Latent variable analysis: Growth mixture modeling and related techniques for longitudinal data. In D. Kaplan (Ed.), *Handbook of quantitative methodology for the social sciences* (pp. 345–368). Newbury Park, CA: Sage.

Muthén, B. (2006). The potential of growth mixture modeling. *Infant and Child Development, 15,* 623–625.

Muthén, B., & Curran, P. (1997). General longitudinal modeling of individual differences in experimental designs: A latent variable framework for analysis and power estimation. *Psychological Methods, 2,* 371–402.

Muthén, B., & Shedden, K. (1999). Finite mixture modeling with mixture outcomes using the EM algorithm. *Biometrics, 55,* 463–469.

Muthén, L. K., & Muthén, B. O. (2005). *Mplus, the comprehensive modeling program for applied researchers user's guide.* Los Angeles: Authors.

Nagin, D. (1999). Analyzing developmental trajectories: Semi-parametric group-based approach. *Psychological Methods, 4,* 139–177.

Nesselroade, J. R., & Cable, D. G. (1974). "Sometimes it's okay to factor difference scores": The separation of trait and state anxiety. *Multivariate Behavioral Research, 9,* 273–282.

Osborne, R. T., & Suddick, D. E. (1972). A longitudinal investigation of the intellectual differentiation hypothesis. *Journal of Genetic Psychology, 121*(1), 83.

Raudenbush, S. W. (2001). Comparing personal trajectories and drawing causal inferences from longitudinal data. *Annual Review of Psychology, 52,* 501–525.

Raykov, T. (1997). Growth curve analysis of ability means and variances in measures of fluid intelligence of older adults. *Structural Equation Modeling, 4,* 283–319.

Raykov, T., & Marcoulides, G. A. (2008). *An introduction to applied multivariate analysis.* Mahwah, NJ: Erlbaum.

Rogosa, D., & Willett, J. B. (1985). Understanding correlates of change by modeling individual differences in growth. *Psychometrika, 50*(2), 203–228.

Shadish, W., Cook, T., & Campbell, D. (2002). *Experimental and quasi-experimental designs for generalized causal inference.* Boston: Houghton Mifflin.

Singer, J., & Willett, J. (2003). *Applied longitudinal data analysis: Modeling change and event occurrence.* New York: Oxford University Press.

Sörbom, D. (1979). An alternative to the methodology for analysis of covariance. *Psychometrika, 43,* 381–396.

Sullivan, E. V., Rosenbloom, M. J., Lim, K. O., & Pfefferman, A. (2000). Longitudinal changes in cognition, gait, balance in abstinent and relapsed alcoholic men: Relationships to changes in brain structure. *Neuropsychology, 14*(2), 178–188.

Wainer, H., & Spence, I. (2004). Graphical presentation of longitudinal data. In B. S. Everitt & D. C. Howell (Eds.-in-Chief), *Encyclopedia of statistics in behavioral science* (pp. 1–10). New York: Wiley.

Walker, A., Acock, A. C., Bowman, S. B., & Li, F. (1996). Amount of care given and caregiving satisfaction: A latent growth curve analysis. *Journal of Gerontology: Psychological Science and Social Science, 51B*(3), 130–142.

Walls, T. A., & Schafer, J. L. (Eds.). (2006). *Models for intensive longitudinal data.* Oxford, UK: Oxford University Press.

Wechsler, D. (1970). *The Wechsler Intelligence Scale for Children.* New York: Psychological Corporation.

Willett, J. B. (1990). Mearsuring change: The difference score and beyond. In H. J. Walberg & G. D. Haertel (Eds.), *The international encyclopedia of education evaluation* (pp. 632–637). Oxford, UK: Pergamon.

Winer, B. J. (1962). *Statistical principles in experimental design.* New York: McGraw-Hill.

Wishart, J. (1938). Growth-rate determinations in nutrition studies with the bacon pig, and their analysis. *Biometrika, 30*(1/2), 16–28.

Wohlwill, J. (1973). *The study of behavioral development.* New York: Academic Press.

CHAPTER 24

Growth Curve Modeling from a Structural Equation Modeling Perspective

KEVIN J. GRIMM
NILAM RAM

Growth curve modeling, as we know it today, was initially developed in the late 1950s (Rao, 1958; Tucker, 1958) and is one of the main analytical techniques for examining and understanding developmental change—how and when it happens, interindividual differences in how and when it happens, and why it happens (McArdle, 2009; McArdle & Nesselroade, 2003). The ability to fit growth curve models in the structural equation modeling (SEM) framework (Meredith & Tisak, 1984, 1990) drastically changed the way psychologists approached longitudinal data because the dynamics of the developmental process became a focus, as opposed to static entities, and true variation in change was separable from error variance (see also Cronbach & Furby, 1970).

In this chapter we highlight some of the ways in which growth curve models are being used to articulate and test theories and specific hypotheses of development. We begin by noting some foundational issues surrounding the use of growth curve models, review the growth curve model as it can be fit into the SEM framework, paying particular attention to modeling nonlinear forms of change, and illustrate the application of these models to longitudinal panel data. We close with some notes on the types of innovations and applications we see on the horizon.

Central Issues

Successful application of growth curve models requires consideration of some central issues and assumptions regarding the constructs and processes underlying their changes. Particularly important are how constructs are measured, the time scale of the developmental process of interest, the form or shape of the hypothesized within-person change process, where between-person differences manifest along that process, and what the determinants of change may be.

Measurement

Typically, the basic data to which growth curve models are applied are repeated measures obtained from multiple individuals. Among the first considerations in modeling such data is how the construct was measured. What are the measurement properties of the instrument? Was the instrument sensitive to and able to capture within-person change? Many tests or scales are highly reliable and valid but may not be useful in measuring change within an individual for several reasons. First, items or scales should measure the same construct at each age, grade, or measurement occasion so that those scores can be quantitatively compared. Measures that capture different constructs at different points in the developmental process are not useful for examining within-person change in a specific construct. To ensure that scores are indeed comparable across the repeated measures, a thorough investigation of *measurement invariance* is needed (see Meredith, 1993; Meredith & Horn, 2001). Second, the scale should adequately represent the entirety of skills at one or more ages, grades, and so forth, so that the full range of growth can be adequately tracked. Violation of the needed representation of abilities may be evident when ceiling (or floor) effects are noted in data—an indication that participants have "grown out" of the range of abilities measured by the scale. Third, the scale should have equal reliability at different levels of proficiency so that both subtle changes and differences can be discriminated. In sum, measurement properties of the scale being used have severe consequences for how much can be learned from investigations of longitudinal change and should be considered thoughtfully before proceeding too far in any growth curve modeling analysis. See Edwards and Wirth (2009) and Meredith and Horn (2001) for a more in-depth discussion of issues surrounding measurement and developmental change.

Time Metrics

A second key consideration for understanding longitudinal change is the choice of an appropriate metric of time. Within the growth curve model, the time variable along which change is tracked serves as a proxy for the underlying change process (e.g., age-related change, school-related change, etc.). To illustrate, Figure 24.1a shows a longitudinal plot of seven time-ordered reading scores obtained from a small subsample of individuals from the Early Childhood Longitudinal Study—Kindergarten cohort (ECLS-K; National Center for Education Statistics, 2001). In this figure, the time metric, the x-axis, is *measurement occasion*. Measurement occasion is often used when studying longitudinal change because it is a straightforward and simple metric for time. Additionally, it may simplify presentation and estimation when fitting growth curves. However, measurement occasion rarely serves as an adequate proxy for the developmental processes being studied. That is, measurement occasion, as a researcher-assigned variable, is an unlikely metric to adequately represent the time scale underlying the developmental processes (except perhaps when examining exposure or practice effects; McArdle & Woodcock, 1997). Figure 24.1b shows the same seven time-ordered reading scores from Figure 24.1a, but with *age* as the time metric used along the x-axis. Here it becomes clearly visible that individuals were measured at different ages, and that there was differential spacing between measurements. The differential spacing is important to consider because it may highlight key features of the developmental processes driving changes in reading abilities that were not apparent when the data were scaled by measurement occasion. Age, as a time metric for understanding developmental processes, can be a very useful tool, as many processes are hypothesized as being age-based, such as changes in height (not, however, that age is the only process underlying changes in height). Figure 24.1c is a third plot of the same data but with *grade in school* as the time metric. Differential spacing is again evident, as the assessments took place in the fall and spring of kindergarten and first grade, as well as in the springs of third, fifth, and eighth grades. For academic variables, grade may be an appropriate time metric for understanding change because changes may be driven by school-related processes—what is taught in school. In our examples we shall use grade in school as the time metric when fitting growth curve models to these data.

It is also possible that the developmental process under study is simultaneously following multiple time metrics. For example, the majority of school-related learning processes may be closely tied to grade level. Additionally, children who are relatively older within their grades and thus further along in their age-related development may be better able to take advantage of schooling opportunities. On top of those processes, practice effects tracked in relation to measurement occasion may also contribute to the observed changes. Unfortunately, due to high collinearity among time metrics (increases in grade are almost always accompanied by correspondent increases in age), the unique contributions of multiple processes and time metrics are difficult to untangle unless tackled in the design phase (see Ferrer, Salthouse, McArdle, Stewart, & Schwartz, 2005; McArdle & Woodcock, 1997; Morrison, Smith, & Dow-Ehrensberger, 1995). In sum, care should be taken to select a time scale and metric that serves as an adequate proxy for the underlying processes of interest. See also Ram, Gerstorf, Fauth, Zarit, and Malberg (2010), Sliwinski, Hofer, Hall, Buschke, and Lipton (2003), and Wohlwill (1973) for more in-depth discussion of issues surrounding choice of time metric.

Within-Person Change

Once an appropriate, and theoretically derived, time metric is chosen, the next critical issue is to determine how the observed scores are related to the time metric at the individual level. Thus the goal is to describe how the developmental process unfolds within each person—within-person or intraindividual change. When examining individual change patterns, like those presented in Figure 24.1, it is necessary to consider what the key characteristics of change are. That is, how should the individual change patterns be summarized? Many descriptions are possible. For example, one way to summarize the repeated-measures data is to describe each child's development using a simple line. Each trajectory, then, could be characterized by two parameters: an intercept, or predicted score at the beginning of kindergarten, and a slope, representing the rate of growth during the observation period. Looking at the plots it is obvious that a linear change pattern would not adequately represent each individual's trajectory; straight lines are a gross oversimplification of the changes in these children's reading achievement from kindergarten through eighth grade. Note that although many nuances of the change trajectories would be lost, linear depictions of growth would still provide some information regarding children's reading ability at school entry and their overall rate of change from kindergarten through eighth grade.

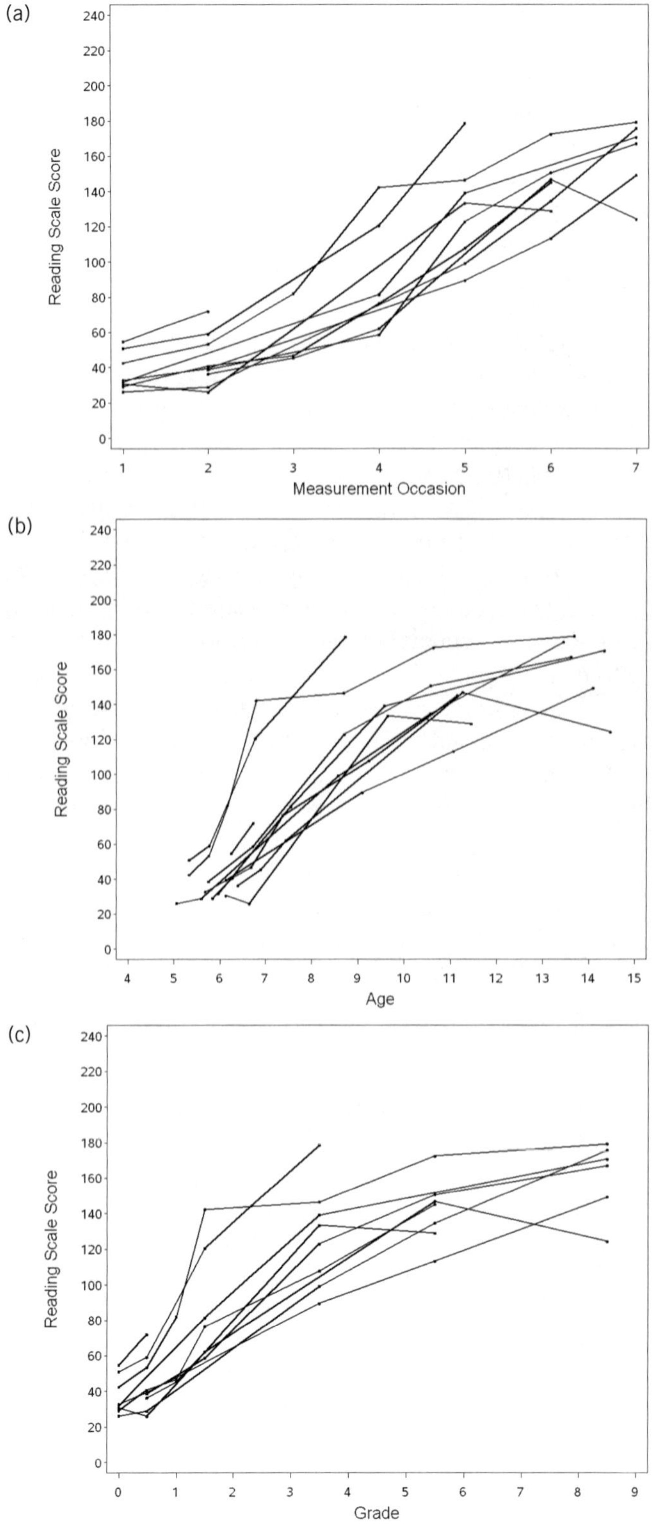

FIGURE 24.1. Longitudinal plot of observed reading achievement scores with (a) measurement occasion, (b) age, and (c) grade as the time metric.

If we are interested in more precise and potentially more informative depictions of development, individual change patterns might alternatively be summarized using mathematical functions that more closely mimic the nonlinear change patterns observed in the individual trajectories. In the empirical illustration to follow, we review a few nonlinear growth curves. Common functions for describing the observed nonlinearities in development include quadratic (and higher order polynomials), exponential, logistic, Gompertz, and Richards curves. Here, a specific and highly structured mathematical function is used to describe the pattern of within-person change. The suitability of the model's description is judged both in relation to statistical fit to the data and to the match between the theoretical notions about the processes guiding development and the parameters of the function. When little is known about the underlying processes, prototypical within-person change patterns can be described using an unstructured curve (McArdle & Epstein, 1987; Meredith & Tisak, 1990). The unstructured, or latent basis, model is often used to decompose the repeated measures into initial-score and total-change components. The key property of this model is that the changes are not structured to follow specific linear or nonlinear functions. Instead, the curve is estimated from the data. Somewhere between these two approaches, another way to summarize within-person change patterns is with a series of splines (see Cudeck & Klebe, 2002; Ram & Grimm, 2007)—a series of lines or curves that connect at specific points in time (knot points). These models are often called *multiphase* models, as the various splines can be used to represent a set of hypothesized phases of development. In this sense, knot points represent points in time at which one phase is ending and another phase is beginning. Spline and multiphase models can be theoretically useful when the process under investigation is thought to be guided by developmental shifts, such as Piaget's stages of development. In sum, a number of possibilities are available for describing within-person changes, each useful for articulating a particular theoretical (or atheoretical) model of development.

Between-Person Differences in Change

No matter the specific within-person change model chosen, the next key issue is where, along the within-person change model, between-person or interindividual differences are manifested. For example, the linear model has two parameters—an intercept and a slope—and in most applications, these two parameters are allowed to vary over persons. Thus between-person differences in these two particular aspects of change thought to guide the underlying developmental process are estimated (variances and covariances). Take, as a second example, the logistic curve, a more complex nonlinear model that has four parameters: (1) a lower asymptote related to preexisting or initial level of attribute, (2) an upper asymptote related to final or potential level of the attribute, (3) an inflection point capturing the timing of change, and (4) a rate of change capturing how quickly an individual moves from the lower to the upper asymptote. All four aspects of change can differ across persons and in certain applications, allowing each of these aspects of change to vary over people is reasonable. However, in specific applications it may not be reasonable to allow people to differ in all aspects of the curve, for theoretical or practical reasons. For example, Marceau, Ram, Houts, Grimm, and Susman (in press) used logistic growth curves to describe between-person differences in the timing and tempo of pubertal development, as measured by the Tanner stages (Marshall & Tanner, 1969, 1970). Given that all individuals progress through five Tanner stages of pubertal development, lower and upper asymptotes of the logistic curve were the same for all individuals. These parameters were thus fixed, and the between-person differences were evident only in the timing and tempo (rate of change). Similarly, Browne and Du Toit (1991) used a Gompertz curve (Gompertz, 1825) to describe within-person changes during a learning task. The Gompertz curve has four parameters describing the within-person change process and could be used to capture between-person differences in change. However, the model was parameterized such that participants differed in the timing, rate of growth, and final upper asymptote, but it did not allow for between-person differences in the lower asymptote. Theoretical notions of key change aspects should drive the location of between-person differences in the model, noting that data constraints may also limit the number and location of between-person differences. In sum, thoughtful consideration is necessary to choose the within-person change model that best captures the process and the between-person model that best captures at what point, along that process, differences are manifested.

Determinants of Change

The growth curve model comprises the within-person change model, along with between-person differences in key change aspects. Once an appropriate growth curve is fit, the focus often turns to the determinants of the change process (see McArdle & Epstein, 1987). Determinants of between-person aspects of change can be evaluated to understand potential reasons that people differ in the developmental process. The latent growth curve with determinants enables researchers to test theoretical notions regarding developmental processes and their determinants.

Conceptual Principles and Statistical Assumptions

Although initially developed in the late 1950s (Rao, 1958; Tucker, 1958), growth curve modeling did not become a key component of longitudinal research until Meredith and Tisak (1984, 1990) showed how the latent growth curve could be fit as a restricted common factor model using available SEM software. Almost at the same time, very similar models emerged from the multilevel (e.g., mixed effects, random coefficient) modeling tradition under the logic that the repeated observations were nested within participants (see Bryk & Raudenbush, 1992; Hox & Boom, Chapter 25, this volume). Multilevel and SEM approaches to fitting growth curves have advantages and disadvantages (see Ghisletta & Lindenberger, 2004) and identical models can be constructed using both approaches (Ferrer, Hamagami, & McArdle, 2004). We consider the SEM and multilevel perspectives simply as more or less practical implementations (depending on one's specific data structure and model) of the same growth curve modeling approach. Here, we review and illustrate the model using an SEM perspective.

Latent Growth Curve as a Structural Model

As a structural model, the latent growth curve is a restricted common factor model, which can be written as

$$\mathbf{y}_i = \nu + \Lambda\eta_i + \mathbf{u}_i \qquad \textbf{(24.1)}$$

where $\mathbf{y}_i$ is a $T \times 1$ vector of the repeatedly measured observed scores for individual i, where T represents the number of repeated assessments based on the chosen time metric, ν is a vector of intercepts that are set equal to zero, Λ is a $T \times R$ matrix of factor loadings defining the major components (i.e., latent factors) of the growth curve (e.g., intercept and slope), where R is the number of components, η_i is an $R \times 1$ vector of latent factor scores (e.g., intercept & slope scores) for individual i, and $\mathbf{u}_i$ is a $T \times 1$ vector of residual or unique scores for individual i. The latent factor scores are written as deviations from the group mean and written as

$$\eta_i = \alpha + \xi_i \tag{24.2}$$

where α is an $R \times 1$ vector of latent factor means and ξ_i is an $R \times 1$ vector of mean deviations for individual i. The expected mean (μ) and covariance structure (Σ) of observed variables are written as

$$\begin{aligned} \mu &= \alpha\Lambda \\ \Sigma &= \Lambda\Phi\Lambda' + \Theta \end{aligned} \tag{24.3}$$

where Φ is an $R \times R$ matrix of latent variable covariances and Θ is a $T \times T$ matrix of residual covariances. Often, an equality constraint is placed on the diagonal elements of Θ and off-diagonal values are fixed at zero. These constraints follow the homogeneity of variance assumption common in repeated-measures ANOVA and force all observed variable covariances to be generated from the latent variables and their covariances. However, among the benefits of fitting growth curves in the SEM framework is the ability to test and evaluate a variety of different residual structures. The choice of residual structures is often made without much thought; however, this decision can have large impacts on convergence, model fit, and latent variable variances and covariances (see Ferron, Dailey, & Yi, 2002; Grimm & Widaman, 2010; Kwok, West, & Green, 2007; Sivo, Fan, & Witta, 2005).

A path diagram of a latent growth curve model with two latent variables is given in Figure 24.2. In path diagrams, squares represent observed variables, circles represent latent variables, and the triangle denotes the unit constant. One-headed arrows represent directional relationships, such as regression coefficients and factor loadings, whereas two-headed arrows represent nondirectional or symmetric relations, such as variances and covariances. Following path diagram tracing rules, the covariance and mean structure of the observed scores is derived from the variances, covariances, and means of the latent and observed variables. The path diagram exactly replicates the necessary matrix algebra given previously.

Specific Growth Curves

We present a series of specific growth curves, such as the linear model, to demonstrate how models are specified in the SEM framework. In each of these descriptions, we present specifications of the Λ matrix because this matrix defines the latent growth components. In these specifications, we assume that there are four equally spaced measurement occasions ($T = 4$).

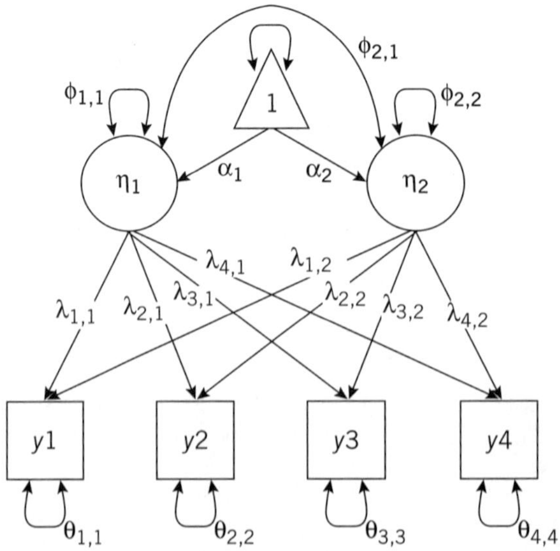

FIGURE 24.2. Path diagram of a latent growth curve with two latent variables.

Linear Change

The linear change model is probably the most commonly fit growth curve in applied research. The linear change model has two latent variables; an intercept, usually centered at an initial point in time; and a linear slope representing the overall rate of change during the observation period. The intercept and slope are allowed to vary over persons and covary with each other. The linear growth model is similar to fitting a linear regression model to each individual's data and then summarizing the estimated intercepts and slopes. In the linear growth model, the Λ matrix is specified as

$$\Lambda = \begin{pmatrix} 1 & \dfrac{1-k_1}{k_2} \\ 1 & \dfrac{2-k_1}{k_2} \\ 1 & \dfrac{3-k_1}{k_2} \\ 1 & \dfrac{4-k_1}{k_2} \end{pmatrix} \quad \textbf{(24.4)}$$

The first column defines the intercept, and the second column defines the linear slope. The constants k_1 and k_2 are chosen to center the intercept and rescale the slope. Often, k_1 is set to 1 to center the intercept at the first occasion and k_2 is set to 1 to scale the slope in terms of the unit of time used in the selected time metric.

Quadratic Change

The quadratic change model is often used when the linear model does not adequately capture the change process and/or nonlinearity is evident in the longitudinal plot. The quadratic model has three latent variables, an intercept, a linear slope, and a quadratic slope. The interpretation of the parameters of the quadratic model can be difficult (see Cudeck & du Toit, 2002) and therefore, although easily implemented, is not often useful from a theoretical perspective. In the quadratic growth model, the Λ matrix is specified as

$$\Lambda = \begin{pmatrix} 1 & 0 & 0 \\ 1 & 1 & 1 \\ 1 & 2 & 4 \\ 1 & 3 & 9 \end{pmatrix} \quad \textbf{(24.5)}$$

if k_1 and k_2 are set equal to 1. As in the linear model, the first and second columns define the intercept and linear slope, respectively. The factor loadings for the third column are squares of the factor loadings of the second column and define the quadratic slope.

Exponential Change

Exponential change, as well as a variety of inherently nonlinear curves, can be fit in the structural modeling framework (see Browne, 1993; Browne & du Toit, 1991). The exponential change model is a useful model for discussion because it has been found to adequately represent change in several learning tasks (e.g., Burchinal & Appelbaum, 1991) and lifespan cognitive development (e.g., McArdle, Ferrer-Caja, Hamagami, & Woodcock, 2002) and is a relatively simple nonlinear model. The complexity of the between-person differences influences how nonlinear models such as this can be fit as structural models (Grimm & Ram, 2009). More specifically, if the between-person differences (latent variables) enter the model linearly (are additive), then the model is easily estimated as a structural model. If the between-person differences enter the model nonlinearly (are multiplicative), then the model can be approximated using a first-order Taylor series (see Browne, 1993; Grimm, Ram, & Hamagami, in press). The Λ matrix in an exponential growth curve with linearly entering between-person differences can be specified as

$$\Lambda = \begin{pmatrix} 1 & 1-e^{-a\cdot(1-k_1)} \\ 1 & 1-e^{-a\cdot(2-k_1)} \\ 1 & 1-e^{-a\cdot(3-k_1)} \\ 1 & 1-e^{-a\cdot(4-k_1)} \end{pmatrix} \quad \textbf{(24.6)}$$

where k_1 centers the intercept (as in the linear model) and a is the estimated rate of approach to the asymptote. Notice that a, the rate of approach, is an estimated *parameter,* as opposed to a latent variable, and does not vary over people.

If the rate of approach is expected to vary over persons, then between-person differences enter the model nonlinearly, and this model can only be approximated (not estimated directly) as a structural model. The approximation method is complex. Thus we present brief details regarding the specification of the Λ matrix and refer readers to thorough descriptions (Browne, 1993; Browne & Du Toit, 1991). In this method, the Λ matrix is adjusted to include a third latent variable representing the rate of approach. The Λ matrix can be specified as

$$\Lambda = \begin{pmatrix} 1 & 1-e^{-\mu_a \cdot (1-k_1)} & \alpha_2 \cdot (1-k_1) \cdot e^{-\mu_a \cdot (1-k_1)} \\ 1 & 1-e^{-\mu_a \cdot (2-k_1)} & \alpha_2 \cdot (2-k_1) \cdot e^{-\mu_a \cdot (2-k_1)} \\ 1 & 1-e^{-\mu_a \cdot (3-k_1)} & \alpha_2 \cdot (3-k_1) \cdot e^{-\mu_a \cdot (3-k_1)} \\ 1 & 1-e^{-\mu_a \cdot (4-k_1)} & \alpha_2 \cdot (4-k_1) \cdot e^{-\mu_a \cdot (4-k_1)} \end{pmatrix} \tag{24.7}$$

As in equation 24.6, the first column defines the intercept and the second defines the asymptote. The third column now defines the rate of approach. The factor loadings for the upper asymptote are the same as in equation 24.6 with a small notation difference, as a was replaced with μ_a to denote this estimate is the mean rate of approach. The factor loadings for the rate of approach factor are the partial derivative of the nonlinear function with respect to the rate of approach and α_2 is the mean of the asymptote factor. Finally, the mean of the rate of approach factor, α_3, is fixed to zero.

Unstructured Change

Unstructured change is a very flexible model that is able to capture a variety of types of nonlinear change patterns because its form is not structured. Instead, factor loadings for the second factor are estimated from the data with the exception of two factor loadings that are fixed for identification purposes. The Λ matrix in the unstructured growth curve can be specified as

$$\Lambda = \begin{pmatrix} 1 & 0 \\ 1 & \lambda_{2,2} \\ 1 & \lambda_{3,2} \\ 1 & 1 \end{pmatrix} \tag{24.8}$$

In this model, the first column defines the intercept and the second defines a *shape* factor. The first factor loading of the shape factor is fixed at 0, the last is fixed at 1, and the middle factor loadings are estimated from the data. Thus the shape factor can take on a variety of change patterns and is interpreted as the total amount of change from the first to the fourth occasion. Thus the unstructured model attempts to decompose the repeated measures into an initial score and a change score (whose rate of change varies according to the data).

Multiphase Change

Multiphase change can be specified in a variety of ways because the type of change model within each phase can vary. For simplicity and illustration purposes, we present a model with two phases and linear change within each phase. The Λ matrix in this growth curve can be specified as

$$\Lambda = \begin{pmatrix} 1 & 0 & 0 \\ 1 & 1 & 0 \\ 1 & 1 & 1 \\ 1 & 1 & 2 \end{pmatrix} \tag{24.9}$$

In this model, the first column defines the intercept centered at the first measurement occasion. The second column defines the first linear phase representing change during the first two measurement occasions and the third column defines the second linear phase representing change from the second to fourth measurement occasions.

Developmental Applications

Growth curves have furthered our understanding of developmental processes in a diverse array of fields. Historically, these models were used to study and simplify obviously growing entities, such as crops, bacteria, humans, and human populations. In social sciences, growth curve approaches have been applied to study various developmental processes. Growth curves have been extensively applied to answer questions regarding the development of cognitive abilities across the entire lifespan (e.g., McArdle et al., 2002) and changes during learning trials (e.g., Browne & Du Toit, 1991), as well as changes in behavior and personality.

A recent interesting application used growth curve models to study changes in behavior before and after an intervention (Van der Velden, Brugman, Boom, & Koops, 2009). In this study, multiple cohorts of students were measured at four measurement occasions. The cohorts differed in the timing of the intervention and the number of occasions before and after the intervention. Van der Velden and colleagues (2009) modeled changes before and after the intervention using linear growth curves even though the first cohort was measured only once before the intervention and the third cohort was measured only once after the intervention. This work highlights the complexity with which growth curves can be applied to answer important questions regarding the effects of interventions.

Illustration

Data

Longitudinal reading data from the ECLS-K cohort (National Center for Education Statistics, 2001) is used for illustrative purposes. The ECLS-K is a nationally representative sample of more than 21,000 children who attended kindergarten in the 1998–1999 school year. These children were followed from the fall of kindergarten to the spring of eighth grade. Reading assessments were administered in the fall and spring of kindergarten and first grade and in the spring of third, fifth, and eighth grade. Achievement scores were vertically linked via an item response model and are appropriate for examining change.

As a first step when studying change processes (once basic univariate and multivariate descriptive statistics have been studied and invariance evaluated), observed scores by grade in school at assessment are plotted in Figure 24.3 for a 1% random sample of participants (plotting data from more than 21,000 participants might prove less informative, as individual trends could not be discerned). From this figure, it becomes obvious that the longitudinal change patterns are not linear; thus models that allow for nonlinear trajectories must be considered. Previous studies of the development of prereading and reading skills have shown nonlinear trajectories (Grimm & Ram, 2009; Pianta, Belsky, Vandergrift, Houts, & Morrison, 2008). Furthermore, Pianta and colleagues (2008) found two unobserved classes of readers: children who develop reading skills early and those who develop their reading skills later on in the developmental process. Pianta and colleagues used a growth mixture model (Muthén & Shedden, 1999) to account for between-person differences in the timing of reading change. Thus a statistical model that allows for variability in this particular aspect of change may be theoretically important and statistically useful.

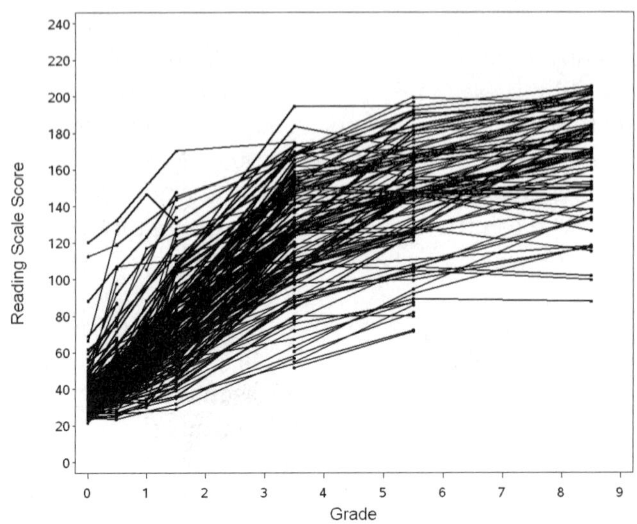

FIGURE 24.3. Longitudinal plot of observed reading achievement scores for a 1% random sample with grade as the time metric.

Models

A series of growth curves were fit to the longitudinal reading data (Mplus input and output scripts can be downloaded from *http://psychology.ucdavis.edu/labs/Grimm/personal/downloads.html*). Growth curves examined here included the linear, quadratic, logistic, Gompertz, unstructured, and unstructured multiphase. All models were fit with unstructured and independent residual variances because of the potential influence of floor and ceiling effects in the reading data. Fit statistics for these models are given in Table 24.1. A benefit of using the SEM framework for growth curves is the availability of absolute fit indices, such as the comparative fit index (CFI), Tucker-Lewis index (TLI), and root mean square error of approximation (RMSEA), which are useful in comparing the model implied covariance (Σ) and mean (μ) structure to the observed covariance (S) and mean (m) structure. CFI and TLI values greater than .90 indicate good fit, and RMSEA values less than .10 and .05 indicate adequate and good fit, respectively.

Results

The linear model showed poor fit based on every indication of model fit. Obviously, based on the individual change patterns, the linear model was an inadequate representation of the changes in reading achievement during this time period, and this was supported by the statistical fit indices. The quadratic was a drastic improvement over the linear model ($\Delta\chi^2$ = 32,522, Δdf = 4); however, the absolute fit indices remained poor, indicating that the quadratic curve was not an adequate representation of the observed changes in reading achievement.

Two inherently nonlinear models were then fit to the observed reading data. Both models have similar elongated *s*-shapes but differ with respect to the symmetry of development. The logistic model is perfectly symmetrical with respect to the inflection point, whereas the Gompertz model is asymmetrical such that ~37% of the total change occurs before the inflection point. These curves each have four parameters: lower asymptote, upper asymptote, rate of change, and timing of changes. In the estimation of these models, the lower asymptote was not allowed to vary over persons, as this parameter represents the level of reading achievement as $t \to -\infty$, at which, theoretically, there should be no variance

TABLE 24.1. Fit Statistics for the Latent Growth Curves Fit to the Longitudinal ECLS-K Reading Measurements

	Linear[a]	Quadratic	Logistic	Gompertz	Unstructured	Unstructured multiphase
$\chi^2(df)$	51,877 (23)	19,355 (19)	10,560 (18)	8,185 (18)	11,804 (18)	3,113 (15)
Parameters	12	16	17	17	17	20
CFI	.340	.754	.866	.896	.850	.961
TLI	.397	.728	.843	.879	.825	.945
RMSEA (CI)	.329 (.326–.331)	.221 (.218–.223)	.168 (.165–.170)	.147 (.145–.150)	.177 (.174–.180)	.099 (.097–.102)

[a]Convergence issues were encountered.

in scores. Thus the timing of changes, rate of change, and total amount of change were allowed to vary over persons. Generally, the logistic and Gompertz models had better fit statistics than the linear and quadratic models. Furthermore, fit indices for the Gompertz model tended to be stronger than those for the logistic model, indicating asymmetry in the development of reading ability; however, note that direct comparisons cannot be made statistically. Thus children tended to accelerate fastest in the earlier stages of reading. Latent variable parameter estimates for the Gompertz model are contained in Table 24.2a. The

TABLE 24.2. Parameter Estimates from the Gompertz and Unstructured Multiphase Growth Curves

	(a) Gompertz growth curve				(b) Unstructured multiphase growth curve		
Parameter	Intercept	Total Change	Rate of Change[a]	Timing of Change[a]	Intercept	Primary Slope	Secondary Slope
Mean (α)	21.080*	144.857*	.564*	1.522*	34.806*	41.595*	90.576*
	(.229)	(.435)	(.001)	(.009)	(.074)	(.144)	(.249)
Factor loadings (Λ)							
$\lambda_{1,.}$	= 1	.094*	−49.113*	−18.212*	= 1	= 0	= 0
		(.001)	(.395)	(.131)			
$\lambda_{2,.}$	= 1	.169*	−44.430*	−24.538*	= 1	.266*	= 0
		(.001)	(.225)	(.097)		(.001)	
$\lambda_{3,.}$	= 1	.261*	−26.506*	−28.665*	= 1	.430*	= 0
		(.001)	(.288)	(.084)		(.002)	
$\lambda_{4,.}$	= 1	.363*	−1.163*	−30.071*	= 1	=1	= 0
		(.001)	(.355)	(.084)			
$\lambda_{5,.}$	= 1	.721*	67.634*	−19.294*	= 1	=1	.548*
		(.001)	(.426)	(.051)			(.002)
$\lambda_{6,.}$	= 1	.899*	54.907*	−7.789*	= 1	=1	.799*
		(.001)	(.617)	(.055)			(.002)
$\lambda_{7,.}$	= 1	.981*	19.319*	−1.562*	= 1	=1	= 1
		(.001)	(.374)	(.023)			
Covariance matrix (Φ)							
	= 0				98.162*		
					(1.139)		
	= 0	546.764*			79.007*	289.452*	
		(10.833)			(1.728)	(4.472)	
	= 0	.899*	.007*		−44.069*	−54.967*	407.741*
		(.048)	(.000)		(2.342)	(4.765)	(8.029)
	= 0	−5.421*	−.014*	.238*			
		(.168)	(.001)	(.005)			

Note. Standard errors contained within brackets, "=" denotes a fixed parameter, "*" denotes that parameter estimate is significantly different from 0 at $p < .01$.

[a]Mean of latent variable not contained within α matrix but estimated as part of model.

mean growth function had a lower asymptote of 21.080, growth was 144.857 points to the upper asymptote, and changes were most rapid toward the spring of first grade. There was significant variation in the total amount of change, the rate of change, and the timing of these changes. Furthermore, there was a negative correlation (r = –.48) between the total amount of change and the timing of changes. Thus, children who showed the most growth in reading tended to change earlier. There was a positive correlation (r = .46) between the total amount of change and the rate of change, suggesting that children who showed more growth tended to grow at a faster rate. Finally, there was a negative correlation (r = –.34) between the rate of change and the timing of changes, suggesting that children who changed earlier tended to change more rapidly. A plot of the mean trajectory based on the Gompertz model, along with a 95% confidence interval on the between-person differences, is contained in Figure 24.4a. The predicted average curve for reading shows a smooth nonlinear trajectory and sizable between-person differences in the key developmental features. The benefits of these nonlinear models is their elegance and the fact that their parameters are interpretable and can be mapped onto theoretical notions regarding development. However, the Gompertz model's level of fit was still less than ideal.

Coming from a more atheoretical perspective, we also fit the unstructured change model. The unstructured model fit better than the linear model ($\Delta\chi^2$ = 40,073, Δdf = 5) and had better absolute fit indices than the quadratic model, but it did not show the level of fit achieved by the logistic and Gompertz models. This indicated that one between-person differences component was not sufficient for capturing individual changes and between-person differences in the development of reading achievement from kindergarten through eighth grade. Following this approach further, we fit a multiphase model with two phases. The first phase modeled changes during kindergarten through the end of first grade, whereas the second phase modeled changes from the end of first grade through eighth grade. The knot point was chosen because it represents the distinction between early and late primary grades. More specifically, children tend to be exposed to a variety of reading strategies during early primary school, whereas, in later primary school, children tend to become more proficient in the skills learned in early primary school. Additionally, the knot point was fixed, a limitation of fitting multiphase models in the SEM framework. Within each phase, an unstructured model was fit because of the obvious nonlinearity in the developmental patterns. Thus this model had an intercept term centered at the fall of kindergarten, one change factor representing growth during kindergarten and first grade, and a second change factor representing growth from the end of first grade through eighth grade. The unstructured multiphase model showed adequate fit based on the CFI, TLI, and RMSEA and thus had the best absolute fit of the models tested.

Latent variable parameter estimates for the unstructured multiphase model are contained in Table 24.2b. The first change factor showed a nonlinear growth pattern such that more change occurred during first grade than during kindergarten. On average, children's reading scores increased 41.595 points from school entry through the end of first grade. The second change factor showed decelerating change, with gradual slowing during the later grades. On average, from the end of first grade to the end of eighth grade, children's reading scores increased 90.576 points. There was significant variation in the intercept and the first and second change factors. Furthermore, the intercept was positively correlated with the first change factor (r = .47) and negatively correlated with the second change factor (r = –.22), whereas the first and second change factors were negatively correlated (r = –.16) with each other. A plot of the mean trajectory and 95% confidence bounds around the

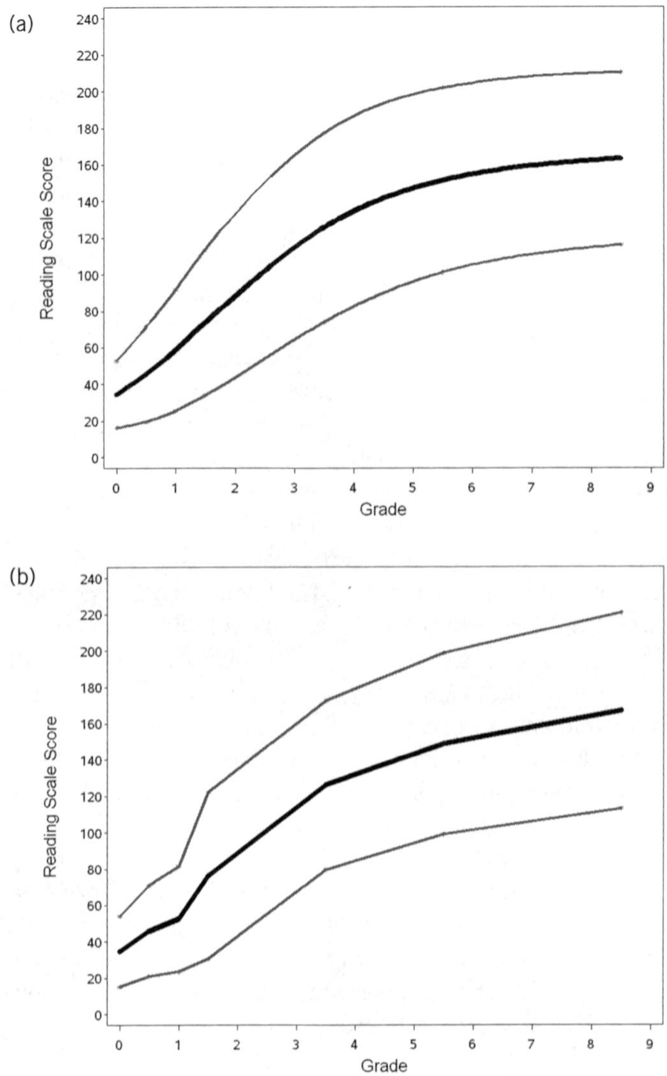

FIGURE 24.4. Predicted mean trajectories with 95% confidence interval of between-person differences based on the (a) Gompertz and (b) unstructured multiphase models.

between-person differences is contained in Figure 24.4b. As discussed earlier, an unstructured model is atheoretical with respect to the change pattern. Thus the curve displayed in Figure 24.4b is not smooth but angular.

Model Choice

When determining the model that best represents the data and the developmental process, there are several points to consider. First, researchers must consider statistical fit: the discrepancy between the model implied and observed mean and covariance structure. Additionally, comparative fit indices, such as the Bayesian information criterion (BIC) and

Akaike information criterion (AIC) are useful for comparing models that are not nested (e.g., logistic and Gompertz models). A second point is theoretical fit, or the match between model components and substantive notions of the developmental process. Third, the interpretability and substantive utility of parameter estimates should be considered. Examining our results in terms of statistical fit, the unstructured multiphase model is the clear favorite. It was the only model with absolute fit indices that could be deemed acceptable. In terms of match to theoretical notions of development, the Gompertz model is the favorite, as timing, rates, and total amounts of change are key features in the development of reading abilities. In terms of interpretability and substantive utility of parameter estimates, the Gompertz model again is the favorite.

Plotting the predicted prototypical developmental trajectories from the Gompertz and the unstructured multiphase models (Figure 24.4) allows additional comparisons and the opportunity to learn a bit more about the data and the hypothesized generating process. Figures 24.4a and 24.4b show striking similarities in terms of the predicted pattern of change and amount of between-person differences. The main difference appears in the early grades as the unstructured model shows greater growth during kindergarten, which is followed by slower change during the summer between kindergarten and first grade. Thus the unstructured multiphase fits better due to its flexibility but is possibly overfitting (modeling error or unique features of the data that would not replicate). The noted differential growth during the academic year and summer is an important aspect of changes in reading achievement (see McCoach, O'Connell, Reis, & Levitt, 2006; Skibbe, Grimm, Bowles, & Morrison, in press) in limited time periods, but it may be of trivial use in understanding the longer term developmental trajectory of reading abilities. In the end, based on the additional substantive understanding and match to developmental theory and an understanding of model differences facilitated by the plots, we concluded that the Gompertz model was an adequate representation of the development of reading achievement from kindergarten through eighth grade for these data.

Future Directions

The latent growth curves described here are the first steps along the path to understanding developmental processes. There are a variety of extensions of latent growth curves for studying multiple groups (McArdle & Hamagami, 1996), latent classes (Muthén & Shedden, 1999), multivariate growth (McArdle, 1988), and lead–lag relationships (McArdle & Hamagami, 2001). Growth curves have also been presented with underlying measurement models (Curran et al., 2008; McArdle, 1988; McArdle et al., 2009) and with a survival model to account for attrition (McArdle, Small, Backman, & Fratiglioni, 2005). Methodologists, in conjunction with substantive researchers, are continually adapting and refining this approach for use with different populations, different types of variables, and different conceptualizations of time.

Key issues that are being and will continue to be addressed in future latent growth curve models and their applications include the incorporation of multiple time metrics, accommodation of missing data, and treatment of measurement error. Observed developmental changes are rarely driven by a single process. Thus, to obtain a more complete understanding of what influences change, further work needs to be done on how combinations of time metrics can be incorporated to examine longitudinal change (Ram et al., 2010;

Sliwinski et al., 2003). Likely, this will require additional consideration of the theoretical and methodological distinctions among within-person change and between-person differences and of how multiple time metrics are purposefully incorporated when designing longitudinal studies.

Every longitudinal study suffers from participant attrition and/or mortality. Researchers must decide how to handle the resulting incompleteness of the data. Often, as was done in the estimation of models presented here, full information maximum likelihood methods (Finkbeiner, 1979; see Enders, 2001, for a primer) are used to include data from all participants under missing-at-random assumptions. However, attrition in longitudinal studies is unlikely to conform to such assumptions. Additional work is needed to study the limitations of how we treat incomplete data in longitudinal studies and how to account for different amounts and types of incomplete data when modeling change.

Returning to measurement concerns, observed scores are typically treated as equally reliable across persons and time, when in fact this is rarely, if ever, the case. In some applications, an underlying measurement model (e.g., factor or item response theory model) can be incorporated into the growth curve model and used to account for differential reliability of observed scores (e.g., McArdle et al., 2009). However, estimation is often cumbersome. Further work is needed to understand how differentially weighting scores based on their reliability may ease the estimation burdens while still addressing changes or differences in error of measurement across persons and time.

More generally, we see in psychology and the social sciences the beginning of a shift from the use of simple linear change models toward the use of complex growth curves that are being used in biology and chemistry to study growth processes commonly found in natural systems. These often nonlinear growth curves may provide more accurate and useful depictions of developmental processes than models currently in use. In the long run, they likely shall guide the way from description to explanation. Key to this shift will be the reformulation of growth curves in terms of difference and differential models in which changes in the rate of change become the key components of development. As the conceptual models get tethered to these change-focused models, a more complete understanding of developmental change processes will surely ensue.

Acknowledgments

Kevin J. Grimm was supported by REECE Program Grant No. DRL-0815787 from the National Science Foundation and Grant No. R305A06021 from the National Center for Research on Early Childhood Education, Institute of Education Sciences, U.S. Department of Education. Nilam Ram was funded by National Institute on Aging Grant Nos. RC1-AG035645, R21-AG032379, and R21-AG033109. The content is solely the responsibility of the authors and does not necessarily represent the official views of the funding agencies. Input and output scripts from Mplus can be found at *http://psychology.ucdavis.edu/labs/Grimm/personal/downloads.html.*

References

Browne, M. W. (1993). Structured latent curve models. In C. M. Cuadras & C. R. Rao (Eds.), *Multivariate analysis: Future directions 2* (pp. 171–198). Amsterdam: North-Holland.

Browne, M. W., & Du Toit, S. H. C. (1991). Models for learning data. In L. Collins & J. L. Horn (Eds.),

Best methods for the analysis of change (pp. 47–68). Washington, DC: American Psychological Association.
Bryk, A. S., & Raudenbush, S. W. (1992). *Hierarchical linear models: Applications and data analysis methods*. Thousand Oaks, CA: Sage.
Burchinal, M., & Appelbaum, M. I. (1991). Estimating individual developmental functions: Methods and their assumptions. *Child Development, 62*, 23–43.
Cronbach, L. J., & Furby, L. (1970). How should we measure "change"—or should we? *Psychological Bulletin, 74*, 68–80.
Cudeck, R., & du Toit, S. H. C. (2002). A version of quadratic regression with interpretable parameters. *Multivariate Behavioral Research, 37*, 501–519.
Cudeck, R., & Klebe, K. J. (2002). Multiphase mixed-effects models for repeated measures data. *Psychological Methods, 7*, 41–63.
Curran, P. J., Hussong, A. M., Cai, L., Huang, W., Chassin, L., Sher, K. J., et al. (2008). Pooling data from multiple longitudinal studies: The role of item response theory in integrative data analysis. *Developmental Psychology, 44*, 365–380.
Edwards, M. C., & Wirth, R. J. (2009). Measurement and the study of change. *Research in Human Development, 6*, 74–96.
Enders, C. K. (2001). A primer on maximum likelihood algorithms available for use with missing data. *Structural Equation Modeling, 8*, 128–141.
Ferrer, E., Hamagami, F., & McArdle, J. J. (2004). Modeling latent growth curves with incomplete data using different types of structural equation modeling and multilevel software. *Structural Equation Modeling, 11*, 452–483.
Ferrer, E., Salthouse, T. A., McArdle, J. J., Stewart, W. F., & Schwartz, B. S. (2005). Multivariate modeling of age and retest in longitudinal studies of cognitive abilities. *Psychology and Aging, 20*, 412–422.
Ferron, J., Dailey, R., & Yi, Q. (2002). Effects of misspecifying the first-level error structure in two-level models of change. *Multivariate Behavioral Research, 37*, 379–403.
Finkbeiner, C. (1979). Estimation for the multiple factor model when data are missing. *Psychometrika, 44*, 409–420.
Ghisletta, P., & Lindenberger, U. (2004). Static and dynamic longitudinal structural analyses of cognitive changes in old age. *Gerontology, 50*, 12–16.
Gompertz, B. (1825). On the nature of the function expressive of the law of human mortality, and on a new mode of determining the value of life contingencies. *Philosophical Transactions of the Royal Society of London, 115*, 513–585.
Grimm, K. J., & Ram, N. (2009). Nonlinear growth models in Mplus and SAS. *Structural Equation Modeling, 16*, 676–701.
Grimm, K. J., Ram, N., & Hamagami, F. (in press). Nonlinear growth curves in developmental research. *Child Development*.
Grimm, K. J., & Widaman, K. F. (2010). Residual structures in latent growth curve analysis. *Structural Equation Modeling, 17*, 424–442.
Kwok, O., West, S. G., & Green, S. B. (2007). The impact of misspecifying the within-subject covariance structure in multiwave longitudinal multilevel models: A Monte Carlo study. *Multivariate Behavioral Research, 42*, 557–592.
Marceau, K., Ram, N., Houts, R. H., Grimm, K. J., & Susman, E. J. (in press). Individual differences in boys' and girls' timing and tempo of puberty: Modeling development with nonlinear growth models. *Developmental Psychology*.
Marshall, W. A., & Tanner, J. M. (1969). Variations in patterns of pubertal changes in girls. *Archives of Disease in Childhood, 44*, 291–303.
Marshall, W. A., & Tanner, J. M. (1970). Variations in patterns of pubertal changes in boys. *Archives of Disease in Childhood, 45*, 13–23.
McArdle, J. J. (1988). Dynamic but structural equation modeling of repeated measures data. In J. R.

Nesselroade & R. B. Cattell (Eds.), *Handbook of multivariate experimental psychology: Perspectives on individual differences* (2nd ed., pp. 561–614). New York: Plenum Press.

McArdle, J. J. (2009). Latent variable modeling of differences and changes with longitudinal data. *Annual Review of Psychology, 60*, 577–605.

McArdle, J. J., & Epstein, D. (1987). Latent growth curves within developmental structural equation models. *Child Development, 58*, 110–133.

McArdle, J. J., Ferrer-Caja, E., Hamagami, F., & Woodcock, R. W. (2002). Comparative longitudinal multilevel structural analyses of the growth and decline of multiple intellectual abilities over the life-span. *Developmental Psychology, 38*, 115–142.

McArdle, J. J., Grimm, K. J., Hamagami, F., Bowles, R. P., & Meredith, W. (2009). Modeling life-span growth curves of cognition using longitudinal data with multiple samples and changing scales of measurements. *Psychological Methods, 14*, 126–149.

McArdle, J. J., & Hamagami, F. (1996). Multilevel models from a multiple group structural equation perspective. In G. Marcoulides & R. Schumacker (Eds.), *Advanced structural equation modeling techniques* (pp. 89–124). Hillsdale, NJ: Erlbaum.

McArdle, J. J., & Hamagami, F. (2001). Latent difference score structural models for linear dynamic analysis with incomplete longitudinal data. In L. Collins & A. Sayer (Eds.), *New methods for the analysis of change* (pp. 137–175). Washington, DC: American Psychological Association.

McArdle, J. J., & Nesselroade, J. R. (2003). Growth curve analyses in contemporary psychological research. In J. Schinka & W. Velicer (Eds.), *Comprehensive handbook of psychology: Vol. 2. Research methods in psychology* (pp. 447–480). New York: Pergamon Press.

McArdle, J. J., Small, B. J., Backman, L., & Fratiglioni, L. (2005). Longitudinal models of growth and survival applied to the early detection of Alzheimer's disease. *Journal of Geriatric Psychiatry and Neurology, 18*, 234–241.

McArdle, J. J., & Woodcock, J. R. (1997). Expanding test–retest designs to include developmental time-lag components. *Psychological Methods, 2*, 403–435.

McCoach, D. B., O'Connell, A. A., Reis, S. M., & Levitt, H. (2006). Growing readers: A hierarchical linear model of children's reading growth over the first two years of school. *Journal of Educational Psychology, 98*, 14–28.

Meredith, W. (1993). Measurement invariance, factor analysis and factorial invariance. *Psychometrika, 58*, 525–543.

Meredith, W., & Horn, J. L. (2001). The role of factorial invariance in modeling growth and change. In L. M. Collins & A. G. Sayer (Eds.), *New methods for the analysis of change* (pp. 203–240). Washington, DC: American Psychological Association.

Meredith, W., & Tisak, J. (1984, July). *"Tuckerizing" curves*. Paper presented at the annual meeting of the Psychometric Society, Santa Barbara, CA.

Meredith, W., & Tisak, J. (1990). Latent curve analysis. *Psychometrika, 55*, 107–122.

Morrison, F. J., Smith, L., & Dow-Ehrensberger, M. (1995). Education and cognitive development: A natural experiment. *Developmental Psychology, 31*, 789–799.

Muthén, B., & Shedden, K. (1999). Finite mixture modeling with mixture outcomes using the EM algorithm. *Biometrics, 55*, 463–469.

National Center for Education Statistics. (2001). *User's manual for the ECLS-K public-use data files and electronic codebook*. Washington, DC: U.S. Department of Education.

Pianta, R. C., Belsky, J., Vandergrift, N., Houts, R., & Morrison, F. J. (2008). Classroom effects on children's achievement trajectories in elementary school. *American Educational Research Journal, 45*, 365–397.

Ram, N., Gerstorf, D., Fauth, E., Zarit, S., & Malberg, B. (2010). Aging, disablement, and dying: Using time-as-process and time-as-resources metrics to chart late-life change. *Research in Human Development, 7*, 27–44.

Ram, N., & Grimm, K. J. (2007). Using simple and complex growth models to articulate developmental change: Matching method to theory. *International Journal of Behavioral Development, 31,* 303–316.

Rao, C. R. (1958). Some statistical methods for comparison of growth curves. *Biometrics, 14,* 1–17.

Sivo, S., Fan, X., & Witta, L. (2005). The biasing effects of unmodeled ARMA time series processes on latent growth curve model estimates. *Structural Equation Modeling, 12,* 215–231.

Skibbe, L. E., Grimm, K. J., Bowles, R. P., & Morrison, F. J. (in press). Literacy growth in the academic year versus summer from preschool through second grade: Differential effects of schooling across four skills. *Scientific Study of Reading.*

Sliwinski, M. J., Hofer, S. M., Hall, C., Buschke, H., & Lipton, R. B. (2003). Modeling memory decline in older adults: The importance of preclinical dementia, attrition, and chronological age. *Psychology and Aging, 18,* 658–671.

Tucker, L. R. (1958). Determination of parameters of a functional relation by factor analysis. *Psychometrika, 23,* 19–23.

Van der Velden, F., Brugman, D., Boom, J., & Koops, W. (2009). EQUIP for educators: The longitudinal effects of a school-based universal prevention program on moral cognitions and antisocial behavior in young adolescents. In *EQUIPping high school students: Effects of a universal preventive intervention on antisocial behavior* (pp. 73–99). Enschede, The Netherlands: Ipskamp Drukkers.

Wohlwill, J. F. (1973). *The study of behavioral development.* New York: Academic Press.

CHAPTER 25

Growth Curve Modeling from a Multilevel Model Perspective

JOOP J. HOX
JAN BOOM

Central Issues

Multilevel or mixed models have become standard tools for analyzing longitudinal or repeated-measures data. The basic multilevel model for longitudinal data views repeated measures as variables nested in individuals, who may or may not be nested in groups. Compared with the classic repeated-measurements multivariate analysis of variance (MANOVA) approach, this approach has several advantages. First, it deals very simply with panel dropout, because in multilevel modeling there is no assumption that each participant must be measured on the same number of occasions. Thus participants with incomplete data are simply retained in the data set for those measurement occasions on which they provided data. The assumption in this approach is that data are missing at random (MAR; Little, 1995), which is weaker than the assumption of missing completely at random (MCAR) that is made in MANOVA using listwise deletion. Second, it is possible to include time-varying covariates in the model. Third, using polynomial functions or piecewise regression, the change over time can be modeled very flexibly. Fourth, the most interesting difference is that, by allowing regression coefficients for the change model to vary across participants, different participants can have their own trajectory of change, which can in turn be modeled by time-invariant participant characteristics. All this makes multilevel modeling of longitudinal data an attractive approach in developmental research.

It is useful to distinguish between repeated measures that are collected at fixed or at varying occasions. If the measurements are taken at fixed occasions, all individuals provide measurements for the same set of occasions, usually regularly spaced, such as once every year. When occasions are varying, measures are collected for different individuals at different points in time. Such data occur, for instance, in growth studies, in which physical or psychological characteristics are studied for a set of individuals at different moments in their development. The data collection could be at fixed moments in the year, but the individuals would be of different ages at that moment, which effectively turns the fixed occasions design into a varying occasions design. For fixed occasion designs, especially when the occasions are regularly spaced and there are no missing data, repeated-measures MANOVA is a viable alternative for multilevel analysis. Another possibility in such designs is using structural equation modeling–based growth analysis known as latent curve models (Bollen & Curran, 2006), or latent variable growth curve modeling (Duncan, Duncan, & Strycker, 2006), and as discussed by Grimm and Ram in Chapter 24 in this volume. For a multilevel analysis of longitudinal data, the difference between fixed and varying occasions is not important. However, for simplicity, this chapter focuses on fixed occasion data (for an example of analyzing varying occasions data, see the chapter on longitudinal multilevel modeling in Hox, 2010a).

Conceptual Principles and Statistical Assumptions

The multilevel regression model for longitudinal data is a straightforward application of the standard multilevel regression model, with measurement occasions within subjects replacing the subjects-within-groups structure. At the lowest level, which contains the repeated measures, we have the following model:

$$Y_{ti} = \pi_{0i} + \pi_{1i}T_{ti} + \pi_{2i}X_{ti} + e_{ti} \tag{25.1}$$

where Y_{ti} is the response at occasion t ($t = 1, \ldots, T_i$) for individual I ($i = 1, \ldots, n$), T_{ti} indicates the measurement occasion, and X_{ti} represents a time-varying predictor variable. The π's are the regression coefficients, intercept and slopes—which in the general model vary across individuals and therefore carry a subscript i for individuals—and e_{ti} is an occasion-level residual error term, which is assumed to have a normal distribution.

Participant characteristics, such as gender, are time-invariant predictors, which enter the equation at the second level:

$$\pi_{0i} = \beta_{00} + \beta_{01}Z_i + u_{0i} \tag{25.2}$$

$$\pi_{1i} = \beta_{10} + \beta_{11}Z_i + u_{1i} \tag{25.3}$$

$$\pi_{2i} = \beta_{20} + \beta_{21}Z_i + u_{2i} \tag{25.4}$$

In these equations, Z is an individual-level, time-invariant predictor variable, such as gender or socioeconomic status. The u are individual-level residuals, which are assumed to have a multivariate normal distribution and to be uncorrelated with the lowest level residuals e_{ti}.

By substitution, we obtain the single equation model:

$$\begin{aligned} Y_{ti} = {} & \beta_{00} + \beta_{10}T_{ti} + \beta_{20}X_{ti} + \beta_{01}Z_i + \beta_{11}Z_iT_{ti} + \beta_{21}Z_iX_{ti} + \\ & u_{1i}T_{ti} + u_{2i}X_{ti} + u_{0i} + e_{ti}. \end{aligned} \tag{25.5}$$

Multilevel modeling relies on the same assumptions as simple multiple regression modeling, such as linear relationships and normality and homoscedasticity of the residuals. Multilevel regression assumes that the residuals at the lowest level have a normal distribution and homoscedasticity and that the residuals at the second level are independent from the residuals at the first level and have a multivariate normal distribution and homoscedasticity. Just as in ordinary multiple regression, multicollinearity is a problem, and when a polynomial function of time is used, it is customary to center the time variable on its overall mean or on a simple value close to the overall mean.

Multilevel models for participants within groups assume that participants from the same group are more similar than participants from different groups. This implies a dependency between the participants who are in the same group, which in an empty model is expressed by the second-level variance component. Generally there is no need to assume a specific structure for this dependency. Participants within the same group are assumed to be exchangeable and the intraclass correlation refers to the average correlation between two randomly chosen participants from the same group. In multilevel models for occasions within participants, the measurement occasions are not freely exchangeable, because they are ordered in time, generally following a data collection design with regularly spaced measurement occasions. In such models, it often makes sense to assume a specific structure for the covariances between measurements across time. A standard multilevel model for repeated measures, without varying slopes, has just one variance term for the intercept at the subject level. The correlation structure for the measurements over time implied by this model is a structure in which all correlations between any two measurement occasions are identical. This is an improbable structure, similar to the sphericity assumption in repeated-measures analysis of variance (ANOVA). A more attractive correlation structure derives from the intuitively plausible assumption that correlations between measures taken at different measurement occasions are higher when these occasions are close to each other in time. This correlation structure is economically represented by an autoregressive model. In contrast, MANOVA for longitudinal data estimates all covariances between occasions, thereby assuming a saturated model for the correlation structure. Multilevel models for repeated measures can also incorporate such a saturated model for the correlations between the measurement occasions. The advantage of a saturated model is that it always fits perfectly, but the disadvantage is that a saturated model estimates a large number of parameters. When multilevel modeling is used for longitudinal data, the goal is often to find a model that is more parsimonious than the saturated MANOVA model but still represents the correlation structure well.

Longitudinal designs in developmental research often concern the analysis of structured change, such as growth or decline over time. The appropriate model for such research problems is a latent curve model, in which change in the outcome variable is modeled as a function of time or age. When polynomials and varying regression coefficients are used, the multilevel model becomes a very flexible analysis tool. Allowing coefficients for time to vary across participants also implies specific dependency structures. Because the focus of this chapter is on modeling individual trajectories, the possibility of specifying specific structures across time is not explored here. For a discussion of different covariance structures, we refer to Hedeker and Gibbons (2006), Hox (2010b), and Raudenbush (2002).

Modeling the dependencies over time can be done implicitly, by allowing random coefficients for the time variable, or explicitly by specifying a specific structure, and these approaches can also be combined. The remainder of this chapter discusses the use of multilevel modeling to specify latent curve models in developmental research and provides an example of multilevel modeling of developmental data and an example of using a combination of elements from an accelerated design and an interrupted time series design to model the effect of an intervention. The discussion takes up the issue of when specific approaches are useful.

Developmental Applications

Growth curve modeling regards change over time in a longitudinal design as a collection of individual underlying trajectories. The pattern of responses over time provides information on individual and average trajectories. Multilevel regression analysis is one way to analyze growth curves. A related but somewhat different approach is latent growth modeling using a structural equation approach, which is discussed elsewhere (Grimm & Ram, Chapter 24, this volume). In a multilevel growth curve model, equation 25.1 for the trajectories over time includes varying regression coefficients π_{0i}, the intercept, and π_{1i}, the slope for the time variable. In an otherwise empty model, these can be modeled by

$$\pi_{0i} = \beta_{00} + u_{0i} \quad \textbf{(25.6)}$$

$$\pi_{1i} = \beta_{10} + u_{1i} \quad \textbf{(25.7)}$$

In this model, β_{00} represents the average initial level of the response variable y, and u_{0i} the individual variation in the initial level of y. Similarly, β_{10} represents the average growth rate and u_{1i} the individual variation in the growth rate. Thus the growth curves of different individuals are characterized by individually different initial levels and rates of growth. If polynomials are used for the time variable, the regression coefficient for the square of time is the average acceleration (or deceleration) and the residual indicates the interindividual variation in the rate of acceleration (or deceleration).

Multilevel modeling of development as a function of time or age is a very flexible tool. Typically, the parameters that describe the individuals' growth curves are modeled by individual characteristics in order to explain individual variations in the growth trajectory. For this to work well, it is important that the occasion-level model is specified in a way that the estimated parameters have a straightforward meaning. One issue here is the metric of time. If measurement occasions are simply counted, the first occasion should be coded as zero. The first occasion must be coded as zero because the meaning of cross-level interactions with the time variable, the intercept variance, and the covariances between slopes and intercept are all defined at the time point zero. If zero is not part of the range of the time variable, all these estimates are essentially meaningless. When the metric of time is given as the individuals' age, the proper zero code is often not their calendar age. Zero in these models is interpreted as the point in time at which the process under study has started. For example, in longitudinal modeling of vocabulary growth, Raudenbush and Bryk (2002) use 12 months as the beginning of the learning process.

A thorough introduction to the multilevel model for change is provided by Singer and Willett (2003). More technical information on multilevel or hierarchical linear models can be found in Raudenbush and Bryk (2002).

Illustration

An Illustration in Development of Mathematical Skill

This example concerns longitudinal data from the Early Childhood Longitudinal Study—Kindergarten cohort (ECLS-K; National Center for Education Statistics, 2001). The ECLS-K is a nationally representative sample of more than 21,000 children who attended kindergarten in the school year 1998–1999. Reading and mathematics tests were administered in the fall and spring of kindergarten and first grade and in the spring of third, fifth, and eighth grade. Achievement scores were equated via an item response model and are appropriate for examining change. These same data are also used as an example in the chapter on growth curve modeling from a structural equation modeling (SEM) perspective (Grimm & Ram, Chapter 24, this volume). In our example, we use the mathematics score as dependent variable. All together, there are 95,076 mathematics measurements taken on 21,409 children, indicating that we have on average data for 4.4 measurement occasions out of a maximum of 7 measurement occasions. The overall mean mathematics score is 69.2 with a standard deviation of 44.40.

Approximately 37% of the measurement occasions are missing. The missing occasions are not MCAR. At the first measurement occasion, 13.0% of the cases are missing the math score. At the last measurement occasion, 56.6% of the cases are missing. The cases that are present at the last measurement have at the first measurement a mean mathematics score of 27.1, whereas the cases that are missing have a mean initial math score of 24.9. The standardized difference is 0.24, a value generally considered small. It is clear that children who have a relatively low score for mathematics have a larger probability of dropping out of the study. Because the observed value for their math scores at earlier occasions is available, we have a variable math score that is both indicative of dropout and that can be predicted well from earlier occasions. The availability of a variable (math score at earlier occasions) that predicts both the missingness and the variable that shows missing values (math score at later occasions) indicates that we may assume that the data are MAR (Schafer & Graham, 2002), which is the assumption made in analyzing incomplete longitudinal data using multilevel modeling.

In general, measurement occasions are represented by consecutive variables in the data file. For a multilevel analysis the data must be restructured to a stacked or "long" data file.

These data illustrate nicely the problem of the metric of time. The measurement occasions are not evenly spaced but spaced at increasing intervals. To even this out, the semesters were coded starting at zero for the fall semester of kindergarten. Consecutive semesters were then counted, including the semesters in which no data collection took place, but excluding the summer season. Finally, the semester codes were divided by 2, so that a difference of 1 unit on the time variable indicates a difference of 1 year.

Figure 25.1 shows a scatterplot for the math variable. It clearly shows that the spacing of the data collection changes. Also, it suggests a nonlinear trend: Math skill is increasing, but the increase evens off at the end. A cubic trend is also significant in these data, but because it explains very little variance, it is ignored. Given the scatterplot, we add a squared term for time to the model (to minimize collinearity with the linear time variable, the median value of 1.5 is subtracted before squaring[1]).

Table 25.1 presents the results of a sequence of multilevel analyses of the ECLS-K data. The first model is the null model that contains only the intercept. The second model contains time and time squared, and the third model adds varying slopes for both time and time squared. All parameter estimates are significant. The development over time is large; in the first year the average math score increases by 17.3, which is 39% of the standard deviation. The negative regression coefficient for time squared indicates that the growth

[1] It is more common to center on the overall mean, but we have chosen the median because this produces simple rounded values for the time codings. The difference from centering on the mean is negligible in most cases.

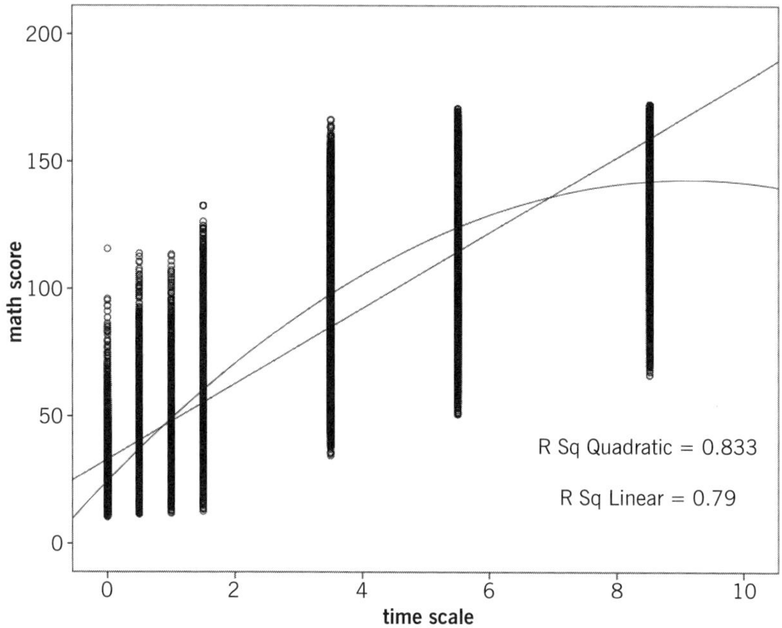

FIGURE 25.1. Scatterplot of math scores, ECLS-K data.

rate for the math score decreases over time. In the last interval, the predicted growth is 7.5, which is considerably less than 17.5.

The sequence of variance estimates shows an apparent anomaly that is typical in multilevel analysis of longitudinal data. In the null model we have no predictors, so the residual variances can be interpreted as error variances. After including the time indicators, the residual error variance at the second level *increases*. Therefore, the time indicators appear to explain negative variance at the second level. Negative variance is obviously impossible. The apparent anomaly occurs because in the empty model the variance is decomposed over

TABLE 25.1. Math Score Development over Time

	Intercept-only	+ Time fixed	+ Time random
Intercept	68.9 (0.17)	27.5 (0.11)	27.9 (0.07)
Time		21.7 (0.03)	21.3 (0.04)
Time^2		–1.5 (0.01)	–1.4 (0.01)
σ^2_e	1832.9 (9.67)	113.1 (0.59)	55.1 (0.36)
σ^2_{u0}	139.2 (6.01)	206.3 (2.30)	160.4 (1.89)
σ^2_{u1}			25.7 (0.39)
σ^2_{u2}			0.43 (0.01)
Deviance	964771.1	745135.4	708587.7

the two levels assuming simple random sampling at both levels. But in these data there is no time sampling; the measurement occasions follow a simple sequential design. If there are no missing values, the time indicators have in fact zero variance at the subject level and therefore cannot explain subject-level variation. The problem of explaining negative variance is described in general terms by Snijders and Bosker (1994) and, specifically for longitudinal data, in Hox (2010a). Hox asserts that we need to have "time" properly included in the model for the variance at the occasion and the subject level to make sense. Hence, not the first but the last model in Table 25.1 is the benchmark model against which to evaluate the explained variance at separate levels. If we want to assess the amount of variance explained by time, we cannot investigate the effect on the occasion and subject levels separately. However, we can assess the explained total variance (the sum of the occasion-level and subject-level variances). A comparison of the empty model with the model with time and time squared included as fixed effects shows that time and time squared explain 83.8% of the total variance, an estimate that is the same as the ordinary least squares (OLS) estimate printed in Figure 25.1. We may conclude that there is a strong process of growth over time.

Table 25.2 repeats the results of the model with the time variables random and then shows the results of models that add the time-varying predictors reading score (grand mean centered) and data collection in fall, then the time invariant predictor child gender, and then the cross-level interactions between child gender and the two time indicators. The parameter estimates in Table 25.2 indicate that reading and being measured in the fall both have an effect. Being measured in the fall is a dummy variable, so the drop after the summer is comparatively small. Reading is on a scale comparable to the mathematics scale, and the regression coefficient of 0.36 indicates that quite a bit of variance is predicted by this variable. In fact, both the time-level variance and the child-level variance drop considerably. In addition, some of the variance of the slopes of the time variable is also explained by the

TABLE 25.2. Math Score Predicted

	Time random	+ Varying predictors	+ Invariant predictor	+ Cross-level interaction
Intercept	36.7 (0.10)	46.6 (0.13)	46.4 (.14)	46.4 (.14)
Time	17.3 (0.03)	11.7 (0.07)	11.6 (.07)	10.7 (.08)
Time^2	-1.4 (0.01)	–0.70 (.01)	–0.70 (.01)	–0.59 (.01)
Reading		0.36 (.00)	0.36 (.00)	0.36 (.00)
In fall		–0.47 (.07)	–0.48 (.07)	–0.47 (.07)
Gender			–0.58 (.11)	–0.83 (.11)
Gender*time				–1.6 (.07)
Gender*time 2				0.22 (.01)
σ^2_e	55.1 (0.36)	52.6 (.35)	52.6 (.35)	52.7 (.35)
σ^2_{u0}	160.4 (1.89)	36.3 (.67)	36.1 (.67)	35.9 (.66)
σ^2_{u1}	25.7 (0.39)	14.8 (.26)	14.7 (.26)	14.0 (.25)
σ^2_{u2}	0.43 (0.01)	0.28 (.01)	0.28 (.01)	0.27 (.01)
Deviance	708587.7	688243.3	688218.0	687743.8

time-varying predictors. Child gender is significant; girls score somewhat lower than boys, but this explains hardly any variance between children. The cross-level interactions are also significant, but again they explain very little slope variation.

The final model in Table 25.2 indicates an increase in mathematics ability over time, with a slower increase at the end of the measurement occasions. Part of the increase can be predicted by the reading score, which also increases over time. That reading explains a considerable amount of between-children variation in the intercept and the slopes implies that the variation in the growth trajectories for reading and mathematics must be quite similar, something that is not explicitly modeled here. Using a multivariate multilevel model would show such covariation between the time slopes for reading and mathematics at the expense of creating a complicated model. We consider this beyond the scope of this chapter; for an example, see Goldstein (2003, Chapter 5). As illustrated in Hox (2010a, Chapter 16), SEM is a more flexible approach for analyzing parallel growth curves.

An Illustration of Evaluation of an Intervention

Our next example concerns evaluating an intervention program by using a longitudinal design that was set up to circumvent the need for a randomized control group. In many developmental and educational research projects, it is not feasible or even possible to set up a proper randomized control study. It is costly to have control groups, and sometimes it is considered unethical not to let the control group profit from a (potentially beneficial) intervention program. When it is possible to set up a longitudinal experiment, an interrupted time series design is a viable alternative to a cross-sectional experimental design (Shadish, Cook, & Campbell, 2002). In our example the interrupted time series design is combined with features from cohort sequential latent curve modeling and piecewise growth modeling (see Singer & Willett, 2003, Chapter 5) to examine the effects of an intervention. The final model also includes time-varying predictors.

EQUIP for Educators (EFE) is an multicomponent educational program designed to motivate and teach students how to think and act responsibly (DiBiase, Gibbs, Potter, & Spring, 2005). In the present study we focus on the effects of EFE on attitude toward antisocial behavior in a sample of 705 students attending prevocational secondary education. Full details on this study can be found in Van der Velden, Brugman, Boom, and Koops (2009).

Seven schools participated, each with 4 measurements spaced 4 months apart. Schools were assigned to three intervention cohorts based on the number of pre- and posttest assessments (see Table 25.3).

The intervention was always done in grade 8, but data collection took place according to various time paths depending on school; data waves were spread over three different academic years (seventh grade to ninth grade). It is often difficult to assign schools and classes randomly to conditions, and in this case it was impossible, because schools were assigned

TABLE 25.3. Overview of Project Design, Data Collection, and Intervention

	M1	Intervention	M2	Intervention	M3	Intervention	M4
Intervention Cohort 1	166	X	166	—	153	—	135
Intervention Cohort 2	381	—	331	X	308	—	322
Intervention Cohort 3	59	—	82	—	81	X	76

TABLE 25.4. Measurement Occasions Aligned on Intervention

	T1	T2	T3	Intervention	T4	T5	T6
Intervention Cohort 1	—	—	M1	X	M2	M3	M4
Intervention Cohort 2	—	M1	M2	X	M3	M4	—
Intervention Cohort 3	M1	M2	M3	X	M4	—	—

to the cohorts according to their logistical possibilities. There were significant differences between cohorts concerning sex ($\chi^2(2) = 8.1, p = .017$), age ($F(2,601) = 7.19, p = .001$) and ethnicity ($\chi^2(2) = 209.7, p = .000$). Sex, age, and ethnicity (Dutch vs. ethnic minority) are included in the analyses as potential predictors. To illustrate the design, it is useful to view the cohorts aligned on intervention; see Table 25.4.

Due to time constraints at assessment, the number of missing values fluctuated on the different measures used in this study. Moreover, for all measures, individual scale scores were computed only if at least 80% of the items were scored. Attrition of scale scores ranged from 0.4% to 4.8% at first assessment, from 0.9% to 3.8% at second assessment, from 0.8% to 2.9% at third assessment, and from 0.8% to 4.1% at fourth assessment. Descriptives are presented in Table 25.5. Attitude is measured as the average over 12 items on a 4-point scale (1–4; low scores indicating a more negative attitude toward antisocial behavior).

We use multilevel modeling to gain insight into the trajectories and longitudinal effects of the intervention (using HLM; Raudenbush, Bryk, Cheong, Congdon, & Du Toit, 2000).

The level 1 model in this case is a combination of two growth trajectories: the baseline part applying to all measurement occasions and the intervention part applying only to the postintervention measurements and different for each cohort, as in a cohort sequential design.

$$Y_{ti} = \pi_{0i} + \pi_{1i}(Slope)_{ti} + \pi_{2i}(Interv.\ Interc.)_{ti} + \pi_{3i}(Interv.\ Slope)_{ti} + e_{ti} \quad \textbf{(25.8)}$$

where Y_{ti} is the response at occasion t ($t = 1, \ldots, T_i$) for individual I ($i = 1, \ldots, n$) as before. The values for the intercept of the baseline (all 1) are implicit in π_{0i}. The values for the slope of the baseline are in $(Slope)_{ti}$. The $(Interv.\ Interc.)_{ti}$ represents the values of the immediate effect of the intervention and are 1 for each postintervention measurement (hence we refer to it as the intercept for the intervention effect). The $(Interv.\ Slope)_{ti}$ represents the longer term effect of the intervention, and the values start at 0 for the first postintervention measurement and increase by 1 for each subsequent postintervention measurement (hence we refer to it as the *slope for the intervention effect*). The last two terms represent time-varying explanatory variables, as indicated with an X in equation 25.1. However,

TABLE 25.5. Attitude toward Antisocial Behavior

	T1		T2		T3		T4	
	M	*SD*	*M*	*SD*	*M*	*SD*	*M*	*SD*
Intervention Cohort 1	2.03	0.52	1.91	0.52	2.00	0.52	2.10	0.54
Intervention Cohort 2	1.85	0.55	1.86	0.53	1.76	0.55	1.78	0.57
Intervention Cohort 3	1.68	0.52	1.68	0.48	1.69	0.51	1.61	0.49

the present parameterization makes it easier to compare our model with an SEM cohort sequential accelerated model.

The π's are the regression coefficients, intercept and slopes, which may vary across individuals and therefore carry a subscript i for individuals, and e_{ti} is an occasion-level residual error term, which is assumed to have a normal distribution.

The final level 2 model is

$$\pi_{0i} = \beta_{00} + \beta_{01}(\text{Sex})_i + \beta_{02}(\text{Ethnicity})_i + u_{0i} \quad \textbf{(25.9)}$$

$$\pi_{1i} = \beta_{11}(\text{Ethnicity})_i + u_{1i} \quad \textbf{(25.10)}$$

$$\pi_{2i} = \beta_{20} + \beta_{21}(\text{Ethnicity})_i + u_{2i} \quad \textbf{(25.11)}$$

$$\pi_{3i} = \beta_{30} + \beta_{31}(\text{Sex})_i \quad \textbf{(25.12)}$$

The intercept (equation 25.9) is influenced by sex and ethnicity and has a random component u_{0i}. The slope (equation 25.10) is zero on average but has a random component and is influenced by ethnicity. The β_{10} term was therefore not required. The immediate effect of the intervention (intervention intercept; equation 25.11) was influenced by ethnicity and had a random component. The subsequent effect of the intervention (intervention slope; Equation 25.12) was influenced by sex only and had no significant random component (perhaps unsurprisingly as only one cohort contributed to information for this effect). Sex and ethnicity were centered at their grand mean to facilitate parameter interpretation. Table 25.6, with the final model in the last column, and Figure 25.2 present the results.

Figure 25.2 represents the average trajectory without the effects of sex and ethnicity. In particular, the drop at virtual measurement occasion 4 is much more pronounced for the Dutch group and persists for Dutch girls, whereas for ethnic minority boys the intervention seems to have resulted in an adverse effect.

Other alignments are possible, too. Some schools started with the premeasurement in grade 7 just before summer break and with intervention (which took 16 weeks) in the beginning of eighth grade, whereas other schools started later and had their intervention at the end of the school year. So it is possible to create a baseline based on time of year in 4-month chunks, from the last quarter of grade 7 onward. It is also possible to test the model by, for example, reversing cohorts 1 and 3 in terms of the intervention effect loadings as a deliberate misaligning on intervention. Indeed, in this case the fit is worse than in the nonintervention models in Table 25.4, implying that there is a genuine effect related to the interventions.

The same model was estimated with a SEM-based latent variable growth curve model with a cohort sequential structure in Van der Velden and colleagues (2010). Effects of the predictors could only be estimated for each cohort separately, and therefore regression coefficients had to be constrained to be equal between cohorts. Assessing the effects of predictors such as sex and ethnicity became complex and confusing and is much more straightforward in the present multilevel approach.

Future Directions

When viewed carefully, multilevel models and structural equation models for change over time are just different representations of the same underlying model. Bollen and Curran (2006) provide a thorough discussion of longitudinal models from a structural equation

TABLE 25.6. Attitude toward Antisocial Behavior Score Predicted

	No intervention		Intervention	
	No predictors	Predictors	No predictors	Predictors
Intercept	1.87 (.021)	1.85 (.018)	1.89 (.021)	1.88 (.020)
Slope	−0.01 (.008)		−0.05 (.010)	—
Interventions Intercept			—	−0.09 (.019)
Intervention Slope			0.12 (.019)	0.05 (.015)
$\text{Sex}_{\text{intercept}}$		−0.14 (.038)		−0.11 (.038)
$\text{Sex}_{\text{slope}}$				
$\text{Sex}_{\text{intervinterc}}$				
$\text{Sex}_{\text{intervslope}}$				−0.10 (.025)
$\text{Ethnicity}_{\text{intercept}}$				−0.22 (.042)
$\text{Ethnicity}_{\text{slope}}$		−0.05 (.014)		−0.05 (.025)
$\text{Ethnicity}_{\text{intervinterc}}$				0.13 (.054)
$\text{Ethnicity}_{\text{intervslope}}$				
σ^2_{u0}	0.202 (.016)	0.198 (.016)	0.206 (.016)	0.194 (.015)
σ^2_{u1}	0.013 (.002)	0.013 (.002)	0.005 (.005)	0.005 (.005)
σ^2_{u2}			0.025 (.027)	0.029 (.027)
σ^2_{u3}				
σ^2_{e}	0.086	0.086	0.081	0.079
Deviance	2374	2346	2328	2261

Note. SE in parentheses.

perspective, and Hedeker and Gibbons (2006) provide a comparable discussion from the multilevel regression perspective. Duncan and colleagues (2006) provide an introduction to longitudinal modeling from both perspectives. The advantage of SEM with longitudinal data is that SEM makes it possible to include distant outcomes, to use growth curve intercept and slopes as predictors, and to examine mediation effects. In multilevel longitudinal analysis, adding more levels for groups and other contextual units is straightforward.

Both in SEM and in the multilevel perspective, incomplete data can be handled in a straightforward manner. If the data collection is based on sampling measurement occasions, as in studies that employ experience sampling, the SEM representation becomes cumbersome, because the varied set of measurement occasions are modeled as missing occasions, and the result is that there are a large number of distinct measurement occasions, most of them missing for any particular subject. Multilevel analysis is a much easier and more direct approach to this situation. Both approaches assume that the missingness process is MAR, which is a much weaker assumption than the MCAR that listwise deletion in MANOVA

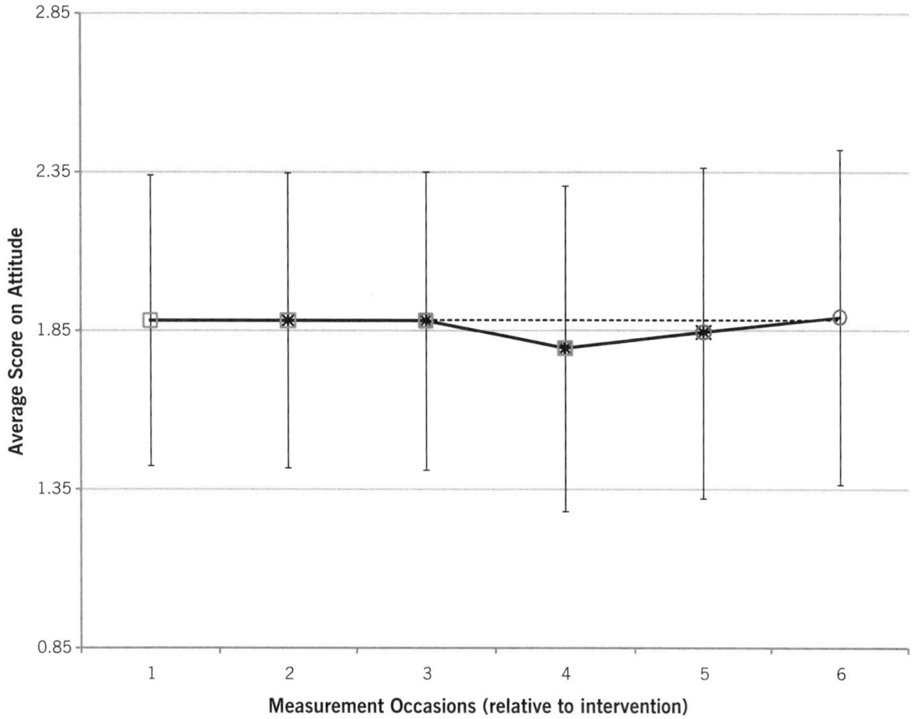

FIGURE 25.2. Trajectory for the three cohorts aligned as in Table 25.2. The heavy line represents the modeled trajectory, the dashed line represents the modeled baseline. Gridlines are one *SD* apart. The intervention was between virtual measurement occasions 3 and 4.

implies. The ability to deal with incomplete data is used in the second example. By using an accelerated design, using only four measurement occasions in each cohort, it is possible to analyze a synthetic sample in which there are up to three measurement occasions before the intervention and up to three measurement occasions following it. This design enables a detailed analysis of the trends in the data, in our case showing an immediate effect of the intervention, which subsequently decreases over time.

Given that the underlying models are very similar if not equivalent, an ongoing trend is that SEM and multilevel analysis are merging. Structural equation modelers have argued that multilevel models are a special case of SEM (cf. Curran, 2003; Mehta & Neale, 2005). In addition, software is appearing that can estimate multilevel SEMs, such as Mplus (Muthén & Muthén, 2009) and Gllamm (Rabe-Hesketh, Skrondal, & Pickles, 2004), which includes the multilevel regression models currently analyzed with mixed modeling software such as HLM or MLwiN. Combining the strength of SEM and multilevel modeling, the multilevel structural equation approach promises an extremely flexible tool with which to analyze longitudinal developmental data.

Acknowledgments

The content is solely the responsibility of the authors and does not necessarily represent the official views of the funding agencies. We thank Kevin Grimm for providing us with the ECLS-K data and

Floor Van der Velden and Daniel Brugman for generously making available parts of the EQUIP data set. Input and output scripts can be found at *www.crmda.ku.edu/Guilford/HDRM*.

References

Bollen, K. A., & Curran, P. J. (2006). *Latent curve models*. Hoboken, NJ: Wiley.

Curran, P. J. (2003). Have multilevel models been structural equation models all along? *Multivariate Behavioral Research, 38*, 529–569.

DiBiase, A. M., Gibbs, J. C., Potter, G. B., & Spring, B. (2005). *EQUIP for educators: Teaching youth (grades 5–8) to think and act responsibly*. Champaign, IL: Research Press.

Duncan, T. E., Duncan, S. C., & Strycker, L. A. (2006). *An introduction to latent variable growth curve modeling* (2nd ed.). Mahwah, NJ: Erlbaum.

Goldstein, H. (2003). *Multilevel statistical models* (3rd ed.). London: Arnold.

Hedeker, D., & Gibbons, R. D. (2006). *Longitudinal data analysis*. Hoboken, NJ: Wiley.

Hox, J. J. (2010a). *Multilevel analysis, techniques and applications* (2nd ed.). New York: Routledge.

Hox, J. J. (2010b). Panel modeling: Random coefficients and covariance structures. In J. J. Hox & J. K. Roberts (Eds.), *Handbook of advanced multilevel analysis* (pp. 85–96). New York: Routledge.

Little, R. J. A. (1995). Modeling the drop-out mechanism in repeated measures studies. *Journal of the American Statistical Association, 90*, 1112–1121.

Mehta, P. D., & Neale, M. C. (2005). People are variables too: Multilevel structural equations modeling. *Psychological Methods, 10*, 259–284.

Muthén, L. K., & Muthén, B. O. (1998–2009). *Mplus user's guide* (6th ed.). Los Angeles: Authors.

National Center for Educational Statistics. (2001). *Kindergarten Class of 1998–1999 (ECLS-K)*. Retrieved August 8, 2011, from *http://nces.ed.gov/ecls/kindergarten.asp*.

Rabe-Hesketh, S., Skrondal, A., & Pickles, A. (2004). Generalized multilevel structural equation modeling. *Psychometrika, 69*, 167–190.

Raudenbush, S. W. (2002). Alternative covariance structures for polynomial models of individual growth and change. In D. S. Moskowitz & S. L. Hersberger (Eds.), *Modeling intraindividual variability with repeated measures data* (pp. 25–57). Mahwah, NJ: Erlbaum.

Raudenbush, S. W., & Bryk, A. S. (2002). *Hierarchical linear models* (2nd ed.). Thousand Oaks, CA: Sage.

Raudenbush, S. W., Bryk, A. S., Cheong, Y., Congdon, R. T., & Du Toit, M. (2004). *HLM 6: Hierarchical linear and nonlinear modeling*. Lincolnwood, IL: Scientific Software International.

Schafer, J. L., & Graham, J. W. (2002). Missing data: Our view of the state of the art. *Psychological Methods, 7*, 147–177.

Shadish, W. R., Cook, T. D., & Campbell, D. T. (2002). *Experimental and quasi-experimental designs*. New York: Houghton Mifflin.

Snijders, T. A. B., & Bosker, R. J. (1994). Modeled variance in two-level models. *Sociological Methods and Research, 22*, 342–363.

Singer, J. D., & Willett, J. B. (2003). *Applied longitudinal data analysis*. New York: Oxford University Press.

Van der Velden, F., Brugman, D., Boom, J., & Koops, W. (2009). EQUIP for educators: The longitudinal effects of a school-based universal prevention program on moral cognitions and antisocial behavior in young adolescents. In *EQUIPping high school students: Effects of a universal preventive intervention on antisocial behavior* (pp. 73–99). Enschede, The Netherlands: Ipskamp Drukkers.

CHAPTER 26

Nonlinear Growth Modeling

SHELLEY A. BLOZIS

Studies of behavioral development have greatly benefited from the application of growth models to improve understanding of development (Card & Little, 2007). Growth models involve fitting a function to a set of data to describe a response variable over time. Two functions that are commonly used in growth models are linear and quadratic functions. A linear function for growth assumes a constant rate of change in a response across a study period. A quadratic function assumes that change is not constant, with the change rate governed by a rate of acceleration. These two forms of growth are simple in their interpretation. Behavioral development does not always follow these forms of change, however, making it necessary in some situations to consider a nonlinear growth model, that is, a growth model based on a nonlinear function. Growth models based on nonlinear functions allow for a wide variety of growth trends. A commonly applied growth model is one based on a negatively accelerated exponential function in which a response may, for example, initially change at a relatively fast pace but then slow, with the response tending toward an unchanging, asymptotic value. In a study of hand function development in children with unilateral cerebral palsy, for instance, a negatively accelerated exponential function was effective in describing the nonconstant rate of change in the measures and providing a means to measure the potential developmental response (Holmefur, Krumlinde-Sundholm, Bergström, & Eliasson, 2010). Other examples of nonlinear change in studies of development include those that follow multiple phases of change, such as a response that first follows a linear trend in the beginning of the study but then shifts to a different linear trend in the latter part of the study. A growth model based on a multiphase function, a model that may be used to capture this type of nonlinear change, was effective, for instance, in capturing a shift in life satisfaction in older individuals (Gerstorf et al., 2008).

Central Issues

Approaches to growth modeling have commonly emphasized mean change across a population of individuals and provided tools for describing population-level trends. Repeated-measures analysis of variance (ANOVA), in which a set of population means is assumed to follow a linear or quadratic trend, is a typical example of a model that emphasizes change at the population level. Importantly, models of this sort assume that change in a response is systematic with time solely at the population level. Although responses within individuals are likely to be correlated due to the nature of repeated-measures data, these dependencies in a repeated-measures ANOVA model are not assumed to be due to change that is specific to the individual. That is, the model does not explicitly account for change in a response that may be unique to the individual.

In contrast to models that emphasize change at the population level, growth models that are defined at the individual level assume that growth for each individual in a population is a systematic function of time (Fitzmaurice, Laird, & Ware, 2004; Singer & Willett, 2003). More specifically, an individual's response is assumed to be due to a growth function that is common to all individuals in the population but is particular to each individual with regard to the coefficients that define the function (Laird & Ware, 1982). Change in a measured response across members of a population may be assumed to follow a linear form of growth over time, for instance, but the intercept and linear rate of change that define the growth trajectory may be unique to each individual. As a result, each individual is assumed to have a growth trajectory that may be completely unique (with regard to the growth coefficients, such as the intercept and slope) from those of other individuals in the population. In developmental research, models that are based on growth defined at the individual level for a population of individuals are commonly referred to as mixed-effects models. Now a widely popular modeling framework, mixed-effects models provide an essential means of characterizing behavioral development.

Linear models, and linear growth models in particular, are often applied in studies of developmental data (e.g., Carlson & Iacono, 2008; Cillessen & Borch, 2006; Marsh, 2007; Solomon & Theiss, 2008). Linear models more generally form a class of models in which the coefficients of the model enter the model in a linear, or additive, manner. In a linear mixed-effects model, the coefficients of the model, whether they are fixed or random, enter the model in a strictly linear manner. Thus the essential feature of a standard linear model or a linear mixed-effects model is that any unknown parameter enters the model linearly (Davidian & Giltinan, 1995). For models of growth, this means that a growth model that is linear in its parameters may represent one of many possible forms of growth, including of course many that are nonlinear in form. Specifically, nonlinear growth forms are possible in a linear model framework through transformations of the measures of time. That is, in contrast to the unknown coefficients of a linear model that must enter a model linearly, measures of time, which are assumed to be fixed and known, may enter a model in a nonlinear manner, such as in a quadratic function in which measures of time are squared. In fact, any nonlinear transformation of time that involves known parameters may be incorporated into a growth model, and the model is still considered linear in its parameters, even though the form of change is nonlinear.

Given the nature of developmental data, there are many behaviors that change at a rate that is not constant across time. There are, in fact, several ways in which a linear growth model may be specified to allow for nonlinear change in a response. Higher order polynomial functions, such as a quadratic or a cubic function, may be applied by defining functions that involve nonlinear (e.g., squared and cubed) transformations of time. An exponential function in which any parameter that appears in the exponent is known, for instance, allows a response to follow a curve that includes an asymptote. This is useful in studies of behaviors that follow a nonlinear form of growth that tends toward an asymptote.

Furthermore, developmental studies that involve behavioral measures obtained during times of transition, such as the period from adolescence through early adulthood, may require other forms of nonlinear growth, such as those defined by multiple functions that may be linked together to allow for multiple phases of change in a response. Multiphase models, models that specify a sequence of behavioral courses that relate to different periods of time, such as one behavioral course followed by a second, may be used to study behaviors that involve transitions (Bates & Watts, 2007). Such models have also been considered under a mixed-effects model framework (Cudeck & Klebe, 2002; Singer & Willett, 2003). Under a two-phase growth model, for instance, average growth during an earlier stage of development may follow one form of change, such as a positive linear trend, and later change course to follow a different trend, such as a decreasing linear trend (e.g., Gerstorf et al., 2008; McArdle & Wang, 2008).

The popularity of linear growth models, that is, models that are linear in their parameters, has likely been due to the availability of commercial statistical software packages that may be used to fit such models. Specialized statistical software programs for structural equation modeling (SEM; e.g., AMOS, LISREL, and Mplus), programs designed especially for multilevel data (e.g., HLM and MLwiN), or more major statistical software packages (e.g., SAS, SPSS, and Systat), for instance, may be implemented in the estimation of mixed-effects models that are linear in their parameters. The particular software package that is used to estimate a model will dictate the particular model features that may be considered in an analysis. Software programs that were designed for multilevel data will typically allow unique times of measurement between individuals, for instance, whereas not all programs designed for estimating linear SEMs will allow for individual-specific times of measurement. Latent basis models, latent growth models that do not specify a particular form of change, are typically fitted within an SEM framework. Multiphase mixed-effects models may be applied using a range of statistical software programs, such as programs developed for estimating multilevel models (Cudeck & Klebe, 2002).

Conceptual Principles and Statistical Assumptions

Statistical software developments have more recently provided increased access to fitting growth models that are nonlinear in their parameters. Nonlinear models are those that include one or more unknown coefficients that enter the model in a nonlinear way. Nonlinear growth models, such as one based on an exponential function that includes an unknown coefficient in the exponent, are particularly important in developmental research because nonlinear models may provide a closer approximation or a more realistic representation of a behavioral growth trajectory. This is due to the fact that specification of growth models that are nonlinear in their parameters is more flexible than of models that are linear in their parameters. In many cases, a nonlinear function may be specified to have parameters that have a simple interpretation and relate directly to the behavior under study. A behavioral response whose growth rate slows over time so that the response approaches an asymptote, for instance, may be best approximated by a negatively accelerated exponential function, where it is the asymptotic value of the response, that is, the potential response, that is of particular interest (e.g., Blozis, Conger, & Harring, 2007).

When a nonlinear growth model involves random effects, one or more of the model parameters may vary across individuals in a population. In a nonlinear mixed-effects model, individual differences in any of the features that describe change in a response may be taken into account by the model, including individual differences in unknown parameters that enter a model in a nonlinear manner. This is an important aspect of nonlinear mixed-effects models that distinguishes them from linear mixed-effects models. Thus, as a class of models, nonlinear mixed-effects models naturally extend the selection of functional growth forms while also allowing for individual differences in aspects of growth that would otherwise need to be assumed constant for individuals in a population under a linear mixed-effects model. Thus growth models that include nonlinear parameters offer many improvements in the ways developmental trajectories may be defined by a statistical model.

Model Formulation

A general model may be used to represent a family of growth models that are nonlinear in their parameters. Models that are linear in their parameters are simply a special case. Defining a growth model in such general terms allows the model formulation to encompass both linear and nonlinear models. Furthermore, a model may contain only fixed effects, only random effects, or a combination of random and fixed effects, with the latter being perhaps most applicable in studies of development. Fixed effects are the effects of predictors (e.g., time) that are constant across individuals in a population and so characterize a behavioral trajectory across individuals of a population. Random effects are effects of predictors that vary across individuals in a population and so characterize a behavioral trajectory for the individual.

In a nonlinear mixed-effects model, an unknown parameter, whether it is fixed or random across individuals in a population, may enter the model linearly or nonlinearly. In cases in which only the fixed parameters of the model may enter nonlinearly and the random effects are restricted to enter only linearly, the model is in a class of what are called partially nonlinear or conditionally linear mixed-effects models (Blozis & Cudeck, 1999). A fully nonlinear mixed-effects model is one in which one or more random coefficients enters the model in a nonlinear manner; fixed effects may enter linearly or nonlinearly. These distinctions among models, that is, among linear mixed-effects models, partially nonlinear mixed-effects models, and fully nonlinear mixed-effects models, are important because complications in obtaining maximum likelihood (ML) estimates arise when random coefficients enter a model in a nonlinear manner (see Blozis, 2007a, for a discussion).

To formulate a nonlinear growth model for repeated measures, first define $\mathbf{y}_i = (y_{i1}, \ldots, y_{in_i})'$ as a set of repeated measures for individual i that has been recorded at different points in time, denoted by a set of values $\mathbf{t}_i = (t_{i1}, \ldots, t_{in_i})'$, for $i = 1, \ldots, N$. The total number of individuals studied is denoted by N, and n_i represents the maximum number of recorded observations for individual i. For the latter, a subscript i indicates that across the sample, individuals may be measured a different number of times. This may occur in practice when some individuals miss a scheduled assessment and so fewer observations were made than were originally planned. Missing data may also occur by design when some missing data are planned for a study (Graham, Taylor, Olchowski, & Cumsille, 2006). Additionally, the specific times at which the response is measured may vary between individuals, and so the particular values of time included in $\mathbf{t}_i$ may be unique to the individual. A growth model that incorporates such flexibility in the recordings of time measures is particularly useful in studies of development in which individuals are often measured at different times, such as in studies involving young children, in which age is the measure of time and children vary in their ages at each assessment. This manner of handling time is also particularly useful in developmental studies in which the spacing between assessments is not the same across individuals in the sample.

In addition to measures of time, a model for a repeated-measures variable may also involve covariates that also change over time, such as time-varying measures of reading ability that are used to predict repeated measures of mathematical ability. Covariates that are invariant with time may also be incorporated into a model. Covariates are invariant with time if they are constant for the individual across the study period. Examples of such variables are an individual's marital status and educational level, assuming such variables do not change over the study period.

Assuming a growth model includes random effects, a mixed-effects model may be specified. Let $\mathbf{X}_i$ denote covariates, whether they change over time or are constant for the individual. A mixed-effects model for $\mathbf{y}_i$ in which $\mathbf{y}_i$ is a function of time, and possibly covariates $\mathbf{X}_i$ may be expressed as

$$\mathbf{y}_i = f(\mathbf{t}_i, \mathbf{X}_i, \beta, \mathbf{b}_i) + \varepsilon_i \quad \textbf{(26.1)}$$

where $f(\bullet)$ is a function, such as an exponential function, hypothesized to characterize the response over time $\mathbf{t}_i$. The coefficients of the model are the set of unknown, fixed effects β and the set of unknown random effects $\mathbf{b}_i$ that vary across individuals. Whereas the growth function is assumed to be common to all individuals in a population, the coefficients of the function may vary between individuals due to the random effects $\mathbf{b}_i$. The set of errors of the model, $\varepsilon_i = (\varepsilon_{i1}, \ldots, \varepsilon_{in_i})'$, represents the discrepancies between $\mathbf{y}_i$ and the hypothesized trajectory.

Assuming change in $\mathbf{y}_i$ is systematic with time only at the population level, for example, a growth model for $\mathbf{y}_i$ may include the fixed coefficient β but not the random effect $\mathbf{b}_i$. Thus change in $\mathbf{y}_i$ would be considered only at the population level, and the model would not be a mixed-effects model. This model would be useful in situations in which all individuals follow the same developmental trajectory, with individual scores possibly varying at random about the mean curve. Dependencies between scores measured within individuals may be addressed by allowing the errors measured within an individual to covary, such as by specifying a pattern of autocorrelation.

Assuming change in $\mathbf{y}_i$ is systematic with time at the individual level, in addition to the population level, the random effect $\mathbf{b}_i$ would be included in a mixed-effects model to allow change in $\mathbf{y}_i$ to be unique to the individual. In this case, a response is assumed to change according to a function that is common to all individuals of a population but of which one or more of the growth coefficients are unique to the individual. As described earlier, a model may also include a set of covariates $\mathbf{X}_i$ whose values change with time or that are fixed for the individual and so remain constant for the study period. Under a mixed-effects model, the effects of time-varying covariates may also be random across individuals in a population.

An important feature of nonlinear growth models is that a great number of functions may be considered in characterizing a longitudinal response. Particular functions may be chosen and formulated so that the coefficients are relevant to particular aspects of growth in a response. In Blozis, Conger, and Harring (2007; see also Blozis, 2007a), for instance, a structured latent curve model was applied to study individual-level change in reading performance using an exponential function. One parameter was defined as the performance level at an early point in the study (as defined by the model's intercept). A second parameter defined the asymptote of the response and so was related to potential reading performance at older ages. A third parameter defined a nonlinear change rate, as the rate of change in reading performance was not thought to be constant across time. In this particular application of an exponential function that included random effects, all three coefficients of the exponential function were allowed to vary across individuals. Given that reading performance could be characterized well by a function that included random coefficients that defined critical aspects of reading development at an individual level, future studies of reading performance may consider potential moderators of these particular aspects of change. That is, future studies may consider questions about how different features that define performance may be due, for instance, to individual or contextual characteristics.

The manner of defining a general growth model as in equation 26.1 allows for a great range in the specification of a growth model. This includes the more popular mixed-effects models that are strictly linear in their parameters (e.g., a linear mixed-effects model). When a mixed-effects model includes one or more parameters that enter the model in a nonlinear manner, there are two subclasses of models to consider. These are the partially nonlinear mixed-effects model (also called the conditionally linear mixed-effects model) and the fully nonlinear mixed-effects model. Partially nonlinear mixed-effects models are those in which any nonlinear coefficient is assumed to be constant across individuals in a population. Random coefficients, on the other hand, are restricted to enter the model in a linear manner. In contrast, fully nonlinear mixed-effects models are models for which a random coefficient may enter the model linearly or nonlinearly. Fixed coefficients may also enter linearly or nonlinearly. This distinction between types of nonlinear mixed-effects models is important due to differences in the computations involved in obtaining ML estimates of model parameters, with fully nonlinear mixed-effects models being the most flexible in terms of model specification but also often being the most difficult to estimate in practice. These two general types of nonlinear mixed-effects models are described next.

Partially Nonlinear Mixed-Effects Models

Partially nonlinear mixed-effects models, also referred to as conditionally linear mixed-effects models, are models in which any coefficient that goes into the model in a nonlinear manner is strictly fixed across individuals (Blozis & Cudeck, 1999; Harring, Cudeck, & du Toit, 2006). Thus any random coefficient may enter the model only in a linear manner. This implies a restriction of this modeling framework in that any coefficient that is nonlinear is specified to be constant for all individuals. A partially nonlinear mixed-effects model based on a growth function that includes a nonlinear change rate, for instance, such as an exponential function, would be assumed to be the same for all individuals. Some allowance for individual differences in nonlinear parameters is possible, however, if such parameters may be specified as functions of individual characteristics, such as a model that includes a nonlinear growth rate that differs strictly as a function of the participant's gender. Otherwise, random variation in nonlinear coefficients is not possible.

An important advantage of the formulation of a partially nonlinear mixed-effects model is that ML estimation of the model parameters may rely on procedures that are commonly used to estimate strictly linear models. For instance, ML estimation of a partially nonlinear mixed-effects model may proceed using algorithms that are typically implemented when estimating linear SEMs, such as the expectation–maximization (EM) algorithm or the Newton–Raphson algorithm. Jennrich and Schluchter (1986) describe ML estimation of a linear mixed-effects model, and Blozis and Cudeck (1999) extend the approach for estimation of a partially nonlinear mixed-effects model. Some commercially available software programs may also be used to estimate partially nonlinear mixed-effects models. Although currently limited to cases in which data are complete, LISREL (beginning with version 8.8) may be used to fit partially nonlinear mixed-effects models within an SEM framework (see Blozis, Harring, & Mels, 2008). In addition to the linear random coefficients of a model, latent covariates may also be included in a partially nonlinear mixed-effects model (also see Blozis, 2004; Blozis & Cudeck, 1999). Mx, a free and downloadable statistical software program for multivariate analyses (Neale, Boker, Xie, & Maes, 2003), may also be used to fit partially nonlinear mixed-effects models and are not restricted to complete data (Blozis, 2007b).

Structured Latent Curve Model

A structured latent curve model is a model that shares technical features with a partially nonlinear mixed-effects model, and so it is reviewed here. A structured latent curve model represents another class of models that may also be considered when characterizing growth in a measured response that follows a nonlinear form of change (Browne, 1993; Browne & du Toit, 1991). Under a structured latent curve model, a growth function that may be a nonlinear function is initially specified for the common response. Examples of functions that may be considered under a structured latent curve model are a logistic function, a Gompertz function, and an exponential function. These three functions share similar qualities with regard to their shapes, and the specific curve chosen for a given problem might depend on what is hypothesized about the behavioral trajectory. A logistic growth function, for example, yields an S-shaped curve. Choi, Harring, and Hancock (2009) provide an extensive discussion of this function in the context of longitudinal data analysis. All three functions are considered, for instance, in an analysis of infant mental development using a twin sample (Neale & McArdle, 2000).

At the individual level, a first-order Taylor polynomial is used to define the response. The polynomial is defined by a linear function of a set of random coefficients that vary across individuals and a set of basis functions. The basis functions are defined by the first-order partial derivatives of the common function taken with regard to each coefficient of the common function. The random coefficients allow for individual differences in the coefficients that characterize the response. Browne and du Toit (1991) provide analytical derivatives for a form of an exponential function, a Gompertz function, and a logistic function.

Unlike a partially nonlinear mixed-effects model, as described previously, a structured latent curve model allows for individual differences in all of the coefficients that describe change in the response, including those that relate to a parameter that enters the model in a nonlinear manner. Due to the manner in which the model is specified at the individual level (i.e., by using a first-order Taylor polynomial), the model is conditionally linear with regard to the random coefficients. That is, the random coefficients enter the model only in a linear manner. Importantly, although individual differences in a nonlinear coefficient may be accommodated, a structured latent curve model is technically similar to the partially nonlinear mixed-effects model in that random coefficients enter the model only linearly, and so estimation of a structured latent curve model may also proceed using methods used to fit strictly linear models (see Blozis, 2007a). Related to this aspect of the model, only functions of a particular kind may be used in a structured latent curve model (see Browne, 1993). Despite this, however, many of the functions that are suitable under this framework, such as those mentioned earlier, are applicable to many kinds of developmental data (e.g., Rast & Zimprich, 2009).

Fully Nonlinear Mixed-Effects Models

Fully nonlinear mixed models are mixed-effects models in which random coefficients may enter a model either linearly or nonlinearly (Davidian & Giltinan, 1995). In the analysis of developmental data, this can be a great advantage in terms of model specification relative to models that are restricted with regard to nonlinear parameters. That is, a fully nonlinear mixed-effects model is more flexible in that any nonlinear function may be specified in the model and that all parameters of the chosen function may vary across individuals, including those parameters that enter nonlinearly, such as a nonlinear change rate. In the context of developmental studies, this implies that the rate of development in a behavior, when assumed to change at a nonconstant rate, may vary across individuals.

Although fully nonlinear mixed-effects growth models can play an important role in studies of developmental data, a difficulty often arises in the estimation of nonlinear mixed-effects models that include nonlinear random effects. Specifically, estimation of a fully nonlinear mixed-effects model becomes increasingly difficult with the addition of random effects that enter the model nonlinearly. Whereas estimation of a partially nonlinear mixed-effects model may rely on common estimation procedures, even though a fixed and unknown nonlinear parameter is included in the model, estimation of a fully nonlinear mixed-effects model must proceed using alternative methods, or the model must be reexpressed in a manner that allows for standard estimation procedures to be used (Davidian & Giltinan, 1995). This is due to the fact that there is not a closed-form solution to the problem of estimating a model that includes random, nonlinear coefficients. A number of solutions to the problem have been proposed, although many are oftentimes difficult to implement in practice (although see du Toit & Cudeck, 2009). Thus, despite the added flexibility in how a model may be specified under a fully nonlinear mixed-effects model, the application of the model may in practice be difficult.

A Quadratic Growth Model as a Nonlinear Model

Behavioral responses that are considered to change at nonconstant rates are very often handled by applying a quadratic growth function. The typical formulation of a quadratic function applied in practice is one in which one parameter denotes the response level when time = 0, a second is the instantaneous rate of change when time = 0, and the third is the rate of acceleration. A different and equivalent formulation of the function is one in which the parameters define very different aspects of the curve. Thus model fit will be identical for the two formulations; only the parameters will have a different interpretation. Cudeck and du Toit (2002) describe two formulations of a nonlinear growth model based on a quadratic function.

In one formulation, for instance, a quadratic function is given as (Cudeck & du Toit, 2002):

$$f(t_i,\beta) = \beta_1 - (\beta_1 - \beta_0)\left(\frac{t_i}{\beta_2} - 1\right)^2$$

where the coefficient β_0 is the expected value of the response when $t_i = 0$. The coefficient β_1 represents the maximum (or minimum) value of the response y expected under the growth function, and β_2 is the value of t_i when the response is at its maximum (or minimum). Although the coefficients β_0 and β_1 enter the function in a linear manner, the coefficient β_2 does not. Under a partially nonlinear mixed-effects model in which β_2 is fixed across individuals but β_0 and β_1 are random, for example, this version of a quadratic function may be applied using an estimation procedure developed for strictly linear models (see Blozis, 2007a). Assuming that the maximum (or minimum) of the response occurs at different times for different individuals, a random effect for β_2 may be necessary, however, in which case estimation must proceed using special procedures for estimation of fully nonlinear mixed-effects models (Davidian & Giltinan, 1995).

Developmental Applications

Nonlinear growth models are naturally applicable to many developmental processes, such as those studied over long periods of time in which changes in behaviors, sometimes complex, are expected to occur. Nonlinear development in children is especially common given that childhood is a phase of development often characterized by relatively dramatic periods of change. Several examples from studies of early development, such as studies of speech and vocabulary development, often describe development as following a nonlinear form of change in which the rate of change in the measured response is not constant but, rather, tends to change at different rates as children mature. In a study of reading skills in native English speakers and English-language learners, Lesaux, Rupp, and Siegel (2007) demonstrated that the development of reading skills from kindergarten through the fourth grade also follows a nonlinear course. Indeed, there are many instances in which a nonlinear growth model has been successfully applied to the study of development. Huttenlocher, Haight, Bryk, Seltzer, and Lyons (1991), for instance, apply a mixed-effects model to the study of early vocabulary development that showed a nonlinear form of change. Blozis et al. (2007) apply a negatively accelerated exponential function using a structured latent curve model to study the development of reading ability in a sample of children. Adolescence, also a period often marked by complex forms of change (e.g., Somerville, Jones, & Casey, 2010), is another area of study that may also benefit from the application of nonlinear growth models.

Studies of human development across the lifespan may be marked by nonlinear forms of change. Studies of relatively short-term duration may also be characterized by nonlinear change. A study carried out by Burke, Shrout, and Bolger (2007), for instance, shows that a nonlinear mixed-effects model may be used to better understand individual differences in individuals' responses to the loss of a spouse. In a different example, Gerstorf and colleagues (2008) demonstrate nonlinear patterns of change in older adults when studying life satisfaction and its decline in older adults.

Illustration

Data are presented from the National Longitudinal Survey of Youth (NLSY) of Labor Market Experience in Youth supported by the U.S. Department of Labor. The sample of 405 children considered here were the children of female respondents of the original sample described in Curran (1997). The data studied are scores measured by the Reading Recognition subtest from the Peabody Individual Achievement Test (PIAT), an instrument designed to assess word recognition and pronunciation ability. Children were selected for study in this subsample if they were between 6 and 8 years old at the first assessment. Scores were obtained every other year over a 6-year period for a total of up to four assessments. Reading scores are a sum of items correctly answered, with a possible range of 0–84. Total test scores were divided by 10 prior to analysis. Approximately 16% of children were missing reading scores on one occasion, 23% on two occasions, and 4% on three occasions. Patterns of missing data are given in Table 26.1. Across the sample, there are eight patterns of missing data. Three patterns (2, 4, and 8) may be representative of participant dropout.

Changes in test scores were studied by considering scores as a function of the child's age. Child's age was available at the first assessment. Subsequent ages were calculated as the expected ages at the following measurement waves. That is, ages at the second, third, and fourth waves were computed as the age at the first assessment plus increments of 2, 4, or 6 years, respectively. To obtain an intercept of the model that was interpretable for the observed age range, child's age was centered to 10 years, which is the approximate age of children at the midpoint of the study. To denote the linear transformation of age, centered values of age are denoted henceforth by *age**. Data for a subset of 10 children with complete data are presented in Figure 26.1, in which observed reading scores are plotted according to age. As can be seen in the plot, reading scores tend to increase as children grow older, with the rate of change possibly slowing as the children grow older. Individual differences are notable in reading performance at 10 years, performance levels in the final assessment period, as well as in the rate of change.

A variety of growth models may be considered that differ in terms of the function used to describe growth in reading performance (see Blozis, 2007a; Blozis et al., 2007). Common choices are linear growth and quadratic growth models. If reading performance is expected to increase at a relatively fast rate when children are young and then slow as children grow older, then reading performance may be expected to follow an exponential function. Thus a likely candidate for a response function is a negatively accelerated exponential function.

Here a mixed-effects model was applied to the data using different response functions to characterize development of reading scores. In each model, the coefficients of the growth function were assumed to be random across individuals. The first model assumed no change in performance scores but allowed for individual differences in performance levels

TABLE 26.1. Patterns of Observed and Missing Data

Pattern	Read1	Read2	Read3	Read3	Frequency	Percentage
1	1	1	1	1	233	57.50
2	1	1	1	0	31	7.65
3	1	1	0	1	28	6.91
4	1	1	0	0	83	20.49
5	1	0	1	1	6	1.48
6	1	0	1	0	5	1.23
7	1	0	0	1	3	0.74
8	1	0	0	0	16	3.95

Note. Read1, Read2, Read3, and Read4 are measures of *Reading* at the four measurement occasions.

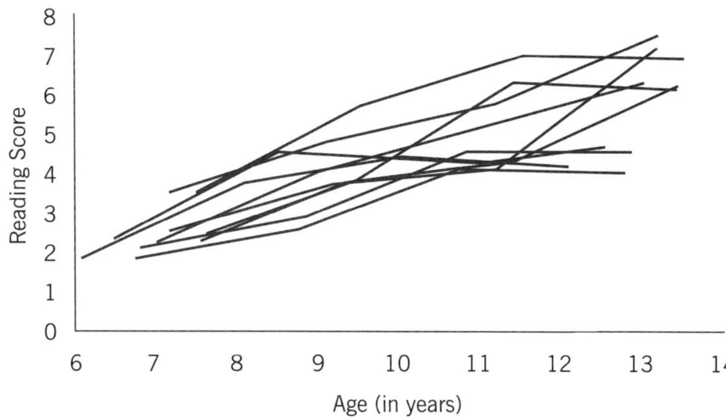

FIGURE 26.1. Subset of reading scores for 10 children with complete data measured at four time points.

by including a random intercept. Subsequent growth models allowed for different forms of change, specifically linear growth, quadratic growth, and exponential growth. Also, under each model, the time-specific errors were assumed to be independent between occasions and to have constant variance across time.

After selecting the relatively best fitting growth model, the variances of the random coefficients were first evaluated to assess whether all random coefficients were necessary to characterize individual differences in the reading trajectories. The assumption of constant error variance was then assessed by fitting an additional model that allowed the error variances to vary by occasion. Finally, given that children varied in age at each measurement occasion, it is possible that a child's mean age could influence reading performance. Thus, child's mean age was calculated across the four time points (even for those children with some missing reading data) and included in the model at the second level as a predictor of the model's intercept. The models fitted to the data are described next.

Model 1 assumed no growth in reading performance:

$$\text{No Growth: } Reading_{ij} = \beta_{0i} + \varepsilon_{ij}$$

where $Reading_{ij}$ is a child's score at age j. The coefficient β_{0i} is the child's expected score across the study period, and ε_{ij} is the error of the growth model for the child at age j. The parameters of the model are β_0, the common intercept; ϕ_0, the variance of the random intercept; and σ^2_ε, the variance of the time-specific errors. Model 1 served as a reference model to others that assumed some form of growth.

Models 2 and 3 assumed that growth in reading performance followed a linear and quadratic function, respectively:

$$\text{Linear Growth: } Reading_{ij} = \beta_{0i} + \beta_{1i}(age^*_{ij}) + \varepsilon_{ij}$$
$$\text{Quadratic Growth: } Reading_{ij} = \beta_{0i} + \beta_{1i}(age^{*2}_{ij}) + \beta_{2i}age^*_{ij}) + \varepsilon_{ij}$$

where in the linear growth model, β_{0i} is the expected performance score for child i at age 10 years and β_{1i} is the expected change in the reading rating for that child across the study period. In the quadratic growth model, β_{0i} is the expected performance level for the child at age 10, β_{1i} is the expected instantaneous rate of change in performance when the child is 10 years old, and β_{2i} is the child's expected rate of acceleration across the study period. The parameters of the linear and quadratic growth models are the fixed growth coefficients (β_0 and β_1 for the linear growth model; β_0, β_1, and β_2 for the quadratic growth model), the unique elements of the covariance matrix of the random effects (Φ), and the unique variance of the time-specific errors. Under the linear growth model, the covariance matrix of the random effects is

$$\Phi = \begin{pmatrix} \phi_0 & \\ \phi_{10} & \phi_1 \end{pmatrix}$$

where ϕ_0 and ϕ_1 are the variances of the random intercept and linear slope, respectively, and ϕ_{10} is their covariance. Under the quadratic growth model, the covariance matrix of the random effects is

$$\Phi = \begin{pmatrix} \phi_0 & & \\ \phi_{10} & \phi_1 & \\ \phi_{20} & \phi_{21} & \phi_2 \end{pmatrix}$$

where ϕ_0, ϕ_1, and ϕ_2 are the variances of the random intercept, instantaneous change rate, and rate of acceleration, respectively, and ϕ_{10}, ϕ_{20}, and ϕ_{21} are the covariances between the random effects.

Model 4 assumed exponential growth in reading performance, with the particular function chosen to have an intercept and asymptote that could differ from zero. Using the formulation of an exponential function given in Meredith and Tisak (1990), a function was fitted that included three parameters:

$$\text{Exponential Growth:} \quad Reading_{ij} = \beta_{1i} - (\beta_{1i} - \beta_{0i})\exp\{-\beta_{2i}(age^*_{ij} + \varepsilon_{ij})\} \quad \textbf{(26.2)}$$

where, for child i, β_{0i} and β_{1i} are the expected performance level at age 10 and asymptotic performance levels, respectively, and β_{2i} is the rate of change. The parameters of the exponential growth model are the fixed growth coefficients (β_0, β_1, and β_2), the unique elements of the covariance matrix of the random effects (Φ), and the variance of the time-specific errors. The covariance matrix of the random effects is

$$\Phi = \begin{pmatrix} \phi_0 & & \\ \phi_{10} & \phi_1 & \\ \phi_{20} & \phi_{21} & \phi_2 \end{pmatrix}$$

where ϕ_0, ϕ_1, and ϕ_2 are the variances of the random intercept, asymptote, and nonlinear change rate, respectively, and ϕ_{10}, ϕ_{20}, and ϕ_{21} are the covariances between the random effects.

An alternative but equivalent formulation of the exponential growth model is one based on a structured latent curve model (Browne & du Toit, 1991), and this was the formulation considered in the current analysis. An advantage of formulating a nonlinear growth model as a structured latent curve model, when it is possible, is that the burden of estimation may be reduced (see Blozis, 2007a). If a nonlinear growth function can be expressed by a first-order Taylor polynomial, as in Browne and du Toit (1991), then there is no longer an issue of a random effect appearing in the model in a nonlinear manner.

Under a structured latent curve model and assuming the exponential growth function in (2), the common reading performance score evaluated at age_j^* was assumed to be

$$\mu_t = f(\beta, age_t) = \beta_1 - (\beta_1 - \beta_0)\exp\{-\beta_2 age_j^*\} \quad \textbf{(26.3)}$$

where μ_t is the common response at age_j^*. The coefficients of the growth function, β_0, β_1, and β_2, have the same interpretation as those coefficients provided in equation 26.2. At the child level, the response is assumed to be a linear combination of a set of basis functions weighted by a set of coefficients that are unique to the child. Each basis function is defined by the first-order partial derivative of the common function in equation 26.3 taken with respect to each of the coefficients of the function, namely β_0, β_1, and β_2 (cf. Browne & du Toit, 1991):

$$\frac{\partial f(\beta, age_j^*)}{\partial \beta_0} = f_0' = \exp\{-\beta_2 age_j^*\} \quad \textbf{(26.4a)}$$

$$\frac{\partial f(\beta, age_j^*)}{\partial \beta_1} = f_1' = 1 - \exp\{-\beta_2 age_j^*\} \quad \textbf{(26.4b)}$$

$$\frac{\partial f(\beta, age_j^*)}{\partial \beta_2} = f_2' = (\beta_1 - \beta_0)(age_j^*)\exp\{-\beta_2 age_j^*\} \quad \textbf{(26.4c)}$$

where $\beta = (\beta_0, \beta_1, \beta_2)'$. Let Λ_i be a matrix with columns defined by the basis functions in equations 26.4a, 26.4b, and 26.4c:

$$\Lambda_i = [\ \mathrm{f}'_{0i} \quad \mathrm{f}'_{1i} \quad \mathrm{f}'_{2i}\ ]$$

where each basis function is now evaluated according to specific values of the child's age at each measurement occasion, as denoted by the subscript i for each basis function (e.g., f_{0i}). A child's set of reading scores across the study period, denoted by $\mathbf{Reading}_i$, for $\mathbf{Reading}_i = (Reading_{i1}, \ldots, Reading_{in_i})'$, is then defined as a first-order Taylor polynomial

$$\mathbf{Reading}_i = \Lambda_i\alpha + b_{0i}^*\mathrm{f}'_{0i} + b_{1i}^*\mathrm{f}'_{1i} + b_{2i}^*\mathrm{f}'_{2i} + \varepsilon_i$$

where the expected values of the child-specific weights, b_{0i}^*, b_{1i}^*,and b_{2i}^*,are equal to zero. Under a first-order Taylor polynomial, a child's set of reading scores is assumed to be the sum of the set of basis functions in Λ_i weighted by the set of fixed coefficients in α and the individual basis functions, f_{0i}, f_{1i} and f_{2i}, each weighted by their respective random effect that is specific to the child, namely b_{0i}^*, b_{1i}^*, and b_{2i}^*, respectively. Now, letting $\mathrm{b}_i = (b_{0i}^*, b_{1i}^*,\text{and } b_{2i}^*)'$ and $\beta_i = \alpha + \mathrm{b}_i$ the data model may be simplified in its expression as

$$\mathbf{Reading}_i = \Lambda_i\beta_i + \varepsilon_i \quad \textbf{(26.5)}$$

where $\alpha = (\beta_0, \beta_1, 0)'$ is obtained by solving the set of linear equations: $f(\beta, \mathbf{age}_i^*) = \Lambda_i\alpha$, where $f(\beta, \mathbf{age}_i^*)$ is the common response function evaluated according to different values of a child's age (see Browne, 1993), with $\mathbf{age}_i^* = (age_{i1}, \ldots, age_{ini})$.

Estimation of the mixed-effects models of no growth, linear growth, and quadratic growth, as well as the structured latent curve model based on an exponential function, was performed using Mx (Neale et al., 2003) with ML. Mx provides ML estimates with likelihood-based confidence intervals (CI) (Neale & Miller, 1997). Here, 95% CI for parameters are reported. Comparisons of model fit were based on likelihood ratio tests and values of the Akaike information criterion (AIC). Assuming that a chi-square statistic for a likelihood ratio test is distributed as chi-square with degrees of freedom equal to the difference in the number of parameters that define the two models to be compared, statistically nonsignificant values indicate that the least complex model is preferred. Smaller values of the AIC among competing models are preferred.

Under a mixed-effects model and a structured latent curve model, ML estimates are considered valid when missing data are missing at random (MAR). Missing data are MAR when the missingness (i.e., whether or not data are missing) is independent of the missing data, although the missingness may depend on the observed data (Little & Rubin, 2002). Here, the assumption that the missing data are MAR implies that whether or not a child is missing data is not related to the child's missing reading data after accounting for any dependence of the missingness on the observed data.

Results

Measures of overall model fit, given by deviance values (–2 log likelihood function values) and AIC values (AIC = –2 log likelihood –2p, where p is the number of model parameters), are provided in Table 26.2. As indicated by the results of the likelihood ratio tests provided and AIC values, the structured latent curve model based on an exponential function (Model 4) provided the best overall fit among the growth models considered. That is, although the

TABLE 26.2. Model Fit Comparisons across Different Growth Models for Reading Scores

Growth function	–2log$L$	p	AIC	Model comparison	$\chi^2(df)$	p-value
1. No change	5051.8	3	5057. 8			
2. Linear growth	3226.8	6	3238.8	1 v 2	1825.0(3)	< .001
3. Quadratic growth	2963.8	10	2983.8	2 v 3	263.0(4)	< .001
4. Exponential growth	2941.5	10	2961.5	1 v 4	2110.3(7)	< .001
4a. Exponential with nonconstant error variance	2939.8	13	2965.8	4 v 4*b*	1.7(3)	0.19
4b. Exponential with age_i	2940.9	11	2962.9	4 v 4*a*	0.6(1)	0.44

Note. N = 405. All models include random growth coefficients. –2log$L$ is –2 times the log of the likelihood function value; p is the number of parameters that define a model; AIC is the Akaike information criterion, calculated as –2log$L$ + 2p; $\chi^2(df)$ is the chi-square statistic and corresponding degrees of freedom for a likelihood ratio test between nested models; $age_{.i}$ moderates the intercept of the model.

linear and quadratic growth functions provided a better fit relative to the no-growth model, the exponential growth model was best overall in terms of the likelihood ratio tests performed and having the lowest AIC value. Maximum likelihood estimates of Model 4 are provided in Table 26.3. For the exponential growth model, the estimated 95% CI for the variances of the random coefficients (not reported) did not include zero as interior points, indicating that there was variation between children in the coefficients of the exponential function. Thus the three random effects were retained in the model.

Next, the assumption that the occasion-specific error variance was constant across the study period was evaluated by fitting an additional model (Model 4a) that allowed the error variance to vary by measurement occasion. A deviance test comparing Models 4 and 4a was not statistically significant at the .05 level ($\chi^2 = 1.7$ (3 *df*), $p = 0.19$)′. Thus the assumption of constant error variance may be reasonable. Next, the mean age of each child across the four planned measurement occasions was computed and entered into the model as a predictor of the child's random intercept. Given that children varied in age at each measurement occasion, it is possible that a child's mean age could also influence reading performance. Thus mean age was calculated across the four time points and specified as a predictor of the random intercept in Model 4b:

$$\beta_{0i} = \gamma_{00} + \gamma_{01}\text{age}^*_{i.} + r_{0i}$$

where $\text{age}_{i.}$ is the mean age of child i across the four planned measurement occasions. The coefficient γ_{00} is the expected reading score for a child when children were at the mean ages across the study period, γ_{01} is the effect of mean age on the intercept, and r_{0i} is the error of the regression. The estimated 95% confidence interval for the effect of $\text{age}_{i.}$ on the random intercept (not reported) suggested that mean age was not an important moderator of the model's intercept. Model 4 was retained as the final model.

TABLE 26.3. Maximum Likelihood Estimates of an Exponential Growth Model for Reading Scores

	Mean structure	
Parameter	MLE	95% CI
θ_0, intercept	4.66	(4.55, 4.77)
θ_1, asymptote	7.34	(6.95, 7.81)
θ_2, change rate	0.188	(0.163, 0.213)
Covariance structure		

$$\text{Level 2: } \hat{\Phi} \begin{bmatrix} 1.08 & 0.27 & -0.64 \\ 0.50 & 3.2 & 0.57 \\ -0.070 & 0.11 & 0.01 \end{bmatrix} \quad \text{Level 1: } \hat{\sigma}^2 = 0.235$$

Note. $N = 405$. Child's age is centered at 10 years. MLE is the maximum likelihood estimate. 95% CI is a likelihood-based 95% confidence interval for the parameter. For the estimated covariance matrix at the second level, $\hat{\Phi}$, the diagonal elements are estimated variances of the random effects, lower diagonal elements are the covariances between the random effects, and upper diagonal elements are the corresponding correlation coefficients.

ML estimates of a mixed-effects model and a structured latent curve model are considered valid when missing data are MAR. When missing data are not missing at random (NMAR), methods that address the missing data process are necessary. The more commonly applied NMAR methods for linear mixed-effects models are detailed in Molenberghs and Kenward (2007). These include selection models, pattern-mixture models, and shared parameter models. Xu and Blozis (2011) describe fitting selection models and pattern-mixture random-effects models for a partially nonlinear mixed-effects model and a structured latent curve model. A pattern-mixture random-effects model, for instance, may be applied to study how patterns of missing data moderate the trajectories of a longitudinal response (Demirtas & Schafer, 2003; Hedeker & Gibbons, 1997).

For the reading data, three patterns of monotonic missing data may suggest participant dropout (see Table 26.1, patterns 2, 4, and 8), with the remaining patterns representing different patterns of missing data. To study the effect of dropout on the reading trajectories, an indicator variable denoting dropout was created ($D = 1$ if the child was dropped from the study between the second and final assessment; $D = 0$ otherwise). Of the 405 children, 130 were classified into a group of study dropouts. The indicator of dropout was incorporated into the structured latent curve model for reading scores by allowing the variable to moderate the intercept of the growth function. The expression for this effect may be represented as

$$\beta_{0i} = \gamma_{00} + \gamma_{01} D_i + r_{0i}$$

A 95% CI for the effect of dropout on the intercept included zero as an interior point, however, suggesting no meaningful difference in performance levels at age 10 between those who remained in the study and those who dropped out. Other patterns of missing data could be considered, as well as the other coefficients of the growth model.

In summary, a nonlinear function was preferred to the models that were based on models that were linear in their parameters, including the model that assumed growth in reading scores followed a quadratic function. Relative to the fit provided by these different models, a structured latent curve model that assumed exponential growth provided the best relative fit to the reading scores. Specifically, scores tended to follow an increasing exponential function, with response levels tending toward an upper asymptote in the latter period of development. Individuals varied in their responses, as evidenced by the need for the random coefficients. Moderators of the growth coefficients, namely the mean age of children and indicator of dropout, were not important in describing the individual growth trajectories.

Future Directions

Longitudinal studies of human development are increasingly relying on growth models to improve understanding of behavioral development. Growth models provide a flexible analytical framework for describing behavioral development. Mixed-effects models in particular allow for the study of how individual or contextual variables may moderate development at the individual level. Individual variables are characteristics of the person, such as gender or education level. Contextual variables are characteristics of the context in which the individuals are measured, such as family or home environment. Growth models based on linear and quadratic functions are among the most commonly applied models in developmental research. Development of some behavioral measures may not, however, follow either one of these forms. Nonlinear growth models offer a more extensive framework for the study of longitudinal development data by increasing the pool of growth functions that may be considered.

Behavioral responses that are studied over time and that are expected to change at a nonconstant rate across a study period may be best represented by a nonlinear growth function. Exponential functions are applicable in many situations in which a response is expected, for example, to slow in its rate of change with time as it tends toward an asymptote. Reading performance is one example in which a measured behavior is expected to increase at a relatively rapid rate when children are young. As children develop and their skills improve, reading performance tends to slow in its rate of change and tend toward a stable level (also see Blozis et al., 2007). Among a set of competing growth models that allowed for individual differences in the coefficients that described change in reading performance, including models based on a linear mixed-effects modeling framework, a negatively accelerated exponential function provided a relatively good fit to the data.

Applications of polynomial functions to describe development in behavioral courses are commonplace. In cases in which a behavioral response is measured over relatively short periods of time, a linear growth function may very well capture change in a response. Conversely, behaviors studied over relatively longer periods of time may be more apt to change at a nonconstant rate, and the need for nonlinear models becomes increasingly important in characterizing longitudinal data. Models that allow for nonlinear change, such as those based on nonlinear functions or those that link together two or more functions in a multiphase model, may serve to better represent developmental data, both in terms of providing a better fit to the data and of improving interpretation of growth coefficients.

Similar to growth models that are linear in their parameters, growth models based on nonlinear functions are most commonly applied to a single measured response. When multiple indicators of a variable are obtained, it may be possible to study change in a response by way of a second-order latent curve model (that is, a curve-of-factors model; McArdle, 1988; Meredith & Tisak, 1990). Under a second-order latent curve model, a latent variable is assumed to be measured by a set of indicator variables measured at the same points in time. Assuming that the measurement structure is invariant across time, change in the latent response may be studied by applying a growth function to the factors (e.g., Hong & Ho, 2005). Second-order latent curve models may also be specified to handle nonlinear growth functions, such as in a partially nonlinear mixed-effects model and structured latent curve model (Blozis, 2006) and a fully nonlinear mixed-effects model (Harring, 2009).

References

Bates, D. M., & Watts, D. G. (2007). *Nonlinear regression analysis and its applications*. Hoboken, NJ: Wiley.

Blozis, S. A. (2004). Structured latent curve models for the study of change in multivariate repeated measures. *Psychological Methods, 9*, 334–353.

Blozis, S. A. (2006). A second-order structured latent curve model for longitudinal data. In K. van Montfort, H. Oud, & A. Satorra (Eds.), *Longitudinal models in the behavioral and related sciences* (pp. 189–214). Mahwah, NJ: Erlbaum.

Blozis, S. A. (2007a). A Newton procedure for a conditionally linear mixed-effects model. *Behavior Research Methods, 39*, 695–708.

Blozis, S. A. (2007b). On fitting nonlinear latent curve models to multiple variables measured longitudinally. *Structural Equation Modeling, 14,* 179–201.

Blozis, S. A., Conger, K. J., & Harring, J. R. (2007). Nonlinear latent curve models for longitudinal data. *International Journal of Behavioral Development, 31,* 340–346.

Blozis, S. A., & Cudeck, R. (1999). Conditionally linear mixed-effects models with latent variable covariates. *Journal of Educational and Behavioral Statistics, 24,* 245–270.

Blozis, S. A., Harring, J. R., & Mels, G. (2008). Using LISREL to fit nonlinear latent curve models. *Structural Equation Modeling, 15,* 346–369.

Browne, M. W. (1993). Structured latent curve models. In C. M. Cuadras & C. R. Rao (Eds.), *Multivariate analysis: Future directions 2* (pp. 171–197). Amsterdam: Elsevier.

Browne, M. W., & du Toit, S. H. C. (1991). Models for learning data. In L. M. Collins & J. L. Horn (Eds.), *Best methods for the analysis of change* (pp. 47–68). Washington, DC: American Psychological Association.

Burke, C. T., Shrout, P. E., & Bolger, N. (2007). Individual differences in adjustment to spousal loss: A nonlinear mixed model analysis. *International Journal of Behavior Development, 31,* 405–415.

Card, N. A., & Little, T. D. (2007). Longitudinal modeling of developmental processes. *International Journal of Behavioral Development, 31,* 297–302.

Carlson, S. R., & Iacono, W. G. (2008). Deviant P300 amplitude development in males is associated with paternal externalizing psychopathology. *Journal of Abnormal Psychology, 117,* 910–923.

Choi, J., Harring, J. R., & Hancock, G. R. (2009). Latent growth modeling for logistic response functions. *Multivariate Behavioral Research, 44,* 620–645.

Cillessen, A. H. N., & Borch, C. (2006). Developmental trajectories of adolescent popularity: A growth curve modeling analysis. *Journal of Adolescence, 29,* 935–959.

Cudeck, R., & du Toit, S. H. C. (2002). A version of quadratic regression with interpretable parameters. *Multivariate Behavioral Research, 37,* 501–519.

Cudeck, R. A., & Klebe, K. J. (2002). Multiphase mixed-effects models for repeated-measures data. *Psychological Methods, 7,* 41–63.

Curran, P. J. (1997, April). *Comparing three modern approaches to longitudinal data analysis: An examination of a single developmental sample.* Symposium presented at the biennial meeting of the Society for Research in Child Development, Washington, DC.

Davidian, W., & Giltinan, D. M. (1995). *Nonlinear models for repeated measurement data.* London: Chapman & Hall.

Demirtas, H., & Schafer, J. L. (2003). On the performance of random-coefficient pattern-mixture models for non-ignorable dropout. *Statistics in Medicine, 22,* 2553–2575.

du Toit, S. H. C., & Cudeck, R. (2009). Estimation of the nonlinear random coefficient model when some random effects are separable. *Psychometrika, 74,* 65–82.

Fitzmaurice, G. M., Laird, N. M., & Ware, J. H. (2004). *Applied longitudinal analysis.* New York: Wiley.

Gerstorf, D., Ram, N., Estabrook, R., Schupp, J., Wagner, G., & Lindenberger, U. (2008). Life satisfaction shows terminal decline in old age: Longitudinal evidence from the German Socio-Economic Panel Study (SOEP). *Developmental Psychology, 44,* 1148–1159.

Graham, J. W., Taylor, B. J., Olchowski, A. E., & Cumsille, P. E. (2006). Planned missing data designs in psychological research. *Psychological Methods, 11,* 323–343.

Harring, J. R. (2009). A nonlinear mixed effects model for latent variables. *Journal of Educational and Behavioral Statistics, 34,* 293–318.

Harring, J. R., Cudeck, R., & du Toit, S. H. C. (2006). Fitting partially nonlinear random coefficient models as SEMs. *Multivariate Behavioral Research, 41,* 579–596.

Hedeker, D., & Gibbons, R. D. (1997). Application of random-effects pattern-mixture models for missing data in longitudinal studies. *Psychological Methods, 1,* 64–78.

Holmefur, M., Krumlinde-Sundholm, L., Bergström, J., & Eliasson, A.-C. (2010). Longitudinal development of hand function in children with unilateral cerebral palsy. *Developmental Medicine and Child Neurology, 52*, 352–357.

Hong, S., & Ho, H.-Z. (2005). Direct and indirect longitudinal effects of parental involvement on student achievement: Second-order latent growth modeling across ethnic groups. *Journal of Educational Psychology, 97*, 32–42.

Huttenlocher, J., Haight, W., Bryk, A., Seltzer, M., & Lyons, T. (1991). Early vocabulary growth: Relation to language input and gender. *Developmental Psychology, 27*, 236–248.

Jennrich, R. I., & Schluchter, M. D. (1986). Unbalanced repeated measures models with structured covariance matrices. *Biometrics, 42*, 805–820.

Laird, N. M., & Ware, J. H. (1982). Random-effects models for longitudinal data. *Biometrics, 38*, 963–974.

Lesaux, N. K., Rupp, A. A., & Siegel, L. S. (2007). Growth in reading skills of children from diverse linguistic backgrounds: Findings from a 5-year longitudinal study. *Journal of Educational Psychology, 99*, 821–834.

Little, R. J. A., & Rubin, D. B. (2002). *Statistical analysis with missing data* (2nd ed.). New York: Wiley.

Marsh, H. W. (2007). Do university teachers become more effective with experience?: A multilevel growth model of students' evaluations of teaching over 13 years. *Journal of Educational Psychology, 99*, 775–790.

McArdle, J. J. (1988). Dynamic but structural equation modeling of repeated measures data. In R. B. Cattell & J. Nesselroade (Eds.), *Handbook of multivariate experimental psychology* (2nd ed., pp. 561–614). New York: Plenum Press.

McArdle, J. J. (2004). Latent growth curve analysis using structural equation modeling techniques. In D. Teti (Ed.), *Handbook of research methods in developmental science* (pp. 340–365). New York: Blackwell.

McArdle, J. J., & Wang, L. (2008). Modeling age-based turning points in longitudinal life-span growth curves of cognition. In P. Cohen (Ed.), *Applied data analytic techniques for turning points research* (pp. 105–127). New York: Routledge/Taylor & Francis Group.

Meredith, W., & Tisak, J. (1990). Latent curve analysis. *Psychometrika, 55*, 107–122.

Molenberghs, G., & Kenward, M. G. (2007). *Missing data in clinical studies*. West Sussex, UK: Wiley.

Neale, M. C., Boker, S. M., Xie, G., & Maes, H. H. (2003). *Mx: Statistical modeling* (6th ed.). (Available from Virginia Commonwealth University, Department of Psychiatry, Box 900126, Richmond, VA 23298)

Neale, M. C., & McArdle, J. J. (2000). Structured latent growth curves for twin data. *Twin Research, 3*, 165–177.

Neale, M. C., & Miller, M. B. (1997). The use of likelihood-based confidence intervals in genetic models. *Behavior Genetics, 27*, 113–120.

Rast, P., & Zimprich, D. (2009). Individual differences and reliability of paired associates learning in younger and older adults. *Psychology and Aging, 24*, 1001–1006.

Singer, J. D., & Willett, J. B. (2003). *Applied longitudinal data analysis: Modeling change and event occurrence*. New York: Oxford University Press.

Solomon, D. H., & Theiss, J. A. (2008). A longitudinal test of the relational turbulence model of romantic relationship development. *Personal Relationships, 15*, 339–357.

Somerville, L. H., Jones, R. M., & Casey, B. J. (2010). A time of change: Behavioral and neural correlates of adolescent sensitivity to appetitive and aversive environmental cues. *Brain and Cognition, 72*, 124–133.

Xu, S., & Blozis, S. A. (2011). Sensitivity analysis of a mixed model for incomplete lonitudinal data. *Journal of Educational and Behavioral Statistics, 36*, 237–256.

CHAPTER 27

Group-Based Trajectory Modeling in Developmental Science

DANIEL S. NAGIN
CANDICE L. ODGERS

Central Issues

Over the past decade there has been an outpouring of studies of developmental trajectories in psychology, medicine, and criminology that apply a method alternatively called group-based trajectory modeling (GBTM) by Nagin (2005, 1999) or growth mixture modeling (GMM) by Muthén (2001). These models are appealing, as they can be applied to chart the development of a wide range of phenomena and provide an empirical means of identifying clusters of individuals following different developmental trajectories. Conceptually, GBTM and GMM have much in common. Although important differences exist between the two classes of models—which will be discussed—for ease of communication we refer to both as *group-based trajectory models* or *group-based models*.

Group-based models have been applied to map heterogeneity in the development of outcomes as varied as physical aggression (Nagin & Tremblay, 1999), cortisol levels (Van Ryzin, Chatham, Kryzer, Kertes, & Gunnar, 2009), Internet usage (Christ, Krishnan, Nagin, & Günther, 2002), obesity (Mustillo et al., 2003), anxiety (Côté et al., 2004), and crime trends at the level of block face (Weisburd, Bushway, Lum, & Yang, 2004). More recently, group-based models have been extended to capture differential treatment responses to clinical and randomized trials and have been leveraged to facilitate causal inference in epidemiological studies in which randomization to treatment conditions is not possible (for a review, see Nagin & Odgers, 2010). Arguably, the most compelling applications of group-based models occur when there are clear expectations regarding the number, size, and shape of groups believed to exist within the population (Bauer, 2007). For example, close to 20 years ago

Moffitt (1993) proposed a developmental taxonomy that outlined expectations regarding the origins, developmental course, and outcomes of two distinct pathways believed to underlie the population distribution of antisocial behavior. To test such taxonomical theories, researchers traditionally applied assignment rules based on theoretically derived criteria. Assignment rules are useful but have limitations and pitfalls. One pitfall is that the existence of distinct trajectories must be assumed beforehand. Second, an assignment rule–based approach provides no basis for calibrating the precision of individual classifications to the groups that compose the taxonomy. For a fuller discussion of these issues see Chapter 1 of Nagin (2005). Research in both criminology and psychology has recently moved away from a classification-based approach and instead is applying group-based models to test Moffitt's predictions (for reviews, see Odgers, Moffitt, et al., 2008; Piquero, 2005).

The introduction of group-based models into developmental research has provided new opportunities for discovery, but their rapid evolution also means that the underlying assumptions and extensions of these models may still be unfamiliar to those working in this area. The purpose of this chapter is to provide a nontechnical overview of the conceptual principles and statistical assumptions underlying group-based modeling alongside illustrations from developmental research. Future directions in group-based methodology are also discussed, along with some preliminary reporting guidelines.

Conceptual Principles and Statistical Assumptions

This section provides a brief overview of three forms of trajectory modeling—growth curve modeling, GMM, and GBTM. Citations to far more complete technical descriptions are provided. Hierarchical modeling (Bryk & Raudenbush, 1987; Goldstein, 1995) and latent curve analysis (McArdle & Epstein, 1987; Meredith & Tisak, 1990; Muthén, 1989; Willett & Sayer, 1994) are two important alternative approaches to group-based trajectory modeling. For our purpose we refer to them as growth curve modeling (GCM). GCM, GMM, and GBTM share a common analytical objective—measuring and explaining differences across population members in their developmental trajectories. What distinguishes GCM, GMM, and GBTM is their approach to modeling individual-level heterogeneity, as each approach makes different technical assumptions about the distribution of trajectories in the population.

GCMs capture interindividual differences in change over time and aggregate repeated measures into relatively few parameters, such as estimates of the average rate of growth across time (Bollen & Curran, 2006). In doing so, GCMs capture mean trends in development (nomothetic aspects of change), as well as individual departures from the average trend (idiographic aspects of change) (Preacher, Wichman, Briggs, & MacCallum, 2008). Although the assumptions underlying hierarchical modeling and latent growth curve analysis differ in important respects, they also have important commonalities (MacCallum, Kim, Malarkey, & Kiecolt-Glaser, 1997; Raudenbush, 2001; Willett & Sayer, 1994). For the purposes of this review one commonality is crucial: Both model the population distribution of individual trajectories based on a *continuous* distribution function and assume that the random effects are continuously distributed throughout the population, usually according to a multivariate normal distribution. More practically speaking, both types of models assume that individuals are drawn from the same population and that development can be captured using one set of parameters. However, if one trajectory shape does not "fit all," then the group-based trajectory models to be described will likely provide a better fit to the research question (for a more complete description of GCM see Grimm & Ram, Chapter 24, this volume; Hox & Boom, Chapter 25, this volume).

Growth Mixture Modeling

GMM is an innovation of Muthén and Shedden (1999) that elaborates on GCM based on a class of statistical models called finite mixture models (McLachlan & Peel, 2004; Titterington, Smith, & Makov, 1985). Finite mixture models are used to analyze data believed to be composed of distinct subpopulations that are not identifiable based on measured characteristics. An example is a case in which the population is composed of two groups, one with versus one without an underlying vulnerability to a disease. If disease vulnerability can be measured, the groups could be analyzed separately. However, if the groups are not measurable, the data will be composed of a mixture of the two groups. In short, finite mixture models are designed to analyze data composed of a mixture of two or more groups whose outcomes are generated by distinct statistical processes. For the disease example, separate components of the mixture would model the outcome (e.g., symptoms over time) for the "genetically vulnerable" versus the "not genetically vulnerable" group. In general, finite mixture models may have more than two components, but the components cannot be infinite.

In the context of group-based modeling, such subpopulations may constitute groups with different unconditional (mean) trajectories that cannot be explained by the interindividual variability provided by the random effects. The innovation of Muthén and Shedden (1999) was to apply finite mixture modeling to GCM so that two or more GCMs are used to model population variability in developmental trajectories. The basic outputs of the model are two or more GCMs interpreted in the same way as a single-group GCM and estimates of the proportion of the population following each GCM. Muthén's writings on GMM imply that he considers each GCM as modeling a separate subpopulation following a different growth curve.

Group-Based Trajectory Modeling

Group-based trajectory modeling is also an application of finite mixture modeling, but the motivation for applying this method is fundamentally different from that for GMM. Finite mixture-based trajectory models assume that the population is composed of a mixture of distinct groups defined by their developmental trajectories. The assumption that the population is composed of distinct groups is likely too strong. Unlike biological or physical phenomena, in which populations may be composed of discrete groups such as different types of animal or plant species, population differences in developmental trajectories of behavior are unlikely to reflect such bright-line differences (although biology has a long tradition of debates concerning classification; see Appel, 1987).

Many taxonomic theories predict different trajectories of development across subpopulations (e.g., Belsky, Steinberg, & Draper, 1991; Kandel, 1975; Loeber, 1991; Moffitt, 1993; Patterson, Debaryshe, & Ramsey, 1989). However, the purpose of such taxonomies is generally to draw attention to differences in the causes and consequences of different developmental pathways rather than to suggest the existence of distinct groups. Group-based modeling can provide a methodological complement to theories that predict differing developmental etiologies and trajectories; that is, group-based models allow one to ask whether the trajectories and etiologies predicted by theory are actually present in the population.

Testing taxonomic theories requires making assumptions about the population distribution of developmental trajectories, which brings us to the fundamental distinction between GBTM and GMM. GMM assumes that the population distribution of trajectories is composed of two or more subpopulations, each following a conventional GCM. In contrast, GBTM takes no stand on the population distribution of trajectories and instead uses the trajectory groups as a statistical device for approximating the unknown distribution of trajectories across population members. In practice, developmental theory rarely provides explicit guidance on how unobserved individual differences in development are distributed in the population.

The application of finite mixture models employed in GBTM aligns with the seminal work of Heckman and Singer (1984), who built on the capability of finite mixture models to approximate the distribution of unobserved individual differences in duration models. The authors observed that social science theory rarely provided theoretical guidance on the population distribution of unobserved individual differences, yet statistical models of duration data were often sensitive to their assumed distributional form. Their proposed estimator finessed the problem of having to specify a distribution of unobserved individual differences by approximating the distribution with a finite mixture model.

Figure 27.1 depicts the use of a finite number of groups to approximate a continuous distribution. Panel A depicts the population distribution of some behavior z. In Panel B, this same distribution is replicated and overlaid with a histogram that approximates its shape. Panel B illustrates that any continuous distribution with finite endpoints can be approximated by a discrete distribution (i.e., a histogram) or alternatively by a finite number of "points of support" (i.e., the dark shaded "pillars"). A higher number of support points yields a discrete distribution that more closely approximates the true continuous distribution.

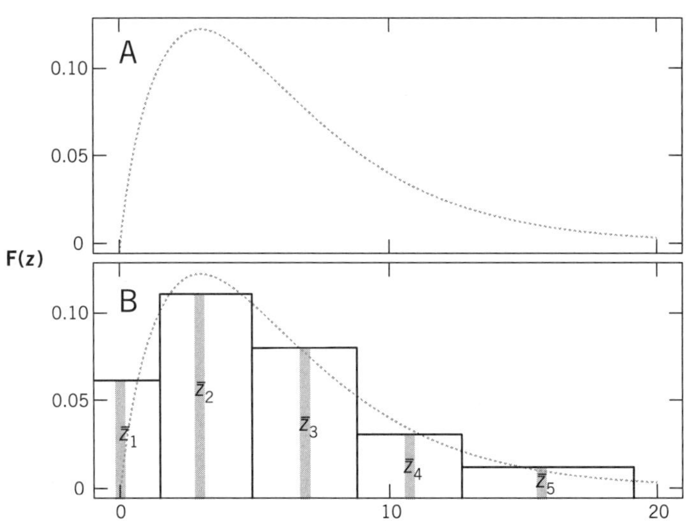

FIGURE 27.1. Using groups to approximate an unknown distribution.

Thus, in GBTM, trajectory groups should be thought of as a statistical device for approximating what is likely a continuous population distribution of trajectories of unknown shapes. The trajectory groups are a convenient statistical device for summarizing trajectories in distinct regions of the distribution. Like contour lines on a topographic map, the groups are not literal entities but, rather, approximations of distinctive regions of the surface. Also, just as a topographic map traces regularly or irregularly varying geographic surface, trajectory groups may suggest a population distribution of trajectories that varies regularly (e.g., all generally rising trajectories) or irregularly (e.g., some rising and others falling). Both are useful pieces of information regarding the contours of the distribution.

From a technical perspective, the difference between trajectory groups across methods is that GMM includes random effects in each group's trajectory model and GBTM does not. The addition of random effects into GMMs allows for within-group variability in individual-level trajectories and can lead to important differences in the way an analysis proceeds, including the use of fewer trajectory groups within the GMM framework. If the groups are thought of as subpopulations following different GCMs, the reduction in number of groups results in a more parsimonious model. By contrast, in GBTM, where groups are used as a device for approximation, increasing the within-group variability of individual-level trajectories is at odds with the objective of reducing within-group variability in development. Stated differently, in GBTM, a group is conceptually thought of as a collection of individuals who follow approximately the same developmental trajectory, the conceptual equivalent of a contour line on a topographic map. Trajectory groups can also be thought of as latent longitudinal strata in which population variability is captured by shape and level differences across groups (Haviland, Nagin, & Rosenbaum, 2007; Haviland, Rosenbaum, Nagin, & Tremblay, 2008).

How Many Groups?

One of the key challenges in group-based modeling is determining the number of groups or latent classes that best represents heterogeneity in developmental trajectories. This issue has been discussed extensively in prior work (McLachlan & Peel, 2004; Muthén, 2004; Nagin, 2005; Nylund, Asparouhov, & Muthén, 2007). Fit indices commonly used to guide model selection include the Bayesian information criteria (BIC; Raftery, 1995; Schwartz, 1978), the Akaike information criterion (AIC; Akaike, 1974), the Lo–Mendell–Rubin likelihood ratio test (Lo, Mendell, & Rubin, 2001), and entropy. However, model selection based on the mechanical and rigid application of a formal statistical criterion may lead to an inferior choice. The strengths and weaknesses of alternative model specifications depend on the substantive questions being asked and the data available. Although the application of formal statistical criteria to the model selection process serves to support and guide theory, there is no escaping the need for judgment; otherwise, insight and discovery will fall victim to the mechanical application of method. The objective of the model selection is typically not the maximization of some statistic of model fit. Rather, the objective is to summarize the distinctive features of the data in the most parsimonious—and useful—fashion.

An often neglected step is testing the adequacy of the selected model. The most basic test of adequacy is whether the final model satisfies the research question. Beyond this important substantive test, Nagin (2005) lays out several statistically oriented criteria for assessing model adequacy, including (1) obtaining a close correspondence between the estimated probability of group membership and the proportion assigned to that group based on the posterior probability of group membership, (2) ensuring that the average of the posterior probabilities of group membership for individuals assigned to each group exceeds a minimum threshold of 0.7, (3) establishing that the odds of correct classification based on the posterior probabilities of group membership exceed a minimum threshold of 5, and (4) observing reasonably tight confidence intervals around estimated group membership probabilities.

Regardless of the criteria used for selection, the choice of the number of groups—and the potential of reifying groups—has been a topic of much discussion and debate in the literature. For example, Bauer and Curran (2003) demonstrated that seemingly modest specification error may result in the overextraction of groups in GMM analyses. Their work serves as a useful caution against the quixotic quest to identify the true number of groups in either GMM or GBTM analyses. Perhaps most important, this work reinforces the need to move away from interpretations of trajectory groups as literally distinct entities. It is our view that trajectory groups are just approximations of a more complex reality. As William Baumol (1992) observes:

> A well-designed model is, after all, a judiciously chosen set of lies, or perhaps more accurately put, partial truths about reality, which have been chosen so as to permit us to reason more effectively about some issue than we otherwise could. The model must be an oversimplification if it is to be tractable analytically. Optimality model constructions must be based on the trade-off between these two desiderata—accuracy of representation of reality and usability in analysis. (p. 55)

Once trajectory groups are understood to be clusters of individuals following similar trajectories, the interesting questions become: Are the trajectory groups distinguishable in terms of preexisting characteristics, subsequent outcomes, treatment response, or their relationship to trajectories for other outcomes or behaviors? If they differ on none of these dimensions, then the clusters no longer serve a useful substantive purpose. However, if group differences exist, then their continued study may have merit by whatever statistical method is chosen.

Developmental Applications

A group-based methodology is responsive to calls for "person-based" approaches to analyzing development (Bergman, 1998; Magnusson, 1998) and methods that are capable of providing a statistical snapshot of the key characteristics of individuals following distinctive developmental pathways. The push for methodological advancement is also driven by a long tradition of group-based theorizing about both normal and pathological development in psychology. Examples include theories of personality development (Caspi, 1998), learning (Holyoak & Spellman, 1993), language and conceptual development (Markman, 1989), mental disorders such as depression (Kasen et al., 2001), eating disorders (Tyrka, Graber, & Brooks-Gunn, 2000), alcoholism (Cloninger, 1987), conduct disorder and delinquency (Loeber, 1991; Moffitt, 1993; Patterson et al., 1989), and anxiety (Cloninger, 1986), as well as the development of prosocial characteristics such as conscience (Kochanska, 1997).

To illustrate the utility of group-based modeling in psychology, consider the four trajectories of physical aggression shown in Figure 27.2. These trajectories, first reported in Nagin and Tremblay (1999), are based on teacher-reported physical aggression from ages 6

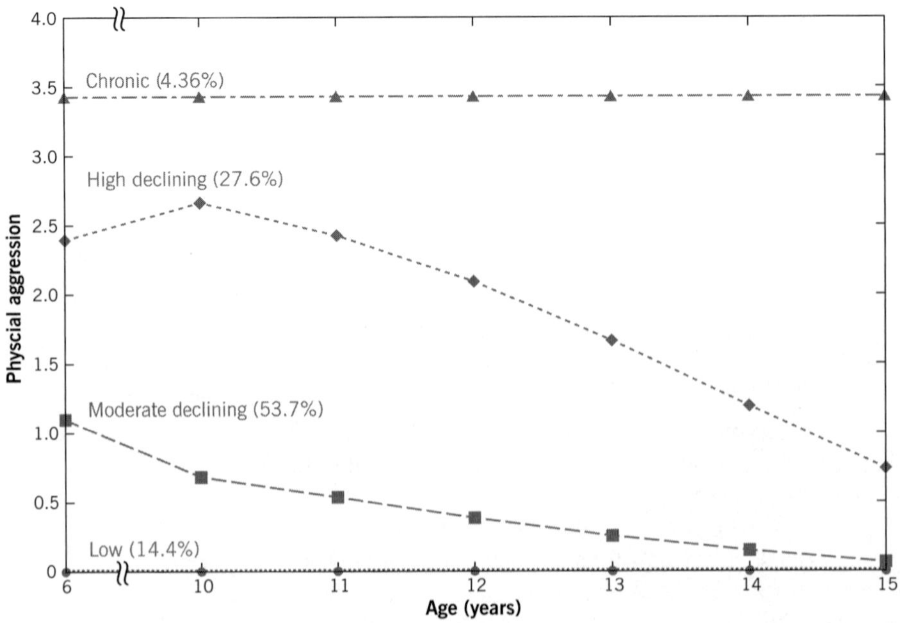

FIGURE 27.2. Trajectories of physical aggression from ages 6 to 15 for males in the Montreal-based longitudinal study.

to 15 among over 1,000 males in Montreal. Table 27.1 displays the characteristics of individuals following the four physical aggression trajectories shown in Figure 27.2. The trajectories and their correlates conform to long-standing findings regarding the predictors and consequences of childhood aggression. For example, individuals in the chronic aggression group tended to have the least educated parents and were most likely to score in the lowest quartile of the sample's IQ distribution. By contrast, individuals in the low aggression group were least likely to suffer from these risk factors. Furthermore, over 90% of the chronic aggression group failed to reach the eighth grade on schedule, and 13% had acquired a

TABLE 27.1. Physical Aggression Group Profiles in Montreal Study

	Group			
Variable	Low	Moderate declining	High declining	Chronic
Years of school for mother	11.1	10.8	9.8	8.4
Years of school for father	11.5	10.7	9.8	9.1
Low IQ (% in lowest quartile)	21.6	26.8	44.5	46.4
Completed eighth grade on time (%)	80.3	64.6	31.8	6.5
Juvenile record (%)	0.0	2.0	6.0	13.3
# of sexual partners age 17[a]	1.2	1.7	2.2	3.5

[a]Number of sexual partners at age 17 within the past year.

juvenile record by age 18. By comparison, only 19% of the low aggression group had fallen behind grade level by the eighth grade, and none had a juvenile record. Results provide an example of how group-based models can be applied to understand heterogeneity in development and to test theories related to etiology and outcomes. This example illustrates two valuable properties of a group versus classification rule-based approach, including the identification of distinct developmental progressions that are not observable using ad hoc classification and the ability to distinguish chance versus real variation across individuals.

Illustrations

This section provides illustrations of two extensions to the basic model. Although the examples are based on GBTM, they could just as well be conducted in the GMM framework. For a more complete description of model extensions, including dual and multitrajectory modeling, see Nagin and Odgers (2010).

Adding Predictors of Trajectory Group Membership

The two most important outputs of the basic model are estimates of the shape of each group's trajectory and the size of the group as measured by the proportion of the population following that trajectory (often referred to as probability of trajectory group membership). One popular model extension is to allow the probability of trajectory group membership to depend on baseline characteristics. For example, data from Farrington and West's (1990) classic study of more than 400 males from a poor neighborhood in London, England, were modeled to account for the relationship between trajectories of convictions from ages 10 to 32 and a variety of psychosocial risk factors. As shown in Figure 27.3, a four-group model best fit the data. The largest trajectory group generally had no convictions and accounted for 69.5% of the population. The three offending trajectories included an adolescent-limited group (12.4% of the population), which peaked sharply in late adolescence and then declined to a near zero rate of offending by age 20; a high-rate chronic trajectory (5.9% of

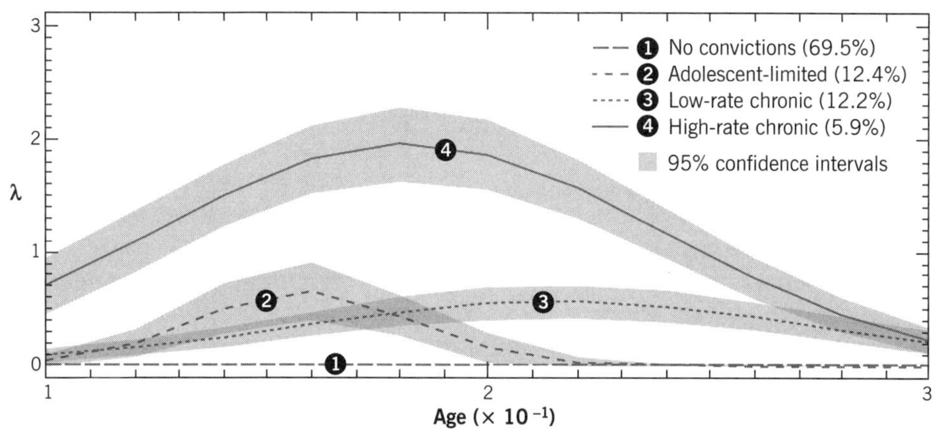

FIGURE 27.3. Trajectories of convictions in the Cambridge Study of Delinquent Development.

the population) with a high-hump shaped trajectory; and a low-rate chronic trajectory that accounted for the remaining 12.2% of the population. Also shown in the figure are 95% confidence intervals around each trajectory.

Results in Table 27.2 illustrate how the probability of trajectory group membership varied with four classic psychosocial risk factors for antisocial behavior (low IQ, high risk-taking behavior, poor childrearing behavior, and parental criminality) based on a multinomial logit model. The coefficients were estimated jointly with the parameter estimates of the trajectories themselves, with the comparison group set as the rare trajectory. For every trajectory group, all coefficient estimates are positive (although not all are statistically significant), which indicates that the majority of these psychosocial characteristics are risk factors for following a trajectory of heightened delinquency.

Adding Time-Varying Covariates and Estimating "Treatment Effects" in GBTMs

Group-based models can also be applied to provide group-specific estimates of whether major life transitions, such as the birth of a child, or clinical interventions, such as counseling or drug treatment, alter the developmental course of the outcome under study. In a very

TABLE 27.2. Predictors of Trajectory Group Membership in the Four-Group London Model

Variable	Coefficient estimate	*Z*-score
Adolescent limited		
Intercept	–2.99	–6.31
Low IQ	0.74	1.50
Criminal parents	1.01	2.19
High risk-taking	1.44	3.29
Poor childrearing	0.79	1.68
Low chronic		
Intercept	–2.79	–7.48
Low IQ	1.15	2.86
Criminal parents	1.38	3.46
High risk-taking	0.72	1.71
Poor childrearing	0.56	1.28
High chronic		
Intercept	–4.97	–8.22
Low IQ	1.33	2.50
Criminal parents	2.08	3.98
High risk-taking	2.21	4.03
Poor childrearing	1.16	2.22

Note. Rare trajectory is the comparison group.

useful set of analyses, Muthén and colleagues (2002) used a similar framework to analyze whether a randomized intervention had differential effects across trajectory groups. Nagin, Pagani, Tremblay, and Vitaro (2003) demonstrated this model extension in the Montreal study by testing whether grade retention and/or separation from biological parents altered a child's trajectory of violence across adolescence. A simplified version of the unconditional trajectories that emerged from these data is presented in Figure 27.4. Two trajectories that made up an estimated 65.4% of the population remained low and also declined throughout adolescence ("low 1" and "low 2"). The "rising" group, estimated to account for 13.4% of the population, began adolescence with low levels of violence but subsequently increased steeply. Two groups began with a high rate of violence but followed very divergent paths: One group declined (and hence is labeled "declining"), whereas the other group (labeled "chronic") remained high through adolescence.

The unconditional model was then expanded to test whether first-time grade retention and/or separation from the participant's biological parents seemed to alter the trajectories, as both of these stressors have been associated with heightened delinquency (Maguin & Loeber, 1996; Nagin et al., 2003; Pagani, Tremblay, Vitaro, Boulerice, & McDuff, 2001). More specifically, the effects of Fail (coded 1 in all periods subsequent to an individual's first being retained at grade level and 0 in periods prior to retention) and Separation (equal to 1 in all periods in which the boy is not living with both of his biological parents and equal to 0 in periods in which he is living with them) on each of the trajectories was estimated. Note that the definition of Fail does not test whether there is an enduring effect of school failure on violence, as it can change value only once (i.e., when and if the boy is retained at a grade level for the first time after the age of 11). Grade retention predicted significant increases in violent delinquency for each trajectory group (see Table 27.3). By contrast, separation from biological parents was associated with a significant increase in violent delinquency for only

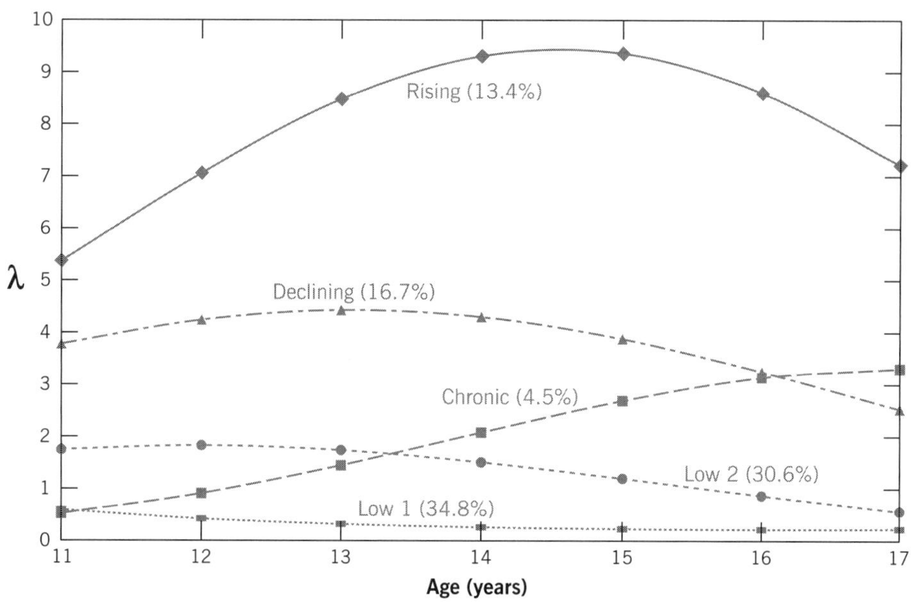

FIGURE 27.4. Trajectories of violent delinquency in the Montreal-based longitudinal study.

TABLE 27.3. Influence of Grade Retention and Family Breakup on Trajectories of Violence

Variable	Coefficient estimate	*Z*-score
Low 1 trajectory		
Intercept	13.26	3.27
Age	–18.95	–3.05
Age 2	5.76	2.47
Grade retention (> 10)	0.37	2.28
Family separation (< 10)	0.39	2.30
Low 2 trajectory		
Intercept	–3.45	–2.10
Age	5.99	2.46
Age 2	–2.52	–2.84
Grade retention (> 10)	0.36	5.79
Family separation (< 10)	–0.05	–0.60
Rising trajectory		
Intercept	–6.56	–3.38
Age	8.70	3.20
Age 2	–2.42	–2.56
Grade retention (> 10)	0.20	2.99
Family separation (< 10)	0.13	1.60
Declining trajectory		
Intercept	–8.52	5.40
Age	15.90	6.66
Age 2	–6.39	–7.15
Grade retention (> 10)	0.27	4.78
Family separation (< 10)	0.08	1.28
Chronic trajectory		
Intercept	–6.29	–5.04
Age	11.64	6.42
Age 2	–4.12	–6.35
Grade retention (> 10)	0.29	5.40
Family separation (< 10)	–0.01	–0.25

one group (Low 1). Thus grade retention in adolescence was associated with subsequent increases in the violent delinquency of each trajectory group, whereas family breakup was not.

Figure 27.5 graphically depicts three scenarios for the rising trajectory. Scenario 1 (labeled "no retention") predicts the expected offending rate from ages 11 to 17 under the assumption that the boy is not retained during this time period. Scenario 2 (labeled "retention at age 14") depicts the expected offending rate assuming the boy is retained at age 14 and thus from age 15 onward is behind grade level. Finally, the third scenario, called the "group average" trajectory, uses the weighted average of the Fail variable to trace out the expected trajectory of individuals following the rising trajectory. Prior to age 14, the group average trajectory lies above the two other trajectories, because a portion of individuals in the group have already been retained, whereas no retention has occurred yet in either of the other two scenarios. After age 14, the group average is sandwiched between the other two trajectories, because it reflects a composite trajectory of individuals who have and have not experienced grade retention.

Future Directions

Group-based trajectory models are emerging as an important set of tools for developmental scientists, particularly for those interested in methodologies that can facilitate causal inference and estimate group-specific treatment effects in situations in which randomization to treatment condition is not feasible. Group-based trajectory modeling has no special

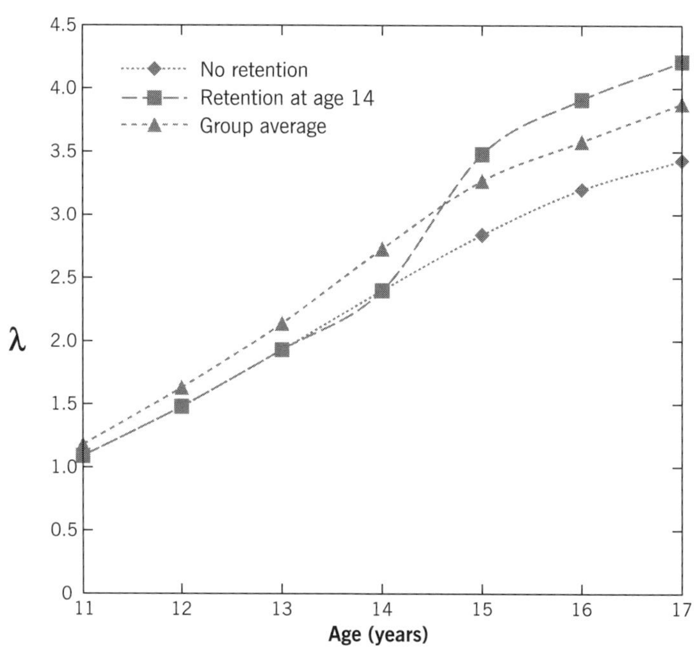

FIGURE 27.5. The impact of grade retention on the rising trajectory in the Montreal-based longitudinal study.

immunity to the hazards of drawing causal inferences from nonexperimental data, but recent work described in Haviland and colleagues (2008), Haviland and Nagin (2005), and Haviland et al. (2007) attempts to reduce this hazard by combining group-based modeling and propensity score matching to recreate the desirable features of experimental designs by creating balance between "treatment" versus "control" groups that have formed naturally over the course of an observational study (Rosenbaum & Rubin, 1983). The combination of group-based modeling and propensity score modeling may offer a number of advantages. First, propensity score matching within trajectory group may create control and treatment groups that are more comparable given that individuals within both groups were following similar developmental pathways prior to treatment. Second, the trajectory groups may represent meaningful subgroups in the population for whom treatment effects may vary. For example, in our previous work we tested whether substance exposure in early adolescence had differential health effects depending on whether children were following a no-conduct-problem versus a conduct-problem-prone trajectory (Odgers, Caspi, et al., 2008).

Despite the increasing number of applications of group-based trajectory models in developmental research, few guidelines exist to assist researchers when reporting model results. The following recommendations are provided to encourage the future presentation of results from group-based models in a transparent, understandable, and replicable fashion. The list that follows includes a nontechnical summary of basic reporting requirements for group-based models and is intended to apply to both GBTM and GMM. We acknowledge that any set of reporting principles will be incomplete and that a consensus on best reporting practices is still evolving. For those conducting group-based analyses in a structural equation modeling framework, we also recommend a review of reporting guidelines and principles summarized by McDonald and Ho (2002).

1. There is no such thing as an all-purpose statistical method. The chosen method must fit the research question and the data being analyzed. Researchers should explicitly articulate their rationale for using group-based models, whether it is testing a taxonomic theory, characterizing population variation in the form of latent developmental strata, or simply exploring the data.

2. Technical issues specific to the application of group-based models should be detailed, including a clear explanation for the choice of the number of groups included in the final model. This choice should not be reduced to a mechanical choice based on a specific fit statistic but rather should be based on a combination of formal statistical criteria, as well as the substantive usefulness and validity of the model as it relates to the research question(s). With that said, the adequacy of the chosen model should be supported by criteria such as those recommended by Nagin (2005), and attention should be paid to the selection of the functional form for each group (e.g., Is the order of the polynomial for each trajectory high enough to match the shapes that theoretically might emerge from the data?).

3. Whenever possible, it is good practice to make programming script available by request or online for those interested in replicating the trajectory solutions in their own data and/or, ideally, to publish the covariance matrix (or matrices) used as input into the models.

4. It is important that researchers adhere to sound reporting guidelines that apply to use of any statistical method, including reporting basic univariate information for the

variables that will be input into the trajectory model, including indices of central tendency, variability, and skew, and describing the amount and type of missing data across assessments. It is also important to describe the type of missing data technique, if any, that was applied in the analysis.

The conceptual appeal of group-based models has resulted in a substantial increase in the number of published studies over the last decade and is currently driving advancements in both developmental theory and methodology. As we continue to learn how group-based models can be applied to answer both basic and applied research questions, caution is also required to avoid the reification of groups, oversimplification of reality, and the application of an appealing method in the absence of theory. Ideally, with a critical eye toward the use of group-based models in psychological research, we can continue to pioneer new ways of understanding and charting development over time.

Acknowledgments

This work was funded in part by the National Science Foundation (Grant Nos. SES-99113700 and SES-0647576), the National Institute of Mental Health (RO1 MH65611-01A2), and the National Institute on Aging (Grant No. R01 AG032282-02). Candice Odgers is a William T. Grant Scholar.

References

Akaike, H. (1974). New look at statistical-model identification. *IEEE Transactions on Automatic Control, 19*(6), 716–723.

Appel, T. A. (1987). *The Cuvier–Geoffroy debate: French biology in the decades before Darwin*. New York: Oxford University Press.

Bauer, D. J. (2007). Observations on the use of growth mixture models in psychological research. *Multivariate Behavioral Research, 42*, 757–786.

Bauer, D. J., & Curran, P. J. (2003). Distributional assumptions of growth mixture models: Implications for overextraction of latent trajectory classes. *Psychological Methods, 8*(3), 338–363.

Baumol, W. (1992). On my attitudes: Sociopolitical and methodological. In M. Szenberg (Ed.), *Eminent economists: Their life philosophies* (pp. 51–59). Cambridge, UK: Cambridge University Press.

Belsky, J., Steinberg, L., & Draper, P. (1991). Childhood experience, interpersonal development, and reproductive strategy: An evolutionary theory of socialization. *Child Development, 62*(4), 647–670.

Bergman, L. R. (1998). A pattern-oriented approach to studying individual development: Snapshots and processes. In R. B. Cairns, L. R. Bergman, & J. Kagan (Eds.), *Methods and models for studying the individual* (pp. 83–121). Thousand Oaks, CA: Sage.

Bollen, K. A., & Curran, P. J. (2006). *Latent curve models: A structural equation approach*. Hoboken, NJ: Wiley.

Bryk, A. S., & Raudenbush, S. W. (1987). Application of hierarchical linear models to assessing change. *Psychological Bulletin, 101*(1), 147–158.

Caspi, A. (1998). Personality development across the life course. In N. Eisenberg & W. Damon (Eds.), *Handbook of child psychology: Vol. 3. Social, emotional, and personality development* (5th ed., pp. 311–388). New York: Wiley.

Christ, M., Krishnan, R., Nagin, D., & Günther, O. (2002, June). *An empirical analysis of web site stickiness*. Paper presented at the European Conference on Information Systems, Gdansk, Poland.

Cloninger, C. R. (1986). A unified biosocial theory of personality and its role in the development of anxiety states. *Psychiatric Developments, 4*(3), 167–226.

Cloninger, C. R. (1987). A systematic method for clinical description and classification of personality variants: A proposal. *Archives of General Psychiatry, 44*(6), 573–588.

Côté, S., Boiven, M., Liu, X., Nagin, D. S., Zoccolillo, M., & Tremblay, R. E. (2004). Depression and anxiety symptoms: Onset, developmental course and prediction during early childhood. *Journal of Child Psychology and Psychiatry, 50*, 1201–1208.

Farrington, D. P., & West, D. J. (1990). The Cambridge Study in Delinquent Development: A prospective longitudinal study of 411 males. In H. J. Kerner & G. Kaiser (Eds.), *Criminality: Personality, behavior, and life history* (pp. 115–138). Berlin: Springer Verlag.

Goldstein, H. (1995). *Multilevel statistical models* (2nd ed.). London: Arnold.

Haviland, A. M., & Nagin, D. S. (2005). Causal inferences with group-based trajectory models. *Psychometrika, 70*(3), 557–578.

Haviland, A. M., Nagin, D. S., & Rosenbaum, P. R. (2007). Combining propensity score matching and group-based trajectory analysis in an observational study. *Psychological Methods, 12*(3), 247–267.

Haviland, A., Rosenbaum, P. R., Nagin, D. S., & Tremblay, R. E. (2008). Combining group-based trajectory modeling and propensity score matching for causal inferences in nonexperimental longitudinal data. *Developmental Psychology, 44*(2), 422–436.

Heckman, J., & Singer, B. (1984). A method for minimizing the impact of distributional assumptions in econometric models for duration data. *Econometrica, 52*(2), 271–320.

Holyoak, K. J., & Spellman, B. A. (1993). Thinking. *Annual Review of Psychology, 44*, 265–315.

Kandel, D. (1975). Stages in adolescent involvement in drug use. *Science, 190*, 912–914.

Kasen, S., Cohen, P., Skodol, A. E., Johnson, J. G., Smailes, E., & Brook, J. S. (2001). Childhood depression and adult personality disorder: Alternative pathways of continuity. *Archives of General Psychiatry, 58*(3), 231–236.

Kochanska, G. (1997). Multiple pathways to conscience for children with different temperaments: From toddlerhood to age 5. *Developmental Psychology, 33*(2), 228–240.

Lo, Y. T., Mendell, N. R., & Rubin, D. B. (2001). Testing the number of components in a normal mixture. *Biometrika, 88*(3), 767–778.

Loeber, R. (1991). Questions and advances in the study of developmental pathways. In D. Cicchetti & S. Toth (Eds.), *Rochester symposium on developmental psychopathology* (Vol. 3, pp. 97–116). Rochester, NY: University of Rochester Press.

MacCallum, R. C., Kim, C., Malarkey, W. B., & Kiecolt-Glaser, J. K. (1997). Studying multivariate change using multilevel models and latent curve models. *Multivariate Behavioral Research, 32*(3), 215–253.

Magnusson, D. (1998). The logic and implications of a person-oriented approach. In R. B. Cairns, L. R. Bergman, & J. Kagan (Eds.), *Methods and models for studying the individual* (pp. 33–64). Thousand Oaks, CA: Sage.

Maguin, E., & Loeber, R. (1996). Academic performance and delinquency. In M. Tonry (Ed.), *Crime and justice: A review of research* (Vol. 20, pp. 145–264). Chicago: University of Chicago Press.

Markman, E. M. (1989). *Categorization and naming in children: Problems of induction*. Cambridge, MA: MIT Press.

McArdle, J. J., & Epstein, D. (1987). Latent growth curves within developmental structural equation models. *Child Development, 58*(1), 110–133.

McDonald, R. P., & Ho, M. H. R. (2002). Principles and practice in reporting structural equation analyses. *Psychological Methods, 7*(1), 64–82.

McLachlan, G., & Peel, D. (2004). *Finite mixture models*. New York: Wiley Interscience.

Meredith, W., & Tisak, J. (1990). Latent curve analysis. *Psychometrika, 55*(1), 107–122.

Moffitt, T. E. (1993). Adolescence-limited and life-course-persistent antisocial behavior: A developmental taxonomy. *Psychological Review, 100*(4), 674–701.
Mustillo, S., Worthman, C., Erkanli, A., Keeler, G., Angold, A., & Costello, E. J. (2003). Obesity and psychiatric disorder: Developmental trajectories. *Pediatrics, 111*(4), 851–859.
Muthén, B. O. (1989). Latent variable modeling in heterogeneous populations. *Psychometrika, 54*(4), 557–585.
Muthén, B. (2001). Second-generation structural equation modeling with a combination of categorical and continuous latent variables: New opportunities for latent class/latent growth modeling. In A. Sayers & L. Collins (Eds.), *New methods for the analysis of change* (pp. 291–322). Washington, DC: American Psychological Association.
Muthén, B. (2004). Latent variable analysis: Growth mixture modeling and related techniques for longitudinal data. In D. Kaplan (Ed.), *Handbook of quantitative methodology for the social sciences* (pp. 345–368). Newbury Park, CA: Sage.
Muthén, B., Brown, C. H., Masyn, K., Jo, B., Khoo, S. T., Yang, C. C., et al. (2002). General growth mixture modeling for randomized preventive interventions. *Biostatistics, 3*(4), 459–475.
Muthén, B., & Shedden, K. (1999). Finite mixture modeling with mixture outcomes using the EM algorithm. *Biometrics, 55*, 463–469.
Nagin, D. (2005). *Group-based modeling of development.* Cambridge, MA: Harvard University Press.
Nagin, D. S. (1999). Analyzing developmental trajectories: A semiparametric, group-based approach. *Psychological Methods, 4*(2), 139–157.
Nagin, D. S., & Odgers, C. L. (2010). Group-based trajectory modeling in clinical research. *Annual Review of Clinical Psychology, 6*(1), 109–138.
Nagin, D., Pagani, L., Tremblay, R. E., & Vitaro, F. (2003). Life course turning points: A case study of the effect of school failure on interpersonal violence. *Development and Psychopathology, 15*(343), 343–361.
Nagin, D. S., & Tremblay, R. E. (1999). Trajectories of boys' physical aggression, opposition, and hyperactivity on the path to physically violent and nonviolent juvenile delinquency. *Child Development, 70*(5), 1181–1196.
Nylund, K. L., Asparouhov, T., & Muthén, B. O. (2007). Deciding on the number of classes in latent class analysis and growth mixture modeling: A Monte Carlo simulation study. *Structural Equation Modeling, 14*(4), 535–569.
Odgers, C. L., Caspi, A., Nagin, D. S., Piquero, A. R., Slutske, W. S., Milne, B. J., et al. (2008). Is it important to prevent early exposure to drugs and alcohol among adolescents? *Psychological Science, 19*(10), 1037–1044.
Odgers, C. L., Moffitt, T. E., Broadbent, J. M., Dickson, N., Hancox, R. J., Harrington, H., et al. (2008). Female and male antisocial trajectories: From childhood origins to adult outcomes. *Development and Psychopathology, 20*(2), 673–716.
Pagani, L., Tremblay, R. E., Vitaro, F., Boulerice, B., & McDuff, P. (2001). Effects of grade retention on academic performance and behavioral development. *Development and Psychopathology, 13*(2), 297–315.
Patterson, G. R., Debaryshe, B. D., & Ramsey, E. (1989). A developmental perspective on antisocial behavior. *American Psychologist, 44*(2), 329–335.
Piquero, A. (2005). *Taking stock of developmental trajectories of criminal activity over the life course.* Washington, DC: National Institute of Justice.
Preacher, K. J., Wichman, A. L., Briggs, N. E., & MacCallum, R. C. (2008). *Latent growth curve modeling.* Thousands Oaks, CA: Sage.
Raftery, A. E. (1995). Bayesian model selection in social research. In P. Marsden (Ed.), *Sociological methodology* (Vol. 25, pp. 111–163). Cambridge, MA: Blackwell.
Raudenbush, S. W. (2001). Comparing personal trajectories and drawing causal inferences from longitudinal data. *Annual Review of Psychology, 52*, 501–525.

Rosenbaum, P. R., & Rubin, D. B. (1983). The central role of the propensity score in observational studies for causal effects. *Biometrika, 70*(1), 41–55.

Schwartz, G. (1978). Estimating the dimension of a model. *Annals of Statistics, 6,* 461–464.

Titterington, D. M., Smith, A. F. M., & Makov, U. E. (1985). *Statistical analysis of finite mixture models*. New York: Wiley.

Tyrka, A. R., Graber, J. A., & Brooks-Gunn, J. (2000). The development of disordered eating: Correlates and predictors of eating problems in the context of adolescence. In J. A. Sameroff, M. Lewis, & S. M. Miller (Eds.), *Handbook of developmental psychopathology* (pp. 607–624). New York: Kluwer Academic/Plenum Press.

Van Ryzin, M. J., Chatham, M., Kryzer, E., Kertes, D. A., & Gunnar, M. R. (2009). Identifying atypical cortisol patterns in young children: The benefits of group-based trajectory modeling. *Psychoneuroendocrinology, 34*(1), 50–61.

Weisburd, D., Bushway, S., Lum, C., & Yang, S. M. (2004). Trajectories of crime at places: A longitudinal study of street segments in the city of Seattle. *Criminology, 42*(3), 283–320.

Willett, J. B., & Sayer, A. G. (1994). Using covariance structure analysis to detect correlates and predictors of individual change over time. *Psychological Bulletin, 116*(2), 363–381.

CHAPTER 28

Longitudinal Mixture Models and the Identification of Archetypes

NILAM RAM
KEVIN J. GRIMM
LISA M. GATZKE-KOPP
PETER C. M. MOLENAAR

Central Issues

Along a variety of fronts there is growing acknowledgment of heterogeneity of persons—individuality or uniqueness. A number of methodologies that explicitly address interindividual differences have been developed and are being used to obtain a greater understanding of when and why individuals differ from one another. For example, multigroup and multilevel models are often used to examine how the observed relations among variables differ among groups or levels of a third variable (Bryk & Raudenbush, 1992; Jöreskog, 1971). Latent structure and finite mixture methods are used to identify, in an exploratory way, subgroups that exhibit different patterns of relations among variables (Lazarsfeld & Henry, 1968; McLachlan & Peel, 2000). Extensions are used to identify subgroups characterized by different means and covariance structures (Arminger, Stein, & Wittenberg, 1999; Collins & Lanza, 2010), factor models (Lubke & Muthén, 2005; Yung, 1997), and trajectories (Muthén & Shedden, 1999; Nagin, 1999). Together, these models offer a variety of possibilities for identifying and characterizing heterogeneity in a sample and, by inference, a population.

There is also an abundance of theoretical perspectives that explicitly acknowledge heterogeneity by making use of phenotypic taxonomies to classify people into categories.

Nowhere is this more formalized than in the *Diagnostic and Statistical Manual of Mental Disorders* (DSM-IV-TR; American Psychiatric Association, 2000). This publication represents decades of effort to capture and quantify heterogeneity within psychopathology. Categorical distinctions, such as autism or schizophrenia, although sometimes inconsistent, are used for prognoses and to guide treatment. Furthermore, within these phenotypic distinctions, each instantiation of the DSM has attempted to differentiate within-phenotype distinctions. Subtype specifiers now exist for most major diagnostic classifications, including depression, schizophrenia, attention-deficit/hyperactivity disorder (ADHD), phobias, and eating disorders.

Phenotypic classifications are also used to explore heterogeneity at the biological level. For instance, individuals appear to vary with regard to their biological stress reactivity in ways that are difficult to discern behaviorally but that have strong implications for physical and psychological development. Stress responsivity research suggests at least two physiological phenotypes (Heim, Elhert, & Hellhammer, 2000; Miller, Chen, & Zhou, 2007, p. 28): The "typical" profile is one in which individuals' cortisol levels rise in response to a stressor, peaking within approximately 10–20 minutes, followed by a gradual recovery to baseline approximately 40 minutes poststress. In contrast, some individuals' cortisol trajectories are marked by normative response but a general failure of recovery. This prolonged elevation of cortisol is associated with both physical and psychological risks related to chronic stress and later development or aging. Because cortisol production is causally related to neural, cardiac, and metabolic physiological processes, the theoretical and empirical evidence suggests a biological model that (1) restricts the range of hypothesized subtypes and (2) allows for the derivation of specific hypotheses about clinical and developmental consequences related to observed heterogeneity in the population. The key point is that theoretically driven approaches provide the opportunity for specificity in hypotheses regarding how many phenotypes there are and how each phenotype is expressed. This specificity has implications for the statistical approach taken to identify underlying phenotypes.

In this chapter we explore how a collection of longitudinal mixture models (latent class longitudinal profile model, latent class growth model, growth mixture model, quasi-simplex mixture model) can be coupled with phenotypic theory. Typically, longitudinal mixture models are used in an exploratory manner, the objective being to identify subgroups of individuals who differ in how they change and develop over time. Outside of model assumptions, the analyses are purposefully devoid of theory. The underlying idea is to "let the data speak." However, in working with these models and observing how they are applied in the literature, we find that the models are used in ways that constrain the types of change and development that can be observed—stories written in a particular genre, so to speak.

Although these constraints might be viewed negatively, we suggest that they provide some unique opportunities to articulate theoretically precise hypotheses about when and where idiosyncratic or archetypal patterns of behavior change manifest. We reframe these "exploratory" methods as "semiconfirmatory" models and use them to articulate phenotypic, person-oriented theory. Our conclusions are that (1) although longitudinal mixture models are typically considered an "exploratory" procedure, they are, in practice, highly constrained explorations of data; and (2) given the constraints inherent in their implementation, such models are useful for articulating particular theoretical hypotheses.

Conceptual Principles and Statistical Assumptions

Stories come in many genres—action-adventure, crime, detective, fantasy, horror, mystery, romance, science fiction, western, and serious literary fiction. Depending on the genre, different archetypes are often used. Detective stories, for instance, often have one or more murderers and a protagonist who is a professional investigator. Westerns often feature rugged, individualistic heroes. Romances typically highlight a man and a woman, heterosexual love, and a happy ending.

Studies that use longitudinal mixture models to describe how behavior proceeds over time also come in many different genres. Generally, mixture models help to identify archetypes and separate individuals into categories described by those archetypes. For example, in developmentally oriented applications, mixture models provide descriptions of developmental phenotypes (e.g., early learners vs. late learners; experimenters vs. life course persisters) and probabilistic classification of individuals into phenotypic categories. Depending on the particular mathematical model being used, different kinds and numbers of archetypes can emerge. The choice of model implicitly or explicitly puts limitations on the particular archetypes or types of characters identified. Thus care should be taken to work within the genre that is best suited for a particular research question or to work across multiple genres.

A complication encountered when using such models is that different descriptions of development can be obtained from the same data. Approached from one genre, or making use of one model, we obtain a different narrative (and phenotypes) than would be obtained when using another genre, or model. To illustrate this, we run the same longitudinal data (shown in Figure 28.1) through a number of longitudinal mixture models and set the emergent stories side by side. As a forewarning, we do not conclude that one model (and the theory it attempts to articulate), is better than another. Rather, our goal is to highlight that, even with analytical techniques that are often considered exploratory and devoid of theory, special care should be taken to select a model that articulates and aligns with one's research goals.

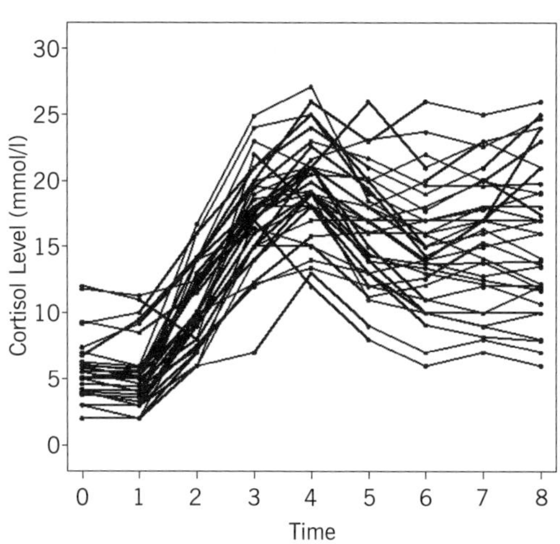

FIGURE 28.1. Cortisol levels obtained from 34 individuals across nine occasions.

A General Framework: Mixtures within SEMs

Mixture models can often be interpreted as multiple-group structural equation models (SEMs) in which a grouping variable, c, is latent or unobserved. For example, consider how the people we encounter over the course of a day are classified into gender categories. In most instances, we use a variety of easily observable characteristics to classify individuals as male or female. By observing their height, weight, physical build, facial features, voice, clothing, hair style, and so forth, we develop multivariate profiles. Then, based on those profiles, we classify people into one or another latent gender category. In principle, we compare the individuals we meet to some theoretical archetypes (e.g., Ken and Barbie) and make probabilistic judgments about who they are more or less like. Quite often we are right in our classifications, but sometimes we are wrong.

In the following sections we outline a selection of longitudinal mixture models that can be used to model how individuals change over time. For precision these are presented in matrix equation form and supplemented with graphical representations (upper panels of Figures 28.2–28.6). The models impose different constraints on the data and thus articulate substantially different theories of change. These differences are most easily identified in the mathematical renditions by noting which and how many Greek letters (e.g., Λ, B, Ψ, Θ) are included or "missing" from each model, or, for readers who are less familiar with the underlying mathematics, by noting which sets of arrows (e.g., one-headed arrows between triangle and squares, or two-headed arrows on and among circles) are included in or missing from each model. After outlining the general and multiple-group SEM frameworks in which the collection of longitudinal mixture models is placed, each model is presented in turn. We highlight the parallels between the diagrams and the matrices as we go.

Basic SEM Framework

Placed within an SEM framework, the mixture model allows great flexibility in identifying subgroups. For example, when working with univariate repeated-measures data, individuals' vector of t repeated scores can be represented generally as a combination of a "measurement model":

$$y_i = \tau + \lambda\eta_i + \varepsilon_i, \tag{28.1a}$$

and a "structural model":

$$\eta_i = \alpha + \beta\eta_i + \zeta_i. \tag{28.1b}$$

In the path diagrams, the ys are rendered as squares, the η's, ε's, and ζ's as circles, the τ's and α's as arrows from the triangle to squares and circles, respectively, the λ's as one-headed arrows between the η circles and squares, and the β's as one-headed arrows between the η circles.

Summarizing across persons, we obtain the mean and covariance expectations of the model. Mean expectations are

$$\mu = \tau + \Lambda(\mathrm{I} - \mathrm{B})^{-1}\alpha \tag{28.2a}$$

where μ is the $T \times 1$ longitudinal vector of the expected means, where τ is a $T \times 1$ longitudinal vector of intercepts (the collection of arrows from the triangle to squares), and α is a $p \times 1$ vector of latent variable means (the collection of arrows from the triangle to circles) that are weighted by the $T \times p$ matrix Λ, which can be thought of as a design matrix, adjusting for any regressions among the latent variables (through $(I - B)^{-1}$). The covariance expectations are

$$\Sigma = \Lambda(I - B)^{-1}\Psi(I - B)^{-1}\Lambda' + \Theta \quad \textbf{(28.2b)}$$

where Σ, the expected $T \times T$ covariance matrix, is a function of Λ, a $T \times p$ design matrix (the collection of one-headed arrows between circles and squares); B, the $p \times p$ matrix of regressions among the latent variables (the collection of one-headed arrows between circles and squares); Ψ, the $p \times p$ (residual) covariance matrix of the latent variables (the collection of two-headed arrows emanating from one set of circles); and Θ, a $T \times T$ residual covariance matrix of the observed variables, ε_{ti} (the collection of two-headed arrows emanating from the other set of "residual ε" circles). Note that in the general model some (identification) constraints must be imposed to identify the model (e.g., keep the number of degrees of freedom equal to or greater than zero).

Multiple-Group SEM

The SEM framework is easily extended to accommodate and examine differences among multiple groups of individuals. We simply introduce a categorical grouping variable, c, with two or more categories to divide the longitudinal data into nonoverlapping, mutually exclusive subsets of data. The model becomes

$$\mu_c = \tau_c + \Lambda_c(I - B_c)^{-1}\alpha_c$$
$$\Sigma_c = \Lambda_c(I - B_c)^{-1}\Psi_c(I - B_c)^{-1'}\Lambda_c' + \Theta_c \quad \textbf{(28.3)}$$

The pervasiveness of the c subscripts indicates that groups can, in principle, differ in all aspects of the model highlighted here. Graphically, each group, $c = 1$ to C, gets its own diagram. This model is extremely flexible in that completely invariant, partially invariant, or completely noninvariant models can be specified to examine the existence of group heterogeneity in any subset of parameters (subset of arrows). Not only may the contents of each matrix differ, but even the dimensions of each matrix can differ among groups. From a substantive perspective, this setup allows for the possibility that the observed and latent variables may be driven by completely different underlying processes within each group.

Mixture SEM

The preceding model assumes that c is an observed characteristic. However, the grouping variable may be a latent or unobserved characteristic. Latent grouping variables are accommodated by incorporating probabilistic classification (similar to a logistic regression). Model expectations become

$$\mu_c = \Sigma_{c=1}^{C} \pi_c[\tau_c + \Lambda_c(\mathrm{I} - \mathrm{B}_c)^{-1}\alpha_c]$$

$$\Sigma_c = \Sigma_{c=1}^{C} \pi_c\left[\Lambda_c(\mathrm{I} - \mathrm{B}_c)^{-1}\Psi_c(\mathrm{I} - \mathrm{B}_c)^{-1\prime}\Lambda_c' + \Theta_c\right] \quad \textbf{(28.4)}$$

where π_c is the proportion of participants in class c (sum of individual probabilities of membership in that class as a proportion of total number of individuals). Individual probabilities of class membership range between 0 and 1 ($0 \leq \pi_{ci} \leq 1$), with the constraint that the sum of individual class probabilities equals 1 ($\Sigma_{c=1}^{C} \pi_{ci} = 1$). All matrices can, in principle, differ across classes.

A Collection of Longitudinal Mixture Models

Within this general framework, a number of interesting longitudinal mixture models can be constructed by imposing additional constraints on the matrices or parameters that differ between classes and/or the probability that particular individuals are in a particular class. These include latent class longitudinal profile models (LCLPM), latent class growth models (LCGM), growth mixture models (GMM), and quasi-simplex mixture models (QSMM). Graphical depictions are given in the upper panels of Figures 28.2–28.6. Note that the path diagrams are shown for only one group. As per the multiple-group conceptualization, additional parallel path diagrams are used to represent and obtain parameters related to each group, $c = 1$ to C.

Latent Class Longitudinal Profile Model

The LCLPM is a simplification of the general SEM mixture framework. This model focuses on between-class differences in the manifest variable intercepts (in this case equivalent to observed variable means), τ_c, and variances, Θ_c. Specifically, by not including any latent variables, model expectations reduce to

$$\mu_c = \Sigma_{c=1}^{C} \pi_c[\tau_c]$$

$$\Sigma_c = \Sigma_{c=1}^{C} \pi_c[\Theta_c] \quad \textbf{(28.5)}$$

with the additional constraint that Θ_c is diagonal (no within-class covariances) and, in most applications, invariant across classes. The model is represented graphically in the upper panel of Figure 28.2. As can be seen, the observed data (squares) are modeled using only a few sets of arrows (matrices). Specifically, the expected means are modeled with one set of arrows directly connecting the triangle (a constant) with the squares (the elements of τ_c), and the expected variances are modeled as being completely accounted for by the two-headed arrows on the unique ε_t variables associated with each of the observed measures (the elements along the diagonal of Θ_c). Note that there are no double-headed arrows between the unique ε_t variables, meaning that they are modeled as independent (no covariances, as per the diagonal nature of Θ_c). The resulting profiles and individual class probabilities provide a description of group-level differences as described by the mean of each class's scores over time.

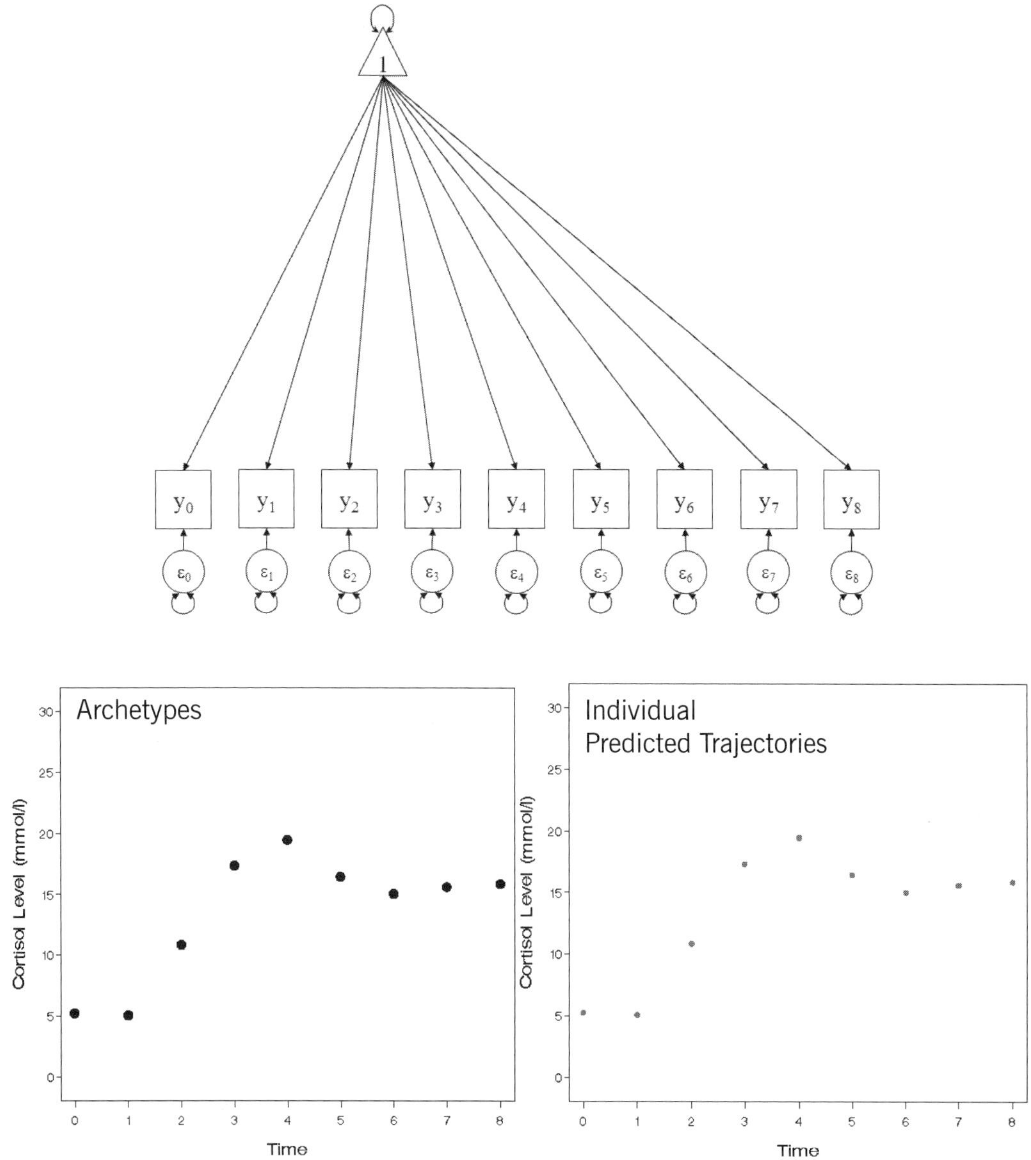

FIGURE 28.2. *Top panel*: Path diagram for the LCLPM. *Bottom panel*: Archetype (left) and individual (right) trajectories obtained from the one-class LCLPM.

Latent Class Growth Model

With interest in interindividual differences in intraindividual change, developmental researchers often make use of growth curve models (see Blozis, Chapter 26, this volume; Bollen & Curran, 2006; Duncan, Duncan, Stryker, Li, & Alpert, 2006; Grimm & Ram, Chapter 24, this volume; McArdle, 2009; Preacher, Wichman, MacCallum, & Broggs, 2008; Ram & Grimm, 2009). These models provide an alternative to the general SEM mixture framework. Instead of focusing on the manifest variable intercepts and means and variances,

LCGMs focus interpretation on latent variable means, α_c, that characterize specific aspects of change trajectories over time (Nagin, 2005; Nagin & Odgers, 2010, and Chapter 27, this volume). Expectations of the LCGM usually take the form

$$\begin{aligned} \mu_c &= \Sigma_{c=1}^{C} \pi_c [\Lambda_c \alpha_c] \\ \Sigma_c &= \Sigma_{c=1}^{C} \pi_c [\Theta_c] \end{aligned} \quad \textbf{(28.6)}$$

with the additional constraint that Θ_c is both diagonal and invariant across classes and that the elements of Λ_c are fixed a priori to define linear, quadratic, or other polynomial trajectories. The model is represented graphically in the upper panel of Figure 28.3. In place of the set of arrows directly connecting the triangle (a constant) with the squares (the elements of τ_c) in the previous model, the expected means are modeled through a set of latent variables (the circles labeled with η). Specifically, paths from the triangle to the observed variables are modeled through a set of one-headed arrows connecting the latent variables to the squares (the elements of Λ_c) and a set of one-headed arrows connecting the triangle to the latent variables (the elements of α_c). Together these arrows are the graphical representation of the multiplication seen in the first line of equation 28.6. Note the assumption that there is no within-class variability in the latent variables. That is, all the elements of Ψ_c are constrained to be zero, represented in the diagram by the absence of any two-headed arrows on or among the latent variables.

Growth Mixture Models

GMMs provide an alternative to the mixture SEM that allows for within-class variability in the latent variables, Ψ_c (Muthén, 2004; Muthén & Muthén, 2000; Muthén & Shedden, 1999). This can be readily noted in Figure 28.4, where now there is a set of two-headed arrows on and among the latent variables (the elements of Ψ_c may be nonzero). Expectations of the GMM can be written as

$$\begin{aligned} \mu_c &= \Sigma_{c=1}^{C} \pi_c [\Lambda_c \alpha_c] \\ \Sigma_c &= \Sigma_{c=1}^{C} \pi_c [\Lambda_c \Psi_c \Lambda_c' + \Theta_c]. \end{aligned} \quad \textbf{(28.7)}$$

This model is written in the most general form such that every matrix has a c subscript to denote that it may be allowed to differ over latent classes. However, in practice, researchers tend to constrain the Λ, Ψ, and Θ matrices to be invariant across latent classes and to keep the focus on the mean differences in the latent variables, α_c. That is, the parameters associated with the one-headed arrows between the latent η variables and the squares, the two-headed arrows among the latent η variables, and the two-headed arrows on and among the residual ε variables are constrained to be equal across groups, whereas the set of arrows between the triangle and the latent η variables are allowed to differ across groups. In some more elaborate implementations, the structure of the design matrix, Λ_c, the latent variable covariance structure, Ψ_c, and the residual covariance structure, Θ_c, are also allowed to differ among classes. As in the previous model, all the elements of Λ_c are usually defined a priori to capture linear, quadratic, higher polynomial, or other patterns of change. However, in some situations it is possible to define Λ_c with minimal identification constraints to obtain interesting nonlinear trajectories (i.e., latent basis growth mixture model used later; see

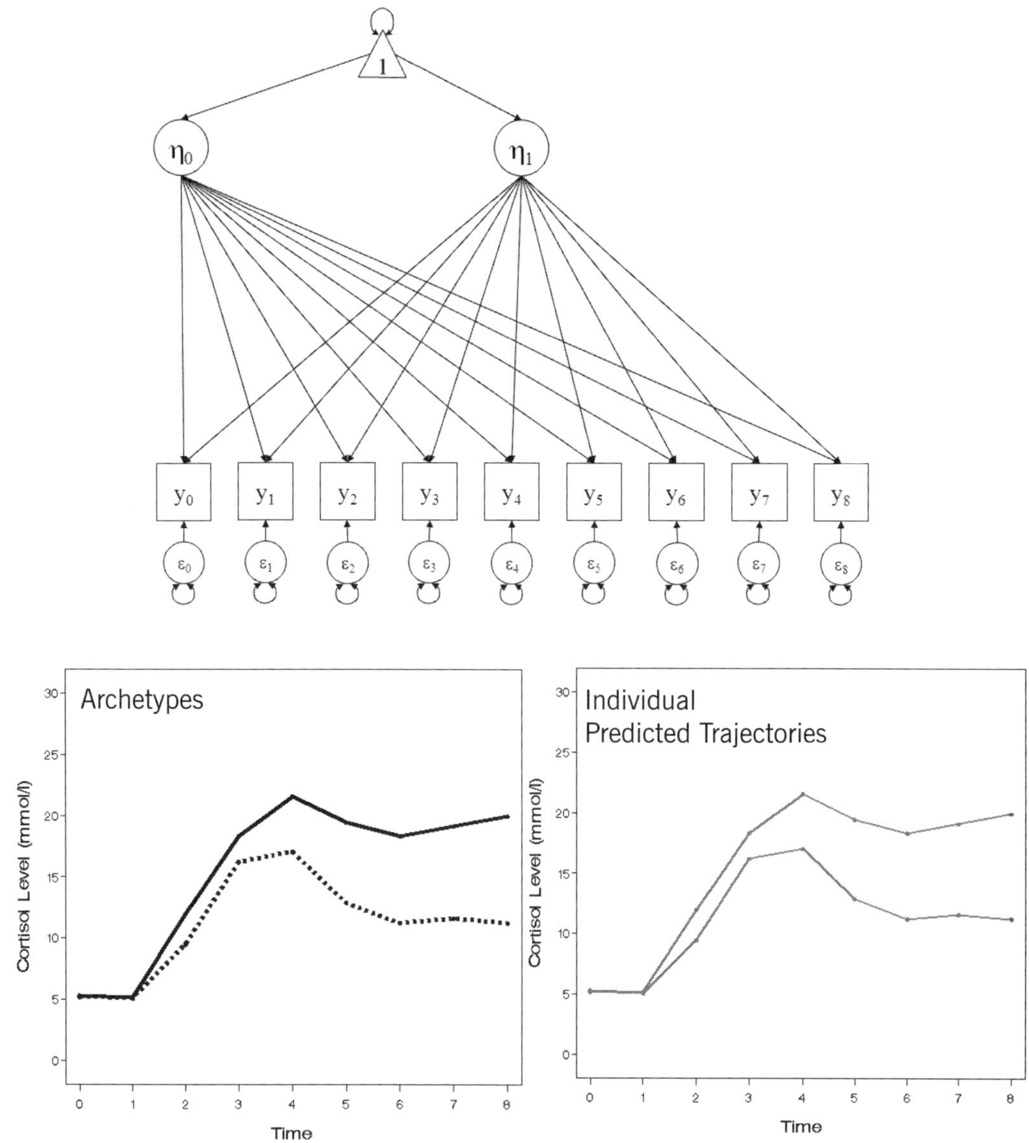

FIGURE 28.3. *Top panel*: Path diagram for the LCGM with no heterogeneity in the latent factors. *Bottom panel*: Archetype (left) and individual (right) trajectories obtained from the two-class LCGM.

also Grimm, Ram, & Estabrook, 2010; Ram & Grimm, 2009). The obtained parameter estimates and individual class probabilities provide a description of group-level differences in prototypical amounts and patterns of within-person change and the between-person differences therein. As in growth curve models more generally, the specifications of Λ_c provide both the flexibility and constraints needed to make specific statements about developmental theory (see Burchinal, Nelson, & Poe, 2006; Grimm & Ram, 2009; McArdle & Nesselroade, 2003; Ram & Grimm, 2007). In our illustration we use two versions of this model: one that captures interindividual differences using two aspects of intraindividual change

(Λ_c is $T \times 2$), as depicted in Figure 28.4 with two latent η variables, and one that captures interindividual differences using three aspects of intraindividual change (Λ_c is $T \times 3$), as depicted in Figure 28.5 with three latent η variables.

Quasi-Simplex Mixture Models

All of the models so far have assumed that there are no directional associations among the repeated measures. In particular, all elements of the B matrix were assumed to be zero.

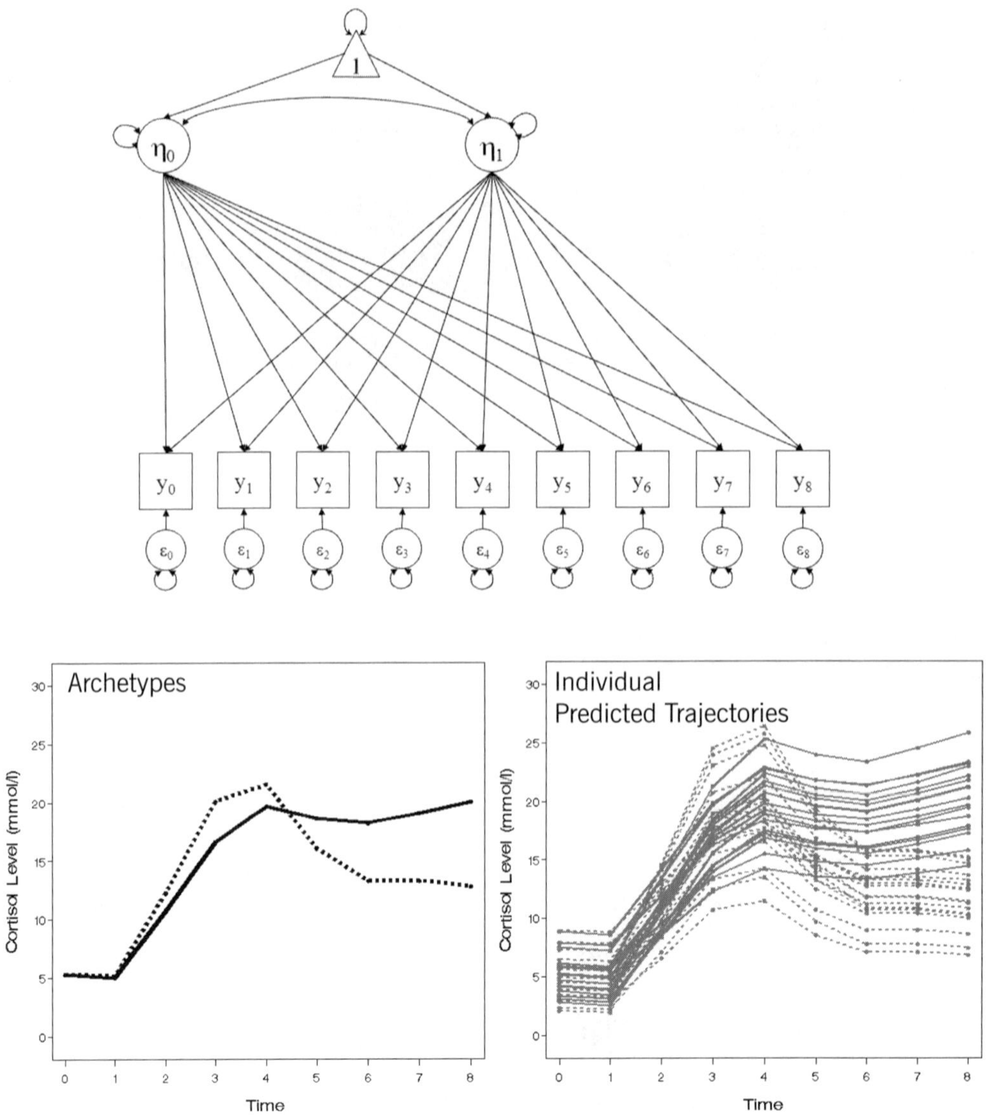

FIGURE 28.4. *Top panel*: Path diagram for the GMM with heterogeneity in the latent factors. *Bottom panel*: Archetype (left) and individual (right) trajectories obtained from the two-class single-phase GMM.

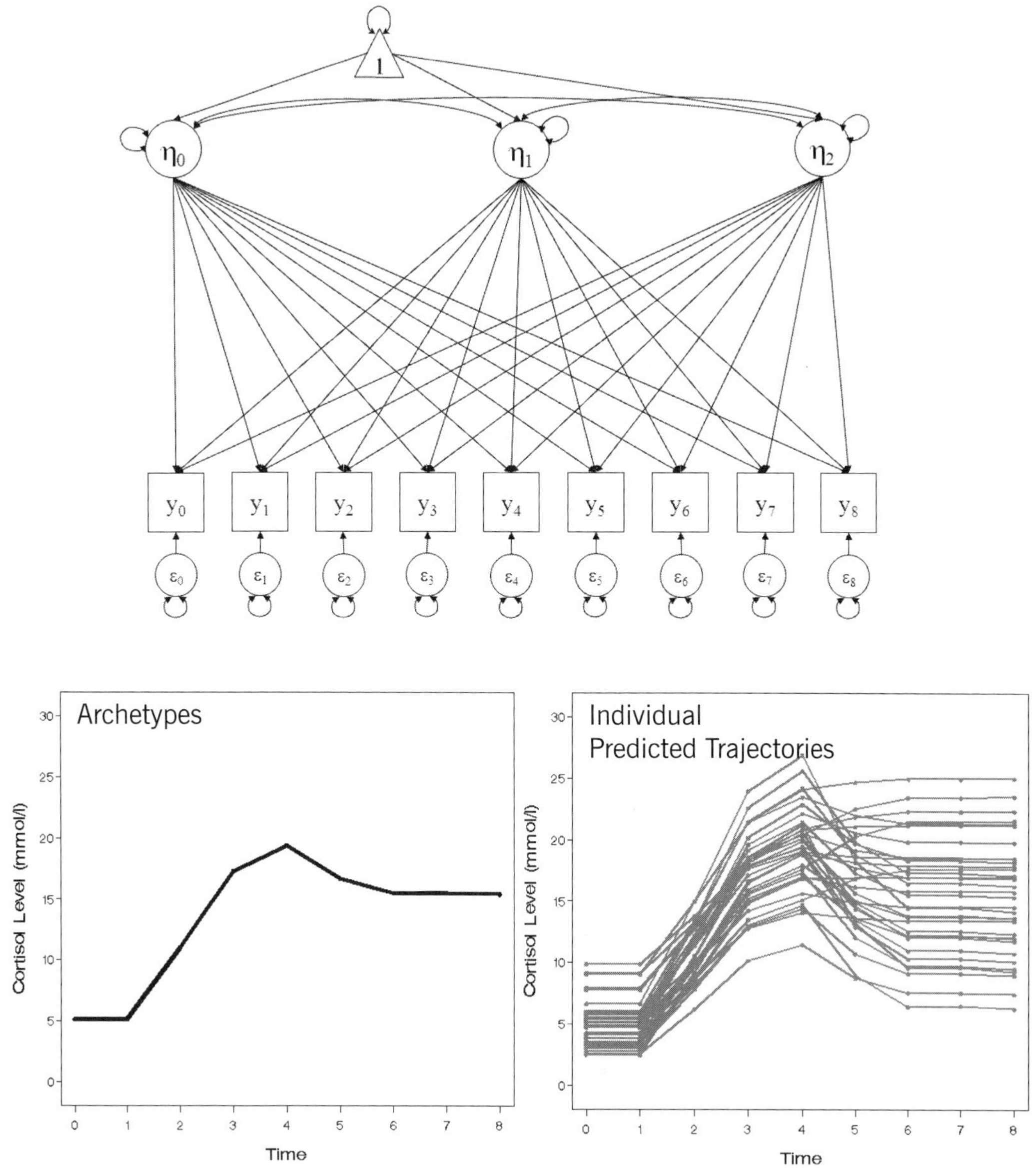

FIGURE 28.5. *Top panel*: Path diagram for the three-phase GMM. *Bottom panel*: Archetype (left) and individual (right) trajectories obtained from the one-class three-phase GMM.

That is, there were no one-headed arrows between any of the latent η variables. Focusing on the occasion-to-occasion relations, the quasi-simplex model provides yet another alternative representation of change over time within the SEM framework. Expectations from the quasi-simplex model can be written as

$$\mu_c = \Sigma_{c=1}^{C} \pi_c[\alpha_c]$$
$$\Sigma_c = \Sigma_{c=1}^{C} \pi_c\left[(I - B_c)^{-1}\Psi_c(I - B_c)^{-1'}\right] \quad \textbf{(28.8)}$$

where the mean structure is saturated, and with the additional constraint that Ψ_c is both diagonal and invariant across classes. The model is depicted graphically in Figure 28.6. Each of the observed variables has a corresponding latent η variable. The means of these variables are modeled by the set of one-headed arrows between the triangle and the latent η variables (the elements of α_c). The variances are modeled by the set of two-headed arrows on each (the diagonal elements of Ψ_c). Carryover from one time to the next is modeled by the one-headed arrows between the latent η variable (the elements of B_c). One can easily see the process orientation of the model by examining how the means and variance carry through from left to right.

The models in equations 28.5–28.8 are simplified or reduced versions of equation 28.4. The path diagrams highlight the mathematical distinctions of the models graphically. In the LCLPM (Figure 28.2), the repeated measures are not connected to each other. In the LCGM (Figure 28.3), change across time is captured by two latent variables that have means but no variance or covariance. In the single-phase growth mixture model (Figure 28.4), change across time is also captured by two latent variables that have means, variances, and a covariance. The three-phase GMM (Figure 28.5) adds complexity to the representation of change by incorporating an additional factor. Finally, in the QSMM (Figure 28.6), change over time results from "injections" of means and variances that carry through from one occasion to the next. All the models presented here constrain one or more matrices, and thus articulate a set of assumptions about how the information contained in the data are structured. The key point is that the models are vastly different and thus provide the opportunity to highlight different aspects of the data. Thus, although the use of a longitudinal mixture model is typically considered an exploratory procedure, it is, in practice, a highly constrained exploration.

Developmental Applications

In the previous sections we described a collection of longitudinal mixture models that can be derived within the general SEM mixture model. Each model places or uses constraints on particular matrices, either in their form (e.g., all the elements of Ψ are zero in the LCGM) or in differences among classes (e.g., usually Λ, Ψ, and Θ are invariant across latent classes in GMM applications). Practically, these constraints are often needed for model identification and are extremely helpful for obtaining numerically tractable solutions; they make it much easier to estimate parameters of the model. At the same time, constraints may make models more or less useful in terms of theoretical tractability. For example, within the LCLPM, the constraint that there are no connections (arrows) among the residual factors, ε_0 to ε_8 (i.e., that Θ_c is diagonal), articulates a theory that there is no autocorrelation over time within each latent class. That is, the model suggests that individuals' scores or, more precisely, the distributions of scores at a given point in time, are completely unrelated to the prior and subsequent scores or distributions—development as a collection of states, not a continuous process.

In each and every model the constraints (i.e., assumptions) can and should be evaluated with respect to their provision of numerical and theoretical tractability. Unfortunately, there are no clear guidelines about how such evaluations should proceed. It is not reasonable to concern ourselves only with theoretically tractable models for which we cannot obtain solutions. Nor is it reasonable to concern ourselves only with numerically tractable models that

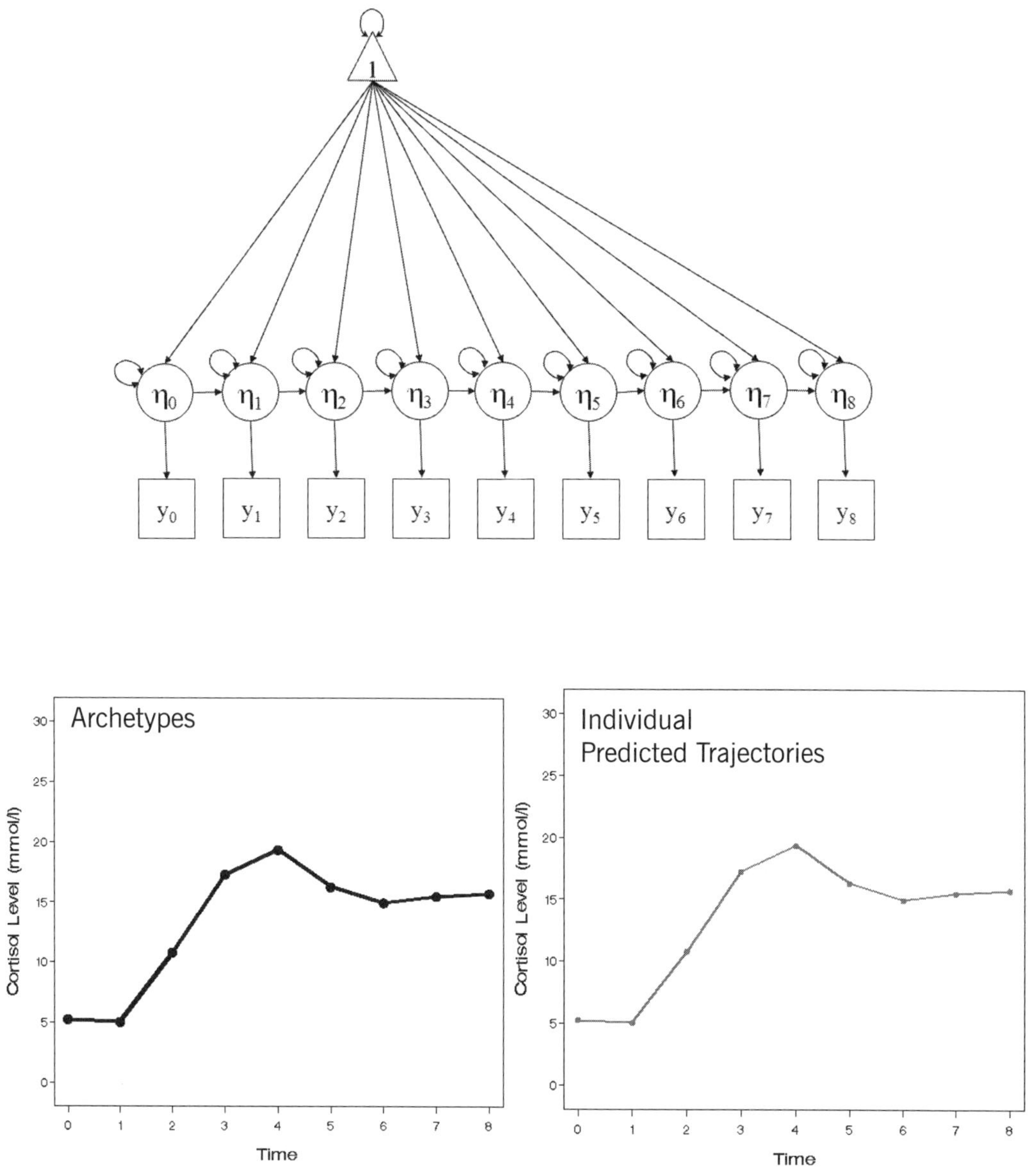

FIGURE 28.6. *Top panel*: Path diagram for the QSMM. *Bottom panel*: Archetype (left) and individual (right) trajectories obtained from the one-class QSMM.

do not align with our theoretical perspectives. Caught in the middle, we can make use of theory and choose the particular genre of model that fits best with one's research questions and underlying assumptions about development.

The general goals of all longitudinal mixture models presented here are to describe patterns of scores for individuals over time (Wohlwill, 1973). However, given the constraints inherent in their implementation, all the models outlined describe the patterns in different ways. The LCLPM describes each group's pattern of scores using a set of occasion-specific means and group-specific variances. Interpretation focuses on the pattern of group-level differences across occasions. Key assumptions regarding development are that the repeated observations are locally independent within class—that is, the ordering of the occasions is immaterial. The LCGM describes the groups' pattern of change using a relatively parsimonious set of change factors that capture each group's level at the first observation, the total amount of change, and the pattern of change across the occasions. The key developmental assumptions are that there is a distinct ordering of occasions and that all individuals within a group follow exactly the same trajectory. Any deviations from that trajectory are assumed to be noise. The GMM assumes, instead, that there are some systematic differences in change within a class—that individuals within a group do not follow exactly the same trajectory. A parsimonious set of change factors will capture each class's average level at the first observation, interindividual differences in that level within each class, the average total amount of change, the extent of interindividual differences in change within each class, and the pattern of change across the occasions. A key assumption is that within classes individuals may differ in initial level or amount of change but have trajectories of precisely the same pattern. The QSMM describes each class's pattern of change using a set of occasion-specific means, occasion-to-occasion regressions, and (residual) variances. Interpretation focuses on progression in group-level averages and rank-ordering of persons across occasions. Key assumptions are that the repeated observations are ordered and that changes in the rank ordering of individuals are indicative of the change process.

Of special note in the interpretation of the models presented is the usual use and dependence (in SEM) on sample-level summaries of the data. Models are written in terms of expectations for the observed *group-level* means and covariances—descriptions, not of any specific individual's data, but of the between-person distributions and relations among those distributions (Robinson, 1950). Thus interpretations of results for within-person change rely on assumptions that between-person differences are also indicative of within-person change (between–within convergence). Mathematically, the within-person and between-person structures are equivalent (i.e., ergodic) only under very strict (and rare) conditions, namely (1) stationarity of variables' attributes and (2) equivalence of the relations among variables for *all* individuals (see Molenaar, 2004). Except in unusual cases, the results of models based on group-level means and covariance cannot be used to make individual-level inferences without committing an ecological fallacy. In sum, care should be taken that the underlying assumptions of the models are kept in mind when interpreting the results with respect to individual-level development. After all, one does not want to be disappointed to find, in the end, that the romance novel one was reading was actually a tragedy.

Illustration

Empirical Data

To illustrate each of the models described herein we use *T*-data (persons × occasions on a single variable) obtained as part of a study of older adults' responses to stress. Using nonlinear growth and GMM (Ram & Grimm, 2007, 2009), we illustrate how these data can be approached from several perspectives. The data were collected as part of the MacArthur Successful Aging Studies to investigate interindividual differences in cortisol production and dispersion in response to a stress-provoking intervention. Nine successive measurements (coded t = 0–8) of cortisol (mmol/l) were obtained over the course of a few hours from 34 older participants. As can be seen in Figure 28.1, these data, collected over a relatively short span of time, are typical developmental data, describing within-person change over time and between-person differences in change. The first two measurements ($t = 0$ and 1) were taken as baseline measurements. Participants then began a driving simulation challenge task (the stress-provoking intervention). Observations 2, 3, and 4 were taken during and directly after the challenge and are indicators of cortisol production or stress response. The remaining observations (5, 6, 7, and 8) were taken during a postchallenge rest period and are viewed as indicators of cortisol dissipation or stress recovery (see Seeman et al., 1995; Seeman, Singer, & Charpentier, 1995, for details of the experimental protocol).

It may be noted that the sample size is relatively small ($N = 34$). The statistical procedures underlying SEM and mixture models are large sample techniques. However, there is not a general rule that precludes using these models to explore data, whether obtained from larger samples (population surveys) or smaller samples (experimental studies). Identification and description of unobserved groups depends on many factors, including the extent of between-group differences, homogeneity of the trajectories, relative group sizes, and reliability of measurement. As in the determination of statistical power for a priori hypothesis testing, the utility of post hoc explorations must be evaluated in relation to the particulars of the research question. The exploratory principles on which longitudinal mixture modeling is based apply to data collected in large panel studies and data collected in small experimental studies.

A Collection of Models

A collection of mixture models was fit to the data. Each set produced a different developmental story. Each included the following procedures: (1) problem definition, (2) model specification, (3) model estimation, and (4) model selection and interpretation (see Ram & Grimm, 2009, for a detailed account of these implementation steps). Scripts for model specification can be found at *www.crmda.ku.edu/Guilford/HDRM*. Here, we highlight interesting aspects of the process with respect to model selection and interpretation.

Model Selection and Interpretation

Fit indices for the collection of mixture models, by genre and number of classes, are given in Table 28.1. Making use of a wide variety of indices (see Masyn, 2009; Muthén, 2004; Nylund, Asparouhov, & Muthén, 2007; Ram & Grimm, 2009), we identified, within each set of mixture models, the best latent class representation of the data (indicated in boldface). When the different fit indices were contraindicated (e.g., for the LCLPM the Akaike information criterion [AIC] and Bayesian information criterion [BIC] pointed toward a four-class solution, and the likelihood ratio tests pointed toward a one-class solution), we selected the more parsimonious model.

Among the LCLPMs, the best model was a one-class model. Among the LCGMs, the best model was a two-class model. When using latent basis GMMs, the single-phase model indicated two classes, whereas the three-phase model indicated only one class. With the QSMM, there was no evidence of multiple classes; only a single class was evident. In sum, the exact same data are characterized by different archetypes when filtered through different models. Choice of genre makes a difference to conclusions about the existence of multiple classes of individuals. With one type of model, we would infer that there is only one

TABLE 28.1. Model Fit of LCLPM, LCGM, GMM (Single-Phase and Three-Phase), and QSMM

Model type	Parameters	AIC	BIC	ABIC	Entropy	Class sizes	VLMR LRT	LMR LRT	Bootstrap LRT
Latent class longitudinal profile model									
1-Class	**18**	**1701**	**1728**	**1672**	—	**34**	—	—	—
2-Class	28	1606	1649	1561	.944	15.7, 18.3	.2470	.2564	< .0001
3-Class	38	1578	1636	1517	.958	13.9, 6.9, 13.1	.2269	.2337	< .0001
4-Class	48	1541	1615	1465	.985	6.0, 6.9, 9.0, 12.1	.3172	.3280	< .0001
5-Class[a]	58	1539	1627	1446	.990	3.0, 13.0, 9.0, 5.0, 4.0	.4578	.4634	< .0001
Latent class growth model									
1-Class	10	1725	1740	1709	—	34	—	—	—
2-Class	**20**	**1600**	**1630**	**1568**	**.949**	**18.2, 15.8**	**.0197**	**.0220**	**< .0001**
3-Class	30	1582	1627	1534	.929	6.6, 14.1, 13.3	.4016	.4112	< .0001
4-Class[b]	40	1555	1616	1491	.962	6.5, 3.0, 12.5, 12.0	.3073	.3142	< .0001
Growth mixture model (single phase)									
1-Class	13	1568	1588	1547	—	34	—	—	—
2-Class	**26**	**1434**	**1474**	**1393**	**.963**	**16.6, 17.4**	**.0244**	**.0262**	**< .0001**
3-Class[(c)]	37	1409	1465	1350	.979	16.0, 10.9, 7.1	.2079	.2139	< .0001
Growth mixture model (3-phase)									
1-Class	**15**	**1411**	**1434**	**1387**	—	**34**	—	—	—
2-Class	29	1411	1455	1365	.966	6.0, 28.0	.5759	.5850	—
Quasi-simplex mixture model									
1-Class	**26**	**1346**	**1386**	**1305**	—	**34**	—	—	—
2-Class[d]	35	1347	1400	1291	.822	10.2, 23.8	.8199	.8268	.6667

Note. AIC, Aikake Information Criteria; BIC, Bayes Information Criteria; ABIC, Adjusted BIC; VLMR LRT, Vuong–Lo–Mendell–Rubin Likelihood Ratio Test; LMR LRT, Lo–Mendell–Rubin LRT.

[a]Model has more free parameters than the 54 unique pieces of information in the observed mean vector and covariance matrix.

[b]Solution was unstable and different results emerged when using different sets of starting values.

[c]Intercept variance was fixed to 0 in class 3, estimated standard errors for this model may not be trustworthy.

[d]The mean for occasion 2 was fixed to 0 in class 2 to obtain a solution.

archetype (homogeneity), whereas with another type of model, we would infer that there are multiple archetypes (heterogeneity).

Within each genre (LCLPM, LCGM, GMM [single-phase], GMM [three-phase], and QSMM), the parameter estimates were used to generate plots of the archetypal trajectories and the individual predicted trajectories. These are plotted in the lower panels of Figures 28.2–28.6. Although there are similarities, there are also nuanced differences. Viewed from a general perspective, all archetypal trajectories follow the baseline, response (increase), and recovery (decrease) pattern—as would be expected from the experimental protocol governing data collection. Examining each model's archetypes and predicted individual trajectories, we see some important differences.

In the LCLPM (Figure 28.2), the sample is composed of a single group defined by a set of occasion-specific means (and variances). The nine occasions are treated as independent; thus the expected values for the archetype are not connected by lines (left panel). Similarly, the predicted cortisol levels for any given individual in the sample are given by the means (right panel). In the LCGM (Figure 28.3), two archetypes emerged. These trajectories (left panel) differ primarily in terms of level (one lower throughout, one higher throughout). The predicted individual trajectories (right panel) clearly show that individuals are expected to follow one of two trajectories, with pure homogeneity within class. The single-phase GMM (Figure 28.4) also had two archetypes. In contrast to the LCGM, these two archetypal trajectories (left panel) are of different shapes. One is characterized by a less steep increase in response to the stressor and a relatively flat recovery, the other by a steeper increase and a relatively pronounced decrease. GMM assumptions about heterogeneity within a class are readily apparent in the predicted individual trajectories (right panel), in which we see a distinct trajectory for all 34 persons (17 in each class). The three-phase GMM has only a single archetype characterized by a flat baseline phase, an increasing response phase, and a declining and leveling recovery phase (left panel). The within-class heterogeneity is clear in the predicted trajectories. It might also be noted that the three-phase GMM with one class (AIC = 1411) fits the data relatively better than the single-phase growth mixture model with two classes (AIC = 1434). Finally, the QSMM (Figure 28.6) also has only a single archetype (left panel), characterized by a process model with a carryover of means and variances from one occasion to the next. As is clear from the individual predicted trajectories, all individuals are expected to follow the archetype exactly. In sum, the different models provide for somewhat different conclusions about the nature and extent of homogeneity and heterogeneity. Choice of genre makes a difference in our conclusions about the change process and the interindividual differences therein.

Future Directions

Our examples highlight how longitudinal mixture models offer multiple narratives from the same data and illustrate how each of these narratives is limited or shaped by the specific bounds imposed during model specification. Much can be learned about possible groups and patterns of change that exist within one's data. However, as with all exploratory procedures, what can be learned is limited by what is looked for. Thus care should be taken that the models used in the exploration both allow for and capture the type and extent of differences in longitudinal change that are expected.

We have touched on only a few of the modeling possibilities. The flexibility of the general

SEM framework in which the mixture model is placed allows for an almost infinite number of longitudinal models. The range of possibilities for articulating theoretically driven ideas about change processes and heterogeneity in those processes is limitless. Problem definitions (initial hypotheses) must be precise enough that informed choices can be made about which models to use. As the field moves forward in its formulations about the nonlinearity of development, complex conceptions of change will emerge. For each process of interest it should be clearly articulated how and when changes proceed, whether those changes manifest at the individual level, at the group level, or at the population level. Constructing precise and testable theories will make the job of choosing an appropriately matched model easier.

New challenges lie ahead in the estimation of mixture models. Currently, little is known about how much and what kind of data are needed to obtain one or another type of story. On the modeling side, we need to learn more about how the models and estimation algorithms react to outliers, missing persons, missing variables, and missing occasions, and/or complexities and anomalies in the parameter space. On the substantive side, we need to learn more about what types of models are most appropriate for representing what types of changes, the time scale on which the processes of interest occur, and where and when the interesting interindividual differences will manifest.

Longitudinal data are often rich and complex. They have much to tell us about the intricacies of development. Longitudinal mixture models provide an opportunity to obtain those stories. Just as a writer determines the genre of his or her manuscript as the characters and the plot are developed, so too the researcher constrains his or her results to one of several possibilities through the choice of models he or she elects to fit. When carefully coupled with phenotypic theory, those choices can be directed toward identification and elaboration of genre-specific archetypes. We look forward to the wide variety of stories that may emerge as data are filtered through different longitudinal mixture models to obtain action-adventures, mysteries, science fiction, fantasies, and above all, romances—because they are bound to have a happy ending.

Acknowledgments

We gratefully acknowledge the support provided by John R. Nesselroade, John J. McArdle, the Longitudinal Research Institute, and Grant No. T32 AG20500 from the National Institute on Aging, which together fostered Nilam Ram's and Kevin Grimm's initial collaborations and development. Current support comes from the National Institute on Aging (Grant No. RC1 AG035645) and the National Science Foundation REECE Program Grant (Grant No. DRL-0815787). Special thanks to Teresa Seeman and Marilyn Albert for graciously providing the example data.

References

American Psychiatric Association. (2000). *Diagnostic and statistical manual of mental disorders* (4th ed., rev.). Washington, DC: Author.

Arminger, G., Stein, P., & Wittenberg, J. (1999). Mixtures of conditional mean- and covariance-structure models. *Psychometrika, 64,* 475–494.

Bollen, K. A., & Curran, P. J. (2006). *Latent curve models: A structural equation perspective.* New York: Wiley.

Bryk, A. S., & Raudenbush, S. W. (1992). *Hierarchical linear models: Applications and data analysis.* Newbury Park, CA: Sage.

Burchinal, M., Nelson, L., & Poe, M. (2006). Growth curve analysis: An introduction to various methods for analyzing longitudinal data. *Monographs of the Society for Research in Child Development, 71*, 65–87.

Collins, L. M., & Lanza, S. T. (2010). *Latent class and latent transition analysis for the social, behavioral, and health sciences*. New York: Wiley.

Duncan, T., Duncan, S., Stryker, L., Li, F., & Alpert, A. (2006). *An introduction to latent variable growth curve modeling*. Mahwah, NJ: Erlbaum.

Grimm, K., & Ram, N. (2009). Nonlinear growth models in Mplus and SAS. *Structural Equation Modeling, 16*, 676–701.

Grimm, K. J., Ram, N., & Estabrook, R. (2010). Growth mixture models with inherently nonlinear change models using Mplus and OpenMx. *Multivariate Behavioral Research, 45*, 887–909.

Heim, C., Elhert, U., & Hellhammer, D. (2000). The potential role of hypocortisolism in the pathophysiology of stress-related bodily disorders. *Psychoneuroendricinology, 25*, 1–35.

Jöreskog, K. G. (1971). Simultaneous factor analysis in several populations. *Psychometrika, 36*, 409–426.

Lazarsfeld, P. F., & Henry, N. W. (1968). *Latent structure analysis*. Boston: Houghton Mifflin.

Lubke, G. H., & Muthén, B. (2005). Investigating population heterogeneity with factor mixture models. *Psychological Methods, 10*, 21–39.

Masyn, K. (2009). Discrete-time survival factor mixture analysis for low-frequency recurrent event histories. *Research in Human Development, 6*, 165–194.

McArdle, J. J. (2009). Latent variable modeling of differences and changes in longitudinal data. *Annual Review of Psychology, 60*, 577–605.

McArdle, J. J., & Nesselroade, J. R. (2003). Growth curve analysis in contemporary psychological research. In J. Shinka & W. Velicer (Eds.), *Comprehensive handbook of psychology: Vol. 2. Research methods in psychology* (pp. 447–480). New York: Wiley.

McLachlan, G. J., & Peel, D. (2000). *Finite mixture models*. New York: Wiley.

Miller, G. E., Chen, E., & Zhou, E. S. (2007). If it goes up, must it come down?: Chronic stress and the hypothalamic–pituitary–adrenocortical axis in humans. *Psychological Bulletin, 133*, 25–45.

Molenaar, P. C. M. (2004). A manifesto on psychology as idiographic science: Bringing the person back into scientific psychology, this time forever. *Measurement: Interdisciplinary Research and Perspectives, 2*, 201–218.

Muthén, B. (2004). Latent variable analysis. Growth mixture modeling and related techniques for longitudinal data. In D. Kaplan (Ed.), *The Sage handbook of quantitative methodology for the social sciences* (pp. 345–368). Thousand Oaks, CA: Sage.

Muthén, B. O., & Muthén, L. K. (2000). Integrating person-centered and variable-centered analysis: Growth mixture modeling with latent trajectory classes. *Alcoholism: Clinical and Experimental Research, 24*, 882–891.

Muthén, B. O., & Shedden, K. (1999). Finite mixture modeling with mixture outcomes using the EM algorithm. *Biometrics, 55*, 463–469.

Muthén, L. K., & Muthén, B. O. (1998–2006). *Mplus user's guide* (4th ed.). Los Angeles: Authors.

Nagin, D. S. (1999). Analyzing developmental trajectories: A semiparametric, group-based approach. *Psychological Methods, 4*, 139–157.

Nagin, D. S. (2005). *Group-based modeling of development*. Cambridge, MA: Harvard University Press.

Nagin, D. S., & Odgers, C. L. (2010). Group-based trajectory modeling in clinical research. *Annual Review of Clinical Psychology, 6*, 109–138.

Nylund, K. L., Asparouhov, T., & Muthén, B. (2007). Deciding on the number of classes in latent class analysis and growth mixture modeling: A Monte Carlo simulation study. *Structural Equation Modeling, 14*, 535–569.

Preacher, K. J., Wichman, A. L., MacCallum, R. C., & Briggs, N. E. (2008). *Latent growth curve modeling*. Thousand Oaks, CA: Sage.

Ram, N., & Grimm, K. (2007). Using simple and complex growth models to articulate developmental change: Matching theory to method. *International Journal of Behavioral Development, 31,* 303–316.

Ram, N., & Grimm, K. (2009). Growth mixture modeling: A method for identifying differences in longitudinal change among unobserved groups. *International Journal of Behavioral Development, 33,* 565–576.

Robinson, W. S. (1950). Ecological correlations and the behavior of individuals. *American Sociological Review, 15,* 351–357.

Seeman, T. E., Berkman, L. F., Gulanski, B., Robbins, R., Greenspan, S., Charpentier, P., et al. (1995). Self-esteem and neuroendocrine response to challenge: MacArthur Successful Aging Studies. *Psychosomatic Research, 39,* 69–84.

Seeman, T. E., Singer, B., & Charpentier, P. (1995). Gender differences in pattern of HPA axis response to challenge: MacArthur Studies of Successful Aging. *Psychoneuroendicrinology, 20,* 711–725.

Singer, J. D., & Willet, J. B. (2003). *Applied longitudinal data analysis: Modeling change and event occurrence*. New York: Oxford University Press.

Wohlwill, J. F. (1973). *The study of behavioral development*. San Diego, CA: Academic Press.

Yung, Y.-F. (1997). Finite mixtures in confirmatory factor-analysis models. *Psychometrika, 62,* 297–330.

CHAPTER 29

Multilevel Structural Equation Modeling

JAMES A. BOVAIRD
LESLIE H. SHAW

Modern research agendas in the developmental sciences are increasingly approached from an ecological perspective (i.e., Bronfenbrenner, 1979). For example, numerous environmental influences have been identified that affect obesity, particularly in children (e.g., availability of food at home, food choices at school, access to physical activity, parental modeling, neighborhood safety; see Gorin & Crane, 2008, for a review). Without understanding the multiple interrelated environmental influences that collectively represent the ecological determinants of childhood obesity, we are unable to develop interventions that are responsive to key factors that fuel the epidemic. Multilevel structural equation modeling (MSEM) is an appropriate analytical framework for such developmental research because it allows flexible and often complex modeling of phenomena within and between multiple ecological contexts.

The statistical framework for considering multiple hierarchical (i.e., children within classrooms within schools) or parallel (i.e., children within schools and neighborhoods) levels of contextual influence *on a single outcome* is available through multilevel modeling (MLM). MLM can also be used in a similar manner to model time-related repeated-measures data for the purpose of evaluating developmental trajectories. Frequently referred to as latent growth modeling (LGM), this approach can be implemented as either a multilevel model (see Hox & Boom, Chapter 25, this volume) or as a multivariate structural equation model (SEM). Oftentimes, however, contextual modeling also requires simultaneous consideration of multiple pathways of influence among multiple outcomes measured at different levels of influence. Evaluations of simultaneous causal paths, multiple outcomes, feedback loops, proximal and distal causes and outcomes, and latent variables and measurement models are all currently possible using SEM. This chapter discusses the integration of SEM and MLM as multilevel structural equation modeling that allows for consideration of complex multivariate modeling in the context of hierarchical levels of influence.

Central Issues

Perhaps the most important issue to address when considering a multilevel model in general is the determination of what constitutes a multilevel model in the first place. Bovaird (2007) broadly defined multilevel models as those containing variables measured at different hierarchically sampled levels. Thus a multilevel data set can arise either if distinct outcomes are measured at multiple levels (i.e., child level and family level) or if an outcome is measured at a particular hierarchical level but the intention is to associate it with information at another level. For instance, when studying multiple children in their family contexts, children may be described as nested within their particular family and multiple families may be further nested within neighborhoods. An appropriate multilevel approximation to this example would then reflect a combination of child-, family-, and neighborhood-level variables. According to Bovaird (2007), although a multilevel model need generally and simply to involve variables measured at multiple organizational levels, the term *multilevel modeling* has become synonymous with the statistical procedures most often used to implement the model itself, including hierarchical linear modeling (HLM), random coefficient modeling (RCM), and linear mixed modeling (LMM).

Two Perspectives on Multilevel Dependency

There are two general situations that most often lead to the need to model a behavioral phenomenon as multilevel: complex sampling and random parameters (Bovaird, 2007; Muthén, 1994). In both situations the overall observed variance among measured variables must be separated into its macro-level contextual source (i.e., between-unit variance at an organizational or group level) and its micro-level individual source (i.e., within-unit variance at the organization- or group-member level). Simply put, if the macro-level organizational unit, or *cluster*, merely serves to provide access to micro-level units and there is not a substantively interesting or necessary phenomenon to model at the macro level, then a complex sampling approach to dealing with the multilevel phenomenon that statistically adjusts for the multilevel dependency may be appropriate (Stapleton, 2006).

If there is a substantively interesting phenomenon at the macro level, *or* if there is a measurement model appropriate at the macro level, *or* if assignment to condition occurs at the macro level (as in cluster-randomized trials), then a random coefficient approach is necessary, and consideration of multiple levels of modeling is essential. That is to say, there can be a general model of interest within each contextual group that is common to all groups, but that model can vary randomly to a degree across groups to take into account characteristics of each organizational group that may affect the expression of the model within each group. The next section discusses four general approaches to modeling multilevel phenomena when the model contains substantive relevance at the macro levels.

Aggregation versus Disaggregation

Bovaird (2007) outlined three general approaches to proceeding with a multilevel data set: disaggregation, aggregation, and multilevel modeling. The *disaggregation* approach focuses on the lower (e.g., micro) level, typically the person, and occurs when the researcher ignores any complex sampling that may have given rise to the data itself by implementing a single-level model. This approach is most often used when the focus of the model is at the micro level, such as when neighborhood characteristics are used to predict child-level participation in extracurricular activities. Disaggregation most often results in underestimated standard errors that then lead to an inflated Type I error rate. In addition, ignoring the presence of clustered data tends to lead to inflated model fit statistics, particularly if there is a large intraclass correlation (ICC), large within-cluster sample sizes, and highly correlated variables (Muthén, 1994).

The reverse approach, *aggregation*, or an *ecological analysis*, focuses on the macro level by using group means or other aggregates of micro-level variables in a macro-level analysis. An example is using aggregates of student-level academic achievement as an indicator of teacher-level performance, as in the so-called value-added accountability systems. Although disaggregation typically suffers from an increased Type I error rate, aggregation may suffer from an increased Type II error rate, or reduced power. Use of aggregation—or disaggregation—often results in an increased chance of committing an *ecological fallacy* in which inferences about micro-level behavior are incorrectly made from inaccurately represented macro-level data, or an *atomistic fallacy* in which inferences about macro-level behavior are incorrectly made from micro-level data (Hox, 2010).

Burstein, Linn, and Cappel (1978) proposed a two-step approach to modeling complex sampling data by developing separate models at each level of the sampling hierarchy, referred to as a *slopes-as-outcomes* approach. This approach also has limitations in that it lacks a simultaneous statistical integration of all hierarchical levels. Consequently, *multilevel modeling* is the preferable approach to analyzing data obtained through complex sampling because it accounts for the nonindependence due to hierarchical nesting, incorporates multiple sample sizes, and allows for *simultaneous* inferences at all organizational levels. Multilevel modeling is most often accomplished through either extension of the general linear model to include random effects, in addition to traditional fixed effects (see Hox & Boom, Chapter 25, this volume), or through an SEM approach (see Grimm & Ram, Chapter 24, this volume).

Isomorphism

Multilevel modeling has the capacity to simultaneously model variables measured at different sampling levels, and several authors have elaborated on the parallels in implementing a multilevel model between MLM and SEM (see Bauer, 2003; Bovaird, 2007; Curran, 2003; Duncan, Duncan, Okut, Strycker, & Li, 2002; Mehta & Neale, 2005; and Muthén, 1994; among others). As a number of these authors have pointed out, there is an isomorphism, or structural equality, in the mathematical systems used to define model parameters in the MLM and SEM frameworks such that LGMs for longitudinal or repeated-measures data, as well as hierarchically nested MLM models, can be parameterized, or mathematically defined, within the SEM framework. Further illustrating the blurred boundaries between these two modeling frameworks, some methodologists have also demonstrated how a measurement model can be implemented in a multilevel model (e.g., Bauer, 2003; Raudenbush, Rowan, & Kang, 1991) or as a multilevel model itself (see Mehta & Neale, 2005). In fact, "many of the differences between MLM and SEM-based approaches are based on tradition rather than the inherent limitations of either model" (O'Connell & McCoach, 2008, p. 135).

Multilevel Structural Equation Modeling

In demonstrating the isomorphism between MLM and SEM formulations of standard LGM for longitudinal data (observations nested within individuals) and the traditional contextual MLM example (students within classrooms), methodologists have taken advantage of SEM's use of a *multivariate* approach to implementing an MLM. In the SEM framework, the unit of analysis is the macro-level unit, and the accompanying data are a t-variate outcome vector, where t is the number of members of each macro-level unit. Thus, a two-level model in the MLM framework is a one-level model in the SEM framework. This leads to the claim that MSEM can consider three levels (kids within classes as one level, within schools as a second level). Bovaird (2007) makes the distinction between this application of MLM as SEM and true MSEM, in which separate models are specified at each level (child, classroom, and school) and those levels are allowed to interact.

Thus perhaps the key conceptual difference between MLM and SEM approaches is the unit of analysis used by the models, which is also logistically made apparent when preparing data for analysis in the respective frameworks. The MLM framework uses a single, univariate outcome variable for all participants nested within a particular cluster, whereas SEM utilizes a multivariate approach. MLM data are often referred to as being in person-period or stacked format, in which each line in the data file represents a micro-level observation with a separate variable representing macro-level group membership. Conversely, SEM data are in wide or multivariate format, in which each row in the data matrix pertains to a macro-level unit and multiple columns for each micro-level unit are nested within each macro-level unit. SEM offers the further advantage of providing model fit estimates and the capability of modeling multiple pathways at different levels, as well as the ability to analyze univariate and multivariate outcomes (Bauer, 2003).

Multilevel Measurement Models

One advantage of modeling complex structures through MSEM is the flexibility to allow different measurement and structural models at the macro and micro levels. Consistent with recommendations to develop portions of the overall model in isolation prior to evaluating the model as a whole (e.g., Anderson & Gerbing, 1988), a researcher should determine whether the macro-level latent factor means the same thing as the same factor measured at the micro level. In addition, if the proportion of observed variance attributed to between-groups sources at the macro level can be calculated for individual indicators, can the same proportion be calculated for the latent factor? Essentially, this presents a measurement invariance problem (see Millsap & Cham, Chapter 7, this volume), but rather than testing invariance between groups or over time, invariance must be assessed across hierarchical levels.

Mehta and Neale (2005) discuss a flexible general–specific model perspective for developing a multilevel confirmatory factor analysis (MCFA) model developed through a four-step process. First, a univariate random-intercepts model is established to determine the extent of between-groups variance on the individual indicators by calculating a univariate ICC. The ICC is the ratio of between-cluster variance to the total variance and is an index of the magnitude of dependency among observations due to clustering. Determination of a significant ICC is typically used to justify the need for a multilevel model. Next, a multivariate random-intercepts model is established to determine the degree of correlation between indicators at both the macro and micro levels and to provide a baseline model for model comparison. This is followed by implementing an MCFA with a measurement model at each level to evaluate whether that measurement model is configurally invariant at each level through model comparison statistics. Finally, multilevel metric invariance is tested. If metric invariance is successfully supported, then a random intercept and a common scale have been established for the latent variable, and a latent variable ICC can be calculated. If between-level metric invariance for the latent variable is not established, then the question remains as to whether the construct has the same meaning at both the macro and micro levels. If this is the case, the researcher must consider either that there is a different construct measured at the macro level than at the micro level or evaluate the theoretical implications of partial metric invariance (see Millsap & Cham, Chapter 7, this volume).

By imposing a specific measurement model at each level, a latent variance can be obtained for both the macro and micro levels. However, if a common scale for the latent variable at both levels is not achieved by establishing configural and metric invariance, the magnitude of the obtained variances cannot be directly compared through calculation of a latent ICC. Assuming a two-level model, the variance of the latent factors at both levels,

$$V(\eta_{gi}) = \Psi_T = \Psi_B + \Psi_W \tag{29.1}$$

can be used to calculate the latent variable ICC:

$$ICC = \Psi_B/(\Psi_B + \Psi_W) \tag{29.2}$$

Bauer (2003) and Curran (2003) presented an alternative approach to conceptualizing a multilevel latent variable through a hierarchical factor structure similar to a factor-of-curves approach. Unfortunately, this approach is quite restrictive in that it requires a set of constraints on factor loadings and residual variances, including configural invariance of the measurement model between levels, metric invariance between macro and micro levels, and zero residual variance at the macro level (Mehta & Neale, 2005).

Conceptual Principles and Statistical Assumptions

It is well known that SEM allows simultaneous consideration of both measurement and structural portions of complex models. Like MLM, the need for MSEM is indicated by sources of variance to be modeled *within* grouping units, or clusters, as well as variance to be modeled *between* grouping units. As in the MLM parameterization, separate micro- and macro-level equations can be specified as either a within- or between-groups model, respectively. MSEM extends traditional SEM by allowing the measurement and structural models to be modeled at multiple hierarchical levels and potentially to differ by level.

Goldstein and McDonald (1988) and Muthén (1989, 1994) demonstrated that it is possible to divide the total variance–covariance matrix into matrices representing the within-groups and between-groups sources of variance to formulate an MSEM. According to Muthén's approach, individual observations, y_{gi}, are decomposed into (1) the aggregated mean of group g of which individual i is a member, y_g, and (2) an individual deviation from the group mean, y_w. Consequently, decomposing the observed variables into within- and between-groups sources leads to the ability to decompose the overall observed covariance matrix into between- and within-groups sources:

$$V(y_{gi}) = \Sigma_T = \Sigma_B + \Sigma_W \qquad \textbf{(29.3)}$$

Muthén (1989, 1994) demonstrated that the pooled within-group sample covariance matrix S_{PW} is the unbiased estimate of the population within-groups covariance matrix (Σ_W), but S_B is the unbiased estimate of the composite matrix ($\Sigma_W + c\Sigma_B$) rather than the population between-groups covariance matrix (Σ_B). The scaling parameter c becomes necessary as an ad hoc estimator roughly equivalent to the average within-groups sample size. As S_B is a weighted sum of Σ_W and Σ_B, it is necessary to model the between- and within-groups models simultaneously in order to model S_B properly. See Muthén (1994) for calculation of Σ_W and Σ_B. The population covariance matrices can then be described by separate models:

$$\Sigma_B = \Lambda_B \Psi_B \Lambda'_B + \Theta_B \qquad \textbf{(29.4)}$$
$$\Sigma_W = \Lambda_W \Psi_W \Lambda'_W + \Theta_W$$

This allows the same measurement and structural model to be hypothesized at both levels or different models to be hypothesized.

Estimating Multilevel Structural Models

Ideally, the best estimation procedure for the variance partitioning approach presented in equation 29.4 is maximum likelihood (ML) because it maximizes "the likelihood that the observed data were drawn from a particular population" (Bovaird, 2007, p. 161). ML estimation accounts for all available data and provides efficient and consistent estimates (Duncan et al., 2002). A number of approaches have been proposed to implement the general model presented in equation 29.4 using ML estimation but with limited degrees of success (e.g., McDonald, 1993; Mehta & Neale, 2005). Consequently, alternative estimation procedures have been developed due to the computational burden of ML estimation procedures, especially with unbalanced or missing data, as well as large sample sizes, variables, or time points.

Muthén (1994) demonstrated that a limited-information maximum likelihood (MUML) estimator could be used to approximate ML estimates when data are balanced or relatively balanced (Duncan et al., 2002; Muthén, 1994). According to Duncan and colleagues (2002), this method greatly simplifies the model specification and offers a degree of utility compared with ML estimation. When within-group sample sizes are balanced, the MUML estimator is equivalent to ML estimation, but it is only an approximation of ML with unbalanced sample sizes. As a contrast to full information, or raw data, maximum likelihood (FIML; Arbuckle, 1996), MUML has been referred to as a limited-information (Hox, 2010) approach largely due to its reliance on the ad hoc group sample size estimator c and its use of Σ_W and Σ_B as input rather than the raw data. Though desirable, FIML is computationally demanding and is available in SEM software only for two-level models.

Muthén's Maximum Likelihood Estimate

Muthén (1989, 1994), showed how MSEM could be implemented with existing SEM software using the MUML estimator for unbalanced data, which is also referred to as the partitioning variance approach. By treating each level of nesting as a unit of analysis and each individual outcome as a separate, cluster-level indicator of a latent variable, standard SEM methods can then be used to model the separate between- and within-cluster variances (Mehta & Neale, 2005). The between- and within-group matrices can be modeled from a multiple-group perspective within most SEM software programs by which one "group" is the within-groups model and the other "group" is the between-groups model. The primary hurdle in a partitioning variance approach to MSEM is the proper estimation of the within- and between-group covariance matrices. For a more thorough introduction than is provided here, see Muthén (1989, 1994).

Other Alternatives

Duncan and colleagues (2002) discuss two alternative ML methods based on data restructuring rather than an alternative estimation method—a factor-of-curves approach and a curve-of-factors approach. A factor-of-curves model (FOC; McArdle, 1988) may be used to model growth among multiple units with a higher order common factor describing the communality across lower order growth model parameters. In contrast, a curve-of-factors approach (COF; McArdle, 1988) is used to fit a higher order growth model on lower order latent factors. Bauer (2003) and Curran (2003) presented generalizations of these applications that also permit cross-sectional multilevel models appropriate for the common children-within-classrooms context.

Following the model specifications outlined in Duncan et al. (2002), a three-level factor-of-curves LGM is presented in Figure 29.1A. The micro level of the FOC model includes repeated observations of each student's individual growth trajectory (level 1) as explained by the student's individual differences in initial status and change over time (level 2). The macro level of the model includes the variation among schools (level 3).

The level 1 within-student growth model is expressed as a $T \times 1$ vector of repeated measures for each student in each school, where T is the number of repeated measures. The level 2 between-student model for individual growth within a school is a 2×1 vector with two latent growth factors per student representing the intercept and slope for each student's growth structure. In the FOC parameterization, a separate two-level growth structure is established for each of n students within a school and organized horizontally in the figure. The latent means for each student's growth structure are fixed to zero for identification, but are estimated at level 3 (although not shown in the diagram). Finally, the level 3 model contains a 2×1 vector of the latent growth means for the two between-school growth parameters and a vector of school-level variation distributed with a zero mean vector and variance–covariance matrix (ϕ) between the growth parameters.

Extending MSEM beyond Two Levels

Most SEM software programs are limited to two-level hierarchical structures (Duncan et al., 2002); thus, modeling data with more than two levels requires either sophisticated programming techniques or substantial data restructuring in order to manage the data in a way that is conducive to MSEM. Several authors (Bauer, 2003; Duncan et al., 2002) have demonstrated the ability to estimate more than two levels within the SEM framework. For instance, Bauer (2003) estimated a three-level MLM of item responses (level 1) nested within teachers (level 2) nested within schools (level 3) as a two-factor MSEM by incorporating equality constraints on factor loadings, residual variances of the items, and variances

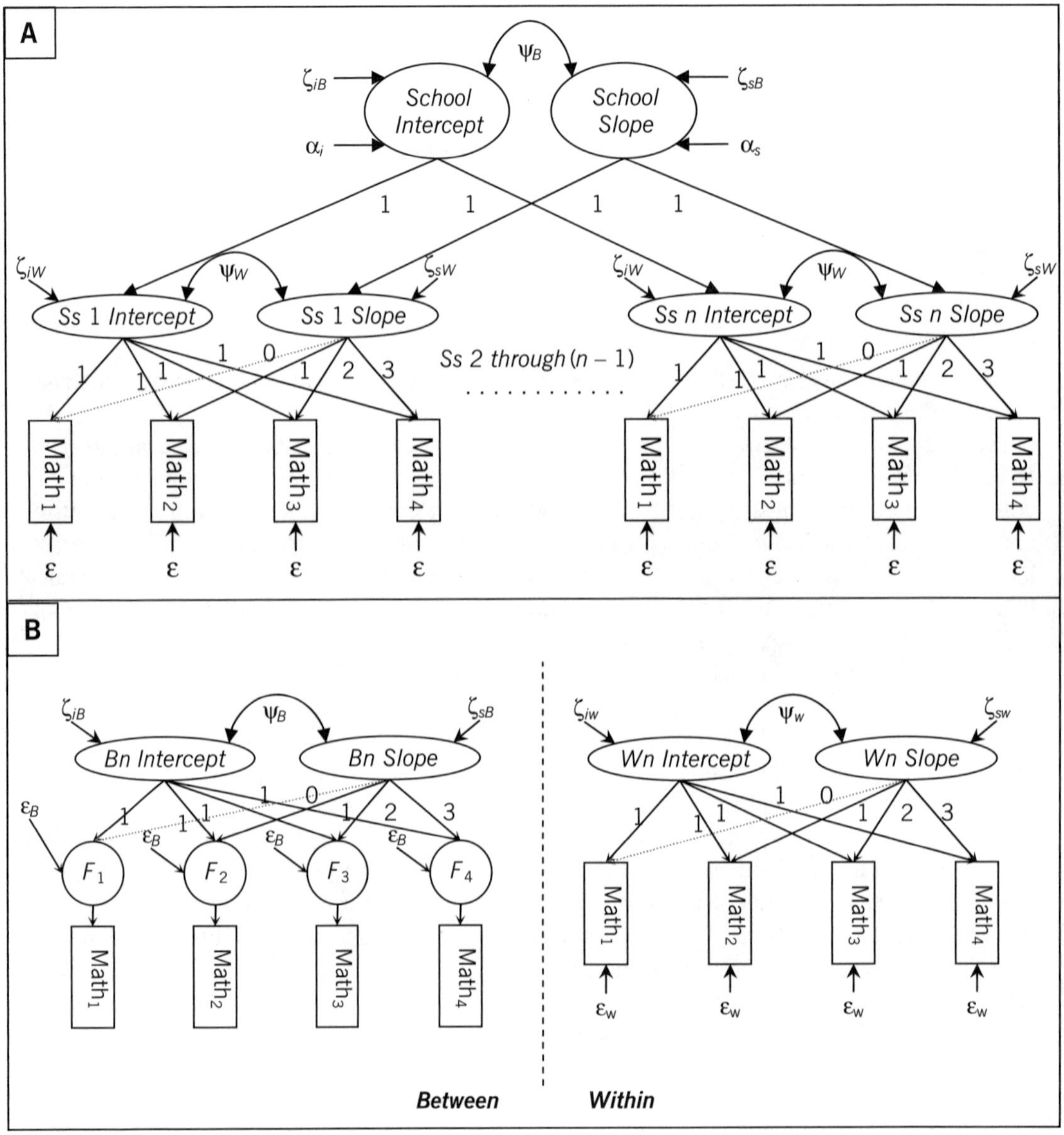

FIGURE 29.1. (A) A three-level factor-of-curves growth model representing the development of mathematics achievement among young school-age children nested within schools. (B) A multilevel latent growth model presented as a two-level MSEM with child development (level 1, within-level, or micro-level) nested within school contexts (level 2, between-level, or macro-level).

and covariances of the factor scores for teachers within a school. The model included a measurement model for two outcome factors and a measurement model for the items within each factor. The data set was structured so that each row represented a school and the first nine entries (variables) in the row contained nine item responses from one teacher from that school. Entries 10–18 contained item responses for a second teacher in each school. This pattern was followed for up to 30 teachers per school, resulting in up to 270 entries per row/school. As not all schools had the same number of teachers, resulting in unbalanced within-school sample sizes, any schools with less than 30 teachers had missing data for the nonobserved item responses. By including two latent variables to capture the nesting of teachers within schools on each measurement factor, the model is then parameterized as a second-order latent variable model. Equality constraints placed on common indicators were repeated over teachers sampled within a school, allowing the common within-school variances for teachers to be drawn into the second-order factor.

Duncan and colleagues (2002) also demonstrated the ability to model more than two levels of nesting in the latent variable model (LVM) framework by estimating a four-level hierarchical model of adolescent substance use over a 1-year period, with adolescents nested within households nested within geographic regions. They demonstrated the comparability of a multilevel model estimated in the SEM framework and a hierarchical linear model using commonly available software. Duncan et al. estimated a three-level latent growth model using an FOC model within a limited-information multilevel latent growth modeling approach to add the fourth level (geographic region), allowing for simultaneous decomposition of the sample covariance matrix into between- and within-level components. They found roughly comparable results for parameters estimated in the SEM and MLM software programs used, yet the different estimation procedures used by these programs may have been responsible for the slight differences found in the random effects estimates.

General Procedural Framework

Three general approaches have been proposed for developing multilevel structural models. The initial framework put forth by Muthén (1994) was a four-step process involving (1) conducting a conventional analysis ignoring the multilevel structure, (2) determining the degree of between-groups variance, (3) exploring the within-groups structure, and (4) exploring the between-groups structure. Hox (2010) outlined a different stepwise procedure for model development, suggesting that the researcher evaluate model fit between a set of nested null, independence, and saturated models. Hox's approach focuses on determining whether there is any meaningful between-groups structure rather than investigating whether individual variables have meaningful between-groups variance. Mehta and Neale (2005) also presented a model comparison perspective for developing MSEMs that follows the common procedures in the MLM literature. They suggest concentrating on determining the degree of between-groups variance, developing the structural or fixed portion of the model, and then clarifying the random components. Interested readers may also consult Peugh and Enders (2010) regarding further suggestions and concerns in developing the between-groups portion of the model when exploration at that level is necessary.

Muthén's (1994) four-step framework mirrors the various multistep procedures recommended for developing standard SEM models that involve considering and developing portions of the overall model in isolation prior to evaluating the model as a whole (see Anderson & Gerbing, 1988). This is not surprising, though, because Muthén's framework was initially presented in the context of the MUML approach, which considers the between and within portions of the model separately by separating Σ_T into Σ_B and Σ_W. Conversely, Hox's approach and the framework employed by Mehta and Neale (2005) are more consistent with the model comparison perspective common in MLM applications.

Ryu and West (2009) suggest that when evaluating model fit for an MSEM, it is important to test level-specific model fit as opposed to standard approaches, which evaluate the entire model. Standard approaches tend to be less sensitive to level-specific misfit, dominated by the within-group model, and to be unable to differentiate the sources of misfit (e.g., it is not clear which level, if not both, is misspecified). The authors also note that misfit on one level might affect estimates at the other level. Rather than evaluating global model fit and assuming invariance across levels in terms of fit, Ryu and West advocate the use of level-specific test statistics in order to pinpoint specific areas of misspecification.

Both approaches may be intuitive to researchers depending on their modeling background (i.e., MLM or SEM) and the intention of the model. Because MSEM is a synthesis of both the MLM and SEM paradigms, a combination of approaches may provide the most utility in developing models. Testing model fit between competing nested models, as espoused by Hox (2010) and Mehta and Neale (2005), is also possible using the four-step framework. Perhaps random coefficient models implemented as structural models may be best developed through the frameworks illustrated by Hox and Mehta and Neale, whereas traditional structural models with meaningful components at both macro and micro levels may be best developed through Muthén's (1994) approach, with either approach utilizing appropriate model fit statistics for decision making.

Developmental Applications

Predictors measured at macro organizational levels in an MLM analytical context are commonly referred to as contextual effects. Context can be defined as "any event or condition outside the organism that is presumed to influence, or be influenced by, the person's development" (Bronfenbrenner & Crouter, 1983, p. 359). Developmental researchers know the ecological importance of considering dynamic *macrosystemic* interactions of cultural, political, and economic systems alongside the *chronosystem* of changes across time, in terms of both individual child development and development of higher level organizational units or even broader systems (Bronfenbrenner, 1979). Perhaps the most significant benefit of MSEM to developmental researchers is its ability to allow complex simultaneous modeling of multiple levels and types of contextual influences on individuals and their development. Snijders and Bosker (1999) outlined several *propositions* that can be used to summarize the types and nature of contextual effects and relationships typically contained within multilevel models. These propositions are presented pictorially in Figure 29.2.

First, *macrounit* propositions (see Figure 29.2A) occur when both predictors and outcomes are not directly observable at the macro level but are instead measured at the micro level. This occurs when level 2 units are themselves aggregates of level 1 units. The need for multilevel modeling is hardly obvious in this scenario but is often still necessary due to the well-known problems (e.g., increased chance of committing an ecological fallacy, decreased power) associated with this example of an aggregation analysis. In contrast, *microunit* propositions (see Figure 29.2B) occur when both predictors and outcomes are measured at the micro level but the data arose from a complex sampling design in which

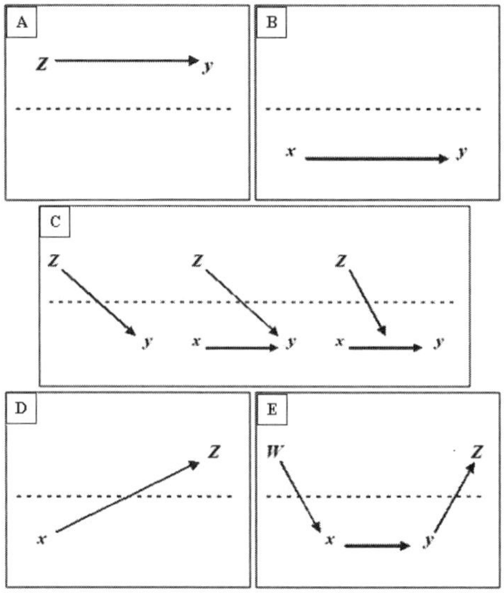

FIGURE 29.2. Examples of types of multilevel relationships. (A) macrounit proposition; (B) microunit proposition; (C) macro–micro propositions; (D) emergent proposition; (E) causal chain proposition.

micro-level units were selected as a result of sampling their respective macro-level units. This represents a less obvious case of the need for multilevel modeling when contextual dependency is a nuisance rather than of substantive interest.

Presenting a more obvious need for multilevel modeling are multilevel propositions in which both macro and micro effects on y may be hypothesized by researchers. Panel C in Figure 29.2 presents three common *macro–micro* propositions. First, perhaps, a given macro variable is presumed to predict a micro-level outcome, as may be the case when the availability of early childhood centers in a community influences whether a child in that community is adequately prepared for kindergarten. Second, perhaps there is a *conditional macro–micro* proposition in which the effect of early childhood centers on school readiness is conditional upon the child's family's socioeconomic status (SES) that also has a known influence on school readiness. Finally, perhaps there is a *cross-level interaction* in that, rather than having an additive effect of community facility availability and socioeconomic status, the type of early childhood center available moderates the impact of SES on readiness. That is to say that availability of Head Start programs may permit enrollment in early childhood programs despite a family's low SES, leading to increased school readiness.

Emergent (micro–macro) propositions (see Figure 29.2D) in which the micro-level predictor has an effect on macro-level outcomes, such as student attitudes affecting teacher stress, present a further need for multilevel models. That is, although one student's attitude may contribute to a teacher's stress level, some aggregate measure of student attitude is the true predictor of a teacher's stress. The notion of an emergent proposition is not new, but consideration of such relationships within the multilevel context without some level of aggregation is more recent. Rather than using a simple within-class average as the predictor (i.e., aggregation), latent variable approaches such as MSEM allow for simultaneous modeling of both within- and between-class variability, which also serves to disattenuate the predictive effect for unreliability of the within-class average (Ludtke et al., 2008).

Finally, leading to a clear need for MSEM are *causal chain* propositions (see Figure 29.2E) in which macro–macro relationships (or micro–micro relationships) may be mediated through micro (or macro) variables. For instance, parenting practices (macro level) influence children's study habits (micro level), which in turn influence the child's achievement. Poor parenting practices that lead to deficient work habits and underachievement by the child may then lead to increased parental stress.

Preacher, Zyphur, and Zhang (2010) point out that the between and within sources of variance in two-level designs are uncorrelated, or orthogonal. As a consequence, between components cannot be used to predict within components, or vice versa, as would be required in macro–micro, emergent, or causal chain propositions. Preacher and colleagues raise this issue as an important one for researchers to consider when they propose multilevel propositions, and especially for those considering mediational hypotheses. Statistically, the effect of one variable on another must be at the same level, as in micro–micro or macro–macro propositions. A predictor at the macro level is constant within all micro-level members of the group; therefore, variability between macro-level units cannot influence variability within a macro-level unit. Thus, although a research hypothesis may suggest that macro-level variables are related to micro-level variables, the actual statistical model implied by cross-level propositions must test whether macro-level variance is related to variance among macro-level aggregates (manifest or latent) of micro-level variables. Appropriate modeling of such cross-level effects is revisited in the second empirical illustration testing a multilevel mediation hypothesis.

Illustrations

Three-Level Model of Mathematics Development

Shaw and Bovaird (2010) sought to extend the work of Bauer (2003) and Duncan and colleagues (2002) by comparing a hierarchical FOC approach to the MUML and FIML approaches for modeling a three-level LGM as an MSEM using mathematics achievement data from the kindergarten cohort of the Early Childhood Longitudinal Study (ECLS-K). ECLS-K is a federally funded longitudinal database from the National Center for Educational Statistics (NCES), which follows the academic achievement of a nationally representative sample of children enrolled in kindergarten during the 1998–1999 school year. Shaw and Bovaird used the first four waves of data (fall and spring kindergarten, fall and spring first grade) from children nested within schools in a midwest region who did not change schools from the fall of their kindergarten year to the spring of first grade. Two samples were considered, based on distribution of children within schools: a balanced sample of $n = 10$ randomly sampled children from each of $k = 56$ schools for a total sample size of $N = 560$ children and an unbalanced sample that averaged $n \sim 13.568$ children per each of $k = 74$ schools for a total sample size of $N = 1{,}006$ children. In order to avoid further sample size imbalance due to nonresponse or attrition (see Bauer, 2003), students with missing data were excluded from the analysis.

Initially, a two-level LGM for mathematics assessment was extended to include students nested within schools by treating the repeated-measures portion of the model as a multivariate measurement model. In this three-level FOC LGM, the first level of the model includes students' individual growth trajectories, the second level models the variation in students' growth within a school, and the third level of the model includes the variation among schools. The baseline three-level LGM was modeled using two estimation procedures: (1) Muthén's MUML limited-information estimator and (2) a FIML estimator.

Three-Level Factor-of-Curves Latent Growth Model

Following the model specifications outlined in Duncan and colleagues (2002), a three-level FOC LGM was implemented as a one-level SEM (see Figure 29.1A, page 508). This structure is similar to a first-order multivariate associative LGM but with two higher order factors hypothesized to explain the variability in lower order growth factor. The first level of the model includes students' individual growth trajectories, the second level models the variation in students' initial status and subsequent growth across kindergarten and first grade within a school, and the third level includes the variation in average status and average change among schools. In this structure and with a balanced sample, the school is the unit of analysis rather than the student, so the data file contains one row for each school in the study ($k = 56$). Each row contains the repeated measures for each student enrolled in that school, so with $n = 10$ students, each with four waves of data, the balanced data file contains 40 columns organized as 10 sets of 4 observations. The unbalanced data file then contains one row per each of the $k = 74$ schools with 88 columns (the largest school size was $n = 22$) organized as 22 sets of 4 observations. For schools (rows) with less than $n = 22$ students, missing data are introduced for each set of four observations less than the maximum within-school sample size.

Limited Information and Full-Information Multilevel Latent Growth Models

This three-level MSEM can also be approached through the variance partitioning method in which the total variance–covariance matrix is divided into between- and within-group matrices, $S_T = S_B + S_W$. Based on this approach, the between- and within-group matrices can be modeled simultaneously either (1) by utilizing a multiple-group perspective with an SEM software program through Muthén's MUML approach by specifying each component (within vs. between) as a separate group in the model or (2) through direct ML as implemented in most commercial SEM programs.

This model is visually depicted in Figure 29.1B on page 508. In contrast to the data structure necessary for an FOC model, the variance-partitioning data file treats each student as the unit of analysis. Consequently, each row contains four repeated observations per student in addition to a school-level identifier used to determine the between-schools variance–covariance matrix.

Table 29.1 presents parameter estimates and standard errors for the three-level MSEM as estimated by (1) a hierarchical FOC model, (2) a limited-information maximum likelihood variance-partitioning model (MUML), and (3) a full-information maximum likelihood variance-partitioning model (ML). As can be seen in Table 29.1, the ML and MUML approaches provide nearly identical parameter estimates and standard errors when the data are balanced, but estimates (and standard errors) vary considerably between the variance-partitioning approaches and the FOC model. The discrepancy is further magnified when the data are unbalanced and is especially apparent in the random effect (variance) estimates relative to the fixed effects. This is not surprising, as the MUML approach is equivalent to

TABLE 29.1. Parameter Estimates and Standard Errors for a Three-Level MSEM of ECLS-K Mathematics Achievement Data by Estimator

	ML		MUML		FOC-ML	
	Est.	*SE*	Est.	*SE*	Est.	*SE*
			Balanced			
Fixed effects						
Intercept	22.72	0.91	22.72	0.92	23.36	0.65
Slope	10.96	0.30	10.96	0.30	10.17	0.22
Random effects						
I (b)	23.72	8.75	24.14	7.43	17.40	4.37
I with S (b)	0.00	—	0.00	—	0.00	—
S (b)	–0.94	0.94	–0.93	0.81	4.10	0.78
I (w)	43.92	4.77	43.89	4.43	50.75	4.36
I with S (w)	13.68	1.54	13.70	1.44	11.65	1.37
S (w)	7.62	0.89	7.61	0.90	7.78	0.83
Residual	23.38	1.70	23.41	1.62	24.53	1.10
			Unbalanced			
Fixed effects						
Intercept	22.81	0.85	22.97	0.74	23.50	0.61
Slope	11.05	0.29	10.94	0.24	10.24	0.22
Random effects						
I (b)	30.36	8.93	27.08	6.25	22.36	4.17
I with S (b)	0.00	—	0.00	—	0.00	—
S (b)	0.04	1.03	1.06	0.72	5.34	0.81
I (w)	39.99	3.34	44.81	5.89	47.57	3.08
I with S (w)	14.11	1.11	13.35	2.52	11.40	1.00
S (w)	7.31	0.67	6.26	1.31	7.92	0.62
Residual	25.27	1.32	18.18	5.58	25.29	0.83

FIML (i.e., it provides ML estimates) under balanced designs and becomes only an approximate ML estimator when the design is unbalanced due to the use of the scaling parameter, *c*, as an ad hoc estimator roughly equivalent to the average within-groups sample size. The FOC model, as a hierarchical factor model similar to the MSEM approach proposed by Bauer (2003), requires further restrictions to the model, including no residual variances at the between level that are allowed in the variance-partitioning approach. As unbalanced cluster sizes are fairly common in applied settings, researchers should implement FIML to achieve ML estimation rather than the MUML procedure. When cluster sizes are balanced, choice of procedure should be based on software familiarity and availability.

Parent–Teacher Relationship as a Mediator of an Intervention Effect on Child Behavior

Sheridan and colleagues (2011) examined whether teacher perceptions of the parent–teacher relationship mediate the positive effect of a behavioral intervention on child social skills among a sample of children identified as expressing disruptive behavior in the classroom. Sheridan et al. originally tested the hypothesized relationship as a multilevel path analysis, which is a special case of MSEM with no measurement model or latent variables. They tested the effect of assignment to the intervention condition (vs. control) on postintervention assessments of the parent–teacher relationship and social skills with preintervention assessments as covariates. This example presents an analysis of simulated data based on parameters reported by Sheridan and colleagues using an LGM structure for change rather than using postintervention assessments with preintervention covariates. Data were simulated for $n = 2–3$ children per each of $k = 75$ classrooms for a total of $N = 225$ children on three measurement occasions, each with no missing data.

In this context, MSEM was necessitated because of a complex sampling paradigm that resulted in 2–3 students being sampled per classroom and because classroom was also the unit of randomization to receive the intervention. Although the complex sampling may have been dealt with through the use of sampling weights (see Stapleton, 2006), assignment of classrooms to receive the intervention constitutes "something interesting" at the classroom level and requires a multilevel model.

This example tests the hypothesis that the behavioral intervention serves to effect positive change in the parent–teacher relationship, which in turn leads to improvements in children's social skills. Based on the Preacher and colleagues (2010) framework, the effect of an improved parent–teacher relationship on change in the child outcome is modeled at the within-classrooms level (level 1), and the effects of assignment to the intervention on classroom-average parent–teacher relationship and classroom-average child social skills will be modeled at the between-classrooms level (level 2). Change in the mediator and the outcome are operationalized as latent change across three assessment waves, as estimated through an LGM structure.

Sheridan and colleagues (2011) previously reported a significant direct effect of the behavioral intervention on several child outcomes, including social skills based on teacher reports. The MSEM presented in Figure 29.3 suggests a significant indirect effect of the intervention on change in social skills as mediated through change in teachers' reports of their relationships with the child's parent(s). The multilevel mediation model demonstrated an excellent fit to the data; $\chi^2(27) = 28.40, p = .39$; $CFI > 0.99$; $RMSEA = .02$; $SRMR_w = .03$, $SRMR_b = .08$. The indirect effect of the intervention on social skills through parent–teacher relationships was significant: indirect $B = 0.21$, $t = 2.79$, $p < .05$. The reported significant direct relationship between the intervention and child social skills (Sheridan et al., 2011) became nonsignificant with the inclusion of the mediating variable ($B = 0.14$, $t = 1.54$, $p > .05$), suggesting that an improved parent–teacher relationship fully mediates the effect of the intervention on children's improved social skills. Parameter estimates based on simulated data with population parameters derived from results in Sheridan and colleagues are presented in the path model in Figure 29.3. Readers are reminded that this example is intended as an illustration and based on simulated rather than empirical data. No substantive implications should be drawn from this example.

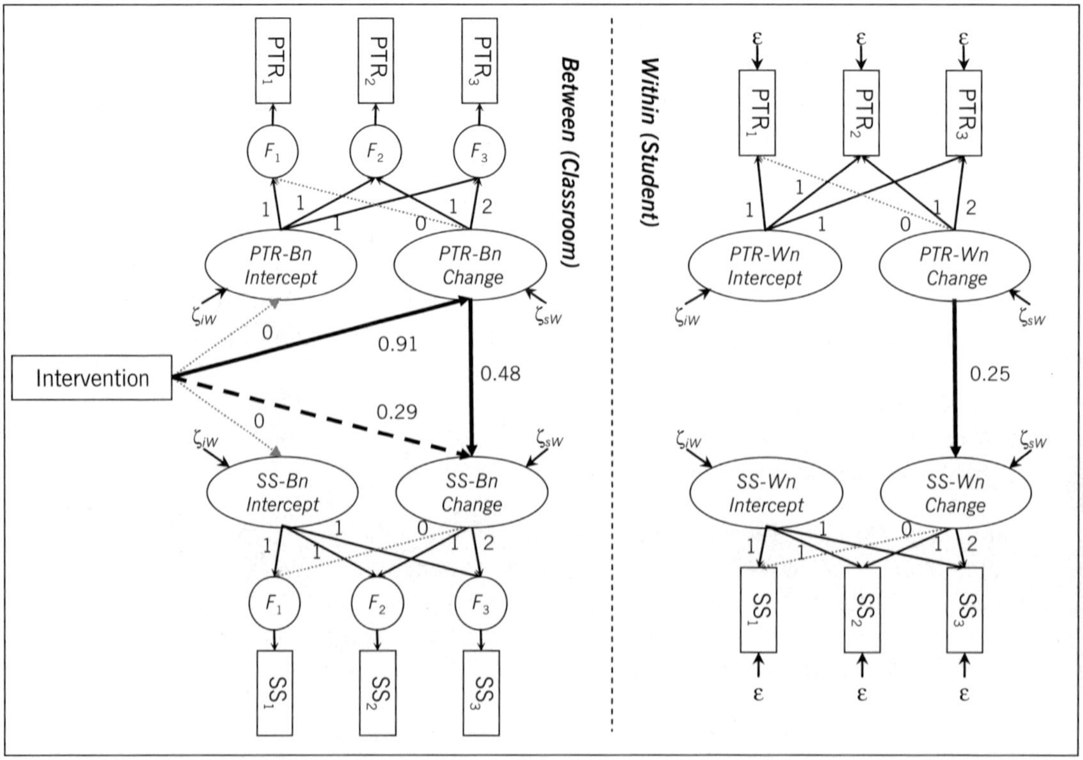

FIGURE 29.3. Path diagram and standardized solution for mediational MSEM. PTR, parent–teacher relationship; SS, social skills; grayed-out, dashed lines, 0.0; solid dashed line, not statistically significant at the $p < .05$ level. Residual variances and exogenous covariances are not shown to enhance diagram readability.

Future Directions

A number of areas within MSEM are still being actively researched by methodologists and statisticians alike, including estimation refinements, determination of the appropriate standardized solution to enhance interpretation, development of additional exact and approximate model fit indices to aid in model development, and clarification of the role of the multiple sample sizes involved in multilevel modeling. Small sample sizes at macro levels can substantially limit the complexity of the overall model (Mehta & Neale, 2005), necessitating a "large" sample size for MSEM, particularly when using ML estimation methods. Oftentimes, recommendations suggest a minimum of at least 50–100 units at the highest organizational level. Additional work in the area of Bayesian estimation of MSEM models, especially in the case of small macro-level sample sizes, is also needed. Bayesian methods have already been shown to be effective with small sample sizes in standard SEM (see Lee & Song, 2004).

MSEM presents several advances over standard SEM and MLM that can be of use to the developmental researcher despite such limitations. Hierarchical data structures (multilevel modeling) are becoming increasingly common, and the need to develop complex latent variable models with the capacity to simultaneously model both multiple structural pathways and multiple latent variables is increasing as well. This is especially true for developmental researchers, as the role of context and ecology continues to be emphasized. Although not illustrated in this chapter per se, the general SEM framework is flexible enough to accommodate a number of the methodologies discussed in this volume as special cases, and theoretically any SEM can be generalized to a multilevel case in the presence of complex sampling.

References

Anderson, J., & Gerbing, D. (1988). Structural equation modeling in practice: A review and recommended two-step approach. *Psychological Bulletin, 103*, 411–423.

Arbuckle, J. L. (1996). Full information estimation in the presence of incomplete data. In G. A. Marcoulides & R. E. Schumacker (Eds.), *Advanced structural equation modeling: Issues and techniques* (pp. 243–277). Hillsdale, NJ: Erlbaum.

Bauer, D. (2003). Estimating multilevel linear models as structural equation models. *Journal of Educational and Behavioral Statistics, 28*, 135–167.

Bovaird, J. A. (2007). Multilevel structural models for contextual factors. In T. Little, J. Bovaird, & N. Card (Eds.), *Modeling contextual effects in longitudinal studies* (pp. 149–182). Mahwah, NJ: Erlbaum.

Bronfenbrenner, U. (1979). *The ecology of human development: Experiments by nature and design.* Cambridge, MA: Harvard University Press.

Bronfenbrenner, U., & Crouter, A. C. (1983). The evolution of environmental models in developmental research. In P. H. Mussen (Series Ed.) & W. Kessen (Vol. Ed.), *Handbook of child psychology: Vol. 1. History, theory, methods* (4th ed., pp. 357–414). New York: Wiley.

Burstein, L., Linn, R. L., & Cappel, F. J. (1978). Analyzing multilevel data in the presence of heterogeneous within-class regression. *Journal of Educational Statistics, 3*, 347–383.

Curran, P. J. (2003). Have multilevel models been structural equation models all along? *Multivariate Behavioral Research, 38*, 529–569.

Duncan, T., Duncan, S., Okut, S., Strycker, L., & Li, F. (2002). An extension of the general latent variable growth modeling framework to four levels of the hierarchy. *Structural Equation Modeling, 9*, 303–326.

Goldstein, H. I., & McDonald, R. P. (1988). A general model for the analysis of multilevel data. *Psychometrika, 53*, 455–467.

Gorin, A. A., & Crane, M. M. (2008). The obesogenic environment. In E. Jelalian & R. G. Steele (Eds.), *Handbook of childhood and adolescent obesity* (pp. 145–161). New York: Springer.

Hox, J. J. (2010). *Multilevel analysis: Techniques and applications* (2nd ed.). New York: Routledge.

Lee, S., & Song, X. (2004). Evaluation of the Bayesian and maximum likelihood approaches in analyzing structural equation models with small sample sizes. *Multivariate Behavioral Research, 39*, 653–686.

Ludtke, O., Marsh, H. W., Robitzsch, A., Trautwein, U., Asparouhov, T., & Muthén, B. (2008). The multilevel latent covariate model: A new, more reliable approach to group-level effects in contextual studies. *Psychological Methods, 13*, 203–229.

McArdle, J. J. (1988). Dynamic but structural equation modeling of repeated measures data. In R. B. Cattell & J. Nesselroade (Eds.), *Handbook of multivariate experimental psychology* (2nd ed., pp. 561–614). New York: Plenum Press.

McDonald, R. P. (1993). A general model for two-level data with responses missing at random. *Psychometrika, 58*, 575–585.

Mehta, P. D., & Neale, M. C. (2005). People are variables too: Multilevel structural equations modeling. *Psychological Methods, 10*, 259–284.

Muthén, B. O. (1989). Latent variable modeling in heterogeneous populations. *Psychometrika, 54,* 557–585.

Muthén, B. (1994). Multilevel covariance structure analysis. *Sociological Methods and Research, 22,* 376–398.

O'Connell, A., & McCoach, B. (Eds.). (2008). *Multilevel modeling of educational data*. Charlotte, NC: Information Age.

Peugh, J. L., & Enders, C. K. (2010). Specification searches in multilevel structural equation modeling: A Monte Carlo investigation. *Structural Equation Modeling, 17,* 42–65.

Preacher, K. J., Zyphur, M. J., & Zhang, Z. (2010). A general multilevel SEM framework for assessing multilevel mediation. *Psychological Methods, 15,* 209–233.

Raudenbush, S. W., Rowan, B., & Kang, S. J. (1991). A multilevel, multivariate model of studying school climate with estimation via the EM algorithm and application to U.S. high school data. *Journal of Educational Statistics, 16,* 296–330.

Ryu, E., & West, S. G. (2009). Level-specific evaluation of model fit in multilevel structural equation modeling. *Structural Equation Modeling, 16,* 583–601.

Shaw, L. H., & Bovaird, J. A. (2010). *Extending multilevel structural equation modeling beyond two levels*. Unpublished manuscript.

Sheridan, S. M., Bovaird, J. A., Glover, T. G., Garbacz, S. A., Witte, A., & Kwon, K. (2011). *A randomized trial examining the effects of Conjoint Behavioral Consultation on disruptive behaviors and the mediating role of the parent–teacher relationship*. Manuscript submitted for publication.

Snijders, T., & Bosker, R. (1999). *Multilevel analysis: An introduction to basic and advanced multilevel modeling*. Thousand Oaks, CA: Sage.

Stapleton, L. M. (2006). An assessment of practical solutions for structural equation modeling with complex data. *Structural Equation Modeling, 13,* 28–58.

PART VI

Nonindependent Data Analysis

CHAPTER 30

Foundational Issues in Nonindependent Data Analysis

WILLIAM L. COOK

Suppose you had a sample of 10 students and for each you had a measure of an independent (predictor) variable and a dependent (outcome) variable. Suppose also that in your small sample there was a fairly large effect of the independent variable on the dependent variable, but not quite large enough to be statistically significant. A power analysis indicates that if you had 10 more participants, the effect would be statistically significant. You consider making a copy of each student's data (both the independent variable and dependent variable) and adding it into the file with the original scores. You change the ID number of these duplicated scores so that now you have what appears to be a sample of 20 students. When you rerun the analysis, the prediction is statistically significant.

Is there something wrong with this approach, beside the fact that it constitutes scientific misconduct? Well, you really have only 10 independent observations. Student 1's outcome score is matched perfectly with student 11's score (i.e., the copy), student 2's outcome is matched perfectly with student 12's outcome (the copy), and so on. These outcome scores are redundant, not independent. Statistical inference (i.e., concluding that something happened more often—or less often—than chance can explain) depends on the number of times some phenomenon is replicated in a sample of *independent* observations. However, when the outcome of one participant provides information about the outcome of another participant (i.e., they are statistically associated), they are nonindependent. In this case, an inference based on the assumption that each observation can be counted as an independent observation would be mistaken.

The degree of nonindependence in actual research is probably never as great as in the example of the duplicated data. However, ignoring the issue can lead to mistaken inferences, and results one thought were reliable may prove to be spurious. In developmental research, in which individuals are observed over time within particular contexts (e.g., family relationships) that influence the individual and that are themselves changing (e.g., as family members develop over time), nonindependence of observations is common. In this chapter I provide a simple and straightforward introduction into "the problem" of nonindependent observations. I discuss the contexts in which it is likely found, how it affects the statistical analyses used to test hypotheses, what types of individual and social processes bring it about, how it is modeled and measured, and why, when handled appropriately, it is an asset rather than a problem for developmental research.[1]

In statistical theory the sample size, or *N*, is assumed to measure independent observations. This is called the "independence assumption." Correlated observations are not independent. The size of the correlation of the outcome scores measures the degree of nonindependence. It does not matter whether the correlation is positive or negative; if the outcomes are correlated, the sample size (i.e., *N*) does not accurately reflect the number of independent observations. In the example of duplicated scores presented earlier, the "true" *N* (i.e., the number of independent observations) was half the size of the *N* after duplication. In the more common case of nonindependent observations, the effective *N* (i.e., the number of independent outcomes) is less than the observed *N*, and how much less depends on the size of the correlation that measures nonindependence.

Why is it necessary to adjust the size of the sample *N*? *N* is used in a number of statistical formulas that provide the basis for making inferences. It is used, for example, in the formula for a variance and in determining the degrees of freedom. Consequently, if the sample *N* does not represent independent observations, especially if it overestimates the number of independent observations, its use in a statistical formula can result in bias. Specifically, there will be bias in the *standard error* of the test statistic and therefore in the *p*-value of the significance test (Kenny & Judd, 1986). If there is serious nonindependence, an analysis that takes nonindependence into account is required. Unlike some assumptions of statistical theory (e.g., normal distribution), which can sometimes be violated without very serious consequences, violation of the independence assumption typically has serious consequences.

When there is some reason to suspect that the observations are not independent, the level of nonindependence should be tested. When should one suspect that one's observations are nonindependent? Nonindependent observations are often found in four common research contexts: observations over time (e.g., longitudinal data), group data (e.g., children within families), data from people in close spatial proximity to each other (e.g., residents of the same neighborhood) (Kenny & Judd, 1986), and social network data. In longitudinal samples (or any over-time design), an individual's past behavior is usually correlated with his or her future behavior. This kind of nonindependence is called *serial dependence*, because each score in a series of scores is correlated with one or more prior scores in the series. Serial dependence can arise because there is stability in a person's personality, or because the behavior is biologically determined, or because social factors maintain the behavior within a certain range of values (Warner, 1992). Serial dependence must be taken into account in statistical analyses because the observed number of over-time observations is not equal to the number of *independent* observations (i.e., there is nonindependence). An excellent introduction to the problem of serial dependency can be found in discussions of the interrupted time-series design (e.g., Cook & Campbell, 1979, Chapters 5 and 6) and the spectral analysis of social behavior (e.g., Warner, 1998).

Nonindependence is also common in data from group members, including two-person groups, or dyads. There is group nonindependence if the scores of group members are

[1]Much of the material in this chapter is covered in Chapters 2, 7, 11, and 15 of *Dyadic Data Analysis* (Kenny, Kashy, & Cook, 2006).

more similar (or dissimilar) to each other than they are to the scores of people who are not members of the same group (Kenny, Kashy, & Cook, 2006, p. 4). Group nonindependence is found among members of a family, members of a clique, students in a classroom, and similar contexts. As discussed later, group nonindependence sometimes—but not always—indicates that the individuals are *interdependent*. Interdependence is a special case of nonindependence that occurs when one person's behavior is contingent on another's. If there is group nonindependence, the scores of group members will be correlated within a given point in time. Of course, if scores are correlated within time, they will usually be correlated across time, as well. In analyses of group relationships observed over time (e.g., dyadic versions of sequential analysis, cross-lagged regression analysis, and some applications of growth curve analysis), both group and serial nonindependence are likely to be present.

Observations of individuals situated within spatial proximity to each other may also be similar. For example, the *nearest neighbor model* reflects the observation that people from the same neighborhood tend to be more similar on variables such as social and economic status. However, neighbors are not typically considered to be members of a group in the way that family members or students in a classroom are. Nonetheless, they are likely to be exposed to some of the same events (e.g., communicable diseases) because people who live in close proximity are likely to have more contact with each other. I return to the topics of group, serial, and spatial nonindependence later in this chapter. However, the primary focus is dyadic nonindependence, because much of what applies to the dyad generalizes to these other contexts.

Sources of Nonindependence in Dyadic Analysis

Within the various contexts in which group nonindependence is found, there are certain processes that are the source of the similarity or nonindependence of scores. Kenny has identified four sources of dyadic nonindependence in dyads (Kenny, 1996; Kenny & Judd, 1986): compositional effects, partner effects, mutual influence, and common fate. *Compositional effects* refer to the situation in which people are similar before they even meet or became paired. A classic example in psychological experiments is the selection of members of the control group to be matched on some variable with someone in the treatment group, the purpose being to control for individual differences. In this case, *matched pairs* have been intentionally created. It is easy to see how this design feature could invalidate the use of an independent samples *t*-test (the Student's *t*) to test the difference between the treatment and control groups. One would need to use a matched pairs *t*-test or some other method of statistical analysis (e.g., mixed-model regression) to compensate for the nonindependence. Compositional effects also arise naturalistically. For example, children who are friends tend to be similar in many ways. This can be due, in part, to the tendency of children to select similar others as friends (Laursen, Popp, Burk, Kerr, & Stattin, 2008).

The interaction history of dyad members can also produce nonindependence in measures of their characteristics. *Partner effects* occur when characteristics of one person affect the outcome of the partner. For example, extremely unresponsive parenting may create learned helplessness in children (Fincham & Cain, 1986), or a mother's playfulness may produce a positive mood in a child that subsequently leads to greater compliance with maternal demands (Lay, Waters, & Park, 1989; Parpal & Maccoby, 1985). *Mutual influence* occurs when each partner's outcome affects the other's outcome or, in other words, there is dyadic feedback. Reciprocity of negativity is perhaps the most common form of mutual influence. One person's negativity is very likely to elicit negativity from a partner, which will itself be reciprocated, creating a positive feedback loop that can be self-perpetuating (Cook, Kenny, & Goldstein, 1991; Gottman, Coan, Carrere, & Swanson, 1998). Partner effects and mutual influence both indicate that the outcomes are *interdependent*, because one person influences the other. *Common fate* is a form of nonindependence that does not imply a process of interpersonal influence. Rather, it occurs when group members are affected by a common factor. For example, children who grew up in the Great Depression had similar attitudes toward investing in the stock market as adults because they had the common experience of the stock market crash in 1929 (Elder, 1999). Children who grow up in the same family may be similar because of shared environmental factors (Moos & Moos, 1981; Olson, Portner, & Lavee, 1985), but siblings can also contribute nonshared factors to each other's environment that may magnify their differences (Cook & Kenny, 2006; Plomin, Asbury, & Dunn, 2001). As is seen later, these different processes imply different *models of nonindependence*.

Measurement of Nonindependence

As mentioned earlier, statistical tests assume that the sample consists of independent replications of the outcome of interest, and nonindependence violates this assumption. If one suspects that there are nonindependent observations in one's data, it is important to check. Therefore, one needs to know how to measure it. The measurement of nonindependence in dyads depends on two key factors: (1) whether the dyad members are *distinguishable* or *indistinguishable* and (2) whether the outcome is measured on a quantitative scale (e.g., marital satisfaction) or a categorical scale (e.g., a "yes" or "no" response). Dyad members are distinguishable if there is some meaningful variable on which they differ. For example, sibling dyads (except twins) are distinguishable on the basis of birth order. Other examples of distinguishability are family roles (e.g., parent vs. child), occupational roles (e.g., supervisor vs. worker), and gender. For distinguishable dyads assessed on a quantitative scale, nonindependence can be measured by the Pearson correlation. However, when the dyad or group members are *indistinguishable*, (e.g., best friends, gay couples, twins), the Pearson correlation will not be correct.

Dyads consist of two people whom we can designate person A and person B. When dyad members are distinguishable, there is no question about the identity of person A (e.g., the mother) and person B (e.g., the infant). When dyad members are indistinguishable (e.g., identical twins), there is no clear way to designate who is person A and who is person B. Consequently, when entering their data for analysis, their scores are arbitrarily assigned to one data column (e.g., column A) or the other (e.g., column B). It is easy to compute a Pearson r that associates the scores in column A with the scores in column B. But given that the assignment to columns was arbitrary, one could take a few of the scores in the A column and exchange them with the corresponding scores from column B and compute the Pearson r again. However, the Pearson r would now have a different value. Consequently, the Pearson r is not a good measure of nonindependence for indistinguishable dyads. For indistinguishable dyad members (assessed on a quantitative scale), nonindependence should be measured by the *intraclass correlation*. The intraclass correlation is not affected by the arbitrary assignment of dyad members to groups.

The analysis of variance (ANOVA) method of calculating the intraclass *r* provides some insight into why the intraclass *r* is unaffected by the arbitrary arrangement of dyad members' scores. In this analysis, each dyad has an identifying number (in additional to subject ID), and this dyad ID is used as the independent variable in an ANOVA. The outcome variable for person A and person B from each dyad is entered on a separate record. So if one has a sample of 50 dyads, there will be 100 records (i.e., the observed *N* will be 100). Members of the same dyad would have different outcome scores, but they will have the same dyad ID number. When dyad ID is used as the independent variable (which has 50 levels!) in a one-way ANOVA, the results for the between-groups factor will indicate how much of the variance is explained by group membership. If people in the same dyad have systematically similar (or dissimilar) scores, then the independent variable (dyad ID) in the ANOVA will explain more of the variance. Specifically, the ANOVA results will provide a measure of the mean square between groups (MS_b) and the mean square within groups (MS_w). The MS_b measures the variance due to dyad (the variance in the dyad means times 2). It would be zero if all the dyad means are the same. The MS_w measures the variance within dyads. It will be zero if, within each dyad, each person has the same score. The ANOVA intraclass *r* is calculated by the following formula:

$$r_I = \frac{MS_B - MS_W}{MS_B + MS_W} \tag{30.1}$$

It measures the proportion of the total variance accounted for by dyad membership. Thus it does not rely on who is person A and who is person B within each dyad. There are different ways to measure the intraclass *r* (Griffin & Gonzalez, 1995; Kenny & Judd, 1986; Kenny, Kashy, & Cook, 2006) besides the ANOVA method.

For distinguishable dyads whose outcomes are categorical, nonindependence is measured by Cohen's kappa (Cohen, 1960). For example, if you wanted to measure nonindependence in the attachment styles (assume four categories) of 100 sibling pairs, one would construct a 4 × 4 table in which the attachment style of one child (e.g., older siblings) defines the columns and the attachment style of the other child (i.e., younger siblings) defines the rows. The diagonal cells of this table will show at what points siblings are similar in their attachment styles, and the off-diagonal cells will indicate how often siblings differ in attachment style. Cohen's kappa tests whether the observed agreements differ from the number of agreements expected by chance, much as in a chi-square test. A kappa of 0 indicates that agreement is exactly what is expected by chance, so there is independence. A kappa of 1.0 indicates perfect agreement. The lower limit of kappa can be less than –1.0, so it cannot be interpreted exactly like a correlation. Kenny and colleagues (2006) provide a detailed introduction to the measurement of nonindependence, including some suggestions for the analysis of nonindependence in categorical scores for the indistinguishable case.

Effect of Nonindependence on Statistical Tests

As noted earlier, it does not matter whether the correlation of dyad members' scores is positive or negative; the fact that they are not independent leads to bias in the statistical test. Negative nonindependence occurs when there are dyadic processes such as compensation (e.g., lenient mother vs. strict father) and social comparison (e.g., a rival's happiness might make one unhappy) and in situations in which the more work one person does, the less there is for the other to do (e.g., division of household labor). The larger the correlation (positive or negative), the smaller the *effective* N (and the correct degrees of freedom). If the correlation of outcomes is perfect (i.e., +1 or –1), the effective N equals the number of dyads. In most cases the effective N will be somewhere between the number of dyads and the number of individuals in the sample (Kenny, Kashy, & Bolger, 1998). Typically, the larger the N, the more power one has to test a hypothesis. By using the observed N rather than the smaller, effective N in a power analysis (Cohen, 1988), one can underestimate the number of participants needed for a particular study. By leading one to collect too small a sample, nonindependence can affect one's study even before the data have been collected.

The effect of nonindependence on a particular analysis depends on whether the correlation for nonindependence is positive or negative and whether the independent variable varies within or between dyads. A *within-dyad* variable is one on which dyad members have different scores (e.g., gender) and a *between-dyad variable* is one on which dyad members have the same score (e.g., years married) but which varies from dyad to dyad. If the independent variable varies between dyads and the two outcomes have a positive correlation, the test will be too liberal (i.e., the p-value would be smaller than it should be, leading to Type I errors). If the independent variable varies between dyads and the outcomes are negatively correlated, the test will be too conservative (i.e., too many Type II errors). If the independent variable varies within dyads and the outcomes are positively correlated, the test will be too conservative, and if the independent variable varies within dyads and the outcomes are negatively correlated, the test will be too liberal. Kenny and colleagues (1998) provide formulas for calculating how much bias is introduced into an analysis by treating individuals as the units of analysis when there is nonindependence of observations. As a general rule, if the p-value for a test of nonindependence is .20 or less, individuals should not be treated as the units of analysis (Myers, 1979). However, the p-value for nonindependence should be estimated while controlling for the independent variables. In other words, nonindependence should be measured on the unexplained variance in dyad members' outcomes. This can be clearly seen in the path diagrams representing common models of dyadic relationships.

Models of Nonindependence in Dyadic Relationships

If the outcome scores of dyad members are not correlated, then one can treat individual outcomes as the unit of analysis and use ordinary statistical models (ANOVA, regression) to test the effects of independent variables. But if observations are nonindependent, treating the individual as the unit of analysis would lead to biased results. In this case, special models that treat the dyad (or group) as the unit of analysis should be used. In this section I present three models of nonindependence from the classic article "Models of Nonindependence in Dyadic Research" (Kenny, 1996). My purpose in presenting these models is not to provide detailed information on their statistical analysis but to illustrate how three different processes produce nonindependent observations in dyadic outcomes. Each model is described in terms of the simplest scenario, one in which there is one predictor variable (X) and one outcome variable (Y) for each member of a dyad, or four variables altogether. In each case, the dyad members are assumed to be distinguishable according to some meaningful categorical variable (e.g., gender or family role). The models are easily modified for use with dyad members who are indistinguishable (e.g., identical twins, same-sex couples; Kenny et al., 2006, Chapter 7).

The Actor–Partner Interdependence Model

The path diagram for the actor–partner interdependence model (APIM; see Figure 30.1) presents in an intuitive manner how characteristics of the partner contribute to nonindependence of observations and how including the partner effects in the model controls for this nonindependence. The simplest version of the APIM consists of two outcomes (Y_1 and Y_2) from two paired individuals (person 1 and person 2) who may have any of several types of relationship to each other (e.g., parent and child, teacher and student, or nontwin siblings). The independent variables (X_1 and X_2) measure some personal characteristic of person 1 and person 2 (e.g., age, attachment style, perceived control in the relationship).

The horizontal path from X_1 to Y_1 measures the actor effect for person 1, and the horizontal path from X_2 to Y_2 measures the actor effect for person 2. An *actor effect* measures the extent to which one's outcome is predicted by one's own characteristics. The diagonal paths from X_2 to Y_1 and from X_1 to Y_2 measure the partner effects. *Partner effects* measure the extent to which a person's outcome is predicted by characteristics of the partner. There are also two important correlations in the model. The double-headed arrows connecting the X variables indicate how similar the partners are on the predictor variables, and the correlation between the error or residual terms (e_1 and e_2). The importance of this residual correlation will become clear momentarily.

Note that in the path diagram, the paths from X_1 to Y_1 and from X_1 to Y_2 are bolded. These paths are highlighted because they illustrate that both Y_1 and Y_2 are affected by X_1. If there is a positive effect of X_1 on both Y_1 and Y_2, then when the X_1 score is high, both the Y_1 and Y_2 scores will tend to be high, and when the X_1 score is low, both the Y_1 and Y_2 scores will tend to be low. In other words, because X_1 affects them both, Y_1 and Y_2 will tend to rise and fall together; they will be positively correlated, and they will be nonindependent. (If both are also affected by X_2, X_2 will also contribute to nonindependence.) By including the effect of X_1 on Y_1 in the analysis, we explain the variance in Y_1 that is due to X_1. If we did not include X_1 as a cause of Y_1 in our model, the variance due to X_1 would become part

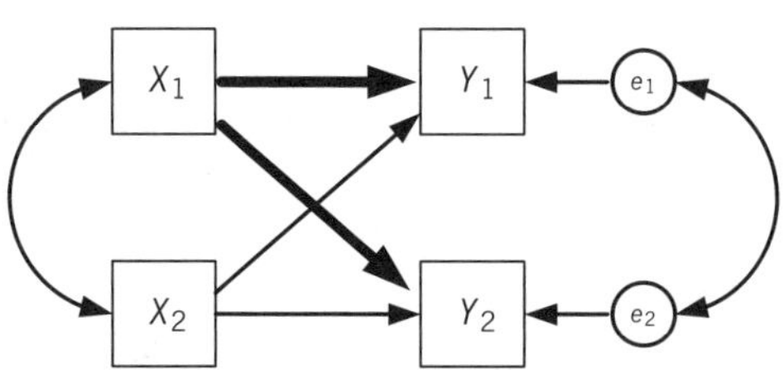

FIGURE 30.1. The actor–partner interdependence model. X_1 and X_2 are independent variables for person 1 and person 2, Y_1 and Y_2 are their respective dependent variables, and e_1 and e_2 are the corresponding residual variances. The effect of a person's X on his or her own Y is an actor effect. The effect of a person's X on the partner's Y is a partner effect. Bolded arrows indicate that Y_1 and Y_2 are both influenced by X_1 and will, therefore, be nonindependent. Correlation (curved arrow) of the residuals indicates that there is nonindependence beyond that explained by the model.

of the residual or unexplained variance in Y_1 (i.e., e_1). We also explain the variance in Y_2 that is due to X_1 by including the X_1 to Y_2 path in our analysis. If we did not include this path in the model, the residual for Y_2 (i.e., e_2) would contain unexplained variance due to X_1. But we have included these paths in our model. Consequently, neither residual contains variance due to X_1, so any correlation between e_1 and e_2 must be due to factors other than X_1. Because X_2 is also a predictor of Y_1 and Y_2, we have removed from the residuals any variance due to X_2. Consequently, we have removed (or controlled for) two sources of nonindependence in the Y_1 and Y_2 scores. Recall that nonindependence actually refers to the correlation between two outcomes that exists after controlling for the independent variables. Thus, if our model has *not* accounted for all the nonindependence in the data, this residual correlation would be significant. By including the outcomes of both people in the analysis, we are able to measure the residual nonindependence.

The assumption of independent observations would not have been violated if we had tested separate models for person Y_1's outcome and person Y_2's outcome. In one model, we could regress Y_1 on X_1 and X_2 to estimate the actor and partner effects predicting Y_1. In a second model, we could regress Y_2 on X_1 and X_2 to estimate the actor and partner effects predicting Y_2. In both models, the sample size will be equal to the number of dyads, so the number of independent observations is not inappropriately large. These analyses would be relatively simple (i.e., ordinary regression analysis), whereas estimating both partner effects and both actor effects in a single model requires more complicated statistical analysis (e.g., multilevel modeling or structural equations modeling). However, being able to estimate the correlation of the residuals gives important additional information about the phenomenon under study, and this cannot be done without both outcome variables in the analysis. This correlation tells us whether there is statistically significant nonindependence in the outcomes, above and beyond the nonindependence we have explained. In other words, it suggests that a factor (or factors) that the dyad members have in common accounts for additional significant variance in each person's outcome. This can be important hypothesis-generating information, guiding our understanding of the phenomenon and our elaboration of the model. For information on the specifics of APIM analysis, see Ackerman, Donnellan, Kashy, and Conger, Chapter 31, this volume, and Chapter 7 in *Dyadic Data Analysis* (Kenny et al., 2006).

The Mutual Influence Model

Like the APIM, the mutual influence model (Kenny, 1996) is a model of interdependence because it models a process of interpersonal influence (see Figure 30.2). In this model, each person's outcome is partially caused by an actor effect. The variable X_1 is a cause of Y_1, and X_2 is a cause of Y_2. In contrast to the APIM, however, the other cause of each person's outcome is not the partner's X variable, but the partner's Y variable. Thus the model specifies that person 2's outcome (Y_2) is a cause of person 1's outcome (Y_1), and person 1's outcome (Y_1) is a cause of person 2's outcome (Y_2). This is how a feedback process is modeled, so I have referred to this model as the dyadic feedback model (Cook, 2003) as a way of distinguishing it more clearly from the APIM, in which there is also mutual influence.

The purpose of the path diagram of the mutual influence model is to identify the aspects of the model that account for the nonindependence of observations. Toward this end, two of the paths in the model have been highlighted by thicker lines. These lines run first from

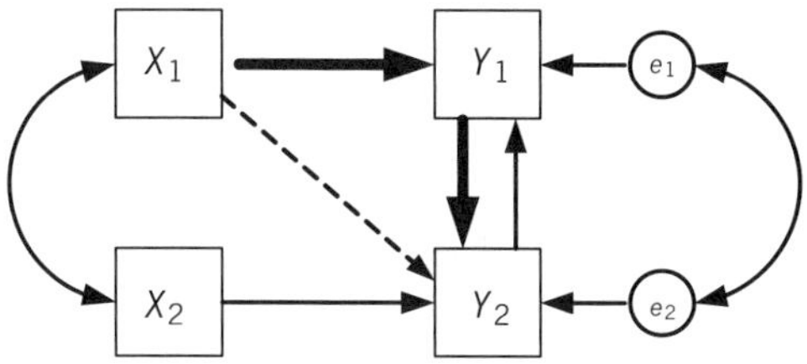

FIGURE 30.2. The mutual influence model. X_1 and X_2 are the independent variables for person 1 and person 2, Y_1 and Y_2 are their respective dependent variables, and e_1 and e_2 are the corresponding residuals. Each person's outcome (Y) influences the other's outcome. The effect of each actor's independent variable on the partner's outcome is mediated by the actor's own outcome (see bolded arrows). The dashed line represents the indirect effect of the actor on the partner. Nonindependence occurs when one independent variable affects both outcomes (Y_1 and Y_2), even though one of the paths (e.g., X_1 to Y_2) is mediated.

X_1 to Y_1, then from Y_1 to Y_2. (We could also have used the paths from X_2 to Y_2 and from Y_2 to Y_1, as the process modeled is the same). This part of the model specifies a *mediational* pathway whereby the effect of X_1 on Y_2 is mediated by its effect on Y_1 (see Baron & Kenny, 1986). If there is a significant path from X_1 to Y_1 and also a significant path from Y_1 to Y_2, then X_1 has a legitimate and significant effect on Y_2, although this effect is entirely indirect (i.e., entirely mediated by Y_1). The dashed line from X_1 to Y_2, which is not directly estimated, represents this indirect effect.

Recall that in the APIM, the reason for the correlated outcomes of person 1 and person 2 was that each of their outcomes was influenced by X_1. In other words, X_1 was a common cause of both Y_1 and Y_2, thus forcing these variables to correlate with each other. In the mutual influence model, the same effect exists. X_1 has a direct effect on Y_1 and an indirect effect on Y_2, thus forcing these variables to correlate with each other. The only difference in the source of nonindependence in this model versus the APIM is that there is mediation. Likewise, X_2 has a direct effect on Y_2 and an indirect effect on Y_1. It is therefore a second source of nonindependence in the outcomes. It is not necessary for both of these mediational submodels to be significant for there to be nonindependence of outcomes. As with the APIM, the correlation of the residual factors (e_1 and e_2) accounts for sources of nonindependence not included in the model. Models in which there are feedback processes require special methods of estimation. For further information on this analysis, see Kenny and colleagues (2006) and Sadler and Woody (2008).

The Common Fate Model

In contrast to the APIM and the mutual influence model, the nonindependence of observations in the common fate model (Kenny, 1996) is not due to *inter*dependence. Interdependence means that the dyad members influence each other. In the case of the common fate model, partners do not influence each other; they are both influenced by some other source that they have in common. The path diagram (see Figure 30.3) should make this clear.

As in the figures for the APIM and mutual influence models, there are four variables: two predictor variables (X_1 and X_2 for person 1 and person 2, respectively) and two outcome

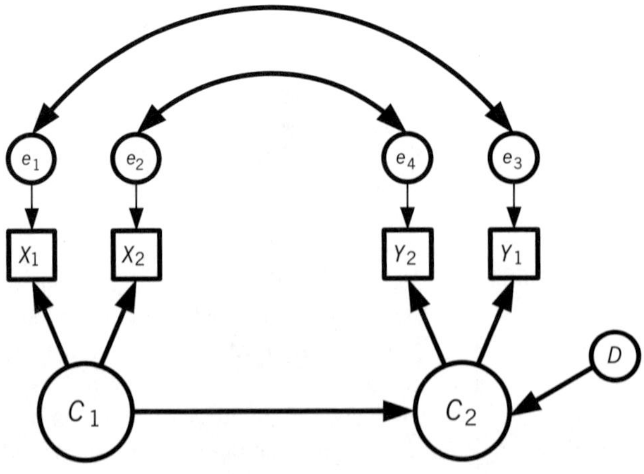

FIGURE 30.3. The common fate model. Each person's observed score on the independent variable (X_1 and X_2) is caused by the same factor, an unobserved (latent) independent variable (C_1). Each person's observed outcome (Y_1 and Y_2) is also influenced by a latent variable (C_2). The latent independent variable (C_1) influences the latent outcome variable (C_2). Because the observed scores are affected by the same factor, they will be nonindependent. Residuals (e.g., e_1 and e_3) are correlated within person. D is the residual or disturbance on the latent outcome variable.

variables (Y_1 and Y_2 for person 1 and person 2, respectively). These are measured (or observed) variables. In the common fate model, X_1 and X_2 (and Y_1 and Y_2) are ratings of the same thing, although from two individual perspectives. Suppose, for example, that X_1 and X_2 are siblings' ratings of family cohesiveness. The depiction of C_1 as a cause of X_1 and X_2 in Figure 30.3 implies that when C_1 is high (a family with high cohesiveness), both X_1 and X_2 will be high, and when C_1 is low, both X_1 and X_2 will be low. In other words, because they are both caused by C_1, they will correlate with each other. So the source for the nonindependence of observations in the common fate model is due to causal factors that individuals have in common.

Another implication of the relations of X_1, X_2, and C_1 is that the shared variance, or covariance, between X_1 and X_2 is an indirect measure of C_1, the "unmeasured" or latent variable. Such latent variable measures can be used as both independent and dependent variables in further analyses. For example, the latent variable C_1 is a predictor of the latent variable C_2 (e.g., the level of coactivity in the family) in Figure 30.3. Because Y_1 and Y_2 are both influenced by C_2 and C_2 is influenced by C_1, the nonindependence between Y_1 and Y_2 is partially due to C_1. To finish the description of the model, the unexplained variance in C_2 is labeled D. The unexplained variances for X_1 and X_2 (residuals e_1 and e_2) include variance due to the respondent's unique perspective (Cook & Goldstein, 1993). Because each person's unique perspective on the X variable may be correlated with his or her unique perspective on the Y variable, the corresponding residuals are allowed to correlate (e.g., e_1 and e_3). If there is a correlation in these residuals, it indicates the presence of a rater effect, which is measured at the individual level of analysis. The C variables, as already noted, reflect something the dyad members have in common, so they are measured at the dyadic level of analysis. Because it contains both individual and dyadic level factors, the common fate model is a *multilevel model*.

The Social Relations Model

Typically, the APIM, mutual influence model, and common fate model are used with data from a *standard dyadic design*. In the standard dyadic design, each person has only one partner. In some designs individuals have more than one partner. For example, Warner, Kenny, and Stoto (1979) introduced an analysis for the round-robin design. A round-robin design is one in which each person in a group provides data (observational or self-report) about his or her relationship with each of the other group members. The data used in this design are called *directed relationship data* because the measure of person A in relationship to person B is not the same as the measure of person B in relationship to person A. Kenny and La Voie (1984) elaborated this approach and named it the *social relations model*. For present purposes we assume that directed relationship data have been collected within a round-robin family design (e.g., Cook, 1994; Kashy & Kenny, 1990). In a two-parent, two-child family, the round robin design will produce 12 relationship-specific measures (4 actors with 3 partners each). The focus of this section is on the multiple sources of nonindependence measured by the social relations model (SRM). For details on the statistical analysis of the SRM, see Card and Toomey (Chapter 32, this volume).

According to the SRM, one person's attitudes, feelings, or behavior toward another person is potentially a function of four systematic sources of variance: an actor effect, a partner effect, a relationship effect, and a group effect.[2] For example, a child's positivity toward his or her mother is determined by the child's general disposition to be positive (an actor effect), the mother's general tendency to elicit positivity from others (a partner effect), the child's positivity to mother that is unique to their relationship (a relationship effect), and the family or group effect (the overall level of positivity in the family). Likewise, the mother's positivity toward the child is a function of the mother's positivity (an actor effect), the child's tendency to elicit positivity (a partner effect), the mother–child relationship effect, and the family effect. Each of these factors is based on multiple observations that have something in common, and that common element causes the observations to correlate with each other. Consequently, each factor accounts for a unique kind of nonindependence.

Actor Nonindependence

In the round-robin family design, one collects data on each person's relationship with each of the other participating family members, so for the mother, we may have observed scores for (1) her positivity toward the children's father, (2) her positivity toward the older of the two children, and (3) her positivity toward the younger of the two children. Suppose now that some mothers are dispositionally more positive than other mothers. As with the APIM, the

[2]Actor and partner effects are found in both the actor–partner interdependence model (APIM) and in the social relations model (SRM). In both cases, an *actor effect* means that a person's outcome is determined by something about him- or herself, and a *partner effect* means that a person's outcome is determined by something about his or her partner. In the APIM, however, actor and partner effects are a function of particular variables, just as a genetic effect is a function of a particular gene. By way of contrast, in the SRM, variance due to actor and partner effects is measured without reference to or identification of any particular causal variable. Statistical significance of SRM actor and partner factors indicates only that *something* about the actor (or partner) affects the person's outcome. This parallels the use of structural equation modeling to identify the role of genetic factors versus shared environmental factors in some behavior genetic research (e.g., Neiderhiser, Reiss, Hetherington, & Plomin, 1999). Genetic factors can be identified as causal of a particular outcome without identifying any particular causal gene.

actor effect means that a person's outcome is predicted by his or her own characteristics. A mother's positive disposition will tend to make her more positive toward all family members, so there should be positive correlations among the mother–father, mother–older child, and mother–younger child scores. Actor nonindependence measures consistency in a person's thoughts, feelings, or behavior across multiple partners. Nonindependence due to actor characteristics is explained and controlled for by specifying a latent variable as a common cause of these scores. In the family SRM, there is an actor factor for each role (i.e., mother, father, older child, and younger child). If the factor for a particular role is significant (i.e., it has reliable variance), it means that families differ in terms of the person's traits as an actor.

Partner Nonindependence

In the round-robin design, each person is also the target or partner in relationship to each of the other family members, so for the older child, there will be measures of (1) mother's positivity toward the older child, (2) father's positivity toward the older child, and the younger sibling's positivity toward the older child. If in the sample of families some stable trait of the child consistently elicits high positivity (or low positivity) from each of the other family members, then the three observed scores should be correlated. By specifying a latent variable that is a common cause of each family member's relationship to the older child, nonindependence due to the partner can be estimated and controlled for. In the family SRM, there is a partner factor for each role (i.e., mother, father, older child, and younger child). If the factor is significant (i.e., it has reliable variance), it means that families differ in terms of the person's ability to elicit a consistent response from other family members.

Group Nonindependence

The hallmark of a personality trait or individual difference is cross-situational consistency in one's thoughts, feelings, attributions (loosely referred to as "perceptions"), or behavior. The actor and partner factors of the SRM meet this criteria because they reflect consistency across multiple relationships. Consistency due to individual differences is common in SRM research, but sometimes there is consistency at the level of the group. In other words, characteristics of the group as a whole may cause the scores of all the individuals within groups or families to be correlated. By specifying a latent variable as a common cause of all 12 directed relationships in a two-parent, two-child family, nonindependence due to the group effect can be estimated. Although there are as many actor and partner factors as there are roles within a group, there is only one group factor. If the factor is statistically significant (i.e., it has reliable variance), it means that families differ in terms of some characteristic that all family members have in common. In groups other than the family, group nonindependence may be caused by compositional effects (i.e., group members were similar before becoming members of the group). For example, in high school cliques, group members may share attitudes or values that attract them to each other (e.g., feelings toward authority, an interest in sports, or a desire to be popular).

Reciprocity Nonindependence

When interdependence exists in a group, it means that one person's behavior has consequences for other people in the group. The reason can be that one person's behavior has a direct consequence—for example, when one family member eats more than his or her share of dessert—or it may have indirect consequences, as when one family member worries about the excessive eating of another (Kelley & Thibaut, 1978). As each person in the group adapts to the behavior of the others, the development of feedback loops is inevitable. Baumrind (1980) expressed it as follows: "Within a reciprocal and interacting system such as the family, individuals produce by their actions the environmental conditions that affect their own as well as others' behavior. One person's behavior is simultaneously a response to environmental stimuli and a stimulus to others' response within the interactive system of social exchange" (p. 640). Such feedback processes are the defining feature of family systems because it is through such processes that the family "self-organizes." The source of nonindependence is the same as in the mutual influence model.

The SRM provides estimates of feedback or reciprocity at both the individual and dyadic levels of analysis. At the individual level it is estimated by the correlation of the actor effect for a particular role (e.g., mother's actor effect) with the partner effect for the same role (i.e., mother's partner effect). Actor–partner reciprocity correlations are estimated for each role in the family (mother, father, older child, and younger child). At the dyadic level of analysis, reciprocity nonindependence is indicated by the correlation of the relationship effects of each person in a dyad (e.g., mother-to-father with father-to-mother).

Nonindependence in Social Network Analysis

Two of the chapters in this volume (Gest & Kindermann, Chapter 33, and Veenstra & Steglich, Chapter 34) describe procedures for social network analysis. The goal of social network analysis is to identify and describe linkages or connections between the nodes in a network and to evaluate how network dynamics affect and are affected by the actions of network members. The nodes may be people, animals, organizations, communities, or other such entities. These linkages between nodes are measured categorically (i.e., present or absent). Nonindependence in the outcomes of network members should be expected when there are repeated interactions between network members (leading to serial dependence), when network members are part of the same subgroup (clique or clan), and when network members are defined on the basis of their spatial proximity (e.g., members of a neighborhood).

The sources of linkages, and thus nonindependence, may also be the same as in other forms of dyadic relationships. For example, in sociometric research, there is a measure of *centrality* (i.e., how central one is within the network) called the *in-degree*. The in-degree indicates how often one is selected or nominated by others (e.g., being chosen as a friend). How often one is selected by others corresponds to partner nonindependence in the SRM insofar as characteristics of the person drive the selection process. Another measure of centrality, the *outdegree*, indicates how many others one selects or nominates according to some criteria (e.g., how many people one nominates as "friend"). The outdegree corresponds to actor nonindependence in the SRM insofar as characteristics of the "chooser" affect who gets chosen. Group nonindependence may also occur in social networks. Identifying with members of one's own subgroup, or identifying negatively with members of another subgroup, may create a sense of belongingness shared by all members of a subgroup. Finally, reciprocity nonindependence is very common in social network analysis. In social network analysis, reciprocity is typically measured by how often one is selected or nominated by those whom one selects or nominates (i.e., mutual selection).

One source of nonindependence found in social networks that is not typically discussed in the context of dyadic data analysis is *transitivity*. According to the notion of transitivity, if person A and person B are friends, and person B and person C are friends, there is an increased probability that persons A and C will be friends. Because transitivity requires three people to be observed, it is a *triadic*—rather than a dyadic—source of nonindependence. Nonindependence is present because knowing about two dyads (AB and BC) provides information about a third dyad (AC). In other words, transitivity is indicative of a higher order of nonindependence. Although the models of nonindependence discussed earlier (e.g., APIM) measure and control for dyadic nonindependence (i.e., correlations in the outcomes of individuals), the presence of higher order sources of nonindependence, such as transitivity, constitutes a violation of the independence assumption for these models.

Conclusion

Nonindependence is a statistical issue that may be of interest to people only when dealing with a particular problem in the analysis of their own data. Of interest to many people, however, is the conceptualization of nonindependence as a reflection of individual and social processes that influence (and that are influenced by) human development. The ability to use statistical analysis to describe these processes—while at the same time controlling for the bias they would otherwise introduce into the data analysis—can provide the basis for elaborating a theory (e.g., by demonstrating the need to include a social dimension) and can extend the generality of one's findings.

In this chapter I have given a brief overview of nonindependence and its relevance to the study of human development. There are particular contexts in which nonindependent observations are especially likely, such as the outcomes of family relationships or students in a classroom or group, observations measured over time, and social networks. Particular processes are likely to give rise to nonindependent observations. For example, personality traits and genes make observations of a person taken at one point in time similar to those taken at later times, accommodation to the behavior of a partner can make one more similar to that partner, and social comparison processes and/or reactions against a partner can make one different from that person. Processes of reciprocity can actually stabilize processes that make individuals similar or lead to exaggerated differences in the behavior of individuals. Processes of selection and rejection can create subgroups of relatively similar people within social networks.

The nonindependence of observations generated by such processes leads to bias in statistical analysis. It is therefore important to know how to detect (i.e., measure) the presence of nonindependent observations, to model the processes that cause it, and, in that way, to remove bias due to nonindependence from a statistical analysis. For many of us, the interpersonal processes that cause nonindependence may themselves become the object of scientific inquiry, such as research describing how reciprocity of negativity affects the development of marital relationships (Gottman, 1979) or the degree to which characteristics of a family member affect one's sense of attachment to that person (Cook, 2000). In this regard, models of nonindependence, which are still relatively new and unexplored, provide not just a means of controlling for statistical bias but also a lens through which new discoveries can be made.

Acknowledgments

I thank David A. Kenny and Connie Woods for their helpful suggestions.

References

Baron, R. M., & Kenny, D. A. (1986). The moderator–mediator variable distinction in social psychological research: Conceptual, strategic, and statistical considerations. *Journal of Personality and Social Psychology, 51*, 1173–1182.

Baumrind, D. (1980). New directions in socialization research. *American Psychologist, 35*, 639–652.

Cohen, J. (1960). A coefficient of agreement for nominal scales. *Educational Psychological Measurement, 20*, 37–46.

Cohen, J. (1988). *Statistical power analysis for the behavioral sciences* (2nd ed.). Hillsdale, NJ: Erlbaum.

Cook, T. D., & Campbell, D. T. (1979). *Quasi-experimentation: Design and analysis issues for field settings*. Boston: Houghton Mifflin.

Cook, W. L. (1994). A structural equation model of dyadic relationships within the family system. *Journal of Consulting and Clinical Psychology, 62*, 500–510.

Cook, W. L. (2000). Understanding attachment security in family context. *Journal of Personality and Social Psychology, 78*, 285–294.

Cook, W. L. (2003). Quantitative methods for deductive (theory-testing) research on parent–child dynamics. In L. Kuczynski (Ed.), *Handbook of dynamics in parent–child relations* (pp. 347–372). Thousand Oaks, CA: Sage.

Cook, W. L., & Goldstein, M. J. (1993). Multiple perspectives on family relationships: A latent variables model. *Child Development, 64*, 1377–1388.

Cook, W. L., & Kenny, D. A. (2006). Examining the validity of self-report assessments of family functioning: A question of the level of analysis. *Journal of Family Psychology, 20*, 209–216.

Cook, W. L., Kenny, D. A., & Goldstein, M. J. (1991). Parental affective style risk and the family system: A social relations model analysis. *Journal of Abnormal Psychology, 100*, 492–501.

Elder, G. H., Jr. (1999). *Children of the Great Depression: Social change in life experience*. Boulder, CO: Westview Press.

Fincham, F. D., & Cain, K. M. (1986). Learned helplessness in humans: A developmental analysis. *Developmental Review, 6*, 301–333.

Gottman, J. M. (1979). *Marital interaction: Experimental investigations*. New York: Academic Press.

Gottman, J. M., Coan, J., Carrere, S., & Swanson, C. (1998). Predicting marital happiness and stability from newlywed interactions. *Journal of Marriage and the Family, 60*, 5–22.

Griffin, S. W., & Gonzalez, R. (1995). Correlational analysis of dyad-level data in the exchangeable case. *Psychological Bulletin, 118*, 430–439.

Kashy, D. A., & Kenny, D. A. (1990). Analysis of family research designs: A model of interdependence. *Communication Research, 17*, 462–482.

Kelley, H. H., & Thibaut, J. W. (1978). *Interpersonal relations: A theory of interdependence*. New York: Wiley.

Kenny, D. A. (1996). Models of nonindependence in dyadic research. *Journal of Social and Personal Relationships, 13*, 279–294.

Kenny, D. A., & Judd, C. M. (1986). Consequences of violating the independence assumption in analysis of variance. *Psychological Bulletin, 99*, 422–431.

Kenny, D. A., Kashy, D. A., & Bolger, N. (1998). Data analysis in social psychology. In D. T. Gilbert, S. T. Fiske, & G. Lindzey (Eds.), *Handbook of social psychology* (4th ed., Vol. 1, pp. 233–265). Boston: McGraw-Hill.

Kenny, D. A., Kashy, D. A., & Cook, W. L. (2006). *Dyadic data analysis*. New York: Guilford Press.

Kenny, D. A., & La Voie, L. (1984). The social relations model. In L. Berkowitz (Ed.), *Advances in experimental social psychology* (Vol. 18, pp. 142–182). New York: Academic Press.

Laursen, B., Popp, D., Burk, W. J., Kerr, M., & Stattin, H. (2008). Incorporating interdependence into developmental research: Examples from the study of homophily and homogeneity. In N. Card, J. Selig, & T. Little (Eds.), *Modeling dyadic and interdependent data in the developmental and behavioral sciences* (pp. 11–37). New York: Taylor & Francis.

Lay, K. L., Waters, E., & Park, K. A. (1989). Maternal responsiveness and child compliance: The role of mood as a mediator. *Child Development, 60*, 1405–1411.

Moos, R. H., & Moos, B. S. (1981). *Family Environment Scale manual*. Palo Alto, CA: Consulting Psychologists Press.

Myers, J. L. (1979). *Fundamentals of experimental design* (3rd ed.). Boston: Allyn & Bacon.

Neiderhiser, J. M., Reiss, D., Hetherington, E., & Plomin, R. (1999). Relationships between parenting and adolescent adjustment over time: Genetic and environmental contributions. *Developmental Psychology, 35*, 680–692.

Olson, D. H., Portner, J., & Lavee, Y. (1985). *Faces III*. St. Paul: University of Minnesota, Family Social Science.

Parpal, M., & Maccoby, E. E. (1985). Maternal responsiveness and subsequent child compliance. *Child Development, 56*, 1326–1334.

Plomin, R., Asbury, K., & Dunn, J. (2001). Why are children from the same family so different? Nonshared environment a decade later. *Canadian Journal of Psychiatry, 46*, 225–233.

Sadler, P., & Woody, E. (2008). It takes two: A dyadic, SEM-based perspective on personality development. In N. A. Card, J. P. Selig, & T. D. Little (Eds.), *Modeling dyadic and interdependent data in the developmental and behavioral sciences* (pp. 139–163). New York: Taylor & Francis.

Warner, R. M. (1992). Sequential analysis of social interaction: Assessing internal versus social determinants of behavior. *Journal of Personality and Social Psychology, 6*, 51–60.

Warner, R. M. (1998). *Spectral analysis of time-series data*. New York: Guilford Press.

Warner, R. M., Kenny, D. A., & Stoto, M. (1979). A new round robin analysis of variance for social interaction data. *Journal of Personality and Social Psychology, 37*, 1742–1757.

CHAPTER 31

Dyadic Data Analyses in a Developmental Context

ROBERT A. ACKERMAN
M. BRENT DONNELLAN
DEBORAH A. KASHY
RAND D. CONGER

Relationships are a fundamental context of human development (Reis, Collins, & Berscheid, 2000), and dyads such as parents and children, teachers and students, and sibling pairs are a ubiquitous feature of many developmental studies. An essential quality of these relationships is that the two individuals are interdependent, such that the thoughts, feelings, and behaviors of one person are related to the thoughts, feelings, and behaviors of the other person. A careful statistical analysis of this interdependence provides important opportunities to better understand relationships, how they develop over time, and their essential role in shaping the course of individual development (see, e.g., Laursen, 2005). Models for dyadic data, such as the actor–partner interdependence model (APIM; Kenny, Kashy, & Cook, 2006) specifically allow researchers to study interpersonal influence processes and can be extended to longitudinal investigations to study such developmentally important concepts as reciprocity in family relationships and issues of peer socialization. The goal of this chapter is to provide an introduction to these models.

Central Issues

Several influential perspectives within developmental psychology highlight the salience of relationships for human development. Transactional perspectives (e.g., Sameroff, 2010), as well as Bronfenbrenner's updated bioecological model (e.g., Bronfenbrenner & Morris,

2006), are predicated on the notion that development is the outcome of a dynamic interplay between the individual and his or her social contexts. A core idea is that all developmentally salient relationships—from friendships to more asymmetrical dyads, such as teachers and students and parents and children—involve reciprocal relations such that the partners in these dyads influence each other. In terms of family relationships, these perspectives have changed the assumption that parents simply exert a unidirectional influence over their children and instead posit that parents and children mutually influence each other (Bell, 1968; Lytton, 1990). In a similar vein, family systems approaches (Cox & Paley, 1997) assert that each member of a family unit is nested within a set of interdependent subsystems (e.g., the sibling relationship, the father–child relationship, and the overall family group). Patterns of influence are argued to involve reciprocal or bidirectional relations between these systems. Taken together, these perspectives remind scholars that interdependence is critical for understanding human development across the lifespan (see also Laursen, 2005).

Despite the prominence of these approaches and the myriad empirical studies that they have generated, researchers have been slow to exploit the rich potential of dyadic data for studying developmental processes. One likely explanation is that the methodological tools and training available to many developmental researchers lag behind the sophistication of their theoretical approaches. Many widely used techniques, such as ANOVA and multiple regression analysis, explicitly assume that the observations used in the analyses are independent of one another. Violations of this assumption result in biased standard errors. Therefore, researchers who work with dyadic data need, at a minimum, statistical tools to model interdependence and correct standard errors.

Although correcting standard errors for nonindependence of observations is important, we believe that the true benefits of dyadic data analysis lie in the types of questions that can be asked of the data that are collected in developmental studies. For example, dyadic models provide researchers with techniques to study influence processes. This is particularly important in longitudinal contexts when it is possible to estimate how strongly changes in one dyad member are associated with changes in the other member. In this chapter, we describe three dyadic data analytical techniques that can be used for advancing developmental research: the standard APIM, the cross-lagged APIM, and the dyadic growth model. We initially focus on a basic dyadic model suitable for cross-sectional investigations: the standard APIM. We then discuss the cross-lagged APIM and briefly comment on the dyadic growth model. Given space constraints, we do not delve into technical details associated with these models. Rather, we present readers with a primer regarding basic conceptual issues and practical advice regarding their application. We provide citations to more detailed accounts throughout. In particular, we highly recommend the monograph by Kenny and colleagues (2006).

Conceptual Principles and Statistical Assumptions

Before describing the statistical models, we first define a few key terms and concepts that are central to the analysis of dyadic data. Familiarity with these terms is essential for understanding the applied methodological literature surrounding dyadic data analysis (see, e.g., Kenny et al., 2006) and properly conducting the analyses described in this chapter. Cook

(Chapter 30, this volume) provides a detailed introduction to these and other foundational issues.

Types of Dyadic Variables

Researchers collect different kinds of variables on dyads. Attributes can vary *between dyads* (i.e., the two dyad members have the same value, but these values vary from dyad to dyad), *within dyads* (i.e., the two dyad members have different scores but the average score, averaging across the dyad members, is the same for every dyad), or both between and within dyads (so-called *mixed* variables; i.e., the two dyad members may have different values and the dyad average score may vary across dyads as well). In a study of siblings raised in the same household, between-dyads variables could include individual difference attributes of the parents, as well as measures of the overall family climate (i.e., these attributes are the same for both siblings). Examples of within-dyads variables could be birth order in a study of nontwin siblings or gender if the study included only opposite-sex sibling pairs (i.e., these attributes will be different for each sibling within the dyad, but all sibling pairs will have an older and younger member or a male and female member). Finally, examples of mixed variables in a sibling study could be temperament traits or drinking (i.e., individuals differ in these attributes both within and across dyads). The nature of a variable can be determined empirically by computing the intraclass correlation between the dyad members' scores on that variable. If the correlation is 1.0, the variable is between dyads, if the correlation is –1.0, it is a within-dyads variable, and if the correlation is somewhere in between 1 and –1, it is a mixed variable.

Distinguishability

A crucial concept in dyadic data analysis is whether dyad members can be meaningfully distinguished by some attribute (usually a within-dyads categorical variable). If the answer is yes, then the dyad members are said to be *distinguishable* on this attribute. Gender is a very common distinguishing variable in research involving heterosexual dyads (e.g., married couples). Family role (e.g., parent, child) is another distinguishing characteristic for many developmental studies. When dyad members cannot be distinguished by a meaningful attribute, then the dyad members are said to be *indistinguishable*. Examples of indistinguishable dyads may include partners in same-sex romantic relationships and identical twins. In many of these cases, the only way to identify dyad members during data collection is through some arbitrary labeling process, such as twin A or twin B. Nonetheless, it should be emphasized that dyads can be distinguishable on a variable other than gender. For instance, same-sex friends could be distinguished by whether they are older or younger (see, e.g., Popp, Laursen, Kerr, Stattin, & Burk, 2008).

Moreover, there is an important distinction between *conceptual distinguishability* and *empirical distinguishability*. Conceptual distinguishability refers to whether dyad members can be classified in a systematic manner according to some variable, whereas empirical distinguishability addresses whether the conceptual distinguishability actually makes a practical difference in the data from the two "types" of dyad members. If means, variances, and covariances do not differ across the distinguishing variable, then the data are empirically indistinguishable. Researchers often treat data from married couples as distinguishable by gender, but in many cases there is little evidence of systematic differences in relationship processes for men and women. Detailed information about testing distinguishability is available elsewhere (Ackerman, Donnellan, & Kashy, 2011; Kashy, Donnellan, Burt, & McGue, 2008; Kenny et al., 2006).

The distinction between distinguishable and indistinguishable data is critical because it affects how models should be specified. In general, there is increased statistical power associated with analyses using indistinguishable dyads (see Kashy et al., 2008). With indistinguishable data, estimates are derived by pooling within dyads, as well as across dyads. In contrast, with distinguishable dyads, separate estimates are derived for each of the two "types" of individuals. Consequently, estimates are derived by pooling across, but not within, dyads. In this chapter we limit our discussion to the distinguishable case given the added complexity of analyses for indistinguishable dyads.

Interdependence, Dependence, and Nonindependent Data

All three terms refer to the idea that data from two linked individuals are likely to be correlated. This interdependence provides the essential starting point for modeling how the linked individuals affect one another (Kashy, Campbell, & Harris, 2006; Kenny et al., 2006). However, the proper analysis of dependent data often requires the use of specialized software packages. Multilevel modeling (MLM) and structural equation modeling (SEM) software programs are both well suited for estimating models that incorporate interdependence, and both can be used for dyadic data analysis. We strongly encourage researchers interested in conducting dyadic data analyses to develop facility with programs stemming from both data analytic traditions. Some analyses are easier to perform with certain kinds of software packages than others. For example, in this chapter, we primarily use MLM for the analyses. However, when presenting the cross-lagged APIM for panel data, we discuss how to conduct the analyses using SEM, as we believe it is easier to estimate this model with this kind of software package.

In general, MLM is very useful when researchers have diary data and indistinguishable dyads (but see Ackerman et al., 2011). MLM software packages can also handle multiple predictors and interaction terms easily. SEM works well for distinguishable dyads and panel data, and it is quite flexible for dealing with complicated patterns of correlated residuals. In addition, SEM also offers the ability to test specific model constraints in a very straightforward fashion and provides omnibus measures of absolute model fit to the underlying data. A potential drawback occurs when using SEM packages with indistinguishable dyads, because this requires special constraints and adjustments to model fit statistics (see Olsen & Kenny, 2006). Thus MLM and SEM packages each have certain advantages and sometimes disadvantages for particular data analytical applications.

Dyadic Data Structures

Data from dyads can be structured in a variety of ways. The three most commonly used for dyadic data include the dyad, individual, and pairwise data formats. Familiarity with these formats is important because different analyses require different structures. Examples of these different data structures are also available in the online appendix for this chapter, available at *www.crmda.ku.edu/Guilford/HDRM*. We use the pairwise data structure when estimating the standard APIM with MLM. Advice on restructuring data sets can be found in Kenny and colleagues (2006).

Developmental Applications and Illustrations

In the following sections we discuss conceptual issues, basic data requirements, and key model parameters for three dyadic models: the standard APIM, the cross-lagged APIM, and the dyadic growth model. Given space constraints, we place most of our focus on the standard APIM and the cross-lagged APIM. To facilitate a better understanding of how to set up and implement the standard APIM and cross-lagged APIM, we supplement each discussion with a concrete empirical example. Readers are encouraged to download the associated deidentified data sets and syntax from *www.crmda.ku.edu/Guilford/HDRM* to gain practice with running the models themselves. We must emphasize, however, that these examples are intended to illustrate data analytical issues and are not intended to advance substantive claims.

Cross-Sectional Data and the APIM

The APIM (Kenny et al., 2006) is a simple but useful model for evaluating questions of dyadic influence in cross-sectional designs (see Cook & Kenny, 2005). Figure 31.1 presents an example of the APIM for distinguishable dyad members—in this case, a mother and her child (for coverage of the indistinguishable case, see Ackerman et al., 2011; Kashy & Donnellan, in press; Kenny et al., 2006; Olsen & Kenny, 2006). In general, the APIM is useful for evaluating how intrapersonal variables (e.g., personality attributes, mental health variables, religiosity) are associated with interpersonal variables (e.g., parenting styles, relationship conflict, relationship satisfaction). In our example, the objective is to model the connections between an individual's neuroticism and her or his observed positive engagement behaviors (i.e., an interpersonal style indicative of effective communication, warmth,

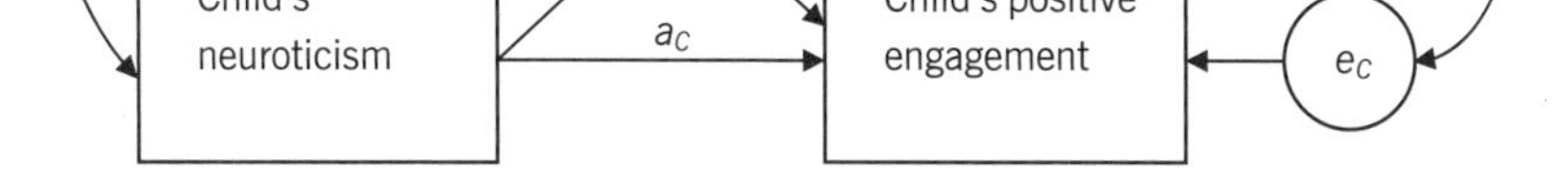

FIGURE 31.1. Illustration of the standard APIM for distinguishable dyad members. a_M, mother's actor effect; a_C, child's actor effect; p_{CM}, mother's partner effect on child; p_{MC}, child's partner effect on mother; e_M, variance in mother's positive engagement not explained by mother's or child's neuroticism; e_C, variance in child's positive engagement not explained by mother's or child's neuroticism; r_x, covariance between predictors; r_y, residualized nonindependence not accounted for by the actor and partner effects in the model.

and support; see Ackerman, Kashy, Donnellan, & Conger, in press) in families. The idea behind this example is that the personality attributes of parents and their children affect their interactional patterns (see, e.g., Donnellan, Conger, McAdams, & Neppl, 2009; Ellenbogen, Ostiguy, & Hodgins, 2010).

Data for this example come from the Iowa Youth and Families Project (Conger & Elder, 1994). The sample includes data from mothers and their teenage children from the 424 families participating in the study in 1991. Trained interviewers met with the families twice each year. Upon the first meeting, families were asked to complete a set of measures that included self-reports of neuroticism using a well-established measure. Approximately 2 weeks later, families were videotaped engaging in a conflict resolution task from which various interpersonal behaviors were later coded. Several of these interpersonal behaviors (i.e., communication, prosocial behavior, warmth, assertiveness, and listener responsiveness) were aggregated to form a composite variable that we call positive engagement.

The parameters of primary interest within the standard APIM are the actor and partner effects. The actor effect refers to the association between a person's *own* predictor variable (neuroticism in this case) and his or her outcome score (observed positive engagement). The partner effect refers to the association between the person's *partner's* predictor score and the person's outcome. Because the dyad in our example is conceptually distinguishable by family role, there may be two actor effects, one for mothers, or a_M, and one for children, or a_C. Likewise, there may be two partner effects, the partner effect for child's neuroticism on the mother's outcome, p_{MC}, and the partner effect for mother's neuroticism on the child's outcome, p_{CM}. As can be seen in Figure 31.1, the other parameters in this model include the covariance between the dyad members' scores on the predictor variable (i.e., r_x), the residual variances for both dyad members (i.e., the residual variance for mothers, e_M, and the residual variance for children, e_C), and the covariance between the residual variances for both dyad members (i.e., r_y). In some cases the covariance between the dyad members' scores on the predictor variable is interesting, as it can convey evidence of similarity (or dissimilarity) on focal constructs. This information is perhaps relevant when considering whether friends and romantic partners have initially similar characteristics (e.g., selection and assortative mating, respectively).

Basic Data Requirements

The standard APIM requires that the same predictor and outcome variables are measured for both members of the dyad. This is not always possible with certain developmental variables (e.g., self-esteem may not be measurable for both the mother and her toddler-age child). Moreover, the outcome variables, as well as any predictor variables for which researchers plan to estimate actor and partner effects, must be mixed variables. In light of this requirement, researchers should think carefully about whether an APIM analysis is appropriate for the types of data that they are collecting.

To use MLM to estimate the standard APIM, the data structure needs to be pairwise (see Table A at *www.crmda.ku.edu/Guilford/HDRM*). Moreover, it is generally prudent to grand mean–center the predictor variables. In our current example, this amounts to computing the grand mean for the actor's neuroticism (across both mothers and children) and subtracting this value from each of the original scores. We would perform the same operation for the partner's neuroticism. It is also advisable to use either dummy coding or effects coding with the distinguishing variable, if one exists.

Specifying the APIM

The distinguishable APIM can be specified in two statistically equivalent ways that differ in how the fixed effects are specified. The first alternative, which we refer to as the *interaction model*, focuses on estimating average intercepts, actor effects, and partner effects (averaging across the two "types" of dyad members), as well as interactions between the distinguishing variable (i.e., role) and each of these effects. Thus the interaction model explicitly tests whether there are significant differences in the size of the intercepts, actor effects, and partner effects as a function of the distinguishing variable. The second alternative has been called the *two-intercept model* in the literature (Raudenbush, Brennan, & Barnett, 1995). In this model, separate intercepts, actor effects, and partner effects are estimated for the two levels of the distinguishing variable. Thus, the two-intercept model does not test whether there are significant differences as a function of the distinguishing variable; instead, it provides tests of whether each of the four key effects (i.e., actor effects for mothers and children and partner effects for mothers and children) differs significantly from zero. As we illustrate later, both of these models provide useful information about the model parameters.

In either specification of the distinguishable APIM, the random effects portion of the model should include separate estimates of the residual variances for mothers and children, as well as the correlation between the unexplained variance in the outcome across dyad members. This residual structure can be achieved using an error structure known as heterogeneous compound symmetry. Moreover, we recommend using restricted maximum likelihood (REML) as the estimation method, as it provides unbiased estimates of the fixed effects parameters (see Snijders & Bosker, 1999, p. 56). To be sure, when the number of level two units is large, then the differences in the estimates produced by REML and maximum likelihood (ML) will be negligible; however, in cases in which researchers have a small number of level two units, ML tends to underestimate the variance components (see Raudenbush & Bryk, 2002). Use of ML is best reserved for cases in which researchers are interested in contrasting the fit of nested models (e.g., testing empirical distinguishability; see Kashy et al., 2008; Kenny et al., 2006).

Interpreting Estimates from the Standard APIM

Table 31.1 presents the results of the APIM analyses using the two alternative specifications. For both of these alternatives, the fixed effects estimates are interpreted as regression coefficients. The left side shows results for the interaction model, and the right side shows the results for the two-intercept model. Looking first at the interaction model results, we see that the average positive engagement score across the whole sample is 1.94. Moreover, the significant role effect suggests that mothers (i.e., role = 1) had significantly higher average positive engagement than children. The statistically significant actor effect indicates that, averaging across mothers and children, for each 1-unit increase in an individual's neuroticism, his or her predicted positive interpersonal behavior decreases by .067 points. The interaction between actor and role estimates and tests whether there is a difference in actor effects for mothers and children. Here we find no such difference. The partner effect indicates that persons higher in neuroticism (averaging over mothers and children) have partners who have slightly lower predicted positive engagement; in this example, however, the partner effect was not statistically significant. Last, the nonsignificant interaction between

TABLE 31.1. Parameter Estimates from the APIM Models Predicting Mother's and Child's Positive Engagement Behavior as a Function of Their Own Neuroticism and Their Partner's Neuroticism

Interaction model			Two-intercept model		
Fixed effects	*b*	*t*	Fixed effects	*b*	*t*
Intercept	1.945	95.87*	Mother intercept	2.206	80.72*
Role main effect	.262	19.85*	Child intercept	1.683	81.83*
Actor neuroticism	–.067	2.34*	Mother actor	–.110	2.27*
Role-by-actor neuroticism	–.043	1.45	Child actor	–.024	.73
Partner neuroticism	–.040	1.44	Mother partner	–.025	.58
Role-by-partner neuroticism	.015	.51	Child partner	–.055	1.50
Random effects		Wald *Z*	Random effects		Wald *Z*
Residual variance mother	.289	13.96*	Residual variance mother	.289	13.96*
Residual variance child	.163	13.96*	Residual variance child	.163	13.96*
Residual correlation	.423	10.18*	Residual correlation	.423	10.18*

*$p < .05$.

partner and role suggests that the effect of the partner's neuroticism on the person's positive engagement is similar for mothers and children.

The right side of Table 31.1 presents the results from the two-intercept model. This model is similar to a simple slopes analysis in "regular" regression with interactions. We find it particularly useful for following up significant interactions found in analyses using the interaction model. In the current example, the mothers' actor effect was statistically significant and negative, indicating that mothers with higher levels of neuroticism exhibited less positive engagement with their children. The children's actor effect, in contrast, was negative but not significant. It is important to be cautious about this last result because the overall interaction between role and actor effect was not statistically significant in the interaction model. Thus there is no direct and compelling evidence that the actor effects differ significantly for mothers and children. The basic logic here is important: The two-intercept model is useful as a follow-up to omnibus interaction tests to get separate estimates for each dyad member distinguished by role. If researchers estimate the two-intercept model without first estimating the interaction model, they may erroneously conclude that the actor and/or partner effects differ by role.

Models for Longitudinal Dyadic Data

The APIM has several extensions to dyadic research in which both individuals are assessed at multiple points in time. Therefore, it can be useful for addressing developmental questions regarding stability and change, as well as interpersonal questions involving reciprocity. One common extension is known as the cross-lagged APIM. In our discussion of cross-lagged models, we detail an SEM approach for studies that include relatively few waves (e.g., panel studies) and an MLM approach for studies that include many waves (e.g., daily diary studies). We note here (and elsewhere) that either approach can be used for either type of data, but in our view, these pairings are a natural fit.

The Cross-Lagged APIM

The key feature of a cross-lagged model is that a person's present behavior is predicted to be a function of that person's past behavior and the person's partner's past behavior. Given this change in the predictor variables, the actor and partner effects are interpreted somewhat differently than in the standard APIM. In the cross-lagged model, the actor effect now estimates stability, or the degree to which a person's current behavior is similar to his or her own past behavior. Similarly, because the partner effects estimate the degree to which the partner's past behavior predicts the person's present behavior, the partner effects can be interpreted as an indication of prospective partner influence.

For example, Popp and colleagues (2008) used a version of the cross-lagged APIM to tease apart the effects of selection and socialization in the development of drinking behavior among teenagers. This is a long-standing issue in developmental studies involving peers, and the cross-lagged APIM was able to bring a fresh analytical perspective to this enduring question. Popp and colleagues showed that at the beginning of friendships, older members in the dyads may socialize their younger friends to drink relatively more over time (i.e., there was a partner effect such that the behavior of one member of the dyad was associated with the future behavior of the other dyad member). In this longitudinal context, actor effects capture the stability of drinking behavior, or the degree to which a person's own past drinking behavior predicts his or her present behavior. In contrast, partner effects capture the cross-person effect, or the extent to which one person's past drinking behavior is connected to his or her friend's present drinking behavior.

CROSS-LAGGED APIM USING SEM

In some research contexts the analysis of dyadic over-time data fits more naturally into an SEM approach. Panel data is a case in point, because researchers who collect this type of data are generally interested in examining developmental processes that occur over a span of years. In other words, the time lags often have special developmental significance. In contrast to diary data, the intervals for panel data are often much longer (e.g., 6 months or a year), and fewer waves of data are collected. Thus the stability and/or cross-partner influence associated with the lag between two waves may have more developmental significance than the lag between 2 days in a daily diary study. As a result, researchers working with panel data may want to allow for the possibility that the actor and partner effects connected with the lags may differ across the time intervals in the study.

This approach to modeling longitudinal data stands in contrast to the standard specification of the cross-lagged APIM for diary data in which the actor and partner effects connected with lags are typically constrained to be the same across the days of the study. In such studies, there are few reasons to expect changes in the strength of the effects from one day (or even week) to the next. Indeed, we should emphasize that all data collection strategies (i.e., days vs. years) should match expectations about the processes under investigation. More details about the planning of longitudinal data collections are available in Donnellan and Conger (2007).

Figure 31.2 shows an example of the cross-lagged APIM applied to panel data for distinguishable dyads involving mothers and sons (see also Popp et al., 2008, for an example). Data for this example come from the Iowa Youth and Families Project. Mothers and sons provided yearly self-reports of their levels of depression, anxiety, and hostility using the Symptom Checklist-90—Revised (SCL-90-R; Derogatis, 1983). An aggregate of these symptoms was used to create a composite variable called "psychological distress." This model therefore looks at the stability and cross-partner influence of psychological distress for mother–son dyads across the years of 1989, 1990, and 1991. This example is similar to a model first considered by Ge, Conger, Lorenz, Shanahan, and Elder (1995); however, those authors did not connect their analytical approach to the APIM, and they used a more complicated latent variable extension of the basic cross-lagged APIM. Nevertheless, they were interested in basic issues of reciprocity in terms of whether the psychological distresses of parents and children were prospectively associated with each other. To be sure, the fact that Ge and colleagues (1995) investigated such a question illustrates the point that issues of dyadic influence are of enduring interest to developmentally oriented researchers.

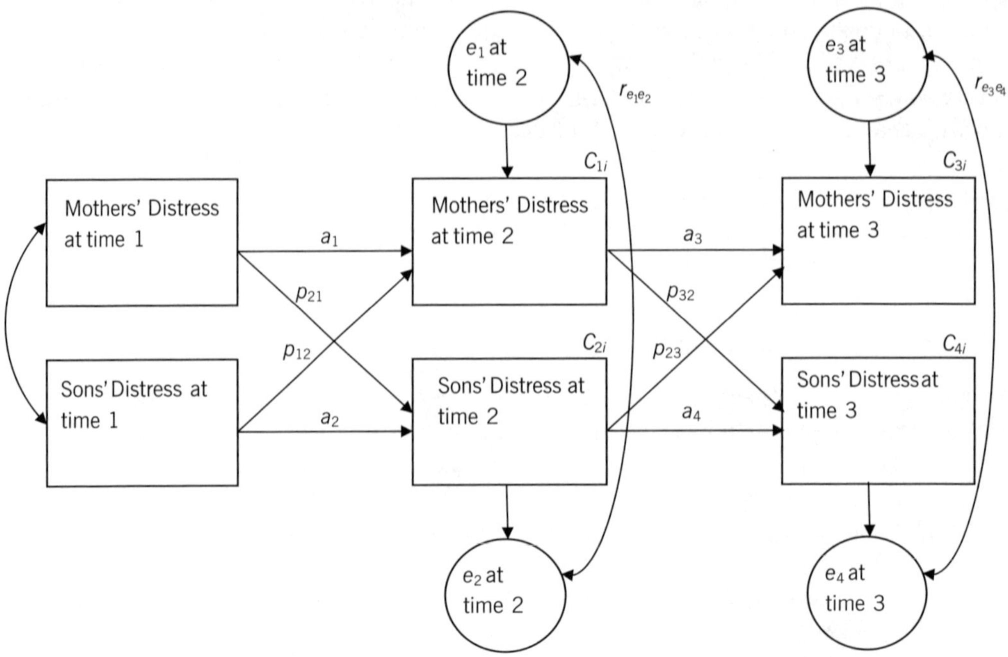

FIGURE 31.2. Panel data illustration of cross-lagged APIM for distinguishable dyad members. a_1, mothers' actor effect from time 1 to time 2; a_2, sons' actor effect from time 1 to time 2; a_3, mothers' actor effect from time 2 to time 3; a_4, sons' actor effect from time 2 to time 3; p_{21}, mothers' partner effect from time 1 to time 2; p_{12}, sons' partner effect from time 1 to time 2; p_{32}, mothers' partner effect from time 2 to time 3; p_{23}, sons' partner effect from time 2 to time 3; C_{1i}, mothers' intercept for time 2; C_{2i}, sons' intercept for time 2; C_{3i}, mothers' intercept for time 3; C_{4i}, sons' intercept for time 3; e_1, residualized variance in mothers' distress at time 2; e_2, residualized variance in sons' distress at time 2; e_3, residualized variance in mothers' distress at time 3; e_4, residualized variance in sons' distress at time 3; r_{e1e2}, residualized time-specific nonindependence at time 2; r_{e3e4}, residualized time-specific nonindependence at time 3.

Basic Data Requirements. The key data requirement for the cross-lagged APIM is that the same variables need to be measured for both partners and available over multiple time points (at least two, but preferably more; see Willett, Singer, & Martin, 1998). Moreover, the variables must be mixed. The data structure required to perform a cross-lagged APIM in SEM is a dyadic over-time data set (see Table B at *www.crmda.ku.edu/Guilford/HDRM*). This data structure is very similar to a dyad data set in that each row includes observations for both members of the data. However, in the dyadic over-time data set there are separate variables designating each person's outcome at each point in time.

Interpreting Estimates from the Cross-Lagged APIM. As seen in Figure 31.2, to specify the cross-lagged APIM for panel data in SEM, we freely estimate separate actor effects for each time interval. Specifically, we freely estimate mothers' and sons' actor effects from time 1 to time 2 (a_1 and a_2, respectively), as well as mothers' and sons' actor effects from time 2 to time 3 (a_3 and a_4, respectively). In doing so, we allow for the possibility that the stability of distress for mothers and sons may become stronger or weaker over time. Likewise, we freely estimate mothers' and sons' partner effects from time 1 to time 2 (p_{21} and p_{12}, respectively), as well as mothers' and sons' partner effects from time 2 to time 3 (p_{32} and p_{23}, respectively). This permits the possibility that the degree of cross-partner influence for mothers and sons may become stronger or weaker over time. This is an inherently developmental issue, as reciprocal influences might be more or less pronounced depending on the salience of a particular relationship at different points in the lifespan. For example, parents and offspring may mutually influence each others' psychological distress more strongly in early adolescence than in emerging adulthood.

In addition to these effects, we also freely estimate the means for mothers' and sons' distress at time 1 (as well as the covariance between these means) and the intercepts for mothers' and sons' distress at time 2 (C_{1i} and C_{2i}, respectively) and time 3 (C_{3i} and C_{4i}, respectively). Moreover, we freely estimate the residuals for mothers' and sons' distress at time 2 (e_1 and e_2, respectively) and time 3 (e_3 and e_4, respectively) and freely estimate the covariances between these time-specific residuals at time 2 (r_{e1e2}) and time 3 (r_{e3e4}).

Estimating this model in AMOS (version 7.0) resulted in the parameter estimates presented in Table 31.2. As can be seen, the actor effects for mothers and sons across both of the time intervals were positive and significant. This indicates that levels of psychological distress were somewhat stable for both mothers and sons, such that higher levels of distress the previous year were associated with higher levels of distress at present. If we wanted to test whether the stability coefficients for each member of the dyad differ across the time intervals, we could constrain the two respective actor effects to be equal and then examine whether the fit of the model significantly worsened. Performing this test for the sons' actor effects resulted in a significantly worse fitting model ($\Delta\chi^2(1) = 4.962, p = .026$). There is thus evidence to suggest that the stability of sons' distress was stronger from time 2 to time 3 than it was from time 1 to time 2. This pattern is developmentally sensible, as there is evidence that individual differences become more consistent with age (see Caspi, Roberts, & Shiner, 2005). Performing this test for the mothers' actor effects also worsened fit ($\Delta\chi^2(1) = 3.866, p = .049$), thereby providing evidence that mothers' actor effects increase significantly over time. In other words, the better fitting model is one that assumes that actor effects increase over time.

Examination of the partner effects in Table 31.2 shows that only the association between the mothers' distress at time 1 and the sons' distress at time 2 was significantly different

TABLE 31.2. Parameter Estimates for the Cross-Lagged APIM for Panel Data

	Waves			
	Time 1 to time 2		Time 2 to time 3	
	b	*t*	*b*	*t*
Mother intercept	.315	3.733**	.240	2.385*
Son intercept	.609	5.398**	.595	5.645**
Mother actor	.672	13.117**	.821	14.156**
Son actor	.371	7.117**	.547	9.907**
Mother partner	.156	2.279*	.024	0.397
Son partner	.057	1.462	.001	0.027

*$p < .05$; **$p < .01$.

from zero. This finding indicates that mothers who reported higher levels of psychological distress in 1989 had sons who reported higher levels of psychological distress in 1990. However, after imposing equality constraints on the partner effects for mothers across the two time intervals, we failed to find evidence that the two partner effects were significantly different from one another ($\Delta\chi^2(1) = 2.166, p = .141$). We then constrained all four partner effects to the same value and found that this model did not fit significantly worse ($\Delta\chi^2(3) = 3.424, p = .331$). More important from a substantive point of view, the partner effects themselves reached significance ($b = .053, t = 2.066, p = .039$). Altogether, this suggests that there may be reciprocal influences over time and that these effects are quite subtle. This point underscores concerns about statistical power in dyadic contexts.

Given these results for partner effects, we urge researchers to try imposing equality constraints on their models. Although doing so may result in a less developmentally interesting story, it provides the literature with parsimony and, in some cases, a more accurate portrayal of dyadic processes. It might well be the case that both mothers and sons exert subtle influences on each other during adolescence. That being said, more sophisticated latent variable models may provide increased power to detect these subtle effects given that such models are able to account for the effects of measurement error.

CROSS-LAGGED APIM USING MLM

We illustrate the MLM approach to a cross-lagged APIM using data from a 2-week daily diary study of dating couples (Campbell, Simpson, Boldry, & Kashy, 2005). In this study both members of 103 heterosexual couples reported on their relationship satisfaction daily for 14 days. The model (see Figure 31.3) is similar in structure to the standard APIM, but there are several important differences. The most obvious difference is that the predictors in the cross-lagged model are the person's and the person's partner's past scores on the outcome. Thus we predict the woman's relationship satisfaction on a particular day as a function of her own satisfaction on the preceding day and her partner's satisfaction on the preceding day. Likewise, the man's relationship satisfaction at one point in time is predicted

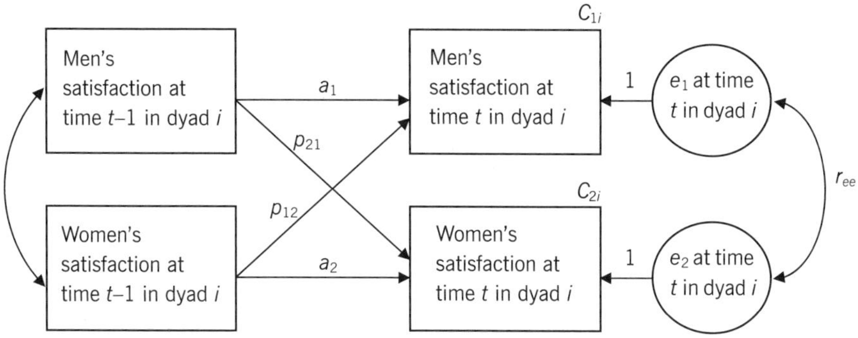

FIGURE 31.3. Diary data illustration of cross-lagged APIM for distinguishable dyad members. a_1, men's actor effect; a_2, women's actor effect; p_{21}, men's partner effect on women; p_{12}, women's partner effect on men; C_{1i}, men's intercept for relationship satisfaction; C_{2i}, women's intercept for relationship satisfaction; e_1, residualized variance in men's satisfaction not explained by men's and women's satisfaction the previous day; e_2, residualized variance in women's satisfaction not explained by men's and women's satisfaction the previous day; r_{ee}, residualized time-specific nonindependence not explained by actor and partner effects in model.

by his own satisfaction and his partner's satisfaction on the previous day. In this case, there are no reasons to suspect that the strength of these lags changes over time.

In this cross-lagged model, the actor effect (a_1 and a_2 for men and women, respectively) estimates the average stability of relationship satisfaction. Therefore, rather than obtaining separate actor effects for each time interval like the cross-lagged APIM using SEM, this model provides an average estimate of the actor effect across all of the time intervals. Similarly, the partner effects (p_{21} and p_{12} for men and women, respectively) estimate the average degree of cross-partner influence. Because we use grand mean–centered values for the lagged predictor variables, the intercepts shown in Figure 31.3 (C_{1i} and C_{2i} for men and women, respectively) represent men's and women's average level of satisfaction across the 14 days.

The other key difference with this cross-lagged APIM is that we are able to estimate a number of random effects, some of which are not evident in Figure 31.3. Indeed, in addition to the previously discussed fixed effects for the intercepts, actor effects, and partner effects, the cross-lagged model in MLM specifies that there are random effects for the intercepts, actor effects, partner effects, and residuals. In other words, in addition to having an average stability coefficient for the women (i.e., the fixed effect estimate of the women's actor effect), the stability coefficients are allowed to vary in size from couple to couple (i.e., the random effect or variance in the actor effect). Thus there are two intercept variances that estimate dyad-to-dyad variation in average satisfaction, two actor effect variances that estimate dyad-to-dyad variation in stability, two partner effect variances that estimate dyad-to-dyad variation in reciprocity or influence, and two residual variances.

The random effects part of the model can also include as many as 16 covariances or correlations. Four of these correlations model similarity in the effects across the two partners: (1) The correlation between the two partners' intercepts estimates the degree to which the two partners' average levels of satisfaction are similar, (2) the correlation between the two partners' actor effects estimates whether partners are similar in their degree of stability,

(3) the correlation between the two partners' partner effects estimates whether partners are similar in their degree of reciprocity or influence, and (4) the correlation between the two partners' residuals (r_{ee} in Figure 31.2) captures the time-specific similarity in relationship satisfaction between men and women that is not accounted for by the other predictors in the model. The remaining covariances include cross-effect within-person covariances (e.g., women's intercept with women's actor effect) and cross-effect between-person covariances (e.g., women's intercept with men's actor effect).

Basic Data Requirements. As was the case with the cross-lagged APIM for SEM, the cross-lagged APIM for MLM requires that researchers collect data on the same mixed variables for both dyad members at multiple points in time. For the cross-lagged APIM with MLM, we recommend that researchers collect as many waves as possible. This is especially important in the typical lagged model used with diary data because the first observation is lost (at time 1 there are no data on the past). Importantly, this model also assumes that the time intervals between data collection waves are constant. In addition, the time lag should match theoretical expectations about the processes under investigation. Put simply, the lags should be long enough so that change can occur on focal variables but not so long as to preclude detecting contingencies that might dissipate over time.

The data structure necessary to perform a cross-lagged APIM in MLM is a person–period pairwise data set (see Table C at *www.crmda.ku.edu/Guilford/HDRM*). In this data structure, each row represents one wave of data for one of the two dyad members. Thus in the present example the study included daily measurements for 14 days on 103 dyads, so each dyad has 28 data rows, 14 for each partner, and the data set as a whole includes 2,884 records.

To prevent problems when creating the lagged variables, researchers should ensure that the same number of intervals exists for each dyad. In cases of missing data, blank rows of data should be inserted to stand in for those intervals in which data were not collected from both members of the dyad. Before creating the lagged variables, researchers should grand mean–center the predictors. After this centering is completed, the lagged variables should be created using the immediately preceding wave (i.e., unless there is a theoretical rationale to do otherwise, researchers should use a lag of 1). Syntax for restructuring dyadic over-time data in SPSS/PASW can be obtained from Ackerman by email request.

Interpreting Estimates from the Cross-Lagged APIM. The first step in interpreting results from a cross-lagged model using MLM is to make sure that the model ran successfully (i.e., it converged and there were no warnings). In this example, the model converged, and we are thus able to interpret the parameter estimates with confidence. The men's intercept for relationship satisfaction was 6.32, and the women's intercept for relationship satisfaction was 6.39. These results indicate that men's and women's average relationship satisfaction levels across the 14 days were rather high considering that the ratings were made on a 1–7 scale.

The actor effect for women was positive and statistically significant, $b = 0.24$, $t(66) = 6.30$, $p < .001$, suggesting that women's satisfaction levels were relatively stable. The actor effect for men was similarly positive and statistically significant, $b = 0.28$, $t(67) = 6.76$, $p < .001$. The partner effects were also positive, but only the partner effect of the man's previous satisfaction on the woman's current satisfaction was even marginally significant (for women, $b = 0.08$, $t(56) = -1.88$, $p = .07$; for men, $b = 0.04$, $t(37) = 1.15$, $p = .26$). This

TABLE 31.3. Correlation Matrix for Cross-Lagged APIM for Diary Data Example

Variable	1	2	3	4	5	6
1. Men's intercept	.14**					
2. Women's intercept	.65**	.09**				
3. Men's actor effect	–.19	.05	.05*			
4. Women's actor effect	–.12	–.70*	–.25	.04*		
5. Men's partner effect	–.12	–.51+	–.22	.77+	.04+	
6. Women's partner effect	.16	.25	.67*	–.37	–.06	.08*

Note. Values along the diagonal represent variances and values off the diagonal represent population estimates of correlations based on variance components.
$+p < .10$; $*p < .05$; $**p < .01$.

suggests that women whose partners were especially happy on one day were themselves happier the next.

In addition to fixed effects, there were also a host of significant random effects to interpret. As Table 31.3 shows, there was significant variance in the intercepts for both men and women. This provides evidence of dyad-to-dyad differences in the average levels of satisfaction for both genders. There was also a strong positive correlation between the intercepts for men and women, suggesting that dating partners' average satisfaction levels were very closely related.

To evaluate whether there were dyad-to-dyad differences in the stability of relationship satisfaction, we examine the variance estimates for men's and women's actor effects. As Table 31.3 shows, there was significant variance in the actor effects for both men and women, indicating that people differed in the stability of their satisfaction levels. However, the small, nonsignificant correlation between the actor effects provides no evidence that individual differences in stability were linked for men and women. Another important question is whether there are dyad-to-dyad differences in the degree of cross-partner influence for men and women. Simply put, do people differ in terms of cross-partner influence for relationship satisfaction? In this example, there was some evidence of variance in the partner effects for both men and women. However, individual differences in cross-partner influence were not correlated for men and women.

A Brief Introduction to Dyadic Growth Curves

Many developmental questions concern whether there are systematic increases or decreases in behavior over time, and this focus can be extended to the dyadic context. For example, Kashy and colleagues (2008) examined twins' reports of conflict with their mothers across adolescence. In this study, the use of dyadic growth curve models revealed evidence of increasing conflict in parent–child relationships, as well as evidence that the two twins' degree of change over time was correlated. The topic of growth models is well covered in this *Handbook* (see Grimm & Ram, Chapter 24; Hox & Boom, Chapter 25; and Blozis, Chapter 26), and more complete coverage of dyadic extensions can be found in Kashy and

Donnellan (2008, in press) and Kashy and colleagues (2008). In this chapter, we provide only a brief discussion of how growth models can be extended to the dyadic context.

The basic idea of a growth model is to determine whether a variable of interest increases or decreases with time in a systematic fashion. Consider as an example the variable of self-esteem in a sample of adolescents measured at four yearly occasions starting at age 13 (i.e., assessments were made at ages 13, 14, 15, and 16). Assuming that time is coded as 0, 1, 2, 3 for the four assessments, respectively, a linear growth model would estimate the "trajectory" of self-esteem as a function of two parameters: an intercept, which is the estimate of the average level of self-esteem at age 13 (when time = 0), and a slope term, which measures the estimated change in self-esteem as age increases by 1 year. In addition to estimating the average intercept and slope, individual growth models also typically estimate variance in the intercepts (i.e., to what extent do 13-year-olds vary in their predicted self-esteem?), variance in the slopes (i.e., to what extent does the linear change in self-esteem vary across adolescents?), and covariance between the intercept and slope (e.g., do adolescents who begin relatively low in self-esteem increase more slowly over time?).

The extension of individual growth curve modeling to the dyadic context is fairly straightforward. Consider as an example a study of heterosexual dating couples in mid-adolescence in which each person reports on the level of conflict in the relationship every week for a 6-week period. In dyadic growth models for distinguishable dyads, there are two intercepts and two slopes (comprehensive treatment of indistinguishable dyads is covered in Kashy et al., 2008). These intercepts and slopes each have variances that can be correlated within person for each type of dyad member (e.g., if the female adolescent starts the study reporting high levels of conflict, does she also tend to report increases in conflict over time?). More important, in the dyadic case, the intercepts and slopes can be correlated between persons. For example, the correlation between the intercepts would estimate whether female adolescents who start the study reporting high levels of conflict have dating partners who also report high levels of conflict at the outset. The correlation between the slopes estimates whether female adolescents who perceive increasing levels of conflict over time have male partners who also perceive that conflict is increasing.

In spite of their growing popularity in developmental research, growth curve models are not suitable for all applications. Growth curve models actually have fairly stringent requirements in terms of measurement. It is essential that "a given value of the outcome on any occasion [represents] the 'same' amount of the outcome on every occasion" (Singer & Willett, 2003, p. 13). Variables that are standardized within each wave are not appropriate, because the value of a "zero" may represent a different absolute level at each time point. This would happen if the actual means fluctuated over time. Beyond simply using the same items with the same response option at each wave, researchers should consider formally testing for measurement invariance to confirm that responses on the composite variable (e.g., the summed responses to our measure of conflict) capture the underlying latent variable in the same way at each occasion (Schmitt & Kuljanin, 2008). Researchers should also recognize that it can be very difficult to detect correlates of change given issues of statistical power (e.g., Hertzog, Lindenberger, Ghisletta, & von Oertzen, 2006). For instance, it can be hard to find a connection between the slopes of two partners in the same relationship. Both the number of waves of data collection and the number of dyads are factors to consider. We recommend aiming for large numbers of both. To be sure, the precision of parameter estimates improves with additional waves of data collection, and this is especially true when researchers collect only a few waves of data (see Figure 4 in Willett et al., 1998).

Dyadic growth models can be estimated using either MLM or SEM. As was the case for cross-lagged models, each data analytical method has its own strengths and weaknesses. MLM is particularly useful when the exact timing of measurement waves differs across participants (e.g., the actual ages in the 13-year-old assessment fall anywhere between 12.5 years and 13.5 years) and when researchers plan to include predictor variables that may moderate the effects of time on the outcome. SEM is very useful when researchers need to specify constraints on the residual variances and correlations and when there is interest in obtaining omnibus tests of fit.

Future Directions

Statistical Power Issues

As with all analyses, statistical power is an important issue for dyadic analyses. Researchers need to think carefully about power and plan to conduct studies that have a reasonable chance of detecting anticipated effects. Partner effects are typically more interesting than actor effects. Kenny and Cook (1999) argued that "the presence of partner effects implies that something relational has occurred in that a person's response depends on some property of the partner" (p. 435). Thus researchers want to be able to find evidence of these important effects. Our experience, however, is that partner effects are harder to detect than actor effects given typical effect sizes (i.e., small effects; see Ackerman et al., 2011). Power is also an issue with longitudinal models, given that the rank-order stability for many constructs is likely to be high so that actor effects may "crowd out" partner effects (see Kashy & Donnellan, in press). It might take a large sample to detect theoretically important partner effects in a longitudinal context given the stability of many constructs. Researchers need to pay careful attention to the timing of data collection.

These concerns ultimately boil down to the practical things that researchers can do to make their studies more powerful. The answer is both simple and daunting. The power of any analysis is a function of the sample size, the true effect size, and the level of statistical significance selected for an investigation (i.e., alpha). The alpha level is set by convention (typically .05), and therefore researchers can basically strive to use good measures to minimize the effects of measurement error and work to increase sample size. (Researchers have no control over the true effect size in nature.) Likewise, increasing the number of measurement occasions can improve power in many longitudinal contexts (see, e.g., Hertzog et al., 2006). Explicit planning for statistical power in dyadic contexts is slightly more complicated than traditional power analyses given the statistical interdependence between individuals. Kenny and colleagues (2006) provide formulas and approximations for power analysis. Nonetheless, the simplest piece of advice that we can give is that more is usually better in terms of number of dyads, measurement reliability, and number of assessments.

On a related note, some researchers are interested in calculating effect sizes that can be contrasted across studies. To our knowledge, this is not something that can easily be done, because the effect sizes are dependent on multiple factors. Thus researchers would have to assume an almost impractical ideal of consistency across studies. For instance, if researchers wish to compare the magnitude of partner effects in the cross-lagged APIM, they must assume that the stability coefficients (i.e., actor effects) across studies are of the same size. Fluctuations in the stability coefficients (which often depend on the time interval of the study and issues of reliability) will influence the size of the partner effect. Aside from this, it is difficult to compare effect sizes across studies, as standardization procedures depend on the variances of the variables, as well as the other variables that are included in the model. If such aspects of the study are not consistent, then researchers may very well be comparing "apples to oranges."

Estimating More Complicated Models: Extensions of the Dyadic Models

The APIM offers a general framework for analyzing dyadic data, and there are a number of extensions that can be added to the basic model. Importantly, we described procedures for estimating the APIM that are suitable for variables that are more or less measured on at least an interval scale. The estimation procedures we outlined are not optimal for nominal or clearly ordinal outcome variables. Common categorical variables in developmental contexts might include whether married partners have contemplated divorce in the preceding month (1 = Yes, 0 = No) or whether parents and children have evidence of passing the threshold for a psychiatric disorder. Researchers interested in extensions with these kinds of variables should consult Kenny and colleagues (2006).

In addition, researchers investigating dyadic processes are often interested in the synergistic effects of the two individuals' attributes. Within the APIM framework, the effects of the ways actor and partner attributes combine to affect individuals' outcomes can be assessed by incorporating interactions between actor and partner effects. For example, it might be the case that mothers and their children who are both high on negative affectivity combine such that their interactions are uniquely devoid of positive engagement. The combination of data from each partner in a dyad can be specified in several ways (e.g., difference scores, profile correlations, and multiplicative terms), and researchers should carefully consider which approach best captures their underlying conceptual model. We refer interested readers to Ackerman and colleagues (2011) and Kenny and colleagues (2006) for more information about these variables (often called dyadic indices in the literature).

Conclusions

Developmental researchers, especially those who focus on social and emotional development, have a long-standing interest in dyadic relationships. Dyadic models applied to both cross-sectional and longitudinal data have the ability to illuminate essential processes of interdependence, mutual influence, socialization, selection, and reciprocity. The three dyadic models described here (i.e., the standard APIM, the cross-lagged APIM, and the dyadic growth curve model) provide researchers with sophisticated tools for investigating central questions that have been the mainstay of developmental research for decades. Ultimately, the use of these kinds of models and their more complicated extensions has the ability to bring the data analyses conducted by researchers in closer accord with contemporary developmental theorizing about relationships. This more intimate coupling of theory and method will help to further improve developmental research about important topics such as interpersonal influence, interdependence, and linked patterns of change over time.

Acknowledgments

Grants from the Eunice Kennedy Shriver National Institute of Child Health and Human Development, the National Institute of Mental Health, and the American Recovery and Reinvestment Act (Nos. HD064687, HD051746, MH051361, and HD047573) helped to partially fund the writing of this chapter. The content is solely the responsibility of the authors and does not necessarily represent the official views of the funding agencies. Some of the data described in this chapter were collected with funds from multiple sources, including the National Institute of Mental Health (Grant Nos. MH00567, MH19734, MH43270, MH59355, MH62989, and MH48165), the National Institute on Drug Abuse (Grant No. DA05347), the National Institute of Child Health and Human Development (Grant No. HD027724), the Bureau of Maternal and Child Health (Grant No. MCJ-109572), and the MacArthur Foundation Research Network on Successful Adolescent Development among Youth in High-Risk Settings.

References

Ackerman, R. A., Donnellan, M. B., & Kashy, D. A. (2011). Working with dyadic data in studies of emerging adulthood: Specific recommendations, general advice, and practical tips. In F. D. Fincham & M. Cui (Eds.), *Romantic relationships in emerging adulthood* (pp. 67–97). New York: Cambridge University Press.

Ackerman, R. A., Kashy, D. A., Donnellan, M. B., & Conger, R. D. (in press). Positive-engagement behaviors in observed family interactions: A social relations perspective. *Journal of Family Psychology*.

Bell, R. Q. (1968). A reinterpretation of the direction of effects in studies of socialization. *Psychological Review, 75* (2), 81–95.

Bronfenbrenner, U., & Morris, P. A. (2006). The bioecological model of human development. In R. M. Lerner (Vol. Ed.), *Handbook of child psychology: Vol. 1. Theoretical models of human development* (6th ed., pp. 793–828). New York: Wiley.

Campbell, L., Simpson, J. A., Boldry, J., & Kashy, D. A. (2005). Perceptions of conflict and support in romantic relationships: The role of attachment anxiety. *Journal of Personality and Social Psychology, 88*, 510–531.

Caspi, A., Roberts, B. W., & Shiner, R. L. (2005). Personality development: Stability and change. *Annual Review of Psychology, 56*, 453–484.

Conger, R. D., & Elder, G. H., Jr. (1994). *Families in troubled times: Adapting to change in rural America*. Hillsdale, NJ: Aldine.

Cook, W. L., & Kenny, D. A. (2005). The actor–partner interdependence model: A model of bidirectional effects in developmental studies. *International Journal of Behavioral Development, 29*, 101–109.

Cox, M. J., & Paley, B. (1997). Families as systems. *Annual Review of Psychology, 48*, 243–267.

Derogatis, L. R. (1983). *SCL-90–R administration, scoring, and procedures manual: II*. Townsen, MD: Clinical Psychometric Research.

Donnellan, M. B., Conger, K. J., McAdams, K. K., & Neppl, T. (2009). Personal characteristics and resilience to economic hardship and its consequences: Conceptual issues and empirical illustrations. *Journal of Personality, 77*, 1645–1676.

Donnellan, M. B., & Conger, R. D. (2007). Designing and implementing longitudinal studies. In R. W. Robins, R. C. Fraley, & R. F. Krueger (Eds.), *Handbook of research methods in personality psychology* (pp. 21–36). New York: Guilford Press.

Ellenbogen, M. A., Ostiguy, C. S., & Hodgins, S. (2010). Intergenerational effects of high neuroticism in parents and their public health significance. *American Psychologist, 65*, 135–136.

Ge, X., Conger, R. D., Lorenz, F. O., Shanahan, M., & Elder, G. H. (1995). Mutual influences in parent and adolescent psychological distress. *Developmental Psychology, 31*, 406–419.

Hertzog, C., Lindenberger, U., Ghisletta, P., & von Oertzen, T. (2006). On the power of multivariate latent growth curve models to detect correlated change. *Psychological Methods, 11*, 244–252.

Kashy, D. A., Campbell, L., & Harris, D. W. (2006). Advances in data analytic approaches for relationships research: The broad utility of hierarchical linear modeling. In A. L. Vangelisti & D. Perlman (Eds.), *The Cambridge handbook of personal relationships* (pp. 73–89). New York: Cambridge University Press.

Kashy, D. A., & Donnellan, M. B. (2008). Comparing MLM and SEM approaches to analyzing developmental dyadic data: Growth curve modeling of hostility in families. In N. A. Card, J. P. Selig, & T. D. Little (Eds.), *Modeling dyadic and interdependent data in the developmental and behavioral sciences* (pp. 165–190). New York: Routledge.

Kashy, D. A., & Donnellan, M. B. (in press). Conceptual and methodological issues in the analysis of data from dyads and groups. In K. Deaux & M. Snyder (Eds.), *The Oxford handbook of personality and social psychology*. New York: Oxford University Press.

Kashy, D. A., Donnellan, M. B., Burt, S. A., & McGue, M. (2008). Growth curve models for indistinguishable dyads using multilevel modeling and structural equation modeling: The case of adolescent twin's conflict with their mothers. *Developmental Psychology, 44*, 316–329.

Kenny, D. A., & Cook, W. (1999). Partner effects in relationship research: Conceptual issues, analytic difficulties, and illustrations. *Personal Relationships, 6*, 433–448.

Kenny, D. A., Kashy, D. A., & Cook, W. L. (2006). *Dyadic data analysis*. New York: Guilford Press.

Laursen, B. (2005). Dyadic and group perspectives on close relationships. *International Journal of Behavioral Development, 29*, 97–100.

Lytton, H. (1990). Child and parent effects in boys' conduct disorder: A reinterpretation. *Developmental Psychology, 26*(5), 683–697.

Olsen, J. A., & Kenny, D. A. (2006). Structural equation modeling with interchangeable dyads. *Psychological Methods, 11*(2), 127–141.

Popp, D., Laursen, B., Kerr, M., Stattin, H., & Burk, W. J. (2008). Modeling homophily over time with an actor–partner interdependence model. *Developmental Psychology, 44*, 1028–1039.

Raudenbush, S. W., Brennan, R. T., & Barnett, R. C. (1995). A multivariate hierarchical model for studying psychological change within married couples. *Journal of Family Psychology, 9*, 167–174.

Raudenbush, S. W., & Bryk, A. S. (2002). *Hierarchical linear models: Applications and data analysis methods* (2nd ed.). Thousand Oaks, CA: Sage.

Reis, H. T., Collins, W. A., & Berscheid, E. (2000). The relationship context of human behavior and development. *Psychological Bulletin, 126*, 844–872.

Sameroff, A. J. (2010). A unified theory of development: A dialectic integration of nature and nurture. *Child Development, 81*, 6–22.

Schmitt, N., & Kuljanin, G. (2008). Measurement invariance: Review of practice and implications. *Human Resource Management Review, 18*, 210–222.

Singer, J. D., & Willett, J. B. (2003). *Applied longitudinal data analysis: Modeling change and event occurrence*. New York: Oxford University Press.

Snijders, T., & Bosker, R. (1999). *Multilevel analysis: An introduction to basic and advanced multilevel modeling*. London: Sage.

Willett, J. B., Singer, J. D., & Martin, N. C. (1998). The design and analysis of longitudinal studies of development and psychopathology in context: Statistical models and methodological recommendations. *Development and Psychopathology, 10*, 395–426.

CHAPTER 32

Applying the Social Relations Model to Developmental Research

NOEL A. CARD
RUSSELL B. TOOMEY

The social relations model (SRM) is a conceptual and analytical approach to identifying individual-, dyad-, and group-level contributions in interpersonal perceptions and behaviors. Originally developed and applied to social psychological data (Kenny, 1994; Kenny & La Voie, 1984), the model has been less often used in developmental research. However, we argue that developmental scientists can fruitfully apply this model to answer important developmental questions, and we hope to demonstrate this potential in this chapter.

We first elaborate on the central issues of the need for a dyadic focus in developmental science and the value of the SRM to advance this focus. We then describe the relevant designs, parameter estimates, and statistical inferences that make up the basic SRM, as well as extensions of this basic SRM in terms of analyzing groups with roles (e.g., families), methods of studying subgroup relations, multivariate extensions of the SRM, and extensions into three or more person data. We then review previous developmental research using the SRM, identifying the advances made by these works, as well as their limitations. Finally, we describe our view of important future directions for using the SRM in developmental research.

Central Issues

Developmental scientists have historically acknowledged the importance of interactions and relationships with others across the lifespan (e.g., Bronfenbrenner, 1979; Bronfenbrenner & Morris, 1998; Collins & Laursen, 1999; Hartup, 1979). To provide just a few examples, there has been extensive research documenting the importance of parenting behaviors and parent–child relationships in infancy and beyond (see Bornstein, 2002), of peer interactions and relationships during childhood and adolescence (see Rubin, Bukowski, & Laursen, 2008), and of spouses and other interactional partners throughout adulthood (see Berscheid, 1994). This focus on social interactions and relationships does not disavow the importance of individual factors, such as genetic influences, on development; instead, it highlights the inextricable social embeddedness of human development, which operates both as a main effect and in interaction with individual-level factors (e.g., Belsky, 2005; Gottlieb, 1998) in shaping development trajectories.

Despite the long-standing acknowledgment of the importance of interpersonal interactions and relationships by developmental theorists and researchers, the vast majority of developmental research has utilized the individual as the fundamental unit of analysis. We suspect that the primary reason for this disconnection between a conceptual focus on social embeddedness and an empirical focus on the individual can be attributed to the limitations of traditional data analytical tools. For instance, a fundamental assumption of statistical inference with traditional analytical approaches (e.g., the general and generalized linear models) is that each case (e.g., person) is independent of other cases. This analytical assumption of independence contrasts with our conceptual expectations of interdependence among people.

Fortunately, analytical tools have emerged over (approximately) the last three decades that allow us to move beyond assumptions of independence to explicitly model interdependence. Currently, several analytical approaches model interdependent data, including the actor–partner interdependence model (see Cook & Kenny, 2005), one-with-many designs and analyses (see Kenny, Kashy, & Cook, 2006, Chapter 10), and various techniques of social network analysis (see Wasserman & Faust, 1994; for encompassing overviews of methods for interdependent data analysis, see Card, Selig, & Little, 2008; Kenny et al., 2006). Therefore, the SRM is not the only method of analyzing interdependent data. However, we view it as a particularly valuable approach in that it explicitly models the relative roles of individuals, dyads, and groups in interdependent phenomena, and extensions of this model provide great flexibility in answering numerous developmental questions. We next describe this model to provide a foundation for discussing how developmental researchers can use this powerful approach.

Conceptual Principles and Statistical Assumptions

The SRM is actually a collection of related approaches to modeling individual and dyadic aspects of data collected when a group of individuals perceives, evaluates, or enacts behavior toward a group of other individuals. The individuals perceiving, evaluating, or behaving toward others are termed *actors* in the SRM framework, whereas the targets of these perceptions, evaluations, or behaviors are termed *partners*.

We next describe variants in the SRM in terms of design and form of data collected. After this, we describe the estimation of basic parameters of SRMs, as well as methods of drawing statistical inferences about these estimates. Finally, we describe more advanced models from this basic SRM framework.

Design and Data Collection

The SRM is not only a method of analysis but also a framework for conceptualizing and designing studies. In this section, we describe the common designs and data requirements for the SRM.

Types of Designs

As mentioned, the general design of the SRM is for one group of actors to evaluate a group of partners. The three basic designs of the SRM differ in whether the actors and partners come from separable groups or the same group. Figure 32.1 displays these three designs, in which data are collected from hypothetical eight-child groups (children A to H) and *X*s represent measured data (see also Kenny, Kashy, & Cook, 2006).

The half-block design (Figure 32.1a) is the simplest method. Here, the actors are members of one group, and the partners are members of a second, nonoverlapping group. For instance, within a group of children categorized as boys or girls, one could investigate the perceptions the boys (actors) have of females (partners). This design allows for estimation of three of the five parameters of the SRM (actor, partner, and relationship variances; described subsequently). The analysis of this design is also straightforward (i.e., evaluated as two-way random-effects analysis of variance [ANOVA], with actors as one factor and partners as a second factor), so we do not discuss it further.

The block (also called full block) design (Figure 32.1b) expands on the half-block design. As with the half block, this model is used when there are two groups of nonoverlapping individuals. However, whereas the half-block uses perceptions, evaluations, or behaviors of only one group toward the other, the block design also uses data of the second group toward the first. Returning to our previous example of perceptions and genders, this design would use data not only about boys' perceptions of girls but also about girls' perceptions of boys. This model would allow the estimation of all five parameters of the SRM, described subsequently.

The round-robin design (Figure 32.1c) is the prototypical design for the SRM. In this design, actors and partners are considered members of a common group, and all individuals in this group (actors) provide data about all other members of this group (partners). Because this round-robin design is the most common design considered by quantitative methodologists, as well as the most commonly used design in substantive (developmental and other) research, we focus attention primarily on this design in this chapter.

Data Requirements

The SRM was originally applied in controlled (i.e., laboratory) social psychology experiments. These origins of the SRM have led to rather strict recommendations for the sorts of data that are needed for the SRM.

First, the SRM was developed with the assumption of continuous (and presumably normally distributed) data. Most applications of the SRM attempt to approximate this by measuring perceptions, evaluations, or behaviors of an actor toward a partner on some Likert-type scale (e.g., 1–5 or 1–7 scale). However, there are some naturalistic applications for which dichotomous measures are used. For example, a study using peer nominations as a measure of interpersonal perceptions of children within a school setting might use the presence or absence of a nomination by one child of another as round-robin data (e.g., Card, Hodges, Little, & Hawley, 2005). Simulation studies have indicated that the SRM is robust to such violations of distributional assumptions, at least to the extent to which they have been studied (e.g., Lashley & Bond, 1997, found that the SRM performed well with dichotomous data up to the most extreme [10%/90%] level tested).

Second, the initial use of SRMs in controlled laboratory studies meant that there were no missing data. Therefore, there have been no efforts to advance methods of missing data management beyond crude methods of listwise deletion.

(a) Half-block design

	A	B	C	D	E	F	G	H
A					X	X	X	X
B					X	X	X	X
C					X	X	X	X
D					X	X	X	X
E								
F								
G								
H								

(b) Block design

	A	B	C	D	E	F	G	H
A					X	X	X	X
B					X	X	X	X
C					X	X	X	X
D					X	X	X	X
E	X	X	X	X				
F	X	X	X	X				
G	X	X	X	X				
H	X	X	X	X				

(c) Round-robin design

	A	B	C	D	E	F	G	H
A		X	X	X	X	X	X	X
B	X		X	X	X	X	X	X
C	X	X		X	X	X	X	X
D	X	X	X		X	X	X	X
E	X	X	X	X		X	X	X
F	X	X	X	X	X		X	X
G	X	X	X	X	X	X		X
H	X	X	X	X	X	X	X	

FIGURE 32.1. Three basic designs of the SRM family.

Parameter Estimation

The basic SRM provides estimates of five parameters, with the possibility of a sixth. The five parameters commonly estimated include three variances (actor, partner, and relationship) and two covariances (actor–partner, also called generalized, and dyadic). The sixth possible estimate is of between-group variance (which is simply the variance in overall means, $M_{\bullet\bullet}$, across groups). We next describe these parameters in turn, describing how each is conceptualized and estimated. To aid interpretation, we refer to Figure 32.2, which contains a hypothetical sociomatrix (i.e., matrix of data) from a six-person round-robin design.

	1	2	3	4	5	6	Total
1	--	X_{12}	X_{13}	X_{14}	X_{15}	X_{16}	$M_{1\bullet}$
2	X_{21}	--	X_{23}	X_{24}	X_{25}	X_{26}	$M_{2\bullet}$
3	X_{31}	X_{32}	--	X_{34}	X_{35}	X_{36}	$M_{3\bullet}$
4	X_{41}	X_{42}	X_{43}	--	X_{45}	X_{46}	$M_{4\bullet}$
5	X_{51}	X_{52}	X_{53}	X_{54}	--	X_{56}	$M_{5\bullet}$
6	X_{61}	X_{62}	X_{63}	X_{64}	X_{65}	--	$M_{6\bullet}$
Total	$M_{\bullet 1}$	$M_{\bullet 2}$	$M_{\bullet 3}$	$M_{\bullet 4}$	$M_{\bullet 5}$	$M_{\bullet 6}$	$M_{\bullet\bullet}$

FIGURE 32.2. Hypothetical sociomatrix of data for univariate SRM.

Actor Variance

This variance refers to the magnitude of interindividual (i.e., between-person) difference in perceiving, evaluating, or behaving toward others. To estimate this variance, it is first necessary to estimate actor effects for each person, using the following equation (see Kenny, 1994):

$$\hat{a}_i = \frac{(n-1)^2}{n(n-2)} M_{i\bullet} + \frac{n-1}{n(n-2)} M_{\bullet i} - \frac{n-1}{n-2} M_{\bullet\bullet} \quad \textbf{(32.1)}$$

Here, $\hat{a}_i$ is the estimated actor effect for person i and is based largely on the row mean (see Figure 32.2) for that person ($M_{i\bullet}$). The second piece of this equation is a correction for the fact that this person did not have the opportunity to have scores toward him- or herself (i.e., the column mean, $M_{\bullet i}$). To illustrate, if the data are liking scores and person i is highly liked by others, this person's row mean is deflated relative to others' given that the others were not scored on likability; this part of the equation corrects this deflation. The third component of this equation subtracts the overall group mean ($M_{\bullet\bullet}$), which results in estimated actor effects being centered at zero (i.e., positive scores result when the person's effect is higher than average for the group, whereas negative scores result when the person's effect is lower). These three components are weighted by functions of the group sample size, n. Because estimation of the overall actor variance involves additional model estimates, we describe this estimation after describing the remaining four variance–covariance components.

Partner Variance

This variance refers to the magnitude of interindividual difference in being perceived, evaluated, or behaved toward by others. As with estimates of actor variance, estimates of partner variance require one to first estimate partner effects for each person (Kenny, 1994):

$$\hat{b}_i = \frac{(n-1)^2}{n(n-2)} M_{\bullet i} + \frac{n-1}{n(n-2)} M_{i\bullet} - \frac{n-1}{n-2} M_{\bullet\bullet} \quad \textbf{(32.2)}$$

From this equation, partner effects for person i ($\hat{b}_i$) are a function primarily of their column mean ($M_{\bullet i}$), corrected for that person's row mean ($M_{i\bullet}$) and centered around the overall group mean ($M_{\bullet\bullet}$).

Relationship Variance

This variance refers to the magnitude of interdyadic difference in a particular actor perceiving, evaluating, or behaving toward a particular partner. To estimate this variance, it is first necessary to estimate relationship effects for each of the $n(n-1)$ directional dyads in the group using the following equation:

$$\hat{g}_{ij} = X_{ij} - \hat{a}_i - \hat{b}_j - M_{\bullet\bullet} \tag{32.3}$$

This equation reveals that the relationship effect for actor i toward partner j ($\hat{g}_{ij}$) begins with the score in that cell (X_{ij}; see Figure 32.2), but subtracts the centered actor effect of person i ($\hat{a}_i$) and the centered partner effect of person j ($\hat{b}_i$), as well as centers around the overall group mean ($M_{\bullet\bullet}$). The subtraction of individual actor and partner effects means that this relationship effect indexes the extent to which person i's perceptions and so forth of person j exceed expectations given i's typical perceptions of others and others' perceptions of j.

It is worth noting that relationship effects, as well as the estimate of relationship variance described subsequently, contain both reliable interdyadic variability and random error. In order to separate these two components to provide unbiased estimates of relationship variance (as well as other parameters, such as disattenuated dyadic covariance), it is necessary to obtain multiple measures (indicators) of variables. These can be multiple measures over short periods of time (i.e., shorter than those in which one expects the underlying construct to change) or else multiple forms of measurement at the same time (e.g., multiple items). Details for analysis of multiple indicators in SRM are described in Kenny (1994).

Actor–Partner Covariance

This association, also called generalized covariance, evaluates the direction and extent to which individuals' actor effects are associated with their partner effects. Positive values indicate that individuals with high actor effects tend to have high partner effects, whereas individuals with low actor effects tend to have low partner effects; for example, a positive actor–partner covariance for liking within a peer group would indicate that children who like their peers tend to be liked by their peers. Negative values indicate that individuals with high actor effects tend to have low partner effects, and vice versa. Estimation of this covariance is described subsequently.

Dyadic Covariance

This association evaluates the direction and extent to which one person's perceptions and evaluations of or behaviors toward a second person are associated with that second person's perceptions and evaluations of and behaviors toward the first person. More formally, this covariance quantifies the association between the relationship effect of person i toward person j ($\hat{g}_{ij}$) and the relationship effect of person j toward person i ($\hat{g}_{ji}$). Considering again the example of liking, a positive association would imply that if Ira highly likes Jane, then Jane tends to also highly like Ira.

Estimates of Variance Components

We have reserved presentation of the equations for estimating each of these variances and covariances until now because the equations involve various combinations of each of these estimates. We note that the equations presented are not necessarily intuitive, but they are straightforward to apply. For space consideration, we make no effort to derive or justify these equations; interested readers can consult Appendix B of Kenny (1994).

Because relationship variance (s_g^2) is used in subsequent equations, we present the equation to estimate this parameter first (Kenny, 1994):

$$s_g^2 = \frac{1}{2}\left(\frac{2\sum\left(\frac{\hat{g}_{ij} + \hat{g}_{ji}}{2}\right)^2}{\left[\frac{(n-1)(n-2)}{2}\right] - 1} + \frac{\sum\left(\hat{g}_{ij} - \hat{g}_{ji}\right)^2}{(n-1)(n-2)} \right) \quad \textbf{(32.4)}$$

The dyadic covariance ($s_{gg'}$) is estimated using a similar equation, with the exception that the second term within the large parentheses is subtracted from, rather than added to, the first (Kenny, 1994):

$$s_{gg'} = \frac{1}{2}\left(\frac{2\sum\left(\frac{\hat{g}_{ij} + \hat{g}_{ji}}{2}\right)^2}{\left[\frac{(n-1)(n-2)}{2}\right] - 1} - \frac{\sum\left(\hat{g}_{ij} - \hat{g}_{ji}\right)^2}{(n-1)(n-2)} \right) \quad \textbf{(32.5)}$$

These two estimates are then used, along with the previously described actor and partner effects for each individual, in the estimation of actor variance (s_a^2), partner variance (s_b^2), and actor–partner covariance (s_{ab}; Kenny, 1994):

$$s_a^2 = \frac{\sum \hat{a}_i^2}{n-1} - \frac{s_g^2(n-1)}{n(n-2)} - \frac{s_{gg'}}{n(n-2)} \quad \textbf{(32.6)}$$

$$s_b^2 = \frac{\sum \hat{b}_i^2}{n-1} - \frac{s_g^2(n-1)}{n(n-2)} - \frac{s_{gg'}}{n(n-2)} \quad \textbf{(32.7)}$$

$$s_{ab} = \frac{\sum\left(\hat{a}_i \hat{b}_i\right)}{n-1} - \frac{s_{gg'}(n-1)}{n(n-2)} - \frac{s_g^2}{n(n-2)} \quad \textbf{(32.8)}$$

Statistical Inference

The previous section presented equations that provide point estimates of the five SRM parameters (three variances and two covariances) within a single group. It is common to attempt to make inferences about these point estimates, either in the form of significance tests (typically null hypothesis tests of whether the parameter is reliably different from 0) or construction of confidence intervals. For either approach, it is necessary to compute standard errors of the point estimate. Although three approaches to computing confidence intervals of SRM parameters have been proposed, two have been shown useful and are common in research (the third, a jackknife procedure, suffers from low power and has no advantages over the other two).

Between-Groups t-Test

A straightforward and widely used method of determining statistical significance of parameters is by performing a *t*-test (with *df* = number of groups – 1) on the parameter estimates across multiple groups (weighting by $n - 1$ when group sizes differ) (Kenny & La Voie, 1984). If the result of this test is significant, then one concludes that the parameter is reliably different from zero. This approach necessarily requires multiple groups.

Within-Group t-Test

Bond and Lashley (1996; Lashley & Bond, 1997) proposed an alternative approach based on mathematically derived equations for parameter estimate of variability within groups. The equations are cumbersome, so we do not reproduce them here. However, they are also straightforward to implement, requiring only the parameter estimates described previously, sample sizes, and number of groups. This approach can be used with either single (Bond & Lashley, 1996) or multiple (Lashley & Bond, 1997) groups.

Comparing Methods of Statistical Inference

The within-group *t*-test approach can be used with either single or multiple groups, whereas the between-group *t*-test approach requires multiple groups. Furthermore, Lashley and Bond (1997) performed a simulation study comparing these approaches, finding that both adequately controlled for Type I error rates but that the within-group *t*-test had slightly greater significant power. Based on these considerations, it might appear clear that the within-group *t*-test is the superior approach. Indeed, in basic SRM, it appears to be superior. However, the major limitation to this approach is that it has not yet been extended beyond the basic SRM design. In these situations, the between-group *t*-test is the best available option. We turn to these more complex approaches to SRM next.

Beyond the Basics: Extensions of the SRM

Although the basic SRM has great potential in developmental research, consideration of some more advanced models opens possibilities for answering even more complex developmental questions. We next briefly describe four of the extensions of the basic SRM.

Matrix Partitioning

Although we earlier described three basic SRM designs, there is a fourth design called the block round-robin (Boldry & Kashy, 1999). This design is essentially a round-robin, but there exist meaningful subgroups within the larger group on which one can partition the larger sociomatrix. For example, a developmental research study might investigate interpersonal perceptions within an entire class of schoolchildren but then partition this larger matrix of data by sex (Card et al., 2005). The result is essentially two smaller round-robin designs (a group of boys and a group of girls) combined with a block design (cross-sex perceptions across boys and girls).

These designs are typically analyzed in components as two round-robin designs and a block design. In the example of partitioning by sex, one would estimate all five SRM parameters within the group of boys, within the group of girls, and for the cross-sex block design. Because the within-group *t*-test method of significance testing has not yet been expanded to block round-robin designs, a between-group *t*-test approach is used for statistical inference. Specifically, one treats the 15 SRM parameters (5 each for boys, girls, and cross-sex in our example) of each group as a "case" that is tested via a *t*-test. However, this basic *t*-test can be expanded into a repeated-measures ANOVA framework to allow comparisons across the partitioning blocks; for example, to compare differences in actor variance across boys, girls, and cross-sex data.

SRM with Roles

The field of dyadic data analysis commonly differentiates between distinguishable and indistinguishable dyads (e.g., Griffin & Gonzalez, 1995; Kenny et al., 2006). In the context of dyads, distinguishable members are those that (1) can be consistently assigned to one of two conceptually defined categories, or roles, across all dyads and (2) are empirically different in their means, variances, and/or covariances among variables (Kenny et al., 2006). For example, dyads of heterosexual romantic relationships can conceptually be distinguished by sex ("roles" of male vs. female), and nontwin sibling dyads can conceptually be distinguished by age (roles of older vs. younger); such dyads would be considered distinguishable if this conceptual distinction was also supported by empirical differences in their data. In contrast, indistinguishable dyads (also referred to as exchangeable dyads) do not have roles that can be meaningfully and consistently assigned to members across dyads. For example, gay and lesbian romantic relationships are not distinguished by sex (given that both members are the same on this variable), and twins cannot be meaningfully distinguished by age (an assignment to older or younger role based on the short interval between births would likely not be meaningful; as mentioned, Kenny et al. [2006] emphasized the need to empirically evaluate the distinguishing feature, with the expectation of finding differences in means, variances, and/or covariances with other variables by role). The classification of dyads as distinguishable or indistinguishable is not an absolute quality but rather one that is specific to the particular variable under consideration (e.g., same-sex friends are indistinguishable on sex but may be distinguishable on other features, such as relative power).

In the SRMs we have considered thus far, individuals are considered indistinguishable (this statement also applies to the half-block and block designs because members within each group are considered indistinguishable). However, the SRM can be extended to consider groups in which members have assignable roles. Developmental science has used this model primarily in the study of family perceptions, evaluations, and behaviors (discussed later). For instance, researchers might collect data from four-person families that all contain a father, mother, older child, and younger child.

These SRMs with roles are typically analyzed as confirmatory factor analytical models. Here, the $n(n - 1)$ scores that serve as data for a traditional round-robin SRM are considered manifest variables (e.g., in the four-person families described above, manifest variables would be the score of the father toward the mother, toward the older child, and toward the younger child; scores of the mother toward the father, older child, and younger child; etc.). Variances in these manifest variables are decomposed into latent variables with fixed loadings to specified manifest variables: for example, the father/actor construct is indicated by manifest variables of father to mother, older, and younger; mother/partner construct is indicated by manifest variables of father, older, and younger to mother; and relationship variances are the residual variances of the manifest variables. Actor–partner and dyadic covariances are accommodated by estimating appropriate covariances (e.g., father/actor–partner covariance is estimated as the association between father/actor and father/partner constructs; older–younger dyadic covariance is estimated as the association between older to younger and younger to older relationship constructs). For further details of these models, see Cook and Kenny (2004).

The SRM with roles provides considerably more results than the traditional SRM. First, the actor, partner, and relationship effects, although still centered around the group (e.g., family) mean, have potentially nonzero values for each role, and it is possible to compare these means across roles (e.g., do fathers or mothers provide more support to family members?). Second, the variance estimates (actor, partner, and relationship) differ in that they now index between-family variance for a particular role (vs. variance between indistinguishable individuals in a group), and these variances can be compared across roles (e.g., are fathers or mothers more variable in their perceptions, etc., of other family members?). Third, the covariances are now specific to role. For the actor–partner covariance, this is within a role (e.g., do older or younger children have a stronger association?). For the dyadic covariance, there are separate estimates for each role pair (are there different magnitudes of father–mother versus older–younger reciprocity?).

Multivariate SRM

The SRMs we have described to this point can be considered univariate in that they analyze one variable (e.g., a particular perception individuals have of each other). Multivariate SRMs expand on this by simultaneously modeling multiple variables and the individual and dyadic links among these variables.

Consider the bivariate SRM of two variables, X and Y, which we might hypothetically consider as perceptions and behaviors of others (respectively) for clarity. Here, it is possible to estimate five parameters (actor, partner, and relationship variances; actor–partner and dyadic covariances) for X (perceptions) and these same five parameters for Y (behaviors). However, it is also possible to estimate six additional parameters across variables. Four of these are at the individual level. The actor–actor covariance indexes the association of individual differences across actor effects of X and Y (e.g., is how children perceive their peers associated with how they behave toward their peers?). The partner–partner covariance indexes the association of individual differences across partner effects of X and Y

(e.g., is how children are perceived by their peers associated with their peers' behavior toward them?). The actor–partner covariance indexes the association of actor effects of *X* with partner effects of *Y* (e.g., is how children perceive their peers associated with how their peers behave toward them?). The partner–actor covariance indexes the association of partner effects of *X* with actor effects of *Y* (e.g., is how children are perceived by their peers associated with how they behave toward their peers?). There are also two covariances at the dyadic level. The intrapersonal covariance indexes the association of relationship effects across *X* and *Y* (e.g., is a child's perception of a particular peer associated with his or her behavior toward that peer?). Finally, the interpersonal covariance indexes the association between directed (*i* toward *j*) relationship effects of *X* and the returned (*j* toward *i*) relationship effect of *Y* (e.g., is a child's perception of a particular peer associated with that peer's behavior toward the child?).

The parameters of the bivariate SRM are estimated similarly to those of the traditional (univariate) SRM. The five parameters estimated for one variable (actor variance, s_a^2; partner variance, s_b^2; relationship variance, s_g^2; actor–partner covariance, s_{ab} dyadic covariance, $s_{gg'}$) are also estimated for the second variable, with different subscripts (actor variance, s_c^2; partner variance, s_d^2; relationship variance, s_h^2; actor–partner covariance, s_{cd}; dyadic covariance, $s_{hh'}$, respectively). The six across-variable covariances are estimated using equations similar to those for the univariate SRM. Specifically, the intrapersonal (s_{gh}) and interpersonal ($s_{gh'}$) covariances are estimated using the following equations (Card, Little, & Selig, 2008; Kenny, 1994):

$$s_{gh} = \frac{\sum\left(\frac{(\hat{g}_{ij}+\hat{g}_{ji})(\hat{h}_{ij}+\hat{h}_{ji})}{4}\right)}{\left(\frac{(n-1)(n-2)}{2}\right)-1} + \frac{\sum(\hat{g}_{ij}-\hat{g}_{ji})(\hat{h}_{ij}+\hat{h}_{ji})}{2(n-1)(n-2)} \quad \textbf{(32.9)}$$

$$s_{gh'} = \frac{\sum\left(\frac{(\hat{g}_{ij}+\hat{g}_{ji})(\hat{h}_{ij}+\hat{h}_{ji})}{4}\right)}{\left(\frac{(n-1)(n-2)}{2}\right)-1} - \frac{\sum(\hat{g}_{ij}-\hat{g}_{ji})(\hat{h}_{ij}+\hat{h}_{ji})}{2(n-1)(n-2)} \quad \textbf{(32.10)}$$

The four individual-level across-variable covariances—actor–actor (s_{ac}), partner–partner (s_{bd}), actor–partner (s_{ad}), and partner–actor (s_{bc})—are estimated with the following four equations (Card et al., 2007; Kenny, 1994):

$$s_{ac} = \frac{\sum \hat{a}_i \hat{c}_i}{n-1} - \frac{s_{gh}(n-1)}{n(n-2)} - \frac{s_{gh'}}{n(n-2)} \quad \textbf{(32.11)}$$

$$s_{bd} = \frac{\sum \hat{b}_i \hat{d}_i}{n-1} - \frac{s_{gh}(n-1)}{n(n-2)} - \frac{s_{gh'}}{n(n-2)} \quad \textbf{(32.12)}$$

$$s_{ad} = \frac{\sum \hat{a}_i \hat{d}_i}{n-1} - \frac{s_{gh'}(n-1)}{n(n-2)} - \frac{s_{gh}}{n(n-2)} \quad \textbf{(32.13)}$$

$$s_{bc} = \frac{\sum \hat{b}_i \hat{c}_i}{n-1} - \frac{s_{gh'}(n-1)}{n(n-2)} - \frac{s_{gh}}{n(n-2)} \quad \textbf{(32.14)}$$

The within-group *t*-test approach to significance testing described earlier for use with univariate SRMs has not yet been adapted to the bivariate SRM (although adaptations to the univariate actor–partner and dyadic covariances would presumably apply to the four individual bivariate and the two dyadic bivariate covariances, respectively; these adaptations have not yet been evaluated). For this reason, the between-group *t*-test is used for statistical inference of bivariate SRM parameters.

Finally, it is worth noting that multivariate models with three or more variables can also be evaluated. These models do not require any special equations beyond those for the bivariate SRM. Instead, one simply estimates the bivariate parameters from all possible two-variable combinations (e.g., for three variables: *X* with *Y*, *X* with *Z*, *Y* with *Z*) and uses these bivariate parameter estimates (along with the univariate estimates) as sufficient statistics for multivariate analysis (Card, 2007).

Higher Dimensional Analyses

The SRMs described to this point use two-person data to model individual and dyadic effects (from two-dimensional sociomatrices). Although this emphasis on two-person phenomena (e.g., perceptions, evaluations, behaviors) already represents advancement beyond individual-focused research, it is likely that many phenomena are even more complex in that they involve more than two individuals. For instance, children may be more or less likely to aggress against a peer depending on the role taken by a third person (see, e.g., Card & Hodges, 2006; Salmivalli, 2001). For three-person phenomena such as these, an extension of the SRM called the triadic relations model (TRM) is appropriate. The TRM (Bond, Horn, & Kenny, 1997) analyzes data cubes (i.e., three dimensions, rather than two-dimensional matrices used by the SRM) that consist of data among three individuals. The concepts are easier to understand through a specific example, so we rely on one of the few uses of the TRM with children, a study that investigated children's perceptions of specific peers aggressing against particular victims (i.e., perceiver–aggressor–victim combinations) (Card, Rodkin, & Garandeau, 2010).

Given its higher dimensionality, the TRM estimates many more variances and covariances. Specifically, the TRM estimates seven variances: three at the individual level (e.g., interindividual differences between perceivers, aggressors, and victims), three at the dyadic level (e.g., interdyadic differences between perceiver–aggressor, perceiver–victim, and aggressor–victim pairings), and one at the triadic level (which consists of reliable intertriadic differences, as well as error; these two components can be separated with multiple indicators). The TRM also estimates 16 covariances: 3 among the individual variances, 9 among the dyadic variances, and 4 among the triadic variances (see Bond et al., 1997; Card et al., 2010). Not all of these will be important to every research situation, but consideration of each offers new insight into the complexity of triadic phenomena.

Each of the extensions of the SRM that we have previously described could, in principle, be applied to the TRM. For instance, the ideas of the block round-robin design, or partitioning of the sociomatrix into four submatrices (for two subgroups), could be applied to the TRM by partitioning the data cube into eight subcubes. It is also conceivable that the confirmatory factor analysis representation of the SRM with roles could be applied to a TRM with roles, though this has not yet been considered. There has been at least one extension of the TRM to multivariate data (Bond, Kenny, Broome, Stokes-Zoota, & Richard, 2000), resulting in 33 across-variable covariance estimates (compared with 6 for the multivariate SRM). Finally, it is possible, at least in principle, to continue the extension from two-dimensional SRM to three-dimensional TRM even further into higher dimensional models, though the number of possible estimates increases drastically and our ability to think of plausible hypotheses decreases with each dimension. However, each of these possibilities is purely speculative, as there is very little work to either apply or evaluate the feasibility (e.g., sample size requirements) of these higher dimensional models.

Developmental Applications

Use of the SRM in developmental studies has been somewhat limited. In this section, we highlight areas of research within the field of developmental science that have utilized this model to address the unique research questions posed by the interdependencies present in developmental science. Given the explicit focus on relationships, it is likely not surprising that the SRM has been primarily used in two aspects of developmental science: the study of peer relations and the study of family relationships.

Applications of the SRM to Studying Peer Relations

Concurrent Studies of Children and Adolescents

The traditional SRM has been used to address several features of peer relationships, including friendship qualities, aggression and victimization, and social status. These investigations have largely utilized adolescent samples (e.g., Betts & Rotenberg, 2008; Card & Hodges, 2010; Malloy & Cillessen, 2008); however, some investigations have taken place during early childhood (e.g., Hawley & Little, 1999; Ross & Lollis, 1989). The majority of peer relations studies using the traditional SRM have been cross-sectional in nature. Strong longitudinal methods to assess social relations within groups are still lacking; however, as discussed subsequently, a few studies have assessed the stability of variance and covariance estimates longitudinally (i.e., Betts & Rotenberg, 2008; Malloy, Sugarman, Montvilo, & Ben-Zeev, 1995). We next highlight studies that analyze social relations within groups, specifically focusing on studies that examine issues or use research methods typical in studies of children and adolescents.

The traditional SRM has been applied to research questions about child and adolescent perceptions about peers and about specific relationships with peers. These perceptions are often gathered using peer nomination inventories in naturalistic studies or observation in play groups with unacquainted peers (Little & Card, 2005). Application of the SRM in these situations allows the investigation of dyadic relationships within group contexts and specific actor, partner, and relationship variance partitioning. Peer perceptions such as *liking* (identified by an item such as "I like these kids") are commonly used to examine mutual liking (friendships; see, e.g., Betts & Rotenberg, 2008). Mutual dislike, or antipathetic relationships, has not been explored using the SRM; however, previous reviews have called for this type of investigation (Little & Card, 2005). Beyond perceptions of liking, researchers have examined other relational characteristics such as aggression and victimization (e.g., see Card & Hodges, 2010; Card et al., 2005; Coie et al., 1999). The research on aggression and victimization using the SRM is growing. As reviewed by Card and Hodges (2010), the study of aggression and victimization has been conducted in observational and naturalistic studies over the past two decades. Both types of studies find that a large percentage of variance is due to interdyadic variability, consistent with previous speculations that aggression is largely a dyadic phenomenon (see Pierce & Cohen, 1995). The new understanding of aggressive behavior among children and adolescents gained by the use of SRM has implications for intervention in peer aggression, namely, a focus on characteristics of the aggressor–victim dyad (e.g., antipathy, conflict resolution difficulties) rather than those of either the aggressor or the victim. Future research, however, is still needed that addresses characteristics of dyadic relationships in larger peer contexts that contain a large amount of aggression and victimization.

In addition to studying aggression, past research using the bivariate SRM has examined associations between dyadic liking and socioemotional problems (e.g., Zimmer-Gembeck, Waters, & Kindermann, 2010). This research goes beyond the partitioning of the variance of a single construct by examining the covariation of actor, partner, and relationship between two constructs. For example, Zimmer-Gembeck and colleagues (2010) found that depressed adolescents perceived their peers to be more negative and perceived themselves to be less accepted by their peers; in addition, these two perceptions covaried with being less liked by their peers. This type of bivariate exploration, for example, could inform the previously described research on aggression by serving as a model to move beyond simple partitioning of the variance of aggression to examine covarying characteristics of aggressors and their victims.

Finally, the SRM has been used to examine such characteristics within children and adolescent peer groups as sociometric status (e.g., acceptance, rejection, popularity). For example, Card and colleagues (2005) found significant generalized and dyadic reciprocity correlations of social preference ("Who do you like to hang out with?") and influence ("Who gets others to go along with what they say?"), such that those with greater perceived levels of social status are also likely to view others as high in social status, and this is also the case in specific dyads. This work, again, could continue to be expanded on by examining longitudinal associations between social status and other relational variables.

Although these uses of the traditional SRM considered phenomena that were salient during the periods of childhood and adolescence, most of these investigations have been cross-sectional and have not examined change or stability over time. As discussed previously, this limitation to the current research is primarily due to the novelty of this model being applied to developmental research—and because of the novelty, there have been no advancements in how applying the SRM to longitudinal data.

Longitudinal Applications

The research has not been exclusively cross-sectional, as there are two exceptions: Malloy and colleagues (1995) and Betts and Rotenberg (2008). First, Malloy and colleagues examined the product-moment coefficients (specifically, the reliability coefficients) of perceiver and target effects over 3 years. Several variables were analyzed in this investigation, including math skills, reading skills, strength, behavior, friendships, popularity, attractiveness, and happiness. Using their longitudinal method, Malloy and colleagues (1995) found that perceiver effects were less consistent over time compared with target effects. In comparison, Betts and Rotenberg examined the stability of the associations between promise keeping, secret keeping, and number of friendships over two waves of data by examining the bivariate correlations of the perceiver and target effects. Their application of the SRM to examine stability of target and perceiver effects over time is novel and a beginning step to using the SRM to examine developmental data.

In sum, the SRM has largely been applied in a research cross-sectional design. Despite this limitation, the findings from this body of research are significant and have implications for future research and practice for those interested in child and adolescent peer relations. Although the majority of the work has taken place in the field of peer relations, this model could be applied to several other contexts of child and adolescent developmental research, such as family or community. In fact, a growing literature uses the family SRM to examine family relationships that include one or more children.

Applications of the SRM to Studying Families

In addition to use of the indistinguishable case SRM to study peer relations, the SRM with roles has been used to examine family relationships. Typically, these studies include three or four family members to investigate dyadic relationships effects over and above the unique family effect. The family SRM is useful in that it can ascertain child effects, parent effects, and relationships effects (Eichelsheim, Dekovic, Buist, & Cook, 2009).

The body of research that utilizes the SRM to study families was recently reviewed by Eichelsheim and colleagues (2009). In their review, the authors categorized the available literature into two categories based on the focus of the study: affectivity and influence. Studies that focused on affectivity examined measures such as support, conflict, or warmth, whereas studies that focused on influence examined measures such as acquiescence, aversive behaviors, or effectance. Eichelsheim and colleagues examined actor, partner, and relationship effects across studies, as well as generalized and dyadic reciprocity across the studies used in their review. Their review of the literature found larger actor effects than partner effects; this finding was also qualified by a secondary finding that children have larger actor variances than parents. This secondary finding suggests that parents are more differential in their relationships with other family members, whereas children experience their relationships with other family members more similarly. Typically, family variance was small and did not account for a significant proportion of the variance in family relationships. There was significant reciprocity in studies of family relationships that focused on affectivity but not on influence.

Future Directions

Although the applications of the SRM to studying peer relations and family interactions represent valuable contributions to developmental science, we believe that further efforts are needed to achieve the full potential of the SRM in this field. We next describe two refinements to the SRM that we believe are most necessary to meet the unique needs of developmental research: improved methods of managing missing data and the development of true developmental models of the SRM.

Expanding Data Management Flexibility

As we described earlier, an obstacle in using the SRM in developmental science is that there have been inadequate efforts to move beyond rather restrictive data requirements of normality and complete data.

There are some phenomena in developmental science that must be measured at non-continuous, non-normal levels, either for pragmatic (e.g., peer nominations are more time efficient than peer ratings) or conceptual (i.e., some developmental phenomena are conceptually categorical or otherwise non-normal) reasons. It will be useful for future research to continue to study, likely through simulation research, the impact that violations of the assumption of continuous, normally distributed variables have on SRM parameter estimation. Of course, if the existing methods of SRM estimation are not robust to violations of this assumption, it will be useful to consider alternative estimation techniques.

Similarly, developmental research commonly faces challenges of missing data. Unlike the context of controlled (i.e., laboratory-based), single-occasion data collection conditions within which the SRM was originally developed, developmental science often relies on naturalistic data, ideally collected over time (discussed later), that invariably contains missing values. As indicated earlier, there are currently no adequate steps for dealing with missing data in the SRM. Currently, researchers using SRM employ the equivalent of listwise deletion by removing data from individuals with missing data. However, contemporary developmental science views listwise deletion as an unacceptable procedure for dealing with missing data (e.g., Graham, Cumsille, & Elek-Fisk, 2003). Modern advancements in missing data approaches include using algorithms to impute the missing information. However, these algorithms are based on linear models derived for individual data that do not take into account the multitude of SRM information that might be used to estimate missing values (actor, partner, and relationship variances, actor–partner and dyadic covariances, within and across variables and occasions). New methods of imputation need to be developed to take into account the full range of information in the SRM.

Need for Truly Developmental Models of the SRM

Although the SRM has been used to study children, adolescents, and adults—as well as within the context of families—we argue that a truly developmental framework for the SRM is generally lacking. Developmental science is fundamentally about the study of change over time, yet the SRM is, with only a few exceptions, used in a static manner. We next describe four potential extensions of the SRM that would allow it to become a more truly developmental model.

Age-Cohort Comparisons

The simplest extension of the SRM would be to deliberately collect round-robin (or other designs) data from groups of individuals of different ages (e.g., in classrooms of first, third, and fifth graders) and then contrast the SRM parameters across these ages. Such contrasts would be readily performed by transforming the between-groups *t*-test approach to significance testing into a between-groups ANOVA (or regression, if the age groups approximate a continuous distribution). As one example, it might be useful to evaluate whether relationship variance in liking increases with age in order to evaluate whether children become more discriminating with age (i.e., rather than liking or disliking everyone, having specific liked or disliked peers).

Longitudinal Univariate Comparisons

Although age-cohort comparisons can be suggestive of developmental differences, they are threatened by the possibility of cohort (rather than developmental) differences (e.g., Baltes, 1968; Schaie, 1965). For this reason, longitudinal comparisons are preferred to allow conclusions of developmental change to be made (longitudinal data are also advantageous because they allow estimates of interindividual stability over time; for recent reviews of the advantages of longitudinal data, see, e.g., Card & Little, 2007; Collins, 2006; Little, Card, Preacher, & McConnell, 2009).

As illustrated in two studies (Betts & Rotenberg, 2008; Malloy et al., 1995), the extension of the SRM to accommodate two-time, one-variable data is possible. The stability of SRM effects (interindividual stability for actor and partner effects; interdyadic for relationship effects) can be estimated using the bivariate SRM to estimate across-time associations among parallel effects (e.g., actor effects at time 1 with actor effects at time 2). Across-time and across-effect associations could also be estimated (e.g., do time 1 actor effects predict time 2 partner effects?). We also speculate that mean-level changes across time could be evaluated by centering actor, partner, and relationship effects on a time-averaged group mean, rather than a time-specific group mean, though this speculation has not been evaluated.

Longitudinal Multivariate Analyses

One of the most useful and widely used longitudinal models is the cross-lag panel analysis (see Selig & Little, Chapter 16, this volume, as well as Little et al., 2009; Little, Preacher, Selig, & Card, 2007). In this model, data from two or more variables (e.g., X and Y) are collected at two or more time points, and analyses evaluate whether earlier values of one variable predict residual change in the other variable (e.g., whether time 2 Y is predicted by time 1 X after controlling for time 1 Y). These cross-lag panel models provide arguably the most informative information regarding causality that can be obtained from naturalistic data (Little et al., 2009).

Although we are unaware of prior attempts to do so, it seems plausible that the multivariate SRM could be analyzed within this panel model framework. To do so, one would estimate all possible bivariate associations among all variables across all times (e.g., actor–actor covariances between time 1 X and time 1 Y, between time 1 X and time 2 X, between time 1 X and time 2 Y, between time 1 Y and time 2 X, between time 1 Y and time 2 Y, and between time 2 X and time 2 Y; with comparable sets of estimates for partner–partner, actor–partner, partner–actor, intrapersonal, and interpersonal covariances). These covariances could then be used as sufficient statistics of multivariate models (e.g., regressions) of interest to the cross-lag panel model (e.g., actor effects of time 2 Y being predicted by actor effects of time 1 X after controlling for actor effects of time 1 Y). We emphasize that this sort of panel model extension of the SRM seems plausible to us but has not yet been fully developed in the quantitative literature nor applied in the developmental literature.

Growth Curve Analyses

Growth curve models of individual-level data estimate average patterns of intraindividual (i.e., within person) change, as well as interindividual variability (i.e., between-person differences) in this change (see Grimm & Ram, Chapter 24, this volume; Hox & Boom, Chapter 25, this volume). There have been no efforts to extend the SRM into a growth curve framework, but this also seems possible in one of two ways. First, it might be possible to estimate all SRM effects for each time point and then use these estimates as data for the growth curve analysis. Alternatively, it might be possible to estimate growth trajectories for each dyad across time and then use these growth parameter estimates (e.g., intercept and linear slope) as data for SRM analyses. Although these strategies seem viable, the exact details would undoubtedly be complex. Clearly, there needs to be considerable quantitative work before such models are a realistic possibility for developmental science.

Conclusions

In this chapter, we have described the basic SRM and extensions of this basic model. We also briefly reviewed the applications of the SRM within developmental science, namely in the areas of peer relations and family research, in which it has been most commonly applied. We also identified some important work that needs to be done to adapt the SRM to the unique demands of developmental research.

We hope that this description has helped you, the reader, glimpse the potential opportunities for the SRM to advance developmental science. At the same time, the future directions we have described constitute as much a wish list as a prediction, and it is likely that developmental applications of the SRM will face these and other challenges for quite some time. Nevertheless, we believe that the opportunities provided by the SRM to study development in the relationship context in which it occurs outweigh the challenges that will arise in this effort.

References

Baltes, P. B. (1968). Longitudinal and cross-sectional sequences in the study of age and generation effects. *Human Development, 11*, 145–171.

Belsky, J. (2005). Differential susceptibility to rearing influence: An evolutionary hypothesis and some evidence. In B. J. Ellis & D. F. Bjorklund (Eds.), *Origins of the social mind: Evolutionary psychology and child development* (pp. 139–163). New York: Guilford Press.

Berscheid, E. (1994). Interpersonal relationships. *Annual Review of Psychology, 45*, 79–129.

Betts, L. R., & Rotenberg, K. J. (2008). A social relations analysis of children's trust in their peers across the early school years. *Social Development, 17*, 1039–1055.

Boldry, J. G., & Kashy, D. A. (1999). Intergroup perception in naturally occurring groups of different status: A social relations perspective. *Journal of Personality and Social Psychology, 77*, 1200–1212.

Bond, C. F., Jr., Horn, E. M., & Kenny, D. A. (1997). A model for triadic relations. *Psychological Bulletin, 2*, 79–94.

Bond, C. F., Jr., Kenny, D. A., Broome, E. H., Stokes-Zoota, J. J., & Richard, F. D. (2000). Multivariate analysis of triadic relations. *Multivariate Behavioral Research, 35*, 397–426.

Bond, C. F., Jr., & Lashley, B. R. (1996). Round-robin analysis of social interaction: Exact and estimated standard errors. *Psychometrika, 61*, 303–311.

Bornstein, M. H. (Ed.). (2002). *Handbook of parenting* (2nd ed.). Mahwah, NJ: Erlbaum.

Bronfenbrenner, U. (1979). *The ecology of human development*. Cambridge, MA: Harvard University Press.

Bronfenbrenner, U., & Morris, A. C. (1998). The bioecological model of human development. In W. Damon (Series Ed.) & R. M. Lerner (Vol. Ed.), *Handbook of child psychology: Vol. 1. Theoretical models of human development* (pp. 793–828). New York: Wiley.

Card, N. A. (2007, May). *Children's perceptions of same- and cross-sex peers' social behavior and social status*. Paper presented at NSF Conference on Social Relations Modeling Approaches to Intergroup Relations, University of Connecticut.

Card, N. A., & Hodges, E. V. E. (2006). Shared targets for aggression by early adolescent friends. *Developmental Psychology, 42*, 1327–1338.

Card, N. A., & Hodges, E. V. E. (2010). It takes two to fight in school, too: A social relations model of the psychometric properties and relative variance of dyadic aggression and victimization in middle school. *Social Development, 19*(3), 447–469.

Card, N. A., Hodges, E. V. E., Little, T. D., & Hawley, P. H. (2005). Gender effects in peer nominations for aggression and social status. *International Journal of Behavioral Development, 29*, 146–155.

Card, N. A., & Little, T. D. (2007). Longitudinal modeling of developmental processes. *International Journal of Behavioral Development, 31*, 297–302.

Card, N. A., Little, T. D., & Selig, J. P. (2008). Using the bivariate social relations model to study dyadic relationships: Early adolescents' perceptions of friends' aggression and prosocial behavior. In N. A. Card, J. P. Selig, & T. D. Little (Eds.), *Modeling dyadic and interdependent data in the developmental and behavioral sciences* (pp. 245–276). New York: Routledge.

Card, N. A, Rodkin, P. C., & Garandeau, C. F. (2010). A description and illustration of the triadic relations model: Who perceives whom as bullying whom? *International Journal of Behavioral Development, 34*, 374–383.

Card, N. A., Selig, J. P., & Little, T. D. (Eds.). (2008). *Modeling dyadic and interdependent data in the developmental and behavioral sciences*. New York: Routledge.

Coie, J. D., Cillessen, A. H. N., Dodge, K. A., Hubbard, J. A., Schwartz, D., Lemerise, E. A., et al. (1999). It takes two to fight: A test of relational factors and a method for assessing aggressive dyads. *Developmental Psychology, 35*, 1179–1188.

Collins, L. M. (2006). Analysis of longitudinal data: The integration of theoretical model, temporal design, and statistical model. *Annual Review of Psychology, 57*, 505–528.

Collins, W. A., & Laursen, B. (Eds.). (1999). *Relationships as developmental contexts*. Mahwah, NJ: Erlbaum.

Cook, W. L., & Kenny, D. A. (2004). Application of the social relations model to family assessment. *Journal of Family Psychology, 18*, 361–371.

Cook, W. L., & Kenny, D. A. (2005). The actor–partner interdependence model: A model of bidirectional effects in developmental studies. *International Journal of Behavioral Development, 29*, 101–109.

Eichelsheim, V. I., Dekovic, M., Buist, K. L., & Cook, W. L. (2009). The social relations model in family studies: A systematic review. *Journal of Marriage and Family, 71*, 1052–1069.

Gottlieb, G. (1998). Normally occurring environmental and behavioral influences on gene activity: From central dogma to probabilistic epigenesis. *Psychological Review, 105*, 792–802.

Graham, J. W., Cumsille, P. E., & Elek-Fisk, E. (2003). Methods for handling missing data. In J. Schinka & W. Velicer (Eds.), *Handbook of psychology: Vol. 2. Research methods in psychology* (pp. 87–114). New York: Wiley.

Griffin, D., & Gonzalez, R. (1995). Correlational analysis of dyad-level data in the exchangeable case. *Psychological Bulletin, 118*, 430–439.

Hartup, W. W. (1979). The social worlds of childhood. *American Psychologist, 34*, 944–950.

Hawley, P. H., & Little, T. D. (1999). On winning some and losing some: A social relations approach to social dominance in toddlers. *Merrill-Palmer Quarterly, 45*, 185–214.

Kenny, D. A. (1994). *Interpersonal perception: A social relations analysis*. New York: Guilford Press.

Kenny, D. A., Kashy, D. A., & Cook, W. L. (2006). *Dyadic data analysis*. New York: Guilford Press.

Kenny, D. A., & La Voie, L. (1984). The social relations model. In L. Berkowitz (Ed.), *Advances in experimental social psychology* (Vol. 18, pp. 142–182). Orlando, FL: Academic Press.

Lashley, B. R., & Bond, C. F., Jr. (1997). Significance testing for round robin data. *Psychological Methods, 2*, 278–291.

Little, T. D., & Card, N. A. (2005). On the use of social relations and actor–partner interdependence models in developmental research. *International Journal of Behavioral Development, 29*, 173–179.

Little, T. D., Card, N. A., Preacher, K. J., & McConnell, E. (2009). Modeling longitudinal data from research on adolescence. In R. M. Lerner & L. Steinberg (Ed.), *Handbook of adolescent psychology* (3rd ed., pp. 15–54). New York: Wiley.

Little, T. D., Preacher, K. J., Selig, J. P., & Card, N. A. (2007). New developments in latent variable panel analyses of longitudinal data. *International Journal of Behavioral Development, 31*, 357–365.

Malloy, T. E., & Cillessen, A. H. N. (2008). Variance component analysis of generalized and dyadic peer perceptions in adolescence. In N. A. Card, J. P. Selig, & T. D. Little (Eds.), *Modeling interdependent data in the developmental and behavioral sciences* (pp. 213–244). New York: Routledge.

Malloy, T. E., Sugarman, D. B., Montvilo, R. K., & Ben-Zeev, T. (1995). Children's interpersonal perceptions: A social relations analysis of perceiver and target effects. *Journal of Personality and Social Psychology, 68*, 418–426.

Pierce, K. A., & Cohen, R. (1995). Aggressors and their victims: Toward a contextual framework for understanding children's aggressor–victim relationships. *Developmental Review, 15*, 292–310.

Ross, H. S., & Lollis, S. P. (1989). A social relations analysis of toddler peer relationships. *Child Development, 60*, 1082–1091.

Rubin, K. H., Bukowski, W. M., & Laursen, B. (Eds.). (2009). *Handbook of peer interactions, relationships, and groups*. New York: Guilford Press.

Salmivalli, C. (2001). Group view on victimization: Empirical findings and their implications. In J. Juvonen & S. Graham (Eds.), *Peer harassment in school: The plight of the vulnerable and victimized* (pp. 398–419). New York: Guilford Press.

Schaie, K. W. (1965). A general model for the study of developmental problems. *Psychological Bulletin, 64*, 92–107.

Wasserman, S., & Faust, K. (1994). *Social network analysis: Methods and applications*. New York: Cambridge University Press.

Zimmer-Gembeck, M. J., Waters, A. M., & Kindermann, T. (2010). A social relations analysis of liking for and by peers: Associations with gender, depression, peer perception, and worry. *Journal of Adolescence, 33*, 69–81.

CHAPTER 33

Analysis of Static Social Networks and Their Developmental Effects

SCOTT D. GEST
THOMAS A. KINDERMANN

At the beginning of the 21st century, a maverick group of social scientists is discovering that all networks—from a cocktail party to a terrorist cell to an international conglomerate—have a deep underlying order and operate according to simple but powerful rules. Knowledge of the structure and behavior of these networks illuminates everything from the vulnerability of economics to the way diseases are spread. . . .

—quoted from Durett (2004, p. 201) as the contemporary press release for Barabási (2002)

Current enthusiasm about the potential of social network methods seems to be approaching the confidence that J. L. Moreno expressed in 1934, when he gave his main volume the exuberant title *Who Shall Survive?* The field is experiencing an explosion of research. Analyses extend to a wide array of phenomena in medicine, economics, sociology, and psychology and promise to explain important outcomes with a power that surpasses other contextual approaches. Highly publicized examples include the spread of obesity in a geographical area (Christakis & Fowler, 2007), the adoption of technology services (Hill, Provost, & Volinsky, 2006), the spread of disease (Cohen, Brissette, Skoner, & Doyle, 2000), and patterns of collaboration in a country (Eagle, Macy, & Claxton, 2010), among companies (Baker & Faulkner, 1993; Mizruchi, 2007), or among scientists (Moody, 2004). Similarly, psychological applications have traced the spread of happiness, loneliness, and suicidal behavior (Bearman & Moody, 2004; Cacioppo, Fowler, & Christakis, 2008; Fowler & Christakis, 2008), of aggression and drug-related behavior (Dijkstra et al., 2010; Kiuru, Burk, Laursen, Salmela-Aro, & Nurmi, 2010; Light & Dishion, 2007; Popp, Laursen, Kerr, Stattin & Burk, 2008; Urberg, Degirmencioglu, Tolson, & Halliday-Scher, 1995), and academic motivation and school dropout (Berndt, Hawkins, & Jiao, 1999; Cairns, Leung, Buchanan, & Cairns, 1995; Hallinan & Williams, 1990; Kindermann, 2003, 2007; Sokatch, 2006).

The contemporary explosion of research on social networks rests on a long history of social and mathematical thinking that has been consolidated in the past two decades in the form of authoritative textbooks and increasingly powerful and accessible software programs. In his fascinating monograph on the development of social network analysis, Freeman (2004) traces the history of network insights across the last centuries, including contributions of Comte, Toennies, Durkheim, Spencer, Hobson, and Galton. He argues that four key premises define all modern approaches to social network analysis: "(1) social network analysis is motivated by a structural intuition based on ties linking social actors, (2) it is grounded in systematic empirical data, (3) it draws heavily on graphic imagery, and (4) it relies on the use of mathematical and/or computational models" (Freeman, 2004, p. 3). Summaries and discussions of the links between social science theories and mathematical graph theory appear in textbooks (Knoke & Yang, 2008; Scott, 2000; Wasserman & Faust, 1994), statements by leading researchers (Borgatti, 2009; Borgatti, Mehra, Brass, & Labianca, 2010; Wellman, 1988), and in a growing number of online resources (Hanneman & Riddle, 2005; *en.wikipedia.org/wiki/Social_network*; *en.wikipedia.org/wiki/Graph_theory*).

In this chapter, we present an overview of the key methods, findings, and promises of social networks analysis. After identifying six central themes in social networks analysis with relevance for developmental research, we review some of the conceptual principles and graph theoretical and statistical assumptions of social networks analysis, describe some of the measures that can be computed in relation to each central theme, highlight potential developmental applications of these measures, and present several illustrations in more detail. We conclude with a discussion of current challenges and future directions for the field. To distinguish our chapter from the subsequent one on dynamic network analysis (Veenstra & Steglich, Chapter 34, this volume), we focus on the analysis of network data collected at a *single point in time* but highlight how descriptive measures derived from "static" social network assessments can be incorporated into developmental research.

Central Issues

Connectivity

In social networks analysis, social connections are seen as based on individual *choices for relationships*, and it is assumed that the *structure* and *organization* of these connections have important developmental consequences. An appealing feature of social networks analysis methods is that they were mainly developed to test long-standing theoretical propositions about group life emerging from the social sciences (Freeman, 2004). Accordingly, many social networks analysis procedures focus on describing the richness and structural cohesion of ties, including basic measures of the density, reciprocity, transitivity, and hierarchical structure of social ties.

Important Individuals

A common intuition about social networks is that some members are more important or influential than others. But what constitutes an important or influential position in a network? For example, does importance stem from an individual's sheer number of social connections (i.e., connections as social capital), or does it arise from serving as a strategic "bridge" between otherwise disconnected parts of the network (i.e., a brokerage perspective)? Social networks analysis has been centrally concerned with developing measures that capture notions of what it means to occupy an important position in a network (Borgatti, 2005; Borgatti & Everett, 2006).

Cohesive Subgroups

A third enduring issue in social networks analysis is the identification of cohesive subgroups within larger social networks. At an intuitive level, *cohesive subgroups* should be characterized by a large number of connections within subgroups and relatively few connections between subgroups. Social networks analysis efforts have centered on the development of algorithms that efficiently identify maximally cohesive subgroups (Kindermann & Gest, 2009).

Social Ties in Relation to Individual Attributes

Social networks analysis has also been concerned with the development of metrics to describe the distribution of individual attributes (e.g., thoughts, behaviors, or demographic characteristics) in relation to the distribution of social ties in a network. Most broadly, this issue centers around the question of homophily (do similar individuals affiliate with one another?), but it includes questions of how to summarize the attributes of each network member's peer group and how to identify behaviors that are positively valued or negatively sanctioned in the network.

Software for Network Analysis and Visualization

The availability of software for the manipulation, analysis, and visualization of social network data has proliferated in the past decade. The programs include stand-alone, general purpose packages (UCINET), open-source platforms (R), and a variety of programs designed to address particular analytical challenges such as identifying cohesive subgroups and visualizing networks.

Network Data Collection Procedures

Finally, an issue that we believe deserves more attention is the variety of methods available to collect social network data. The dominant approach has been to collect information about social ties that are either present or absent—in developmental research, typically the presence or absence of feelings of friendship or liking from one child to another. Because the focus is on individual preferences, analyses are based on children's self-reports.

However, there are also alternative methods for collecting data regarding the strength of social ties. One method that has been gaining acceptance is *sociocognitive mapping (SCM)*. The method has been developed by Robert Cairns and colleagues, and it follows observational strategies in which children themselves, as expert observers about peer affiliations, report about all groups of age-mates whom they see "hanging out" with one another on a regular basis. This approach is based less on interpersonal attraction and more on observable affiliations. One specific advantage of observational methods is that not each and every member of a network needs to participate in assessments in order to construct reliable peer group maps (Cairns & Cairns, 1994); it is sufficient if many peers report that a nonparticipating child is a group member. This alternative permits and sometimes requires different analysis approaches because of interindividual differences in frequencies of observations (see Kindermann & Gest, 2009).

Conceptual Principles and Statistical Assumptions

Several key principles distinguish social network analysis from other quantitative approaches in the social and behavioral sciences (Freeman, 2004; Scott, 2000; Wasserman & Faust, 1994; Wellman, 1988). Most fundamentally, social networks analysis is centrally concerned with the *relations between* interacting individuals rather than with the individuals per se. Wasserman and Faust (1994) list four additional principles of social networks analysis: (1) individuals and their actions are interdependent rather than independent; (2) social ties between individuals are the conduits through which social or material resources flow or are transferred; (3) the network structure is seen as constraining opportunities for individual action; and (4) network structures can be studied as lasting patterns of relations among individuals.

Mathematical Graph Theory and Its Application to Social Networks Analysis

Mathematical graph theory and its applications in social networks analysis involve a relatively small set of core concepts that are the building blocks of all of the measures described in this chapter. A graph is defined as a set of points and the set of lines that connect the points. Points (also called nodes or vertices) are typically called *actors*, and the lines that connect the actors are described as social relations or *social ties*. Two basic properties of graphs have implications for how they can be analyzed. First, graphs are *directed* if social ties may be asymmetrical (for at least some A and B, $A \rightarrow B \neq B \rightarrow A$); they are *nondirected* if the ties are always symmetrical. In directed graphs, it is conventional to refer to the sender of a tie as the *ego* and the receiver of that tie as the *alter.*

Second, graphs are *nonvalued* if social ties are measured on a binary scale (0 = absent, 1 = present); they are *valued* if ties can take on a broader range of values representing gradations in the strength of a social tie. These two properties of graphs can exist in any combination. For example, in a study of classroom friendships, a researcher could choose to analyze (1) a nonvalued directed graph (often abbreviated as a *digraph*) summarizing which youths named each other as friends; (2) a valued directed graph that summarizes how close each youth feels to each of his or her friends (e.g., rated on a Likert-type scale); (3) a nonvalued, nondirected graph by restricting attention to reciprocated friendship choices; or (4) a valued nondirected graph by characterizing the closeness of each dyad (e.g., as the average ratings provided by the two youths).

In general, quantitative methods for analyzing graphs are much more fully developed for nonvalued graphs than for valued graphs and are more fully developed for directed graphs than for nondirected graphs (Wasserman & Faust, 1994). In all cases, the graph can be represented as an $n \times n$ matrix, where n is the number of actors in the network. In the discussion that follows, we focus mostly on nonvalued digraphs but highlight some developmental applications of other types of graphs.

Social Ties

Many quantitative procedures in social networks analysis build on three simple ways to characterize the social ties that connect actors in a network. A *walk* is a sequence of adjacent actors and the ties that connect them, with the length of a walk defined as the number of ties traversed (e.g., the walk A→C→B→D→C→E has length 5 because 5 social ties were crossed to get from A to E). A *path* is a walk in which no actor is visited more than once (e.g., A→C→B→D→E). A *geodesic path* (also called graph-theoretic distance or geodesic distance) has the special quality of being the shortest possible path between two actors (e.g., A→C→E). The formulas for calculating many network indices (e.g., the importance of an actor's position in the network) differ depending on whether one considers walks, paths, or geodesics, so, as discussed later, one should choose the formula that best captures the process by which one expects the phenomenon of interest to move through a network (see also Borgatti, 2005).

Analysis of Data

Hypothesis testing in social networks analysis presents challenges due to the nonindependence of observations and the unknown distributional properties of many network statistics. The interdependence of actors means that a core assumption of inferential statistics based on the general linear model (i.e., independent error terms) is violated. Interdependencies result in artificially low standard errors that increase the risk of Type II errors (i.e., falsely rejecting the null hypothesis). Most critically, the extent and sources of nonindependence are not always known and thus cannot be modeled as they are in multilevel modeling.

Consequently, hypothesis testing in social networks analysis makes use of nonparametric permutation tests (Borgatti, Everett, & Freeman, 2002; Wasserman & Faust, 1994). Permutation testing involves three steps. First, one calculates the network statistic of interest. Second, one permutes a randomly selected row or column of the network graph and recalculates the network statistic, then repeats this process many times (e.g., 500, 1,000, 2,000) to derive a sampling distribution of the test statistic across different permutations of the network graph. Third, one compares the original statistic to the empirically derived sampling distribution to determine in which percentage of cases the statistic was as large as or larger than the one obtained; the percentage is the p-value for the obtained statistic. The advantage of this approach is that the sampling distribution is constructed for networks with the same distributional properties as the originally observed network.

Some Key Structural Indices Derived from Social Network Analysis

A useful feature of graphs is the ability to extract subgraphs consisting of a subset of actors and their relations. This means that identical or conceptually similar indices can be computed both for the network as a whole and for conceptually interesting subsets. Common subgraphs of interest in social networks analysis include the cohesive subgroups within the network (e.g., cliques within a classroom) and each actor's *ego network* (i.e., the subset of actors who have social ties to that actor). Ego network ties can be defined as those sent by the ego, those received by the ego, or the union or intersection of the two. In the following summary of measures emerging from the central themes of social networks analysis we highlight some but not all of these possibilities.

Connectivity

Three simple measures describing basic patterns of connectivity among actors in a network are density, reciprocity and transitivity. *Density* is defined as the proportion of possible ties that exist (i.e., in a network with N actors, $N(N-1)$ directional ties are possible), capturing the volume of actors' connections. *Reciprocity* is the proportion of all directional ties sent by an ego that are reciprocated by the alter, and *transitivity* captures the extent to which "friends of friends are friends." These indices can be computed over the entire network, separately for each subgroup within a network, or separately for each actor's ego network.

Patterns of connectivity at the triad level play a critical role as a point of intersection between social-psychological theories and social network analytical strategies. Heider's (1946) cognitive balance theory, for example, directly motivated early efforts to formalize social-psychological theories of small-group dynamics into graph-theoretic terms (Cartwright & Harary, 1956). This eventually led to the proof that structural balance dynamics at the triad level can produce distinctive patterns of connectivity at the network level (Holland & Leinhardt, 1971). Network-level patterns of connectivity are often summarized in terms of the *triad census*, which enumerates the frequencies of different patterns of ties among all possible triads. For example, in a directed network of three members, any given dyad can display 16 possible patterns of ties, ranging from no ties among any actors to reciprocal ties among all actors. Each of these patterns implies a distinct mixture of "local dynamics" (e.g., reciprocity, transitivity, intransitivity, hierarchy). For example, a triad pattern in which there are two reciprocated friendship dyads (e.g., $A \leftrightarrow B$, $A \leftrightarrow C$) but no ties between the third dyad implies a dynamic favoring reciprocity but not transitivity. The relative frequency of the triad patterns, and especially the degree to which a given pattern occurs more often than expected by chance, provides a succinct summary of the degree to which different sorts of local network dynamics may be occurring inside the network. In this sense, even a static snapshot of network structure can provide hints regarding the developmental processes that may have given rise to it.

Two other indices capture broader patterns of connectivity in a network. First, networks vary in the extent to which social ties are evenly or unevenly distributed across actors. In some networks, a small number of actors participate in many ties, whereas many actors receive few or none; in other networks social ties are more evenly distributed. This hierarchical-versus-egalitarian feature of networks can be described by a *centralization* index (Wasserman & Faust, 1994) that reaches a theoretical maximum of 1.0 when a single actor receives all of the ties and a theoretical minimum of zero when all actors receive the same number of ties. Centralization can also be computed as a feature of a subgroup or an ego network. Second, Moody and White (2003) introduced a measure of *structural cohesion* that is anchored in formal properties of graph theory, capturing the extent to which a network is prevented from splitting into distinct unrelated subgroups by few versus many individuals whose friendship ties connect the subgroups (weak vs. strong cohesion). Structural cohesion depends on the entire pattern of social ties across all members. Thus it provides a broad, network-level picture of how strongly all members are linked to each other through multiple indirect paths of "friends of friends." In addition, it is possible to characterize each individual actor's relative *nestedness* in the network (Moody & White, 2003) so that variations in the number of different levels of nestedness within a given network can be interpreted as an index of the degree of network hierarchy (Ahn, Garandeau, & Rodkin, 2010).

Important Individuals

In a classic social networks analysis paper, Freeman (1979) described three notions and accompanying measures of *network centrality*. He reasoned that an actor may be important by virtue of being connected to many other actors, so he defined *degree centrality* as the actor's total number of social ties, with common variations being *indegree* centrality (ties received from others) and *outdegree* (ties sent to others). Readers will recognize that within developmental research on children's peer relations, the dominant paradigm for defining peer status (i.e., tallying how many times each actor is named as "liked most" or named as a friend) corresponds to Freeman's definition of indegree centrality. An actor may also be important by linking otherwise disconnected actors, so Freeman operationalized *betweenness centrality* in terms of the number of geodesic paths in a network that passes through a given actor. Finally, Freeman suggested that actors could be important by being generally near to other actors in the network, so he quantified an individual's *closeness centrality* in terms of the summed geodesic distances between that individual actor and all other actors in the network. Bonacich (1987) extended the notion of degree centrality by devising a way to give extra weight to actors having ties to other well-connected actors (*eigenvector centrality*). Additional variations and refinements to these basic notions are described elsewhere (Wasserman & Faust, 1994).

As noted earlier, Borgatti (2005) emphasizes the importance of choosing a centrality measure with computational underpinnings that match the nature of the network process one is studying. For example, in defining important airports, it may make sense to presume a rationally planned system by focusing on airports that lie along many geodesic (shortest) paths. In contrast, to define middle school youths who are important in the spread of rumors, it may be better to identify youths who fall along many walks, because rumors do not necessarily travel along geodesic paths and may instead "circle back" and reach the same individuals many times through multiple routes. Borgatti and Everett (2006) place centrality measures in the context of mathematical graph theory, arguing that *radial* measures (e.g., degree and eigenvector) quantify an actor's overall volume of ties and make the most sense when a network has a single core, whereas *medial* measures (e.g., betweenness) quantify an actor's involvement in bridging otherwise disconnected members and are informative when the network is composed of two or more relatively distinct cores (e.g., genders in an elementary school classroom or racial/ethnic groups in a racially segregated high school). As a practical matter, correlations among seemingly similar indices are often constrained by distributional issues (see Valente, Coronges, Lakon, & Costenbader, 2008, for an empirical comparison of intercorrelations among centrality measures).

Cohesive Subgroups

Researchers are often interested in identifying cohesive subgroups within a larger network, and several distinct social networks analysis traditions have developed methods designed to achieve this goal (see summaries in Gest, Moody & Rulison, 2007; Kindermann & Gest, 2009). Early researchers used principal components analysis or centroid factor analysis to identify subgroups (factors). Recently, researchers have used a variety of correlation-based algorithms to identify peer groups (e.g., Bagwell, Coie, Terry, & Lochman, 2000; Cairns, Cairns, Neckerman, Gest, & Gariepy, 1988; Cairns, Perrin, & Cairns, 1985; Rodkin, Farmer, Pearl, & Van Acker, 2000). These approaches, which have links to block modeling traditions in social networks analysis (White, Boorman, & Breiger, 1976), share the premise that groups can be conceptualized as individuals whose patterns of social ties are similar (i.e., correlated).

Other approaches rely on specific patterns of graph connectivity to identify subgroups (for a review, see Moody, 2001). The strictest approach is to find *n-cliques*: subgroups of size *n* in which each actor has direct social ties with *all* other actors. But criteria can be relaxed to identify subgroups that meet any specified level of connectivity. These approaches can be computationally intensive in large networks and often produce groups that overlap heavily. An alternative graph-theoretic strategy is to employ iterative algorithms that optimize a function that produces subgroups with relatively high within-group density and relatively low between-group density (e.g., UCINET factions; Borgatti et al., 2002). A third approach relies on statistical modeling, reassigning nodes across subgroups until the probability of within-group ties is maximized (Frank, 1995). As the number of alternative grouping algorithms proliferates (Porter, Onnela, & Mucha, 2009), a common way to compare solutions is with measures of *modularity* (Newman & Girvan, 2004), summarizing the degree to which ties fall within groups rather than between groups.

We conclude with three points about subgroups. First, there is little empirical research comparing the results of different grouping algorithms applied to the same data. In one study (Gest, Moody, & Rulison, 2007), valued graphs based on Cairns's SCM data collection procedure yielded highly comparable solutions across a variety of grouping approaches, whereas the same grouping approaches applied to nonvalued directed graphs based on friendship nominations yielded significantly lower comparability. A conclusion is that researchers should choose a grouping procedure from a tradition that matches their conceptual notion of what constitutes a group but should check the robustness of substantive findings with respect to variations in grouping algorithms. Second, none of the approaches to group identification definitively solves the "number of subgroups" issue: The investigator must apply judgment in arriving at a number of subgroups that is theoretically sensible and useful for the task at hand. Third, identifying distinct subgroups is not a necessary step in conducting rigorous network analyses. For example, Kindermann (1993, 2007) proposed a strategy (described more fully later) to identify the key peers for each individual member of a network, with no assumption that each child belongs to one and only one subgroup or that the larger network is composed of subgroups that are distinct and nonoverlapping.

Software for Network Analysis and Visualization

The number of statistical software packages available to conduct the network analyses described here has expanded rapidly in the past decade (for a list, see *en.wikipedia.org/wiki/Social_network_analysis_software*). Historically, the most comprehensive and widely used social networks analysis program in the social sciences is the University of California Irvine NETwork analysis program (Borgatti et al., 2002). UCINET includes a wide range of powerful and flexible matrix manipulation and transformation tools and can calculate virtually all of the indices described in this chapter and many more. The chief limitation of UCINET is that it does not support batch processing, making it cumbersome to compute the same network index across multiple networks. More recently, several powerful libraries of network analysis tools have been added to the R statistical platform (social networks analysis, networks, statnet, igraph). Taken together, these libraries support nearly all of the network indices historically provided by UCINET, plus many additional ones. Three key advantages of R are its price (free), cross-platform support (Windows, Mac OS, Linux), and the ability to write scripts for batch processing, a virtual necessity when a large number of networks must be analyzed. The chief disadvantage of the R platform is the learning curve required to master the scripting language and the uneven documentation of specific algorithms that underlie some procedures.

A variety of other software packages exist for specific social networks analysis purposes. Several programs specialize in the identification of cohesive subgroups: Well known are NEGOPY (Richards, 1995) and its newer expanded version MULTINET (Seary, 2005) and KliqueFinder (Frank, 2004). Several programs exist to analyze data generated by the SCM data collection method. The classic program (SCM; *www.cds.unc.edu/biogs/leung.htm*) forms a co-occurrence matrix and identifies groups from similarities in conomination patterns (using intercorrelations of the columns of the matrix and applying decision rules for accepting ties). NETWORKS (Kindermann & Kwee, 2009) and NETJAWS (a Java version; Mehess & Kindermann, 2009; available at *web.pdx.edu/~thomas*) use binomial z tests and Fisher's exact tests to identify significant dyadic connections from the co-occurrence matrix. NETWORKS includes procedures that estimate average observer reliability with the overall map of identified ties.

Multiple programs exist to visualize social networks. NetDraw is linked to the UCINET package. Pajek (De Nooy, Mrvar, & Batagelj, 2005) was designed with special features to facilitate visualization of very large networks but has been enhanced to allow the calculation of many of the network indices described in this chapter. In recent years, new programs for stochastic modeling of social networks have also emerged. SIENA (Simulation Investigation for Empirical Network Analysis; Snijders, Steglich, Schweinberger, & Huisman, 2007; *stat.gamma.rug.nl/siena.html*) and statnet (Handcock, Hunter, Butts, Goodreau, & Morris, 2003) implement the most recent options for specifying p^* models, and SIENA also implements a simulation method for studying the coevolution of network structures and individual behavior over time (see Veenstra & Steglich, Chapter 34, this volume).

Developmental Applications

To date, discussions of network measures have focused largely on structural characteristics of networks, that is, indices based on the social ties among actors in a network. For social networks analysis to be useful to developmental researchers in answering questions about peer selection and peer influence, however, this information needs to be considered in relation to the substantive attributes of the actors who make up a person's network. Adding information about the characteristics of the affiliates allows researchers to examine (1) the composition of the network and individual peer groups, (2) the nature of peer environments, and (3) the psychological meaning of features of networks.

Homophily and the Composition of Peer Networks

Homophily concerns the degree to which individuals with similar attributes affiliate with one another (McPherson, Smith-Lovin, & Cook, 2001). Although homophily is ubiquitous, important developmental questions can focus on variations in the strength of homophily across different attributes over developmental time and across contexts. If the attribute is categorical (e.g., sex, race), homophily can be quantified with Freeman's *network segregation index* (Freeman, 1972), calculated as the difference between the number of observed cross-group ties and the number of randomly expected cross-group ties, divided by the number of randomly expected cross-group ties. When the segregation index is 1.0, all ties fall within separate groups; when the value is 0, ties are distributed randomly across groups.

When the attribute is approximately continuous (e.g., ratings on a Likert-type scale), the most general way to quantify homophily is to compute a spatial correlation relating distance in the social network to differences on the individual attribute; for example, Moran's I (Moran, 1950) ranges from –1.0 to +1.0, with positive values indicating a tendency for individuals with similar levels of the attribute to be close to each other in the network. At the level of subgroups, homophily may be quantified by an analysis of variance that documents the degree to which between-group variations in the attribute are larger than within-group variations (e.g., summarized by an intraclass correlation). Because social networks analysis offers precise metrics to describe the degree to which the networks of members of different sociodemographic groups are integrated, it can be a powerful tool in the study of sociodemographic and behavioral homophily or segregation, whether based on gender, race/ethnicity, or patterns of behavior (e.g., aggression, antisocial behavior, school motivation, academic achievement).

Sex Differences in Peer Relations

An extensive literature exists that focuses on sex differences in friendship patterns (Rose & Rudolph, 2006; Underwood, 2007). Key questions have included whether there are sex differences in the density of friendship ties, the salience or distinctiveness of friendship groups (vs. dyadic relations), and the salience of status hierarchies (Gest, Davidson, Rulison, Moody, & Welsh, 2007). Social networks analysis methods for identifying cohesive subgroups and characterizing connectivity could provide strong tests of these issues.

Peer Relations of Aggressive Youths

Extensive research has focused on differences in the peer experiences of aggressive and nonaggressive youths (Rubin, Bukowski, & Parker, 2006). Key questions have been whether aggressive youths have less extensive or more loosely connected friendship groups, whether aggressive youths occupy influential or peripheral positions within the network, and the extent to which aggressive youths selectively affiliate with one another (Cairns et al., 1988). Social networks analysis methods can be employed more extensively in this area to identify cohesive subgroups, to characterize the network centrality of aggressive youths (both within the network and within their cohesive subgroups), and to characterize levels of homophily and patterns of connectivity within these subgroups.

Developmental Change in Segregation and Integration

Perhaps most interesting for developmental researchers are questions focusing on how segregation according to gender, race, ethnicity, or behavior emerges over time and in different settings. Freeman's segregation index can be used to chart normative developmental changes in (and perhaps in setting level correlates of) gender segregation; similar indices could help to clarify the correlates of different degrees of friendship integration across racial/ethnic groups (Rodkin et al., 2000). More generally, the behaviors or attitudes that are most salient in a given network can be identified by computing spatial correlations that quantify the extent to which similarity on the attribute is associated with proximity in the network.

Network Diversity

In studies of peer influence, the dominant paradigm has been to create peer profile scores based on the average scores of a youth's peers. The diversity of contacts within a person's network has only recently received attention. People with more diverse networks seem to be less affected by contagion of the common cold (e.g., Cohen et al., 2000) and economically better off in a country (Eagle et al., 2010). Diversity can be operationalized in several ways: Eagle and colleagues use topological diversity (entropy in a person's overall phone contacts) and geographic diversity (spread across geographical regions). Highly diverse networks imply that an individual splits his or her time more evenly among various social ties and across geographical regions (Eagle et al., 2010, p. 1030) and receives more useful information. Cohen and colleagues (2000) define diversity as diversity of social roles (i.e., relationships with different partners, e.g., parents, children, neighbors, or workmates; higher diversity denotes more variety in relationships) and see diversity as a factor that can make people susceptible to negative influences. Such findings may extend to children and adolescents.

Capturing the Nature of the Peer Environment

Network descriptors are often based on the personal characteristics of the members in people's networks. Aggregate descriptors can have the form of composition proportions (with dichotomous variables, e.g., the number of obese or delinquent people in a person's network; Christakis & Fowler, 2007; Haynie, 2002) or the form of aggregated peer profile scores in psychological characteristics ($N - 1$ averages, so that each member has a group context denoted by the central tendency of his or her group members; e.g., Kindermann, 1993, 2007).

A common method for capturing each actor's "peer environment" is to calculate a score for each actor that is the arithmetic average of the actor's peers on an attribute in question. The set of relevant peers to include in these calculations is up to the investigator: It may be each actor's self-reported peers, the members of the actor's cohesive subgroup (excluding the actor her- or himself), or peers identified via probabilistic strategies (e.g., Kindermann, 2007). Typically, each actor's peers are characterized by their arithmetic mean on the attribute as a measure of the group's central tendency. Other approaches may depend on a researcher's theory or question (e.g., the proportion of peers above some designated threshold on a variable), but little is known about alternative ways to summarize the attributes of actors' peers.

Psychological Meaning of Network Centrality and Connectivity

Several studies illustrate the application of social networks analysis measures of network connectivity. At the level of the entire network (or a cohesive subgroup), individual attributes can be identified that are correlated with network centrality. Correlates of centrality can be interpreted as indicating the degree to which the members positively value or negatively sanction the attribute. For example, two networks may be characterized by similar levels of homophily in academic achievement, but achievement may be correlated positively with centrality in one network and correlated negatively with centrality in the other network. In the context of research on social norms, this index can be a measure of *norm salience* (i.e., the consequence of the behavior for adjustment in the setting; Cialdini, Kallgren, & Reno, 1991), in contrast to descriptive norms (the degree to which the behavior is common or typical in the setting) and injunctive norms (the degree to which individuals state that they approve of or disapprove of the behavior).

Network Centrality and Attachment to School

Empirical studies testing the correlates of individual nestedness within cohesive groups (Moody & White, 2003) are also emerging. Recall that the structural cohesiveness of a network can be quantified in terms of the maximum number of ties that must be broken to separate the network into distinct parts and that an individual's nestedness is defined by the number of ties that must be broken to separate him or her from the network. In their original study, Moody and White (2003) calculated the nestedness of each youth in the Add Health study in his or her school's friendship network, hypothesizing that youths who were deeply nested in the friendship network (i.e., for whom many ties must be broken to separate them from the core of the network) would feel more strongly attached to school. Consistent with expectations, school attachment was associated with individual nestedness, even after controlling for potential correlates of attachment such as individual attributes (e.g., school size, gender, grade point average) and measures of network centrality (degree, betweenness).

Ahn and colleagues (2010) built on this by using variability in the degree of nestedness experienced by students as an indicator of classroom hierarchy (i.e., more hierarchical classrooms showed a greater range of nestedness). In a sample of 42 third- and fourth-grade classrooms, aggressive children were found to achieve the highest levels of perceived popularity when they attended relatively hierarchical classrooms with high friendship density. These studies underscore that social networks analysis indices that capture broad patterns of connectivity in networks can contribute to our understanding of individual differences in functioning in social contexts.

Network Connectivity and Gender Differences

Gest, Davidson, and colleagues (2007) examined sex differences in patterns of friendship connectivity in a sample of 427 fifth-grade and seventh-grade youths. Girls' and boys' networks were analyzed separately. Friendship nominations were used to derive cohesive subgroups, and friendship and "like most" nominations were used to derive measures of density, reciprocity, transitivity, and centralization (hierarchy). Freeman's segregation index was used to measure the distinctiveness of the cohesive subgroups (i.e., in a girls' network, a high segregation index indicates that friendships across subgroups were rare). Potential sex differences were explored at both the whole- and same-sex network levels. Boys' groups were somewhat larger than girls' groups, but there were no systematic differences in the social networks analysis indices, providing little evidence for "two cultures" views of gender differences in friendships.

Illustrations

The use of social networks analysis in developmental research can be illustrated with studies in which social networks analysis methods are used to derive peer profile scores that capture central features of each individual's peer environment, scores that are used in longitudinal models to examine evidence for peer influence effects. As illustrations, we use our own research on the effects of peer aggression on the development of social-psychological adjustment (Rulison, Gest, Loken, & Welsh, 2010) and on the effects of peers' academic engagement on the development of children's engagement in the classroom (Kindermann, 2007).

Aggressive Peer Environments and the Adjustment

Rulison and colleagues (2010) studied the influence of peer aggression on social-psychological adjustment over a 5-year period (third–seventh grades), using Cairns's SCM data collection method (Cairns et al., 1988), in which youths are asked which of their classmates "hang around together a lot." Responses were aggregated into a co-occurrence (conomination) matrix in which each cell value gives the number of respondents who named that dyad as belonging to the same group. Cohesive subgroups were identified using principal components analysis, based on the premise that peers who do not share a direct dyadic connection may nonetheless influence each other if they are part of a cohesive subgroup that shares and reinforces a common set of behavioral norms. Peer aggression profile scores for each youth were calculated as the average score for the members of each youth's subgroup.

Next, a series of multilevel models examined between-person and within-person effects of peer aggression profile scores in relation to several measures of social-psychological adjustment. In this analytical framework, robust within-person effects (especially when manifested in cross-lag associations) would constitute stringent evidence that deviations from the typical peer environment are influential, with each person essentially serving as his or her own control. However, Rulison and colleagues (in press) found primarily between-person effects: Typically, affiliating with aggressive peers was associated with higher aggression for all youths but was associated with poorer adjustment (lower social preference and self-esteem, higher victimization) only for girls. The preponderance of between-person effects does not clarify whether these are due to selection, socialization, or some combination of the two.

Peer Environments and Academic Development

Kindermann (2007) examined peer influence on academic engagement from the beginning to the end of the sixth-grade school year. The study also used Cairns's data collection method and the co-occurrence matrix, but binomial z tests were employed to identify sixth graders from the conomination matrix who were observed (named) together as members of the same group more often than expected by chance. This strategy is dyadic in the sense that all peer partners were included who had a dyadic connection to an individual (i.e., the equivalents of "friends of friends" were not considered if they had no direct connection to a child, and direct connections were included even when the specific partners were not connected to one another but only to the target child). The focus on direct connections reflects the author's theoretical premise that direct interactions are the primary mechanisms of social influence.

Peer profile scores were computed for each individual by calculating the average teacher-rated academic engagement score across all significant partners of the individuals (excluding the target child). The group profile scores in fall were used in a structural equation model to predict changes in students' teacher-rated engagement from fall to spring, with an extensive set of control variables that were standardized for a variety of characteristics that can be confounded with group influences (e.g., size, gender composition, and stability of groups; academic achievement; teacher and parent involvement). The model indicated that peer engagement profiles predicted changes in individual engagement over and above the controls, consistent with expectations of peer influence effects.

Future Directions

In this chapter we have focused on descriptive measures of social networks and on their developmental implications. The reasons are that descriptive approaches have dominated network research in multiple disciplines and that social networks analysis concepts and measures can play an important role in testing long-standing developmental theories about peer relationships. Nonetheless, one of the most rapidly advancing areas of social networks analysis is statistical modeling of networks using the exponential family of random graph models (ERGM or p^* models; Handcock et al., 2003). For example, de la Haye, Robins, Mohr, and Wilson (2010) tested ERGMs to clarify how obesity-related behaviors were distributed in three adolescent friendship networks. Among other findings, they determined that friends were similar in levels of organized physical activity in two of the three networks, even after modeling the behavioral similarity that may have resulted from network dynamics related to reciprocity and transitivity. The rapid advancement of statistical techniques for examining the interplay between people's (static or changing) social networks, the characteristics of these networks, and their own individual development over time (e.g., Snijders, Steglich, & Schweinberger, 2005) may, by itself, be one of the most important trends in the field.

Improving Designs and Methods to Support Causal Inferences

However, amid enthusiasm for the burgeoning research on peer networks, it is easy for researchers (or interventionists) to assume that the connections found between networks and individuals are the product of peer influences. None of the social networks analysis indices described to this point can overcome the logical obstacles to inferring a causal role of peer influences. Beyond the usual cautions about inferring causality from cross-sectional data, special concerns arise in making causal inferences about the role of peers (see also Kindermann, 2008). Key issues center on individual confounds when influences are studied from people who are highly similar to target subjects under study, as well as on environmental and developmental confounds.

Assortativeness

Assortativeness (or selection) effects refer to the fact that people tend to join peers and peer groups that are similar to themselves. These effects have traditionally been a problem for all kinds of studies on social influences (e.g., Kandel, 1978), because the correlations between individuals and their peer networks are just as likely to be the effect of selection as of influence. Longitudinal designs are one strategy, because they allow researchers to examine change in individuals as a consequence of their (prior) peer network interactions when controlling for their own initial similarity to network members. Use of additional control variables is a second strategy.

For example, in his study of peer effects on school motivation, Kindermann (2007) found that students who were initially more motivated (engaged) tended to be affiliated with similar peers and remained comparably stable in their motivation over time, whereas students who were initially less motivated affiliated with less motivated peers and showed decreases in their motivation. The study suggested several additional individual controls: Children's sex was used to make sure that effects that look like peer effects are not just outcomes of the fact that girls tend to do better in school and to affiliate with similar girls; academic achievement (mathematics) was controlled to make sure that effects are not just effects of the intellectual potential of highly achieving students; and network size and stability were controlled to make sure that effects existed for an average network with an average length of individual exposure.

Contextual Confounds

Tighter controls may be needed. By themselves, longitudinal designs may not be sufficient because there are likely to be confounding third variables that can lead *both* to initial similarity *and* to parallel changes over time. Several kinds of *contextual confounds* can affect members of a network in the same way. We take an illustration from a study by Aral, Muchnik, and Sundararajan (2009). Friendship networks among Internet users appeared extremely predictive of users' choices to adopt specific services. However, this was largely an outcome of the fact that people with specific characteristics were similarly targeted by advertising campaigns. Because friends tend to have similar interests, to be of similar age, and to be online at similar times and may live close to one another, they can encounter similar environmental influences. Failing to account for such third variable influences can inflate estimates of influence effects. Based on their Internet data, Aral and colleagues argue that using traditional methods to infer social influences from networks can result in overestimations by 300%–700%.

At least two kinds of contextual confounds can be distinguished. First, there is *physical and temporal location*: People who attend the same school, live in the same neighborhood, or do the same things at the same time may experience common environmental influences (e.g., a math curriculum that influences achievement, food options that influence physiological processes, an unsafe neighborhood that influences outdoor exercise). Similarity in experiences contributes to both initial person-to-network similarities and to correlated patterns of developmental change. In Bronfenbrenner and Morris's (2006) terms, these are *exosystem* or *macrosystem* effects. Known location confounds (e.g., school, neighborhood) can be controlled in multilevel models, but unknown confounds (e.g., academic tracking within a school or curricula, food options that covary with socioeconomic status across neighborhoods) may produce findings that suggest peer influence effects when peers are not the real cause.

The second contextual confound is *developmental synchrony*, denoted by personal factors that lead people to meet at a certain point in time and to follow similar trajectories.

The same factors that led to initial peer similarity (and to formation of a network) may, over time, also lead to movement along similar pathways. For example, Cohen-Cole and Fletcher (2008) applied several common influence-modeling strategies to the Add Health data set and found (weak) evidence of "network influence" effects on variables for which there should be none (such as body height or acne). Similarity in maturation may be a feature around which peer networks are organized (see Moffitt, 1993), and synchrony can lead to developmental pathways that can look like peer influences. Developmental confounds may also be able to explain the almost paradoxical spread of loneliness across networks (Cacioppo et al., 2009). Instead of "social contagion," the spread may be an outcome of the fact that people seek out others who are in similar life circumstances (e.g., divorced people may seek out other divorcees instead of married acquaintances) and then show synchrony in their developmental paths.

MECHANISMS OF TRANSMISSION

One key strategy to counter suspicions of confounds in studies on network influences is to examine *mechanisms* of how transmission from peer groups to people comes about. Kindermann (2008) discusses some common mechanisms (e.g., reinforcement, modeling, persuasion), and Sage and Kindermann (1999) used classroom observations to examine reinforcement contingencies in peer networks as a mechanism for peer influence effects on school motivation. Berndt, Laychak, and Park (1990) conducted observations of discussions among friends to identify persuasion mechanisms in peer groups. If mechanisms of peer transmission can be identified, contextual confounds may still exist, but they would exist in addition to direct peer influences in a setting.

MATCHED CONTROLS

The second strategy for eliminating alternative explanations for peer network effects is to form samples of *matched controls*. These would consist of individuals matched on an array of variables that show high person-to-group similarity (so that control participants are similar to target children on as many assortative variables as possible), with the exception of those that are being tested as alternatives to peer influences.

Several kinds of control groups are possible. Controls may be participants who are similar to target participants but are themselves unaffiliated and not connected to the individuals under study. If the goal is to rule out maturational synchrony (e.g., Moffitt, 1993), connected people of the same age should have higher network influence effects than unaffiliated people of the same age (see also Popp et al., 2008). Controls may also be matched (unconnected) people who are members of peer networks that are located in different contexts or develop under different conditions. Thus, if controls who live in a different area, are at a different age, attend a different school, have different teachers, or are measured at different points in time still show similar effects of network influences, this will corroborate assumptions of genuine network effects (see Christakis & Fowler, 2007, for a discussion of geographical confounds; Aral et al., 2009, for a discussion of dynamic matched sampling). Finally, statistical approaches to controlling for many of the confounds may be possible; such approaches are the focus of other chapters in this volume (see Ackerman, Donnellan, Kashy, & Conger, Chapter 31; Card & Toomey, Chapter 32; Veenstra & Steglich, Chapter 34). Overall, efforts to examine alternative competing explanations can be implemented in various ways and at different levels of complexity. Choices for control strategies may be best justified by the specific target phenomenon under study.

Conclusions

We started this chapter by highlighting some of the diverse areas of social science research in which social network methods have led to insights into the role of social contexts in individual development. Because the next chapter in this volume focuses on a social network analytical strategy that is designed to model the dynamic coevolution of social networks and individual behaviors over time, we have focused on foundational concepts in network analysis and on the simplest descriptive measures that emerge from these concepts. Developmental researchers are often hesitant to incorporate social network methods into their studies because they require specialized measurement and data processing procedures, as well as relatively unfamiliar nonparametric statistical tests due to the nonindependence of network data.

Nonetheless, we believe there is much to be gained from a thoughtful integration of even very simple network indices because they are anchored in centuries of social thinking about group social life (Freeman, 2004), they have broad applicability to questions of central interest to developmental researchers, and there is a rapidly expanding set of textbooks and software tools to facilitate their calculation and thoughtful application. Moreover, we have suggested how such measures assessed at single points in time can be productively analyzed in the context of developmental research designs to address questions about developmental change. In doing so, we have touched on the difficult issue of how to support causal inferences regarding network influences on individual behavior.

References

Ahn, H.-J., Garandeau, C. F., & Rodkin, P. C. (2010). Effects of classroom embeddedness and density on the social status of aggressive and victimized children. *Journal of Early Adolescence, 30*, 76–101.

Aral, S., Muchnik, L., & Sundararajan, A. (2009). Distinguishing influence-based contagion from homophily-driven diffusion in dynamic networks. *Proceedings of the National Academy of Sciences, 106*, 21544–21549.

Bagwell, C. L., Coie, J. D., Terry, R. A., & Lochman, J. E. (2000). Peer clique participation and social status in preadolescence. *Merrill-Palmer Quarterly, 46*, 280–305.

Baker, W. E., & Faulkner, R. R. (1993). The social organization of conspiracy: Illegal networks in the heavy electrical equipment industry. *American Sociological Review, 58*, 837–860.

Barabási, A.-L. (2002). *Linked: The new science of networks*. Cambridge, MA: Perseus.

Bearman, P. S., & Moody, J. (2004). Suicide and friendships among American adolescents. *American Journal of Public Health, 94*, 89–95.

Berndt, T. J., Hawkins, J. A., & Jiao, Z. (1999). Influences of friends and friendships on adjustment to junior high school. *Merrill-Palmer Quarterly, 45*, 13–41.

Berndt, T. J., Laychak, A. E., & Park, K. (1990). Friends' influence on adolescents' academic achievement motivation: An experimental study. *Journal of Educational Psychology, 82*, 664–670.

Bonacich, P. (1987). Power and centrality: A family of measures. *American Journal of Sociology, 92*, 1170–1182.

Borgatti, S. M. (2005). Centrality and network flow. *Social Networks, 27*, 55–71.

Borgatti, S. M. (2009). *NetDraw*. Lexington, KY: Analytic Technologies.

Borgatti, S. P., & Everett, M. G. (2006). A graph-theoretic framework for classifying centrality measures. *Social Networks, 28*, 466–484.

Borgatti, S. P., Everett, M. G., & Freeman, L. C. (2002). *UCINET for Windows: Software for social network analysis*. Harvard, MA: Analytic Technologies.

Borgatti, S. P., Mehra, A., Brass, D. J., & Labianca, G. (2010). Network analysis in the social sciences. *Science, 323*, 892–895.

Bronfenbrenner, U., & Morris, P. A. (2006). The bioecological model of human development. In W. Damon (Series Ed.) & R. M. Lerner (Vol. Ed.), *Handbook of child psychology: Vol. 1. Theoretical models of human development* (6th ed., pp. 793–828). New York: Wiley.

Cacioppo, J. T., Fowler, J. H., & Christakis, N. A. (2009). Alone in the crowd: The structure and spread of loneliness in a large social network. *Journal of Personality and Social Psychology, 97*, 977–991.

Cairns, R. B., & Cairns, B. D. (1994). *Lifelines and risks: Pathways of youth in our time*. New York: Cambridge University Press.

Cairns, R. B., Cairns, B. D., Neckerman, H. J., Gest, S. D., & Gariepy, J. L. (1988). Social networks and aggressive behavior: Peer support or peer rejection? *Developmental Psychology, 24*, 815–823.

Cairns, R. B., Leung, M.-C., Buchanan, L., & Cairns, B. D. (1995). Friendships and social networks in childhood and adolescence: Fluidity, reliability, and interrelations. *Child Development, 66*, 1330–1345.

Cairns, R. B., Perrin, J. E., & Cairns, B. D. (1985). Social structure and social cognition in early adolescence: Affiliative patterns. *Journal of Early Adolescence, 5*, 339–355.

Cartwright, D., & Harary, F. (1956). Structural balance: A generalization of Heider's theory. *Psychological Review, 63*, 277–292.

Christakis, N. A., & Fowler, J. H. (2007). The spread of obesity in a large social network over 32 years. *New England Journal of Medicine, 357*, 370–379.

Cialdini, R. B., Kallgren, C. A., & Reno, R. R. (1991). A focus theory of normative conduct. *Advances in Experimental Social Psychology, 24*, 201–234.

Cohen, S., Brissette, I., Skoner, D. P., & Doyle, W. J., (2000). Social integration and health: The case of the common cold. *Journal of Social Structure, 1*(3), 1–7.

Cohen-Cole, E., & Fletcher, J. M. (2008). Detecting implausible social network effects in acne, height, and headaches: Longitudinal analysis. *British Medical Journal, 337*, a2533. Retrieved from *www.bmj.com/content/337/bmj.a2533.full*.

de la Haye, K., Robins, G., Mohr, P., & Wilson, C. (2010). Obesity-related behaviors in adolescent friendship networks. *Social Networks, 32*, 161–167.

De Nooy, W., Mrvar, A., & Batagelj, V. (2005). *Exploratory social network analysis with Pajek*. New York: Cambridge University Press.

Dijkstra, J. K., Lindenberg, S., Veenstra, R., Steglich, C., Isaacs, J., Card, N. A., et al. (2010). Influence and selection processes in weapon carrying during adolescence: The roles of status, aggression, and vulnerability. *Criminology, 48*, 187–220.

Durett, R. (2004). The new science of (random) networks. *Notices of the American Mathematical Society, 50*, 201–204.

Eagle, N., Macy, M., & Claxton R. (2010). Network diversity and economic development. *Science, 328*, 1029–1031.

Fowler, J. H., & Christakis, N. A. (2008). Dynamic spread of happiness in a large social network: Longitudinal analysis over 20 years in the Framingham Heart Study. *British Medical Journal, 337*, a2338. Retrieved from *www.bmj.com/content/337/bmj.a2338.full*.

Frank, K. A. (1995). Identifying cohesive subgroups. *Social Networks, 17*, 27–56.

Frank, K. A. (2004). KliqueFinder. Available at *www.msu.edu/~kenfrank/social%20network/kfuserguid.pdf*.

Freeman, L. C. (1972). Segregation in social networks. *Sociological Methods and Research, 6*, 411–430.
Freeman, L. C. (1979). Centrality in social networks: Conceptual clarification. *Social Networks, 1*, 215–239.
Freeman, L. C. (2004). *The development of social network analysis: A study in the sociology of science*. Vancouver, BC, Canada: Booksurge.
Gest, S. D., Davidson, A. J., Rulison, K. L., Moody, J., & Welsh, J. A. (2007). Features of groups and status hierarchies in girls' and boys' early adolescent peer networks. In P. C. Rodkin & L. D. Hanish (Eds.), *New directions for child and adolescent development: Social network analysis and children's peer relationships* (Vol. 18, pp. 43–60). San Francisco: Jossey-Bass.
Gest, S. D., Moody, J., & Rulison, K. L. (2007). Density or distinction?: The roles of data structure and group detection methods in describing adolescent peer groups. *Journal of Social Structure, 4*. Available at *www.cmu.edu/joss/content/articles/volume8/GestMoody/*.
Hallinan, M. T., & Williams, R. A. (1990). Students' characteristics and the peer-influence process. *Sociology of Education, 63*, 122–132.
Handcock, M. S., Hunter, D. R., Butts, C. T., Goodreau, S. M., & Morris, M. (2003). Statnet: An R package for the modeling of social networks. Available at *www.csde.washington.edu/statnet*.
Hanneman, R. A., & Riddle, M. (2005). *Introduction to social network methods*. Riverside: University of California, Riverside.
Haynie, D. L. (2002). Friendship networks and delinquency: The relative nature of peer delinquency. *Journal of Quantitative Criminology, 18*, 99–134.
Heider, F. (1946). Attitudes and cognitive organization. *Journal of Psychology, 21*, 107–112.
Hill, S., Provost, F., & Volinsky, C. (2006). Network-based marketing: Identifying likely adopters via consumer networks. *Statistical Science, 21*, 256–276.
Holland, P. W., & Leinhardt, S. (1971). Transitivity in structural models of small groups. *Comparative Groups Studies, 2*, 107–124.
Kandel, D. B. (1978). Homophily, selection, and socialization in adolescent friendships. *American Journal of Sociology, 84*, 427–436.
Kindermann, T. A. (1993). Natural peer groups as contexts for individuals' development: The sample case of children's motivation in school. *Developmental Psychology, 29*, 970–977.
Kindermann, T. A. (2007). Effects of naturally existing peer groups on changes in academic engagement in a cohort of sixth graders. *Child Development, 78*, 1186–1203.
Kindermann, T. A. (2008). Can we make causal inferences about the influences of children's naturally existing social networks on their school motivation? In N. A. Card, J. P. Selig, & T. D. Little (Eds.), *Modeling dyadic and interdependent data in the developmental and behavioral sciences* (pp. 343–368). New York: Routledge.
Kindermann, T. A., & Gest, S. D. (2009). Assessment of the peer group: Identifying naturally occurring social networks and capturing their effects. In K. H. Rubin, W. Bukowski, & B. Laursen, *Handbook of peer interactions, relationships, and groups* (pp. 100–117). New York: Guilford Press.
Kindermann, T. A., & Kwee, R. (2009). *NETWORKS 6.5* [Computer program]. Portland, OR: Portland State University, SOcial NETworks Research Group. Available at *www.web.pdx.edu/~thomas*.
Kiuru, N., Burk, W. J., Laursen, B., Salmela-Aro, K., & Nurmi, J.-E. (2010). Pressure to drink but not to smoke: Disentangling selection and socialization in adolescent peer networks and peer groups. *Journal of Adolescence, 33*, 801–812.
Knoke, D., & Yang, S. (2008). *Social network analysis*. Thousand Oaks, CA: Sage.
Light, J. M., & Dishion, T. J. (2007). Early adolescent antisocial behavior and peer rejection: A dynamic test of a developmental process. *New Directions for Child and Adolescent Development, 117*, 77–89.
McPherson, M., Smith-Lovin, L., & Cook, J. M. (2001). Birds of a feather: Homophily in social networks. *Annual Review of Sociology, 27*, 415–444.

Mehess, S., & Kindermann, T. A. (2009). *NETJAWS*: A Java program to identify peer network members in socio-cognitive mapping data [Computer program]. Portland, OR: Portland State University, Department of Psychology. Available at *www.web.pdx.edu/~thomas*.

Mizruchi, M. S. (2007). Political economy and network analysis: An untapped convergence. *Sociologica, 2,* 1–27.

Moffitt, T. E. (1993). Adolescence-limited and life-course-persistent antisocial behavior: A developmental taxonomy. *Psychological Review, 100,* 674–701.

Moody, J. (2001). Peer influence groups: Identifying dense clusters in large networks. *Social Networks, 23,* 261–283.

Moody, J. (2004). The structure of a social science collaboration network: Disciplinary cohesion from 1963 to 1999. *American Sociological Review, 69,* 213–238.

Moody, J., & White, D. R. (2003). Social cohesion and embeddedness: A hierarchical conception of social groups. *American Sociological Review, 68,* 103–127.

Moran, P. A. P. (1950). Notes on continuous stochastic phenomena. *Biometrika, 37,* 17–23.

Moreno, J. L. (1934). *Who shall survive?: A new approach to the problem of human interrelations.* Washington, DC: Nervous and Mental Disease Publishing.

Newman, M. E., & Girvan, M. (2004). Finding and evaluating community structure in networks. *Physical Review E, 69,* no. 026113. Available at *http://link.aps.org/doi/10.1103/PhysRevE.69.026113*.

Popp, D., Laursen, B., Kerr, M., Stattin, H., & Burk, W. J. (2008). Modeling homophily over time with an actor–partner interdependence model. *Developmental Psychology, 44,* 1028–1039.

Porter, M. A., Onnela, J.-P., & Mucha, P. J. (2009). Communities in networks. *Notices of the American Mathematical Society, 56*(9), 1082–1097.

Richards, W. D. (1995). NEGOPY 4.30 manual and user's guide. Vancouver, BC, Canada: Simon Fraser University, School of Communication. Available at *www.sfu.ca/~richards/Pdf-ZipFiles/negman98.pdf*.

Rodkin, P. C., & Ahn, H.-J. (2009). Social networks derived from affiliations and friendships, multi-informant and self-reports: Stability, concordance, placement of aggressive and unpopular children, and centrality. *Social Development, 18,* 556–576.

Rodkin, P. C., Farmer, T. W., Pearl, R., & Van Acker, R. (2000). Heterogeneity of popular boys: Antisocial and prosocial configurations. *Development Psychology, 36,* 14–24.

Rose, A. J., & Rudolph, K. D. (2006). A review of sex differences in peer relationship processes: Potential trade-offs for the emotional and behavioral development of girls and boys. *Psychological Bulletin, 132,* 98–131.

Rubin, K. H., Bukowski, W., & Parker, J. G. (2006). Peer interactions, relationships, and groups. In W. Damon & R. M. Lerner (Series Eds.) & N. Eisenberg (Vol. Ed.), *Handbook of child psychology: Vol. 3. Social, emotional, and personality development* (6th ed., pp. 571–645). New York: Wiley.

Rulison, K. L., Gest, S. D., Loken, E., & Welsh, J. A. (2010). Rejection, feeling bad, and being hurt: Using multilevel modeling to clarify the link between peer group aggression and adjustment. *Journal of Adolescence, 33,* 787–800.

Sage, N. A., & Kindermann, T. A. (1999). Peer networks, behavior contingencies, and children's engagement in the classroom. *Merrill-Palmer Quarterly, 45,* 143–171.

Scott, J. (2000). *Social network analysis: A handbook.* Thousand Oaks, CA: Sage.

Seary, A. J. (2005). *MultiNet: An interactive program for analysing and visualizing complex networks.* Vancouver, BC, Canada: Simon Fraser University, Department of Applied Science.

Snijders, T. A. B., Steglich, C. E. G., & Schweinberger, M. (2005). *Modeling the co-evolution of networks and behavior.* Groningen, The Netherlands: University of Groningen, ICS, Department of Sociology.

Snijders, T. A. B., Steglich, C. E. G., Schweinberger, M., & Huisman, M. (2007). *Manual for SIENA version 3.1.* Groningen, The Netherlands: University of Groningen, ICS, Department of Sociology.

Sokatch, A. (2006). Peer influences on the college-going decisions of low socioeconomic status urban youth. *Education and Urban Society, 39*(1), 128–146.

Underwood, M. (2007). Gender and children's friendships: Do girls' and boys' friendships constitute different peer cultures, and what are the trade-offs for development? *Merrill-Palmer Quarterly, 53*, 319–324.

Urberg, K. A., Degirmencioglu, S. M., Tolson, J. M., & Halliday-Scher, K. (1995). The structure of adolescent peer networks. *Developmental Psychology, 31*, 540–547.

Valente, T. W., Coronges, K., Lakon, C., & Costenbader, E. (2008). How correlated are network centrality measures? *Connections, 28*, 16–26.

Wasserman, S., & Faust, K. (1994). *Social network analysis*. Cambridge, UK: Cambridge University Press.

Wellman, B. (1988). Structural analysis: From method and metaphor to theory and substance. In B. Wellman & S. D. Berkowitz (Eds.), *Social structures: A network approach* (pp. 19–61). Cambridge, UK: Cambridge University Press.

White, H. C., Boorman, S. A., & Breiger, R. L. (1976). Social structure from multiple networks. *American Journal of Sociology, 81*, 730–780.

CHAPTER 34

Actor-Based Model for Network and Behavior Dynamics

RENÉ VEENSTRA
CHRISTIAN STEGLICH

Central Issues

Social relations can have a profound impact on human development in all life stages, be it positive relations such as friendship, support, and trust or negative relations such as dislike, envy, and bullying. The totality of relationships of a given type, measured in a meaningfully delineated social group, can be represented by a *social network*. When networks are used for explaining individual development, it needs to be considered that they also can develop over time. Together with the individual characteristics that change over time, the network change constitutes a mutually dependent feedback process. On one hand, characteristics of individuals and pairs of individuals, and structural positions of individuals within networks, can affect the evolution of the network. The best known example of such dependencies for *selection processes* may be the *homophily* process: the formation of a relationship based on the similarity of two individuals (Lazarsfeld & Merton, 1954; McPherson, Smith-Lovin, & Cook, 2001). On the other hand, networks can affect the individual characteristics and behavioral development of their members. These latter dependencies can be summarized as *influence processes*. A prominent example is the *assimilation* process, by which socially connected individuals become increasingly similar over time (Friedkin, 1998). Because homophily and assimilation result in the same empirical phenomenon (similarity of connected individuals), developmental researchers have long known that the study of influence requires the consideration of selection and vice versa (Billy & Udry, 1985; Cohen, 1977; Kandel, 1978).

Any attempt to analytically separate selection and influence processes is complicated by the fact that network data are inherently interdependent. Whether two individuals are connected in a network can crucially depend on their relations to third parties (Cartwright & Harary, 1956; Feld & Elmore, 1982; Heider, 1946). Only a few statistical methods are capable of mapping (or at least controlling for) such network dependencies. Among these, the prominent tool for the analysis of longitudinal network data is stochastic actor-based modeling (Snijders, 1996, 2001, 2005). A recently developed extension of this method can be used for analyzing simultaneously selection and influence processes, accounting for the mutual feedback between the two (Snijders, Steglich, & Schweinberger, 2007; Snijders, Van de Bunt, & Steglich, 2010; Steglich, Snijders, & Pearson, 2010). In this chapter, we portray this method by first deriving some methodological requirements for analyzing peer influence, then giving a brief sketch of the model and indicating how it meets these requirements. Next, developmental applications and an illustration of the method are given. Underlying model assumptions are presented, as well as analytical options for data that deviate from the example. We finish with an outlook on future developments of this approach.

Conceptual Principles and Statistical Assumptions

Limits of Traditional Approaches

A first methodological point to consider is that selection processes can be an alternative explanation for the outcome of influence processes. In order to tell the difference, *longitudinal data* need to be collected, which at least conceptually opens up the opportunity to study both processes in parallel. Under the stochastic actor-based approach, this is achieved by the construction of a multivariate coevolution model, in which the feedback between network change and behavior change is explicitly incorporated. Note that we use the term *behavior* as shorthand for endogenously changing ("dependent") individual characteristics, although these could also be attitudes, cognitions, performance, and so on.

The second methodological requirement is that, in studying peer selection and peer influence, *complete network data* are needed. The reason for this requirement is that in order to identify the determinants of selection, it does not suffice to know who *was* selected as network partner; it also needs to be known who *was not* selected. Only when the pool of available candidates is known does this become possible. Likewise, in identifying peer influence effects, it needs to be known what the absence of influence looks like, referring to how behavior changes in the absence of opportunities for influence. In earlier studies (Ennett & Bauman, 1994; Kandel, 1978), this was typically acknowledged by comparing a sample of dyads in which the individuals were (and stayed) connected to each other in the network with a matched sample of dyads in which the individuals were (and stayed) unconnected. However, under this approach, the crucially important control for selection processes is impossible. Under the stochastic actor-based approach, no reduction of the data to subsamples of dyads is made, but the total network structure in a fixed group of actors is used for analysis. This implies that the network boundary needs to be fixed by the researcher, who has to decide which social settings or contexts to focus on when collecting the data. There is another far-reaching implication of the necessity to study complete network data. Because many dependencies between actors in networks exist, it is not warranted to apply many commonly used statistical procedures. It is necessary to apply special procedures such as stochastic actor-based modeling, in which network dependencies are explicitly acknowledged and part of the modeling.

As a third methodological requirement, we point out that in studying peer selection and peer influence, *continuous time* needs to be considered. By research tradition, complete network data typically are assessed in discrete-time panel studies as a sequence of "snapshots." However, the changes that are reflected in these discrete time data typically accrue over the unobserved periods between the observation moments, in continuous time and as a consequence of continuous time processes. The importance of this consideration becomes clear when looking at the transitions depicted in Figure 34.1.

Suppose, at the first observation, individual *i* considers *j* a friend but is not behaviorally similar to *j* (configuration on the left), whereas at the second observation, *i* again considers *j* to be a friend but now is behaviorally similar to *j* (configuration on the bottom). In previous literature (Billy & Udry, 1985; Ennett & Bauman, 1994; Kandel, 1978; Popp, Laursen, Kerr, Stattin, & Burk, 2008), such a dynamic pattern is typically considered as influence, as actor *i* adjusting his or her behavior to become similar to friend *j*, as empirical evidence that transition (a) in Figure 34.1 has happened. However, such a conclusion is premature and predicated on the assumption that the friendship remained intact during the whole unobserved period. In most data collection designs, it is not known what happened between the two observations. It is entirely possible that the transitions (b), (c), and (d) happened instead of transition (a). The initial friendship between *i* and *j* may have ended (transition to the configuration on top), and *i* may have changed his or her behavior in the absence of a relationship with *j* (subsequent transition to the configuration on the right). After the behavior of *i* changed, *i* may have renewed the friendship with *j*, which leads to the configuration measured at the second observation. In this alternative scenario, the change in behavior occurred when the relationship between *i* and *j* was absent. The observed dynamic pattern therefore should not be counted as unequivocal evidence for transition (a), referring to influence of *j* on the behavior of *i*. On the contrary, transitions (d) and (b) in the alternative scenario suggest that selection processes can play a role as well. More generally, statistical methods that ignore the possibility of unobserved changes (and hence treat absence of evidence as evidence of absence) are prone to deliver biased results. An adequate test of selection and influence effects should therefore take into account the possibility of such unobserved changes in order to avoid these biases. For the researcher, this implies either continuous time data collection or—if data are measured at discrete moments—at least continuous time modeling. Stochastic actor-based modeling, as explained in this chapter (and as facilitated by the SIENA software), takes the latter approach of taking discrete time data as input but working "behind the scenes" with a continuous time change process when interpreting them.

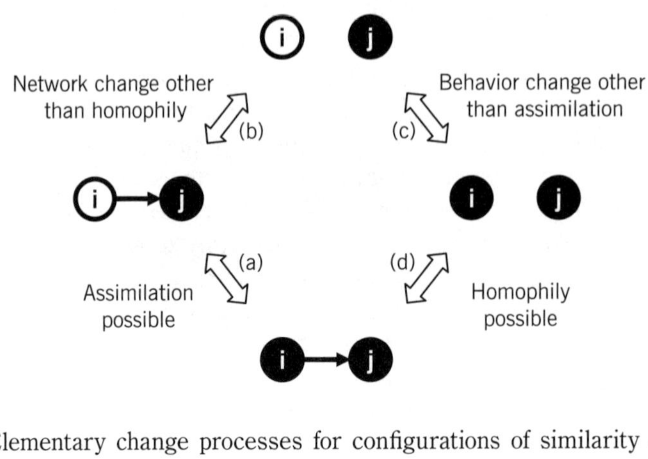

FIGURE 34.1. Elementary change processes for configurations of similarity and friendship in a dyad.

These three methodological requirements are hurdles that are, collectively, not taken by any of the earlier attempts to separate selection from influence processes. As detailed by Steglich, Snijders, and Pearson (2010), these studies tend to err methodologically or statistically by failing to sufficiently control influence for selection or vice versa, analyzing complete networks under clearly violated independence assumptions or disregarding the continuous time process generating observed changes. A particularly important shortcoming from the perspective of network analysis is the neglect of structural (network-inherent, endogenous) selection processes in these earlier studies. Several of these effects are known to play a strong role in the dynamics of friendship networks. For example, it is widely known that friendships are more likely to be established when persons share a common friend (Davis, 1970). Hence, transitivity, rather than similarity in behavior, might account for friendship formation between similar individuals. Not controlling for such structural network tendencies in the analyses can lead to biases of homophily effects, which, in turn, will affect the estimates for assimilation effects by failing to filter out homophily effects in a statistically sound way (Steglich, Snijders, & Pearson, 2010). As its origin in dynamic network analysis suggests, the stochastic actor-based approach presented in this chapter has no difficulty controlling for such effects. How the model does this is explained in a nontechnical way in the next section. For technical details on the model mechanics and estimation, we recommend the descriptions that can be found in Snijders and colleagues (2007).

Stochastic Actor-Based Model

As prerequisites for stochastic actor-based modeling, we assume that the empirical data consist of a sequence of at least two observations of a social network and a behavioral variable, measured at time points $t_1, t_2, \ldots, t_m$ on a given set of actors such as classmates or colleagues. *Ties* are the bilateral constituents of relations such as friendship, trust, or cooperation, directed from one actor to another. In principle, the ties are under control of the sending actor. The tie variables are binary variables, denoted by x_{ij}. A tie from actor i to actor j, denoted $i \rightarrow j$, is either present or absent (x_{ij} then having values 1 and 0, respectively). The tie variables constitute the network, represented by its $n \times n$ adjacency matrix $x = (x_{ij})$ (self-ties are excluded), where n is the total number of actors. The codependent behavior variables are assumed to be discrete and ordinal—for instance, levels of delinquency measured on a Likert-type scale—that are represented by a vector $z = (z_i)$.

Figure 34.2 illustrates the correspondence between a network-behavior configuration and its representation as adjacency matrix and behavior vector. The dependent variable in an actor-based analysis is the time series of observed matrices and behavior vectors, $(x,z)(t_1), (x,z)(t_2), \ldots, (x,z)(t_m)$.

The actor-based model interprets this discrete time series of data as the cumulative result of an unobserved (and therefore not uniquely identifiable) sequence of elementary changes, resulting from decisions made by the actors between observation moments. As such, the approach does justice to the fact that, typically, the underlying change process has not been observed and can be inferred only from modeling. To be able to do so with some statistical power, two rather far-reaching assumptions are made.

The first far-reaching assumption is that of *decomposability into smallest possible changes*. The unobserved change process is assumed to take place as gradually as possible, by "microsteps" that consist of either a tie swap (one network tie being broken or created) or a unit change in behavior. For a single actor, this enforces gradual change. When abrupt

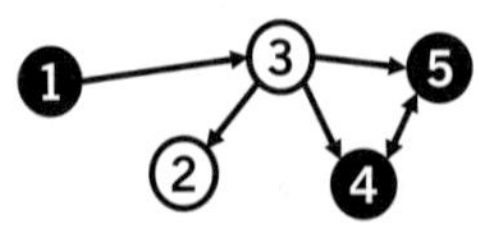

$$x = \begin{pmatrix} 0 & 0 & 1 & 0 & 0 \\ 0 & 0 & 0 & 0 & 0 \\ 0 & 1 & 0 & 1 & 1 \\ 0 & 0 & 0 & 0 & 1 \\ 0 & 0 & 0 & 1 & 0 \end{pmatrix}, \quad z = \begin{pmatrix} 1 \\ 0 \\ 0 \\ 1 \\ 1 \end{pmatrix}$$

FIGURE 34.2. Scheme of a binary social network with binary behavioral variable and its notation as adjacency matrix x and behavior vector z.

changes are known to occur in the data (say, an adolescent drops his or her friendship ties to a whole group at the same moment), the decomposability assumption is violated. When considering the actions of multiple actors, coordinated change is ruled out. A whole group of adolescents starting to smoke at the same moment also violates decomposability.

The second far-reaching assumption is that of *conditional sequential independence*. It is assumed that at any moment in time, the current state of the evolution process (referring to the network and the behavior configuration at this moment) is sufficiently informative, meaning that the history of the process is fully mediated by the current state. This Markov assumption implies that some potentially important quantities (such as the age of a network link or information on whether a behavior level was approached from higher or from lower levels) are not naturally included in the model. In practice, this means that relevant information from the past needs to be included in exogenous predictor variables.

By enforcing a sequential nature on the decisions that accumulate to the observed changes, parameter estimation is facilitated (Holland & Leinhardt, 1977) and the interdependence of the ties and individual behavior that is typical for network data is enacted through feedback processes in continuous time. Ties are formed or broken, and behavior is adjusted upward or downward, in response to the existence of other ties and the behavior of other actors in the network. The dependencies at the beginning of an unobserved period are taken as the starting value of the change process, and later changes naturally depend on these and the occurrence of earlier changes in the sequence. By repeatedly imputing sequences of microsteps, the model allows us to differentiate the strength of multiple contributing mechanisms to observed longitudinal patterns, as discussed in the context of Figure 34.1. This way, any microstep is embedded in a localized decision-making context, and the modeling can be split up into the timing of the actors' opportunities to make a microstep and the decision rules they follow when actually making it, which are addressed later. Due to the unobserved nature of the exact sequence of changes connecting observation moments, simulation-based inference becomes necessary for estimating the model parameters (Snijders, 2001, 2005; Snijders et al., 2007; Snijders, Van den Bunt, & Steglich, 2010).

The basic coevolution model has four parts, expressing the amount of change (rate functions) and the direction of change (objective functions), each for decisions about network change and behavior change. Any imputed sequence amounts to the repeated identification of a focal actor (ego) who gets the opportunity to make a change and the identification of the change outcome. The determination of ego is modeled by the so-called *rate functions* λ, which indicate the frequency of opportunities for behavior and network changes. These functions jointly parametrize an exponential distribution of waiting times. They can depend on individual characteristics of the actors, including features of their network position. In accordance with the selected combination of the focal actor (ego) and decision domain (network or behavior), ego then may change one outgoing tie (either create or break a tie), change his or her own behavior (going one step up or down on the behavior scale), or do nothing (keep the status quo). The outcome probabilities of these decisions depend on the *objective functions f* for behavior and network changes. Objective functions parametrize a multinomial logit choice model. They indicate how attractive it is for an actor to go from an old to a new state. These functions summarize the information actors use to adjust their positions in the network and on the behavior scale. Potential components of this function can be structure-based (endogenous) effects, such as the tendency to form reciprocal relations, or attribute-based (exogenous) effects, such as the preference for similar others. It is assumed that actors have full information about the total network structure and can accurately assess the consequences of their decisions. Based on their evaluations of these consequences, they try to move in a direction of higher values on their objective functions, subject to the constraints of the current network structure and the current behavior of all actors in the network, the changes made by others in the network, and random influences.

Rate and objective functions alike can be expressed as parameter-weighted sums of actor- and domain-specific statistics, $\sum_k \beta_k s_{ik}(x,z)$. The effect statistics s_{ik} express features of the network neighborhood of actor i, and the weights β_k are estimated from the data, expressing the impact of the corresponding statistic on either the amount of change (rate functions) or the direction of change (objective functions). Formally, the total model describes a continuous time Markov chain, with the time parameter t taking values in the continuous interval $[t_1, t_m]$.

Developmental Applications

The actor-based model has been used to study a range of behaviors, such as externalizing problems (aggression, delinquency, weapon carrying), internalizing problems (anxiety, depression, loneliness), and substance use (alcohol, cannabis, cigarettes). The main research questions of these studies were whether adolescents *select* friends based on similarity in behavior and whether adolescents are *influenced* by their friends' behavior.

In an application of the actor-based model, Mercer and DeRosier (2010) reported that lonely children were more likely to select other lonely children as friends. Van Zalk, Kerr, Branje, Stattin, and Meeus (2010) found the same for depressed adolescents. Thus there is support for a greater likelihood of friendship formation among children with similar levels of internalizing problems. The greater likelihood may be the result of fewer overall opportunities for friendship formation due to peer rejection and of active searching for similar friends.

Influence processes offer an alternative explanation for adolescents being similar to their peers in internalizing symptoms. Anxious and depressive feelings and thoughts may increase through reinforcement of negative cues in interactions with friends with internalizing symptoms. Mercer and DeRosier reported indeed that friends' anxiety, depression, and loneliness influenced children's own internalizing problems. These peer influence processes regarding depressive symptoms turned out to be stronger for girls than boys (Van Zalk et al., 2010).

All studies on the coevolution of network and behavior dynamics report clear sex similarity in friendships. Voluntary sex segregation begins in early childhood, peaks in middle childhood, and is to some extent still present in adolescence (see also Maccoby, 1998). Several studies also report selection similarity for age and ethnicity and thus a preference for friends of the same age and same ethnicity. There is also strong support for a selection similarity effect for delinquency and smoking (Baerveldt, Völker, & Van Rossem, 2008; Burk, Kerr, & Stattin, 2008; Mercken, Snijders, Steglich, & De Vries, 2009).

With respect to behavior dynamics, some studies provide evidence for influence effects of friends' behavior, whereas other studies do not. For example, the influence effect of smoking was found in only two out of six countries in the study by Mercken and colleagues (2009). Differences between studies seem to be related to the context in which peer influence is studied. For example, the influence effect of delinquency was found in studies that looked at the effects of grademates or townmates (Baerveldt et al., 2008; Burk et al., 2008) but was absent in studies that looked at the effects of classmates (Knecht, 2008; Light & Dishion, 2007). This suggests that the behavior of out-of-class friends influences delinquency more than does the behavior of classmates.

Beyond the question of whether similarity is due to selection or influence, developmental applications of the actor-based model have led to more insight into the mechanisms underlying network and behavior dynamics. In an exemplary study, Kiuru, Burk, Laursen, Salmela-Aro, and Nurmi (2010) compared selection and influence mechanisms for alcohol use and smoking. It turned out that selection played a greater role than influence in explaining similarity between smoking behavior of friends, whereas both selection and influence played a significant role in explaining similarity in drinking behavior. This finding is consistent with the idea that tobacco use is an addictive activity and that once adolescents have started smoking, the social influence on smoking may become less important for smoking progression. Thus peer influence plays less of a role in the dynamics of smoking behavior. Spatial segregation provides an explanation for the relatively stronger effect of selection compared with influence with regard to smoking. For example, it may be that as society separates smokers from nonsmokers (referring to smoking-designated areas), smokers may be more likely to establish new contacts with other smokers and then affiliate with each other. In addition, Kiuru and colleagues found that adolescents with high levels of smoking tended to receive more peer nominations than those who did not smoke, and smoking was accordingly seen as cool.

In another exemplary study, Dijkstra and colleagues (2010) compared selection and influence mechanisms for weapon carrying. They found that in early adolescence, weapon carrying was quite stable over a 1-year period. Using social network data from 207 Latino male adolescents in New Jersey, they found no support for a selection mechanism on the basis of weapon carrying. However, associating with friends who carry weapons increased the level of weapon carrying over the course of a year. Thus selection plays no role, whereas influence does for the development of weapon carrying. In addition, Dijkstra and colleagues found that adolescents with high levels of problem behavior tended to be not only more popular, referring to the number of nominations received, but also less active, referring to the number of nominations given, than others with low levels of problem behavior. Thus weapon carriers were seen by others as popular and were themselves more selective than others in the number of friendships that they mentioned.

Illustration

We now proceed to an illustration of the method that will further explicate how stochastic actor-based modeling works. The data analyzed are taken from the Teenage Health and Lifestyle Study (West & Sweeting, 1996). A description of the data set is given in Table 34.1. In applications of actor-based modeling, the number of actors in a network is usually between 20 (referring to the size of a small school class) and a few hundred (referring to a complete elementary school, a school grade in secondary education, or a small neighborhood). These numbers are in line with the implicit assumption that each actor is a potential network partner for any other actor. It is possible to combine several networks into one fixed effects analysis, which can be particularly helpful when analyzing multiple small (but independent) networks that of themselves do not yield enough information for estimating parameters. The extra assumption is that all networks follow dynamics with the same parameter values in the objective function.

In our study, we analyze the friendship network in a school cohort ($n = 160$) of Glasgow secondary school students, which was assessed at three time points (1995–1997, roughly equidistant) when students were aged 13–15. Table 34.1 shows that there is a limited amount of missing data, which can be accommodated by the software. A simulation study by Huisman and Steglich (2008) using a network size of 50 suggested that the results will not be biased as long as the missing information is not exogenously imputed. Standard errors will remain reasonably small (and allow detection of significance) as long as a fraction of 20% missing is not exceeded. Also, the number of students who enter the network late or

TABLE 34.1. Description of the Sample and the Variables per Observation Moment (Left) and Longitudinal Transitions between Observation Moments (Right)

	T1	T2	T3		T1–T2	T2–T3	T1–T3
Cohort size	153	151	139	Number leavers	7	15	18
Respondents missing	3	5	2	Number joiners	5	3	4
Fraction females	45.8%	46.4%	45.3%	Number stayers	146	136	135
	Friendship				Friendship change		
Average outdegree	3.91	4.01	4.28	Distance	557	470	591
SD outdegree	1.70	1.64	1.79	Jaccard index	27.5%	31.4%	20.1%
SD indegree	2.40	2.38	2.14				
Density	2.6%	2.7%	3.1%				
Reciprocity	56.3%	53.9%	63.6%				
Transitivity	35.9%	31.2%	43.8%				
Three-cyclicity	28.5%	24.8%	37.7%				
Same sex	88.6%	90.1%	90.1%				
	Hanging				Hanging change		
Average males	2.58	2.73	2.72	Distance	86	88	93
Average females	2.94	3.20	3.11	Fraction stable actors	65.0%	63.4%	60.0%
SD males	1.37	1.35	1.29				
SD females	1.32	1.21	1.20				
	Autocorrelation						
Moran's *I*	0.221	0.280	0.255				

leave early (discussed later in more detail) should not be large. The number of observation moments should in general be at least 2 and is usually less than 10. It should be noted that the model assumes temporal homogeneity of the change process, which may be violated in data sets with many observations (Lospinoso, Schweinberger, Snijders, & Ripley, 2010; Steglich, Sinclair, Holliday, & Moore, in press).

Students nominated around four friends. Due to the restriction to maximally six nominations, the outdegree distribution is truncated—which is not optimal but quite common in network research due to considerations of respondent burden. In Table 34.1, this may have affected the discrepancy between the standard deviations of indegree (higher) and outdegree (lower), which substantially means that the cohort is more differentiated according to popularity (friendship nominations received) than according to activity (friendship nominations given). The network is typical in the sense that it has, first of all, a low density, referring to the proportion of friendship nominations that are actually given in a network. Second, it has a high degree of reciprocity, referring to the proportion of friendship nominations that are mutually confirmed. Third, it has a high degree of triangulation, mapping the tendency to share friends. This triangulation is expressed in the indices for transitivity, which gives the proportion of indirect friendship nominations (friends' friends) who are also directly nominated as friends, and three-cyclicity, referring to the proportion of indirect friendship nominations that are reciprocated with a direct one.

The probability indices for reciprocity, transitivity, and three-cyclicity are conditional probabilities for friendship to exist, given a specific structural embedding. They are identified as "high" relative to the density, which is the unconditional probability for friendships to exist. The probability index for same sex gives the fraction of friendships that are among students of the same sex and is not directly comparable to the other percentages. The fraction of same-sex friendships is high, which is quite normal during childhood and adolescence.

The behavioral dimension that we analyze as a coevolving dependent variable is hanging around the streets, a lifestyle item that ranges from 1 (less than once a month) to 4 (most days). Table 34.1 reveals that throughout the study, female students on average tended to hang around the streets more often than their male schoolmates.

Preconditions for an Analysis

To find out whether it makes sense to analyze the data with an actor-based coevolution model, we first need to check whether there is any association between the network and the behavioral variable, referring to whether the phenomenon we want to explain with selection and influence effects can be found in the data at all. Second, we need to check whether the data are sufficiently informative to allow for identification of effects.

Addressing the first issue, we take a look at Moran's network autocorrelation coefficient, which is a measure of the degree to which friends show the same hanging behavior. Like other correlation coefficients, it can in theory range from –1 to +1, with values close to 0 indicating independence between friendship and hanging behavior, and the values +1 or –1 indicating identity or perfect complementarity of the hanging behaviors of two friends. The positive Moran's I values in our data show that friends tend to exhibit the same hanging behavior. As argued previously, such a result begs the question of causality. On one hand, social influence processes could be responsible: Students might acquire their hanging behavior from their friends. On the other hand, social selection processes could be responsible: Students might select their friends based on similar hanging behavior, for example, because the street is a context for meeting new friends.

To get a rough impression of the statistical power, the second issue, it is possible to examine the descriptive quantifications of the amount of change and the degree of stability in the network and in the behavior. The relevant information is given in the right panel of Table 34.1, which renders change statistics for the periods of analysis (T1–T2 and T2–T3) and for the whole period under study (T1–T3). The attrition and recruitment related to students leaving or joining the cohort is relatively small, which means that there is a reasonably sized core group of students for whom the change processes could be studied. For details about the handling of joiners and leavers, we refer the reader to Huisman and Snijders (2003) and the software manual (Snijders, Steglich, Schweinberger, & Huisman, 2010).

For the group of stayers in a given period, change and stability of the friendship network can be quantified. In general, the total number of changes between consecutive observations should be large enough to provide the information for estimating parameters. More changes will give more information and, thereby, allow more complicated models to be fitted. However, a complete turnover of friendship nominations would call into question the assumption that the waves are consecutive observations of a gradually changing network. If the stable part of the network is very small, the consecutive observations are probably too far apart. This implies that, when designing a study, the researcher needs to have a reasonable estimate of the expected change. For instance, to study the development of a friendship network of a group of initially mutual strangers (e.g., freshmen in high school), it may be good to plan the observation moments to be separated by only a few weeks in the beginning and to enlarge the period between observations after a couple of months.

The Hamming distance is the number of friendship nominations for which change in the period could be observed, referring to the sum of new nominations (friends at the end of the period but not yet at the beginning) and lost nominations (vice versa). It is a lower boundary for the number of microsteps needed to get from one network observation to the next, and as such it gives an indication about the statistical power for identifying parameters for the network evolution part of the model. The observed Hamming distances, around 500 for subsequent observations and almost 600 for the period T1–T3, are reasonably large for identifying medium-sized network models (20–25 parameters).

The Jaccard index, on the other hand, is the fraction of stable friendship nominations among the new, lost, and stable ones in the period (and it disregards stable absence of friendship). Without a good fraction of stability in the data, an initial measurement of the network is uninformative for the evolution process toward the next measurement, and the two measurement points might better be analyzed separately. Based on experience with the method, Jaccard indices around 30% commonly indicate sufficient stability, so the periods T1–T2 and T2–T3 seem sufficiently stable.

Table 34.1 also reports the amount of change in terms of absolute differences in individual hanging behavior from the beginning to the end of the period (distance) and the fraction of actors who do not change their hanging behavior. Because behavior data are fewer than network data (vector vs. matrix), the distances are naturally lower than for the network, here around 90. Therefore, the specification of the behavior dynamics part of a model should be considerably more parsimonious than that of the network dynamics part.

Model Specification

In the following, we give a model specification for an actor-based analysis of our data that allows assessing friends' influence on the respondents' hanging-around-the-streets behavior. In the illustration, most of the analytical results are addressed right away, as are possible modifications of the modeling that some research questions or data formats might require.

A number of effects can be considered for inclusion in the objective and rate functions. When specifying a selection of these for estimation, the researcher should make sure that known features of the data are sufficiently captured in the selected effects. As is illustrated, failure to do so can bias results of the other parameters. The results of our illustrative analyses are reported in Table 34.2. There are results for two model specifications, one corresponding to what we would call the required way of modeling (the triad effects model) and one in which information about interdependence on the triad level is neglected (the dyad effects model). In the descriptions that follow, formulae are given for a few effects to illustrate the principle. The majority of effects are described only conceptually; a complete list of formulae is given in Snijders, Van de Bunt, and Steglich (2010) and Steglich and colleagues (in press). In our example, the relation under study is friendship, so the existence of a tie $i \rightarrow j$ will be described as i calling j a friend, and the behavior in question is hanging around the streets. The fact that behavioral changes are assumed to be by 1 unit in a single

TABLE 34.2. Estimation Results for the Network and Behavior Objective and Constant Rate Function Parameters

	Dyad effects model			Triad effects model		
	Estimate	*SE*	*p*	Estimate	*SE*	*p*
Objective function "friendship"						
Outdegree	–3.11	009	< 0.00	–2.89	0.12	< 0.00
Reciprocity	2.50	0.09	< 0.00	2.27	0.13	< 0.00
Transitive triplets	—			0.39	0.06	< 0.00
Transitive ties	—			0.83	0.12	< 0.00
Three-cycles	—			–0.06	0.12	0.62
Indegree activity	—			–0.22	0.04	< 0.00
Sex (F) alter	–0.20	0.09	0.02	–0.16	0.10	0.08
Sex (F) ego	0.16	0.09	0.08	0.03	0.10	0.74
Same sex	0.99	0.08	< 0.00	0.67	0.08	< 0.00
Hanging alter	–0.00	0.05	0.94	0.014	0.05	0.77
Hanging ego	–0.18	0.05	0.00	–0.08	0.05	0.15
Hanging ego × hanging alter	0.12	0.04	0.00	0.08	0.03	0.00
Objective function "hanging around"						
Linear shape	–1.19	0.25	< 0.00	–1.16	0.36	0.00
Quadratic shape	0.63	0.07	< 0.00	0.63	0.06	< 0.00
Friendship indegree	0.00	0.09	0.92	0.05	0.05	0.37
Friendship outdegree	0.08	0.10	0.44	0.04	0.09	0.67
Average hanging of friends	0.27	0.13	0.04	0.26	0.13	0.04
Effect from sex (F)	0.11	0.13	0.37	0.12	0.13	0.35
Rates of change						
Friendship (period 1)	10.18	0.68		13.17	1.21	
Friendship (period 2)	8.86	0.65		10.70	0.97	
Hanging around (period 1)	6.26	1.48		6.29	2.04	
Hanging around (period 2)	8.05	1.69		8.11	2.70	

time point implies that a "natural" application of the model requires that the total number of scale values of the behavioral outcomes is usually 4 to 10.

Network Dynamics

The following section discusses the parameters in the network objective function for which empirical estimation results are provided in Table 34.2. Significance of these estimates is derived from the approximately normal distribution of the t-ratio, calculated as the ratio of the parameter by its standard error.

Outdegree (Density)

The outdegree effect corresponds to the count of friends an actor nominates, $s_i = \sum_j x_{ij}$. It is an intercept effect that reflects the basic tendency to name friends at all, and as such models the density of the network. Because the objective function parameters refer to a logistical scale, empirical densities of much less than 50% (as we have them in our data set) are reflected in a negative estimate for the outdegree parameter, which can be seen in Table 34.2 as well.

Reciprocity

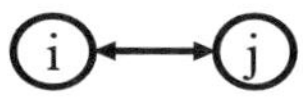

Another basic effect is the tendency toward reciprocation of choices, referring to mutual ties: i chooses j and j chooses i. It is expressed by statistic $s_i = \sum_j x_{ij}x_{ji}$. The parameter will be zero when the (conditional) probability for reciprocation is identical to the (unconditional) probability for any tie to exist. Results for our friendship network show significant positive evidence for reciprocity in the friendship data, which is no surprise because friendship tends to be governed by norms of reciprocation.

Triad Structure

Effects incorporating structural information involving three or more actors are a crucial advance of social network analysis over purely dyad-based approaches (Kenny, Kashy, & Cook, 2006; Popp et al., 2008). A score type test (Snijders et al., 2010), which compares the goodness of fit of different model specifications, assessed that the triad effects model is an improvement ($\chi^2 = 1778.9$, $df = 4$) of the dyad effects model.

TRANSITIVITY

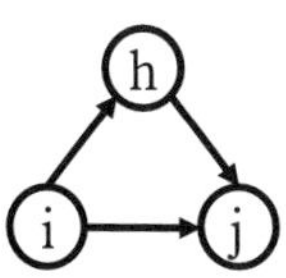

An essential feature of peer group structure is the tendency toward transitivity or transitive closure. Friends of friends become friends (Davis, 1970; Holland & Leinhardt, 1971).

Several effect statistics have been formulated to operationalize transitivity in stochastic actor-based models. Depending on the amount of effort the researcher wants to spend on accurately capturing group structure, either just one or several of these should be included when modeling data that contain endogenous group formation. The most straightforward formulation is the transitive triplets statistic $s_i = \sum_j x_{ij} \sum_h x_{ih} x_{hj}$. This effect measures transitivity for an actor i by counting the number of configurations (i, h, j) in which all three ties $i \to h$, $h \to j$, $i \to j$ are present (and irrespective of whether there are also other ties between these three actors). The tie $i \to j$ becomes increasingly likely the more indirect connections (two-paths) $i \to h \to j$ there are.

Another way of measuring transitivity is the transitive ties effect, expressed by the statistic $s_i = \sum_j x_{ij} \max_h x_{ih} x_{hj}$. It measures transitivity for actor i by counting the number of other actors j for which there is at least one intermediary h forming a transitive triplet. The transitive ties effect expects that given that one intermediary exists, extra intermediaries will not further contribute to the tendency to forming the tie $i \to j$. The results in Table 34.2 report a stronger effect for transitive ties than for transitive triplets, which indicates that the first triplet closing a transitive triangle is much more important for tie formation and stability than subsequent triangles are, which also are closed by the same tie. A third and often used statistic expressing transitivity is $s_i = \sum_j (1 - x_{ij}) \max_h x_{ih} x_{hj}$, which represents the tendency for actors to keep others at a sociometric distance of two, and thus to avoid friendship with friends of friends. This measure is the converse of transitive closure. For that reason, a negative parameter estimate is usually obtained. Note that irrespective of the operationalization chosen, transitivity in a directed network is always in line with a hierarchical ordering, because it allows distinguishing and ordering the three involved actors according to the number of ties they receive and send.

THREE-CYCLES

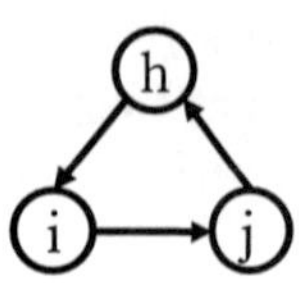

This measure represents the number of three-cycles $i \to j \to h \to i$ that actor i is involved in. Three-cycles are intrinsically nonhierarchical, and a positive three-cycle effect can be interpreted as a tendency toward generalized exchange (Bearman, 1997). In many social networks, there is a tendency to have a hierarchical ordering with relatively few three-cycles; this typically leads to a negative estimate for the three-cycle parameter. In our friendship network, the effect is estimated as negative, but it falls short of significance—presumably because the other hierarchy measure included (indegree activity, discussed next) expresses the hierarchical tendencies in the friendship network more accurately.

Degree Distribution

Indegrees and outdegrees are primary characteristics of the position in a network. The *indegree* is the number of ties directed at an actor, referring to the amount of received nominations. The *outdegree* is the number of ties going from an actor, referring to the amount of provided nominations. When the degree information is used as an endogenous predictor of social ties, in fact, again triadic structure is assessed—as is illustrated in the diagrams in the following.

POPULARITY ALTER

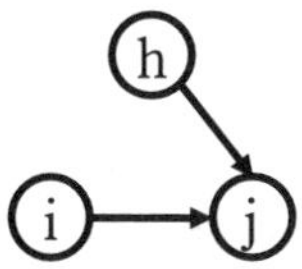

The popularity effect models the tendency to form ties to actors who have high indegrees already, referring to a Matthew effect (Merton, 1968) or the cycle of popularity (Eder, 1985): If lower status peers seek affiliation with higher status peers but face difficulty in affiliating with them, higher status adolescents become increasingly attractive. The effect is not included in our model specification because, when fitting our model in a forward model selection procedure (Snijders et al., 2007), its inclusion was identified as not improving model fit any further after controlling for the more important activity ego effect. In a different model specification for the same friendship network, Steglich and colleagues (in press) estimate the effect, however, and find a significant positive result.

ACTIVITY ALTER AND POPULARITY EGO

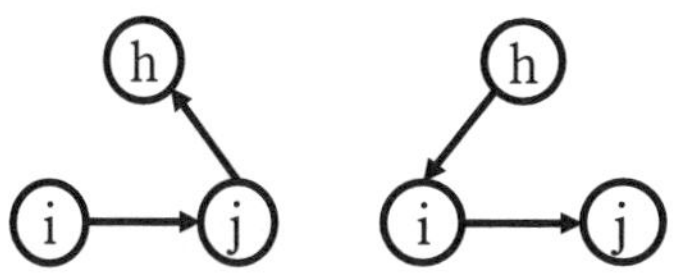

The activity alter effect models the tendency to form ties to actors who have high outdegrees. The popularity ego effect models tendencies of actors with high indegrees to form ties to anyone. As can be seen in the diagrams, both effects allocate agency over the configuration differently: friendship nominations provided by alter *j* versus friendship nominations received by ego *i*.

ACTIVITY EGO

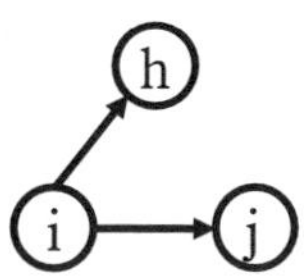

This effect measures self-reinforcing tendencies in the nomination of others. In our empirical example, we find a significant negative effect of indegree-activity ego, which means that receiving a high number of friendship nominations tends to make people send fewer friendship nominations to others—a sign of a global hierarchy, with popular actors on top of the hierarchy and unpopular actors at the bottom. Transitivity effects can also represent hierarchy between actors in the network, but in a different way from these degree-related effects. Transitivity effects represent *local hierarchy*, referring to the ordering of the three involved actors in a triad. To differentiate between local and global hierarchical processes, it is generally recommended to estimate models with both triadic and degree-related effects.

Covariates: Actor-attribute Effects

For an actor attribute, there are two basic effects: the *ego* effect (covariate-related activity effect; sender effect)

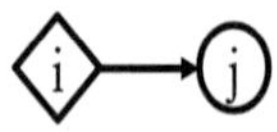

measuring whether actors with higher attribute values (depicted by the diamond shape) tend to nominate more friends and hence have a higher outdegree; and the *alter* effect (covariate-related popularity effect; receiver effect)

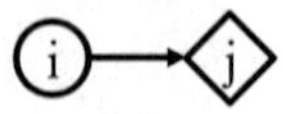

measuring whether actors with higher attribute values tend to be nominated more often and hence have higher indegrees. Actor covariates may be constant, such as sex or ethnicity, or subject to change, such as opinions, attitudes, or behaviors. In our analyses, we identify a marginally significant negative effect of sex alter, meaning that girls are less popular than boys in this network.

Next, there are effects that combine information of sender and receiver, illustrated as

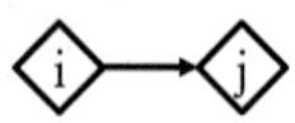

The *similarity* (homophily) effect measures whether ties tend to occur more often between actors with similar values on an attribute. In our analyses it turned out that the network is sex segregated, as indicated by a highly significant same-sex (sex similarity) parameter. What is important to notice is that the same-sex effect drops sharply in effect size from the dyad effects model to the triad effects model—in fact so sharply that confidence intervals for the effect do not overlap between the two models. This illustrates the danger of reporting results when overlooking important structural features in the data. Thus part of the association between sex segregation and the evolution of the network is due to global hierarchy (activity ego) and local hierarchy (transitivity) processes.

Another effect that combines information of sender and receiver is the *ego × alter interaction*. We found that students who hang around the streets a lot show a significantly higher preference for friends who also hang around the streets a lot (significant positive interaction effect ego × alter).

It may occasionally be interesting to summarize the information contained in sender, receiver, and combined effects in a table or a graphic. An explanation of how to do this is provided by Snijders and colleagues (Snijders et al., 2010; Snijders, Van de Bunt, & Steglich, 2010). A summary of the impact of hanging around the street on the friendship network is given in Figure 34.3. What can be seen is that for students who hang around the streets once a month or less (scale scores 2 and 1), the evaluation of friendship decreases with increasing hanging behavior of the candidate friend, whereas for students who hang around the streets once a week or more often (scores 3 or 4), this likelihood increases.

For a dyadic covariate, referring to a variable defined for pairs of actors, there is just one basic effect

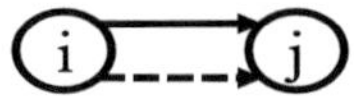

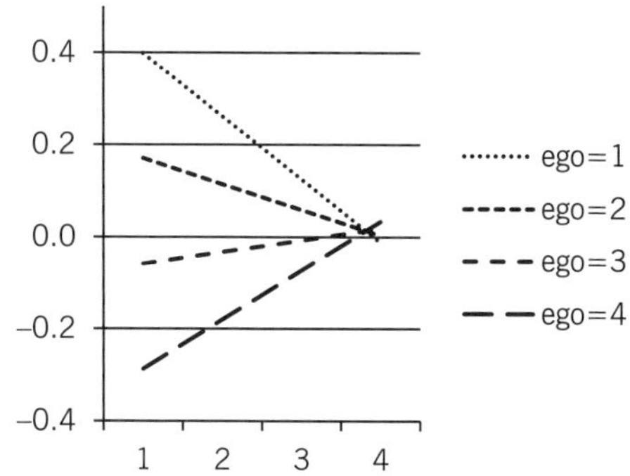

FIGURE 34.3. Joint contributions of ego, alter, and ego × alter effects of the hanging-on-the-street behavior to the network objective function (*Y*-axis) in the triad effects model. The four functions indicate how ego (with four levels of hanging behavior) evaluates alter (with hanging behavior on the *X*-axis).

expressing the extent to which a tie between two actors is more likely when the dyadic covariate (expressed by the dotted line) is larger. Dyadic covariates likewise may be constant, such as the geographical distance between the homes of two actors or the number of years two actors know each other, or changing over time, such as a bully–victim relationship or the number of hours two actors spent together (changing covariates require at least three observation moments). In our example, we did not include such dyadic covariate information.

Interactions

As in other statistical models, interactions can be important to express theoretically interesting hypotheses. In the actor-based framework, it may be natural to hypothesize that the strength of certain effects depends on attributes of the focal actor. For example, girls might have a greater tendency toward transitive closure than boys. This can be modeled by the interaction of the ego effect of sex and the transitive triplets effect.

Behavior Dynamics

Linear and Quadratic Shape Effects

Basic distributional features of the behavior variable are expressed by two shape parameters that should be estimated as control variables. The *linear* shape parameter plays the role of an intercept, whereas the *quadratic* shape parameter controls for underdispersion (regression to the mean, when the parameter is negative) or overdispersion (polarization, when the parameter is positive). Together the two shape effects can be interpreted as expressing the relative prominence of the specific values z_i on the behavior scale (referring to the distribution of z). In the special case in which the behavior variable is dichotomous, the quadratic shape effect is collinear with the linear shape effect and must not be included in the model. However, when the behavior variable contains three or more possible values, it is generally recommended to include the quadratic shape effect. If the overall distributional shape cannot be approximated by a quadratic function (which rarely is the case), higher order shape effects might be necessary to control for. In our empirical example, we see that the coefficient of the quadratic term is positive. The shape contribution to the objective function is then U-shaped, suggesting that changes in the behavior are drawn to the extremes of the range, with actors already low on the behavior to lower values and actors already high on the behavior to higher values. The hanging-around-the-street variable has modes at the extreme ends.

Influence Effects

The actor-based model can represent social influence, referring to influence of alters' behavior on ego's behavior (friends stay similar but behavior changes), in various ways. First, by the *average similarity* effect, expressing the preference of actors to be similar in behavior to their alters in such a way that the total influence of alters is the same regardless of the number of alters (referring to ego's outdegree). Second, by the *total similarity* effect, expressing the preference of actors to be similar in behavior to their alters in such a way that the total influence of the alters is proportional to the number of alters. Third, by the *average alter* effect, expressing that actors whose alters have a higher average value of the behavior also have a stronger tendency toward high values on the behavior themselves. The choice between these different representations of social influence has to be made on theoretical grounds or (in the absence of specific theory) can be facilitated by comparing different model specifications with a score type test (Snijders et al., 2007). In our empirical example, the average alter effect, which we found to be positive, gave the best model fit to the data.

Position-Dependent Effects

In addition to this type of social influence, network position itself could also have an effect on the behavior dynamics. A positive effect of the actor's indegree and outdegree may indicate that those who are more active (higher outdegree) and popular (higher indegree) have a stronger tendency to display higher values of the behavior over time. In our analysis, these effects were included in the estimated models but turned out not to be significant contributors to the behavior dynamics.

Effects of Other Actor Variables

For each actor-dependent covariate (and also if there are multiple behavioral outcomes for each of the other behavior variables), a main effect on the behavior can be included, representing the influence of this actor variable on behavior changes. In addition, it is possible that actor-dependent covariates moderate the influence effect, leading to an interaction between the covariate and the influence effect.

Rate Functions

The objective functions discussed previously refer to which decision actor i makes. The rate functions refer to how frequently in a given period an actor can make a decision. Depending on actor attributes and network position, actors might change their ties at different frequencies. For example, it might be that younger individuals change their friendship ties more often than older individuals. In our analysis, we included only the basic rate of change: We assume that all students differ neither in terms of the number of opportunities per period for changing their networks (indicated by the basic rate for friendship change in Table 34.2) nor in terms of the number of opportunities for changing their behavior (indicated by the hanging rates in the same table). In the quite egalitarian school context and the homogeneous age group we study, this assumption seems to make sense. What we find is that friendship change slows down over time, whereas changes in hanging behavior speed up a bit.

Goodness of Fit and Model Convergence

Goodness of fit for stochastic network models is generally based on a comparison of model-based simulations of network data sets (and the distributions these imply for a host of summarizing statistics) with the observed network data on which the model was estimated (Hunter, Goodreau, & Handcock, 2008). For each individual statistic, the percentile at which the observed value is located in the distribution of simulated values serves as a test; for example, observed values below the 2.5th and above the 97.5th percentiles of simulated values indicate significant departure of the model from the observed data at a 5% significance threshold. Obviously, for effects included in a model, goodness of fit should be perfect on the corresponding statistics; the observed value of the statistic should be in the center of the simulated distribution. Commonly it is recommended to consider estimation results as reliable only when for all model parameters the difference between observed statistic and simulated average statistic is smaller than 10% of the standard deviation of simulated statistics (Snijders et al., 2010). For well-behaved data sets, it is quite common to obtain this convergence in one, maybe two or three estimation runs with successively improved starting values. In our data, we obtained convergence already after the first run.

Future Directions

This chapter has given an introduction to the use of the actor-based model for analyzing the joint interdependent dynamics of networks and behavior. These models can be used to test hypotheses concerning network and behavior dynamics and represent the strength of various tendencies driving the dynamics by estimating parameters. To be useful in this way for statistical inference, the models must be able to give a good representation of the dependencies between network ties, network positions, and behavior of the actors. The models also have to contain parameters that can express theoretical considerations about tendencies driving network and behavior change. Furthermore, the models must be flexible enough to represent several different explanations of change and test these against each other or controlling one for the other. These goals are accomplished by the stochastic actor-based model in which the central model components are the objective functions, analogous to the linear predictor in generalized linear modeling (Long, 1997). The models can be estimated by a software package called SIENA (Simulation Investigation for Empirical Network Analysis), for which the manual is Snijders and colleagues (2010). The program and documentation can be downloaded freely at *stat.gamma.rug.nl/siena.html*. Recently, SIENA also became available as a package in the R statistical programming environment, under the name RSiena (Ripley, Snijders, & Lopez, 2011). Older versions of the software (up to version 3, facilitated in the Stocnet program package) will not be supported in the future.

The actor-based model is relatively new and more complicated than many other statistical models that social scientists are used to. Applications are starting to be published, but more experience is needed to get a better understanding of their applicability and the interpretation of the results. A technical extension would be the possibility of employing a real multilevel model instead of a meta-analytical approach to examine behavior and network dynamics in several networks. Although higher level effects (e.g., school characteristics) can already be included in the meta-analytical approach, such a multilevel extension would increase the statistical power of the analysis. Other issues are the development of an effect size measure (Sijtsema et al., 2010; for two attempts, see Dijkstra et al., 2010) and the development of models for valued ties (for an ordinal scale of relationship strength, see Labun, Wittek, Steglich, & Wielers, 2010).

The actor-based model has proven to be a useful analytical tool for questions about selection (friends change but behavior stays similar) and influence (friends stay similar but behavior changes) effects. The strengths of the model are that it models unobserved changes between observation points, controls for network structure effects, and takes dependencies in the data into account. However, not all assumptions are always realistic. For example, a basic assumption is that actors act independently from each other and cannot coordinate their actions. This means that these models may not adequately model group phenomena, such as co-offending or the effect of collective norms (Baerveldt et al., 2008).

The default in models of network dynamics is that breaking a tie is just the opposite of creating one. This is not always a good representation of reality. It is conceivable, for example, that the loss when terminating a reciprocal tie is greater than the gain in creating one or that transitive closure works especially for the creation of new ties but hardly guards against termination of existing ties. This can be modeled by having two components of the objective function: the *evaluation function*, which considers only the network that will be the case as a result of the change to be made, and the *endowment function*, which is a component that operates only for the termination of ties and not for their creation. Van Zalk and colleagues (2010) tested hypotheses about deselection processes in relation to adolescent depressive symptoms. Deselection offered an alternative explanation for adolescents' tendencies to be similar to their peers.

In this chapter we have tried to represent the current knowledge about the specification of longitudinal network-behavior coevolution models in a concise but more or less complete way, but we hope that this knowledge will expand rapidly. Various extensions of the model are a topic of research. All these developments are tracked at the SIENA website mentioned earlier.

Acknowledgments

Christian Steglich was funded by the Netherlands Organization for Scientific Research (NWO) under Grant No. 461-05-690 (ECRP EUROCORES scheme). We thank the Chief Scientist's Office of the Scottish Home and Health Department for funding data collection carried out by Patrick West and Lynn Michell of Glasgow University.

References

Baerveldt, C., Völker, B., & Van Rossem, R. (2008). Revisiting selection and influence: An inquiry into the friendship networks of high school students and their association with delinquency. *Canadian Journal of Criminology and Criminal Justice, 50,* 559–587.

Bearman, P. (1997). Generalized exchange. *American Journal of Sociology, 102,* 1383–1415.

Billy, J. O. G., & Udry, R. (1985). Patterns of adolescent friendship and effects on sexual behavior. *Social Psychology Quarterly, 48,* 27–41.

Burk, W. J., Kerr, M., & Stattin, H. (2008). The co-evolution of early adolescent friendship networks, school involvement, and delinquent behaviors. *Revue Francaise de Sociologie, 49,* 499–522.

Cartwright, D., & Harary, F. (1956). Structural balance: A generalization of Heider's theory. *Psychological Review, 63,* 277–293.

Cohen, J. M. (1977). Sources of peer group homogeneity. *Sociology of Education, 50,* 227–241.

Davis, J. A. (1970). Clustering and hierarchy in interpersonal relations: Testing two graph theoretical models on 742 sociomatrices. *American Sociological Review, 35,* 843–851.

Dijkstra, J. K., Lindenberg, S., Veenstra, R., Steglich, C., Isaacs, J., Card, N. A., et al. (2010). Influence and selection processes in weapon carrying during adolescence: The roles of status, aggression, and vulnerability. *Criminology, 48,* 187–220.

Eder, D. (1985). The cycle of popularity: Interpersonal relations among female adolescents. *Sociology of Education, 58,* 154–165.

Ennett, S. T., & Bauman, K. E. (1994). The contribution of influence and selection to adolescent peer group homogeneity: The case of adolescent cigarette smoking. *Journal of Personality and Social Psychology, 67,* 653–663.

Feld, S. L., & Elmore, R. (1982). Patterns of sociometric choices: Transitivity reconsidered. *Social Psychology Quarterly, 45,* 77–85.

Friedkin, N. E. (1998). *A structural theory of social influence.* Cambridge, UK: Cambridge University Press.

Heider, F. (1946). Attitudes and cognitive organization. *Journal of Psychology, 21,* 107–112.

Holland, P. W., & Leinhardt, S. (1971). Transitivity in structural models of small groups. *Comparative Groups Studies, 2,* 107–124.

Holland, P. W., & Leinhardt, S. (1977). Dynamic model for social networks. *Journal of Mathematical Sociology, 5,* 5–20.

Huisman, M., & Steglich, C. (2008). Treatment of non-response in longitudinal network studies. *Social Networks, 30,* 297–308.

Huisman, M. E., & Snijders, T. A. B. (2003). Statistical analysis of longitudinal network data with changing composition. *Sociological Methods and Research, 32,* 253–287.

Hunter, D. R., Goodreau, S. M., & Handcock, M. S. (2008). Goodness of fit of social network models. *Journal of the American Statistical Association, 103,* 248–258.

Kandel, D. B. (1978). Homophily, selection, and socialization in adolescent friendship pairs. *American Journal of Sociology, 48,* 427–436.

Kenny, D. A., Kashy, D. A., & Cook, W. L. (2006). *Dyadic data analysis.* New York: Guilford Press.

Kiuru, N., Burk, W., Laursen, B., Salmela-Aro, K., & Nurmi, J.-E. (2010). Pressure to drink but not to smoke: Disentangling selection and socialization in adolescent peer networks and peer groups. *Journal of Adolescence, 33,* 801–812.

Knecht, A. (2008). *Friendship selection and friends' influence: Dynamics of networks and actor attributes in early adolescence.* Utrecht, The Netherlands: Interuniversity Centre for Social Science Theory and Methodology.

Labun, A., Wittek, R., Steglich, C., & Wielers, R. (2010). *Where does reputational power in organizations come from?* Unpublished manuscript.

Lazarsfeld, P. F., & Merton, R. K. (1954). Friendship as social process. In M. Berger, T. Abel, & C. Page (Eds.), *Freedom and control in modern society* (pp. 18–66). New York: Octagon.

Light, J. M., & Dishion, T. J. (2007). Early adolescent antisocial behavior and peer rejection: A dynamic test of a developmental process. *New Directions for Child and Adolescent Development, 118*, 77–89.

Long, J. S. (1997). *Regression models for categorical and limited dependent variables*. Thousand Oaks, CA: Sage.

Lospinoso, J. A., Schweinberger, M., Snijders, T. A. B., & Ripley, R. M. (2011). Assessing and accounting for time heterogeneity in stochastic actor oriented models. *Advances in Data Analysis and Classification, 5*, 147–176.

Maccoby, E. E. (1998). *The two sexes: Growing up apart, coming together.* Cambridge, MA: Belknap.

McPherson, M., Smith-Lovin, L., & Cook, J. M. (2001). Birds of a feather: Homophily in social networks. *Annual Review of Sociology, 27*, 415–444.

Mercer, S. H., & DeRosier, M. (2010). Selection and socialization of internalizing problems in middle childhood. *Journal of Social and Clinical Psychology, 29*, 1032–1059.

Mercken, L., Snijders, T. A. B., Steglich, C. E. G., & De Vries, H. (2009). Dynamics of adolescent friendship networks and smoking behavior: Social network analyses in six European countries. *Social Science and Medicine, 69*, 1506–1514.

Merton, R. K. (1968). The Matthew effect in science. *Science, 159*, 56–63.

Popp, D., Laursen, B., Kerr, M., Stattin, H., & Burk, W. J. (2008). Modeling homophily over time with an actor–partner interdependence model. *Developmental Psychology, 44*, 1028–1039.

Ripley, R. M., Snijders, T. A. B., & Lopez, P. P. (2011). *Manual for SIENA version 4.0*. Oxford, UK: University of Oxford, Department of Statistics.

Sijtsema, J. J., Ojanen, T., Veenstra, R., Lindenberg, S., Hawley, P. H., & Little, T. D. (2010). Forms and functions of aggression in adolescent friendship selection and influence: A longitudinal social network analysis. *Social Development, 19*, 515–534.

Snijders, T. A. B. (1996). Stochastic actor-oriented models for network change. *Journal of Mathematical Sociology, 21*, 149–172.

Snijders, T. A. B. (2001). The statistical evaluation of social network dynamics. *Sociological Methodology, 31*, 361–395.

Snijders, T. A. B. (2005). Models for longitudinal network data. In P. J. Carrington, J. Scott, & S. Wasserman (Eds.), *Models and methods in social network analysis* (pp. 215–247). New York: Cambridge University Press.

Snijders, T., Steglich, C., & Schweinberger, M. (2007). Modeling the coevolution of networks and behavior. In K. Van Montfort, J. Oud, & A. Satorra (Eds.), *Longitudinal models in the behavioral and related sciences* (pp. 41–71). Mahwah, NJ: Erlbaum.

Snijders, T. A. B., Steglich, C. E. G., Schweinberger, M., & Huisman, M. (2010). *Manual for SIENA version 3.2*. Groningen, The Netherlands: University of Groningen, Department of Sociology.

Snijders, T. A. B., Van de Bunt, G. G., & Steglich, C. E. G. (2010). Introduction to stochastic actor-based models for network dynamics. *Social Networks, 32*, 44–60.

Steglich, C., Sinclair, P., Holliday, J., & Moore, L. (in press). Actor-based analysis of peer influence in A Stop Smoking in Schools Trial (ASSIST). *Social Networks, 32*.

Steglich, C., Snijders, T. A. B., & Pearson, M. (2010). Dynamic networks and behavior: Separating selection from influence. *Sociological Methodology, 40*, 329–393.

Van Zalk, M. H. W., Kerr, M., Branje, S. J. T., Stattin, H., & Meeus, W. H. J. (2010). It takes three: Selection, influence, and de-selection processes of depression in adolescent friendship networks. *Developmental Psychology, 46*, 927–938.

West, P., & Sweeting, H. (1996). *Background, rationale and design of the West of Scotland 11 to 16 Study* (Working Paper No. 52). Glasgow, UK: MRC Medical Sociology Unit.

PART VII

Special Topics in Data Analysis

CHAPTER 35

Configural Frequency Analysis in Developmental Research

ALEXANDER VON EYE
EUN-YOUNG MUN
RICHARD M. LERNER
JACQUELINE V. LERNER
EDMOND P. BOWERS

Central Issues

The effects of caffeine are well known. Caffeine is a psychoactive stimulant of the central nervous system. Its effects are ergogenic (they include the temporary suppression of drowsiness and the restoration of alertness). Interestingly, caffeine can also have just the opposite effect. A sizable percentage of the population (about 15%) reports what is known as *paradoxical effects* of caffeine. These individuals report increased sleepiness after consuming caffeine. In addition, the so-called *caffeine nap*, a 15- to 20-minute nap immediately after caffeine consumption, seems to have stronger and longer lasting effects on alertness than caffeine alone.

This example shows that generalizations that are based on statistical data analysis often describe trends that can be found in the population but are inadequate to describe individuals, or even the majority of the population. For example, von Eye and Bergman (2003) showed that the aggregate-level autocorrelation pattern that was found for the drinking behavior of a sample of alcoholics did not describe a single individual validly. Similarly, von Eye, Bogat, and Rhodes (2006) found that, in a large sample of adolescents, negative parental attitudes toward alcohol consumption are predictive of a reduction of the amount of alcohol consumed over a span of 3 months. However, although this trend was significant both overall and in the subpopulation of females, it described less than 50% of the female respondents. Naturally, it failed to describe those who indicated that they did not drink any alcohol at all, as well as those who increased their alcohol consumption over the observation period. In the male subpopulation, this trend describes barely over 50% of the respondents.

Based on these and similar observations, proponents of *person-oriented* research have proposed analyzing data such that justice is done to subpopulations that show different patterns of parameters (Bergman & Magnusson, 1997; Bergman, von Eye, & Magnusson, 2006; von Eye & Bogat, 2006). According to Bergman and colleagues (2006), *configural frequency analysis* (CFA; Lienert, 1968; von Eye & Gutiérrez Peña, 2004; von Eye, Mair, & Mun, 2010) is one of the most suitable statistical methods for data analysis from a person-oriented perspective.

This applies to both cross-sectional and longitudinal research. CFA allows one to determine whether particular patterns of scores occur more often or less often than expected with reference to a base model. The *CFA base model* is a statistical chance model that provides the frame of reference for the statement that a pattern was observed more often or less often than expected or conforms with expectation. In other words, the base model allows one to answer the questions, With respect to what? or What did you expect? when declaring a pattern frequency as deviating from expectation. Different base models can result in different statements about the nature of a pattern frequency as extreme.

In longitudinal research, the patterns that are inspected by using CFA describe aspects of constancy and change over time. For example, a pattern that stands out could describe the development of children who turn out resilient to the effects of domestic violence (Bogat, Levendosky, DeJonghe, Davidson, & von Eye, 2004) or the development of adolescents who engage in heavy drug use at an early age (Tubman, Vicary, von Eye, & Lerner, 1991). In both cases, the base model that is used to evaluate patterns would state that these developmental patterns will occur at random rates (see the section "The CFA Base Model"; see also von Eye, 2004).

In the following sections of this chapter, we present an overview of methods of CFA, with a focus on longitudinal base models and designs. Each of the models is illustrated using a large data set from a cohort-sequential study on positive youth development, the 4-H Study of Positive Youth Development (Lerner et al., 2005, 2009; Phelps et al., 2009).

Conceptual Principles and Statistical Assumptions

In this section, we present basics of CFA, focusing on the CFA null hypothesis, CFA base models, significance testing, and the protection of the significance threshold, α. Sample base models for longitudinal research and sample analyses of empirical data follow.

The CFA Null Hypothesis

To determine which of the cells in a cross-classification deviate from expectation, exploratory CFA needs to examine every cell. Confirmatory CFA focuses on an a priori specified selection of cells. In this chapter, we focus on exploratory CFA, which has found far more applications than confirmatory CFA. In each application, exploratory CFA determines for each cell in a cross-classification whether its frequency allows one to reject the cell-specific null hypothesis H_0:

$$E[m_r] = \hat{m}_r$$

where r indexes the cells of the cross-classification, $\hat{m}_r$ is the expected frequency for cell r, m_r is the observed frequency for cell r, and E is the expectancy (von Eye & Gutiérrez Peña, 2004). There are two possibilities why this null hypothesis may be rejected. First, for a sample of size N, the null hypothesis may be rejected because (using the binomial test for an example) the binomial probability is

$$B_{N,\pi_r}(m_r - 1) \geq 1 - \alpha$$

where π_r is estimated from the sample, and the cell contains more cases than expected. In this case, cell r (also called *configuration*) is said to constitute a *CFA type*. If, in contrast, the null hypothesis is rejected because (again using the binomial test)

$$B_{N,\pi_r}(m_r) \leq \alpha$$

cell r contains fewer cases than expected. In this case, Cell r is said to constitute a *CFA antitype*.

Protecting α in CFA

A well-known characteristic of statistical null hypothesis tests is that the specified threshold of $\alpha = 0.05$ (or 0.01) can be guaranteed only for the first test in a given data set. Even if tests are completely independent, multiple tests, performed on the same data, imply an increase in α. Consider a researcher who performs 10 tests on the same data under the a priori specified $\alpha = 0.05$. The α risk that one of these tests suggests an erroneous decision concerning the null hypothesis is 0.315. The probability that none of these tests suggests an erroneous decision is 0.599 (instead of 0.95).

In most applications of exploratory CFA, the number of tests performed is equal to R, the number of cells in a cross-classification (in confirmatory CFA applications, this number typically is smaller than R). Therefore, it is routine to protect α (this can be seen as parallel to protecting α in analysis of variance [ANOVA] post hoc tests). The most popular method for α protection is the *Bonferroni procedure*. It keeps the protected α^* level constant. Another method, originally proposed by Holm (1979; a combination of these two procedures was proposed by Hommel, 1988), allows α^* to vary depending on the number of tests already performed that led to a rejection of the cellwise H_0.

Specifically, let α be the a priori specified significance threshold for the cellwise CFA tests and α^* the protected threshold ($\alpha^* < \alpha$). Then the protected threshold that results from the Bonferroni procedure is

$$\alpha^* = \alpha/R$$

Clearly, this threshold can suggest extremely conservative statistical decisions when a table contains many cells. Less conservative is Holm's procedure, which proceeds in three steps. First, the tail probabilities of the cellwise test statistics are ranked, in ascending order. Second, the tail probabilities are evaluated, beginning with rank 1, with respect to

$$\alpha_r^* = \frac{\alpha}{R - r + 1}$$

with $r = 1, \ldots, R$. Third, the evaluation of the tail probabilities ends as soon as the first H_0 prevails.

For the first test, the Holm procedure is as conservative as the Bonferroni procedure. Beginning with the second test, the Holm procedure uses less extreme thresholds, and, for the last test under the Holm procedure, $\alpha^* = \alpha$. Alternative procedures and special cases have been proposed (e.g., Perli, Hommel, & Lehmacher, 1985; see von Eye, 2002), all with the goal of protecting α without resulting in a threshold that is prohibitively extreme.

Significance Tests for CFA

The number of tests for the evaluation of the cellwise CFA null hypothesis is large. Every test statistic that is available for residual analysis of log-linear models can be used. In addition, exact tests, such as the binomial and the hypergeometric tests, are suitable. A number of tests specifically designed for CFA have been proposed, also. For the purposes of this chapter, we present three tests that differ in characteristics. The first is the exact binomial test. It can be applied under any sampling scheme. The second test is the z test. It is more powerful than the binomial test and can also be applied under any sampling scheme. The z statistic is asymptotically normally distributed. For this characteristic to apply, the cell size must be reasonable large (see von Weber, von Eye, & Lautsch, 2004). The third test is the *standardized Pearson residual test*. It is more powerful than the other three tests discussed here. It approximates the normal distribution. The test statistic is known from residual analysis and has been proposed for use in CFA by von Eye and Mair (2008).

For the binomial test, let N be the sample size; m the observed frequency of the configuration under examination, r; and p the probability of that configuration. Then the exact binomial test is

$$B_{N,p_r}(m) = \sum_{j=0}^{m} \frac{N!}{j!(N-j)!} p_r^j (1-p_r)^{N-j}$$

with $0 \leq m \leq N$; the probability p_r is the estimate of π_r, which is usually estimated from the sample.

When the sample is large enough, or when $Np \geq 10$ (Osterkorn, 1975), the standard normal

$$z_r = \frac{m_r - Np_r}{\sqrt{Np_r q_r}}$$

approximates the standard normal distribution well, where p_r is, again, the estimate of π_r, $q = 1 - p$, and r indicates the rth cell. Usually, p_r is estimated from the data.

A residual measure that was proposed for use in CFA (von Eye & Mair, 2008) is the *standardized Pearson residual*, z'_r. It is defined as

$$z'_r = \frac{m_r - \hat{m}_r}{\sqrt{\hat{m}_r(1-h_r)}}$$

where h_r is the rth diagonal element of the well-known *hat matrix*, which is defined by

$$H = W^{1/2}X(X'WX)^{-1}X'W^{1/2}$$

The elements of the diagonal matrix W are the estimated expected cell frequencies, $\hat{m}_r$. The standardized Pearson z'_r has the characteristic that, if $m_r = \hat{m}_r$, no standard error can be estimated. This is typically the case when an observed cell frequency is exactly estimated, for example in a saturated model, or when cell r is blanked out. Each of these cases is possible in CFA applications and will not affect the validity of the solution. In addition, if one of the variables is dichotomous, corresponding cells can come with exactly the same z'_r.

The CFA Base Model

Two conditions must be fulfilled for a configuration to be interpreted as constituting a CFA type or antitype. The first is that the observed frequency be more extreme than compatible with the protected level α. The second is that a suitable base model was used for the estimation of the expected cell frequencies. A suitable CFA base model has the following four characteristics (von Eye, 2004; von Eye & Schuster, 1998; von Eye et al., 2010).

1. *Uniqueness of interpretation of types and antitypes.* There must be only one reason for the existence of types and antitypes. For example, the base model for prediction CFA must be specified such that types and antitypes can emerge only if relationships between predictors and criteria exist, but not because of relationships among the predictors or among the criteria.

2. *The base model contains only and all of those effects of a model that are not of interest to the researcher.* If, under this condition, types and antitypes emerge, they reflect only the relationships the researcher is interested in. In the example of prediction CFA, the base model includes all main effects and interactions among the predictors and all main effects and interactions among the criteria. Therefore, types and antitypes can emerge only if relationships among predictors and criteria exist.

3. *Parsimony.* A CFA base model must be as parsimonious as possible.

4. *Consideration of sampling scheme.* This criterion is of importance in particular when marginal probabilities are determined or known before data collection (product–multinomial sampling). The marginals of those variables that were observed under a product–multinomial sampling scheme must be reproduced. By implication, the CFA base model must contain the effects that allow one to reproduce these marginals. This applies accordingly when multivariate product–multinomial sampling took place. Base models that do not contain these effects are not admissible.

Most CFA base models can be specified in terms of log-linear models. There exist base models that are not log-linear, but here we focus on log-linear base models. We give two examples of base models here; additional examples follow when we discuss data applications. The first base model is first-order CFA. This model proposes that the variables under study are independent of each other. This proposition has a clear-cut implication: If variables are specified as independent, only interactions among these variables can be the causes of types and antitypes. These are interactions of any order (not just first-order interactions, as in factor analysis or standard structural equation modeling).

To give an example, consider the four variables A, B, C, and D. The first-order CFA base model for these variables is

$$\log \hat{m} = \lambda + \lambda_i^A + \lambda_j^B + \lambda_k^C + \lambda_l^D$$

where *log* represents the natural logarithm used for log-linear modeling, $\hat{m}$ is the vector of estimated expected cell frequencies, the λs are the model parameters, the subscripts indicate the variable-specific parameters, and the superscripts indicate the variables. Each of the subscripted λs in this model specifies a main effect. Therefore, this model can be contradicted and thus yield types and antitypes only when interactions of first, second, or third order exist.

For the second example, we use the base model for multiple-group CFA (Lienert, 1971; von Eye, 2002). Using this base model, researchers attempt to determine whether the groups under study differ in the space of discriminating variables. The base model makes the two assumptions that main effects, as well as interactions of any order, may exist among the discriminating variables and that the discriminating variables are independent of the grouping variable. If these assumptions are contradicted, the model is rejected, and types and antitypes can result. These types and antitypes necessarily reflect associations between the grouping and the discriminating variables. Using the four variables, *A, B, C,* and *D* again, let *D* be the grouping variable, and *A, B,* and *C* the discriminating variables. The base model for this example is

$$\log \hat{m} = \lambda + \lambda_i^A + \lambda_j^B + \lambda_k^C + \lambda_l^D + \lambda_{ij}^{AB} + \lambda_{ik}^{AC} + \lambda_{jk}^{BC} + \lambda_{ijk}^{ABC}$$

Clearly, this model contains all main effects and all possible interactions among the discriminating variables. If any of the interactions of the discriminating and the grouping variables exist, the model fails, and types and antitypes are bound to emerge. These are the interactions [*A, D*], [*B, D*], [*C, D*], [*A, B, D*], [*A, C, D*], [*B, C, D*], and [*A, B, C, D*].

Developmental Applications and Illustration

In this section, we combine the introduction of CFA base models and the illustration of these models using empirical data examples. We use the term *longitudinal research* whenever observations are made at different points in time. There will be a focus on designs in which the same individuals are repeatedly observed on the same or on different variables. Although CFA can be applied in the analysis of time-lag data, the empirical examples in this chapter use data from the same respondents, repeatedly observed over up to six points in time.

The same data set will be used for all illustrations in this chapter—the 4-H Study of Positive Youth Development (see Lerner et al., 2005; Lerner, von Eye, Lerner, & Lewin-Bizan, 2009; Lerner, von Eye, Lerner, Lewin-Bizan, & Bowers, in press). The 4-H Study was designed to test the idea that when the strengths of youths are aligned across adolescence with family, school, and community resources (and, in particular, resources provided by community-based, out-of-school time youth development programs, such as 4-H, Boys & Girls Clubs, Big Brothers/Big Sisters, YMCA, and scouting), positive youth development (operationalized by the "Five Cs" of competence, confidence, character, connection, and caring) and, as well, youth community contributions (the "sixth C" of positive youth development) will occur (Lerner, 2004, 2007; Lerner et al., 2005). The full details of the method of the 4-H Study have appeared in numerous developmental journals across the past five years (e.g., see Lerner et al., 2009, and Lerner et al., in press). Accordingly, we provide here, in the following paragraphs, only a summary of the design and sample of the study.

Supported by grants from the National 4-H Council, the 4-H Study of Positive Youth Development began in 2002 with a sample of about 1,700 fifth-grade youths and about 1,100 parents from 13 states in the United States. The study uses a form of cohort sequential longitudinal design and, as such, the sample size increases across successive waves of testing. Specifically, data from fifth graders were gathered in wave 1 of the study (the 2002–2003 school year), and these fifth graders were the initial cohort in the study. To maintain at least initial levels of power for within-time analyses and to assess the effects of retesting, subsequent waves of the study involved the addition of a "retest control" cohort of youth (and a sample of their parents). Participants in the added "retest control" cohort were then followed longitudinally. In wave 2, the grade level of the initial cohort was grade 6. As such, a "retest control" group of sixth graders was added to the study, and these youths became members of the second longitudinal cohort, cohort 2. Both the original cohort of fifth graders and the added cohort of sixth graders were followed into grade 7, where, in addition to retesting initial grade 5 and initial grade 6 participants, a new cohort of seventh graders was added to the sample (along with a sample of their parents). In subsequent waves of testing this process was followed.

At this writing, with the beginning collection of grade 12 data, the 4-H study includes more than 6,000 youths (about half of whom have been assessed two or more times) and about 3,000 parents from 43 states. Participants reside in rural, suburban, and urban areas in different parts of the country and represent a diverse variety of racial, ethnic, and religious backgrounds and a range of socioeconomic levels. The number of repeated assessments of the participants makes the design especially sensitive to the detection of trajectories of intraindividual change in the structure and function of virtues. The data set affords a unique opportunity to assess the nature, bases, and import of the development of thriving in adolescence with more waves of data than available in any other data set pertinent to this domain of adolescent development.

Cross-Sectional CFA

In the first illustration of CFA, we ask a question that has not been addressed in the structural models estimated for the data from the 4-H Study of Positive Youth Development. We ask whether patterns of positive youth development can be predicted from patterns of gender (G) and race (R). To assess features of positive youth development, we use the variables selection (S), optimization (O), and compensation (C) as observed at the first observation point.

Selection involves identifying and selecting a subset of activities on which to focus and into which to invest resources. *Optimization* involves attempts at maximizing developmental gains. *Compensation* involves dealing with developmental losses by focusing on alternative activities. These three concepts were originally proposed for research on adult development (Freund & Baltes, 2000). Results from the 4-H project suggest that these concepts can also be fruitfully applied in research on adolescent development.

To answer the preceding question, we perform prediction CFA (see von Eye, Mair, & Bogat, 2005; von Eye, Mun, & Bogat, 2009). Prediction CFA includes, in its base model, all main effects, interactions of any order among the predictors, and interactions of any order among the criterion variables.

In the present example, we use gender and race as predictors and selection, optimization, and compensation as criterion variables. For these variables, the prediction CFA base model can be expressed as

$$\log \hat{m} = \lambda + \lambda_i^G + \lambda_j^R + \lambda_k^S + \lambda_l^O + \lambda_m^C \\ + \lambda_{ij}^{GR} + \lambda_{kl}^{SO} + \lambda_{km}^{SC} + \lambda_{lm}^{OC} + \lambda_{klm}^{SOC}$$

If this base model fails, types and antitypes can emerge, and we know that variability exists that needs explanation and where these discrepancies are located. For the present application, each of the variables *S*, *O*, and *C* was dichotomized as close as possible to the median. Because of the skew in these variables, this procedure resulted in variables with unequal probabilities for the two categories. Gender was scored as female = 1 and male = 2. Race was scored using eight categories: Native American = 1, Asian or Pacific Islander = 2, African American = 3, Latino/a = 4, white = 5, multiracial = 6, other = 7, and inconsistent = 8. Crossing these five variables yields the $2 \times 8 \times 2 \times 2 \times 2$ contingency table with 128 cells that is given in the supplemental material found online at *www.crmda.ku.edu/Guilford/HDRM*. For the cell-specific tests, we used the z test, and we adjusted α using the Bonferroni procedure, which resulted in $\alpha^* = 0.05/128 = 0.00039$. The likelihood ratio χ^2 (LR–χ^2) for this base model is 463.29 ($df = 105$; $p < 0.01$). Thus we expect types and antitypes to emerge.

In spite of the extreme significance threshold, prediction CFA resulted in a total of 9 types and 6 antitypes. Counting by gender, 5 types and 1 antitype were found for the male respondents and 4 types and 5 antitypes for the female respondents. The types in the male population are constituted by configurations 1121, 3221, 8121, 8211, and 8212. The antitype in this population is constituted by configuration 4222. In the female respondent population, the four types are constituted by configurations 3221, 4122, 5222, and 7111. The five antitypes are constituted by configurations 5111, 5121, 5211, 5221, and 8221. In standard CFA applications, researchers interpret every type and antitype. In the present context, we present instead sample interpretations for one type and one antitype each in the female and male respondent populations.

Female Population

- *Type 3221* suggests that, for female African American respondents, it can be predicted that they display above-average scores in selection and optimization but below-average scores in compensation. One hundred three individuals were observed with this pattern, but only 66.54 had been expected under the assumption that the two predictors, *G* and *R*, are independent of the three criteria, *S*, *O*, and *C*.
- *Antitype 5111* shows that, for female white respondents, it can be predicted that it is

very unlikely that they exhibit below-average scores on all three SOC scales. One hundred and twenty respondents were observed showing this pattern, which is over 25% less than the 164.55 that had been expected.

Male Population

- *Type 3221* suggests that, for male African American respondents, it can be predicted that they display above-average scores in selection and optimization but below-average scores in compensation. Seventy-seven individuals were observed with this pattern, but only 48.99 had been expected. This type mirrors the one that is constituted by the same pattern in the female African American population. Therefore, we can conclude that this type is not gender specific.
- *Antitype 4222* shows that, for male Latino respondents, it can be predicted that it is particularly unlikely that they display above-average scores on all three SOC scales. One hundred and eighteen were observed displaying this pattern, but 163.94 had been expected.

This example allows us to highlight some of the characteristics of CFA results (von Eye et al., 2010). Specifically, this example shows, first, that results from CFA are expressed in terms of configurations (cells of a table) that are observed at different rates than expected under some base model. Second, CFA tables are interpreted, in virtually all cases, only after the base model is rejected. A rejected base model is not a guarantee that types and antitypes will result. However, if the base model describes the data well, there is no need to search for types and antitypes that indicate the location of significant discrepancies between model and data.

Third, this example shows that only a selection of cells (configurations) emerges as type- and antitype-constituting. The remaining cells do not deviate from the base model. Types and antitypes thus indicate where, in the table, the action of interest is; specifically, where the interactions among the variables that span the table under study manifest in the form of types and antitypes.

Finally, in the frequency table in the supplemental material found at *www.crmda.ku.edu/Guilford/HDRM*, the largest cells do not constitute types, and the smallest do not constitute antitypes. This is not always the case. Cells of any size can constitute types or antitypes (of course, to constitute a type, a cell must have an observed frequency of $m_r > 0$). The main reason for this characteristic of CFA is that the method focuses on *discrepancies from expectation* instead of sheer size (zero-order CFA being the only exception; see von Eye, 2002). Even relatively small cells can contain more cases than expected, and relatively large cells can contain fewer cases than expected.

CFA of Longitudinal Data Example I: Autoregression

In many longitudinal studies, the same variables are observed at each observation point. For example, to study the longer term effects of an intervention, the dependent variable needs to be observed repeatedly. Now, it is a well-known result of repeated observation studies that the associations among time-adjacent observations are often the strongest effects in a repeated-observation study. These associations manifest in the form of autocorrelations, autoregressions, or autoassociations.

From a person-oriented research perspective, it is questionable that these relationships apply to everybody in a population in the same form and strength. To identify those subgroups for which these relationships do apply and those for which they do not apply, researchers can use the tools of CFA. The base model to use is that of autoregression CFA (von Eye et al., 2009). This base model takes into account all main effects of the repeatedly observed variables, all possible interactions among the repeatedly observed variables and the time-constant or time-varying covariates, but none of the possible interactions among the multiple observations of individual, repeatedly observed variables.

If this base model is rejected, there can be only one reason for types and antitypes. This reason is the autoassociation among the multiple observations of individual, repeatedly observed variables.

Data Example

To describe the autoregression CFA base model more specifically, we present a data example. We again use the data from the 4-H Study of Positive Youth Development (Lerner et al., 2005, 2009, in press). We ask three questions. First, does the usual autocorrelation pattern exist according to which time-adjacent observations show the strongest correlations and correlations become weaker as the distance in time between observations increases? Second, are there particular configurations that carry these correlations in the form of types and antitypes? Third, are types and antitypes solely due to associations between time-adjacent observations? To answer these questions, we use the variable optimization, which was observed at each of the six waves of the 4-H Study of Positive Youth Development.

Before working on these questions, we prepare the data for CFA. Specifically, we dichotomize the observations separately for each observation point in time. (Note that dichotomizing is not a standard procedure of CFA application; often, more than two categories are created or data are categorical to begin with.) As a cutoff, we use the grade-specific median. This method prevents us from analyzing the overall trend (it is positive; scores increase). However, it will allow us to examine the cross-time associations. The correlations among the dichotomized scores appear in Table 35.1.

To answer the first question, we examine the correlations in Table 35.1. Indeed, the correlations right below the diagonal are always the largest in their respective columns. In addition, the correlations in the bottom row of the table are the smallest in their columns.

TABLE 35.1. Cross-Time Correlations among Six Observations of Optimization (O_1–O_6; Dichotomized Variables Used)

	O_1	O_2	O_3	O_4	O_5	O_6
O_1	1.000					
O_2	0.267	1.000				
O_3	0.243	0.545	1.000			
O_4	0.187	0.421	0.479	1.000		
O_5	0.218	0.428	0.468	0.424	1.000	
O_6	0.140	0.334	0.364	0.305	0.322	1.000

We therefore conclude that the correlations between time-adjacent observations are, as expected, the largest. Interestingly, the sizes of these correlations also indicate that there may be systematic variance that the autocorrelations cannot explain. To explore this possibility, we address the second of the preceding questions. We apply autoregression CFA.

In a first run, we perform a standard first-order CFA (a CFA under the base model of variable independence). Labeling the variables O_1–O_6, this base model proposes

$$\log \hat{m} = \lambda + \lambda^{O_1} + \lambda^{O_2} + \lambda^{O_3} + \lambda^{O_4} + \lambda^{O_5} + \lambda^{O_6}$$

This model can be contradicted only if any of the first-, second-, . . . , and fifth-order associations among the six observations exist. Specifically, these are the first-order associations $[\underline{O_1, O_2}]$, $[O_1, O_3]$, $[O_1, O_4]$, $[O_1, O_5]$, $[O_1, O_6]$, $[\underline{O_2, O_3}]$, $[O_2, O_4]$, $[O_2, O_5]$, $[O_2, O_6]$, $[\underline{O_3, O_4}]$, $[O_3, O_5]$, $[O_3, O_6]$, $[\underline{O_4, O_5}]$, $[O_4, O_6]$, $[\underline{O_5, O_6}]$; the second-order associations $[O_1, O_2, O_3]$, . . . , $[O_4, O_5, O_6]$, . . . ; and the fifth-order association $[O_1, O_2, O_3, O_4, O_5, O_6]$. These associations do include those between time-adjacent observations (underlined). We will come back to these associations when we answer Question 3.

For the following CFA run, we use the z test and the Bonferroni-adjusted $\alpha^* = 0.05/64 = 0.00078$. The 2^6 cross-tabulation of the six observations of optimization appears in the supplemental material found at *www.crmda.ku.edu/Guilford/HDRM*. The likelihood ratio χ^2 (LR–χ^2) for this model is 7910.61, which indicates significant model–data discrepancies ($df = 57$; $p < 0.01$). We therefore expect types and antitypes to emerge. The results of first-order CFA are summarized in Table 35.2.

Table 35.2 shows that 43 out of the 64 configurations constitute types or antitypes. Conversely, 21 configurations (only one of them empty) support the base model of variable independence. We can, therefore, conclude that the result according to which the cross-time autocorrelations among the six observations of optimization are strong is carried only by a strong portion of the population. Still, subpopulations may exist that systematically develop counter to the general trend.

Instead of interpreting each of these types and antitypes, we now describe the most extreme configurations. By far the most extreme, type-constituting configuration is the one in which the adolescents stay below the median in optimization throughout the observation period. These respondents are found in configuration 111111. It was expected that 3.77 cases would show this pattern, but 258 did show it. The corresponding z score is 130.93. Clearly far more respondents than expected are consistently below average in optimization. Similarly extreme is the type-constituting configuration 211111. These are the respondents who score above average in optimization at time 1 but regress and stay below average for the rest of the observation period. The expectation was 36.56 cases, but 596 did show this pattern. The corresponding z score is 92.53. Configurations 222221 and 222222 are also extreme and type constituting.

The most extreme antitype-constituting configuration is 221221. These are adolescents who are generally above average in optimization but regress twice to below average, at times 3 and 6. The expectation was 329.05 for this pattern, but only 86 were found showing it. The corresponding z score is –13.40. The next most most extreme antitype-constituting configuration is 212221. These are adolescents who also slip twice below the average of optimization at observation points 2 and 6. It was expected that 293.85 would be in this cell, but only 88 were found. The corresponding z score is –12.01. With a z score of –11.92, similarly extreme is configuration 222121. It also constitutes an antitype.

TABLE 35.2. First-Order CFA of the Cross-Classification of Six Consecutive Observations of Optimization in 6,450 Adolescents

Configuration $O_1O_2O_3O_4O_5O_6$	m	$\hat{m}$	z	p	Type/antitype?
111111	258.00	3.770	130.9338	.000000	Type
111112	9.00	3.278	3.1601	.000789	
111121	29.00	9.724	6.1813	.000000	Type
111122	7.00	8.456	–.5007	.308294	
111211	32.00	6.200	10.3615	.000000	Type
111212	3.00	5.391	–1.0299	.151533	
111221	22.00	15.992	1.5024	.066499	
111222	11.00	13.906	–.7793	.217902	
112111	16.00	7.144	3.3132	.000461	Type
112112	.00	6.212	–2.4925	.006343	
112121	8.00	18.427	–2.4291	.007568	
112122	3.00	16.024	–3.2535	.000570	Antitype
112211	2.00	11.749	–2.8442	.002226	
112212	3.00	10.216	–2.2577	.011982	
112221	11.00	30.304	–3.5067	.000227	Antitype
112222	13.00	26.352	–2.6009	.004648	
121111	18.00	8.000	3.5355	.000204	Type
121112	2.00	6.957	–1.8792	.030106	
121121	13.00	20.635	–1.6807	.046407	
121122	7.00	17.943	–2.5834	.004891	
121211	3.00	13.156	–2.8001	.002555	
121212	1.00	11.440	–3.0867	.001012	
121221	3.00	33.935	–5.3103	.000000	Antitype
121222	7.00	29.508	–4.1435	.000017	Antitype
122111	3.00	15.160	–3.1231	.000895	
122112	1.00	13.182	–3.3553	.000396	Antitype
122121	18.00	39.103	–3.3747	.000370	Antitype
122122	6.00	34.002	–4.8022	.000001	Antitype
122211	.00	24.931	–4.9931	.000000	Antitype
122212	1.00	21.679	–4.4413	.000004	Antitype
122221	18.00	64.305	–5.7744	.000000	Antitype
122222	75.00	55.917	2.5519	.005357	
211111	596.00	36.557	92.5280	.000000	Type
211112	21.00	31.788	–1.9135	.027844	
211121	183.00	94.292	9.1353	.000000	Type
211122	46.00	81.993	–3.9750	.000035	Antitype
211211	85.00	60.118	3.2091	.000666	Type
211212	11.00	52.277	–5.7089	.000000	Antitype
211221	106.00	155.066	–3.9403	.000041	Antitype
211222	74.00	134.840	–5.2394	.000000	Antitype

(cont.)

TABLE 35.2. *(cont.)*

Configuration $O_1O_2O_3O_4O_5O_6$	m	$\hat{m}$	z	p	Type/antitype?
212111	65.00	69.274	–.5135	.303807	
212112	14.00	60.238	–5.9575	.000000	Antitype
212121	85.00	178.682	–7.0083	.000000	Antitype
212122	56.00	155.375	–7.9724	.000000	Antitype
212211	20.00	113.923	–8.7996	.000000	Antitype
212212	20.00	99.063	–7.9436	.000000	Antitype
212221	88.00	293.847	–12.0084	.000000	Antitype
212222	169.00	255.519	–5.4125	.000000	Antitype
221111	138.00	77.572	6.8609	.000000	Type
221112	24.00	67.454	–5.2909	.000000	Antitype
221121	139.00	200.086	–4.3185	.000008	Antitype
221122	65.00	173.988	–8.2626	.000000	Antitype
221211	37.00	127.569	–8.0188	.000000	Antitype
221212	28.00	110.930	–7.8738	.000000	Antitype
221221	86.00	329.047	–13.3987	.000000	Antitype
221222	164.00	286.128	–7.2200	.000000	Antitype
222111	64.00	146.997	–6.8456	.000000	Antitype
222112	48.00	127.824	–7.0603	.000000	Antitype
222121	147.00	379.158	–11.9227	.000000	Antitype
222122	350.00	329.703	1.1178	.131819	
222211	91.00	241.741	–9.6952	.000000	Antitype
222212	188.00	210.209	–1.5318	.062783	
222221	1066.00	623.535	17.7194	.000000	Type
222222	1573.00	542.205	44.2681	.000000	Type

In overview, we see that, as expected, the two configurations that indicate stability (configurations 111111 and 222222) describe far more respondents than expected under the assumptions of independence of the six observations. Each of the antitypes in this example indicates lack of stability. However, there are interesting exceptions. Consider configuration 211111. These individuals, larger in number than expected, show development that, in comparison with their peers, comes to a standstill below the median of the population. Correspondingly, configuration 222221 also describes the larger-than-expected number of respondents who slip toward the end of the observation period, when most other respondents show yet another increase in optimization.

It is also interesting to note that the configurations that would describe patterns of development that suggest a leap in optimization from below to above median, with consistent scores before and after the leap, do not stand out. These are configurations 111112, 111122, 111222, 112222, and 122222. None of these was observed more (or less) often than expected. We conclude that the autocorrelations found in Table 35.1 are mostly carried by the strong pattern of consistent optimization scores 111111 and 2 2 2 2 2 2.

We now proceed to question 3. This question asks whether the patterns that stand out can be explained by first-order autoassociations. This question is important for two reasons. First, the associations between time-adjacent observations are the strongest, as is shown in Table 35.1. Second, if types and antitypes remain or different types and antitypes emerge, there is systematic variation in these observations that cannot be explained by standard statistical models such as simplex models, autoregression models, or structural or lag models, which all model the covariation between pairs of variables. Instead, higher order relationships must exist that may be worth examining.

To answer the third question, we perform another variant of autoregression CFA. The base model of this variant takes into account the main effects of all variables and all first-order interactions between time-adjacent measures.

For the present data set, the autoregression CFA base model thus becomes

$$\log \hat{m} = \lambda + \lambda^{O_1} + \lambda^{O_2} + \lambda^{O_3} + \lambda^{O_4} + \lambda^{O_5} + \lambda^{O_6} + \lambda^{O_1,O_2} + \lambda^{O_2,O_3} + \lambda^{O_3,O_4} + \lambda^{O_4,O_5} + \lambda^{O_5,O_6}$$

For autoregression CFA, we use the z test and the Bonferroni-adjusted $\alpha^* = 0.00078$ again. The 2^6 cross-tabulation of the six observations of optimization is the one in the supplemental material found at *www.crmda.ku.edu/Guilford/HDRM*. The likelihood ratio χ^2 for this model is 2226.38. This represents a significant improvement over the main effect model, but it still indicates significant model–data discrepancies ($df = 52$; $p < 0.01$). We therefore expect types and antitypes to emerge.

The autoregression CFA run yields 34 types and antitypes. Of these, eight had not been designated as types or antitypes by first-order CFA. The vast majority, 26, had been types and antitypes in the prior run. Nine z scores of the repeat types and antitypes now come with a different sign: they have changed from being types to antitypes, and vice versa. The reason for this change is that a different base model was employed. In other words, the frame of comparison has changed, and each observed frequency is compared with a different expected cell frequency (Mellenbergh, 1996). Still, in spite of the significant improvement in overall model fit, the majority of the emerging types and antitypes is constituted by the same cells as in the prior run. Therefore, we conclude that taking into account the associations between time-adjacent observations takes us closer to the data. However, the discrepancies between the base model and the data remain largely where they were before.

Most notably, the two types of stability, 111111 and 222222, still exist. The same applies to the surprisingly large group of individuals who, from the first to the second observation, slip from above-average optimization to below and stay there—still members of a type (211111). Also as before, all of the antitypes are constituted by patterns of change, and patterns of consistent increases in optimization scores do not constitute types or antitypes.

The most dramatic change was observed for configuration 212121. Under the base model of first-order CFA, this configuration constituted an antitype (85 observed vs. 178.68 expected; $z = -7.01$). Here, under the base model of autoregression CFA, this configuration constitutes a type, with only 19.73 expected cases ($z = 14.70$). Of the configurations that are extreme now but did not stand out in first-order CFA, the two most extreme are now

222122 and 222212. Both configurations now constitute types with z scores in excess of 10.

From these results, we conclude that this data set is so complex that standard models, in particular those that consider no more than log-linear first- and second-order moments, are unable to do the data justice. CFA or log-linear models that include higher order interactions are needed to identify the effects in the table and their location. (One hierarchical log-linear model that describes these data well [LR–$\chi^2 = 6.75$; $df = 10$; $p = 0.75$] involves the five-way interactions [O_1, O_2, O_3, O_4, O_6], [O_2, O_3, O_4, O_5, O_6] and the four-way interactions [O_1, O_2, O_3, O_5], and [O_1, O_3, O_4, O_5].) From the perspective of longitudinal developmental research, we note that the idea that all individuals can validly be described using the same model may be problematic because subpopulation-specific patterns of development may be missed.

CFA of Longitudinal Data Example II: Relating Series of Repeated Measures to Each Other

The example given in the last section was important because it illustrated that (1) change over time is not necessarily uniform across all members of a population; (2) data can be complex to the extent that CFA may be the only method that allows researchers to identify where, in a cross-classification, "the action is"; and (3) autoregression CFA is a suitable method for the analysis of longitudinal data. However, in this data example, only one variable was studied. Considering that virtually all empirical research is multivariate, we present, in this section, a method that allows researchers to identify relationships among two or more repeatedly observed variables. As before, results are expressed in the form of types and antitypes and interpreted with reference to a particular base model.

The base model to be considered here needs to include all effects that do not link the series to each other whose relationships are of interest. If this model is rejected, types and antitypes indicate where in the table relationships between the series under study exist. More specifically, the base model takes into account all main effects of all variables that span the table, interactions of all possible orders that include measures within each repeatedly observed variable, but no interactions that contain measures from different variables.

If this base model is rejected, at least one of the terms that were not included must exist. These are the terms that link the series of measures. Consider, for example, variable X, which was observed three times, with measures X_1, X_2, and X_3, and variable Y, observed at the same three times, with measures Y_1, Y_2, and Y_3. The base model that allows one to create types and antitypes that indicate relationships between these two series of measures is

$$\begin{aligned}\log m = \lambda + \lambda^{X_1} + \lambda^{X_2} + \lambda^{X_3} + \lambda^{X_1X_2} + \lambda^{X_1X_3} + \lambda^{X_2X_3} + \lambda^{X_1X_2X_3} \\ + \lambda^{Y_1} + \lambda^{Y_2} + \lambda^{Y_3} + \lambda^{Y_1Y_2} + \lambda^{Y_1Y_3} + \lambda^{Y_2Y_3} + \lambda^{Y_1Y_2Y_3}\end{aligned}$$

After the constant, λ, the first line of this equation shows the main effects and all possible interactions among the three X measures. In parallel, the second line shows all main effects and all possible interactions among the Y measures. The effects that are not included in this model are all those that link X measures to Y measures in the form of 2-, 3-, 4-, 5-, and 6-way interactions. Specifically, the following interactions are not part of the base model:

- *2-way interactions*: $[X_1, Y_1]$, $[X_1, Y_2]$, $[X_1, Y_3]$, $[X_2, Y_1]$, $[X_2, Y_2]$, $[X_2, Y_3]$, $[X_3, Y_1]$, $[X_3, Y_2]$, and $[X_3, Y_3]$;
- *3-way interactions*: $[X_1, X_2, Y_1]$, $[X_1, X_2, Y_2]$, $[X_1, X_2, Y_3]$, $[X_1, X_3, Y_1]$, $[X_1, X_3, Y_2]$, $[X_1, X_3, Y_3]$, $[X_2, X_3, Y_1]$, $[X_2, X_3, Y_2]$, $[X_2, X_3, Y_3]$, $[X_1, Y_1, Y_2]$, $[X_1, Y_1, Y_3]$, $[X_1, Y_2, Y_3]$, $[X_2, Y_1, Y_2]$, $[X_2, Y_1, Y_3]$, $[X_2, Y_2, Y_3]$, $[X_3, Y_1, Y_2]$, $[X_3, Y_1, Y_3]$, and $[X_3, Y_2, Y_3]$;
- *4-way interactions*: $[X_1, X_2, X_3, Y_1]$, $[X_1, X_2, X_3, Y_2]$, $[X_1, X_2, X_3, Y_3]$, $[X_1, X_2, Y_1, Y_2]$, $[X_1, X_2, Y_1, Y_3]$, $[X_1, X_2, Y_2, Y_3]$, $[X_1, X_3, Y_1, Y_2]$, $[X_1, X_3, Y_1, Y_3]$, $[X_1, X_3, Y_2, Y_3]$, $[X_2, X_3, Y_1, Y_2]$, $[X_2, X_3, Y_1, Y_3]$, $[X_2, X_3, X_2, Y_3]$, $[X_1, Y_1, Y_2, Y_3]$, $[X_2, Y_1, Y_2, Y_3]$, and $[X_3, Y_1, Y_2, Y_3]$;
- *5-way interactions*: $[X_1, X_2, X_3, Y_1, Y_2]$, $[X_1, X_2, X_3, Y_1, Y_3]$, $[X_1, X_2, X_3, Y_2, Y_3]$, $[X_1, X_2, Y_1, Y_2, Y_3]$, $[X_1, X_3, Y_1, Y_2, Y_3]$, and $[X_2, X_3, Y_1, Y_2, Y_3]$; and
- *6-way interaction*: $[X_1, X_2, X_3, Y_1, Y_2, Y_3]$.

These interactions, 49 in all, share the characteristic that they each contain both X and Y measures. If any of these interactions exist, the base model is bound to be rejected, and types and antitypes indicate where the series of measures are related to each other, how, and for whom.

Data Example

In the following empirical example, we use data from the 4-H Study of Positive Youth Development again. For the following analyses, we use the variables optimization and compensation, both observed at the first, third, and fifth points in time. Both were dichotomized as closely as possible to their grade-specific medians. Crossed, the six dichotomous variables span a 2^6 contingency table with 64 cells. This table is constructed in a fashion parallel to the last example given previously.

We ask three questions. First, can the data be sufficiently explained based on only the main effects of all variables and those interactions that reflect first- and second-order autoassociations? Second (if the answer to the first question is no), are there configurations that stand out in the form of types or antitypes when the preceding base model is used (the model that sets only the interaction terms to zero that link the two series of measures to each other)? In other words, we ask whether the two series of observations are related to each other. Third, are there gender differences in those configurations that indicate relationships between these two series? To answer this question, we run the CFA separately for the female and the male respondents. The frequency tables for the two runs appear in the supplemental material found at *www.crmda.ku.edu/Guilford/HDRM.*

For the female respondents, we calculate a LR-$X^2 = 1432.96$, which indicates significant data–model discrepancies ($df = 49$; $p < 0.01$). For the male respondents, the corresponding values are LR–$\chi^2 = 940.89$ ($df = 49$; $p < 0.01$, which also indicates significant data–model discrepancies. Therefore, we expect that types and antitypes emerge in both samples. For the search for types and antitypes, we use the z test and the Bonferroni-protected $\alpha^* =$

0.05/64 = 0.00078. Indeed, for the female population, we find 14 types and 11 antitypes, and for the male population, we find 12 types and 9 antitypes. Instead of interpreting each of these in detail (in a substantively oriented study, researchers interpret every type and antitype), we present, in Table 35.3, a selection of types and antitypes. In this example, we focus on the most extreme cells (by z score) for males and females.

The results of this analysis show that there are strong local associations between the two series of measures. Interestingly, these associations do not suggest that corresponding patterns always go hand in hand, as could be expected based on the assumption of synchronous development of optimization and compensation. In fact, of the six most extreme types, only two show optimization and compensation patterns that are the same (111 and 111, as well as 211 and 211 for girls; optimization scores listed first). The table in supplemental material found at *www.crmda.ku.edu/Guilford/HDRM* shows also that these are not even the most frequent patterns. The most frequent pattern in the female sample has pattern 222 for optimization and 221 for compensation. Of the 3,900 girls, 980 showed this pattern; 838.54 respondents had been expected to show this pattern. Therefore, this pattern constitutes a type (z = 4.89; $p < \alpha^*$), but clearly not the most extreme type (extremity ranking based on z scores). Therefore, it is not listed in Table 35.3.

The most extreme type in the female population has pattern 212 for optimization and 211 for compensation (right panel of Table 35.3). This pattern indicates that these girls are above their age-specific median in both optimization and compensation at the first observation, during eighth grade. At the third observation (tenth grade), these girls score below the grade-specific median, and at the fifth observation, they score above the median in optimization and still below the median in compensation. In other words, more girls than expected under the preceding base model with the optimization pattern 212 also show the compensation pattern 211. A total of 171 girls show this combined pattern, but only about 54 had been expected.

The most extreme antitype in the female population has the combined pattern 222 and 211. We conclude that it is particularly unlikely that girls score above their grade-specific

TABLE 35.3. The Most Extreme Types and Antitypes That Indicate Relationships between Three Observations Each of Optimization and Compensation in the Populations of Female and Male Adolescents

Males					Females				
$O_1O_3O_5$	$C_1C_3C_5$	m	$\hat{m}$	z	$O_1O_3O_5$	$C_1C_3C_5$	m	$\hat{m}$	z
Types									
111	121	120	61.64	7.43	111	111	37	6.41	12.08
212	211	90	35.51	9.14	211	211	115	45.00	10.44
222	221	569	413.85	7.63	212	211	171	53.83	15.97
Antitypes									
111	221	5	60.73	−7.15	212	222	18	95.18	−7.91
211	222	9	79.56	−7.91	222	211	39	122.73	−7.56
222	111	11	76.11	−7.46	222	211	71	244.00	−11.08

medians in optimization at all three observation points but slip below the median in compensation at time 3 and stay there.

In the male population (left panel of Table 25.3), the combined pattern 222 and 221 is the second among the most extreme type-constituting configurations. This pattern appeared for 569 boys. The largest positive *z* score was found for patterns 212 and 211. This is the same type that already was the most extreme in the female population. Similarly, the most extreme antitype is also the same in the male and the female populations. It is constituted by the combined configuration 222 and 211. In all, two of the three most extreme types and one of the three most extreme antitypes are the same in the male and the female populations. Still, most of the types and antitypes that were found in the present analyses are gender specific.

From these results, we draw six conclusions. First, strong local associations between the two series of scores of optimization and compensation exist. Second, for the two series of optimization and compensation scores, corresponding patterns (these are the patterns that are the same for the two behavior domains) are not the most frequent. Note that this statement is not a result of configural analysis. This result simply reflects a characteristic of the observed frequency distribution in the cross-classification. Third, for the two series of optimization and compensation scores, patterns that indicate stability for the two behavior domains (these are patterns 111 and 111, as well as 222 and 222) are not the most frequent; the same applies to stable shifts from below- to above-median scores. Fourth, stability patterns constitute types in both populations, but other patterns constitute more extreme types. Fifth, all antitypes are constituted by patterns of instability; and sixth, all types of instability suggest that development in optimization that is not matched by development in compensation is particularly unlikely.

It is interesting to compare these results with those published earlier. The earlier results are all based on structural equation modeling of the development of the selection, optimization, and compensation components of the SOC measure (e.g., Gestsdóttir & Lerner, 2007; Gestsdóttir, Lewin-Bizan, von Eye, Lerner, & Lerner, 2009). The published reports provide a depiction of the extent to which the three components of SOC exist as global and undifferentiated structures or as differentiated facets of intentional self-regulation within and across grades. However, these analyses do not provide knowledge of how the SOC components are differentially linked within people, how they may be manifested differentially within different groups (types) of youths as they develop across the adolescent years, or how the function of one facet of SOC (e.g., optimization) is contingent on the function of another facet of SOC (e.g., compensation) within individuals as they traverse the adolescent period. However, if one's interest is in person-oriented questions, that is, in how variables may function within people across their development, the latter CFA analyses are preferable.

Where Does It All End?: Predicting the Endpoint of Development

Not only from a teleological perspective, but also in intervention research, it can be of interest to ask whether a particular point of development can be reached or predicted based on previous development. For example, one can ask whether alcohol consumption that is followed by cigarette smoking is predictive of later leisure drug use, or one can ask whether a series of intervention steps is predictive of a desired outcome, or whether parental educational style is predictive of adult behavior patterns. Each of these questions relates configurations of series of measures or events to outcome configurations.

In the present context, we discuss CFA base models that allow one to answer questions concerning the point of development reached at the end of an observational period. To illustrate such a base model, consider a series of three events, X_1, X_2, and X_3, that precedes the point in time at which the question concerning the status of development, denoted by Y, is asked. Each of the events, as well as Y, can be a single category but also a configuration of categories. Then the CFA base model that allows one to answer the question concerning the predictive value of the preceding events for the outcome is

$$\log m = \lambda + \lambda^{X_1} + \lambda^{X_2} + \lambda^{X_3} + \lambda^{Y}$$
$$+\lambda^{X_1X_2} + \lambda^{X_1X_3} + \lambda^{X_2X_3} + \lambda^{X_1X_2X_3}$$

This model proposes that all main effects can exist (first row of the equation), that interactions of any order of the preceding events can exist (second row of the equation), and that the preceding events are independent of the outcome event.

If this base model is rejected, one or more of the effects must exist that link the preceding with the outcome events. Types and antitypes will tell us which pattern of preceding events are linked to which pattern of outcome events. The effects that can constitute a link between preceding and outcome events are $[X_1, Y]$, $[X_2, Y]$, $[X_3, Y]$, $[X_1, X_2, Y]$, $[X_1, X_3, Y]$, $[X_2, X_3, Y]$,and $[X_1, X_2, X_3, Y]$. Each of these terms contains at least one of the preceding events and Y. It is important to repeat that CFA does not aim at stating results in terms of variable relationships. Instead, results are stated in terms of configurations that constitute types and antitypes because they contradict the base model. Therefore, logistic regression and multinomial logit models cannot be used to answer the question posed here (von Eye et al., 2005, 2010).

Data Example

In the following data example, we ask whether, over the course of adolescent development, scores above or below the grade-specific median of compensation at a particular point in time can be predicted from a series of scores above and below the age-specific median scores in optimization. Specifically, we ask whether (1) the first three of the six observations of optimization in the 4-H Study of Positive Youth Development are predictive of the sixth observation of compensation and (2) whether these predictions are specific to the self-reported race of the adolescent respondents.

To answer these questions, a 2 (optimization at time 1) × 2 (optimization at time 2) × 2 (optimization at time 3) × 2 (compensation at time 6) cross-classification was created separately for five of the eight race categories already used in the first example in this chapter. The numbers of respondents from the Native American, Pacific Islanders, and Other categories were too small for this configural analysis. For each of the resulting six tables, the base model specified previously was estimated. The tables are reproduced in the supplemental material found at *www.crmda.ku.edu/Guilford/HDRM*. The exact binomial test was used along with the Bonferroni-protected $\alpha^* = 0.05/16 = 0.003125$. Table 35.4 displays the results for the white respondents. Table 35.5 summarizes results for the six race groups.

In its last three rows, Table 35.5 shows that, for each of the racial/ethnic groups, the base model is rejected. Therefore, we expect types and antitypes to emerge. The table shows that only one configuration, 2 1 1 1, consistently constitutes a type for each population

TABLE 35.4. CFA Predicting Compensation (C_6) from Three Consecutive Observations of Optimization (O_1, O_2, and O_3) in a Sample of 4,498 White Adolescents

Configuration $O_1O_2O_3C_6$	m	$\hat{m}$	p	Type/antitype?
1111	136	55.20	$< \alpha^*$	T
1112	92	172.80	$< \alpha^*$	A
1121	8	7.26	.44	
1122	22	22.74	.41	
1211	6	8.23	.83	
1212	28	25.77	.36	
1221	1	18.40	$< \alpha^*$	A
1222	75	57.60	.02	
2111	308	166.33	$< \alpha^*$	T
2112	379	520.67	$< \alpha^*$	A
2121	58	74.33	.02	
2122	249	232.67	.14	
2211	75	109.43	$< \alpha^*$	A
2212	377	342.57	.03	
2221	497	649.82	$< \alpha^*$	A
2222	2187	2034.18	$< \alpha^*$	T

in the study. It suggests that more individuals than expected under the assumption of independence of the precursor pattern and the outcome start above their age-specific median in optimization, slip to below average for the following two observation periods, and display, at time 6, below-median scores in compensation. Each of the other types and antitypes is shown either by a selection of groups only or by just one group.

Interesting from the expectation of consistency is that the type that indicates that individuals who score below median in optimization at all three points in time will also show below-median scores in compensation at time 6 (configuration 1111) does not appear in the multiracial group. The probability for the frequency in this cell to constitute a type is 0.044. This value is remote from the critical $\alpha^* = 0.003125$. Even more dramatic is that the type that suggests consistent above-median scores in optimization and an above-median outcome in compensation is found only in the white sample. In each of the racial groups, this configuration contains the largest number of cases, but it constitutes a type only in the white group.

From the perspective of equifinality (see, e.g., Gottlieb, Wahlsten, & Lickliter, 1998), it is worth noting that, in the white population, below-median scores in compensation are more likely to be obtained than expected from the optimization patterns 111 and 211. There is an above-chance probability of obtaining above-median scores in compensation if optimization pattern 222 was observed. Conversely, optimization patterns 122 and 222 come with significantly reduced chances of reaching a below-median compensation score, and optimization pattern 111 comes with significantly reduced chances of reaching an

TABLE 35.5. CFA Predicting Compensation (C_6) from Three Consecutive Observations of Optimization (O_1, O_2, and O_3) in Samples of 4,498 White, 345 Inconsistently Responding, 701 Latino/a, 189 Multiracial, and 474 African American Adolescents (Type/Antitype Configurations Indicated)

	Race				
Configuration $O_1O_2O_3C_6$	White	Inconsistent responders	Latino/a	Multiracial	African American
1111	T	T	T		T
1112	A				A
1121					
1122					
1211					
1212					
1221	A				
1222					
2111	T	T	T	T	T
2112	A		A		
2121		A			
2122					
2211	A				
2212					
2221	A		A		A
2222	T				
LR–χ^2	373.7	63.19	113.18	33.08	76.72
df	7	7	7	7	7
p	< .01	< .01	< .01	< .01	< .01

above-median compensation score. The results in Table 35.5 suggest similar statements for the other racial/ethnic groups.

Future Directions

CFA is a method that enables researchers to find out where, in a cross-classification, the action is. In contrast to the vast majority of statistical methods, CFA expresses results not in terms of parameters and their significance but, instead, in terms of types and antitypes that are constituted by individual cells or patterns of cells (the latter issue was not discussed in this chapter; see von Eye, 2002). In other words, CFA is applied with the goal of identifying extreme, outlandish cells (cells that constitute types and antitypes). In accordance with this goal of CFA application, researchers specify base models not with the intention to craft a well-fitting model. Instead, CFA base models are specified such that types and antitypes reflect the effect researchers hope to find in a table.

Residual analysis of log-linear models uses methods that are similar to those used by CFA. However, again, the goals of log-linear residual analysis and CFA differ in a fundamental way. The goals of residual analysis concern the validity of a model and, if needed, model improvement. Log-linear models are specified to explain data at the level of variables. In contrast, CFA aims at rejecting cellwise null hypotheses, and it operates at the level of individual cells, also called configurations.

As are most methods of statistics, CFA is in the process of being further developed (see von Eye et al., 2010). Recent developments include autoregression CFA and the prediction of endpoints, both presented in this chapter; mediation CFA; and moderator CFA. Still, there are many issues that are waiting for solutions. In the following paragraphs, we discuss three issues and future developments.

Protection of the Significance Threshold α

In most applications of CFA, the number of significance tests is known a priori. Procedures for α protection under this condition are well known. This applies to both exploratory and confirmatory applications. Recently, a new class of CFA models has been proposed that allows one to identify the role that individual effects of log-linear models play in the emergence of types and antitypes. This class of CFA models (called *functional CFA*; von Eye & Mair, 2008) has the characteristic that the number of tests that are performed is not known before the analysis is complete. Therefore, methodologists need to devise procedures that allow one to protect α when the number of tests is unknown a priori.

Latent Variable CFA

The development of methods of latent variable analysis has made most impressive progress (see, e.g., Skrondal & Rabe-Hesketh, 2004). The analysis of categorical variables and the specification of categorical latent variables is no longer a problem. However, configural approaches in the context of latent variable analysis have yet to be proposed. Three lines of research are being discussed. The first involves the search for types and antitypes using latent variable scores on categorical latent variables (latent traits or latent classes). The second involves the analysis of relationships among categorical latent variables. The third involves the specification of latent variable models as CFA base models.

CFA of Other Parameters Other than Location

The majority of CFA models, so far, focus on location parameters. The questions asked concern the number of cases in particular sectors of the variable space. So far, there exist only two attempts to subject other parameters to CFA. The first of these attempts allows researchers to analyze correlations in longitudinal data sets from a configural perspective (von Eye, 1990). The second attempt subjects polynomial parameters of time series to CFA (von Eye & Nesselroade, 1992). Many other parameters exist, and configural models for the analysis of these parameters have yet to be devised.

In conclusion, CFA is the only method of statistical analysis that allows one to examine cross-classifications with the goals of person-oriented research. In developmental research, the virtues of CFA include the possibility of studying trajectories at the level of configurations instead of associations among variables. Trajectories can be related to each other, they can be predicted, they can be used as predictors, and time-stable as well as time-varying covariates can be taken into account. CFA opens the door to answering research questions that, before the development of CFA, could not be answered.

References

Bergman, L. R., & Magnusson, D. (1997). A person-oriented approach in research on developmental psychopathology. *Development and Psychopathology, 9*, 291–319.

Bergman, L. R., von Eye, A., & Magnusson, D. (2006). Person-oriented research strategies in developmental psychopathology. In D. Cicchetti & D. J. Cohen (Eds.), *Developmental psychopathology* (2nd ed., pp. 850–888). London: Wiley.

Bogat, G. A., Levendosky, A. A., DeJonghe, E., Davidson, W. S., & von Eye, A. (2004). Pathways of suffering: The temporal effects of domestic violence on women's mental health. *Maltrattamento e Abuso all'infanzia, 6*, 97–112.

Freund, A. M., & Baltes, P. B. (2000). The orchestration of selection, optimization, and compensation: An action-theoretical conceptualization of a theory of developmental regulation. In W. J. Perrig & A. Grob (Eds.), *Control of human behavior, mental processes, and consciousness* (pp. 35–58). Mahwah, NJ: Erlbaum.

Gestsdóttir, S., & Lerner, R. M. (2007). Intentional self-regulation and positive youth development in early adolescence: Findings from the 4-H Study of Positive Youth Development. *Developmental Psychology, 43*, 508–521.

Gestsdóttir, S., Lewin-Bizan, S., von Eye, A., Lerner, J. V., & Lerner, R. M. (2009). The structure and function of selection, optimization, and compensation in middle adolescence: Theoretical and applied implications. *Journal of Applied Developmental Psychology, 30*, 585–600.

Gottlieb, G., Wahlsten, D., & Lickliter, R. (1998). The significance of biology for human development: A developmental psychobiological systems view. In R. M. Lerner (Ed.), *Handbook of child psychology* (5th ed., pp. 233–273). New York: Wiley.

Holm, S. (1979). A simple sequentially rejective multiple test procedure. *Scandinavian Journal of Statistics, 6*, 65–70.

Hommel, G. (1988). A stagewise rejective multiple test procedure based on a modified Bonferroni test. *Biometrika, 75*, 383–386.

Lerner, R. M. (2004). *Liberty: Thriving and civic engagement among American youth*. Thousand Oaks, CA: Sage.

Lerner, R. M. (2007). *The good teen: Rescuing adolescents from the myths of the storm and stress years*. New York: Crown.

Lerner, R. M., Lerner, J. V., Almerigi, J., Theokas, C., Phelps, E., Gestsdóttir, S., et al. (2005). Positive youth development, participation in community youth development programs, and community contributions of fifth-grade adolescents: Findings from the first wave of the 4-H Study of Positive Youth Development. *Journal of Early Adolescence, 25*(1), 17–71.

Lerner, R. M., von Eye, A., Lerner, J. V., & Lewin-Bizan, S. (2009). Foundations and functions on thriving in adolescence: Findings from the 4-H Study of Positive Youth Development. *Journal of Applied Developmental Psychology, 30*, 567–648.

Lerner, R. M., von Eye, A., Lerner, J. V., Lewin-Bizan, S., & Bowers, E. P. (in press). Individual and contextual bases of thriving in adolescence: Findings from the 4-H Study of Positive Youth Development. *Journal of Youth and Adolescence.*

Lienert, G. A. (1968). *Die "Konfigurationsfrequenzanalyse" als Klassifikationsmethode in der klinischen Psychologie* [Configural frequency analysis as a classification method in clinical psychology]. Paper presented at the conference of the German Psychological Association, Tübingen.

Lienert, G. A. (1971). Die Konfigurationsfrequenzanalyse III. Zwei- und Mehrstichproben KFA in Diagnostik und Differentialdiagnostik [Configural frequency analysis III. Two- and multiple group CFA in diagnostics and differential diagnostics]. *Zeitschrift für Klinische Psychologie und Psychotherapie, 19*, 291–300.

Mellenbergh, G. J. (1996). Other null model, other (anti)type. *Applied Psychology: An International Review, 45*, 329–330.

Osterkorn, K. (1975). Wann kann die Binomial- und Poissonverteilung hinreichend genau durch die Normalverteilung eresetzt warden? [When can one substitute the binomial and the Poisson distributions by the normal distribution?] *Biometrische Zeitschrift, 17*, 33–34.

Perli, H.-G., Hommel, G., & Lehmacher, W. (1985). Sequentially rejective test procedures for detecting outlying cells in one- and two-sample multinomial experiments. *Biometrical Journal, 27*, 885–893.

Phelps, E., Zimmerman, S., Warren, A. E. A., Jelicic, H., von Eye, A., & Lerner, R. M. (2009). The structure and developmental course of positive youth development (PYD) in early adolescence: Implications for theory and practice. *Journal of Applied Developmental Psychology, 30*, 571–584.

Skrondal, A., & Rabe-Hesketh, S. (2004). *Generalized latent variable modeling*. Boca Raton, FL: Chapman & Hall.

Tubman, J. G., Vicary, J. R., von Eye, A., & Lerner, J. V. (1991). Qualitative changes in relationships between substance use and adjustment during adolescence. *Journal of Substance Abuse, 3*, 405–414.

von Eye, A. (1990). Configural frequency analysis of longitudinal multivariate responses. In A. von Eye (Ed.), *Statistical methods in longitudinal research* (Vol. 2, pp. 545–570). New York: Academic Press.

von Eye, A. (2002). *Configural frequency analysis: Methods, models, and applications*. Mahwah, NJ: Erlbaum.

von Eye, A. (2004). Base models for configural frequency analysis. *Psychology Science, 46*, 150–170.

von Eye, A., & Bergman, L. R. (2003). Research strategies in developmental psychopathology: Dimensional identity and the person-oriented approach. *Development and Psychopathology, 15*, 553–580.

von Eye, A., & Bogat, G. A. (2006). Person orientation: Concepts, results, and development. *Merrill-Palmer Quarterly, 52*, 390–420.

von Eye, A., Bogat, G. A., & Rhodes, J. E. (2006). Variable-oriented and person-oriented perspectives of analysis: The example of alcohol consumption in adolescence. *Journal of Adolescent Research, 29*, 981–1004.

von Eye, A., & Gutiérrez Peña, E. (2004). Configural frequency analysis: The search for extreme cells. *Journal of Applied Statistics, 31*, 981–997.

von Eye, A., & Mair, P. (2008). Functional configural frequency analysis: Explaining types and antitypes. *Bulletin de la Société des Sciences Médicales, Luxembourg, 144*, 35–52.

von Eye, A., Mair, P., & Bogat, G. A. (2005). Prediction models for configural frequency analysis. *Psychology Science, 47*, 342–355.

von Eye, A. A., Mair, P., & Mun, E.-Y. (2010). *Advances in configural frequency analysis*. New York: Guilford Press.

von Eye, A., Mun, E. Y., & Bogat, G. A. (2009). Temporal patterns of variable relationships in person-oriented research: Prediction and auto-association models of configural frequency analysis. *Applied Developmental Science, 13*, 172–187.

von Eye, A., & Nesselroade, J. R. (1992). Types of change: Application of configural frequency analysis to repeated observations in developmental research. *Experimental Aging Research, 18*, 169–183.

von Eye, A., & Schuster, C. (1998). On the specification of models for configural frequency analysis: Sampling schemes in prediction CFA. *Methods of Psychological Research Online, 3*, 55–73.

von Weber, S., von Eye, A., & Lautsch, E. (2004). The Type II error of measures for the analysis of 2 × 2 tables. *Understanding Statistics, 3*, 259–282.

CHAPTER 36

Cluster Analysis and Latent Class Clustering Techniques

CHRISTINE DiSTEFANO

Much of the research conducted with human development has utilized a variable-oriented approach to data analysis in which the focus is on identification of relations among or investigation of mean differences. Although variable-oriented approaches are useful for studying interindividual differences, they are less useful for understanding intraindividual dynamics (Bergman & Magnusson, 1997). In order to address intraindividual differences, more attention has been devoted to the use of person-oriented analyses, such as cluster analysis and latent class clustering procedures (Bergman, Magnusson, & El-Khouri, 2003). These approaches focus on classification of individuals in order to better study intraindividual variation.

Person-oriented analysis methods are well suited to the study of human development because these methods focus on understanding the characteristics of an individual's developmental profile or developmental pattern as compared with his or her peers (Laursen & Hoff, 2006). This strategy appears congruent with dynamic systems theories of human development (Kamphaus & Frick, 2002). Methodologies that consider the unique characteristics of an individual as part of the analysis are critical to ensure that intricacies of an individual's developmental patterns are not overlooked or masked by averaging scores across many individuals. Therefore, a multidimensional person-oriented approach can help describe and classify developmental patterns more clearly and accurately than can variable-oriented systems (Bergman, 1998).

Central Issues

By definition, classification refers to the process of dividing a large heterogeneous group into smaller homogeneous groups in which members are similar to each other and different from cases in other groups (Gordon, 1981). The objective is to identify groups underlying a larger set of data, with the number of groups unknown at the outset. Once created, groups can be thought of as possessing like patterns of characteristics, and cases within the same group may be treated similarly.

Classification systems may be especially useful within the study of human development, in which the goal is often to explain, assist, intervene, and treat individuals who suffer from behavioral, cognitive, physical, and/or emotional problems. Such classification systems may be useful in developmental psychology for several research and clinical purposes, including differentiating individuals by etiology (Cantwell, 1996), identifying individuals' risk or adjustment status (Kagan, 1997), and tracking individual developmental pathways (Richters, 1997). This chapter focuses on two popular methods often used by developmental scientists to create classification systems: cluster analysis and latent class cluster analysis. Each method is discussed in turn.

Conceptual Principles and Statistical Assumptions

Cluster Analysis

Cluster analysis refers to a family of procedures that group cases in order to uncover homogeneous groups underlying a data set (Aldenderfer & Blashfield, 1984; Blashfield & Aldenderfer, 1988; Everitt, 1993). The collection of scores for each case creates a multivariate profile, which is used in analyses to identify like cases. Profiles for each case may be evaluated to gauge the "elevation" (the magnitude of the scores) and the "shape" (the pattern of peaks and troughs) across the set of variables.

As with any statistical method, there are assumptions and considerations underlying cluster analysis. First, the choice of variables is of primary importance. Because each case's multivariate profile is considered when creating the groups, the variables included in the cluster analysis should be the most relevant to the situation under study. Groups identified from a cluster analysis may differ markedly if different variables are included. For cluster analysis, variables are assumed to be both independent and uncorrelated, and cases are assumed to be independent.

A second consideration is that variables used in cluster analyses are thought to be at the observed, rather than latent, level. Therefore, the variables can be considered as directly measured and do not necessarily refer to underlying latent variables. Typically, cluster analysis requires data that are on the same metric level. For cluster analysis, data may be of any scale type (e.g., nominal, ordinal, interval, or ratio); however, the metric level of the data will affect the choice of index used to describe relations between cases (i.e., proximity measure). Data are also scale dependent, meaning that variables with both large mean differences and/or standard deviations may suppress the influence of other variables (Everitt, 1993). If the variables have large standard deviations or are measured on different scales, the variables may be standardized to achieve a common metric before clustering (Aldenderfer & Blashfield, 1984; Everitt, 1993; Milligan, 1996). Standardizing will remove any undue influence of metric or variability (Milligan, 1996); however, it may also have the disadvantage of masking differences on variables that best differentiate the groups (Everitt, 1993). Overall, researchers should be aware that clustering results may differ if standardization is (or is not) carried out.

Proximity Indices

Cluster analysis requires an index to use to join cases. A proximity measure transforms the multivariate raw data, via a mathematical formula, into a matrix that is used to evaluate how alike cases are (Everitt, 1993). There are two general types of proximity measures, similarity indices and dissimilarity indices, within which elements of the data matrix vary based on the direction of the relation between the cases. For dissimilarity indices, *smaller* values indicate that two cases are more alike; for similarity indices, *larger* values indicate that two cases are more alike. Dissimilarity indices are discussed because they are more widely used with cluster analysis (Blashfield & Aldenderfer, 1988).

Dissimilarity indices illustrate how different two cases are from each other across the set of variables. Two highly dissimilar cases would receive a higher value, or greater distance, between cases, whereas highly similar cases receive a low value, showing a smaller distance (Everitt, 1993). Distance measures have a minimum of zero, with no upper bound, so the scores are hard to interpret. These measures are also scale dependent and sensitive to fluctuations in variability across the variables used with clustering.

One popular distance measure used with cluster analysis is the Euclidean distance. From Aldenderfer and Blashfield (1984), the Euclidean distance between two cases, i and j, is described as

$$d_{ij} = \sqrt{\sum_{k=1}^{p} (x_{ik} - x_{jk})^2} \qquad \textbf{(36.1)}$$

where d_{ij} is the distance between case i and case j, x_{ik} is the value of the kth variable for the ith case, and x_{jk} is the value of the kth variable for the jth case. For a multivariate profile, x_{ik} is represented as a vector, and differences between variables are summed over all variables used in the clustering procedure. When calculating a Euclidean distance, two case profiles, a case and a group centroid (i.e., the average profile for a cluster) or two group centroids can be considered. To eliminate the square root, the value is often squared, and $d_{ij}{}^2$ is reported as the squared Euclidean distance.

Distance measures are often criticized because a computed value may be affected by the elevation of the profiles. This means that two profiles with similar shapes but at different elevations may be considered dissimilar. Also, variables with large standard deviations and size differences can overpower the effects of variables with smaller size differences or standard deviations. Finally, distance indices are affected by transformations of scale, such as standardization of variables. Even given these caveats, distance measures are frequently used with cluster analysis.

Clustering Algorithms

There are many choices of clustering algorithms to use to join cases. When choosing an algorithm, the method should be compatible with the purpose for clustering, the level of the variables, and the choice of similarity matrix. Each method represents a different perspective and could produce different results, even when applied to the same data set. At the most basic level, there are seven major families of procedures that cluster cases according to a general method (see Aldenderfer & Blashfield, 1984, pp. 35–53). The two most popular families used with developmental research (Bergman et al., 2003) are discussed: hierarchical agglomerative methods and iterative partitioning methods. Several different clustering techniques underlie each of these families of clustering methods.

Hierarchical Algorithms

Hierarchical agglomerative methods have been the most popular methods used with cluster analysis (Aldenderfer & Blashfield, 1984). These methods examine the proximity matrix and sequentially join cases that are the most similar. After all cases are joined, the proximity matrix is reexamined. A total of $N - 1$ steps are made through a data set, grouping cases from singletons to one large data set of N cases (Lorr, 1983). The most popular hierarchical agglomerative method used in the social sciences (Aldenderfer & Blashfield, 1984) is Ward's method (Ward, 1963). This procedure creates groups that are highly homogeneous by optimizing the minimum variance, or error sum of squares (ESS), within clusters. The ESS formula, as stated in Everitt (1993), is

$$ESS = \sum_{i=1}^{n} (\mathbf{X}_i - \overline{\mathbf{X}})^2 \qquad \textbf{(36.2)}$$

where $\mathbf{X}_i$ is the case (or group) in question and $\overline{\mathbf{X}}$ is the cluster centroid. In the formula, summing from $i = 1$ to n, the n may refer to the total number of cases (at the start of the process) or the number of groups (as the clustering process proceeds). At the first step of the process, each case is its own cluster, and the ESS among groups is 0. Cases are joined into clusters that produce the smallest increase of ESS, computed as a sum over all clusters. Although Ward's (1963) method is popular, it is also sensitive to the elevation of the profiles and may group cases into different clusters based on elevation, even if the shapes of the profiles are similar.

There are caveats to the use of hierarchical agglomerative methods. One major problem is that cases joined at an earlier step cannot be reassigned—even if a case has a closer association with a different group by the end of the assignment process. In other words, a poor start to the clustering process cannot be overcome because only one pass is made through the data set to assign cases. Second, hierarchical agglomerative methods do not have "stopping" rules that state the number of clusters underlying a data set. The researcher can plot the union of cases through the clustering process by using a dendrogram plot (Everitt, 1993). Dendrograms visually represent the merging of cases at each step, from the lowest level (where each of N cases forms its own group) to the highest level (with all cases forming one large group of N cases). Plots may be examined for suggestions of the number of clusters underlying the data set by looking for the large divisions or steps in the graph. A third consideration is that groups created using hierarchical agglomerative methods are nested. This means that the clusters do not overlap, and each cluster can be subsumed as a member of a larger, more inclusive group at later steps in the process. Finally, hierarchical methods may not provide stable groupings. A researcher may obtain different results if a data set is reordered, reshuffled, and reclustered. To overcome this drawback, researchers should use various procedures to cluster a set of data and should interpret only clusters that appear in multiple samples (Bergman et al., 2003).

Iterative Partitioning Methods

Iterative partitioning methods are another clustering algorithm option. As with hierarchical methods, many procedures and choices underlie this family of methods. In this family, clustering is conducted by completing the following series of steps (Aldenderfer & Blashfield, 1984; Everitt, 1993):

1. An initial cut or partition of the data set into *k* clusters is made, with *k* specified by the researcher. The centroid, or the arithmetic mean of values across the set of variables, is computed for each of the *k* clusters. If group information is unknown, the initial partition may be conducted arbitrarily. For example, one choice may be to allow the first *k* cases to serve as the cluster centroids for the *k* groups or to randomly choose *k* cases to serve as the initial group means.
2. Individual cases are assigned to the cluster with the nearest centroid. This assignment is typically conducted using distance measures (e.g., squared Euclidean) in the proximity matrix, assigning cases to the cluster with the smallest distance to a given centroid.
3. Once all cases in the data set are assigned, the centroids of the *k* clusters are recomputed. The data set is reexamined to see whether any cases are now closer to a different cluster centroid than to the centroid of the initial cluster assignment. Cases with smaller distances to different groups are reassigned.
4. Steps 2 and 3 are repeated by making "passes" or iterations through the data set until no cases change cluster assignment.

In developmental research, the *k*-means procedure is the best known of the iterative partitioning methods (Bergman et al., 2003). Although not explicitly stated, the *k*-means procedure tries to minimize the trace of the pooled within covariance matrix (i.e., **trW**; Aldenderfer & Blashfield, 1984). The trace can be computed as the sum of the diagonal elements. This criterion is similar to what is used with Ward's method, because minimizing the trace of the within-group sum of squares matrix is equivalent to minimizing the sum of squared Euclidean distances between cases and the cluster centroid (Everitt, 1993). The hierarchical process is optimized within *k*-means to identify the best (global) solution underlying a data set (Steinley, 2003). However, the minimization of **trW** is scale dependent and may produce different solutions even if raw data and standardized data from the same data set are clustered.

Iterative partitioning methods are not without problems. These procedures are sensitive to the initial cut in the data and may not be able to fully overcome a poor initial partition (Steinley, 2003). As with hierarchical methods, *k*-means may produce a suboptimal solution if the initial cut is poor. This is known as finding a local optimal solution, rather than a global solution, for the entire data set (Steinley, 2003). To avoid problems arising from a poor starting point, centroid values or seed values may be used, whereby the input for the initial partition are *k* centroids based on prior knowledge or previous analyses. Another strategy that has been recommended is to use the final solution from Ward's (1963) hierarchical agglomerative method as the starting point for the iterative partitioning procedure (Bergman et al., 2003; Huberty, DiStefano, & Kamphaus, 1997). When using the Ward's final solution as the initial starting point for the *k*-means procedure, the researcher gains the benefits of both clustering algorithms.

Identifying and Interpreting a Solution

Heuristic criteria may be used to suggest the optimal number of clusters. Three statistics, cubic clustering criterion, pseudo *F*, and pseudo *t*-square, can be plotted by the number of possible clusters (maximum of *N* clusters) to judge the number of groups underlying a data set (Aldenderfer & Blashfield, 1984; Sarle, 1983). Graphs are examined to determine large changes in the level of the plot to suggest the number of clusters underlying the data set (Everitt, 1993). With hierarchical methods, dendrogram plots can be examined. Researchers should use the suggested number of clusters as a starting point and evaluate a range of cluster solutions above and below this point.

Cluster analyses are evaluated on two dimensions. First, the centroid information is considered for each cluster (Aldenderfer & Blashfield, 1984; Everitt, 1993). Cluster centroid values are used to identify subgroups of the population. Second, supporting information about each cluster's demographic characteristics may be considered. For example, when studying children's behavioral development, demographic characteristics may include gender distributions, racial/ethnic membership, and cluster size relative to the total sample. A cluster is named by comparing the centroid information and demographic characteristics to existing theoretical perspectives and prior research. This information can be evaluated and compared across a range of solutions to determine which one fits the data best. Additionally, measures of cluster homogeneity can be computed within clusters to evaluate the average ESS for cases within a group (Bergman et al., 2003).

After the final cluster solution is identified, internal validation and external validation of the solution are recommended. Internal validation procedures capitalize on investigations that use the same data set. These procedures may be conducted by shuffling the data set and reclustering to see which cluster definitions are stable (Bergman et al., 2003). Another method that is useful if the data set is sufficiently large is to randomly split the data set into half samples. One half sample may be used to build a classification rule using predictive discriminant analysis techniques that is then applied to the second half sample (Huberty et al., 1997). This treats the second sample as ungrouped cases, and cases are assigned into the cluster with the closest association (Huberty, 1994). Concordance between the two sets may be assessed by examining the initial group classification and cluster membership predicted by the classification rule. Another internal validation check may be conducted with leave-one-out procedures (Huberty, 1994). Here, each case in the data set may be withheld in turn and the other cases used to build a prediction rule. This rule is used to predict cluster membership for the withheld case(s). This process may be conducted up to *N* times, leaving out different case information at each iteration until all cases have been classified.

External classification procedures focus on using independent data sets to recover the solution. Validation of a cluster solution is paramount to illustrating that the obtained typology is an optimal solution (Bergman et al., 2003). Replication with independent samples is an important criterion, not only to determine the appropriate number of clusters but also to ensure that the agreed-upon solution holds the same meaning in other samples from the same population (Aldenderfer & Blashfield, 1984). Validation procedures may also be conducted by determining whether there are differences between groups on important variables that were *not* used to group cases into clusters (Milligan, 1996).

Latent Class Cluster Analysis

An alternative approach to grouping cases via cluster analysis is to use latent class clustering methods (Clogg, 1995; Collins & Lanza, 2010; Everitt, 1993; Heinen, 1993; Muthén & Muthén, 2007; Vermunt & Magidson, 2002). Latent class cluster analysis has been called other names in the literature, such as finite mixture modeling (McLachlan & Peel, 2000), model-based clustering (e.g., Banfield & Raftery, 1993), and mixture likelihood clustering (Everitt, 1993). These methods use the same general model and include techniques such as latent class analysis, latent profile analysis, mixed-mode clustering, and latent transition analysis. Although the latent class methods have been available for many years (e.g., Gibson, 1959; Lazarsfeld & Henry, 1968), the techniques are enjoying increased popularity through improved computer capabilities and available software (Vermunt & Magidson, 2002). Despite similarities between latent class cluster analysis and cluster analysis, there are also distinctions between the two methods.

Latent class cluster (LCC) analysis has an overarching goal similar to that of cluster analysis: to classify cases into groups such that members within a group are similar to each other and different from individuals in other groups (Vermunt & Magidson, 2002). Similarly, cases are thought to belong to one of K groups underlying the data set in which the number of groups is unknown a priori. The difference is that group membership in LCC is represented as a categorical latent variable.

A central assumption of LCC is the notion that the data used in the analyses come from a mix of populations that have different probability distributions. Therefore, the population consists of homogenous subpopulations (i.e., clusters or classes), in which the groups are discrete and mutually exclusive (Clogg, 1995; Heinen, 1993). Individuals within a certain class have the same probability distribution with respect to the categorical latent variable. Because the set of groups is nonoverlapping, together, all classes account for 100% of the population. In other words, the set of class proportions sums to 1.

A second central assumption in LCC is the assumption of local independence. This assumption states that there is no relation between the observed variables; all relations between the indicators can be explained by the influence of the latent class on an individual's observed scores (Clogg, 1995; Muthén, 2001; Vermunt & Magidson, 2002). This means that the correlations between variables within each class are assumed to be zero. Put another way, when considering the total sample, the latent class variable is the driving force relating the observed variables (Muthén, 2001). This premise is shared with factor analysis, in which the latent factor is influencing relations among the observed variables and is similar to the assumption of local item independence in item response theory. If the latent class variable is removed, there would be no relation between the observed variables within the same class.

As noted by Vermunt and Magidson (2002), the general form of an LCC model is

$$f(\mathbf{y}_i \mid \theta) = \sum_{k=1}^{K} \pi_k f_k(\mathbf{y}_i \mid \theta_k) \qquad \textbf{(36.3)}$$

where $\mathbf{y}_i$ denotes the profile of scores for case i across the set of variables, K is the number of underlying groups or clusters, θ is the set of model parameters, and π_k denotes the probability of belonging to a specific class, k. Here, $f(\mathbf{y}_i|\theta)$ is the mixture of the class-specific density functions, $f_k(\mathbf{y}_i|\theta_k)$. Because the group variable is considered to be measured at the latent level and a model-based procedure is used, measurement error in the observed indices can be partitioned and is reflected in estimates of the within-class residual variance. The vector of model parameters, θ, represents the unique parameters estimated for each class (e.g., centroid values μ_k and variance–covariance matrices, Σ_k).

It is relatively easy to deal with variables measured on different scales using model-based clustering methods. In contrast to cluster analyses, in which variables on differing metric levels should be standardized prior to clustering, latent clustering methods may utilize a mixture of continuous and categorical variables in the same analysis. Finally, LCC procedures follow a probabilistic approach. This means that although each case is grouped into only one class, K, the model recognizes that there may be uncertainty in the classification. Therefore, each case is given a probability value (or mixing value) of belonging to *each* of the K groups, represented by π_k in equation 36.3. The distribution of the indicators ($\mathbf{y}_i$) is a weighted mixture of the K distributions, each distinguished by unique class parameters. Values for the weights range between 0 and 1 per class and sum to 1 across classes.

LCC analysis subsumes both latent class analysis and latent profile analysis. These techniques are similar; measured variables are categorical within latent class analysis and on a continuous metric with latent profile analysis (Muthén & Muthén, 2000). Also, latent class clustering can be considered a probabilistic or model-based variant of nonhierarchical clustering methods (Vermunt, 2004). In fact, the most restrictive form of latent class clustering is comparable to traditional iterative partitioning methods, such as k-means (Everitt, 1993; Vermunt & Magidson, 2002). However, a primary distinction is that k-means clustering considers a case to be a member of a class with certainty, whereas the probabilistic nature of LCC recognizes uncertainty in the classification process.

Model Restrictions

Latent clustering methods allow a more flexible framework than permitted under cluster analysis. Researchers can relax restrictions to determine which parameters should be estimated (i.e., freed) or constrained (i.e., fixed). Imposing different model restrictions allows the evaluation of different solutions to determine which model provides optimal fit to the data in terms of parsimony, fit indices, and interpretability. There are two primary reasons that restrictions are imposed in LCC (Collins & Lanza, 2010). The first is for purposes of identification. As model-based procedures, LCC methods need to set a balance between the number of parameters to be estimated and the amount of information available to use in the estimation process. The number of parameters to be estimated includes the total number of class mixture weights, the number of variables in each class centroid, and freed elements from each class's variance–covariance matrix. A model that is estimating fewer parameters relative to the amount of available information is said to be identified and will produce parameter estimates and fit information for evaluation.

A second reason for imposing restrictions is to test different types of models. This may include testing relations among classes or examining differences when characteristics are relaxed or restrictions are placed on model parameters. Several restrictions concerning μ or Σ may be conducted within LCC. For instance, the mean vector may be freely estimated for all indicators but constrained across groups. This would test whether the groups had the same level of association between the observed and latent indicators. This is similar to invariance testing situations in structural equation modeling (see Bollen, 1989, for more information on invariance tests within the structural modeling framework).

It is more common to freely estimate the centroids for each class for use in defining the group. Most restrictions are concerned with elements of the variance–covariance matrix (Σ_k) (Vermunt, 2004). The Σ_k matrix represents the homogeneity of the observed variables (indicator variances; represented on the diagonal of Σ_k) and the relations between variables beyond what is accounted for by the latent variable (indicator covariances; represented on the off-diagonal elements of Σ_k). Restrictions include imposing the assumption of local independence, conducted by constraining Σ_k to be diagonal and class dependent (i.e., variances estimated for all indicators and unique within a class; all off-diagonal elements fixed to zero). The assumption of local independence may be relaxed by allowing indicators, or subsets of indicators, to be related by freeing selected off-diagonal parameters. Equality of variance–covariance matrices across latent classes is another constraint that may be of interest (Vermunt, 2004). This restriction tests the homogeneity of indicators across classes and may be parameterized by allowing item variances to be different across indicators but constrained to be equal across groups. Constraining variances within a cluster to be equal across groups with no relations among variables is typically assumed with cluster analysis. Specifying this parameterization of Σ_k and running both LCC analysis and k-means will produce similar results. In general, models that are too restrictive are thought to overestimate the number of clusters underlying a data set (Vermunt & Magidson, 2002). In other words, k-means clustering will typically find more groups underlying a data set than will LCC using the same data set without strict parameterizations of Σ_k.

Vermunt and Magidson (2002) note the importance of working with different types of models, in particular considering relations between variables. It is often not realistic to assume that variances are equal across classes or that relations between variables are zero. An advantage to LCC is that different parameterizations of the variance–covariance matrix can be specified and evaluated.

Researchers should test different LCC models by imposing different restrictions on the variance–covariance matrix. A typical set of models may include (1) constraining variances to be equal across classes, with relations between variables constrained to zero; (2) allowing class-dependent variances, constraining covariance terms to zero (i.e., local independence); (3) allowing class-dependent variances and selected covariances (e.g., related scales or variables), constraining values to be equal across classes, and (4) modeling class-dependent variances and freely estimating selected covariances within class.

Estimation

To fit an LCC model to a data set, the model parameters of interest must be estimated. Here, an estimation method is used to classify cases into groups. The method estimates the likelihood of a case belonging to group K, given the profile of individuals' scores across the set of observed variables. The two main estimation methods used are the maximum likelihood (ML) method and the maximum posterior method. Both techniques use likelihood functions derived from the underlying probability density function to identify optimal parameter estimates that produce the highest likelihood (Vermunt & Magidson, 2002). The procedures use iterative estimation techniques (i.e., a version of an expectation-maximization algorithm) to maximize the likelihood function for the requested K-class model.

Conceptually, the estimation process begins by identifying a set of initial parameters. These initial parameters are compared with a second set of estimated parameters to determine which set produces the better estimates. Each time that parameters are estimated, they are assigned a likelihood value, which is the probability of observing the sample data assuming that set of parameters. Through the iterative process, the parameters are reestimated until the optimal parameters with a large likelihood value are obtained. Once the model is obtained, the parameters estimates are interpreted. These estimates are the values most likely to have produced the data.

Iterative estimation procedures need stopping rules to conclude estimation and to determine the final parameter estimates. Typically, two different criteria are used in LCC (Collins & Lanza, 2010). First, the maximum number of iterations may be set. This value states the maximum number of times that the parameters may be reestimated from the data set. Software programs typically conduct a default number of iterations. Second, it is common for researchers to use a convergence criterion. This index allows estimation to stop when the difference between parameters obtained on successive iterations is so small that it is considered trivial.

When running LCC analysis, sometimes a solution cannot be obtained. Nonconvergence may occur if the maximum number of iterations is reached before the convergence criterion stopping rule is met. If this occurs, researchers may increase the maximum number of iterations to allow for a better chance of convergence. Alternatively (or even concurrently), the convergence criterion difference may be relaxed to accept a difference that is less stringent; however, reducing the convergence criterion threshold may lead to less precise parameter estimates (Collins & Lanza, 2010).

Start values are initial estimates of the parameters used to begin estimation. These values are analogous to using various seed values as the starting point for a k-means analysis. In LCC analysis, researchers may vary the number of starts (Collins & Lanza, 2010). Different starting values should be used to ensure that the parameter estimates that are obtained are the best estimates (Heinen, 1996). Most computer programs have a minimum number of random starting values. If the obtained parameters converge to the same solution under the multiple starting points, researchers may have greater confidence that parameter estimates reflect the characteristics of a latent class (Collins & Lanza, 2010).

Identifying and Evaluating a Solution

When conducting LCC analyses, researchers need to determine how many latent classes are optimal. The most common way to uncover the number of underlying groups is to test the fit of various models with increasing numbers of latent classes. In other words, within a certain model specification (e.g., local independence model), a range of class solutions are run and interpreted (e.g., 2–6 classes). For each model, the number of classes extracted is increased until solutions do not converge (Vermunt & Magidson, 2002). The researcher then compares the obtained solutions to determine which model best fits the data.

There are more techniques available to evaluating solutions obtained from latent clustering methods than from cluster analysis. LCC employs model fit criteria to assist with choosing an optimal solution (Clogg, 1995; Vermunt & Magidson, 2002); however, the fit criteria are largely heuristic. The logarithmic log-likelihood value is a global fit index that illustrates how well the K-class model fits the data overall. The larger the log-likelihood ratio value, the greater the evidence that the model fits the data. Nested tests also help to identify differences between models specifying the same number of groups. To allow comparisons, models need to be subsets of each other and differ only in terms of the model parameterization (i.e., the simpler model must be a direct subset of the more complex model). For example, a nested test may be conducted between a model allowing class-dependent variances to be freely estimated for all indicators (complex) and a model that restricts the variances to be equal across classes (simple). More complex models (those with more parameters freed to be estimated) will always fit the data better than models that are simpler (those with fewer parameters to be estimated). When models are nested, the difference in likelihood values can be computed to test whether there is a difference in model fit. The difference value is distributed as a χ^2 test with degrees of freedom equal to the difference in the degrees of freedom between the two models. If the value is significant, it means that the restrictions are detrimental to model fit, suggesting a preference for the model with more freed parameters.

Relative fit indices are useful to determine which model provides a better fit to the data. These indices may be used to compare models that differ in the number of groups identified and/or the model specifications. The Akaike information criteria (AIC) and the Bayesian information criteria (BIC) offer comparative evidence to evaluate different solutions (Muthén & Muthén, 2000; Vermunt & Magidson, 2002). The AIC and BIC are parsimony criteria used to compare different model solutions (i.e., different numbers of groups underlying the data) to determine which model fits the data best. For these indices, the more parameters that are estimated, the higher the value. Both statistics are adjusted for the number of parameters in the model (Akaike, 1977), but BIC also adjusts for sample size, yielding larger values as sample size increases, all other factors held constant. With AIC and BIC, comparatively lower values indicate better fitting models. Beyond just comparing values, researchers may look for significant changes in these values across different models.

Other LCC fit indices measure the degree of uncertainty in the classification. These methods require that individuals are grouped to determine how well the model works to classify cases. Posterior probabilities denote the probability of class membership and are computed using both the model characteristics across the set of K classes and patterns of observed scores (Vermunt & Magidson, 2002). In LCC analyses, cases may associate with more than one group through the mixing weight and thus can have fractional group membership across the set of groups. To judge model uncertainty, a case is typically assigned to the one group with which it has the highest posterior probability of association. This type of classification is termed *modal assignment*.

Posterior probability information is used to create a classification table that illustrates how well the model classifies cases across an entire class. The classification table is a $k \times k$ table that summarizes the average posterior probability values by class. This value is computed by averaging the posterior probability values for all cases assigned to a given group. For example, if LCC identified a three-class solution, the first row of the table would provide the average posterior probabilities of membership in classes 1, 2, and 3 for those cases classified (by modal assignment) as members of class 1. The largest average posterior probability should be found along the diagonal of the classification table, providing information about how similar cases are within the group. A good-fitting solution will have high classification rates (i.e., few cases that are difficult to classify) for each class, interpreted as a greater certainty of classification. Perfect classification is indicated by probability values of 1 for each class.

Entropy is a measure of uncertainty or randomness in the classification procedure. It provides a summary of the information presented in a classification table with one index (Pastor, Barron, Miller, & Davis, 2007). Within LCC analyses, entropy values indicate how well the model predicts class memberships (Akaike, 1977). Values range from 0 to 1, and entropy values closer to 1 illustrate better prediction (Vermunt & Magidson, 2002). Entropy is the maximum of the probability density distribution underlying the LCC model (Akaike, 1977), calculated from posterior probability information, as well as the number of classes K modeled and sample size N.

Each class solution should be evaluated using multiple criteria (e.g., low AIC and BIC values, high entropy, and high average posterior probability values). The estimated class parameters and descriptive information are also evaluated for each group. As with cluster analysis, an optimal solution can be named by interpreting patterns of high and low parameter estimates within each class, considering theory and ensuring that each class has substantive meaning (Muthén & Muthén, 2000).

After selecting a model, an LCC solution can be validated by examining relations between groups on variables that were not used in the classification process. As with cluster analysis, this may be conducted using analysis of variance (ANOVA) to determine whether there are mean differences between classes on external variables. An additional method for validation may be to incorporate the final LCC model within a structural equation modeling framework. Covariates that may help to predict class membership may be added into the model, and, similarly, outcome variables related to the latent class variable and/or indicators may be included. For example, if considering child behavior in school, covariates, such as intelligence scores or family income, may be used to assist in the classification of children to groups. Outcome variables (e.g., standardized test scores) may be assessed to determine whether latent groups yield differences with regard to academic performance. Such investigations extend the nomological network of relations tested beyond classification.

Table 36.1 provides a summary of cluster analysis and LCC analysis. Both methods have strengths and limitations that should be considered.

Developmental Applications

It can be argued that methods of person-oriented analysis are more appropriate than variable-based methods for the study of individual development (Bergman & Magnusson, 1997; Bergman et al., 2003). Person-oriented methods focus on characteristics of individuals that allow the identification and subsequent study of important developmental types that may be present. Cluster analysis and LCC can be used, either separately or in combination with other procedures, to study developmental change (Bergman et al., 2003).

One area of potential confusion arises because cluster analysis and latent class analysis are often conducted as cross-sectional analyses. That is, the methods focus on the identification of groups underlying a set of data at one time point. This practice sheds little light on development, which is the study of how behavioral characteristics are stable (or changing) over time. The following focuses on strategies that use person-oriented methods to study maturation and development.

TABLE 36.1. Comparison of Common Characteristics of Cluster Analysis and Latent Class Cluster Analysis

Characteristics	Cluster analysis	Latent class cluster analysis
Grouping variable	At observed level	At latent level
Assumptions	Variables both independent and uncorrelated (no flexibility in relaxing assumption) Cases are assumed to be independent	Requires an underlying model Data from a mix of populations which have different probability distributions. Local independence (i.e., latent class influences observed scores; no correlation between what is left unexplained [error terms])
Data requirements	Requires standardization if variables are measured on different scales or if variables have large standard deviations	Can use a mix of variables on different metrics without standardization
Grouping methods	Groups formed based on clustering algorithm coupled with proximity index	Uses an estimation procedure to estimate parameters Flexible framework allowing researchers to impose/relax restrictions when estimating parameters
Case assignment	Cases assigned to one group	Cases given a probability value of belonging to each group
Determining results	Results obtained by examining solution using descriptive statistics, supporting information, measures of group homogeneity	Results obtained by examining solution using descriptive statistics Fit indices available to help arrive at a final solution
Longitudinal study	Additional methods required to study longitudinal change (e.g., cross-classifying results, LICUR, ISOA)	Models available to study development over time (i.e., latent transition)
Notes	May produce a greater number of groups with finer detail	Can incorporate variables into a broader model (covariates, distal outcomes, additional latent variables and structural relations) Tends to produce fewer, broadly defined groups

Note. LICUR, linking of clusters after removal of residue; ISOA, I-states as objects analysis.

Cluster analysis involves various procedures for studying development across time. One strategy involves descriptive evaluation of group information (e.g., centroids, variances) across solutions. If different people are assessed at two different time points, underlying groups may be identified and compared to see whether the same groups were present at each time (e.g., DiStefano, Kamphaus, & Mindrila, 2010). Such analyses are termed *investigations of structural stability* (Bergman et al., 2003). For example, behavioral characteristics of students in elementary schools may be examined for change over a 10-year period (DiStefano et al., 2010). Results from this type of investigation would be important for teachers, administrators, and school-based mental health professionals who are interested in the general behavioral types of students in school so that they can plan interventions and provide assistance. Such strategies may also be conducted using individuals of different ages, as well as investigations of developmental change over time or within different cultures, to study developmental similarities and differences for individuals of different background characteristics.

Another strategy for investigating developmental change using cluster analysis links cross-sectional analyses over time. One method involves a procedure termed *linking of clusters after removal of residue* (LICUR; Bergman, 1998; Bergman et al., 2003). The method is appropriate in situations in which there are longitudinal data for individuals at multiple points in time (e.g., measurements of children at different ages). LICUR procedures are beneficial when both the shape and the level of an individual's profile are relevant and when relatively homogeneous groups are desired (Bergman, 1998). The methods can be conducted in a series of steps (Bergman et al., 2003). First, extremely unusual profiles or outlier cases, called residues, are identified at each age group and removed from the data set. Second, hierarchical cluster analyses, using procedures discussed earlier, are conducted separately for each age group. It is important to note that the clustering is done independently at each age period, allowing for the possibility of different numbers of clusters at different time points (Bergman, 1998). In the final step, results of cluster analyses are linked across time by cross-tabulating classifications for adjacent age groups. This involves examining cluster centroids to see which group definitions match across time. The different types may be tested for significance to see whether the frequency of group membership has a probability level greater than chance (Bergman et al., 2003).

The I-states as objects analysis (ISOA) method may also be used to study developmental patterns (Bergman & El-Khouri, 1999). This procedure focuses on the I-state, defined as an individual's profile of information at a specific point in time (Bergman & El-Khouri, 1999, p. 753). The ISOA method can be used to investigate different individuals who are at the same state (i.e., possess a similar pattern of information) at different time points or it may be used to determine the state of one individual at different points in time. Measures at multiple time points are often used with this method. ISOA differs from LICUR in that ISOA analyzes information from the same participants at multiple time points in the same analysis, whereas separate analyses are conducted for each time point in LICUR (Bergman et al., 2003; Bergman & El-Khouri, 1999).

To conduct the longitudinal classification under ISOA, a dissimilarity matrix is computed for all variables across individuals and time points. After the removal of residue cases, the data matrix is clustered. Each individual is assigned to one group using cluster analysis procedures, where groups describe individual stability as well as change over time. The group may be either a developmental type (occurring at levels greater than chance) or an antitype (occurring at levels less than chance) (Bergman & El-Khouri, 1999).

If model-based procedures are used, such as latent class or latent profile analysis, and measurements exist for the same individuals at more than one time point, then a latent transition analysis could be conducted. Under the family of latent clustering methods, latent transition analysis uses longitudinal data to test whether cases switch class membership over time. This type of analysis can provide considerable information about the stability and movement of class assignment. The method is a longitudinal classification strategy, in which the model is used to predict the class in which a individual will belong at a later time period. Because the longitudinal methods recognize the individual in the process, these methods may be preferable to comparisons of cross-sectional data for evaluating change (Bergman & Magnusson, 1997).

Illustration

This example uses scores from the Teacher Rating Scale—Child (TRS-C) of the Behavior Assessment System for Children (BASC; Reynolds & Kamphaus, 1992). Teacher rating data were obtained for children attending a mid-sized public elementary school in northeast Georgia. Data were collected from a sample of 240 kindergarten students. A second report of students' emotional and behavioral characteristics was collected 1 year later, after the transition to first grade.

Items on the TRS-C are organized into 14 subscales of behavior from four overriding dimensions: Externalizing Problems, Internalizing Problems, School Problems, and Adaptive Skills (Reynolds & Kamphaus, 1992). Externalizing Behaviors measures the tendencies for students to display aggressive or hyperactive behaviors, and the Internalizing Problems dimension reports tendencies for students to show feelings of anxiety, worry, or stress. School Problems measures difficulties with learning and schoolwork. Finally, Adaptive Skills measures positive behaviors in the domain of social development and interaction with peers and authority figures. Teacher ratings for each subscale are transformed to a *T*-score (mean of 50, standard deviation of 10). For scales from the Externalizing Problems, Internalizing Problems, and School Problems dimensions, higher scores represent greater levels of problematic behavior. The Adaptive Skills scales report the presence of positive skills; lower scores represent more maladaptive behaviors.

First, cluster analysis was run using the *k*-means procedure using subscales from two areas: internalizing problems and externalizing problems. Variances for the subscales were assumed to be equal across classes, and no covariance terms were allowed (i.e., conditional independence). This model can also be run within an LCC framework. To begin clustering, plots and dendrograms were run with SAS software (version 9.2). The plots suggested that two to five clusters may be underlying the data set. To evaluate the cluster solutions, group centroids were examined and matched to theoretical knowledge of child behavior and psychopathology, as well as prior research. The size of the cluster relative to the total sample and the gender membership in the cluster was used to help identify characteristics of the groups. To validate the final solution, an ANOVA was run on the total scores for the two dimensions that were not used in the cluster analysis, Adaptive Skills and School Problems.

Second, latent profile analysis (LPA) and latent transition analysis (LTA) were employed. Latent profile analysis is of interest because the six teacher rating subscales used as input for the analysis were continuous. The LPA provides a cross-sectional view of emotional and behavioral development; LTA provides information about children's change across the 1-year time period. The following example of LTA briefly illustrates the process; greater detail can be found in texts devoted to the study of change (e.g., Collins & Lanza, 2010).

For the LCC analyses, each class solution was first evaluated using multiple criteria: statistical indices, classification quality, ease of interpretability, and match to theory. Fit indices, log-likelihood values, and the BIC were compared across the different class solutions. Second, the classification quality of the solution was determined through examination of a classification table of posterior probability information and entropy. Third, the interpretability of the solution was examined. This involved a consideration of the pattern of means among the set of teacher-rated subscales, matching the patterns to theory, and evaluating the usefulness of the class solution for practice. Finally, to provide information about children's development, an LTA was run to assess stability and change of group membership over the 1-year period. All analyses were conducted using MPlus 6.0 software (Muthén & Muthén, 2007), and the ML estimator was used to uncover the latent classes.

In the cluster analysis, a two-cluster solution produced two large general clusters that did not show distinct differences between the groups. The five-cluster solution reported one group with two members, suggesting that five groups may be too many to extract from the data. Therefore, comparisons focus on differences between three- and four-cluster solutions.

Cluster centroids for both solutions are presented in Table 36.2. The three-cluster solution produced one large cluster with values that are not significantly different from the mean of 50. This group is also roughly evenly split by gender. The other two clusters show

TABLE 36.2. Cluster Analysis of BASC TRS-C Scale Scores, Kindergarten Sample

Variables	Cluster 1 (n = 145)	Cluster 2 (n = 49)	Cluster 3 (n = 46)	Cluster 1 (n = 47)	Cluster 2 (n = 16)	Cluster 3 (n = 135)	Cluster 4 (n = 42)
Externalizing Problems							
Aggression	45.8	49.5	**69.2**	**66.0**	**65.1**	45.4	47.1
Conduct problems	47.1	47.7	**64.7**	**62.4**	58.3	46.8	46.8
Hyperactivity	45.3	49.2	**64.2**	**62.6**	**62.6**	44.7	46.5
Internalizing Problems							
Anxiety	47.2	56.4	53.3	52.3	**62.9**	46.7	54.2
Depression	44.7	53.4	57.9	55.5	**66.1**	43.3	50.1
Somatization	44.7	**72.9**	49.8	46.5	**73.6**	44.2	**71.4**
Demographic characteristics							
Percent of total	60.4	20.4	19.2	19.6	6.7	56.3	17.5
Percent male	55.2	28.6	67.4	66.0	43.8	54.8	31.0
Percent female	44.8	71.4	32.6	34.0	56.3	45.2	69.0
External validation							
Adaptive skills				42.5^1	45.4^1	54.3^2	53.9^2
School problems				57.0^1	60.3^1	47.2^2	48.7^2

Note. N = 240. Values that differ from the mean by 1 standard deviation or more (regardless of direction) are printed in **boldface**. Mean values with the same superscript are not significantly different.

elevated patterns (i.e., significant *T*-values) of somatization tendencies and externalizing problems, respectively. There also appear to be distinctions among the groups, with gender distributions following expected patterns.

The four-cluster solution was evaluated in the same manner. This solution also produced one large cluster (Cluster 3) with values that are not significantly different from the mean of 50, with an approximately equal distribution of boys and girls. The solution yielded a cluster with evidence of externalizing problems, and, as expected, this group possessed more male members. Cluster 4 provided the same information about a somatizing group of students with predominantly female membership. The second cluster differs from any produced in the three-cluster solution in that it included a group of children suffering from internalizing and externalizing problems. This group is roughly evenly split by gender and, as expected, is small in size relative to the total group. A cluster of children with high levels of emotional and behavioral problems has been noted in previous literature (e.g., Kamphaus, Hubert, DiStefano, & Petoskey, 1997), and so the model including this group may be considered the better choice. The clusters are labeled based on information from the centroids and gender distributions as Externalizing Problems (Cluster 1), General Problems (Cluster 2), Average (Cluster 3), and Internalizing Problems (Cluster 4).

The validation information provides a unique perspective on the using Adaptive Skills and School Problems Scores groups. Children in the Externalizing Problems and General Problems groups were not significantly different from each other on Adaptive Skills, but both groups showed significantly lower levels of these skills than did children in the Average or Internalizing Problems groups. There were no differences between means of students in the Average or Internalizing Problems groups. The same pattern was seen with School Problems. Here, the two clusters exhibiting elevated levels of externalizing subscales showed significantly more problems with adjusting to the school environment than did students in the other two clusters.

Table 36.3 details the fit information for the latent profile analysis solutions. Two different models converged: two- and three-class solutions with variances constrained to be equal and a two-class solution with free variances. The two-class solution with free variances had a lower entropy value but the lowest BIC and the log-likelihood value closest to zero. However, the variable Somatization had to be removed from the analysis for this model solution to produce a solution. Because all six subscales could not be included in the analysis, this solution was not considered further.

TABLE 36.3. Latent Class Cluster Analysis Fit Indices—BASC TRS-C Data, Kindergarten Sample

	Two classes, variances equal	Three classes, variances equal	Two classes, free variance
Global fit			
Log likelihood	–5120	–5006	–4014
Relative fit			
BIC	10344	10155	8069
Uncertainty			
Entropy	.938	.911	.902

Considering the two- and three-class solutions with equal variances, the three-class solution had the lower BIC and higher log-likelihood value. However, one of the classes in this solution was very small, the centroid information was hard to interpret, and the centroid results did not produce a class that matched to prior theory. The two-class solution provided an adequate BIC value and a log-likelihood value that was close to the value reported for the three-class solution. This solution had a high degree of certainty in the classification, as seen by the entropy information and the classification table presented at the top of Table 36.4. As an example of how to interpret the values in a classification table, the relative certainty in the modal assignments shows high values in the diagonal. There were relatively few classification problems, as seen from the low off-diagonal elements. Also, the distinction between groups can be observed. For example, Class 1 has an average prior probability of .987 for children assigned to this group and a low prior probability of group membership in Class 2 (roughly 3%). Besides acceptable fit and uncertainty information, the two-class solution produced estimated parameters for classes of child behavior, which were interpretable and matched prior theory; therefore, this solution was thought to best represent the data. The two-class LPA solution represents two broad classes of behavioral adjustment: typical adjustment and functionally impaired adjustment. Table 36.4 also provides the average centroid information for the classes.

To test developmental stability and change of group membership, an LTA was run using data from the kindergarten and first-grade years and employing the two-class model with variances equal across classes. It is noted that some children had missing data at

TABLE 36.4. Latent Profile Analysis of BASC TRS-C Norm Data: Estimated Parameters

	Class 1: Typical Adjustment (N = 186)	Class 2: Functionally Impaired (N = 54)
Prior probability of class membership		
Class 1	**.987**	.013
Class 2	.033	**.967**
Mixing weight	.78	.22
TRS-C subscales		
Externalizing Problems		
Aggression	46.3 (7.0)	**67.2 (7.0)**
Conduct	47.0 (8.1)	**62.7 (8.1)**
Hyperactivity	45.7 (6.4)	**63.2 (6.4)**
Internalizing Problems		
Anxiety	48.6 (7.1)	55.5 (7.1)
Depression	46.0 (6.8)	59.1 (6.8)
Somatization	50.6 (13.5)	54.0 (13.5)

Note. Variances provided in parentheses next to mean values. **Bolded** values are significant T-values.

the second time point, increasing the sample size for LTA to 194 cases. First, the two-class solution was tested independently in each sample, to ensure that groups with similar definitions were present. These groups (though not reported here) were examined using the same procedures as previously (e.g., examination of parameters and fit) to ensure that similar groups were found. Table 36.5 provides the number of children classified into each of the two classes at each time point. Similar numbers of students were assigned to each class at each time point.

The LTA can examine classification over time by examining transition probabilities (Muthén & Muthén, 2007). These values state the probability of being in a class with a similar definition after the transition point, here noted as the move from kindergarten to first grade. Only one model was tested here, assuming that the transition probability for each class was stable across time; however, much greater flexibility is available in LTA. As with LCC, LTA can accommodate different models, include covariates, relax restrictions with error structures, and recognize different probabilities of class membership over time. Similar fit information is provided with LCC analyses and LTA, so only one model was tested here.

Besides fit information, LTA produces a matrix of transition probabilities that report the probability that an individual is categorized in a class with a similar definition at successive time points. Also reported is the probability of changing class membership over time. This information is presented in a $K \times K$ matrix, where K is the number of latent classes identified at each of the different time points.

The bottom half of Table 36.5 reports the transition probability matrix for behavioral stability and change over the transition period from kindergarten to first grade. Note that table rows sum to a probability of 1, accounting for placement in either category as children are placed into groups between time 1 and time 2. As shown in the table, there is an 87% probability that members in the Typical Adjustment class will remain in that class and a 52% probability that students classified as Functionally Impaired will remain in this class at time 2. Those children who move from one class to another during the 1-year period should

TABLE 36.5. LTA Results, Classification of Children over Time

Number of children classified in each class, by year in school

	Class assignment	
	Typical adjustment	Functionally impaired
Kindergarten	146	46
First grade	151	43

Transitional probabilities of class membership over time

	First grade	
Kindergarten	Typical adjustment	Functionally impaired
Typical adjustment	.87	.13
Functionally impaired	.48	.52

Note. $N = 194$.

be examined with greater detail. For example, 13% of children who were given a rating of Typical Adjustment in kindergarten moved to the Functional Impairment class at time 2. These children may be assessed closer to determine if problems exist, such as difficulties adjusting to the school environment, changes in home environment, or school-related problems, such as learning difficulties or bullying. Similarly, 48% of the children who were classified as Functionally Impaired moved to the Typical Adjustment class in first grade. These students should also be examined to determine whether the changes are due to factors such as greater familiarity with school routines or behavioral and emotional growth.

Future Directions

The need to group individuals with similar characteristics has had a long history in the study of development. One limitation of this chapter is that the viability of solutions in the presence of missing data was not discussed. It is beyond the scope of the chapter to discuss the treatment of missing data in cluster analysis. Methods to treat missing data come with known caveats (e.g., Enders, 2010), and if too much data are lost or imputed, the accuracy of the groups is questionable. As model-based procedures, LCC methods have more flexibility and rigor in the treatment of missing data when compared with cluster analyses. The full information maximum likelihood (FIML) estimator may be applied, so that cases with complete data and cases with missing data are analyzed together and model parameters are adjusted on the basis of all the available information. The area of missing data in person-oriented research holds promise for future study in classification research. For example, techniques may be compared to determine how various methods to treat missing data and different types of missing data perform when various person-oriented analysis strategies are utilized.

Sample size requirements for classification methods have not been specified in detail (Dolnicar, 2003). While the number of cases required will be related to the number of variables included, researchers have yet to determine the variable-to-cases ratio necessary to achieve a stable solution. A recommendation that may hold for both latent class and cluster analyses is to ensure that the minimal sample size is no less than 2^k cases (where k = number of variables), and preferably more than $5*2^k$ (Formann, 1984, as cited in Dolnicar, 2003). Future studies could investigate sample size requirements only over an entire data set, relative to the numbers of variables, a mix of variables from different metrics, and/or using unequal group sizes to provide more detailed recommendations for person-oriented methods.

Additionally, not much is known about the performance of the fit indices in LCC analysis under situations in which the data violate distributional assumptions, include mixed-mode data, or estimate models that vary by sample size or model complexity. Simulations concerning the performance of fit indices and other model selection criteria under LCC models are needed.

In summary, classification methods can be valuable tools in the exploration of human development. Organizing data into subgroups can help researchers identify patterns present in the data. Furthermore, these methods may be used to examine groups at one time point and to determine how individuals change over time. Such analyses have proved useful for describing, predicting, treating, and studying the complexities of human development. Application of classification procedures with empirical research requires care because there are many choices to be made, and criteria for evaluating results are open to interpretation. Careful analysis and execution of the decisions underlying classification will help these methods fulfill their potential as efficient and useful tools for the study of human development.

References

Akaike, H. (1977). On the entropy maximization principle. In P. R. Krishnaiah (Ed.), *Applications of statistics* (pp. 27–41). Amsterdam: North-Holland.

Aldenderfer, M. S., & Blashfield, R. K. (1984). *Cluster analysis*. Beverly Hills, CA: Sage.

Banfield, J. D., & Raftery, A. E. (1993). Model-based Gaussian and non-Gaussian clustering. *Biometrics, 49*, 803–821.

Bergman, L. R. (1998). A pattern-oriented approach to studying individual development: Snapshots and processes. In R. B. Cairns, L. R. Bergman, & J. Kagan (Eds.), *Methods and models for studying the individual* (pp. 83–121). Thousand Oaks, CA: Sage.

Bergman, L. R., & & El-Khouri, B. M. (1999). Studying individual patterns of development using I-states as objects analysis (ISOA). *Biometrical Journal, 6*, 753–770.

Bergman, L. R., & Magnusson, D. (1997). A person-oriented approach in research on developmental psychopathology. *Development and Psychopathology, 9*, 291–319.

Bergman, L. R., Magnusson, D., & El-Khouri, B. M. (2003). *Studying individual development in an interindividual context: A person-oriented approach*. Mahwah, NJ: Erlbaum.

Blashfield, R. K., & Aldenderfer, M. S. (1988). The methods and problems of cluster analysis. In J. R. Nesselroade & R. B. Cattell (Eds.), *International handbook of multivariate experimental psychology* (pp. 311–359). New York: Plenum Press.

Bollen, K. A. (1989). *Structural models with latent variables*. New York: Wiley.

Cantwell, D. P. (1996). Classification of child and adolescent psychopathology. *Journal of Child Psychology and Psychiatry, 37*, 3–12.

Clogg, C. C. (1995). Latent class models. In G. Arminger, C. C. Clogg, & M. E. Sobel (Eds.), *Handbook of statistical modeling for the social and behavioral sciences* (pp. 311–359). New York: Plenum Press.

Collins, L. M., & Lanza, S. T. (2010). *Latent class and latent transition analysis*. Hoboken, NJ: Wiley.

DiStefano, C., Kamphaus, R. W., & Mindrila, D. L. (2010). A typology of teacher-rated child behavior: Revisiting subgroups over 10 years later. *School Psychology Quarterly, 25*, 143–187.

Dolnicar, S. (2003). Using cluster analysis for market segmentation: Typical misconceptions, established methodological weaknesses and some recommendations for improvement. *Australasian Journal of Market Research, 11*, 5–12.

Enders, C. K. (2010). *Applied missing data analysis*. New York: Guilford Press.

Everitt, B. S. (1993). *Cluster analysis* (3rd ed.). New York: Wiley.

Gibson, W. A. (1959). Three multivariate models: Factor analysis, latent structure analysis, and latent profile analysis. *Psychometrika, 24*, 229–252.

Gordon, A. D. (1981). *Classification*. New York: Chapman & Hall.

Heinen, T. (1993). *Discrete latent variable models*. Tilburg, The Netherlands: Tilburg University Press.

Huberty, C. J. (1994). *Applied discriminant analysis*. New York: Wiley.

Huberty, C. J., DiStefano, C., & Kamphaus, R. W. (1997). Behavioral clustering of school children. *Multivariate Behavioral Research, 32*, 105–134.

Kagan, J. (1997). Conceptualizing psychopathology: The importance of developmental profiles. *Development and Psychopathology, 9*, 321–334.

Kamphaus, R. W., & Frick, P. J. (2002). *Clinical assessment of child and adolescent personality and behavior* (2nd ed.). Needham Heights, MA: Allyn & Bacon.

Kamphaus, R. W., Huberty, C. J., DiStefano, C., & Petoskey, M. D. (1997). A typology of teacher rated child behavior for a national U.S. sample. *Journal of Abnormal Child Psychology, 25*, 453–463.

Laursen, B., & Hoff, E. (2006). Person-centered and variable-centered approaches to longitudinal data. *Merrill-Palmer Quarterly, 52*, 377–389.

Lazarsfeld, P. F., & Henry, N. W. (1968). *Latent structure analysis*. Boston: Hougton Mifflin.

Lorr, M. (1983). *Cluster analysis for social scientists: Techniques for analyzing and simplifying complex blocks of data*. San Francisco: Jossey-Bass.

McLachlan, G., & Peel, D. (2000). *Finite mixture models*. New York: Wiley.

Milligan, G. W. (1996). Clustering validation: Results and implications for applied analyses. In P. Arabie, L. J. Hubert, & G. De Soete (Eds.), *Clustering and classification* (pp. 341–375). River Edge, NJ: World Scientific.

Muthén, B. O. (2001). Latent variable mixture modeling. In G. A. Marcoulides & R. E. Schumacker (Eds.), *New developments and techniques in structural equation modeling* (pp. 1–33). Hillsdale, NJ: Erlbaum.

Muthén, B. O., & Muthén, L. K. (2000). Integrating person-centered and variable-centered analyses: Growth mixture modeling with latent trajectory classes. *Alcoholism: Clinical and Experimental Research, 24*, 882–891.

Muthén, L. K., & Muthén, B. O. (2007). *Mplus: User's guide* (5th ed.). Los Angeles: Authors.

Pastor, D. A., Barron, K. E., Miller, B. J., & Davis, S. L. (2007). A latent profile analysis of college students' achievement goal orientation. *Contemporary Educational Psychology, 32*, 8–47.

Reynolds, C. R., & Kamphaus, R. W. (1992). *Behavior Assessment System for Children*. Circle Pines, MN: American Guidance Service.

Richters, J. E. (1997). The Hubble hypothesis and the developmentalists' dilemma. *Development and Psychopathology, 9*, 193–229.

Sarle, W. S. (1983). *Cubic clustering criterion* [SAS Technical Report No. A-108]. Cary, NC: SAS Institute.

Steinley, D. (2003). Local optima in *K*-means clustering: What you don't know may hurt you. *Psychological Methods, 8*, 294–304.

Vermunt, J. K. (2004). Latent profile model. In M. S. Lewis-Beck, A. Bryman, & T. F. Liao (Eds.), *The Sage encyclopedia of social sciences research methods* (pp. 554–555). Thousand Oaks, CA: Sage.

Vermunt, J. K., & Magidson, J. (2002). Latent class cluster analysis. In J. A. Hagenaars & A. L. McCutcheon (Eds.), *Applied latent class analysis* (pp. 89–106). Cambridge, UK: Cambridge University Press.

Ward, J. H. (1963). Hierarchical grouping to optimize an objective function. *Journal of the American Statistical Association, 58*, 236–244.

CHAPTER 37

Meta-Analysis in Developmental Science

MARINUS H. VAN IJZENDOORN
MARIAN J. BAKERMANS-KRANENBURG
LENNEKE R. A. ALINK

Central Issues

Why Meta-Analysis?

More scientists are currently conducting research than the cumulative number of researchers who contributed to social and natural sciences before the middle of the 20th century, and the number of scientific papers published each year is much larger than the total number of papers published by the end of the 19th century. Price proposed that the growing number of scientists, journals, and papers would be best described by an exponential growth curve (Price, 1976). For the number of journals he suggested that the constant involved in this exponential growth is 15 years for a doubling, and for the number of papers he proposed a 10-year period of doubling (Price, 1976). For individual scientists living in the third millennium it has become impossible to keep track of all publications even in their narrow fields of expertise, let alone in the wider area of their (inter)disciplines. Important knowledge is lost from sight before it can influence the course of science or affect policy or practice. Reinvention of lost findings or, worse still, replication of studies without any promise of contributing to science is a costly enterprise.

Meta-analysis is indispensable in an era that is witnessing an overwhelming amount of scientific information. Meta-analysis enables scientists to get easy access to the state of the art in a specific field of inquiry. It also helps to avoid replicating what has already been done more than enough. If the number of similar studies to be done to reject a specific hypothesis runs into thousands—as might be uncovered by Rosenthal's "fail-safe number" (discussed later)—spending scarce resources on another similar investigation is unwarranted (see Bar-Haim, Lamy, Pergamin, Bakermans-Kranenburg, & van IJzendoorn, 2007, for an example). Most important, meta-analysis opens new vistas for theory building and research, as it may show holes in the existing knowledge base and point to critical but neglected areas of investigation.

Meta-analysis is the analysis and synthesis of (primary) empirical studies testing a specific substantive hypothesis or theory. It is a quantitative method to systematize existing experimental, cross-sectional, or longitudinal studies; to present the state of the art in a research domain; and to offer grounded hypotheses for further empirical work. In their authoritative *Handbook of Research Synthesis*, Cooper and Hedges (1994) briefly define meta-analysis as a quantitative synthesis of empirical research for the purpose of creating generalizations (see also Mullen, 1989). Petticrew and Roberts (2006) add the purpose of meta-analysis and define it as a scientific tool to summarize, appraise, and communicate the results and implications of otherwise unmanageable quantities of research. We define meta-analysis in a more formal way as the quantification of the central tendency (combined effect) of a set of study outcomes focusing on a specific hypothesis, the identification of variability in the set, and the explanation of this variability in terms of moderators (study characteristics).

A Brief History of Meta-Analysis

The history of meta-analysis is short and long at the same time. More than a century ago, Karl Pearson (1904) was the first to publish a brief meta-analysis as he reported on a meta-analytical combination of four medical studies on typhus vaccinations. But it would take a long time before meta-analysis was fully endorsed by the medical sciences. The current popularity of meta-analysis in the area of evidence-based medical treatments is reflected in the worldwide Cochrane collaboration of meta-analytic researchers (Grimshaw, Santesso, Cumpston, Mayhew, & McGowan, 2006), which can make or break a new medical intervention or drug. Only 35 years ago, the term *meta-analysis* was introduced in the educational and behavioral sciences by the educational scientist Glass (1976). He performed one of the most controversial meta-analyses ever published. In this meta-analysis on the effectiveness of psychotherapy in 375 studies with 833 study outcomes, Smith and Glass (1977) found that, although psychotherapy was effective (there was a 0.68 standard deviation superiority of the treated group over the control group), there was no significant difference between different types of psychotherapy. Long-term psychoanalysis was as effective as short-term behavior therapy, there was no effect for the kind of training or level of therapeutic experience, and placebo treatment appeared also effective. The findings supported the provocative Dodo bird verdict from *Alice's Adventures in Wonderland*: "*Everybody* has won, and all must have prizes" (Carroll, 1870, Chapter 3).

During the past two decades, the use and impact of meta-analysis have increased a great deal (Figure 37.1). Meta-analysis is used to test scientific theories in an increasing number of disciplines. For example, meta-analysis has become indispensable in molecular genetics (e.g., Guerra & Goldstein, 2010), as well as in cognitive science using fMRI (e.g., Visser, Jefferies, & Ralph, 2010). Some research foundations have started to require a meta-analysis to show that a proposed study is new and pathfinding instead of a superfluous replication of earlier work. Meta-analysis also facilitates the use and interpretation of scientific findings by practitioners, professionals, and policymakers outside the scientific arena. For example, policymakers have to rely on a sound base of empirical findings, and meta-analysis is an outstanding method to integrate and structure the increasing number of

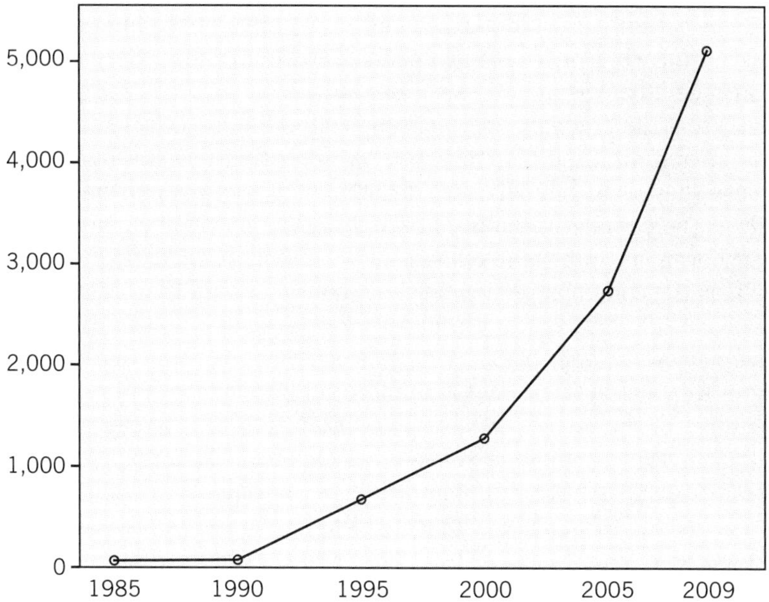

FIGURE 37.1. Number of meta-analyses per year in Web of Science (from 1985 to 2009). A literature search was performed in Web of Science for each of these years using the search term *meta-analy**.

scientific publications (e.g., Reschly, Busch, Betts, Deno, & Long, 2009). Thus the call for evidence-based treatments is becoming louder not only in the medical sciences but also in the behavioral disciplines.

Narrative versus Meta-Analytic Syntheses

Why bother to conduct meta-analyses when the oldest and most established method of integrating scientific literature—the narrative review—is less technical and easier to conduct? In fact, most Ph.D. dissertations still start with an introductory narrative review, and the majority of literature reviews in the developmental disciplines are narrative, sometimes for good reasons. Narrative and quantitative syntheses are surprisingly similar. In many ways narrative and quantitative syntheses serve the same goals and follow the same steps or stages to reach these goals. They both aim at integrating a vast literature from the perspective of a specific theory or hypothesis, and they both try to collect all pertinent studies in a systematic way. Narrative reviews and meta-analyses diverge, however, in the stage of coding the studies and analyzing the data derived from the primary reports. The emphasis in meta-analysis is on replicable procedures for coding the main characteristics of a study and on replicable statistical procedures to analyze the data, taking into account unavoidable sampling errors in testing a hypothesis.

Meta-analyses lead to more reliable, valid, and replicable findings than narrative reviews. In an experimental study Rosenthal (1991) found that narrative reviews may lead to misleading conclusions. He assigned 41 reviewers randomly to two conditions: a group that got basic training in meta-analysis and a comparison group with some training in narrative reviewing. The set of seven empirical studies that these reviewers were asked to synthesize pertained to gender differences in task persistence. The hypothesis was that females would perform boring tasks more persistently than males. Only 27% of the narrative reviewers concluded that the hypothesis was confirmed, whereas 68% of the meta-analysts correctly found that the studies as a whole supported the hypothesis. Narrative reviewers may more often commit Type II errors, that is, accepting the null hypothesis although it is false, because they focus on individual, mostly small studies with small effects, whereas in meta-analysis the cumulative nature of scientific evidence is emphasized. When several small studies show nonsignificant trends, a simple enumeration of these null findings might be misleading, as the combination of studies is more powerful than each individual investigation.

Narrative reviewers not only may be misled by studies with nonsignificant findings based on small samples but also might be more impressionable to or easily influenced by irrelevant features of the studies involved. For example, in their overall conclusions, they might (involuntarily) stress findings from studies conducted at famous research universities or by well-known scientists. They might also be more open to tendentious or provocative titles of papers, leading to an availability bias (Tversky & Kahneman, 1973). Bushman and Wells (2001) asked 280 participants to review 20 fictional studies on the relationship of similarity between people with attraction. Half of the participants were trained in meta-analysis. Although there were some inconsistencies across the studies, there was a positive overall association. The authors manipulated the salience of the titles that the papers carried ("Birds of a Feather Flock Together" vs. "Research Examines Similarity as Source of Liking"), as well as the serial order in which the studies were presented, without changing the results. Participants without meta-analysis training (narrative reviewers) were influenced by the salience manipulation and gave estimates that were biased toward the studies that had salient titles. The rather mechanical process of meta-analysis prevents such human decision-making biases from emerging. Incidentally, the study by Bushman and Wells (2001) also shows the remarkable impact of choice of title on the way findings enter the memory system of the research community.

Meta-analyses thus have great advantages over narrative reviews, but this does not mean that narrative reviews would be obsolete. A meta-analysis is feasible only if the primary studies of interest are empirical rather than theoretical, produce quantitative results rather than qualitative findings, examine the same constructs and relations, have findings that can be configured in a comparable statistical form (e.g., correlation coefficients, odds ratios), and are "comparable" given the question at hand (Petticrew & Roberts, 2006). In many areas of developmental inquiry, these requirements for meta-analysis are not (yet) fulfilled. For example, studies on the development of attachment in middle childhood are not only limited in number but also quite heterogeneous in their use of methods to assess attachment in school-age children. In such a case a critical but balanced narrative approach to this scattered literature may serve the field better than a premature meta-analysis.

The Role of Meta-Analysis in Scientific Research

Primary empirical studies usually test a hypothesis by collecting and analyzing data in a systematic and replicable way. The hypothesis is typically derived from a clearly outlined theory and is often of the following type: Variable *X* (e.g., the quality of parenting) is (causally) related to variable *Y* (e.g., problem behavior of the child). If the result of this primary analysis is disputed because of its unexpected direction or because of alleged flaws in design or statistical methods, secondary analysis of the data may be required. Secondary analysis utilizes the raw data as collected in the original study. By recoding these data or using different strategies for statistical analysis, the original results are put to the test. Secondary analysis may result in a revision of the original results. For example, based on his secondary analysis of Burt's data on the heritability of intelligence in twins, Kamin (1974) concluded that Burt had made up some of the data. However, in many cases, raw data are not available for secondary analysis. This situation creates the need for replication studies, testing the same hypothesis in different participants with slightly different methods, and also for examining the limits of a specific finding in terms of method of measurement, age range, social context, culture, and so forth.

If the number of replication studies increases and if the characteristics of these replication studies slightly differ (but not too much), meta-analysis is possible. Whereas secondary analysis uses raw data, meta-analysis is based on the published outcomes of different studies. In meta-analysis the mean effect size of all studies testing the same hypothesis is investigated. In addition, meta-analysis can test to what extent the variations in study characteristics (i.e., sample and design characteristics) can explain differences in effect sizes and trace these differences back to, for example, developmental processes. For example, Alink and colleagues (2008) found that cortisol levels were positively related to externalizing behavior in preschoolers, but this relation was negative in school-age children.

Meta-analysis combines the strengths of many individual studies. However, meta-analyses need to be replicated as well. Numerous decisions about the collection, coding, and analyses of primary effect sizes are made in the process of a meta-analysis. It is even possible that replication results in different findings due to an error in the original meta-analysis (see De Wolff & van IJzendoorn, 1997, for an example). Even if replication yields similar results, meta-analysis is not the end of the scientific research process. A fruitful meta-analysis generates new research, with new hypotheses on a higher level of specification and precision than could be obtained before the earlier findings had been combined meta-analytically. An example of the heuristic value of meta-analysis is the discovery of the so-called "transmission gap" in studies on intergenerational transmission of attachment (van IJzendoorn, 1995a, 1995b). A meta-analytic combination of studies on the associations between parental attachment representation, parenting behavior, and children's attachment security showed that parental sensitivity could explain only one-fifth of the association between parents' and children's attachment. This "transmission gap" has been the target of numerous studies on attachment in the past decade (e.g., Fonagy & Target, 2005). Figure 37.2 presents a process model of the different steps in scientific research.

Conceptual Principles and Statistical Assumptions

The different stages of meta-analytic research greatly resemble those of primary empirical research (Cooper & Hedges, 1994). Primary studies consist of the following stages: formulating a hypothesis, collecting data, coding raw data, analyzing data, and interpreting and publishing the findings. The stages of meta-analysis run parallel to the empirical research stages: formulating a hypothesis and conducting a quantitative conceptual analysis if needed, systematically collecting the pertinent literature in various databases with different strategies; coding raw data into effect sizes and moderator variables (study characteristics); analyzing data, taking into account the specific nature of meta-analytic data derived

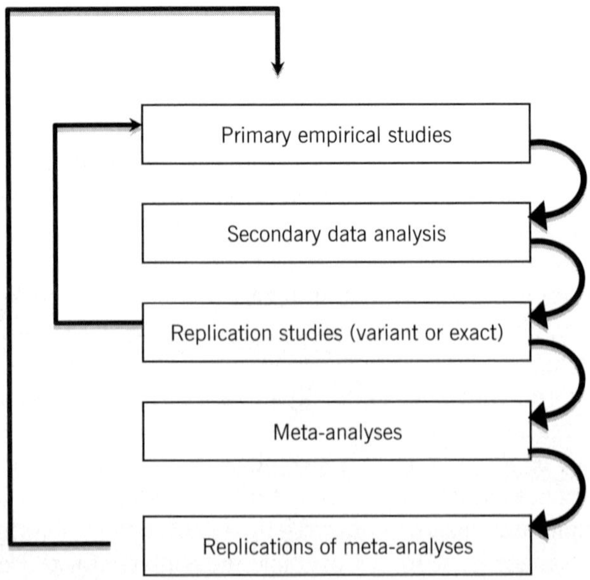

FIGURE 37.2. Process model of studies and analyses.

from samples with varying sizes; and interpreting and publishing the findings. Similar to empirical studies, all stages have to be followed in a systematic and replicable way. Independent research teams going through the meta-analytic stages in a systematic fashion should be able to come to the same conclusions. For example, a coding system is used to quantify the information derived from the empirical papers, resulting in quantitative variables that can be used as moderators in the meta-analyses. Similar to primary empirical research, sufficient intercoder reliability should be established for coders using the coding system to guarantee its replicability.

There are three main steps in the data analysis (Mullen, 1989). First, the combined effect across all studies is computed. Second, the variability of individual effect sizes around the combined effect size is determined and outliers and homogeneous subsets of study outcomes are explored. Third, an attempt is made to explain the variability in effect sizes: Which (moderator) variables from the coding system are responsible for the variability in study outcomes? In turn, interpretation of these results can lead to new hypotheses for future research.

Formulating a Hypothesis, Conceptual Analysis

A crucial step in performing a meta-analysis is formulating a specific hypothesis. This hypothesis needs to be significant to a broad (research) audience (Rosenthal, 1991, 1995), and it needs to cover a domain that would be difficult to explore without a meta-analysis. For example, it is difficult to imagine a single empirical study using both a dot probe and a Stroop paradigm in order to test priming effects in anxious children of various ages. Only meta-analysis allows for comparisons of such diverging paradigms across many studies (Bar-Haim et al., 2007). However, another important feature of the hypothesis is specificity, because the results need to contribute to the rejection, acceptance, or adaptation of a specific theory. For example, it would be less interesting to test whether interventions in general are effective (Lipsey & Wilson, 1993) than to test which types of family interventions would be effective in which types of families at what stage in child development—for example, a video feedback intervention or a purely supportive program (Bakermans-Kranenburg, van IJzendoorn, & Juffer, 2003).

Conceptual analysis may be a prerequisite for a meta-analysis. The questions to be addressed in an early stage of the meta-analysis are what belongs to the domain of the meta-analysis and, within that domain, how can it be carved up in subdomains so that focused analyses can be conducted? For example, in a meta-analysis on parenting styles and relational aggression in children, 76 different parenting constructs were identified in the studies that were selected for inclusion. This is a bewildering variety of potentially relevant dimensions of parenting styles that needs to be condensed into a manageable set of related constructs. Therefore, each construct was described on a separate card, and 15 experts in the field of parenting (at graduate level or above and actively involved in research on parenting) were asked to sort the cards into 10 groups. Each of the groups had to contain at least one card. The same numerical code was given to parenting constructs that were sorted in the same group by a specific expert. Constructs that were sorted into different groups received different numerical codes. A multiple correspondence analysis and a subsequent two-step cluster analysis resulted in four different clusters of related parenting constructs. Separate meta-analyses were conducted for each of these four clusters in order to provide precise answers to the question of what parenting style (e.g., harsh parenting or permissive parenting) is most effective in elevating or decreasing the level of aggression in children (Kawabata, Alink, Tseng, van IJzendoorn, & Crick, in press).

Collecting Data: Studies and Effect Sizes

The second phase in a meta-analysis is the collection of relevant effect sizes reported in papers, book chapters, dissertations, and so forth. Collecting these effect sizes needs to be done systematically, and future researchers need to be able to replicate this process (see the MOOSE criteria for publishing meta-analyses; Stroup et al., 2000). Multiple methods should be used to collect a data set of effect sizes, and thus studies, that is as complete as possible. As a rule of thumb, at least three different methods of data collection might be applied. The most common methods are the digital search in the electronic library, the "snowball" method, and the "expert" method. The digital method utilizes databases such as ERIC, PsycLIT, MEDLINE, Dissertation Abstracts, Google Scholar, and citation indices such as Social Sciences Citation Index (SSCI), Science Citation Index (SCI; emphasis on journal articles), and Publish or Perish (PoP; also including books and book chapters). The snowball method refers to searching reference lists of literature reviews, previous meta-analyses, and empirical papers in order to find references that did not appear in the electronic search. Finally, experts can be consulted about the latest developments in the specific research field. For example, experts can inform the meta-analytic researcher about papers in preparation, conference presentations, dissertations, and other unpublished data. The digital method is the most sound and systematic method that covers the largest time period. Its main limitation concerns the emphasis on journal papers and contributions in English in the digital data files.

The most difficult issue in this phase of the data collection is the "file drawer problem" (Rosenthal, 1991). Researchers know that it is more likely that a paper will be published in which significant findings in the expected direction are reported as compared with a paper reporting nonsignificant or unexpected results, even though the quality of the research is similar. As a consequence, the majority of the relevant studies may end up in the disappointed researchers' file drawers, whereas only a small percentage of the available studies are published because these studies report on significant results. In such a situation a meta-analysis generates skewed results if the unpublished studies are not taken into account. A meta-analysis without these studies may reject the null hypothesis (based on the significant and thus published results), whereas in reality the combined effect size might not be significant, and the null hypothesis should not be rejected. Hence it is extremely important to collect as many unpublished studies as possible, even if the quality of these studies is sometimes questionable. The quality of the research can be included as a moderator variable in the coding system and in the analyses to test the effect of the research quality on study outcomes.

As a matter of fact, researchers should deal with the file drawer problem at its root. It would be helpful if journal editors and reviewers would base their decisions to accept or reject a paper on the hypotheses, research design, and methods, without information about the results (Cooper & Hedges, 1994), but this type of "blind review" most certainly will encounter opposition from journals and their publishers in search of headlines in the media about positive findings. With the emergence of electronic journals, the ideal reviewing procedure might become an attainable goal.

Given the current publication policies, meta-analytic researchers should try to estimate the number of unpublished studies with nonsignificant results that would be needed to reduce the meta-analytic result to nonsignificant (the "fail-safe number"; Rosenthal, 1991). Rosenthal (1991) proposed to use the criterion of $5k + 10$ to evaluate the fail-safe number. If the fail-safe number were smaller than 5 times the number of studies in the meta-analysis plus 10, the chance of the meta-analytic outcome being significantly affected by missing studies would be too large. Orwin (1983) refined this approach by suggesting a higher threshold for the original nonsignificance criterion of Rosenthal, creating the possibility of computing the fail-safe number on the basis of a specific just relevant effect size.

A more recent statistical approach to estimating the influence of the file drawer problem is the so-called "trim and fill" method (Duval & Tweedie, 2000a, 2000b) to calculate the effect of potential data censoring ("missing data") on the outcome of meta-analyses. Using this method, a funnel plot is constructed of each study's effect size against the sample size or the standard error. These plots should be shaped like a funnel if no data censoring is present. However, because smaller or nonsignificant studies are less likely to be retrieved, studies in the bottom left-hand corner of the plot are often missing (Sutton, Duval, Tweedie, Abrams, & Jones, 2000). Therefore, the k right-most studies considered to be symmetrically unmatched are trimmed. The trimmed studies are replaced and their missing counterparts imputed or "filled" as mirror images of the trimmed outcomes. This allows the computation of an adjusted overall combined effect size and confidence interval (Gilbody, Song, Eastwood, & Sutton, 2000; Sutton et al., 2000; see van IJzendoorn, Juffer, & Klein Poelhuis, 2005, for an example of the "trim and fill" method in a meta-analysis on IQ, school achievement, and language in adopted and nonadopted children).

Fortunately, the effect of unpublished manuscripts is usually rather small. Unpublished studies do not considerably differ from published papers. Rosenthal (1991) found differences in combined effect sizes of only 0.07 (Cohen's d) between meta-analyses that did include unpublished results and ones that did not. Dissertations appeared to be responsible for the largest difference. They frequently show modest and nonsignificant effect sizes, and as a result they often do not get published, although the research is generally of sufficient quality. Leaving dissertations out of a meta-analysis can result in a difference in effect sizes of $d = 0.20$, indicating that dissertations generally show considerably lower effect sizes than published studies. It is thus important to include dissertations in a meta-analysis.

Coding System

A coding system for moderators and statistical information is an indispensable part of each meta-analysis. At least four different types of variables should be included. First, substantive issues related to the hypothesis should be covered. For example, in developmental meta-analyses, the age of the participants is critical information, as well as the developmental domain covered by a particular study. Second, the source of the information should be included, that is, whether the study was published in a journal or a dissertation. Third, design features might be important, for example, whether the study was cross-sectional or longitudinal and whether and to what percentage attrition occurred. Fourth, characteristics of outcome measures (e.g., self-report or observational) and statistical information about the outcome (sample size, effect size) should be included. Coding systems should be quantitative, providing either well-defined categories or continuous scales (close-ended items). The intercoder reliability should be established in terms of chance-corrected statistics such as kappas (for categorical moderators) and intraclass correlations (for continuous moderators).

An important question is whether coders should rate quality of the studies. Of course, meta-analysis is dependent on the quality of the primary studies, and the validity of its conclusions cannot go beyond the validity of the findings in the original studies. If the quality of the synthesized studies is bad or insufficient, a meta-analysis cannot produce much more than GiGo (Garbage-in-Garbage-out) bytes of information. Some meta-analysts even argue that a meta-analysis should be based only on the most valid studies, leaving out less than optimally designed studies. Slavin (1995), for example, opted for a "best evidence" synthesis in educational research, selecting studies on design quality.

The problem, however, is how to evaluate quality of empirical studies. Peters and Ceci (1982) showed how subjective quality ratings can be in behavioral disciplines. They selected one paper from each of 12 APA journals, published about 2 years earlier. The papers were above average in terms of their impact (number of citations). They changed the papers slightly by replacing the authors' names with fictitious names and did the same with the institutional affiliations. Then they resubmitted the papers. Remarkably, only 3 of 12 papers were detected as resubmissions. Most surprisingly, 8 out of the remaining 9 papers were rejected because of "serious methodological flaws." Only 13% of the 30 reviewers and editors recommended publication.

This experiment shows the low intercoder agreement for study quality. We recommend including in the coding system proxies for study quality that might indicate some aspect of quality but to avoid rating study quality in more general terms. For example, it might make a difference for study quality whether or not the paper was published in a peer-reviewed journal (even with the flawed procedures just described), what impact status the journal has, and whether specific features of the design (such as random sampling) are in place. These variables can be used as moderators to test whether they have a significant effect on the meta-analytic outcome. For example, in our meta-analyses of studies examining the effects of the Holocaust on first-, second-, and third-generation survivors, we found that the effects were systematically biased when studies used convenience sampling—that is, when participants were recruited from membership lists of Holocaust memorial or support groups instead of randomly drawn from municipality registers (van IJzendoorn, Bakermans-Kranenburg, & Sagi-Schwartz, 2003). Thus bad studies may inflate meta-analytic findings, but we should try to quantify this bias instead of rejecting bad studies a priori.

Statistical Analyses

This section presents some essential meta-analytic procedures to deal with a set of study outcomes and addresses some basic assumptions of meta-analysis and some decisions about the data that have to be made in the meta-analytic process. This section does not pretend to provide sufficiently detailed guidelines for the statistical analysis of meta-analytic data sets. We discuss some basic assumptions and preferred analytical approaches and refer the reader to more detailed treatises of meta-analysis for further guidance (e.g., Lipsey & Wilson, 2001).

The raw data for meta-analysis are the outcomes reported in the pertinent studies. An essential difference between statistical analyses of primary empirical data (derived from a sample of participants) and meta-analysis (based on the outcomes of primary studies) is the variety of effect sizes and sample sizes that constitute meta-analytic data. If sample sizes differ, the precision of the estimates derived from the studies varies, and meta-analytic techniques should take this variety into account by weighting more precise estimates more heavily than less precise estimates. Furthermore, in many domains of inquiry a variety of methods are used, from experimental designs to correlational studies, and the various statistics derived from these studies have to be transformed into a common effect size that is comparable across different designs.

Weighting Study Outcomes

An effect size based on 100 participants is a more "precise" estimate of the population effect size than is an effect size based on 10 participants. Therefore, larger studies should carry more weight in meta-analyses than smaller studies. A simple approach would be to weight each effect size by its sample size. And, in fact, the conventional weighting of correlations used as effect size is $N - 3$ (Lipsey & Wilson, 2001). A statistically more broadly applicable approach is to weight the effect size of a study by the inverse variance. In principle, any weight would do if there are good arguments for using it; for example, in some cases smaller samples may even generate more valid effect sizes than large samples and thus might be weighted more heavily because of quality considerations. But for the inverse variance a statistical theory has been developed (e.g., Cooper & Hedges, 1994), and this has become a unique convention in meta-analytic approaches.

Common Ground for Various Study Outcomes

The issue of a common denominator for various outcomes of individual empirical studies has been addressed by choosing a set of effect sizes that are independent of sample size and can be transformed into each other easily. There are many types of effect size measures, each suited to different research situations. Each type of effect size may also have multiple methods of computation. Three effect sizes are especially popular in the field of developmental research: standardized mean difference (Cohen's *d* or Hedges's *g* [for small samples]), odds ratio, and the correlation coefficient. The standardized mean difference is characteristic of group contrast studies, such as experiments, case-control designs, or comparisons between naturally occurring groups (e.g., gender). The outcome variables are continuous. In the case of dichotomous outcome variables, the odds ratio is the preferred effect size. Correlation coefficients are used in nonexperimental studies with continuous variables. If one of the variables is dichotomous, the preferred statistics at the level of the primary study are the Student *t* or the Fisher *F* ratio, but both can and should be transformed into a correlation coefficient as the common denominator across studies with different designs. *F* and *t* are highly dependent on sample size, and only a transformation to the correlation coefficient via the associated *p*-value and sample size allows these statistics to be entered as effect sizes into meta-analysis. Correlations should be transformed into Fisher *Z* when they are used in multivariate analyses and a well-distributed variable is required: Fisher *Z* has better distributional characteristics than Pearson correlations (Mullen, 1989). Effect sizes such as Cohen's *d* or Pearson correlation can be compared across studies with varying sample sizes and thus can be used as genuine effect sizes.

A Preference for Random Models

Combining individual effect sizes into an overall combined effect size for the total set of studies is rather straightforward. It is the average of the weighted effect sizes for which a standard error and confidence interval can be computed. How the confidence interval is computed depends on the homogeneity of the set of studies. Fixed effects models are based on the assumption that effect sizes observed in a study estimate the corresponding population effect with random error that stems only from the chance factors associated with subject-level sampling error in that study (Lipsey & Wilson, 2001; Rosenthal, 1995). This assumption is not made in random effects models (Hedges & Olkin, 1985). Random effects models allow for the possibility that there are random differences between studies that are associated with variations in procedures, measures, and settings that go beyond subject-level sampling error and thus point to different study populations (Lipsey & Wilson, 2001). Whether fixed or random models can be used depends on the homogeneity of the set of effect sizes. To test the homogeneity of the overall and specific sets of effect sizes, a *Q*-statistic can be computed, although this *Q* has been shown to be rather conservative for small sets of studies (Borenstein, Rothstein, & Cohen, 2005). In general, Borenstein, Hedges, Higgins, and Rothstein (2009) recommend choosing the safe way and always applying the random effects model because fixed and random models converge as long as study sets are homogeneous, whereas in cases of heterogeneous sets the random estimates are more adequate.

It is crucial to include each study and each study participant only once in a meta-analysis. For example, when multiple measures of externalizing behaviors are used within one study, first a meta-analysis on the effect sizes for the different measures of externalizing behavior within the study should be conducted, and then the combined effect size of the study should be included in the final meta-analytic data set. On the other hand, when papers report results separately for boys and girls, it might be advisable to include them separately in the meta-analytic data set. Gender might be tested as an important moderator. This approach might still guarantee that independent outcomes are used in the meta-analysis if one assumes that boys and girls received independent treatments or assessments. Of course, if studies use idiosyncratic procedures, the subset of boys and of girls within the same study may differ less than similar gender groupings across studies, and in that case creating a moderator to indicate whether gender is potentially nonindependent and testing whether this affects the meta-analytic findings is necessary. A similar caveat and procedure is advisable in case of multiple subsets of participants or study outcomes within the same investigation.

Moderator Analysis Is Central to Meta-Analysis

Explaining the variability in effect sizes across individual studies is a major goal of meta-analysis, and a more important one than the goal of providing an overall combined effect size. Moderators such as age, ethnicity, or gender of the participants might explain why in some studies effect sizes are generally small and in other subsets larger. Heterogeneous sets of studies cannot adequately be represented by a single combined effect size, as this may hide bimodal or otherwise skewed distributions of effect sizes. Such heterogeneous data sets leave room for a search for significant moderators. Ideally a moderator divides a heterogeneous set of studies into different homogeneous subsets, for example by splitting a bimodal distribution of effect sizes into two unimodal parts (e.g., one for children who were adopted before 12 months of age and one for children who were adopted after their first birthdays). The combined effect sizes for each of the subsets adequately represent the major trend within those subsets.

To test the influence of categorical moderators, meta-analysis uses an analog to the regular analysis of variance. For example, if gender is a potentially important moderator, the variation of the effect sizes within each subset of studies—boys, girls, mixed—is computed with the Q-statistic. The total variance Q_{total} is partitioned into Q_{between} and Q_{within}. Q_{total} is the variance with any grouping factors ignored, and Q_{within} for each group refers to the variances in the three specific subsets of studies (boys, girls, and mixed). $Q_{\text{between}} = Q_{\text{total}} - Q_{\text{within}}$ and is tested for significance using the chi-square distribution (Borenstein, Hedges, Higgins, & Rothstein, 2009). A significant Q-value for the comparison indicates that the variation between subsets of studies is larger than that within a subset of study outcomes and that the difference in effect size between subsets of studies is significant.

To test the (combined) influence of continuous moderators, transformation of effect sizes into Fisher's Z scores or similar well-distributed effect sizes is needed, and these should be used in multivariate metaregression. Metaregression is based on weighted least squares regression analysis (Borenstein et al., 2009; Lipsey & Wilson, 2001) that takes the specific nature of meta-analytic data into account. Weight is the inverse of the variance for Fisher Z. Weighted regression leads to the same parameter estimates (R-squared, B-weights, etc.) as a regular regression, but the regular regression F-tests, t-tests, and associated probabilities and standard errors are incorrect statistics for metaregression. In weighted regression correct standard errors for B are computed by dividing the standard error by the square root of the mean square residual. In a last step a z test for significance can be conducted by dividing the unstandardized B by the corrected standard error (see Lipsey & Wilson, 2001, for computational examples).

Developmental Applications

Although meta-analysis has not frequently been used to address specific developmental issues, somewhat narrowly defined as the development of specific traits and abilities across larger stretches of the lifespan, this approach can certainly be brought to bear on a variety of critical developmental questions. Of course, in such developmental applications time is a crucial moderator, and meta-analysis can cover a time span that almost no single empirical longitudinal study can manage, simply because of limited funding and restricted human resources. Meta-analysis may serve as a surrogate cross-sequential investigation that combines cross-sectional and longitudinal methods to cover a longer part of the lifespan.

A nice example of this use of meta-analysis is provided by Ferguson's (2010) investigation on the question of whether personality, both normal and disordered, can change significantly or is mainly stable across the lifespan. Ferguson found 47 studies on the stability of personality and temperament (e.g., the Big Five) in children and adults (N = 30,990). The studies each covered varying but restricted periods of development, and meta-analysis used this variety to create a picture of personality development from 0 to 83 years of age. Examining stability trends over the lifespan, the author showed that personality is moderately stable during childhood, increases in stability in the teen years, peaks in stability around age 30, and remains stable from that point forward.

Several meta-analyses that included age as a moderator or potential predictor of variation in effect sizes between studies found no significant age effects. Because of the large power of meta-analyses that contain dozens of studies and thousands of participants, these null findings are developmentally informative as well. In a meta-analysis on antipathetic relationships, or relationships based on mutual dislike, Card (2010) collected 26 studies consisting of over 23,000 children and adolescents and found that the prevalence of antipathetic relationships was about 35% in children and adolescents. Age of assessment was not associated with prevalence rate, indicating that prevalence does not increase or decrease across the time frame studied. Similarly, in a meta-analysis of 69 samples (N = 5,947) on insecure and disorganized attachments as risk factors for externalizing problems, Fearon, Bakermans-Kranenburg, van IJzendoorn, Lapsley, and Roisman (2010) found that age did not moderate the association between disorganized and insecure attachment and level of externalizing behaviors and that the time period between the assessments of attachment and externalizing behavior did not predict variation in effect sizes either. The authors concluded that disorganized and insecure attachment influence externalizing behaviors both in the short and long run.

Meta-analysis might also be used to examine the developmental (dis)continuity of associations between developmental variables. The literature on cortisol production and externalizing behavior shows contrasting associations, although the prevailing hypothesis proposes an inverse relation between cortisol (re)activity and externalizing behavior. Externalizing behaviors would be associated with hypo(re)activity of the physiological systems, including the hypothalamic–pituitary–adrenal (HPA) axis, as aggression and other forms of externalizing behavior would have the function of "jazzing up" the system so that individuals with low activity of the physiological stress systems are aroused, which gives them a pleasant feeling and at the same time lowers the threshold for undertaking risky activities. Alink and colleagues (2008) tested this hypothesis in two meta-analyses, one for basal cortisol (k = 72 studies, N = 5,480) and one for cortisol reactivity to a stressor (k =

29 studies, $N = 2{,}601$). Overall, the meta-analyses showed that there was a small but significant relation between basal level of cortisol and externalizing behavior, whereas cortisol reactivity was not consistently associated with externalizing behavior. However, children's age was a significant moderator of the relation between cortisol and externalizing behavior in our meta-analysis on basal cortisol and externalizing behavior. The association between cortisol and externalizing behaviors in the subset of studies with children of preschool age was significantly different from the one in the subset of school-age studies. Higher levels of externalizing behavior were associated with higher basal levels of cortisol (hyperactivity) in preschoolers and with lower basal levels of cortisol (hypoactivity) in school-age children. There was no significant relation between cortisol and externalizing behavior in adolescents (Alink et al., 2008). Meta-analytically, this intriguing pattern of results could not be explained by the available moderators. In single, short-term longitudinal studies, however, this developmental reversal of the association between cortisol and externalizing would have remained hidden. In this case meta-analysis generates new hypotheses to be investigated in the next generation of developmental studies.

In developmental applications of meta-analysis, age is one of the central moderators, as is evident from the examples just discussed. It is, however, not always easy to classify studies according to the age of their participants and to deal with the unavoidable heterogeneity in age ranges between the various studies. One might argue that age should be coded in a categorical way, to cover specific stages of development, if the meta-analyst wants to test a developmental stage perspective. In contrast, one might decide to use age as a continuous moderator because development is assumed to be a continuous process. Such principled decisions often are wrecked by the limitations of the data at hand. In most cases the pragmatics of a real-life meta-analysis lead to categorizing age into sets of studies that contain a sufficient number of effect sizes (minimally four) in order to have sufficient power to test age differences statistically. If studies report on several assessments across time, and if it is of interest to examine a developmental phenomenon across the largest possible age range, it is logical to choose the first and the last assessments in a study for inclusion in two meta-analyses (comparing the 85% confidence intervals of the effect sizes because the data are not independent) or the largest possible time difference between a predictor and outcome in a longitudinal study. Often the set of pertinent studies is too small and heterogeneous in terms of design and timing of assessments to be able to choose between various alternatives for the meta-analytic treatment of age.

Illustrations

Example 1: Parental Antecedents of Infant Attachment Security

The meta-analysis on parental antecedents of infant attachment security (De Wolff & van IJzendoorn, 1997) illustrates not only the fruitful combination of a quantitative conceptual analysis and a meta-analysis but also the influence of such an endeavor on the field: The study has been cited almost 500 times since its publication (Web of Science, June 8, 2010) without decline over time; for example, it was referred to 65 times in 2008 alone. The aim of the study was to quantify the association between parenting behavior and infant attachment. Ever since the conception of attachment theory, maternal sensitivity had been considered an important condition for the development of a secure attachment relationship between infant and parent, but the various empirical studies used different operationalizations of the concept "sensitivity." Thus we conducted a conceptual analysis. We identified the different operationalizations or constructs of sensitivity used in the total set of studies relating maternal behavior to infant attachment, and we asked experts in the field to sort those constructs that were not self-evident. The sorting task consisted of 40 cards, each describing a specific construct but without information about the source or the empirical findings related to that construct. The experts were instructed to sort the cards into groups of relatively similar operationalizations of sensitivity. These sortings were analyzed with homogeneity analysis (HOMALS; see also SPSS CATPCA). This analysis makes use of a distance model; concepts that are sorted more frequently into the same group are depicted close to each other in a graphical configuration. In the next step, hierarchical cluster analysis was used to distinguish five clusters, each consisting of sensitivity constructs that (according to the experts) were closely related. These clusters or domains of sensitivity could be characterized as, in order, Synchrony, Mutuality, Support, Positive Attitude, and Stimulation. Synchrony, for instance, reflects the extent to which interactions are reciprocal and mutually rewarding (Isabella, Belsky, & Von Eye, 1989), whereas Stimulation can be described as any action on the part of the mother directed to the baby (Miyake, Chen, & Campos, 1985). Based on this conceptual analysis, the studies were grouped according to the domain of sensitivity measured in the specific study, resulting in subsets of studies with similar types of parenting behavior.

In the meta-analysis, we were now able to compute the strength of the association between parenting and attachment for each domain of maternal behavior without mixing apples and oranges (De Wolff & van IJzendoorn, 1997, p. 573). Because some studies included more than one parenting dimension, it was necessary to randomly select one effect size per study for the overall effect size, which was $r = .19$ (95% CI, .16–.22). It was shown that samples with older infants showed stronger effects than samples with younger infants. Comparing the conceptually homogeneous sets of studies that followed from the conceptual analysis, it could be shown that the correlation between maternal behavior and infant attachment security was highest for the set of studies in the cluster Mutuality ($r = .32$, 95% CI, .18–.46), which refers mainly to the mother's skill at modulating the baby's arousal (Kiser, Bates, Maslin, & Bayles, 1986). The meta-analysis also showed that the quality and quantity of physical contact between mother and child and the mere promptness of mother's response to the infant's signals showed relatively weak associations with infant attachment security—important results to take into account when developing interventions to promote secure attachment relationships.

It should be noted that although this meta-analysis presented correlational and not causal evidence for the association between maternal sensitivity and infant attachment security, the direction of the effect was supported in a different meta-analysis: Interventions that were more effective in enhancing parental sensitivity turned out to be also more effective in enhancing attachment security (Bakermans-Kranenburg et al., 2003). Interestingly, interventions starting 6 months after birth or later were more effective in enhancing maternal sensitivity and attachment security than interventions that started prenatally or earlier in the infant's life. This might imply that interventions have the most impact when they are implemented in the period of the formation of a selective attachment relationship (Bakermans-Kranenburg, van IJzendoorn, & Juffer, 2005).

Example 2: Dopamine-Related Genes as Susceptibility Factors

Our second example concerns a meta-analysis testing gene-by-environment (G × E) interaction effects. This is a relatively young branch of science, but, booming as the number of G × E studies is, meta-analysis is necessary to keep track of the progress and to show which results are replicated and which are not. Kim-Cohen and colleagues (2006), for instance, showed meta-analytically that the famous Caspi and colleagues (2002) result that the monoamine oxidase A (MAOA) genotype moderated associations between adverse environment and antisocial outcomes held when combined with the results of four other pertinent studies. The combined effect size for the association between maltreatment and later mental health problems was larger for individuals for whom the MAOA genotype conferred low levels of the MAOA enzyme than for individuals with a high-activity MAOA genotype.

In our own study we tested the role of dopamine-related genes as a susceptibility factor interacting with the rearing environment "for better and for worse"; that is, increasing children's susceptibility to both the adverse effects of unsupportive environments and the beneficial effects of supportive rearing (Belsky, Bakermans-Kranenburg, & van IJzendoorn, 2007; Boyce & Ellis, 2005). The dopaminergic system is engaged in attentional, motivational, and reward mechanisms (Robbins & Everitt, 1999); lower dopaminergic signaling impedes negative feedback-based learning (Klein et al., 2007) and is related to stronger preference for immediate reinforcers (Tripp & Wickens, 2008). We collected all G × E studies on children up to 10 years of age involving dopamine-related genes (*DRD2, DRD4, DAT1*). The cumulative negative effects of these "risk genes" and adverse rearing environments have been stressed, but potentially cumulative positive effects of these same genes interacting with positive rearing environments have remained largely unnoticed. We identified 15 pertinent effect sizes, providing data for two meta-analyses (Bakermans-Kranenburg & van IJzendoorn, 2011). Nine effect sizes concerned vulnerability, that is, moderation by dopamine-related "risk alleles" (*DRD2-A1, DAT-10repeat, DRD4–7repeat*) of the association between adverse rearing environment and behavioral disturbance, such as externalizing behavior, sensation seeking, and attention-deficit/hyperactivity disorder (ADHD). Six effect sizes pertained to the relation between supportive contexts (e.g., warm, responsive parenting) and positive behavioral outcomes such as effortful control or prosocial behavior—enabling a focus on the "bright side."

The combined effect size for vulnerability, that is, behavioral disturbance in the presence of adverse rearing influences, amounted to $r = .37$ (95% CI, .20 ~ .51) for carriers of the "risk alleles," whereas the combined effect size for the comparisons without the "risk alleles" was $r = .10$ (95% CI, –.07 ~ .26). The difference was significant, supporting the idea that carriers of the "risk alleles" were more vulnerable to environmental adversity. However, on the bright side, that is, the association between parental support and better adaptation, we also found a combined effect size of $r = .31$ (95% CI, .16 ~ .44) for carriers of the putatively "risk alleles" and a combined effect size for children without the "risk alleles" of $r = -.03$ (95% CI, –.14 ~ .07). These effect sizes were also significantly different. Children with genotypes that in adverse contexts put them at risk for behavioral disturbances benefited significantly more from parental support than their counterparts.

Studies could contribute to the meta-analysis of vulnerability studies *and* the meta-analysis of the bright side when they reported negative as well as positive environmental or outcome measures. Although the same result was never used twice, children could be included in both meta-analyses and, as a result, it was impossible to directly compare effect sizes across the two sets (i.e., to test whether children with the "risk alleles" were more susceptible to negative rearing effects compared with supportive rearing effects). Therefore, the 85% confidence intervals for the point estimates of the combined effect sizes were computed: Nonoverlapping 85% CIs suggest a significant difference between combined effect sizes that nevertheless are not independent (Goldstein & Healy, 1995; van IJzendoorn et al., 2005). The 85% confidence intervals for negative and positive outcomes for children with the "risk alleles" were overlapping, indicating no difference between the combined effect sizes. In other words children with the putative risk alleles were equally susceptible to negative and supportive influences.

Thus, although based on a relatively small number of studies, our meta-analysis provided support for the hypothesis that seemingly "vulnerable" individuals are actually more susceptible to the environment for better *and* for worse. Incidentally, for our meta-analyses we distilled several effect sizes that in the context of their primary studies were not considered particularly relevant or interesting, as these studies focused on genetic risks. They enabled us, however, to show that dopamine-related genes that, through their influence on attention and reward mechanisms, make children more vulnerable to negative parenting may in fact turn out to be susceptibility genes that in supportive environments promote optimal development.

Future Directions

For several reasons, the role of meta-analysis in human development research will become increasingly important in the near future. First of all, research in this area is often very labor-intensive and time-consuming because observations and field experiments are used, and therefore these studies are usually small scaled. As a result, the statistical power is limited, and there is a risk of accepting the null hypothesis even if this null hypothesis proves to be false in case of a larger sample size. Meta-analysis combines the strength of the relatively small-scale studies and increases the value of research yielding nonsignificant results because of small sample sizes.

Second, meta-analysis is of critical importance for policymakers and professionals working in the area of psychology and education. Policymakers often search for a scientific base for their ideas, for example, regarding the implementation of a new system for preschool education. These types of decisions need to be based on sound scientific evidence. Evidence-based developmental practice will be highly appreciated or even mandated by funding agencies and patients. Meta-analyses are needed to provide this much-needed scientific evidence.

In order to make meta-analysis more effective in summarizing and analyzing trends in developmental studies, we need to pay explicit attention to age as a moderator that might explain variation in study outcomes. With the increase in numbers of cross-sectional and short-term longitudinal studies across many developmental domains, ever more opportunities emerge for meta-analytic researchers to contribute to developmental science in substantial ways. Because in many studies age is included just by convenience, the meta-analyst may work with unbiased age-related data that are not contaminated by assumptions or preconceptions of researchers or participants. The archives of empirical studies that included age on a routine basis might turn out to be a genuine gold mine of meta-analytic data and hypotheses. A concerted effort to exploit this gold mine might be needed, parallel to the Cochrane network (*www.thecochranelibrary.com*) of meta-analytic researchers working in the medical sciences (Grimshaw et al., 2006). As a start we might embark on a meta-analysis of meta-analyses (Wilson & Lipsey, 2001) to dig out the age effects across a large variety of developmental domains to address the variability in developmental continuity across domains, contexts, cultures, and gender.

References

Alink, L. R. A., van IJzendoorn, M. H., Bakermans-Kranenburg, M. J., Mesman, J., Juffer, F., & Koot, H. M. (2008). Cortisol and externalizing behavior in children and adolescents: Mixed meta-analytic evidence for the inverse relation of basal cortisol and cortisol reactivity with externalizing behavior. *Developmental Psychobiology, 50*, 427–450.

Bakermans-Kranenburg, M. J., & van IJzendoorn, M. H. (2011). Differential susceptibility to rearing environment depending on dopamine-related genes: New evidence and a meta-analysis. *Development and Psychopathology, 23*, 39–52.

Bakermans-Kranenburg, M. J., van IJzendoorn, M. H., & Juffer, F. (2003). Less is more: Meta-analyses of sensitivity and attachment interventions in early childhood. *Psychological Bulletin, 129*, 195–215.

Bakermans-Kranenburg, M. J., van IJzendoorn, M. H., & Juffer, F. (2005). Disorganized infant attachment and preventive interventions: A review and meta-analysis. *Infant Mental Health Journal, 26*, 191–216.

Bar-Haim, Y., Lamy, D., Pergamin, L., Bakermans-Kranenburg, M. J., & van IJzendoorn, M. H. (2007). Threat-related attentional bias in anxious and nonanxious individuals: A meta-analytic study. *Psychological Bulletin, 133*, 1–24.

Belsky, J., Bakermans-Kranenburg, M. J., & van IJzendoorn, M. H. (2007). For better and for worse: Differential susceptibility to environmental influences. *Current Directions in Psychological Science, 16*, 300–304.

Borenstein, M., Hedges, L. V., Higgins, J. P. T., & Rothstein, H. (2009). *Computing effect sizes for meta-analysis*. Chichester, UK: Wiley.

Borenstein, M., Rothstein, H., & Cohen, J. (2005). *Comprehensive meta-analysis: A computer program for research synthesis* [Computer software]. Englewood, NJ: Biostat.

Boyce, W. T., & Ellis, B. J. (2005). Biological sensitivity to context: I. An evolutionary-developmental theory of the origins and functions of stress reactivity. *Development and Psychopathology, 17*, 271–301.

Bushman, B. J., & Wells, G. L. (2001). Narrative impressions of literature: The availability bias and the corrective properties of meta-analytic approaches. *Personality and Social Psychology Bulletin, 27*, 1123–1130.

Card, N. A. (2010). Antipathetic relationships in child and adolescent development: A meta-analytic review and recommendations for an emerging area of study. *Developmental Psychology, 46*, 516–529.

Carroll, L. (1870). *Alice's adventures in Wonderland*. Boston: Lee & Shepard.

Caspi, A., McClay, J., Moffitt, T. E., Mill, J., Martin, J., Craig, I. W., et al. (2002). Role of genotype in the cycle of violence in maltreated children. *Science, 297*, 851–854.

Cooper, H., & Hedges, L. V. (1994). *Handbook of research synthesis*. New York: Russell Sage Foundation.

De Wolff, M. S., & van IJzendoorn, M. H. (1997). Sensitivity and attachment: A meta-analysis on parental antecedents of infant attachment. *Child Development, 68*, 571–591.

Duval, S., & Tweedie, R. (2000a). A nonparametric "trim and fill" method for accounting for publication bias in meta-analysis. *Journal of the American Statistical Association, 95*, 89–98.

Duval, S., & Tweedie, R. (2000b). Trim and fill: A simple funnel-plot-based method of testing and adjusting for publication bias in meta-analysis. *Biometrics, 56,* 455–463.

Fearon, R. P., Bakermans-Kranenburg, M. J., van IJzendoorn, M. H., Lapsley, A. M., & Roisman, G. I. (2010). The significance of insecure attachment and disorganization in the development of children. *Child Development, 81,* 435–456.

Ferguson, C. J. (2010). A meta-analysis of normal and disordered personality across the life span. *Journal of Personality and Social Psychology, 98,* 659–667.

Fonagy, P., & Target, M. (2005). Bridging the transmission gap: An end to an important mystery of attachment research? *Attachment and Human Development, 7,* 333–343.

Gilbody, S. M., Song, F. J., Eastwood, A. J., & Sutton, A. (2000). The causes, consequences and detection of publication bias in psychiatry. *Acta Psychiatrica Scandinavica, 102,* 241–249.

Glass, G. V. (1976). Primary, secondary, and meta-analysis of research. *Educational Researcher, 5,* 3–8.

Goldstein, H., & Healy, M. J. R. (1995). The graphical presentation of a collection of means. *Journal of the Royal Statistical Society: Series A. Statistics in Society, 158,* 175–177.

Grimshaw, J. M., Santesso, N., Cumpston, M., Mayhew, A., & McGowan, J. (2006). Knowledge for knowledge translation: The role of the Cochrane collaboration. *Journal of Continuing Education in the Health Professions, 26,* 55–62.

Guerra, R., & Goldstein, D. R. (2010). *Meta-analysis and combining information in genetics and genomics.* London: Chapman & Hall.

Hedges, L. V., & Olkin, I. (1985). *Statistical methods for meta-analysis.* New York: Academic Press.

Isabella, R. A., Belsky, J., & Von Eye, A. (1989). Origins of infant–mother attachment: An examination of interactional synchrony during the infant's first year. *Developmental Psychology, 25,* 12–21.

Kamin, L. J. (1974). *The science and politics of IQ.* Potomac, MD: Erlbaum.

Kawabata, Y., Alink, L. R. A., Tseng, W., van IJzendoorn, M. H., & Crick, N. R. (in press). Maternal and paternal parenting styles associated with relational aggression in children and adolescents: A conceptual analysis and meta-analytic review. *Developmental Review.*

Kim-Cohen, J., Caspi, A., Taylor, A., Williams, B., Newcombe, R., Craig, I. W., et al. (2006). MAOA, maltreatment, and gene–environment interaction predicting children's mental health: New evidence and a meta-analysis. *Molecular Psychiatry, 11,* 903–913.

Kiser, L. J., Bates, J. E., Maslin, C. A., & Bayles, K. (1986). Mother–infant play at 6 months as a predictor of attachment security at 13 months. *Journal of the American Academy of Child and Adolescent Psychiatry, 25,* 68–75.

Klein, T. A., Neumann, J., Reuter, M., Hennig, J., Von Cramon, D. Y., & Ullsprenger, M. (2007). Genetically determined differences in learning from errors. *Science, 318,* 1642–1645.

Lipsey, M. W., & Wilson, D. B. (1993). The efficacy of psychological, educational, and behavioral treatment: Confirmation from meta-analysis. *American Psychologist, 48,* 1181–1209.

Lipsey, M. W., & Wilson, D. B. (2001). *Practical meta-analysis.* Thousand Oaks, CA: Sage.

Miyake, K., Chen, S. J., & Campos, J. J. (1985). Infant temperament, mothers' mode of interaction, and attachment in Japan: An interim report. *Monographs of the Society for Research in Child Development, 50,* 276–297.

Mullen, B. (1989). *Advanced BASIC meta-analysis.* Hillsdale, NJ: Erlbaum.

Orwin, R. G. (1983). A fail-safe *n* for effect size in meta-analysis. *Journal of Educational Statistics, 8,* 157–159.

Pearson, K. (1904). Report on certain enteric fever inoculation statistics. *British Medical Journal, 2,* 1243–1246.

Peters, D. P., & Ceci, S. J. (1982). Peer-review practices of psychological journals: The fate of accepted, published articles, submitted again. *Behavioral and Brain Sciences, 5,* 187–195.

Petticrew, M., & Roberts, H. (2006). *Systematic reviews in the social sciences: A practical guide.* Malden, MA: Blackwell.

Price, D. D. (1976). A general theory of bibliometric and other cumulative advantage processes. *Journal of the American Society for Information Science, 27*(5), 292–306.

Reschly, A., Busch, T., Betts, J., Deno, S. L., & Long, J. D. (2009). Curriculum-based measurement oral reading as an indicator of reading achievement: A meta-analysis of the correlational evidence. *Journal of School Psychology, 47,* 427–469.

Robbins, T. W., & Everitt, B. J. (1999). Interaction of the dopaminergic system with mechanisms of associative learning and cognition: Implications for drug abuse. *Psychological Science, 10,* 199–202.

Rosenthal, R. (1991). Meta-analysis: A review. *Psychosomatic Medicine, 53,* 247–271.

Rosenthal, R. (1995). Writing meta-analytic reviews. *Psychological Bulletin, 118,* 183–192.

Slavin, R. E. (1995). Best evidence synthesis: An intelligent alternative to meta-analysis. *Journal of Clinical Epidemiology, 48,* 9–18.

Smith, M., & Glass, G. (1977). Meta-analysis of psychotherapy outcome studies. *American Psychologist, 32,* 752–760.

Stroup, D. F., Berlin, J. A., Morton, S. C., Olkin, I., Williamson, G. D., Rennie, D., et al. (2000). Meta-analysis of observational studies in epidemiology: A proposal for reporting. *Journal of the American Medical Association, 283,* 2008–2012.

Sutton, A. J., Duval, S. J., Tweedie, R. L., Abrams, K. R., & Jones, D. R. (2000). Empirical assessment of effect of publication bias on meta-analyses. *British Medical Journal, 320,* 1574–1577.

Tripp, G., & Wickens, J. R. (2008). Research review: Dopamine transfer deficit: A neurobiological theory of altered reinforcement mechanisms in ADHD. *Journal of Child Psychology and Psychiatry, 49,* 691–704.

Tversky, A., & Kahneman, D. (1973). Availability: Heuristic for judging frequency and probability. *Cognitive Psychology, 5,* 207–232.

van IJzendoorn, M. H. (1995a). Adult attachment representations, parental responsiveness, and infant attachment: A meta-analysis on the predictive validity of the Adult Attachment Interview. *Psychological Bulletin, 117,* 387–403.

van IJzendoorn, M. H. (1995b). Of the way we were: On temperament, attachment, and the transmission gap: A rejoinder to Fox (1995). *Psychological Bulletin, 117,* 411–415.

van IJzendoorn, M. H., Bakermans-Kranenburg, M. J., & Sagi-Schwartz, A. (2003). Are children of Holocaust survivors less well adapted?: A meta-analytic investigation of secondary traumatization. *Journal of Traumatic Stress, 16,* 459–469.

van IJzendoorn, M. H., Juffer, F., & Klein Poelhuis, C. W. (2005). Adoption and cognitive development: A meta-analytic comparison of adopted and nonadopted children. *Psychological Bulletin, 131,* 301–316.

Visser, M., Jefferies, E., & Ralph, M. (2010). Semantic processing in the anterior temporal lobes: A meta-analysis of the functional neuroimaging literature. *Journal of Cognitive Neuroscience, 22,* 1083–1094.

Wilson, D., & Lipsey, M. (2001). The role of method in treatment effectiveness research: Evidence from meta-analysis. *Psychological Methods, 6,* 413–429.

CHAPTER 38

Evaluating Gene–Environment Interplay

MARA BRENDGEN
FRANK VITARO
ALAIN GIRARD

Central Issues

Until recently, social scientists have exclusively focused on identifying the specific environmental factors implicated in human development. However, there is virtually unanimous consensus that almost all aspects of human development are shaped by both environmental and genetic influences. What's more, genetic and environmental influences likely operate in an interdependent fashion. For example, individuals vary greatly in their behavioral and emotional response to stressful experiences such as physical abuse, peer rejection, divorce, or job loss, and genetic factors may play at least some role in explaining this heterogeneity in response to environmental stressors (Rutter, 2007). Similarly, individuals are believed to play a pivotal role in shaping their own environments (Lerner, 1982; Scarr & McCartney, 1983), and because many of the personal characteristics and behaviors that shape environmental experiences are partly heritable, the environment may itself be influenced by genetic factors. Methodological advances over the past decade have recently made it possible for social scientists to incorporate tests of different types of gene–environment interplay in their developmental models. In this chapter, we describe one way to use genetically informed research to examine how genetic and environmental factors work together to shape human development.

Genetically informed research can be categorized in two broad categories: quantitative genetic research and molecular genetic research. To date, empirical tests of genetic effects on human development have mostly relied on quantitative genetic studies (Johnson, Turkheimer, Gottesman, & Bouchard, 2009). Whereas molecular genetic studies aim to identify specific genes that influence the developmental outcome of interest, quantitative genetic studies do not explicitly measure specific genes. Often, they do not include specific measures of the environment, either. Rather, the relative strength of genetic and environmental influences on the observed developmental outcome (also called the *phenotype*) is statistically inferred by examining the phenotypic similarity of family members who differ in their genetic relatedness. To this end, quantitative studies can use different designs, such as the classical twin design (or twins-raised-together design), which compares the degree of similarity between identical twin pairs with the degree of similarity between nonidentical twin pairs, or the classical adoption design, which examines the phenotypic similarity between children who were adopted at birth and their biological parents or siblings. Other designs are usually variations or extensions of these two approaches, such as the twins-reared-apart design, which is a special version of an adoption design, or the cascade model, which includes other biological and nonbiological relatives of twins (Keller et al., 2009). A description of all available designs would go beyond the scope of this chapter. Perhaps the most widely used behavioral genetic design is the classical twin design. Its popularity is likely due to the fact that twins raised together are relatively easy to find, as twins constitute around 2% of the population and most of them grow up together in the same family. In contrast, the use of other behavioral genetic designs, such as the classical adoption design or the twins-raised-apart design, is often hampered by recruitment difficulties (e.g., with the biological parents in international adoptions) or by the fact that in many local adoptions the biological mother keeps in contact with her child and the adoptive parents, thus confounding estimates of genetic similarity with environmental effects.

Common to all quantitative genetic designs is the premise that phenotypic differences between individuals can be explained by three principal sources of variance: *genetic* (or heritable) factors, *shared* (or common) environmental factors, and *nonshared* (or unique) environmental factors (Petrill, 2002). Genetic effects encompass *additive* (or direct) *genetic effects*, as well as interaction effects between genes. Shared environment effects refer to environmental factors that make members of the same family who live together similar to each other. Notably, shared environment refers not only to family-related characteristics (e.g., socioeconomic status, parental education) but also to features outside the family, such as neighborhood characteristics (e.g., housing density), school-related characteristics (e.g., academic track), or any other feature of the physical and social environment to which family members are jointly exposed. In contrast to shared environmental factors, nonshared environmental factors encompass those experiences—either within or outside the family—that make members of the same family dissimilar. Just like the shared environment, the nonshared environment may refer to experiences within the family or outside the family. For example, siblings may be treated differently by their parents, which, in turn, may be related to differences in siblings' behavior (Conger & Conger, 1994; Dunn, Stocker, & Plomin, 1990; McHale, Crouter, McGuire, & Updegraff, 1995). The most important nonshared environmental influences, however, are likely those experienced outside the family (Dunn & Plomin, 1990). During childhood and adolescence, experiences with peers may be a particularly important source of nonshared environmental influence, as siblings often do not affiliate with the same friends (Thorpe & Gardner, 2006). Depending on the specific design used, quantitative studies apply different statistical approaches to estimate genetic, shared environmental, and nonshared environmental effects on a measured phenotype.

Conceptual Principles and Statistical Assumptions

Genetic modeling using the classical twin design is based on the comparison of identical or monozygotic (MZ) twins and fraternal or dizygotic (DZ) twin pairs, in which both members of a given twin pair are raised together in the same family. Monozygotic twinning occurs when one egg is fertilized by one sperm and then splits after conception into two genetically identical halves. As such, MZ twins are assumed to share 100% of their genes and are of the same sex. Dizygotic twinning occurs when two eggs are fertilized by two separate sperm. DZ twins share approximately 50% of their genes and can be the same sex or different sexes. Genetic, shared environmental, and nonshared environmental sources of interindividual differences are estimated by comparing the intrapair similarity of MZ twins with the intrapair similarity of DZ twins (Falconer, 1960). Notably, because sex differences might foster dissimilarity between members of mixed-sex DZ pairs, estimation of genetic, shared, and nonshared environmental effects rests mainly on the comparison of MZ twins, who are necessarily always of the same sex, and same-sex DZ twins (Neale & Cardon, 1992). However, if the intrapair correlations of same-sex DZ twins and mixed-sex DZ twins are equivalent, and if no mean differences are observed between the two DZ groups, they can be combined in a single DZ group in quantitative genetic analyses.

Genetic effects are represented by the broad heritability coefficient h^2_B. In the classical twin design, genetic effects are indicated when the intrapair similarity (i.e., intrapair correlation) of MZ twin pairs is larger than the intrapair similarity of DZ twin pairs and can be approximated with $h^2_B = 2\ (r_{MZ} - r_{DZ})$. Thus, if the intrapair correlation of MZ twins is $r = .80$ and the intrapair correlation between DZ twins is $r = .50$, the genetic effect h^2_B on the measured phenotype can be estimated as $2\ (.80 - .50) = .60$. In other words, approximately 60% of the phenotypic variability is determined by genetic influences. Shared environmental influences, which are represented by the statistical term c^2, are indicated when there is a substantive intrapair correlation that is comparable for MZ twin pairs and DZ twin pairs. Shared environmental effects can be approximated by subtracting the MZ correlation from twice the DZ correlation, $c^2 = (2r_{DZ}) - (r_{MZ})$. In our example, c^2 would thus be estimated as $(2 \times .50) - .80 = .20$, indicating that approximately 20% of the phenotypic variability is explained by shared environmental influences. Finally, because MZ twins are genetically identical and are jointly exposed to shared environmental influences, any remaining intrapair differences among MZ twins can only be explained by nonshared environmental influences e^2. Nonshared environmental influences can be approximated by the extent to which the MZ intrapair correlation is less than 1, $e^2 = 1 - r_{MZ}$. Using our example, the nonshared environment effect e^2 would thus be estimated as $1 - .80 = .20$, indicating that around 20% of the phenotypic variability is explained by nonshared environmental factors.

Of note, e^2 also includes any measurement error that may have decreased the similarity between the two members of a twin pair, such as when unexpected background noise leads to slightly different testing conditions in a lab task for one twin than for the other. Because measurement error leads to inflated estimates of nonshared environmental effects, it also has a direct bearing on the estimation of shared environmental and/or genetic effects and may result in an underestimation of one or both of these latter effects. One way to reduce the risk of biased estimates associated with measurement error may be through the use of multiple indicators or repeated measures of the phenotype under study (e.g., Arseneault et al., 2003). However, the increased number of variables also results in a substantial increase in model complexity and requires very large samples.

The comparison of intrapair correlations across MZ and DZ twins can provide rough approximations of the relative contributions of genetic, shared environmental, and nonshared environmental factors to a given phenotype. A more precise parameter estimation that also includes the estimation of confidence intervals, and hence of the statistical significance of the estimated parameters, can be achieved through structural equation modeling using a maximum likelihood fit function (Neale & Cardon, 1992). At the simplest level, univariate modeling of variance decomposition provides estimations of the contribution of latent additive genetic (A), latent shared environmental (C), and latent nonshared environmental (E) factors to the observed variance of a given phenotype. This basic ACE model, which is illustrated in Figure 38.1, can be readily estimated using the Mplus software version 5.2 following the script provided at *www.crmda.ku.edu/Guilford/HDRM*. The model is fitted to the data in a two-group model, where correlations of A between the two twins in a pair are fixed to 1.0 for MZ twins and to .5 for DZ twins, correlations of C between the two twins in a pair are fixed to 1.0 for MZ twins and DZ twins, and correlations of E between the two twins in a pair are fixed to 0 for MZ twins and DZ twins. The estimated coefficients a, c, and e, which are fixed to be equal across the two twins in a pair and across MZ and DZ twins, are the factor loadings that provide information about the relative contribution of the latent factors A, C, and E to the total variance (V_t) of each phenotype (P), with $V_t\,(\mathrm{P}) = a^2 + c^2 + e^2$. If one of these coefficients is estimated to be close to zero and not statistically significant, the full ACE model can then be compared with a model in which this parameter is fixed to zero (e.g., an AE or CE model) using a nested χ^2 comparison to determine the most parsimonious model given the pattern of correlations observed within twin pairs.

Notably, the ACE model tests the hypothesis that a specific genetic mechanism—for example, additive genetic effects—is operating for the phenotype under study. In other words, it is assumed that the genetic estimate A reflects the sum of all genetic effects implicated in the trait under study and that the effect of each gene is independent of the effect of other genes. However, traits can also be influenced by genetic interaction effects, such

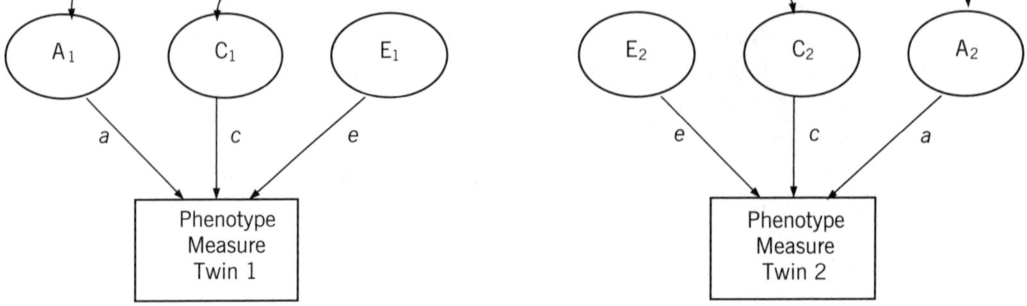

FIGURE 38.1. Univariate ACE model.

as the effect of a recessive gene inherited from one parent being suppressed by the effect of a dominant gene inherited from the other parent. A dominance genetic effect occurs, for example, when a dominant gene for brown eye color is inherited from one parent and a recessive gene for blue eye color is inherited from the other parent. In this case, only the dominant gene is expressed in the trait "eye color," and the individual will have brown, not blue, eyes. In the classical twin design, a dominance genetic effect (D) would be indicated when the size of the intrapair correlation in MZ twins is *more* than twice the size of the intrapair correlation in DZ twins. In contrast, an additive genetic effect (A) is indicated when the size of the MZ correlation is *less* than twice the size of the DZ correlation (Rhee & Waldman, 2002). So far, dominance genetic effects seem to be the exception rather than the rule with respect to many aspects of human social behavioral development studied to date, specifically externalizing and internalizing behavior problems during childhood and adolescence (Burt, 2009a, 2009b; Rhee & Waldman, 2002).

The classical twin design also relies on other assumptions that must be met in order to produce valid estimates of genetic and environmental effects (Keller & Coventry, 2005). First, it is assumed that twins are representative of the general population and should thus be comparable to children from single births (so-called singletons). Comparison studies have shown that twins indeed resemble singletons in regard to most aspects of psychosocial development (e.g., Laffey-Ardley & Thorpe, 2006; Lamarche et al., 2007; Pulkkinen, Vaalamo, Hietala, Kaprio, & Rose, 2003; Thorpe, 2003). Nevertheless, twins are at greater risk of congenital anomalies and birth complications, and phenotypes that are confounded with these complications such as cognitive delays are more common in twins than in singletons. Therefore, twins with obstetric complications are routinely excluded from twin analyses. The violation of the representativeness assumption has important implications for the external validity of the findings, but it does not directly affect the reliability of the estimates of genetic and environmental effects. One assumption that is crucial in this regard, however, is that MZ twins are indeed genetically identical. This notion has been challenged by recent findings of variations in the DNA sequences of identical twins, in which one twin showed signs of dementia or Parkinson's disease and the other did not (Bruder et al., 2008). It has been suggested that the frequency of such copy–number variations (i.e., the presence of additional or missing segments of chromosomes) may be as high as 10% per twin pair (Bruder et al., 2008). Although copy–number variations have been associated with some diseases such as cancer (Dear, 2009), it is unclear to what extent they explain interindividual differences in regard to psychosocial development. Nevertheless, the recent findings of genetic differences between MZ twins suggest that genetic effects may be underestimated at least to some degree in quantitative genetic studies.

Another assumption, which also has a direct bearing on the statistical estimation of effects, dictates that features of the environment shared by twins influence MZ and DZ twins to the same extent. This so-called equal-environment assumption implies, for example, that MZ twins are not treated by their parents or by other people in their social environment more similarly than are DZ twins. Otherwise, a larger intrapair correlation of MZ twins compared with DZ twins in the phenotypic outcome may be partially due to environmental, rather than genetic, influences. Evidence suggests that the equal-environment assumption often may not be tenable, as MZ twins are treated by their parents more similarly than DZ twins, more often share playmates, share the same room, and dress more alike than same-sex DZ twins (Loehlin & Nichols, 1976). However, several studies have shown that the greater similarity in environmental experiences of MZ compared with DZ twins does not necessarily translate into a greater similarity with respect to behavioral outcomes, such as internalizing and externalizing psychiatric disorders, aggression, drug use, personality traits, vocational interests, sexual orientations, and interpersonal relationships (Borkenau, Riemann, Angleitner, & Spinath, 2002; Derks, Dolan, & Boomsma, 2006; Hettema, Neale, & Kendler, 1995; Kendler, Neale, Kessler, Heath, & Eaves, 1993, 1994). These findings have led scholars to the conclusion that even violations of the equal-environment assumption do not invalidate the parameter estimates derived from the classical twin design. Nevertheless, if data are available, it is prudent to examine whether the equal-environment assumption is violated and, if so, whether this violation causes biased model parameters (for more detailed information, see Derks et al., 2006).

An additional assumption is that no assortative mating occurs, which means that individuals do not systematically select a mate with a similar genotype. If their parents are genetically similar, DZ twins will share more than the assumed 50% of genetic information. This, in turn, would reduce the difference between MZ and DZ correlations, thus leading to an underestimation of genetic effects and an overestimation of shared environmental effects. Empirical evidence suggests that spouses resemble each other with respect to a wide variety of characteristics. Because this similarity may at least in part be explained by active selection for a similar partner, the random mating assumption may be violated. Thus, although estimates of shared environmental influences so far have been found to be rather small for many psychosocial aspects of human development (Burt, 2009b; Turkheimer, 2000), the possibility of at least some bias due to assortative mating needs to be considered, especially when large effects of C are found (Loehlin, Harden, & Turkheimer, 2009).

In addition to the assumptions mentioned previously, estimation of effects in a simple ACE model presumes that genetic and environmental influences are independent of each other. This is perhaps the most criticized assumption of the simple ACE model (Collins, Maccoby, Steinberg, Hetherington, & Bornstein, 2000; Lerner, 2006), because estimations of simple effects ignore any possible interplay between genes and the environment. Although gene–environment interplay is a rather general term that covers different concepts (Rutter, Moffitt, & Caspi, 2006), two genetic–environmental mechanisms that may be of specific relevance for developmental researchers are gene–environment interactions and gene–environment correlations.

Gene–environment interaction (or G × E) refers to a situation in which the effect of genes on a developmental outcome varies depending on environmental conditions or the effect of the environment on a developmental outcome varies depending on the individual's genetic disposition (Shanahan & Hofer, 2005). For example, a child's genetic vulnerability for obesity is more likely to manifest itself (i.e., to have a significant effect) in an environment with limited access to regular physical activities and healthy food than in an environment that fosters sports involvement and a balanced diet. Alternatively, consumption of lactose food products can lead to serious mental retardation and brain damage in children with a genetic risk for phenylketonuria, but not in children who do not carry the risk gene. Mathematically, it is irrelevant whether the environment moderates the effect of genes or whether genes moderate environmental effects. However, because genetic effects in quantitative studies are usually conceptualized as latent (i.e., nonmeasured) variables, researchers have mostly interpreted G × E in terms of environmental moderation of genetic effects (for an alternative approach, see Brendgen et al., 2008; Jaffee et al., 2005).

Gene–environment correlation (or *r*GE) refers to a situation in which specific genotypes are associated with specific environments. One way for *r*GE to arise is through environmental influences on genes, such as when a specific environment favors the occurrence of specific genotypes over others (e.g., through evolutionary processes such as natural selection). *r*GE can also arise through genetic influences on the environment, such as when an individual's genetically determined traits influence the kind of environment he or she will experience (e.g., individuals with a genetic vulnerability to depressed mood may withdraw from social activities, lose friends, and become socially isolated). As a result, the environmental variable (lack of friends) becomes correlated with the depressiogenic genotype. Again, although the directionality of effects is inconsequential from a mathematical standpoint, social scientists have been particularly interested in *r*GE that reflects genetic influences on the environment.

As demonstrated by Purcell (2002), the (undetected) presence of either G × E or *r*GE may result in biased genetic, shared environmental, and nonshared environmental effects. Thus an interaction between genetic and shared environmental factors may lead to an inflated genetic estimate A, whereas an interaction between genetic and nonshared environmental factors may lead to an inflated nonshared environmental estimate E. The correlation between genetic and shared environmental factors can inflate the shared environmental estimate C, whereas the correlation between genetic and nonshared environmental factors can inflate the genetic estimate A. It is therefore of critical importance to include G × E and/or *r*GE in the genetic model when one or both types of gene–environment interplay are suspected.

Developmental Applications

For almost all aspects of human development, G × E can be expected to be more common than simple additive effects of genetic and environmental factors because of the principle of natural selection (Rutter et al., 2006). Natural selection proposes that genes are involved in the adaptation of organisms to environmental conditions. Specifically, organisms belonging to the same species often vary considerably in their response to the same environment, and this variability can at least partly be explained by genetic differences. G × E may arise through four different processes (Shanahan & Hofer, 2005). A *diathesis–stress* process occurs when an environmental stressor triggers or exacerbates an individual's genetic predisposition for a specific developmental outcome, or when an environmental stressor is more likely to lead to a specific developmental outcome in individuals with a genetic predisposition. For example, in a diathesis–stress process of G × E a child's genetic disposition to aggression would be more likely to manifest itself when the child suffers physical abuse from parents than when the child is raised in a loving home. In contrast, a *compensation* process is indicated when the presence of a positive environment prevents or reduces the expression of a genetic disposition. For example, a genetic vulnerability to depression may be less likely to manifest itself when an individual receives a high level of social support from others. Of note, when an environmental variable incorporates both positive and negative features at the two different ends of its spectrum, diathesis–stress and compensation processes may reflect opposite poles of a continuum. An example of such a variable is social preference (Coie, Dodge, & Coppotelli, 1982), high levels of which indicate acceptance by peers and low levels indicate rejection. A third possible G × E mechanism is a *suppression* process, which occurs when a restrictive environment reduces the role of genetic influences, such that the same developmental outcome is observed regardless of individuals' genetic dispositions. A suppression process may involve clearly negative environmental conditions, such as environmental toxins that lead to disease in most individuals. It may also, however, involve positive environmental conditions such as social norms or structural constraints that limit the expression of a genetic disposition to undesirable developmental outcomes such as aggression or substance use. Positive environmental features also play a role in the fourth possible G × E mechanism, that is, an *enhancement* process. Here, beneficial environmental conditions facilitate the expression (or effect) of genes that predispose to exceptionally high levels of developmental functioning. A case in point is the provision of special education services that allow gifted students to maximize their genetically determined potential. In contrast to the previously described G × E mechanisms, which concern promotion or prevention of negative developmental outcomes, the enhancement process thus refers to gene–environment interplay toward positive development.

Like G × E, *r*GE is an integral mechanism of all aspects of human development, perhaps particularly so for aspects concerning psychosocial functioning. Thus developmental theorists have suggested for several decades that individuals play a critical role in creating their own environments (Bell, 1968; Lerner, 1982; Scarr & McCartney, 1983). Many—if not most—of the personal characteristics and behaviors that may influence environmental experiences are partly heritable. As a result, the environment may become itself influenced, albeit indirectly, by genetic factors. Plomin and colleagues (Plomin, DeFries, & Loehlin, 1977) have described three different forms of *r*GE: passive, evocative, and selective *r*GE. *Passive r*GE arises when the environment parents provide for their children (e.g., via their parenting style) is influenced by the parents' own genetically determined characteristics (e.g., externalizing or internalizing problems). This type of *r*GE is called *passive* because the child's environmental experiences are not shaped by the child's own characteristics but by parental characteristics that are genetically influenced. As a result, the child's genotype, which is inherited from the parents, is correlated with the environment in which he or she is raised. Whereas passive *r*GE is brought about by parents' genetically influenced characteristics, evocative *r*GE and active *r*GE involve environments that are shaped by an individual's own genetically determined characteristics. *Evocative* (or reactive) *r*GE occurs when the individual's genetically influenced characteristics provoke a specific reaction from the environment. For example, aggressive behavior, which is to a large part determined by genetic factors (Burt, 2009a), may lead to rejection and reciprocated hostility from others. *Selective* (or active) *r*GE arises when individuals, based on their genetically influenced personal characteristics, deliberately select or actively model their own environments. Selective *r*GE would be indicated, for example, when aggressive individuals deliberately choose friends with similar behavioral characteristics.

Although G × E and *r*GE have usually been investigated independently, the two processes can and often do co-occur, such that the same environmental factors may simultaneously be involved in both G × E and *r*GE with respect to a given phenotype (Eaves, Silberg, & Erkanli, 2003; Purcell, 2002). Environmental features that are proximal to the child are most likely to be simultaneously implicated in G × E and *r*GE (Shanahan & Hofer, 2005). For example, quantitative genetic studies provide evidence for G × E (Feinberg, Button, Neiderhiser, Reiss, & Hetherington, 2007) and *r*GE (Narusyte, Andershed, Neiderhiser, & Lichtenstein, 2007) linking aggressive behavior in youths and a problematic relationship with parents. If G × E and *r*GE co-occur, independent estimation of one without simultaneous consideration of the other can result in biased conclusions (Purcell, 2002). For instance, the finding of a greater genetic effect on aggression in an abusive environment than in a supportive environment may reflect true G × E. However, the same result could also stem from the fact that individuals with a particular risk genotype are most likely to experience an abusive environment, reflecting *r*GE. As such, the (undetected) presence of *r*GE may lead to false positive conclusions of G × E. On the flip side, it is also possible that the multicollinearity arising from a correlation between genetic and environmental factors may reduce the statistical power for detecting interactions. Thus a nonsignificant finding of G × E may reflect a true absence of a gene–environment interaction, or it may reflect an undetected *r*GE. For these reasons, G × E and *r*GE should be considered simultaneously in examinations of gene–environment interplay (Purcell, 2002).

Illustrations

In order to assess G × E and *r*GE, one needs to have a measure of the environmental variable that is thought to moderate genetic influences on a developmental outcome or that is thought to be influenced by genetically determined traits. When assessing gene–environment interplay in the classical twin design, the first question that arises is whether the environmental variable of interest is measured at the family—that is, pair—level (e.g., parental divorce) or whether it is measured at the child level (e.g., maternal behavior toward each child). When a variable is measured at the family level, it is necessarily equivalent for the two twins in a pair. Therefore, it is not possible to partition such a variable into genetic and environmental components that explain within-pair differences. As a result, *r*GE involving such variables cannot be examined (Turkheimer, D'Onofrio, Maes, & Eaves, 2005). It is possible, however, to examine whether a variable measured at the family level moderates the latent genetic, shared environmental, and nonshared environmental effects on a measured phenotype. To do so, we expand the basic ACE model to allow each of the three latent variance components to interact with the putative environmental variable measured at the family level, thus leading to the structural equation $P = s\text{FV} + (a + \beta_a\text{FV})A + (c + \beta_c\text{FV})C + (e + \beta_e\text{FV})E$, where *a*, *c*, and *e* are the main effects of A, C, and E, respectively, and β_a, β_c, and β_e represent the interactions of A, C, and E with the family-level variable FV. The *s* coefficient represents the main effect of the family-level variable FV on the measured phenotype P. This model, which is illustrated in Figure 38.2, can be readily estimated using the Mplus software version 5.2 following the script provided at *www.crmda.ku.edu/Guilford/HDRM.*

Using this approach, Turkheimer and colleagues examined the potential moderating effect of family socioeconomic status on the genetic, shared, and nonshared environmental effects on IQ scores in a sample of 319 seven-year-old twin pairs (Turkheimer, Haley, Waldron, D'Onofrio, & Gottesman, 2003). The results showed that the proportion of interindividual differences in IQ attributable to genetic and environmental factors varied with the socioeconomic status (SES) of the family. Specifically, in the poorest families, 60% of the variance in children's IQ was explained by shared environmental factors, and the remaining variance was explained by nonshared environmental factors, whereas the contribution of genetic factors was essentially zero. The reverse pattern was seen in the most affluent families, in which basically all of the interindividual variance of IQ was explained by genetic factors.

As stated by Turkheimer and his colleagues (2003), intuitively the most obvious interpretation of these findings would be that family SES is indeed a measure of the environment

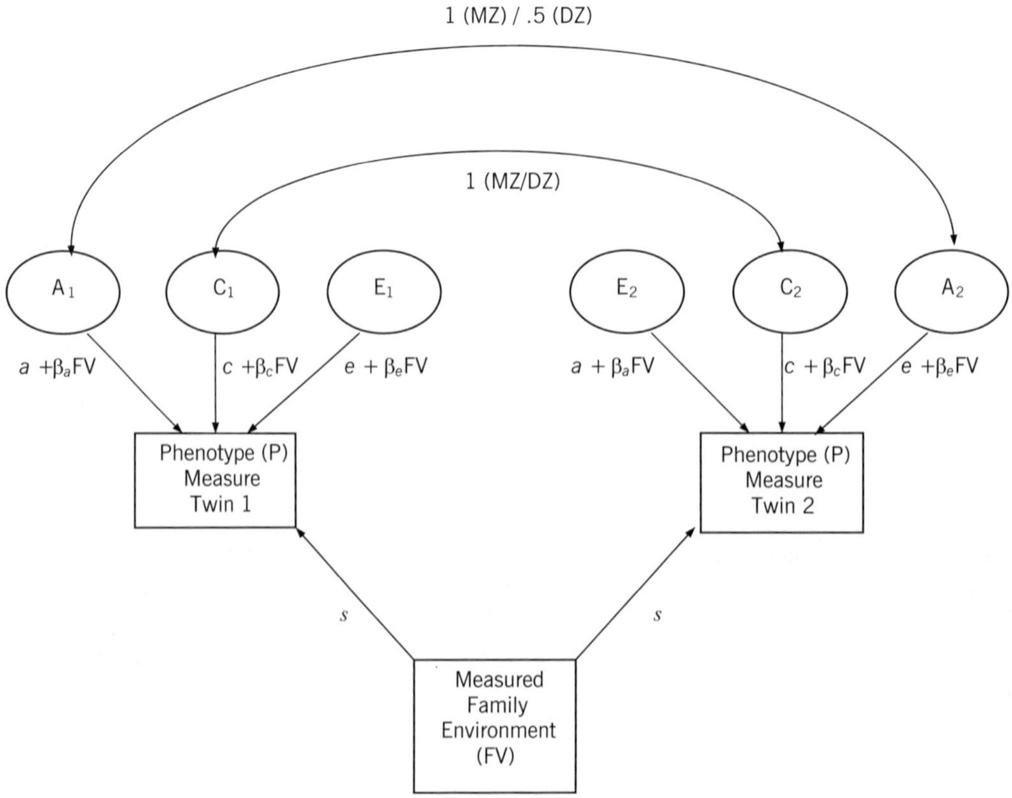

FIGURE 38.2. ACE model including interactions with an environmental variable measured at the family level.

to which the twins are jointly exposed. Genetic differences among individuals in regard to IQ may express themselves more easily in favorable environments, whereas poor environments may restrict individuals from reaching their full genetically determined cognitive potential. The authors also point out, however, that it would be imprudent to interpret SES as a purely environmental variable, because many variables traditionally considered as indicators of environmental experiences are likely—at least to some extent—correlated with individuals' genetic dispositions (Plomin & Bergeman, 1991). At least theoretically, the authors argue, it is conceivable that children growing up in low-SES households differ from more affluent children both environmentally and genetically. However, family-level measures such as SES are necessarily the same for the two twins in a pair. As such, it is impossible to determine in the classical twin design whether family SES has any genetic component and, if so, whether it is the environmental or the genetic component of SES that is responsible for the observed interactions. In other words, it is not clear whether the findings reflect a true gene–environment interaction or a gene–gene interaction instead. As noted by Turkheimer and colleagues (2003), these restrictions considerably limit the interpretation of the findings.

A genetic effect on the putative environmental variable may also introduce bias in the estimation of G × E itself. For example, smaller genetic effects on IQ in more affluent environments might indeed indicate true G × E. However, the same finding could be due to less overall genetic variability—resulting from a greater frequency of individuals with a particular genotype—in affluent environments, which would reflect *r*GE. The undetected presence of *r*GE could thus produce a false finding of G × E (Rutter & Silberg, 2002). A further problem relates to the fact that multicollinearity arising from *r*GE (i.e., a correlation between genetic effects influencing the putative environmental variable and genetic effects influencing the phenotype) may reduce the statistical power for detecting interactions between the environmental variable and the remaining genetic component on the phenotype (Purcell, 2002). In other words, both the presence and the absence of a finding of G × E may be caused by an undetected *r*GE. To minimize bias associated with *r*GE, it is imperative to examine potential genetic effects on putative environmental variables. If genetic effects are found, and if these genetic effects are correlated with those predicting the phenotype under study—indicating the presence of *r*GE—this gene–environment correlation has to be included in models estimating G × E.

The joint estimation of both *r*GE and G × E requires that the environmental variable of interest is measured at the child level (i.e., with separate measures of each member of a twin pair). In this case, the putative environmental variable can be analyzed like any other phenotype. Specifically, using univariate genetic modeling, interindividual differences in regard to the measured environmental variable are first partitioned into genetic, shared environmental, and nonshared environmental sources of influence. Subsequent multivariate modeling then allows an examination of potential gene–environment interplay between the measured behavior or trait and the measured environmental variable.

This approach is illustrated in one of our recent studies of depression in young children (Brendgen et al., 2009). Previous research with adolescents had found that genetic risk for depression may increase the likelihood of exposure to environmental stressors (indicating *r*GE). Exposure to environmental stressors has also been found to moderate the effect of genes on depression (indicating G × E). Relating these processes to a peer-related stressor in childhood, we examined (1) whether genetic risk for depression in children is related to higher levels of rejection by the peer group (*r*GE) and (2) whether peer rejection exacerbates the effect of genetic factors on children's depression (G × E). The research questions were addressed using a sample of 336 twin pairs (196 MZ pairs and 140 same-sex DZ pairs). When the children were in kindergarten, teacher ratings provided a continuous score for each twin's level of depression, and classmate sociometric ratings provided a continuous score for each twin's level of peer acceptance or rejection. Preliminary analyses showed that the phenotypic correlation between peer acceptance or rejection and depression was $r = -.23$. Moreover, within-pair correlations were higher for MZ twins than for DZ twins both in regard to peer acceptance or rejection ($r = .45$ for MZ twins; $r = .31$ for DZ twins) and in regard to depression ($r = .34$ for MZ twins; $r = .18$ for DZ twins).

Using the Mplus software package (Muthén & Muthén, 2004), two separate univariate ACE models were fitted to the data to estimate the additive genetic, shared environmental, and nonshared environmental effects on peer acceptance or rejection and depression, respectively. The results from the univariate models revealed that 30% of the variance in peer acceptance or rejection was explained by additive genetic factors, another 15% of the variance was explained by shared environmental factors, and the remaining 55% of the variance was due to nonshared environmental influences. Of the variance of depression, 30% was explained by additive genetic factors, 3% was explained by shared environmental sources, and the remaining 67% was due to nonshared environmental influences.

Potential *r*GE and G × E in the link between peer acceptance or rejection and depressive behavior were examined next. To this end, a bivariate Cholesky model was specified in which the covariance structure of peer acceptance or rejection and depression was partitioned into (1) "common" latent factors A_C, C_C, and E_C that influence both variables and (2) "unique" latent factors A_U, C_U, and E_U that influence only depression. This bivariate model, which is illustrated in Figure 38.3, can be readily estimated using the Mplus software version 5.2 following the script provided at *www.crmda.ku.edu/Guilford/HDRM*. All model paths are fixed to be equal for the two twins in a pair and for MZ and DZ twins. Paths a_R, c_R, and e_R are the factor loadings of peer acceptance–rejection (R) on the common latent factors. Paths a_C, c_C, and e_C are the factor loadings of depression on the common latent factors. Paths a_U, c_U, and e_U are the factor loadings of depression on the unique latent factors. A significant effect of the "common" latent genetic factor A_C on depression indicates *r*GE. The size of the gene–environment correlation can be calculated as

$$rGE = a_R a_C \Big/ \sqrt{a_R^2 (a_C^2 + a_U^2)}$$

In order to test for G × E, we also included interaction terms for each path predicting depression in the model. A significant interaction between the "common" genetic factor A_C and Peer Acceptance/Rejection ($\beta_{A_C}R$) would mean that the same genes are involved in both *r*GE and G × E. A significant interaction between the "unique" genetic factor A_U and

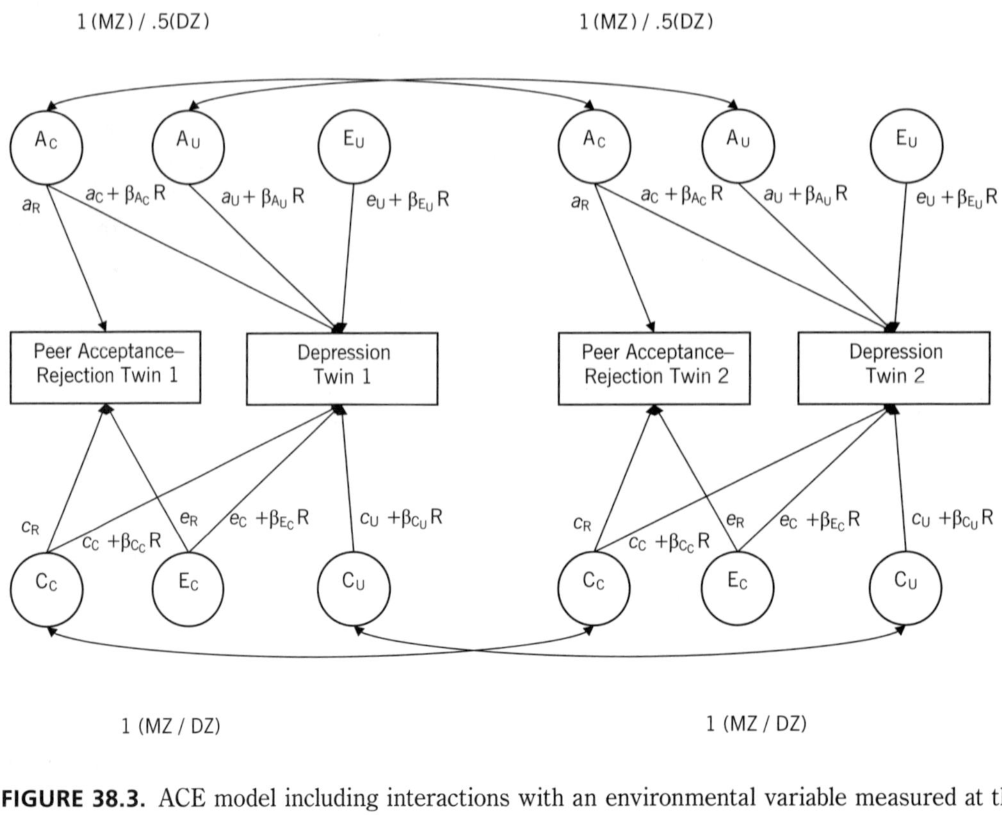

FIGURE 38.3. ACE model including interactions with an environmental variable measured at the individual level.

Peer Acceptance/Rejection ($\beta_{A_U}R$) would mean that different genes are involved in G × E than in *r*GE. In addition, interaction terms between the shared environmental factors C_C and C_U and Peer Acceptance/Rejection ($\beta_{C_C}R$ and $\beta_{C_U}R$, respectively) and between the nonshared environmental factors E_C and E_U and Peer Acceptance/Rejection ($\beta_{E_C}R$ and $\beta_{E_U}R$, respectively) were added to this model. The inclusion of such environment–environment interactions (E × E) is important, because the finding of G × E may in fact reflect an undetected E × E (Purcell, 2002). As such, the total variance (V_T) of depression as a function of peer acceptance or rejection (R) can be expressed as

$$V_T \mid R = (a_C + \beta_{A_C}R)^2 + (a_U + \beta_{A_U}R)^2 + (c_C + \beta_{C_C}R)^2 + (c_U + \beta_{C_U}R)^2 + (e_C + \beta_{E_C}R)^2 + (e_U + \beta_{E_U}R)^2$$

The results from the bivariate model are shown in Table 38.1. Of note, classical fit indices such as χ^2 and root mean square error of approximation (RMSEA) are not available for models including interaction terms. However, such models can be compared with other, more or less complex models using the –2Log Likelihood difference test, which is equivalent to a nested χ^2-difference test (Purcell, 2002). As can be seen in the table, 45% (i.e., $-.30^2/(-.30^2 + .33^2)$) of the genetic variance of children's depression was explained by genetic factors that also influenced peer acceptance/rejection. This corresponds to a

TABLE 38.1. Summary of Bivariate Model Results

Parameter	Estimate	95 % confidence interval
Peer acceptance/rejection		
a_R	.62	(.42; .82)
c_R	.33	(.04; .61)
e_R	.68	(.61; .75)
Depression		
Common effects		
a_C	–.30	(–.52; –.09)
β_{A_C}	.06	(–.23; .35)
c_C	.23	(–.11; .57)
β_{C_C}	–.02	(–.44; .41)
e_C	–.14	(–.25; –.03)
β_{E_C}	.02	(–.13; .18)
Unique effects		
a_U	.33	(.03; .63)
β_{A_U}	.21	(.01; .42)
c_U	–.27	(–.64; .11)
β_{C_U}	.08	(–.43; .59)
e_U	.75	(.68; .83)
β_{E_U}	–.17	(–.31; –.02)

Note. Model –2LL = 3741.18. Parameters are significant when the respective confidence interval does not include zero.

gene–environment correlation of rGE = –.67 (i.e., $(.62\times-.30)/\sqrt{.62^2(-.30^2+.33^2)}$) linking depression and peer acceptance–rejection. There was also a small but significant correlation between the nonshared environmental influence on depression and peer acceptance–rejection of rEE = –.18 (i.e., $(.68\times-.14)/\sqrt{.68^2(-.14^2+.75^2)}$). Shared environmental effects could not overlap because there were no significant shared environmental effects on depression.

The results also showed a significant interaction of peer acceptance–rejection with the latent genetic factor A_U that was unique to depression ($\beta_{A_U}R$ = .21), but not with the latent genetic factor A_C that was common to peer acceptance–rejection and depression ($\beta_{A_C}R$ = .06). These findings indicate that the genetic influences on depression that are involved in rGE with peer acceptance–rejection are not the same as those that are involved in G × E with peer acceptance–rejection. There was no significant interaction of peer acceptance–rejection with the latent shared environmental factors C_C and C_U ($\beta_{C_C}R$ = –.02 and $\beta_{C_U}R$ = .08) or with the latent nonshared environmental factor E_C ($\beta_{E_C}R$ = .02). However, peer acceptance–rejection significantly interacted with the latent nonshared environmental factor E_U that was unique to depression ($\beta_{E_U}R$ = –.17). The moderating effect of peer acceptance–rejection on the genetic and environmental variance components of depression is illustrated in Figure 38.4. As can be seen, the total variance of depression is lower when peer acceptance–rejection is below the mean of 0 (i.e., when children are rather rejected) than when peer acceptance–rejection is above the mean of 0 (i.e., when children are rather popular). Moreover, genetic factors contribute relatively less, whereas nonshared

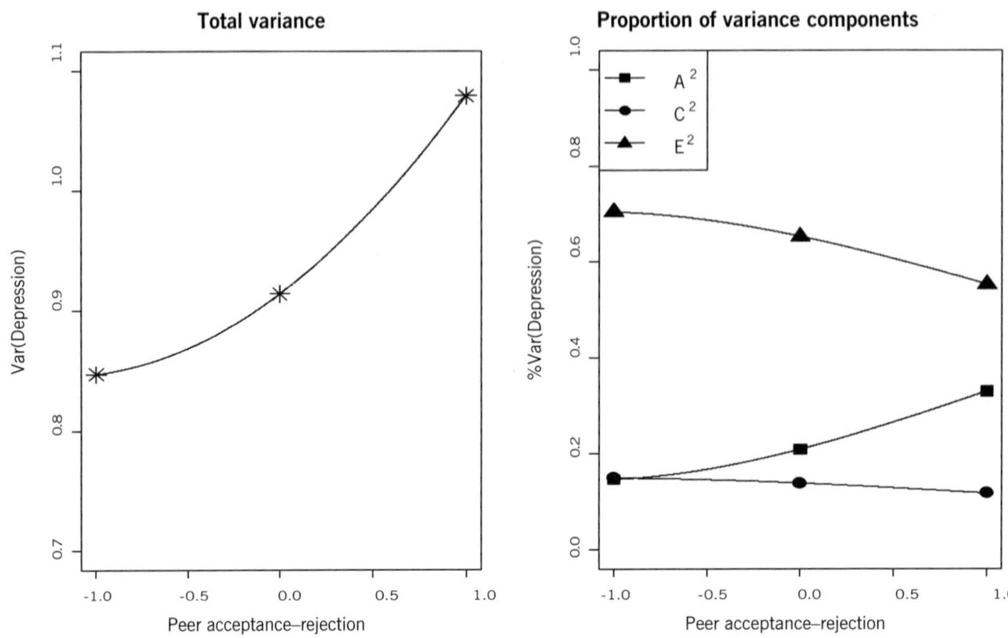

FIGURE 38.4. Illustration of the moderating effect of peer acceptance/rejection on the total variance and on the genetic (A^2), shared environmental (C^2), and nonshared environmental (E^2) variance components of depression.

environmental factors contribute relatively more, to interindividual differences in depression the more rejected children are by peers.

How should these findings be interpreted? The finding of *r*GE, indicating that a significant portion of the genetic factors influencing depression also predicted peer acceptance–rejection, is in line with other findings that youths with genetic risk for depression are at risk for experiencing negative life events (Lau & Eley, 2008). Of course, there is no "gene" that predisposes an individual to peer rejection. However, rejection by peers may be elicited by genetically influenced maladaptive behavior such as a high level of conflict and a lack of collaboration, which has been found to be more frequent in depressed than in nondepressed children (Altmann & Gotlib, 1988). Controlling for *r*GE, the results also provide evidence for G × E, such that individual differences in depression are better explained by genetic factors when children enjoy positive peer relations than when they are rejected. Moreover, interindividual variability of depression was lower and the mean level of depression was higher under conditions of peer rejection than under conditions of popularity. Together, these results suggest that peer rejection constitutes an important source of stress that can foster depressive symptoms even in children without a genetic disposition for depression. Notably, these results are not consistent with a diathesis–stress process of G × E. Rather, they are in line with a suppression process of G × E, in which a restrictive environment reduces the role of genetic influences such that the same developmental outcome is observed regardless of individuals' genetic disposition.

Future Directions

Over the past decade, findings from genetically informative research have provided evidence not only that both genetic and environmental influences are at play in virtually all aspects of human development but also that these effects do not operate independently from each other. As such, the finding of a significant genetic effect does not mean that genes "cause" a specific behavior or trait in a deterministic fashion. Instead, a person's particular genetic makeup predisposes that individual to a certain range of possible behavioral or other characteristics that may affect the environmental circumstances the individual is exposed to. These environmental circumstances, in turn, affect the extent to which the individual's—genetically influenced—behavioral and other characteristics are expressed. Still, much remains to be learned about the role of genes and their interplay with environmental influences on human development.

One important issue concerns the fact that genetic and environmental influences, as well as the specific nature of their interplay, can change at different points during development. Thus certain genes may be turned on or off over the course of developmental maturation (Gottlieb, 1998). Similarly, the same environmental experiences may have different effects at different stages of development. Quantitative genetic studies increasingly employ longitudinal data to assess changes in broad genetic and environmental effects on developmental outcomes. For example, a recent meta-analysis of longitudinal quantitative genetic studies showed a significant increase of genetic effects from adolescence to young adulthood with respect to a variety of internalizing and externalizing problems (Bergen, Gardner, & Kendler, 2007). This increase of genetic effects might at least in part be explained by an increasing importance of selective *r*GE over the course of development. For example, as older children have more autonomy over their friendship choices than younger children, *r*GE underlying the link between individuals' own characteristics and those of their peer group may become stronger with age. To address this issue, future genetically informed studies will need to employ a developmental perspective to assess changes in the interplay between genetic factors with specific, measured environmental context variables.

Although quantitative genetic studies will remain an important instrument for the testing of psychological theories of development and of gene–environment interplay for some time, recent advances in molecular genetics and the completion of the DNA sequencing of the human genome (Collins, Morgan, & Patrinos, 2004) have made it possible to identify specific genes associated with specific phenotypes. As such, scientists are increasingly beginning to include molecular genetics in developmental research (e.g., Burt, 2008; Caspi et al., 2002; Dick et al., 2009). Findings from molecular genetic studies are not always consistent, however. Moreover, because many developmental features—particularly complex social behaviors—are likely determined by multiple genes, specific measured genes typically explain no more than 1% of the variance of quantitative behavioral traits (Kendler, 2005). Nevertheless, molecular genetic studies are an essential tool to help validate findings of gene–environment interplay from quantitative genetic studies.

Molecular genetic studies that examine the interplay between specific measured genes and specific measured environmental variables can also make important contributions to applied issues, such as the development and evaluation of psychosocial intervention programs. Not every treatment is equally beneficial for every individual, and molecular genetic studies can help uncover what type of treatment may be most effective depending on the individual's genetic propensity (Jang, 2005). This was recently shown in a study that tested whether genetic differences moderate the effect of a randomized intervention to reduce externalizing behavior in toddlers (Bakermans-Kranenburg, van IJzendoorn, Pijlman, Mesman, & Juffer, 2008). The intervention, which consisted of parental training to promote positive parenting, was effective in decreasing oppositional behavior only in children with the long variant of *DRD4*, a gene polymorphism related to sensitivity to environmental stimuli. The intervention did not reduce oppositional behavior in children without the long *DRD4* variant, however, although it did improve the parenting behavior of these children's mothers. Although in need of replication, this finding illustrates the invaluable role of research on gene–environment interplay not only in furthering our understanding of human development but also in guiding efforts to improve developmental outcomes.

References

Altmann, E. O., & Gotlib, I. H. (1988). The social behavior of depressed children: An observational study. *Journal of Abnormal Child Psychology, 16*(1), 29–44.

Arseneault, L., Moffitt, T. E., Caspi, A., Taylor, A., Rijsdijk, F. V., Jaffee, S. R., et al. (2003). Strong genetic effects on cross-situational antisocial behavior among 5-year-old children according to mothers, teachers, examiner-observers, and twins' self-reports. *Journal of Child Psychology and Psychiatry, 44*, 832–848.

Bakermans-Kranenburg, M. J., van IJzendoorn, M. H., Pijlman, F. T. A., Mesman, J., & Juffer, F. (2008). Experimental evidence for differential susceptibility: Dopamine D4 receptor polymorphism (*DRD4 VNTR*) moderates intervention effects on toddlers' externalizing behavior in a randomized controlled trial. *Developmental Psychology, 44*(1), 293–300.

Bell, R. Q. (1968). A reinterpretation of the direction of effects in studies of socialization. *Psychological Review, 75*(2), 81–95.

Bergen, S. E., Gardner, C. O., & Kendler, K. S. (2007). Age-related changes in heritability of behavioral phenotypes over adolescence and young adulthood: A meta-analysis. *Twin Research and Human Genetics, 10*(3), 423–433.

Borkenau, P., Riemann, R., Angleitner, A., & Spinath, F. M. (2002). Similarity of childhood experiences and personality resemblance in monozygotic and dizygotic twins: A test of the equal environments assumption. *Personality and Individual Differences, 33*(2), 261–269.

Brendgen, M., Boivin, M., Vitaro, F., Dionne, G., Girard, A., & Pérusse, D. (2008). Gene–environment interactions between peer victimization and child aggression. *Development and Psychopathology, 20,* 455–471.

Brendgen, M., Vitaro, F., Boivin, M., Girard, A., Bukowski, W. M., Dionne, G., et al. (2009). Gene–environment linkages between peer rejection and depressive symptoms in children. *Journal of Child Psychology and Psychiatry, 50*(8), 1009–1017.

Bruder, C. E. G., Piotrowski, A., Gijsbers, A. A. C., Andersson, R., Erickson, S., Diaz de Ståhl, T., et al. (2008). Phenotypically concordant and discordant monozygotic twins display different DNA copy–number–variation profiles. *American Journal of Human Genetics, 82*(3), 763–771.

Burt, S. A. (2008). Genes and popularity: Evidence of an evocative gene–environment correlation. *Psychological Science, 19*(2), 112–113.

Burt, S. A. (2009a). Are there meaningful etiological differences within antisocial behavior? Results of a meta-analysis. *Clinical Psychology Review, 29*(2), 163–178.

Burt, S. A. (2009b). Rethinking environmental contributions to child and adolescent psychopathology: A meta-analysis of shared environmental influences. *Psychological Bulletin, 135*(4), 608–637.

Caspi, A., McClay, J., Moffitt, T. E., Mill, J., Martin, J., Craig, I. W., et al. (2002). Role of genotype in the cycle of violence in maltreated children. *Science, 297,* 851–854.

Coie, J. D., Dodge, K. A., & Coppotelli, H. (1982). Dimensions and types of social status: A cross-age perspective. *Developmental Psychology, 18,* 557–570.

Collins, F. S., Morgan, M., & Patrinos, A. (2004). The Human Genome Project: Lessons from large-scale biology. *Science, 300,* 286–290.

Collins, W. A., Maccoby, E. E., Steinberg, L., Hetherington, E. M., & Bornstein, M. H. (2000). Contemporary research on parenting: The case for nature and nurture. *American Psychologist, 55*(2), 218–232.

Conger, K. J., & Conger, R. D. (1994). Differential parenting and change in sibling differences in delinquency. *Journal of Family Psychology, 8,* 287–302.

Dear, P. H. (2009). Copy–number variation: The end of the human genome? *Trends in Biotechnology, 27*(8), 448–454.

Derks, E. M., Dolan, C. V., & Boomsma, D. I. (2006). A test of the equal environment assumption (EEA) in multivariate twin studies. *Twin Research and Human Genetics, 9,* 403–411.

Dick, D. M., Latendresse, S. J., Lansford, J. E., Budde, J. P., Goate, A., Dodge, K. A., et al. (2009). Role of *GABRA2* in trajectories of externalizing behavior across development and evidence of moderation by parental monitoring. *Archives of General Psychiatry, 66*(6), 649–657.

Dunn, J., & Plomin, R. (1990). *Separate lives: Why siblings are so different.* New York: Basic Books.

Dunn, J., Stocker, C., & Plomin, R. (1990). Nonshared experiences within the family: Correlates of behavior problems in middle childhood. *Development and Psychopathology, 2,* 113–126.

Eaves, L., Silberg, J., & Erkanli, A. (2003). Resolving multiple epigenetic pathways to adolescent depression. *Journal of Child Psychology and Psychiatry, 44*(7), 1006–1014.

Falconer, D. S. (1960). *Introduction to quantitative genetics.* Edinburgh, UK: Oliver & Boyd.

Feinberg, M. E., Button, T. M. M., Neiderhiser, J. M., Reiss, D., & Hetherington, E. M. (2007). Parenting and adolescent antisocial behavior and depression: Evidence of genotype × parenting environment interaction. *Archives of General Psychiatry, 64*(4), 457–465.

Gottlieb, G. (1998). Normally occurring environmental and behavioral influences on gene activity: From central dogma to probabilistic epigenesis. *Psychological Review, 105*(4), 792–802.

Hettema, J., Neale, M., & Kendler, K. (1995). Physical similarity and the equal-environment assumption in twin studies of psychiatric disorders. *Behavior Genetics, 25*(4), 327–335.

Jaffee, S. R., Caspi, A., Moffitt, T. E., Dodge, K. A., Rutter, M., Taylor, A., et al. (2005). Nature × nurture: Genetic vulnerabilities interact with physical maltreatment to promote conduct problems. *Development and Psychopathology, 17*(1), 67–84.

Jang, K. L. (2005). *The behavioral genetics of psychopathology: A clinical guide*. Mahwah, NJ: Erlbaum.

Johnson, W., Turkheimer, E., Gottesman, I. I., & Bouchard, T. J. (2009). Beyond heritability: Twin studies in behavioral research. *Current Directions in Psychological Science, 18*(4), 217–220.

Keller, M. C., & Coventry, W. L. (2005). Quantifying and addressing parameter indeterminacy in the classical twin design. *Twin Research and Human Genetics, 8*, 201–213.

Keller, M. C., Medland, S. E., Duncan, L. E., Hatemi, P. K., Neale, M. C., Maes, H. H. M., et al. (2009). Modeling extended twin family data: I. Description of the cascade model. *Twin Research and Human Genetics, 12*(1), 8–18.

Kendler, K. S. (2005). "A gene for . . . ": The nature of gene action in psychiatric disorders. *American Journal of Psychiatry, 162*(7), 1243–1252.

Kendler, K. S., Neale, M. C., Kessler, R. C., Heath, A. C., & Eaves, L. J. (1993). A test of the equal-environment assumption in twin studies of psychiatric illness. *Behavior Genetics, 23*(1), 21–27.

Kendler, K. S., Neale, M. C., Kessler, R. C., Heath, A. C., & Eaves, L. J. (1994). Parental treatment and the equal-environment assumption in twin studies of psychiatric illness. *Psychological Medicine, 24*, 579–590.

Laffey-Ardley, S., & Thorpe, K. (2006). Being opposite: Is there advantage for social competence and friendships in being an opposite-sex twin? *Twin Research and Human Genetics, 9*, 131–140.

Lamarche, V., Brendgen, M., Boivin, M., Vitaro, F., Dionne, G., & Pérusse, D. (2007). Do friends' characteristics moderate the prospective links between peer victimization and reactive and proactive aggression? *Journal of Abnormal Child Psychology, 35*, 665–680.

Lau, J. Y. F., & Eley, T. C. (2008). Disentangling gene–environment correlations and interactions on adolescent depressive symptoms. *Journal of Child Psychology and Psychiatry, 49*(2), 142–150.

Lerner, R. M. (1982). Children and adolescents as producers of their own development. *Developmental Review, 2*(4), 342–370.

Lerner, R. M. (2006). Another nine-inch nail for behavioral genetics! *Human Development, 49*(6), 336–342.

Loehlin, J., Harden, K., & Turkheimer, E. (2009). The effect of assumptions about parental assortative mating and genotype–income correlation on estimates of genotype–environment interaction in the National Merit Twin Study. *Behavior Genetics, 39*(2), 165–169.

Loehlin, J., & Nichols, R. (1976). *Heredity, environment and personality*. Austin: University of Texas Press.

McHale, S. M., Crouter, A. C., McGuire, S., & Updegraff, K. A. (1995). Congruence between mothers' and fathers' differential treatment of siblings: Links with family relations and children's well-being. *Child Development, 66*, 116–128.

Muthén, L. K., & Muthén, B. O. (2004). *Mplus user's guide* (3rd ed.). Los Angeles: Authors.

Narusyte, J., Andershed, A.-K., Neiderhiser, J., & Lichtenstein, P. (2007). Aggression as a mediator of genetic contributions to the association between negative parent–child relationships and adolescent antisocial behavior. *European Child and Adolescent Psychiatry, 16*(2), 128–137.

Neale, M. C., & Cardon, L. R. (1992). *Methodology for genetic studies of twins and families*. Dordrecht, The Netherlands: Kluwer Academic.

Petrill, S. A. (2002). Examining social behavior and relationships using genetically sensitive designs: An introduction. *Marriage and Family Review, 33*(1), 3–10.

Plomin, R., & Bergeman, C. S. (1991). The nature of nurture: Genetic influence on "environmental" measures. *Behavioral and Brain Sciences, 14*(3), 373–427.

Plomin, R., DeFries, J. C., & Loehlin, J. C. (1977). Genotype–environment interaction and correlation in the analysis of human behavior. *Psychological Bulletin, 84*, 309–322.

Pulkkinen, L., Vaalamo, I., Hietala, R., Kaprio, J., & Rose, R. J. (2003). Peer reports of adaptive behavior in twins and singletons: Is twinship a risk or an advantage? *Twin Research, 6*(2), 106–118.

Purcell, S. (2002). Variance components models for gene–environment interaction in twin analysis. *Twin Research, 5*(6), 554–571.

Rhee, S., & Waldman, I. D. (2002). Genetic and environmental influences on antisocial behavior: A meta-analysis of twin and adoption studies. *Psychological Bulletin, 29*, 490–529.

Rutter, M. (2007). Gene–environment interdependence. *Developmental Science, 10*(1), 12–18.

Rutter, M., Moffitt, T. E., & Caspi, A. (2006). Gene–environment interplay and psychopathology: Multiple varieties but real effects. *Journal of Child Psychology and Psychiatry, 47*(3/4), 226–261.

Rutter, M., & Silberg, J. (2002). Gene–environment interplay in relation to emotional and behavioral disturbance. *Annual Review of Psychology, 53*(1), 463–490.

Scarr, S., & McCartney, K. (1983). How people make their own environments: A theory of genotype–environment effects. *Child Development, 54*(2), 424–435.

Shanahan, M., & Hofer, S. (2005). Social context in gene–environment interactions: Retrospect and prospect. *Journal of Gerontology: Series B, 60*, 65–76.

Thorpe, K. (2003). Twins and friendship. *Twin Research, 6*(6), 532–535.

Thorpe, K., & Gardner, K. (2006). Twins and their friendships: Differences between monozygotic, dizygotic same-sex and dizygotic mixed-sex pairs. *Twin Research and Human Genetics, 9*(1), 155–164.

Turkheimer, E. (2000). Three laws of behavior genetics and what they mean. *Current Directions in Psychological Science, 9*(5), 160–164.

Turkheimer, E., D'Onofrio, B. M., Maes, H. H., & Eaves, L. J. (2005). Analysis and interpretation of twin studies including measures of the shared environment. *Child Development, 76*(6), 1217–1233.

Turkheimer, E., Haley, A., Waldron, M., D'Onofrio, B., & Gottesman, I. I. (2003). Socioeconomic status modifies heritability of IQ in young children. *Psychological Science, 14*(6), 623–628.

CHAPTER 39

Epidemic Models of the Onset of Social Activities

Applications to Adolescent Sexuality, Smoking, Drinking, and Religious Involvement

JOSEPH LEE RODGERS
ANDREY KOVAL

This chapter provides an overview of epidemic models of the onset of social activities—EMOSA models—including a description, discussion of assumptions, and review of past work. We also present the conceptual framework and a brief empirical demonstration of a new category of EMOSA applications. EMOSA models have been in development since the late 1980s and have been applied in a number of studies within the purview and interest of developmental researchers. Their mathematical structure is nonlinear and dynamic, and so they have the capability to account for more complex developmental processes than many linear model–based methods. They apply, specifically, to developmental domains in which change in behavior over time depends at least in part on social influence from within the friendship network. There are two types of these models, social contagion and general diffusion models, which can be defined in such a way that they compete as explanatory of adolescent developmental behaviors. Social contagion models reflect processes transmitted from one person to another, through an explicit behavioral contagion process. General diffusion models reflect processes that involve broader and less specific social influences, such as those that pass through advertising, general word-of-mouth, television shows and movies, or behavioral modeling by famous people. The two can be distinguished both empirically and theoretically, and this distinction has both research and policy implications.

Central Issues

Methodology and Theory

It is easiest to understand EMOSA models with reference to their original research purpose and their psychological intention. The title represented by the EMOSA acronym, "epidemic models of the onset of social activities," was originally defined to reflect both social contagion ("epidemic" and "social") and the first initiation of a behavior such as smoking or drinking ("onset"). Originally, EMOSA models were developed to explain and predict the way that the onset of certain behaviors spread through an intact adolescent network. Sexual behavior, smoking, and drinking were the three domains for which EMOSA models were originally developed.

EMOSA models represent both a methodology and a theory. In fact, many mathematical models that are developed for a specific scientific purpose have accompanying theories. Rodgers (2010) distinguished between mathematical/statistical models designed to apply broadly in many different settings and those designed for a specific research purpose. Examples of the former are regression, ANOVA, structural equation modeling, and multilevel models, each of which provides a statistical/methodological answer to questions asked very broadly across many research domains. On the other hand, many mathematical models are designed to represent a very specific research domain. Early memory models provide an excellent example (e.g., Atkinson & Shiffrin, 1968). Such models are usually a mathematical representation of memory processes and also imply (or often explicitly define) a psychological theory. EMOSA modeling was originally developed to match a specific purpose, and each new EMOSA application has been built to achieve certain specific goals. In this chapter we describe the origins of EMOSA models by reviewing past work and also demonstrate their potential breadth by proposing an EMOSA model in a new and conceptually different research domain.

Illustration

We illustrate the EMOSA concept with reference to smoking behavior. Smoking spreads, at least in part, through social contagion. Unlike sexual behavior, there is nothing biologically "natural" about smoking (though this statement does not argue against a strong biological component involved in both onset and continuation of smoking). The simple process of taking a "stick" that includes paper rolled around leaves, lighting it on fire, and breathing the smoke does not appear on the face of it to be a behavior that would spontaneously develop very often. Social influence, rather than biological drive, stimulates adolescents to try their first cigarette. That influence may come from parents, siblings, or friends. It may come from proximate influences such as direct acquaintances or from more distal sources such as media and literature (see Burt, 1987, and Rodgers, 2007, for specification of the methodological distinctions between these different types of social influence). EMOSA models were originally defined to explain the transmission of direct social influence from one adolescent to another (i.e., social contagion), though they have been adapted in a number of settings to account for more indirect social influences as well (i.e., general diffusion).

Thus, for example, we can imagine a group of five 12-year-old boys spending a summer afternoon together. Only one of them has ever smoked a cigarette, having done so recently with his older brother because they saw a cowboy on television who was smoking and they wanted to emulate his behavior. The boy brought a pack with him and wants his friends to try their first cigarette. He lights a cigarette, takes a puff, and offers it to the boy next to him. For dozens of subtle yet important psychological reasons, this boy considers and declines, but with some embarrassment. The boy with the cigarette then offers it to another boy, who for his own different reasons eagerly inhales and immediately begins to cough violently. After the laughter subsides, the second smoker passes it on to another boy, who eagerly tries the cigarette without complication. The last boy in the group comments, "You'll never get me to smoke one of those things, look what it did to John [the cougher]."

This constructed though realistic anecdote (loosely based on an actual event in my [J. L. R.] adolescence years ago) contains many of the processes that EMOSA models attempt to explain. The first boy and his brother were influenced to try their first cigarette through a general diffusion process. In contrast, within this story, a direct social contagion process—the immediate social influence and facilitation of a friend—caused two of the boys to become "smokers" (in the sense that they would answer "yes" to the survey question, "Have you ever smoked a cigarette, meaning you inhaled the smoke into your mouth and/or lungs?"). One of the boys appeared interested, but resisted; his "transition probability" is obviously lower than for the other boys but probably nonzero. (Note that a transition probability is a measure of the likelihood that a respondent will make the transition from one to another behavioral category, in this case from never having tried a cigarette to having tried one, during the course of a relevant time unit.) Another of the boys had no interest and even implied that he would never smoke under any condition. In the language of EMOSA models, the contagious behavior, smoking, had spread to two of the boys; one other boy had a likely nonzero future transition probability; and one was quite possibly "immune" from smoking, implying a fixed and constant transition probability of zero.

Borrowing Modeling Strategies

The analogy between behavioral contagion and biological contagion is obvious in this case. The onset of smoking behavior spread from one boy to another, and then to a third, in a process analogous to the spread of the cold virus, or swine flu, or HIV. Like a biological disease, some members were more susceptible to the contagious spread than others. Obviously, public health experts would like to understand the correlates, causes, and dynamics of the transmission of onset of smoking, just as they would like to understand the correlates, causes, and dynamics of the spread of HIV, the common cold, and other contagious diseases. Some behaviors become behavioral epidemics for periods of time, just as some diseases do.

The transmission of contagious biological disease is well studied in the epidemiological and medical literature, and sophisticated models exist to account for causes, correlates, and dynamics (see, e.g., May & Anderson, 1987, for careful and sophisticated specification of a whole class of these models). One of the advantages of viewing behavioral contagion as analogous to biological contagion is that the methodological approaches from epidemiology and medical science can be borrowed to study the spread of smoking (and other social) behaviors. This is the basic starting point of EMOSA modeling. We have published many papers since EMOSA models were first proposed in the late 1980s (Rowe, Rodgers, & Meseck-Bushey, 1989), each of which takes advantage of the concept of social or behavioral contagion to study an adolescent process relevant to public health settings. In fact, the medical/epidemiological models use principles from the innovation diffusion literature (Mahajan & Peterson, 1985), from which we can also borrow methodological models and principles.

In the following sections, we review EMOSA models for sexual behavior and pregnancy, for smoking, and for drinking. These models all reflect past work. Following these, we propose a new EMOSA application, to religious behavior among middle and late adolescents, including early college students. The social contagion component of this new domain is obvious. However, the challenges associated with this new modeling exercise are different from those associated with sexuality, smoking, and drinking, although some past stagewise models of sexuality and smoking are useful in the current application. We will fit the new EMOSA model to a longitudinal set of religious involvement data from the National Longitudinal Survey of Youth 1997 data set (NLSY97).

Conceptual Principles and Methodological Assumptions

The original and other, earlier EMOSA models have been reviewed several times before. Rodgers, Rowe, and Buster (1998) and Rodgers (2003) reviewed EMOSA sexuality models, and Rodgers and Johnson (2007) and Rodgers (2007) reviewed EMOSA smoking and drinking models. In this chapter, we illustrate previous EMOSA models within the two separate domains—sexuality models and smoking/drinking models—that build in complexity.

EMOSA Smoking and Drinking Models

Smoking and drinking models are treated together because the forms of the mathematical models are virtually identical for the two domains (though some past results have diverged in substantive interpretation). Rowe and Rodgers (1991a) defined the first EMOSA model of smoking and drinking. That model assumes an intact community of adolescents who act as social influences on one another during the course of a year. Each year (or grade), the model posits that an adolescent is paired (randomly or purposively) with another adolescent whose smoking/drinking status is either "I have never done this behavior" or "I have done this behavior." Obviously, this is a model of *onset*, rather than intensity or continuation of the behavior (though such continuation models do fall within the domain of more complex EMOSA models).

There are four possible pairings. If two nonexperienced adolescents are paired, with some transition probability they can spontaneously engage in the behavior together (e.g., two boys who have never smoked decide to try a cigarette together). We refer to this type of transition as "nonepidemic" transition. If Adolescent A is experienced and Adolescent B is not, or vice versa—the second and third types of pairings—then, with some (different) transition probability, the experienced adolescent "transmits the behavior" through social influence to the other. This type of transition is called "epidemic transition." The fourth type of pairing, between two experienced adolescents, is irrelevant for the increase in the behavior. The model is defined through simple difference equations. These equations are fit to yearly prevalence measures as the variable input values, and parameters in the model (transition probabilities) are estimated by fitting the system of difference equations to the prevalence measures using computer-based optimization routines based on a specified loss function (e.g., least squares, chi-square, or Akaike information criteria [AIC]). The starting point for a social contagion model (see Rowe & Rodgers, 1991b) is a model that ignores nonepidemic transition, using a single difference equation:

$$P_{t+1} = P_t + T(1 - P_t) * P_t \qquad \textbf{(39.1)}$$

where P_t is the prevalence of the behavior in time (year or age) t (i.e., the proportion of adolescents who had ever engaged in the behavior) and T is the transition probability. In this model, $(1 - P_t) * P_t$ captures the proportion of adolescent pairs in which one experienced and one inexperienced adolescent are combined, and with transition probability T, the inexperienced adolescent becomes experienced. The model states that the proportion who have ever done the behavior at time $t + 1$, P_{t+1}, is composed of those who had already done the behavior at time t (P_t), added to those who were inexperienced at time t ($1 - P_t$) but who made the transition through epidemic transmission of the behavior. Rowe and Rodgers fit this model to smoking and drinking prevalence measures from the ADSEX data set, collected in high schools in North Carolina and Florida, and to smoking and drinking data from inner-city Baltimore. Models were fit overall and separately by race–gender subsets, and the different transition parameters were interpreted.

Rowe, Chassin, Presson, Edwards, and Sherman (1992) expanded the EMOSA smoking model into a stagewise model. Within this model, there were categories for the nonsmoker (for those who had never smoked a cigarette), for the experimental smoker (for those who had smoked but who were not smoking regularly), for the smoker (for those who were smoking regularly), and for the reformed smoker (for those who had been smokers but were not currently smoking). With similar contagion processes, captured by several equations similar to equation 39.1, adolescents (or adults) were paired up with another individual during the year, and their joint smoking status provided potential for influence to transition in theoretically meaningful ways among the categories. They fit their model to data from sixth to twelfth graders in an Indiana county school system.

EMOSA models are defined at the aggregate level because they are fit to aggregate prevalence statistics indicating the proportion of a population who have engaged in a certain behavior or not. An important adjustment to equation 39.1 (see Rodgers, 2007; Rodgers & Johnson, 2007) accounts for nonepidemic transition as follows:

$$P_{t+1} = P_t + T_e\,(1 - P_t) * P_t + T_n\,(1 - P_t) * (1 - P_t) \qquad \textbf{(39.2)}$$

where T_e is the transition parameter for epidemic transmission, as in equation 39.1, and T_n is the transmission parameter for nonepidemic transmission. The T_n parameter applies to the proportion of the population of pairs who are both inexperienced in the behavior, $(1 - P_t) * (1 - P_t)$.

Different forms of EMOSA models can compete (e.g., Rodgers & Johnson, 2007; Rowe, Chassin, Presson, & Sherman, 1996). A simpler model, with a different interpretation from equation 39.1, is the following:

$$P_{t+1} = P_t + T(1 - P_t) \qquad \textbf{(39.3)}$$

In this model, the prevalence of those who had performed a behavior is irrelevant, and the transmission parameter simply measures the proportion of inexperienced respondents who made the transmission from time t to time $t + 1$. We refer to this model as "non-prevalence-driven" transition, or "general diffusion." Burt (1987) referred to the first type of process in Equations 39.1 and 39.2 as a "social cohesion process" or, in our language, "social contagion" or "prevalence-driven diffusion." The second term in equation 39.3 he called a "structural equivalence process," whereas we refer to this as "general diffusion." Importantly, Burt showed that the first process, social contagion, would produce an S-shaped prevalence curve, whereas the second would produce a negatively accelerated exponential curve. Rodgers (2007) adapted Burt's two models into a single model, with a parameter estimating the proportion of the two processes that were at work. In the equation

$$P_{t+1} = P_t + T(1 - P_t) * P_t^C \qquad \textbf{(39.4)}$$

the parameter C has the effect of creating equations 39.1 and 39.3 as special cases of a more general model. Equation 39.1 is the model for social contagion and geometrically produces an S-shaped prevalence curve; this model is obtained when $C = 1$. Equation 39.3 is a general diffusion model and geometrically produces a negatively accelerated exponential curve; this model is obtained when $C = 0$. When we estimate C as a proportion between 0 and 1, we are conceptually identifying how much of the diffusion process is associated with social contagion and how much is associated with general diffusion. In other words, C can be estimated from the data and is then informative about the type of process that generated the data. The first estimation of a C parameter was presented in Rodgers (2007) using college student smoking and drinking data from University of Oklahoma students in 2003; using standard optimization methods and PROC NLIN (a nonlinear optimization routine in SAS), C values were estimated to be $C = .80$ for smoking and $C = 1.0$ for drinking, suggesting that both onset processes were strongly associated with social contagion.

Besides the obvious research value obtained from estimating structural and substantively interesting parameters, such an estimate also has policy implications. Intervention programs designed to intervene in smoking, drinking, or adolescent pregnancy programs would be highly informed by knowledge of how the behavior spreads through an adolescent network. If the behavior spreads primarily through face-to-face contact, intervention efforts would naturally focus on pairwise social exchange of knowledge, information, and influence among adolescents. If the behavior spreads primarily through general diffusion processes, intervention efforts would naturally focus on media channels and higher level communication patterns. See Rodgers (2003) for more detailed discussion of how estimating EMOSA models can inform policy.

Of relevance to EMOSA modeling is that most of the data curves to which EMOSA models have been previously fit were clearly S-shaped curves, supporting that at least part of the process involved did indeed emerge from an individual person-to-person social contagion process. In two papers noted earlier, Rodgers (2007) and Rodgers and Johnson (2007), we compared results from the simple aggregate model in equation 39.1 with individual-level smoking and drinking onset data from University of Oklahoma college students. The transition probabilities closely matched the proportion of college students who indicated through short verbal stories that social influence was an important component in their first smoking or drinking experience.

EMOSA Sexuality Models

Rowe and colleagues (1989) defined the first EMOSA sexuality model. Sexuality models are distinguished theoretically from smoking–drinking models because they are inherently two-gender models, with separate prevalence equations defined for males and females (and each gender equation refers to the prevalence measure of the other gender). The first EMOSA sexuality model was similar to equation 39.2:

$$Pm_{t+1} = Pm_t + Tm^* (1 - Pm_t) * Pf_t + k^* (1 - Pm_t) * M_t^* (1 - Pf_t)$$

$$Pf_{t+1} = Pf_t + Tf^* M_t^* (1 - Pf_t) * Pm_t + k^* (1 - Pm_t) * M_t^* (1 - Pf_t) \qquad \textbf{(39.5)}$$

The parameters to be estimated by fitting the model to empirical prevalence data for males and females are *Tm, Tf,* and *k*. The first two are epidemic transition parameters for males and females, respectively, and *k* is a nonepidemic transition parameter that is automatically shared by the male and female. As before, the model assumes that two (in this case opposite-sex, assuming focus on heterosexual behavior) adolescents are paired each year. There are four types of pairs. When both adolescents have previously had intercourse, there is no potential for change in *Pm* or *Pf*, and the first term in each equation accounts for the carryover proportions who had ever had intercourse at the previous time period *t* (year, in most cases). The second and third type of pair occur when an experienced female is paired with an inexperienced male or when an experienced male is paired with an inexperienced female. In these pairs, with transition probability *Tm* or *Tf*, a male or female is added to the proportion of experienced adolescents in the relevant equation for the next year. The fourth type of pair occurs when two inexperienced adolescents are paired, in which case, with transition probability *k*, they each make the transition to being sexually experienced. Besides the two-gender model that requires two equations, this model is different for the smoking–drinking model in equation 39.2 because there is a maturity filter included in the model, M_t. M_t is a measure (a measured variable, not an estimated parameter) of the proportion of females who have reached pubertal maturity at a given time/age *t*. When it is multiplied by $(1 - Pf_t)$, it "filters" out from eligibility to make the transition to being sexually experienced those adolescent females who have not yet reached pubertal maturity. We discovered that such pubertal maturity filters substantially improve the fit of the model when they are applied to female prevalence curves but have no effect for the males (a finding that also matches previous empirical research; see Rowe et al., 1989, for discussion). This model was fit to the ADSEX data, collected from students ages 12–16 in schools across three rounds in Raleigh, North Carolina, and two rounds in Tallahassee, Florida. Parameter estimates were highly interpretable, when compared with empirical results from previous studies. For example, the nonepidemic transition probability was relatively low (*k* ranged from .08 to .14 across race subgroups) compared with the epidemic transition probabilities, and the epidemic probability for males was notably higher than for females (*Tf* ranged from .22 to .33 across races, and *Tm* ranged from .78 to 1.0 across races), suggesting that an experienced female was quite likely to convert an inexperienced male, whereas an experienced male had a lower probability of converting an inexperienced female.

Rodgers and Rowe (1993) extended the EMOSA sexuality model to a five-stage model, predicting onset behavior from complete inexperience to kissing, touching (petting) above the waist, touching below the waist, and sexual intercourse. They used the ADSEX data, from which prevalence estimates for all five categories were obtained, and once again found highly interpretable parameter estimates. Rodgers et al. (1998) further expanded this stagewise model by adding maturity filters (maturity rates were estimated from national medical data), and, importantly, pregnancy probabilities were added to the model as a potential female outcome once a female became sexually experienced. This more complex model was fit to the pregnancy rates estimated from Guttmacher Institute data and to national sexuality prevalence curves estimated from the National Longitudinal Survey of Youth (NLSY). Again, sexuality parameter estimates were interpretable (and similar to those from other data sets), and pregnancy transition rates were similar at older ages to ones already estimated from empirical data and were revealing about younger pregnancy probabilities (see Rodgers et al., 1998, for a summary of the several surprising but interpretable findings, some of which are reviewed briefly in a later section of this chapter).

Assumptions of EMOSA Models

A great deal of attention has been given in past work to the assumptions of these kinds of models. We summarize several of those here (see Rodgers & Johnson, 2007, for more elaborate discussion). First, Rowe and Rodgers (1994) expanded the original EMOSA sexuality model to an "intercohort contagion model" by relaxing the assumption that pairing only occurred within single-year age cohorts and allowing pairings between older and younger adolescents. In that study, we also evaluated the assumption of random pairing by linking adolescents according to their sexual experience status, as well as other features of the social environment. This work demonstrated that, though it appears to violate intuition, the random mixing assumption is actually quite reasonable, as the model is robust to naturally occurring violations of the assumptions (also see Dodd, 1955, for theoretical support for the value of random mixing). Next, we have evaluated the assumption of homogeneous mixing in several ways. Procedurally, this assumption can be relaxed by estimating separate models across subgroups (e.g., race or gender) and testing for differences; we routinely find that race subgroups differ from one another in EMOSA sexuality models, and genders often (but not always) differ in EMOSA smoking and drinking models. To push this investigation further, we also condition on other factors as well. For example, Rowe et al. (1996) fit different smoking models to adolescents whose parents smoked than to those whose parents did not smoke, just as Rodgers and Johnson (2007) found that different mathematical models fit the onset of smoking behavior for those adolescents for whom social contagion was a component of the process, compared with those for whom it was not.

The assumption that social contagion is the only process involved in the onset of these behaviors has been handled by comparing models like those in equations 39.1 and 39.2 to those in equation 39.3. But of more importance, the work reported in Rodgers (2007) that treated each type of process as a special case of a broader model allowed us to estimate the proportion of the two types of processes (social contagion and general diffusion) as they contribute to a particular process.

Developmental Applications of EMOSA Modeling

Past EMOSA Findings

We highlight several past EMOSA findings. The first type of result has already been noted; EMOSA parameter estimates have consistently been reasonable, with excellent face validity, and also have been consistent with other research results, supporting concurrent validity. Furthermore, the individual-level results presented in Rodgers and Johnson (2007) and Rodgers (2007) matched and cross-validated with the aggregate-level EMOSA results when they were applied to interpretations at the individual level. Three other findings will also be reviewed, ones that were not predicted and that were, furthermore, surprising when first identified but then interesting and valuable upon interpretation. These findings fall into the category of surprising or unpredictable results that emerge from a theoretical orientation, one of the notable and valuable features of a successful theory (see Roberts & Pashler, 2000, and Rodgers & Rowe, 2002, for further discussion of such results that emerge from a theory). Such results are valuable because they explicitly push both the theoretical and empirical import of a theoretical orientation. Many examples of such theoretical surprises exist in the hard sciences (e.g., in physics and astronomy) and are used routinely to signal the maturity and success of such scientific enterprises. For example, Einstein's relativity equations made surprising predictions about the nature of matter when it approaches the speed of light, which were later corroborated. Bode's law predicted the location of a "missing" planet, which subsequently resulted in the discovery of Uranus. Social and behavioral scientists are often criticized for "identifying the obvious"; in these less mature behavioral scientific arenas, such findings can help move the field forward.

The first such unpredictable EMOSA result was identified in Rowe and colleagues (1989) and developed and explained in Rowe and Rodgers (1994). In the latter paper, we fit separate models across race to national sexuality prevalence curves estimated from the NLSY data. The surprising finding was that transition parameters were virtually identical for white and black respondents, both in the local ADSEX data in Rowe and colleagues, and in the national data from the NLSY. Previous empirical studies identified substantial differences between black and white adolescents at a given age, with substantially more black males and females having had intercourse than white males and females. What appeared at first to run counter to this finding had a straightforward explanation. We included maturity filters in these models. Black females reach pubertal maturity on average several months earlier than white females (e.g., Harlan, Harlan, & Grillo, 1980). Once this maturational difference was accounted for within the model and given the nonlinear feature of our EMOSA models that allowed small early differences to be magnified over time, the race differences were fully accounted for. This interpretation suggests that past efforts to explain these differences with social and cultural theories that have not accounted for biological differences in maturation (e.g., Furstenberg, Morgan, Moore, & Peterson, 1987; Washington, 1982; Weinberg & Williams, 1988) may have missed a critical and important explanatory process.

The second unpredictable EMOSA result emerged from Rodgers and colleagues (1998; reviewed previously). There we found that the probability of pregnancy, given onset of sexual behavior, was approximately constant across age. This finding appeared counterintuitive, as older adolescent females (and partners) likely use contraceptives more effectively than younger adolescents. Our interpretation, however, is that this result reflects both differences in contraceptive efficacy and also differences in coital rates, which may approximately balance one another in defining probability of pregnancy. In other words, older adolescents almost certainly do use contraceptives more reliably on average than younger and less experienced adolescents, but they also have higher rates of coital activity as well.

The third unpredictable EMOSA result, which comes from Rowe and colleagues (1996), should perhaps not even be called a surprise, because the finding is quite interpretable, yet very revealing. The primary finding in that study was that the transition from a nonsmoker to an experimental smoker was driven by a social contagion process, yet the transition from an experimental smoker to a regular smoker was a constant-rate diffusion process, not dependent on others within the social network. This is quite interpretable within a theoretical framework accounting for nicotine dependence as a critical component of the transition to regular smoker. But the other important and intriguing part of that finding was that children with smoking parents made the transition from nonsmoker to experimental smoker more quickly than those with nonsmoking parents. In other words, the likelihood of social influence from within the friendship network was leveraged by parental smoking status. This finding contextualizes other EMOSA research, suggesting that although the social influence passing from friend to friend may be the proximate process that accounts for the contagious spread of behavior, the more distal causes of such behaviors can certainly originate at home or in other social settings.

Summary of EMOSA as a Developmental Methodology

As developed in the first sections of this chapter, EMOSA models have certain attractions and advantages for developmental researchers, including, in particular, developmental methodologists. The mathematical equations used in EMOSA models are identical in form to both epidemiological models of contagious disease spread and models of innovation diffusion. However, EMOSA models are explicitly developmental. They are built to match a specific developmental process, the onset of a specified behavior that spreads (at least in part) through a social contagion/social influence process.

They are, further and importantly, also naturally nonlinear and dynamic, as most developmental processes are as well. The title of the Rodgers and Johnson (2007) chapter captures this feature: "Nonlinear Dynamic Models of Nonlinear Dynamic Behaviors." Rodgers and colleagues (1998) emphasized that, although most statistical models are linear, the world is decidedly nonlinear—especially developmental processes. Furthermore, linear models such as regression and ANOVA have no natural real-world interpretation but, rather, are simply predictive. EMOSA models are also predictive, and furthermore, they are explanatory in relation to the processes that they model. Though EMOSA models simplify the real world (as all models must, by definition), they account for the interaction of individuals within a friendship network, the social influence that passes through that network, and the changing status of adolescents as they grow, mature, and engage in new behaviors.

Future Directions: A New EMOSA Application

Previous EMOSA models have been developed for adolescent problem behaviors (see Rodgers & Rowe, 1993, for discussion and a taxonomy of mildly and severely deviant behaviors from an EMOSA perspective). But there is nothing inherent within EMOSA models that restricts their use to this domain. Rather, funding histories and grant availability and past research momentum on adolescent problem behaviors have been the primary reasons for such focus. In presenting and describing EMOSA models, we often refer to their potential in regard to socially positive and important behaviors in adolescents, such as the initiation of playing in the school band or taking a particular course in school, such as geometry or a foreign language. In each case, the "onset" of the behavior can be captured using the conceptual models developed in the previous sections. In this section, we develop a new EMOSA application, one that not only is a specific new research domain but that also breaks new ground in terms of broadening their application beyond problem behaviors. We present here an EMOSA model of religious activity during the transition from middle to late adolescence to young adulthood.

The conceptual orientation for this new application involves the recognition that older adolescents, as they transition into the workforce or college, suddenly are confronted with an expanded behavioral repertoire. As they enter a new physical and social environment and build new friendship networks, they may shift behaviors that were firmly established in high school. One student may begin to take dancing classes that she never had time to take in high school; another may drop dancing in favor of more informal social activities. Another student may join a club soccer team, whereas another may shift from soccer to karate. The social networks available in modern settings for adolescent students are remarkable, including Facebook and other networking sites, online poker, and dating services, as well as the more traditional college/young adult parties and sporting events. At least part of the explanation for the shifts into and out of certain social activities is likely to emerge from social influences passed through their new friendship network, which is the type of influence explicitly accounted for by EMOSA models.

Religious behavior is of particular interest during this transition, because many young adults and new (or continuing) college students have an expanded behavioral repertoire in relation to religion. College is particularly easy to describe in an EMOSA context. Whereas younger adolescents were likely to be strongly influenced by family and high school friends in previous church attendance and religious involvement, when they go to college, they may express shifts in that behavior. Those shifts may move in either direction, toward more involvement or toward less involvement. Some of those shifts in behavior may emerge from underlying deeply held religious beliefs. Others may reflect a fairly pure social influence from friends. When a new college student invites his roommate to attend a church service with him, this process reflects a relatively classic form of social contagion, similar in form (though different in outcome, obviously) to that defined early in this chapter in relation to cigarette smoking. This same potential shift in religious behavior can also occur during the transition into workplace activity, following either high school or college graduation.

We identified religious involvement data in the National Longitudinal Survey of Youth 1997 (NLSY97) cohort, which was based on a probability sample of U.S. adolescents between the ages of 12 and 16 on December 31, 1996; first interviews occurred in 1997, when respondents ranged in age from 12 to 17, and then yearly since then. We extracted a subsample of N = 1,150 out of the approximately 9,000 total respondents; the subsample contained all respondents who had answered the religious involvement question in every year between 2000 and 2008 and who were cohort-defined to be age 16 in 2000, age 17 in 2001, and so forth. The seven response outcomes and proportions are included in Table 39.1 and graphed in Figure 39.1. We collapsed these into three categories of religious involvement: goers (active attenders), doubters (irregular attenders), and nongoers. These are shown in Table 39.2, as they were constructed from the original seven response categories.

Within the NLSY97, we actually have individual-level data on the transitions among these categories. However, we build and fit EMOSA models to these transitions through aggregate-level prevalence curves, which do not reflect individual-level changes between the categories. Ultimately, in future research, we will compare the estimates that emerge from the EMOSA models to those obtained from individual-level data analysis to evaluate the performance of the EMOSA models and to test some of the assumptions of the models. In this chapter, we operationalize a set of EMOSA models of religious involvement during late adolescence and early adulthood. We fit one of the models to the NLSY97 religious involvement data and interpret the parameters within that data set. We do not have space in this chapter to present a more expansive evaluation of this particular form of the EMOSA model, and so we introduce it here and save extended empirical evaluation of the model for future research publications.

The basic form of our three-category EMOSA model is shown in Figure 39.2. This portrayal is based on the usual EMOSA conceptualization that each member of the intact

TABLE 39.1a. Prevalence Percentages of the Original Response Categories, NLSY97 Data on Religious Attendance

Year	2000	2001	2002	2003	2004	2005	2006	2007
Age	16	17	18	19	20	21	22	23
Every day	0.87	0.61	0.26	0.17	0.09	0.26	0.17	0.43
Several times a week	12.35	10.26	6.35	5.04	4.26	4.00	4.35	4.61
About once a week	26.96	23.30	18.17	16.52	13.30	12.17	10.96	10.70
About twice a month/24 times	5.65	7.04	7.13	10.26	8.26	7.22	6.70	6.87
About once a month/12 times	6.26	5.65	7.48	8.17	6.87	8.17	6.43	6.78
Less than once a month/3–12 times	10.96	12.70	14.43	12.00	12.87	12.00	10.09	11.57
Once or twice	19.39	20.09	20.70	21.48	25.48	23.83	25.22	24.87
Never	17.57	20.35	25.48	26.35	28.87	32.35	36.09	34.17

Note. $N = 1{,}150$.

TABLE 39.1b. Prevalence Percentages of the Collapsed Modeling Categories, NLSY97 Data on Religious Attendance

Year	2000	2001	2002	2003	2004	2005	2006	2007
Age	16	17	18	19	20	21	22	23
Goers	40.17	34.17	24.78	21.74	17.65	16.43	15.48	15.74
Doubters	22.87	25.39	29.04	30.43	28.00	27.39	23.22	25.22
Nongoers	36.96	40.43	46.17	47.83	54.35	56.17	61.30	59.04

Note. $N = 1{,}150$.

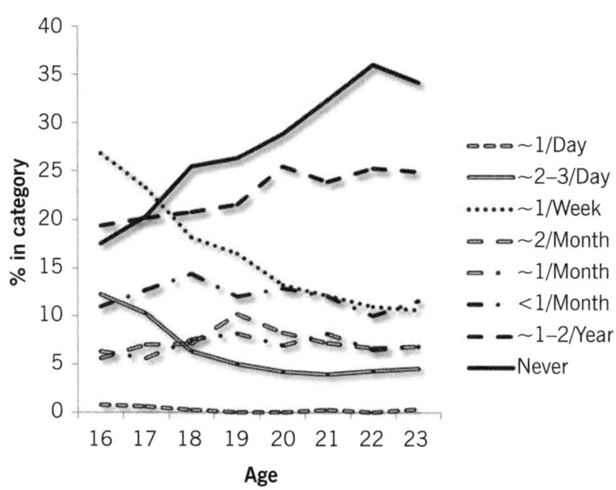

FIGURE 39.1a. Prevalence curves for the eight initial categories in Table 39.1a.

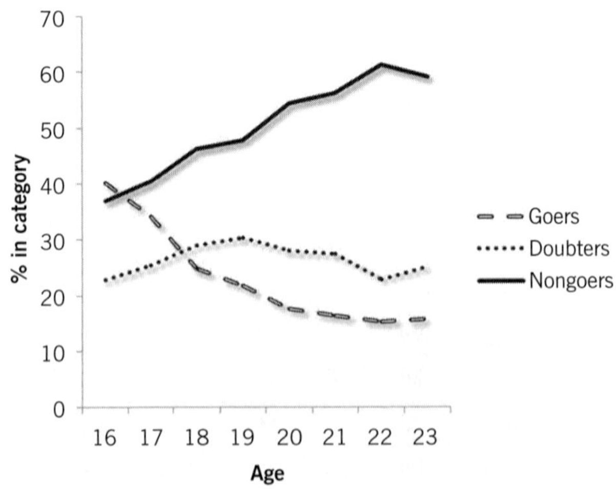

FIGURE 39.1b. Prevalence curves for the three aggregate categories in Table 39.1b.

social community is paired with another member at each time unit (e.g., each year), and that pairing probabilistically reflects the available respondents from the various categories. In this model, we assume that all interactions are contagious, although ultimately we will compare models and model fits for both social contagion and general diffusion (equivalently, social cohesion and structural equivalence, in the language of Burt, 1987). Our EMOSA religion model is similar to the Rowe and colleagues (1996) smoking model in that social influence can move a respondent back and forth between categories (as opposed to pure "onset models," in which an ever-performed behavior stays that way in perpetuity). Thus, a goer who encounters a doubter may be influenced to attend religious services less often (and thus becomes a doubter), whereas a doubter who encounters a goer may begin to attend more often (and thus becomes a goer). Our portrayal in Figure 39.2 accounts for all

TABLE 39.2. Collapsing of the Original Seven Categories into the Three Used in Our EMOSA Model, Yearly Frequency of Attendance at Religious Services

Original response category	Collapsed modeling category
Never	Nongoers
Once or twice	
Less than once a month/3–12 times	
About once a month/12 times	Doubters
About twice a month/24 times	
About once a week	
Several times a week	Goers
Every day	

possible transitions. The transition arrows above and between the circles (categories) can be conceptualized as paths that lead subjects from time t to time $t + 1$. Letters inside the arrows represent possible social encounters along the way. Indices above the letters would then represent and quantify the influence of the social encounter in arriving at the category at the end of the arrow (time $t + 1$). The figures to the outside of each category indicate those who stay in the category from time t to time $t + 1$, and each of their three possible pairings is accounted for. The arrows between categories show both the transition and also the pairings from which the transition emerged. Some of these possible pairings and transitions are not theoretically meaningful. For example, it is difficult to reconcile how a nongoer paired with a doubter would become a goer (at least within the simplification reflected in the conceptual scheme defined previously; other, more complex religious modeling could account for such a shift, e.g., if religious reactance were being evaluated). Or a goer paired with a goer would seem unlikely to become either a doubter or a nongoer. Furthermore, it is necessary to constrain some of these possible pairings and links to be zero (such constraints can be represented by erasing the letters inside arrows), so that the model can be statistically specified, fit, and evaluated.

Within the simplified model that we use to demonstrate this EMOSA application, we assume that the pairing can only influence a respondent to move to the category from which the pairing occurred. Thus, a goer paired with a doubter will either stay a goer or will become a doubter. A nongoer paired with a doubter will either stay a nongoer or will become a doubter. These constraints are reflected in the revised model shown in Figure 39.3. This model shows that the force of the current status can be maintained against any influence, that is, that a goer can stay a goer when paired with any other respondent. This part of the model would assume religious behavior that is relatively impervious to social influence (as much religious behavior is likely to be). As a result, the arrows above each category are not constrained. In other words, a goer can stay a goer whether he or she is paired with a goer, a doubter, or a nongoer. (However, we note that when we estimate the model, any of these freely estimated parameters can be empirically estimated as zero.)

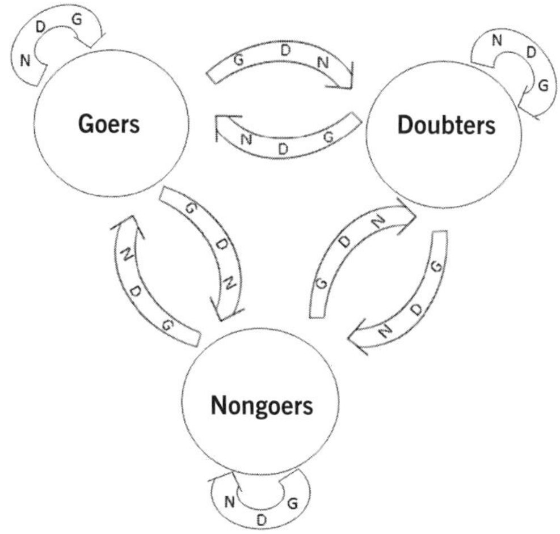

FIGURE 39.2. The overall EMOSA model, before constraints.

The equations that account for this transitions are the following:

$$P_g = P_g\text{Lag}*P_g\text{Lag}*R_{ggg} + P_g\text{Lag}*P_d\text{Lag}*R_{ggd} + P_g\text{Lag}*P_n\text{Lag}*R_{ggn} + P_d\text{Lag}*P_g\text{Lag}*N_{dgg} + P_n\text{Lag}*P_g\text{Lag}*N_{ngg} - P_g\text{Lag}*P_d\text{Lag}*T_{gdd} - P_g\text{Lag}*P_n\text{Lag}*T_{gnn}$$

$$P_d = P_d\text{Lag}*P_d\text{Lag}*R_{ddd} + P_d\text{Lag}*P_n\text{Lag}*R_{ddn} + P_d\text{Lag}*P_g\text{Lag}*R_{ddg} + P_g\text{Lag}*P_d\text{Lag}*T_{gdd} + P_n\text{Lag}*P_d\text{Lag}*N_{ndd} - P_d\text{Lag}*P_g\text{Lag}*N_{dgg} - P_d\text{Lag}*P_n\text{Lag}*T_{dnn}$$

$$P_n = P_n\text{Lag}*P_n\text{Lag}*R_{nnn} + P_n\text{Lag}*P_g\text{Lag}*R_{nng} + P_n\text{Lag}*P_d\text{Lag}*R_{nnd} + P_d\text{Lag}*P_n\text{Lag}*T_{dnn} + P_g\text{Lag}*P_n\text{Lag}*T_{gnn} - P_n\text{Lag}*P_g\text{Lag}*N_{ngg} - P_n\text{Lag}*P_d\text{Lag}*N_{ndd} \quad \textbf{(39.6)}$$

The P_gLag, P_dLag, and P_nLag variables are P_g, P_d, and P_n at the previous year. The *R*, *T*, and *N* terms are the estimated parameters within the model, shown in Figure 39.3. This model was estimated using PROC NLIN in SAS, a modification of the SAS coding presented in Rodgers and Rowe (1993) to fit the multistage sexuality model. The estimation optimized a chi-square objective function, in which chi-square = 8.99 against $df = 6$ (21 proportions as raw data, minus 15 estimated parameters); this chi-square is relatively small (not much bigger than its *df*s), suggesting an adequate fit of the model to the data. We note that we used the data at age 16 as the starting proportions in our estimation routine, and so these are not raw data (which explains why we had 21 data points instead of the 24 implied by Table 39.2).

The parameter estimates are shown in Figure 39.3. We fixed the upper range of the estimates to be 25, so that these are not strictly interpretable as probabilities. Rowe and colleagues (1996) discussed the interpretation of transition parameters as probabilities versus effective contacts. An effective contact interpretation suggests that a given respondent can "convert" more than one other respondent during the course of the year. Thus a few of the parameters are estimated to be bigger than 1.0 (but not much bigger, and relatively few).

The interpretable features of these parameter estimates include the following. First, goers are relatively difficult to influence; most of them stay goers. Furthermore, goers virtually never become nongoers directly but rather are much more likely to become doubters (who then may become nongoers at a future year); note that $T_{gnn} = .01$, whereas $T_{gdd} = .99$. Second, the doubter category appears to be quite attractive during this age period; there are many more of both goers and nongoers who become doubters than vice versa. Third, it is very hard to move nongoers (i.e., the *R* parameters are large relative to the *N* parameters), somewhat difficult to move goers (i.e., the *R* parameters are large relative to the *T* parameters), and easier to move doubters (who only become nongoers in the transition each year). Fourth, once a respondent becomes a doubter, the only path back to a goer is through the nongoer category. Obviously, during these ages and during the time period in which these data were collected, there is overall net movement out of religious attendance (see the general patterns shown in Table 39.1), and this feature of the parameter estimates appears requisite to account for this out-migration from regular attendance.

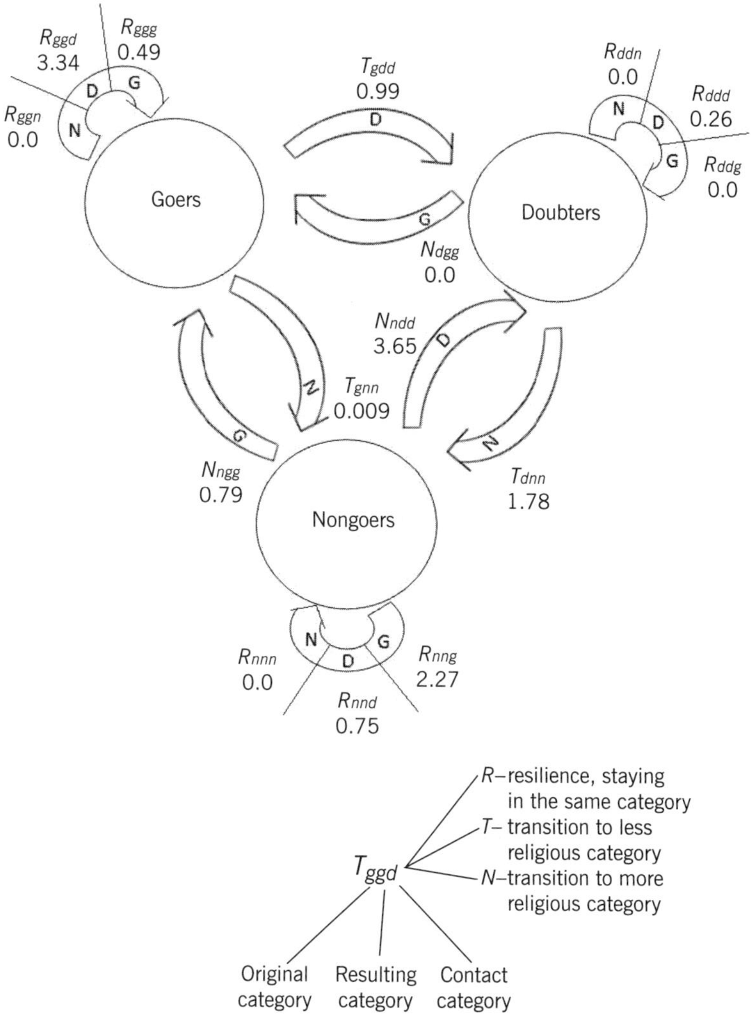

FIGURE 39.3. The constrained EMOSA model, with estimated parameter values included.

We note several caveats. First, we have estimated only a few models and have chosen this one to present because its assumptions and constraints are both straightforward and conceptually meaningful. There are dozens of other models that are interesting and reasonable that will be evaluated in future research. Second, this model has not been compared in any systematic way with other models using statistical criteria to allow them to compete, and there may well be better models than the one we present in Figure 39.3 (though the chi-square supports the idea that this model is itself interesting to interpret). As a corollary to the second point, there is the possibility of competitor models that are equivalent statistically but differ in interpretation from the one we present here (e.g., MacCallum, Wegener, Uchino, & Fabrigar, 1993). Third, among the most interesting questions is whether the different transitions are based on social contagion or on general diffusion; the model in Figure 39.3 assumes social contagion for all transitions, and this assumption needs to be carefully evaluated. To illustrate, we note that the interesting results in the Rowe and colleagues (1992, 1996) studies depend on this distinction. Finally, we are uncertain that our three-category definitions are necessarily the best way to parse these data. For example, inspection of Table 39.1 would lead some to define four categories—the religiously "passionate," religious "regulars," religious "irregulars," and "nonattenders." We will further inspect this definition in future research.

In summary, the preceding model-fitting exercise is illustrative of a new and potentially valuable domain in which EMOSA models may be fit. The NLSY97 survey provides excellent data to which the EMOSA formulation can be fit and to evaluate some of the critical assumptions of the EMOSA model. In future work we will estimate a number of forms of this model to attempt to identify the processes that are required to make each form work in an optimal sense. Then we will compare these results with the actual transition probabilities that can be obtained directly from the NLSY97 data, as a kind of cross-validation between the EMOSA results inferred to the individual level and those actually observed.

We note that in the context of this chapter, our discussion of social contagion in relation to religious involvement is illustrative of the breadth of potential EMOSA applications. EMOSA models can be developed to predict and explain changes in aggregate-level prevalence patterns in any setting in which a diffusion process—either social contagion or general diffusion or perhaps some combination of both—can be reasonably expected to apply. Obviously, this type of application is not limited to adolescent problem behaviors. Other examples of domains in which EMOSA models could be developed include many educational settings. Transition to another grade level, at least in most school settings, would not be especially interesting, because transition is normative and only a relative few do not make the transition at the end of the year. But transition into certain extracurricular events—e.g., playing in the school band or playing an organized sport—would have an EMOSA interpretation underlying this process. Furthermore, transition between political categories among a specified group of politicians would also reflect EMOSA processes. The stages could be "having ever run for a public office," "having held a local office," and "having held an office at a higher level than local." Finally, and returning to religious behavior, switching behavior between different denominations could be modeled from an EMOSA. The General Social Survey (GSS) routinely collects information to construct prevalence curves for involvement in different denominations (see Doughty & Rodgers, 1998, for a different kind of modeling approach applied to the religious switching information in the GSS).

Conclusion

EMOSA models have been shown in the past to have considerable breadth of application. The original EMOSA models—defined to explain onset of adolescent problem behaviors—were expanded to account for transition across categories, resulting in stagewise models of behavioral transition. We discussed and illustrated those types of processes in the section reviewing EMOSA models. In the previous section, we began the process of broadening the EMOSA perspective from focused attention to a few specified adolescent problem behaviors to a broader domain of empirical applications. We illustrate this broadened perspective in relation to a particular domain that appears at face value to have considerable social influence involved, religious attendance behavior, and we fit a simplified form of a general EMOSA conceptualization to illustrate this application. The result had an adequate fit and was interpretable, though we emphasize that there is a great deal more work to be done to demonstrate the utility of the EMOSA approach in relation to religious involvement in late adolescence (or at other ages as well, for that matter). This exercise was designed to be illustrative, however, of the potential for broadening the EMOSA perspective to include quite a number of other socially influenced behaviors.

In this broader developmental context, there are dozens of developmental processes that are fully defined, partly defined, or at least moderated by the social influences that occur within a social network. Building models of these processes that distinguish between and test for the dynamics associated with these processes can help inform both researchers and policymakers (see Rodgers, 2003, for elaboration). EMOSA models are quite transparent in terms of their methodology, the associated psychological theory, and the assumptions involved. This transparency contributes to their value at both a methodological and a theoretical level.

References

Atkinson, R. C., & Shiffrin, R. M. (1968). Human memory: A proposed system and its control processes. In K. W. Spence & J. T. Spence (Eds.), *The psychology of learning and motivation: Advances in research and theory* (Vol. 2, pp. 89–195). New York: Academic Press.

Burt, R. S. (1987). Social contagion and innovation: Cohesion versus structural equivalence. *American Journal of Sociology, 92*, 1287–1335.

Dodd, S. C. (1955). Diffusion is predictable: Testing probability models for laws of interaction. *American Sociological Review, 20*, 392–401.

Doughty, D., & Rodgers, J. L. (1998). Multidimensionality and asymmetry in religious switching behavior. *Journal of Applied Social Psychology, 28*, 609–638.

Furstenberg, F. F., Morgan, S. P., Moore, K. A., & Peterson, J. L. (1987). Race differences in the timing of adolescent intercourse. *American Sociological Review, 52*, 511–518.

Harlan, W. R., Harlan, E. A., & Grillo, G. (1980). Secondary sex characteristics of girls 12 to 17 years of age: The U.S. Health Examination Survey. *Journal of Pediatrics, 96*, 1074–1078.

MacCallum, R. C., Wegener, D. T., Uchino, B. N., & Fabrigar, L. R. (1993). The problem of equivalent models in applications of covariance structure analysis. *Psychological Bulletin, 114*, 185–199.

Mahajan, V., & Peterson, R. A. (1985). *Models for innovation diffusion*. Beverly Hills, CA: Sage.

May, R. M., & Anderson, R. M. (1987). Transmission dynamics of HIV infection *Nature, 326*, 137–142.

Roberts, S., & Pashler, H. (2000). How persuasive is a good fit? A comment on theory testing. *Psychological Review, 107*, 358–367.

Rodgers, J. L. (2003). EMOSA sexuality models, memes, and the tipping point: Policy and program implications. In D. Romer (Ed.), *Reducing adolescent risk: Toward an integrated approach* (pp. 185–192). Newbury Park, CA: Sage.

Rodgers, J. L. (2007). The shape of things to come: Using developmental curves from adolescent smoking and drinking reports to diagnose the type of social process that generated the curves. In T. D. Little, J. A. Bovaird, & N. A. Card (Eds.), *Modeling contextual effects in longitudinal studies* (pp. 343–362). Mahwah, NJ: Erlbaum.

Rodgers, J. L. (2010). The epistemology of mathematical and statistical modeling: A quiet methodological revolution. *American Psychologist, 65*, 1–12.

Rodgers, J. L., & Johnson, A. (2007). Nonlinear dynamic models of nonlinear dynamic behaviors: Social contagion of adolescent smoking and drinking at aggregate and individual levels. In S. M. Boker & M. J. Wenger (Eds.), *Data analytic techniques for dynamical systems* (pp. 213–242). Mahwah, NJ: Erlbaum.

Rodgers, J. L., & Rowe, D. C. (1993). Social contagion and adolescent sexual behavior: A developmental EMOSA model. *Psychological Review, 100*, 479–510.
Rodgers, J. L., & Rowe, D. C. (2002). Theory development should begin (but not end) with good empirical fits: A comment on Roberts and Pashler (2000). *Psychological Review, 109*, 599–604.
Rodgers, J. L., Rowe, D. C., & Buster, M. (1998). Social contagion, adolescent sexual behavior, and pregnancy: A nonlinear dynamic EMOSA model. *Developmental Psychology, 34*, 1096–1113.
Rowe, D. C., Chassin, L., Presson, C. C., Edwards, E., & Sherman, S. J. (1992). An "epidemic" model of adolescent cigarette smoking. *Journal of Applied Social Psychology, 2*, 261–285.
Rowe, D. C., Chassin, L., Presson, C. C., & Sherman, S. J. (1996). Parental smoking and the "epidemic" spread of cigarette smoking. *Journal of Applied Social Psychology, 36*, 437–454.
Rowe, D. C., & Rodgers, J. L. (1991a). Adolescent smoking and drinking: Are they epidemics? *Journal of Studies in Alcohol, 52*, 110–117.
Rowe, D. C., & Rodgers, J. L. (1991b). An "epidemic" model of adolescent sexual intercourse. *Journal of Biosocial Sciences, 23*, 211–219.
Rowe, D. C., & Rodgers, J. L. (1994). A social contagion model of adolescent sexual behavior: Explaining race differences. *Social Biology, 41*, 1–18.
Rowe, D. C., Rodgers, J. L., & Meseck-Bushey, S. (1989). An "epidemic" model of sexual intercourse prevalences for black and white adolescents. *Social Biology, 36*, 127–145.
Washington, A. C. (1982). A cultural and historical perspective on pregnancy-related activity among U.S. teenagers. *Journal of Black Psychology, 9*, 1–28.
Weinberg, M. S., & Williams, C. J. (1988). Black sexuality: A test of two theories. *Journal of Sex Research, 25*, 197–218.

CHAPTER 40

Dynamic Systems

PAUL VAN GEERT

Central Issues

Dynamic Systems in Developmental Methodology

The primary aim of applying dynamic systems theory to developmental psychology is to provide a dynamic explanation of the particular process of long-term change we call development, for instance, the developmental process of language or of theory of mind, in relation to other developmental variables. Development is concerned with long-term change, for instance, change over the course of years or decades. These long-term changes can be observed in the form of events on the short-term time scale, namely the developing person's actions. Change on the long-term time scale (i.e., developmental change) occurs in individuals. In the generic sense, the term *individual* can refer to an individual person, a particular dyad (e.g., a parent–child dyad), a particular group such as a family, or a particular person–environment coupling (e.g., a child–family coupling). It is assumed that the individuals to which the dynamic model is applied have a lifespan that is long enough to show long-term change or development. The processes of change that form the topic of developmental study are complex. If we observe a particular child acting in a context, we are, in fact, observing a complex, intertwined multivariate stream, involving motor activity, perception, emotions, language, and so forth. This stream implies a constant coupling with an environment that is affected by and, in turn, affects these events. However, we believe that we can meaningfully reduce this complexity to a few variables of interest. This reduction is grounded in the assumption that in the variables of choice, the complexity of the system is in a sense preserved or represented. To put it somewhat metaphorically, it is possible to extract some variables out of a complex system, but it is not possible to extract the complex system out of the variables.

An important methodological question is whether it is possible to use interindividual aggregations of data in order to arrive at models that pertain to processes that occur in individuals. According to Molenaar (Molenaar & Campbell, 2009), this is in general not possible, a conclusion based on the ergodicity property. Ergodicity implies that the analysis of the interindividual variability yields the same statistical properties as an analysis of intraindividual variability. The following example illustrates this principle. Suppose that we have a test measuring cognitive level that we administer to a great number of persons of all possible ages. The differences between the test scores can be analyzed, among others, as a function of age of the respondents. This will result in a statistical model that assigns a number of different scores to each possible age (calendar year). For each year we can calculate the average score and a standard deviation. The averages will trace a particular developmental trajectory over the lifespan, including a bandwidth of variability. If ergodicity applies to this particular case, this population-based developmental trajectory plus the variability assigned to it can be treated as a potential description of all individual developmental trajectories (in this case, cognitive level). All individual trajectories will run parallel to the trajectory based on the group data, plus or minus purely random deviations. Their distance from the average trajectory will be given by the possible distances specified in the group-based bandwidth of variability. If ergodicity does not apply, the form of individual trajectories can be widely different from the group-based trajectory, and it is even possible that there exists no individual trajectory that runs parallel to the group-based trajectory.

The ergodicity condition is very rarely met in behavioral data that pertain to processes of change and development. Almost any available data set containing sufficiently large numbers of individual developmental trajectories illustrates how great the differences from a central tendency, such as average growth curves, may be. This variation cannot be reduced to random fluctuation around a common "real" pattern. It originates because individuals are complex dynamic systems whose temporal trajectories are self-organizing patterns unique to the system at issue (which does not preclude the possibility that there exist cases in which many such self-organizing patterns are quite similar to one another). Hence, validating dynamic systems models of change and development requires individual time serial data, collected with a frequency and total duration that is sufficient to capture the properties of the dynamics (Boker, 2002; Steenbeek & van Geert, 2005).

What Is a Dynamic System?

The State Space

In order to construct a dynamic system, a number of components are needed. First, one must be able to describe the states of a dynamic system at any moment in time. One can do that by means of a *state space*, which is a model of all possible states the dynamic system can eventually occupy (some authors use the term *phase space*). By way of example, I refer to the child's development of theory of mind. In the simplest possible case, the state space can consist of a limited number of possible states. For instance, if it were so that a particular child either has a theory of mind or does not, the state space describing theory of mind development consists of two possible states, present or not present. More interesting state spaces consists of variables or dimensions. For instance, if a child's theory of mind can occupy any value between 0 (not present) and 1 (fully present), development of theory of mind can be described by means of a one-dimensional state space consisting of a continuous dimension ranging from 0 to 1. At any moment in time, an imaginary child occupies one point on this theory of mind dimension, which specifies the child's current state of theory of mind development.

It is not implicitly assumed that states in the state space must be single points in the underlying state space. It is much more likely that states of complex, real systems, such as children, occupy fuzzy regions in the state space instead of single points. Finally, the state space representation is a methodological tool, not a theory of the phenomenon. For instance, theorists of embodied cognition might claim that theory of mind does not exist and that it is in fact a large collection of context-specific actions and verbal explanations. In that case, the state space representation must encompass the entire range of possible contexts, including the possible variations in motor and verbal behavior that correspond with this particular conceptualization of theory of mind.

For most cases, one-dimensional continuous state spaces will not be very illuminating. For instance, a developmentalist might be interested in the relations of theory of mind with language development and environmental input. This developmentalist has defined a three-dimensional state space. Note that, at any time, a particular child has a particular level of theory of mind development, of language development, and of environmental support. These are three specific coordinates, specifying the child's current position in the three-dimensional state space.

Time

In order to construct a dynamic system, one needs *time*. At each point in time, the system, for instance a particular child, occupies a point (or fuzzy cloud) in the state space. With the passage of time, the system will follow a sequence of such points (i.e., a trajectory through a state space). Change over time is represented by a line connecting all the successive states in the space it occupies. A trajectory can also be a single point in the space, which occurs if the system settles down on a stable state. Note that in a dynamic system, stability does not imply that change in the abstract sense of the word has stopped; stability means that the system produces a next state that is equal to the preceding one (i.e., the system actively maintains a particular state). In dynamic systems, time can be treated either in a discrete way or in a continuous way. In a discrete dynamics, time is treated as chunks, for instance a second, a day, a week, or a year. The trajectory in the state space consists of discrete hops from one point in the state space to another over each successive chunk of time. If time is continuous, the trajectory in the state space is defined for any arbitrarily chosen point in time, and the trajectory takes the form of a flow or trajectory. Flows can be continuous or discontinuous. In a continuous flow the next step of the trajectory is always arbitrarily close to the preceding step of the trajectory for any arbitrarily small amount of elapsed time. Discontinuous trajectories show leaps, sudden change as from one state of the system to another state of the system, with a range of impossible (nonoccupied) states in between, where the discontinuity lies.

The Dynamic Rule or Evolution Term

The third ingredient of a dynamic system is the *dynamic rule*, also known as the evolution term or time evolution law. A dynamic rule specifies the immediate next state of the system for any point in the state space (this is irrespective of whether we define the next step in continuous or discrete terms).

For instance, let x_t be the state of a system—a particular child described in the 3D-state space of theory of mind, language, and environmental input—at time t and x_{t+1} the state of the system at some immediate later state. Because each state is described by three coordinates, any change in the state space between t and $t + 1$ will be represented by changes in each of these three coordinates. The nature of this change is described by the dynamic rule or evolution term, which takes the form of a mathematical function giving a new value for each of the coordinates after a time lapse 1.

In order to clarify the nature of this dynamic rule, we assume that the three variables that constitute the dimensional state space are mutually related (i.e., they are influencing one another). Change in theory of mind is supposed to be determined by the child's current levels of theory of mind, of language development, and of current environmental input (e.g., some form of social support or reaction from the adult). Change in the child's current level of language development is supposed to be determined by the child's current levels of language development, of theory of mind, and of social support. Finally, change in the current level of social support is supposed to be determined by the child's current levels of social support, of theory of mind, and of language development. In this particular case, the dynamic rule will take the form of three coupled differential or difference equations. It is important that these mathematical functions should be theoretically meaningful; they must represent theoretically plausible mechanisms of change pertaining to the change in relations between the three variables.

If we start at the position of the system at time t, then apply the three coupled equations, we arrive at the system's position or state in the state space at time $t + 1$. If we then apply the three coupled equations to the system's position at time $t + 1$, we arrive at its position or state at time $t + 2$; apply it to $t + 2$ and we arrive at the position at $t + 3$; and so forth up to a position at $t + n$. We have thus iteratively applied the dynamic rule to arrive at state $t + n$, starting from state t. *Iterative* means that we apply the dynamic rule to any preceding state to arrive at an immediate next state. This iterative application of the dynamic rule is what constructs the system's trajectory through the state space, given that the trajectory is the succession of states occupied by the system over time. The iterative nature of the dynamics makes clear why stability is just as dynamic as highly visible changes. The dynamics consists of the fact that there is a point at which the application of the dynamic rule to a state t generates a new state at $t + 1$ that is exactly similar to the state at time t, that then on the basis of $t + 1$ generates a state at $t + 2$ that is similar to the state at $t + 1$. Iterative, coupled dynamic systems inherit a number of interesting properties. They tend to show self-organization, a spontaneous increase in order, nonlinearity, and complexity of behavior (van Geert, 2008; van Geert & Steenbeek, 2005).

It is important to note that dynamic systems do not comply with the axioms of the general linear model, so dynamic systems cannot be studied with methods based on the linear model. The difference between dynamic systems and the general linear model can be explained as follows. Take a simple general linear model of the effects of practice on learning. According to this model, the learning effect y is equal to some constant value (b_0) plus the effect of practice time (x is the amount of practice time, and b_1 is how much practice time contributes to the learning effect, plus or minus an amount of error, which specifies chance or unknown influences). The model describes a set of observations of people with different amounts of practice and different learning effects, all of which are described by the equation "learning effect = constant plus (amount of practice times a particular effect strength)." According to this model, the learning effect in a person who practiced for 6 hours is (on average) equal to the sum of the learning effect in a person who practiced for 2 hours and the learning effect in another person who practiced for 4 hours (plus or minus the error term, which we have now chosen to neglect for the sake of simplicity). However, in a dynamic model, practicing is treated as an iterative process that takes place over the course of time and in a particular individual. For some people, practice works best if it occurs in short but frequent chunks of time. For these people the effect of practicing six times for about an hour is considerably bigger than the effect of practicing once for 6 hours. Others, for whom effects slowly build up during an extended period of practice and who need a considerable warming-up time, the effect of practicing six times for 1 hour may be virtually zero, whereas practicing once for 6 hours has a very considerable effect. All these effects are typically nonlinear and cannot be represented by an additive rule.

Conceptual Principles and Statistical Assumptions

General Methodological Reflections on Dynamic Systems in Development

Theory-Based Nature of Dynamic Rules

It is important to note that the definition of the dynamic rule must be based on theory. A dynamic rule must entail some theoretically plausible mechanism of change. In the first section, I stated that the primary aim of dynamic systems theory is to provide a dynamic explanation of a particular process of long-term change, for instance, the developmental process of theory of mind, language, and cognition in relation to other developmental variables. It is a causal explanation in the sense that a dynamic system employs well-established theoretical principles or mechanisms in order to show, by deductive use of these theoretical principles, how an immediate next state of the system follows from immediately preceding states in the system.

The notion of causality employed here is that of process causality, which defines causality in terms of continuity (Cartwright, 2004; Dowe, 2010). An example of process causality is a ball moving through the air; any preceding position of the ball is the cause of its next position. In dynamic systems, the first goal is deductive; given a theory of some developmental change, a dynamic system is a way to transfer this theory into a state space and a dynamic rule and then to deductively determine, given some sort of starting point, which trajectory through the state space results from the given dynamic rule.

Dynamic Systems and Latent Variables

The term *latent variables* denotes properties that are inferred on the basis of similarities and differences among observable variables, such as a child's retrieving a hidden object. Latent variables represent the dimensions of the state spaces within which development can be situated. In psychology, latent variables are often seen as evidence for some underlying, real mechanism, which is the underlying cause or generator of the observable phenomena (Borsboom, 2008). For instance, babies will not retrieve objects if these objects are hidden under a piece of cloth. A few months later in their development, they will still be fooled if the hiding place is changed while they watch (the famous A-not-B error). This developmental sequence is traditionally interpreted as evidence of an underlying mental mechanism, the object concept, which is the cause of the actual searching and retrieving behavior. Some prominent representatives of developmental dynamic systems theory argue that this interpretation is incorrect (Smith, Thelen, Titzer, & McLin, 1999; Thelen & Smith, 1994). The cause of the statistical similarity among observable events, for instance the retrieval of hidden objects at different ages, lies in the total structure of the system, which in this case comprises not only the brain but the whole body and the environment—the objects and spatial layout—that the embodied agent, the baby, acts on (Smith, 2005; van Geert & Fischer, 2009).

The dynamic systems definition of latent variable is comparable to the definition of order parameters in synergetics, a field of research dealing with spontaneous or self-organizing pattern formation (Haken, 2006). Order parameters are similarities across many different events or actions (e.g., a baby's lack of success in retrieving a particular kind of hidden object). Higher order similarities emerge out of interactions among lower level components of the system (the perceptions, the object manipulations, and the ways the object transforms or resists manipulation). According to Haken (2006), these higher order properties exert causal influences on the lower level patterns, and, as such, the higher order properties have a causal influence on their self-maintenance.

One important consequence of this dynamic systems approach to latent variables is that one cannot use the latent variable to statistically separate the person from the context, for instance, in order to determine how much of the variance in a phenomenon is due to the context and how much to the person. In the developmental process, person and environment stand in a relationship of reciprocal determination, and it is this that the dynamic systems theorist seeks to understand (Steenbeek & van Geert, 2007, 2008).

The Issue of Generalization

Generalization is an important criterion for judging the importance of empirical findings. What is general is often compared with what is individual, and knowledge that pertains only to a particular individual is assumed to be inferior to knowledge that refers to the general. The plea from dynamic systems researchers for individual-based research methodology might seem to move developmental psychology away from general knowledge. However, in the behavioral sciences, the notion of generalizability often refers to specific questions about the extent to which certain sample-based estimations (e.g., an average or a difference between groups) are also true for the population (Lee & Baskerville, 2003; Yin, 2009). Instead, generalizability should refer to the relation between data and theory, theory being the broadest statements about a phenomenon. If we have a theory of development as it occurs in an individual (a theory we have expressed in the form of a dynamical system), the only kind of data that actually refer to that theory must be developmental or change data from an individual. Individual data generalize to theories in the sense that they can either validate or refute the change mechanisms postulated by the theory.

Models based on statistical samples of the population are not generalizable to individual trajectories and vice versa. In order to arrive at general theories, one must first collect many individual cases and start with a model of each individual case separately. The field of language development has several examples of this process.

Dynamic Systems Models as Models of "Individual" Processes: The Methodology of Dynamic Model Building

Classical Dynamic Systems: (Coupled) Differential Equations Models

A classical dynamic systems representation of a developmental process is a mathematical expression of fundamental principles of developmental change, as described by some existing theory or theory of acquisition, learning, or development. Developmental processes can be represented by a network of coupled variables, each of which changes in accordance with two simple principles (for further discussion, see van Geert, 1991, 1994, 2003). First, on the level of single variables, development is defined as an increase or decrease in the variable's level in proportion to the level already attained. Second, the variable's change is assumed to depend on available resources that are limited. For instance, a resource factor for lexical growth (L) is determined by the language spoken in the environment and also by the properties of the child's brain required to process the rapidly changing acoustic signals. The total amount of available resources in the system is the carrying capacity of the system, defined as the level at which a process must stabilize. Given that resources are limited, growth approaches a zero limit as the level of L approaches the level that is sustained by the available resources (e.g., the lexicon of the environment, which limits the number of lexical items that can be learned by a child living in that environment) for K the limit level of L, or the carrying capacity.

$$\frac{\Delta L}{\Delta t} = rL\left(1 - \frac{L}{K}\right)$$

In developmental networks consisting of coupled variables, the change in L may depend on the level (or eventually the rate of change) of other supporting or competing variables in the developmental network. In the case of early language development, cognition or concept formation may represent a supporting variable (van Geert, 1991, 1994, 2003). Equations of this sort permit dynamic models of developmental growth to be constructed and compared with available data, which may be used to estimate the value of the model parameters.

Modeling the change in single variables by means of a differential equation can be extended to more complicated cases, which may have greater theoretical significance. One such extension concerns the use of coupled differential equations. For instance, it is likely that the growth of the lexicon in an infant is a supporting factor for the growth of grammatical complexity of the infant's language. In turn, the growth of grammatical complexity is a supporting factor for the growth of the lexicon (up to a certain age). This type of model can be expressed by coupling the differential equations (e.g., see Kunnen & Bosma, 2000; Lichtwarck-Aschoff, van Geert, Bosma, & Kunnen, 2008; Robinson & Mervis, 1998; van Geert, 1991, 1994; van Geert & Steenbeek, 2005).

Another extension relevant to developmental psychology is the use of differential equation models in *dynamic fields*. For instance, in a simple object search task in an object permanence experiment, a major variable is the spatial position of the objects and their hiding places. For each point on this spatial dimension, there exists a variable, a particular activation value, which, in the case of the current example, would mean a likelihood that the child reaches at this particular point in space in order to retrieve the hidden object. The activation values change over the short- and long-term time course (Schöner, 2009). Dynamic field models can also be specified for more abstract properties of the developmental state space, summarizing real-time performance over longer time frames (van Geert, 1998).

Intraindividual Variability as a Representation of the State of the System

If we repeatedly measure or observe a particular developmental variable over the course of days or weeks, we will observe a considerable amount of fluctuation in the measured levels (de Weerth, van Geert, & Hoijtink, 1999; van Dijk & van Geert, 2007; van Geert & van Dijk, 2002, 2003). According to the classical viewpoint, these fluctuations do not reflect real change in the underlying latent variable or cause. The variability is due to added accidental causes, which must be filtered out in order to arrive at the true change in the underlying variable. However, we have seen that according to dynamic systems theory of real-time action, the cause of the phenomenon is a property of the entire developmental system, which consists of the embodied subject embedded in a particular environment. According to the dynamic explanation of performance, intraindividual variability or contextual variability of some ability, skill, or performance is an intrinsic property of the ability or skill, because the skill as such is a property of the total system (Boker & Nesselroade, 2002; Thelen & Smith, 1994; van Dijk & van Geert, 2005, 2007). As a real property of the total system, variability in the sense of fluctuation can change over the course of developmental time and can provide valuable information about the underlying developmental processes or mechanisms (Van der Maas & Molenaar, 1992; van Geert & van Dijk, 2002). Local peaks in variability can be indicative of developmental transitions, as in the case of language development (Bassano & van Geert, 2007).

The bandwidth of fluctuation that characterizes a particular developmental system can be represented as a *fuzzy set* of characteristic performance levels (van Geert, 2002). An advantage of this fuzzy logic representation is that it is possible to represent systems that are in bimodal or even multimodal states. This is particularly interesting in the case of developing systems, whose states are often not clearly defined and depend on the varying contexts in which they function (Fischer & Bidell, 2006; van Geert & Fischer, 2009). Multimodal states are particularly important around a developmental transition, during which different developmental levels are expressed in different behavioral modalities (e.g., verbal and gestural; Goldin-Meadow, 2006).

Model Fitting, Occam's Razor, and Theoretical Plausibility

The aim of model building is to arrive at the best possible explanation of the available data. However, this aim is often narrowed down to the question of model fitting, which involves generating a description that matches the data. Among the models that produce a similar match with the data, simpler models are preferred to more complex ones. This preference is justified by the principle of parsimony, or the principle known as Occam's razor: "entities are not to be multiplied beyond necessity" (Baker, 2010). However, necessity must be defined by the total of available theoretical and empirical knowledge about a phenomenon under investigation. Although it will always be possible to reduce developmental data in a way that favors some simple model, the data set should be *descriptively relevant* in the sense that it covers a time interval that is long enough to capture the relevant long-term changes (Lichtwarck-Aschoff, Kunnen, & van Geert, 2009).

The difference between using models for explanation and using them for description can be illustrated with the following example. A major issue in the study of lexical growth concerns the occurrence—or nonoccurrence—of an early spurt. Ganger and Brent (2004) argue that the spurt is far from universal and that the observed trajectories can be specified by means of different mathematical models, which can be fitted to the data. The implicit understanding is that the most parsimonious of the better fitting models provides the best possible window onto the underlying process of growth.

In principle, the simplest possible time-dependent model describing the change of a variable L is the linear model. The next simplest model is the quadratic model. The model of change, implicit in the quadratic model, can be inferred by taking the first derivative from the quadratic model, which is

$$\Delta L = b + 2ct.$$

This model says that the change in the lexicon (i.e., the actual learning of words) amounts to adding a constant number of words per unit time (b) and a variable number of words ($2ct$), which reflect twice the time elapsed (if this were an observation model, a symmetrical error term would also be included). As a model of change, the mathematical equation has serious problems. The first problem is that learning is conceived as independent of what has already been learned (the constant factor), which is highly unlikely. This assumption implies that if you put a baby in a university lecture room, the baby could acquire an understanding of quantum physics. The nature of the linear addition is implicitly adapted to the learner's possibilities, in which case the b parameter contains a reference to the learner's level and no longer represents a linear model. The quadratic model is also problematic. The second problem is that in real development, the speed of growth of new words will level off at a more or less constant level. If the c parameter has a positive value, the quadratic model will predict a continuously increasing speed of growth, which is against the known facts. If the c parameter has a negative value, it will predict the observed decline in speed of growth. However, as soon as the temporal parameter, t, is great enough to make $b < 2ct$, the pattern of growth will turn into a pattern of decline (a loss of words and a decrease in vocabulary), which is also against the known facts. Hence, as an explanatory model of lexical growth, the quadratic model can be rejected on the grounds that it generates demonstrably wrong predictions if the time frame covers the entire development of the lexicon.

The logistic growth model explained earlier is a more theoretically plausible model of lexical growth. In terms of empirical coverage, the logistic model can fit linear, quadratic, asymptotic, and S-shaped trajectories, which is an important advantage to explaining a phenomenon in which each of these trajectories can occur, depending on which moments in development the researcher focuses on. The logistic model is the simplest possible growth model if one takes into account its empirical coverage and its relations to an explanatory model of developmental change. Thus an indiscriminate application of Occam's razor to the relations between models and data can lead to results that are implausible from the point of view of developmental dynamics.

Developmental Applications

Collecting Data: Observation of Individual Time Series

Because developmental processes occur in individuals, the data needed to validate a dynamic system must be in the form of a time series. The time series must be long enough to cover the significant properties of the dynamics. For instance, if a dynamic model predicts an S-shaped curve, the duration of the observation must be long enough to capture the qualitative properties of the S-shape. The measurement interval also must be appropriate to the nature of the dynamics studied. Unfortunately, we do not always know the duration and frequency of an empirical developmental process in advance, and they must often be determined inductively. To find characteristic frequencies of intraindividual variation, van Geert and van Dijk (2002) recommend designs with variable measurement intervals. For instance, observations of language development may be done on the basis of 2-week intervals, with intermittent periods in which the observations are done every day or every other day.

Inductive Approaches: Exploring Properties of the State Space

Categorical State Space Grids

The state space is one of the fundamental notions in dynamic systems, and the analysis of trajectories in the state space is one of its most important methodological tools. The *state space grid technique* is based on a state space consisting of observed categorical variables (Hollenstein, 2007). I illustrate this technique with a study of the development of prepositional phrases (e.g., "*on* the mat") and mean length of utterance (MLU). The study follows the language development of two children acquiring Dutch as their first language (25 measurements between ages 18 and 30 months). The simplest construction is that of a prepositional element only (PE alone). The correct strategy is the preposition followed by an obligatory noun phrase (PE–NP). There are two other strategies in which the obligatory element is missing. The first involves a noun phrase that is not the object of the prepositional element, (x–PE). The second involves no nouns but only a verb to complement the prepositional element (PE–V). These two forms are already somewhat more grammatical in comparison to the PE-alone strategy. Finally, there is a category for the uncodable utterances.

The number of words in the utterance and the type of prepositional construction are used as the two dimensions of the state space. The categories are spatially ordered in such a way that meaningful combinations are spatially close to one another. The categorical state space is only an approximation of a space in the ordinary sense of the word. Some parts of the space are in fact nonexistent (e.g., prepositions only are by definition one-word sentences).

Figure 40.1 shows the language production of one of the children during six observation sessions at 2-month intervals. Every utterance with a preposition occupies a particular position in the state space of each observation session. The arrows represent the sequence of utterances. When several arrows are confined to one block in the space, the child has repeated a particular construction (e.g., the PE–V/three-word sentence construction). The state space grid shows that constructions from one state space grid to another are fairly

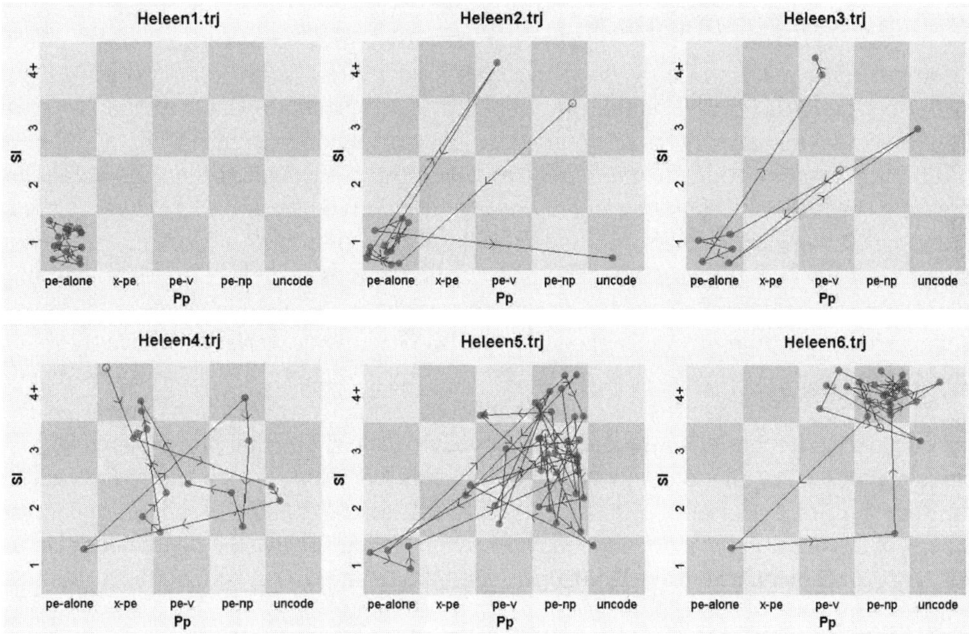

FIGURE 40.1. State space grids of the strategy of the prepositional phrase (horizontally) and sentence length (vertically) for the six sessions of Heleen.

variable. The succession of state space grids provides a good visual representation of the long-term developmental pattern. All properties of the state space grid, such as the amount of scatter of the points across the grid, can be quantified and used for further statistical processing (Hollenstein, 2010).

State Space Modeling, Dynamic Factor Analysis, and Recurrence Analysis

In the state space grids, the dimensions of the state space are a given: They consist of the variables that the researcher uses to code the observations. In certain multivariate data sets, however, the number of variables is too great for an efficient application of the state space grid technique. In this case the researcher can try to reconstruct an underlying state space by means of dynamic factor analysis (Molenaar, 1985; see also Molenaar & Lo, Chapter 20, this volume.

Recurrence analysis also can be used to uncover the properties of an unknown underlying state space. Dynamic factor analysis should be used when there are too many variables. Recurrence analysis should be used when there are too few and their pattern is highly irregular (see Assmann, Romano, Thiel, & Niemitz, 2007; Dale & Spivey, 2006). Recurrence refers to a similarity between a particular observation and some later point in the observed series. By plotting the total structure of recurrences, the researcher can also visually retrieve the underlying structure of the data and use various statistical criteria to reconstruct the nature of the underlying state space (*www.recurrence-plot.tk*).

Dynamic Developmental Model Fitting

The empirical validation of a dynamic systems model often focuses on two issues. First, how closely does the model match the empirical data? Second, what are the most likely values of the model parameters or properties, given a particular empirical data set?

The first issue pertains to the extent to which the model can predict the data. Developmental processes are characterized by properties such as stepwise changes, temporary regressions (*U*-shaped change), discontinuities and continuities in change, and inverted *U*-shaped change (van Geert, 1991, 1998). Dynamic systems models of development, in particular, network models of connected variables, can generate such phenomena fairly easily. Given particular parameter values, the model will generate trajectories that have these qualitative properties. Unfortunately, there are few time series data sets that are detailed enough to show how such phenomena occur in individual cases (language developmental data might be an exception). Recently, a number of authors have made significant progress in identifying techniques for the estimation of dynamic parameters from time series (e.g., Molenaar, Sinclair, Rovine, Ram, & Corneal, 2009; von Oertzen & Boker, 2010). Further details concerning methods of model fitting can be found in recently published specialized handbooks (Boker & Wenger, 2007; Molenaar & Newell, 2010; Valsiner, Molenaar, Lyra, & Chaudhary, 2009).

Illustration

Parent–Child Adaptation in Early Language Development

When speaking to young children, adults tend to adapt their language to that of the child. It is likely that this "child-directed speech" is the result of a transactional process of dynamic adaptation between the child and the adult. The adult adapts child-directed language to the language spoken by the child, which means that the adult simplifies language and then gradually makes it more complex as the child progresses in language acquisition. The child learns from the language presented, which means that the child adapts his or her language to that of the adult.

The data for my illustration (Bassano et al., 2011; van Dijk et al., 2010) consisted of samples of longitudinal speech from three monolingual children in conversation with their parents: one girl learning Dutch (Jessica), one boy learning Austrian German (Jan), and one girl learning French (Pauline). Jessica was studied from roughly age 1 year 7 months to 2 years 10 months; Jan from 1 year 3 months to 3 years; and Pauline from 1 year 2 months to 3 years. Analyses of the transcripts are based on two weekly samples confined to 60 utterances (25 observation sessions for Jessica, 39 for Jan, and 38 for Pauline). Data were collected for MLU, for vocabulary lemmas (the number of word types used in a particular speech sample), and for determiners (e.g., "the," "a"; the structure of determiners in Dutch and German is more complex than in English).

The next step consisted of building a dynamic systems model of language acquisition for each of the three variables and for the corresponding input from the adult (the corresponding child-directed speech). The major variables in the model are the child's output of a particular linguistic variable (e.g., MLU produced during a particular 2-week observation session) and the parent input on the same variable during the same observation session. We simplified the data set by means of a smoothing procedure (comparable to a moving average procedure), discarding information about the variability.

Constructing and Fitting the Dynamic Model

Mathematically, the learning curve is modeled on the basis of a logistic growth equation, with a particular initial value, a growth rate, and a carrying capacity. Recall that the carrying capacity is the sum of available resources, which determines the stable state of the growth equation. In language development, a major component of the carrying capacity is the language of the environment. We assumed that the carrying capacity, which represents the stable state of the growth model, was proportional to the input level (van Dijk et al., 2010). The second major variable, the linguistic variable (e.g., MLU), as presented in the parent's child-directed speech, was conceived of as a derivation first of the parent's habitual level for the variable (e.g., the parent's habitual MLU in informal adult-directed speech), second of the child's current level of the variable, and third of an underlying and unobserved variable that we identify as this particular parent's tendency to adapt his or her language to the language level of the child. Hence the parent's actual adaptation to the language of the child can be expressed as

$$I_t = I_H + s\, A_t\, (L_t - I_H)$$

where I_H is the parent's habitual level in adult-directed speech, L_t is the child's current level of the linguistic variable, A_t is the parent's current tendency to adapt her language to that of the child, and s is a simple damping parameter.

Finally, we assumed that the parent's tendency to adapt child-directed speech, represented by the A_t parameter, is not a fixed property but a parameter that changes in function of the actual acquisition rates of the child. Assume that the child makes only little progress in the learning of the linguistic variable, in spite of the parent's adaptation. In that case, the parent is likely to increase the tendency to adapt and thus will tend to bring his or her language closer to the level of the child's language (a generalization from dynamic scaffolding theory; van Geert & Steenbeek, 2006). The equation expressing the eventual change in the parent's tendency to adapt is

$$\Delta A_t = a\, A_t\, (1 - \Delta L_t/S)$$

where a is a damping parameter and S is a scaling parameter. Finally, the logistic equation for the child's output variable is

$$\Delta L_t = r\, L_t^p\, (1 - L_t/(q\, I_t))$$

where p is an exponent modifying the effect of the level of L on its own growth and q is a proportion specifying the extent to which the child can currently approach the parent's actual input level, I_t. Methodologically speaking, this is a lot of equations and a lot of parameters for a time series consisting of about 38 measurements. However, as stated earlier, the dynamic systems model is supposed to represent a particular underlying theory of language learning and language adaptation, and this theory should thus be reflected in the parameters and relationships from which the model has been built. Given the smoothed curves of the child's output and the parent's input (see Figure 40.2), the parameters can now be relatively easily fitted by means of standard optimization procedures (Hood, 2010).

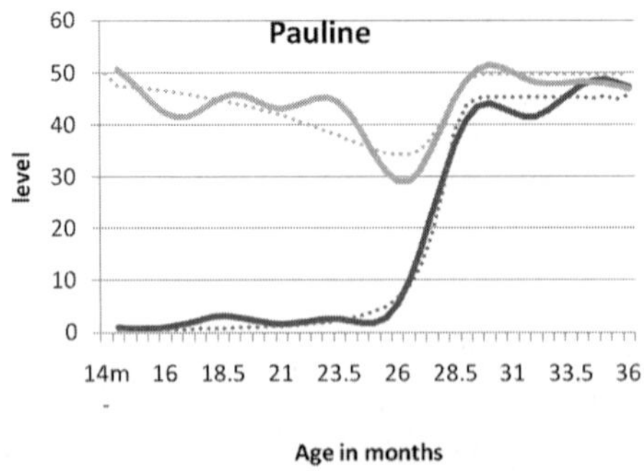

FIGURE 40.2. An example of smoothed data of determiner use in the child and in the parent, compared with the curves based on the dynamic adaptation model (dotted lines).

The model fit obtained with the estimated parameters was good, which may not be very surprising given the great number of parameters used in the dynamic model. However, it is certainly not the case that any smoothed data set can be fitted. In some cases the observed trajectories differ quite substantially from the modeled curves. Such differences can help the researcher to refine the underlying theoretical and dynamic models.

Future Directions

Dynamic systems theory provides a general framework for conceptualizing developmental change and offers a rich toolbox of methods for studying processes of change. Nothing would be more appropriate than a happy marriage between the two. However, marriages, even the potentially happy ones, cannot be arranged at will. To continue with the metaphor, developmental psychology has so far been relatively reluctant to make the acquaintance of this potential partner, for various reasons. One reason lies in the nature of the collection of dense individual time series. This method of data collection is quite unpopular: it is labor intensive; it is often highly demanding on the researcher, as well as on the respondents; it is often met with suspicion on grounds that single cases are not generalizable. Furthermore, the variability and fluctuation that naturally occur with real processes are difficult to handle in a methodological framework in which fluctuation is interpreted as measurement error. The statistical methods required for processing these data look rather forbidding and are relatively unknown. Furthermore, there is a lack of theory formation focusing on mechanisms of change. Researchers are not used to thinking in terms of processes as continuing streams of events, and books on dynamic systems theory are either of the "big-story bestseller" type or are full of outlandish equations. A different kind of reason that dynamic systems theory has not been wholeheartedly embraced by developmental psychology is that dynamic systems–inspired authors in developmental psychology—and I am aware of my own sins in this regard—have presented dynamic systems theory as something entirely new and basically incompatible with the way developmentalists have practiced their trade for the last 50 years or so. Telling people that they will have to throw everything overboard is not the best recipe for acceptance.

What should be done to give dynamic systems theory a more prominent place in developmental psychology? The first step is to convince potential users of the theory that the study of real-time processes of change and the study of distributions and associations of characteristics across populations are complementary and must be integrated into one theoretical meta-framework. Second, it is important to present dynamic systems theory as an approach or meta-method and not as a unique theory of development. Third, developmental psychologists must begin to rethink fundamental methodological issues regarding the nature of theory building and its relation with data collection and the meaning of generalizability and causal explanation. Fourth, researchers should be encouraged to experiment with the techniques developed by the as yet relatively small flock of dynamic systems enthusiasts, alongside the techniques they are familiar with, in order to see what can be learned from the combination.

References

Assmann, B., Romano, M., Thiel, M., & Niemitz, C. (2007). Hierarchical organization of a reference system in newborn spontaneous movements. *Infant Behavior and Development, 30*(4), 568–586.

Baker, A. (2010). Simplicity. In E. N. Zalta (Ed.), *Stanford encyclopedia of philosophy*. Available at *plato.stanford.edu/archives/spr2010/entries/simplicity*.

Bassano, D., Maillochon, I., Korecky-Kröll, K., van Dijk, M., Laaha, S., Dressler, W. U., et al. (2011). A comparative and dynamic approach to the development of determiner use in three children acquiring different languages. *First Language, 31*(3), 253–279.

Bassano, D., & van Geert, P. (2007). Modeling continuity and discontinuity in utterance length: A quantitative approach to changes, transitions and intra-individual variability in early grammatical development. *Developmental Science, 10*(5), 588–612.

Boker, S. M. (2002). Consequences of continuity: The hunt for intrinsic properties within parameters of dynamics in psychological processes. *Multivariate Behavioral Research, 37*(3), 405–422.

Boker, S. M., & Nesselroade, J. (2002). A method for modeling the intrinsic dynamics of intraindividual variability: Recovering the parameters of simulated oscillators in multi-wave panel data. *Multivariate Behavioral Research, 37*(1), 127–160.

Boker, S. M., & Wenger, M. J. (2007). *Data analytic techniques for dynamical systems*. Mahwah, NJ: Erlbaum.

Borsboom, D. (2008). Latent variable theory. *Measurement: Interdisciplinary Research and Perspectives, 6*(1–2), 25–53.

Cartwright, N. (2004). Causation: One word, many things. *Philosophy of Science, 71*, 805–819.

Dale, R., & Spivey, M. (2006). Unraveling the dyad: Using recurrence analysis to explore patterns of syntactic coordination between children and caregivers in conversation. *Language Learning, 56*(3), 391–430.

de Weerth, C., van Geert, P., & Hoijtink, H. (1999). Intraindividual variability in infant behavior. *Developmental Psychology, 35*(4), 1102–1112.

Dowe, P. (2010). Causal process theories. In H. Beebee, C. Hitchcock, & P. Menzies (Eds.), *Oxford handbook of causation* (pp. 213–233). Oxford, UK: Oxford University Press.

Fischer, K. W., & Bidell, T. R. (2006). Dynamic development of action and thought. In W. Damon (Ed.), *Handbook of child psychology: Vol. 1. Theoretical models of human development* (6th ed., pp. 313–399). Hoboken, NJ: Wiley.

Ganger, J., & Brent, M. R. (2004). Reexamining the vocabulary spurt. *Developmental Psychology, 40*(4), 621–632.

Goldin-Meadow, S. (2006). Talking and thinking with our hands. *Current Directions in Psychological Science, 15*(1), 34–39.

Haken, H. (2006). Synergetics of brain function. *International Journal of Psychophysiology, 60*(2), 110–124.

Hollenstein, T. (2007). State space grids: Analyzing dynamics across development. *International Journal of Behavioral Development, 31*(4), 384–396.

Hollenstein, T. (2010). Gridware: State Space Grids. Available at *http://www.statespacegrids.org*.

Hood, G. (2010). Poptools. Available at *http://www.cse.csiro.au/poptools/*.

Kunnen, E. S., & Bosma, H. A. (2000). Development of meaning making: A dynamic systems approach. *New Ideas in Psychology, 18*(1), 57–82.

Lee, A. S., & Baskerville, R. L. (2003). Generalizing generalizability in information systems research. *Information Systems Research, 14*(3), 221–243.

Lichtwarck-Aschoff, A., Kunnen, E. S., & van Geert, P. (2009). Here we go again: A dynamic systems perspective on emotional rigidity across parent–adolescent conflicts. *Developmental Psychology, 45*(5), 1364–1375.

Lichtwarck-Aschoff, A., van Geert, P., Bosma, H., & Kunnen, E. S. (2008). Time and identity: A framework for research and theory formation. *Developmental Review, 28*(3), 370–400.

Molenaar, P. C. (1985). A dynamic factor model for the analysis of multivariate time series. *Psychometrika, 50*(2), 181–202.

Molenaar, P., & Newell, K. (2010). *Individual pathways of change: Statistical models for analyzing learning and development*. Washington, DC: American Psychological Association.

Molenaar, P., Sinclair, K., Rovine, M., Ram, N., & Corneal, S. (2009). Analyzing developmental processes on an individual level using nonstationary time series modeling. *Developmental Psychology, 45*(1), 260–271.

Molenaar, P. C. M., & Campbell, C. G. (2009). The new person-specific paradigm in psychology. *Current Directions in Psychological Science, 18*(2), 112–117.

Robinson, B. F., & Mervis, C. B. (1998). Disentangling early language development: Modeling lexical and grammatical acquisition using an extension of case-study methodology. *Developmental Psychology, 34*(2), 363–375.

Schöner, G. (2009). Development as change of system dynamics: Stability, instability and emergence. In J. Spencer & M. S. C. Thomas (Eds.), *Toward a unified theory of development: Connectionism and dynamic systems theory re-considered* (pp. 25–48). Oxford, UK: Oxford University Press.

Smith, L. (2005). Cognition as a dynamic system: Principles from embodiment. *Developmental Review, 25*(3–4), 278–298.

Smith, L., Thelen, E., Titzer, R., & McLin, D. (1999). Knowing in the context of acting: The task dynamics of the A-not-B error. *Psychological Review, 106*(2), 235–260.

Steenbeek, H., & van Geert, P. (2005). A dynamic systems model of dyadic interaction during play of two children. *European Journal of Developmental Psychology, 2*(2), 105–145.

Steenbeek, H., & van Geert, P. (2007). A theory and dynamic model of dyadic interaction: Concerns, appraisals, and contagiousness in a developmental context. *Developmental Review, 27*(1), 1–40.

Steenbeek, H., & van Geert, P. (2008). An empirical validation of a dynamic systems model of interaction: Do children of different sociometric statuses differ in their dyadic play? *Developmental Science, 11*(2), 253–281.

Thelen, E., & Smith, L. B. (1994). *A dynamic systems approach to the development of cognition and action*. Cambridge, MA: MIT Press.

Valsiner, J., Molenaar, P., Lyra, M., & Chaudhary, N. (2009). *Dynamic process methodology in the social and developmental sciences*. New York: Springer Science & Business Media.

Van der Maas, H., & Molenaar, P. C. (1992). Stagewise cognitive development: An application of catastrophe theory. *Psychological Review, 99*(3), 395–417.

van Dijk, M., & van Geert, P. (2005). Disentangling behavior in early child development: Interpret-

ability of early child language and its effect on utterance length measures. *Infant Behavior and Development, 28*, 99–117.
van Dijk, M., & van Geert, P. (2007). Wobbles, humps and sudden jumps: A case study of continuity, discontinuity, and variability in early language development. *Infant and Child Development, 16*(1), 7–33.
van Dijk, M., van Geert, P., Korecky-Kröll, K., Maillochon, I., Laaha, S., Dressler, W. U., et al. (2010). *Adaptation between child directed speech and early child language: A developmental perspective.* Manuscript submitted for publication.
van Geert, P. (1991). A dynamic systems model of cognitive and language growth. *Psychological Review, 98*, 3–53.
van Geert, P. (1994). *Dynamic systems of development. Change between complexity and chaos*. New York: Harvester.
van Geert, P. (1998). A dynamic systems model of basic developmental mechanisms: Piaget, Vygotsky and beyond. *Psychological Review, 105*(4), 634–677.
van Geert, P. (2002). Developmental dynamics, intentional action and fuzzy sets. In N. Granott & J. Parziale (Eds.), *Microdevelopmental clues: Transition processes in development and learning* (pp. 319–343). Cambridge, UK: Cambridge University Press.
van Geert, P. (2003). Dynamic systems approaches and modeling of developmental processes. In J. Valsiner & K. J. Conolly (Eds.), *Handbook of developmental psychology* (pp. 640–672). London: Sage.
van Geert, P. (2008). Nonlinear-complex-dynamic-systems in developmental psychology. In S. Guastello, M. Koopmans, & D. Pincus (Eds.), *Chaos and complexity in psychology: The theory of nonlinear dynamical systems* (pp. 242–281). Cambridge, UK: Cambridge University Press.
van Geert, P., & Fischer, K. W. (2009). Dynamic systems and the quest for individual-based models of change and development. In J. Spencer & M. S. C. Thomas (Eds.), *Toward a unified theory of development: Connectionism and dynamic systems theory re-considered* (pp. 313–336). Oxford, UK: Oxford University Press.
van Geert, P., & Steenbeek, H. (2005). Explaining after by before: Basic aspects of a dynamic systems approach to the study of development. *Developmental Review, 25*(3–4), 408–442.
van Geert, P., & Steenbeek, H. (2006). The dynamics of scaffolding. *New Ideas in Psychology, 23*(3), 115–128.
van Geert, P., & van Dijk, M. (2002). Focus on variability: New tools to study intra-individual variability in developmental data. *Infant Behavior and Development, 25*, 340–374.
van Geert, P., & van Dijk, M. (2003). The problem of inter-observer reliability in ambiguous observation data. *First Language, 23*(3), 259–284.
von Oertzen, T., & Boker, S. (2010). Time delay embedding increases estimation precision of models of intraindividual variability. *Psychometrika, 75*(1), 158–175.
Yin, R. K. (2009). *Case study research: Design and methods* (4th ed.). Thousand Oaks, CA: Sage.

CHAPTER 41

Planned Missing Data Designs for Developmental Research

STEPHEN A. MISTLER
CRAIG K. ENDERS

Central Issues

Missing data handling techniques have received considerable attention in the methodological literature in the last 30 years. Much of this research has focused on maximum likelihood estimation and multiple imputation. These so-called "modern" analytical approaches have a strong theoretical foundation, and a large body of empirical research supports their use. The advent of sophisticated missing data handling techniques has led methodologists to develop research designs that feature planned missing data (e.g., Graham, Hofer, & MacKinnon, 1996; Graham, Taylor, & Cumsille, 2001; Graham, Taylor, Olchowski, & Cumsille, 2006). Unlike attrition-related missingness, intentional missing values are completely benign. Planned missing data designs exploit this fact by using missing values to solve important practical problems. In particular, incorporating planned missingness can reduce research costs while simultaneously minimizing respondent burden. With careful planning, these benefits can be realized with minimal (and perhaps no) loss of statistical power.

Used in conjunction with modern missing data handling procedures, planned missing data designs are important tools for developmental research. The purpose of this chapter is to describe planned missingness designs and illustrate their use, with a strong emphasis on longitudinal applications. In order to effectively implement these designs, researchers must integrate the missing data in a way that maximizes power (or minimizes the power loss). Doing so requires tools for obtaining a priori power estimates for different configurations of missing data. To this end, a good deal of the chapter is devoted to illustrative analyses that demonstrate how to use the Mplus software package to evaluate the power of different designs.

Conceptual Issues and Statistical Assumptions

This section describes the foundational issues associated with planned missing data designs. We begin with a brief overview of missing data theory, as described by Rubin and colleagues (Little & Rubin, 2002; Rubin, 1976). This theory provides a theoretical rationale for planned missingness designs because it ensures that the missing values are incapable of introducing bias. Next, we give a very brief overview of two modern missing data handling methods, maximum likelihood estimation and multiple imputation. Implementing a planned missingness design is possible only in conjunction with these analysis approaches. Finally, we describe a basic planned missing data design for cross-sectional data. This design provides the basis for the longitudinal designs that are the primary focus of this chapter.

Types of Missing Data

Researchers are often wary of planned missing data designs because they assume that the missing values will negatively affect their results. In truth, the extent to which missing data are capable of introducing bias depends on the reasons for missingness. Rubin and colleagues (Little & Rubin, 2002; Rubin, 1976) proposed a classification system that describes three potential sources of missingness. In practical terms, these so-called missing-data mechanisms serve as assumptions that dictate the performance of a missing-data analysis. This section gives a conceptual overview of Rubin's mechanisms, and additional technique details are available elsewhere in the literature (Enders, 2010a; Little & Rubin, 2002; Schafer & Graham, 2001).

To begin, data are consistent with a missing completely at random (MCAR) mechanism when the propensity for missing values on a variable Y is unrelated to other variables in the data set, as well as to the values of Y itself. To illustrate, consider a school-based study that examines antisocial behavior in teenagers. An MCAR mechanism would hold if the propensity for a missing behavior score is unrelated to other measured variables, as well as to the unseen antisocial behavior scores (e.g., a child is missing for haphazard reasons such as an illness, family vacation, or relocation to another school district). From a practical perspective, MCAR missing values are completely benign because the observed data are a simple random sample of the hypothetically complete data.

Next, the missing at random (MAR) mechanism allows the propensity for missing data on variable Y to be related to other variables in the analysis, but not to the values of Y itself. Returning to the antisocial behavior example, suppose that children from single-parent households are more likely to have a missing behavioral assessment than children from two-parent households. This scenario would satisfy an MAR mechanism if the propensity for missing data is unrelated to behavior after controlling for family composition (e.g., within the subsample of single-parent families, the probability of a missing value is unrelated to antisocial behavior). The modern missing data handling techniques assume an MAR mechanism and thus produce unbiased estimates under both MCAR and MAR. In contrast, most traditional approaches (e.g., deleting incomplete cases) are prone to bias with MAR data.

Finally, a missing not at random (MNAR) mechanism holds when the propensity for missing data on Y is related to the unseen values of Y, even after controlling for other potential sources of missingness. This situation would arise when children with elevated antisocial behavior scores have a higher likelihood of missing data on the behavioral assessment (e.g., because they skip class, are suspended from school, or are incarcerated). An MNAR mechanism is problematic because even the modern analytical approaches are likely to produce biased parameter estimates. Interested readers can consult Enders (2010a, 2010b) for an overview of MNAR models for longitudinal analyses.

In most situations, researchers have no way of knowing why the data are missing, because there is no way to empirically assess the MAR and MNAR mechanisms (e.g., demonstrating that the propensity for missing data on Y is unrelated to the Y scores requires knowledge of the missing values). Fortunately, the planned missing data designs in this chapter produce MCAR data, by definition. From a practical perspective, this implies that intentional missing values are completely benign and are incapable of introducing bias. The only potential drawback of planned missingness is a loss of power. However, with careful planning, these designs can be implemented with minimal (and perhaps no) loss of statistical power.

Modern Missing Data Handling Techniques

The methodological literature generally recommends the use of two modern missing data handling techniques, maximum likelihood estimation and multiple imputation. Maximum likelihood (also known as full information maximum likelihood, or FIML) uses an iterative algorithm to audition different sets of plausible parameter values until it locates the particular estimates that maximize fit to the data. Importantly, the estimation process incorporates all of the available data without actually filling in (i.e., imputing) the missing values. Consequently, even cases with a single observed data point can contribute to a longitudinal analysis. In contrast, multiple imputation uses a regression-based procedure to generate plausible replacement values for the missing scores. As its name implies, the procedure creates multiple copies of the data set (e.g., 20 is a good rule of thumb), each of which contains different filled-in values. The researcher subsequently analyzes each data set separately and then combines the estimates and the standard errors into a single set of results. Relative to traditional missing data handling methods (e.g., discarding incomplete cases), maximum likelihood and multiple imputation are advantageous because they yield unbiased estimates under an MCAR or an MAR mechanism and because they maximize power. These methods are widely available in popular statistical software packages, and we later show how to use the FIML estimator in Mplus (Muthén & Muthén, 2010) to evaluate the power of different planned missingness designs. Additional details on maximum likelihood estimation and multiple imputation are available elsewhere in the literature (Enders, 2010a; Little & Rubin, 2002; Schafer, 1997; Schafer & Graham, 2002).

The Three-Form Design

Having established some necessary background information, we now describe a simple planned missing data design for cross-sectional research. Although this design may be less applicable to developmental research studies, its basic features generalize to the longitudinal designs that we discuss in the next section. Graham and colleagues (1996) proposed the three-form design as a mechanism for reducing respondent burden in cross-sectional studies that utilize large questionnaire batteries. The basic strategy is to administer a subset of the questionnaire items to each respondent. Specifically, the three-form design is composed

TABLE 41.1. Missing Data Patterns from a Three-Form Design

	Item sets			
Form	X	A	B	C
1	O	M	O	O
2	O	O	M	O
3	O	O	O	M

Note. O, observed; M, missing.

of four item sets (X, A, B, and C) that are allocated across three questionnaire forms. Table 41.1 shows the allocation of item sets in a prototypical three-form design. As seen in the table, each form includes the X set but is missing either the A, B, or the C set. Note that the composition of the item sets is flexible, such that a given set could include a single questionnaire, multiple questionnaires, or combinations of items from different questionnaires.

To illustrate the impact of the three-form design on respondent burden, consider a study that examines correlates of antisocial behavior in teenage children. Suppose that the X set consists of a 10-item demographic questionnaire and a 10-item antisocial behavior inventory. Furthermore the A, B, and C sets consist of 20 items each that measure a variety of different constructs (e.g., quality of parental relationships, risk-taking behavior). In this scenario, the three-form design yields data on 80 questionnaire items, although each participant responds to only 60 of the items. Importantly, modern missing data handling techniques allow the researchers to perform the same analyses that they would have performed had the data been complete.

Returning to Table 41.1, it is clear that the three-form design introduces a substantial amount of missing data. For example, 33% of the scores are missing for every X–A variable pair, and 66% of the scores are missing for each A–B variable pair. It is important to reiterate that the missing values are incapable of introducing bias because they are consistent with an MCAR mechanism. Consequently, a loss of power is the primary disadvantage of the three-form design. Interestingly, the drop in power is generally not commensurate with the missing data rate (or even close to it). For example, if the X–A relationship is moderate in magnitude (e.g., $r = .30$), a 33% missing data rate may decrease power by only 1%. With the same effect size, a 66% missing data rate may reduce power by approximately 10% (Enders, 2010a; Graham et al., 2006). This somewhat counterintuitive result owes to the fact that modern missing data handling approaches salvage power by borrowing information from the observed data.

Developmental Applications

Longitudinal designs are difficult to implement because they create logistical challenges for researchers and because they impose a substantial burden on participants. Planned missing data designs can mitigate both of these problems by reducing the number of assessments that each participant completes. The cohort-sequential design (Duncan, Duncan, & Hops, 1996; Nesselroade & Baltes, 1979) is appropriate for situations in which the goal is to examine age-related changes in an outcome variable. This design has a long history in the methodological literature and has enjoyed frequent use in substantive research studies. The cohort-sequential design allows researchers to estimate a single developmental trajectory by piecing together short-term longitudinal studies from different age cohorts. For example, Duncan and colleagues (1996) examined teenage alcohol use over a 6-year span by combining 3 years of data from four different age cohorts. Table 41.2 shows the missing data patterns from their design. Notice that each age cohort has missing data at three age points; the 12-year-old cohort has missing scores at ages 15, 16, and 17; the 13-year-old cohort is missing at ages 12, 16, and 17; and so on. Consistent with the three-form design, the missing values are benign. Although the cohort-sequential design is well suited for longitudinal data analyses (e.g., a FIML growth model), it has limited utility for estimating bivariate associations. For example, the correlation between alcohol use scores at ages 13 and 17 is inestimable because these variables are concurrently missing.

Graham and colleagues (2001) proposed a class of planned missingness designs that extend the logic of the three-form design to longitudinal data. These designs are flexible because they are not limited to situations in which age-related change is the substantive focus. Graham's designs consist of a number of random subgroups, each of which is missing at one or more data collection waves. To illustrate, Table 41.3 shows the missing data patterns from a six-wave design in which each participant completes four assessments. This design incorporates every combination of two missing assessments, but other variations are possible. For example, excluding patterns with missing data at the first wave may be a good strategy, particularly when the goal is to examine associations between baseline measures and individual growth rates. Also, the patterns need not be equally weighted when logistical constraints require an unequal allocation of respondents across the missing data patterns. Later in the chapter, we focus on designs that always include the first and the last wave because this configuration tends to maximize power.

Consistent with the three-form design, the longitudinal design in Table 41.3 introduces a substantial proportion of missing data. Again, bias is not a concern, but power is. Interestingly, a carefully executed planned missingness design may not reduce power at all, particularly when the total number of assessments is fixed by budgetary constraints. To illustrate, suppose that a grant budget can accommodate a total of 1,000 assessments, each costing \$100 to administer. Given a fixed number of assessments, Graham and colleagues (2001) showed that certain planned missing data designs can actually achieve higher power than a corresponding complete-data design. That is, collecting incomplete data from 240 participants may be better than collecting complete data from 200 participants. This conclusion is

TABLE 41.2. Cohort-Sequential Design with Four Age Cohorts

	Age at time of data collection					
Cohort	12	13	14	15	16	17
12	O	O	O	M	M	M
13	M	O	O	O	M	M
14	M	M	O	O	O	M
15	M	M	M	O	O	O

Note. O, observed; M, missing.

TABLE 41.3. Longitudinal Planned Missing Data Design with Every Combination of Two Waves Missing

	Data collection wave						
Pattern	1	2	3	4	5	6	Percentage of sample
1	O	O	O	O	M	M	6.7%
2	O	O	O	M	O	M	6.7%
3	O	O	M	O	O	M	6.7%
4	O	M	O	O	O	M	6.7%
5	M	O	O	O	O	M	6.7%
6	O	O	O	M	M	O	6.7%
7	O	O	M	O	M	O	6.7%
8	O	M	O	O	M	O	6.7%
9	M	O	O	O	M	O	6.7%
10	O	O	M	M	O	O	6.7%
11	O	M	O	M	O	O	6.7%
12	M	O	O	M	O	O	6.7%
13	O	M	M	O	O	O	6.7%
14	M	O	M	O	O	O	6.7%
15	M	M	O	O	O	O	6.7%

Note. O, observed; M, missing.

not uniformly true and depends, in part, on the distribution of the missing values across the data collection waves. For example, a design with missing data at the first or the last wave will tend to have lower power than a design with missing values in the middle waves. The remainder of the chapter addresses this issue in more detail.

Illustration

In order to effectively implement planned missingness designs, researchers must distribute the missing data in a way that maximizes power. In particular, determining which assessments should be missing and deciding how to allocate the sample across the missing data patterns are key considerations. Because study-specific features (e.g., number of data collection waves, functional form of the growth curve, effect size) and logistical constraints (e.g., budget, staff availability, geographical distribution of participants) often affect design decisions, researchers need ways to obtain a priori power estimates for different configurations of missing data. Monte Carlo computer simulations are an ideal tool for this purpose because there is no way to derive analytical power estimates from such a complex design. Throughout the remainder of the chapter, we use the Mplus software package (Muthén & Muthén, 2010) to evaluate the power of different planned missingness designs. Mplus is ideally suited for this task because it has built-in computer simulation facilities that readily incorporate missing data. We provide a brief description of Monte Carlo simulations in this section, and more detailed accounts of the process are available elsewhere in the literature (Muthén & Muthén, 2002; Paxton, Curran, Bollen, Kirby, & Chen, 2001). To facilitate the subsequent discussion, Appendix 41.1 on *www.crmda.ku.edu/Guilford/HDRM* gives an Mplus input file from a Monte Carlo simulation that investigated power for the design in Table 41.3. We refer to this program throughout the remainder of this section.

Executing a Monte Carlo Simulation

The basic goal of a Monte Carlo simulation is to generate a large number of artificial data sets (e.g., 5,000) from a population with a hypothesized set of parameter values. Choosing a reasonable set of parameters is the most difficult part of the process. For illustrative purposes, we used linear growth curve estimates from Odgers and colleagues' (2009) study of antisocial behavior as the basis for our power simulations. The population growth model expresses the outcome variable as a function of a temporal predictor (e.g., age), as follows:

$$Y_{ti} = \beta_0 + \beta_1(TIME_{ti}) + b_{0i} + b_{1i}(TIME_{ti}) + \varepsilon_{ti} \qquad \textbf{(41.1)}$$

where Y_{ti} is the outcome score for case i at time t, $TIME_{ti}$ is the number of years since the initial assessment (e.g., in a six-wave study, *TIME* takes on integer values between 0 and 5), β_0 represents the average initial status score (i.e., the intercept), and β_1 is the average growth rate (i.e., the slope). As a starting point, we set β_0 and β_1 at values of 20.67 and –0.66, respectively. Turning to the so-called random effects, b_{0i} and b_{1i} are residual terms that capture individual differences in the intercepts and slopes, respectively, and ε_{ti} is a time-specific residual. The growth curve model yields a variance estimate for each residual term, as well as a covariance between intercept and slope residuals. We fixed the variance of b_{0j} and b_{1j} at values of 191.55 and 3.30, respectively, and set the covariance between these terms at –7.92 (this corresponds to a correlation of $r = -.32$ between the intercepts and slopes). Finally, we specified the variance of ε_{ti} to be 169. Turning to Appendix 41.1 on *www.crmda.ku.edu/Guilford/HDRM*, the command lines in the MODEL POPULATION section of the Mplus program specify these population parameters. As an aside, it is fairly straightforward to calculate an effect size from the growth model parameters. The difference between the model-predicted means from the first assessment and the final assessment provides an estimate of overall change. The square root of the sum of the intercept variance and the residual variance is the baseline standard deviation. Dividing the estimated change score by the baseline standard deviation results in the effect size expressed on a metric that is roughly equivalent to Cohen's *d*. For our population, the expected change is equal to 3.30, and the baseline standard deviation is 18.99, resulting in an effect size of –.17. This is just shy of Cohen's (1988) small-effect-size benchmark.

Having specified a set of population parameters, the next step is to generate a large number of artificial data sets from the population. The Mplus MONTECARLO command dictates a variety of simulation features. Considering the program in Appendix 41.1 on *www.crmda.ku.edu/Guilford/HDRM*, the NAMES ARE subcommand lists the variable names (e.g., Y1–Y6 are the simulated repeated-measures variables), the NOBSERVATIONS subcommand specifies the sample size, and NREPS determines the number of artificial data sets. Unless otherwise specified, Mplus generates normally distributed variables.

Simulating missing values can be a difficult aspect of a power simulation, but Mplus makes this step rather easy, particularly for planned missingness designs. Returning to Appendix 41.1 on *www.crmda.ku.edu/Guilford/HDRM*, the PATMISS command specifies the configuration of missing data for each of the six patterns in the design; note that a value of 0 represents a complete observation and a value of 1 denotes missing data. Finally, the PATPROBS command specifies the proportion of cases in each pattern. The program in Appendix 41.1 on *www.crmda.ku.edu/Guilford/HDRM* distributes the sample equally across the missing data patterns, but this is not a requirement. Experimenting with unequal weighting schemes is usually a good idea because this distribution can affect power.

The final step of a computer simulation is to estimate a statistical model (e.g., the linear growth curve model from equation 41.1) on each artificial data set. The MODEL portion of the Mplus program in Appendix 41.1 on *www.crmda.ku.edu/Guilford/HDRM* specifies a linear growth model with homoscedastic error terms (i.e., equality constraints on the residual variances). Mplus is flexible because the data-generating model and the analysis model need not be the same. For example, you could use summary statistics and correlations as population parameters in the MODEL POPULATION command and use a growth curve model to analyze each artificial data set in the MODEL command. Finally, note that Mplus implements maximum likelihood missing data handling by default, so invoking this estimator requires no additional steps.

The product of a computer simulation is an empirical estimate of power. Because we generated the data from a population with nonzero growth (i.e., the null hypothesis that the slope equals zero is false), the proportion of samples that produced a statistically significant slope estimate is an estimate of power. Mplus reports the proportion of significant estimates as part of its standard output, so no additional effort is required. Although it sounds tedious to use computer simulations to estimate power, Mplus automates the entire process. In fact, the simulation program in Appendix 41.1 on *www.crmda.ku.edu/Guilford/HDRM* took less than 1 minute to execute. Specifying reasonable values for the population parameters is the most time-consuming part of the process; however, this is true for any power analysis. The advantage of computer simulations is that you can quickly evaluate the impact of missing data on power. This is impossible with standard analytical power approaches (e.g., Cohen, 1988).

Two Scenarios: Fixed Number of Assessments versus Fixed Sample Size

Having outlined the procedural details of a computer simulation, we use the rest of the chapter to evaluate the power of various longitudinal missing data designs. Our simulations are by no means comprehensive, and we limit the subsequent discussion to just two planned missing data designs. The primary goal of this section is to illustrate the process of evaluating these designs rather than to systematically evaluate a variety of different options. Readers who are interested in a broader discussion of different missing data designs can consult Graham and colleagues (2001).

In our experience, substantive researchers often find themselves in one of two situations when planning a study. In the first scenario, budgetary constraints limit the total number of assessments that can be administered, but the total sample size is flexible. For example, at $100 per assessment, the grant budget might accommodate a total of 1,500 assessments, but the sample size needed to produce that number of assessments can vary (e.g., incomplete data from 375 participants vs. complete data from 250 participants). In the second scenario, logistical constraints limit the total sample size, but the number of assessments is flexible. For example, due to the geographical distribution of participants, the research team may be able to track only 250 participants, irrespective of the number of assessments per participant. As you will see, implementing a planned missingness design in the first scenario can increase power, but missing data in the second scenario decreases power. However, this loss of power can be rather small, depending on the configuration of the missing values.

Linear Growth Models

To illustrate the effect of planned missingness on power, we ran Monte Carlo simulations for three separate designs, keeping the total number of assessments fixed (i.e., scenario 1). All three designs were tested for their power to detect linear growth in a six-wave longitudinal study. The simulation's population parameters are the same as those from Appendix 41.1 on *www.crmda.ku.edu/Guilford/HDRM*. The first design consisted of complete data for 250 participants (250 participants each given 6 assessments, for a total of 1,500 assessments). The complete data design correctly detected the linear effect in 83% of the 1,000 artificial data sets (i.e., the empirical power estimate was .83). This value provides a useful benchmark for assessing the impact of planned missing data on power. The second design consisted of incomplete data for 375 participants (375 participants each given 4 assessments, for a total of 1,500 assessments). Every participant was missing two assessments such that every combination of two assessments missing was represented equally across participants. Table 41.3 gives the missing data patterns for the simulation. This design correctly detected the linear effect in 81% of the samples. Stated differently, the planned missing data design produced a power estimate that was 97.5% as large as that of the complete data design. The final design also consisted of incomplete data for 375 participants (375 participants each given 4 assessments, for a total of 1,500 assessments), but the first and the last assessments were complete for all participants. Table 41.4 gives the missing data patterns from the design. This design was included because it was expected to maximize power for detecting linear effects. In ordinary least squares regression, the standard error of a regression slope is inversely proportional to the standard deviation of the predictor (Cohen, Cohen, West, & Aiken, 2003, p. 42). Because the relationship between the standard deviation of the predictor and the standard error of the linear term also holds in a growth model, including complete data at the first and the last assessments should increase the standard deviation of the predictor variable (i.e., age), thereby decreasing the standard error for the linear slope term. The simulation results confirmed this expectation, as the third design correctly detected the linear effect 92% of the time. The previous examples

TABLE 41.4. Longitudinal Planned Missing Data Design with First and Last Assessments Always Included

	Data collection wave						
Pattern	1	2	3	4	5	6	Percentage of sample
1	O	O	O	M	M	O	16.7%
2	O	O	M	O	M	O	16.7%
3	O	M	O	O	M	O	16.7%
4	O	O	M	M	O	O	16.7%
5	O	M	O	M	O	O	16.7%
6	O	M	M	O	O	O	16.7%

Note. O, observed; M, missing.

demonstrate that a planned missing data design can result in little or no loss in power when the number of assessments is held constant. In fact, relative to a complete data design, the planned missing data design with complete endpoints (i.e., the configuration in Table 41.4) actually increased power by nearly 10%.

We next ran Monte Carlo simulations for the same three designs but kept the total number of cases fixed at 250 (i.e., scenario 2). Other than the change to the number of participants in each simulation, the designs are the same as those in Tables 41.3 and 41.4. As before, the power estimate for the complete data design was .83. The second design (i.e., every combination of two missing assessments represented equally across participants) correctly detected the linear effect in 64% of the artificial data sets (i.e., a 23% decrease in power). The syntax for this design is included in Appendix 41.1 on *www.crmda.ku.edu/Guilford/HDRM*. Finally, the design in which the first and the last assessments were complete correctly detected the linear effect 77% of the time (i.e., a 7% decrease in power). As seen from these simulations, implementing a planned missing data design with the number of participants held constant leads to a decrease in power, but this loss in power can be minimized through choosing an appropriate design. In particular, the design with complete endpoints produced a relatively modest decrease in power. This decrease may be quite tolerable in light of the cost savings associated with the design.

It is important to note that the designs in Tables 41.3 and 41.4 are just two of the many different possibilities. A number of factors come into play when implementing planned missing data designs (e.g., the number and the spacing of the repeated-measures variables, the shape of the developmental trajectory, the effect size), and it is generally necessary to investigate power for a variety of plausible scenarios. In particular, the substantive research questions may require alterations to the design. For example, in the fixed endpoints design from Table 41.4, every participant is assessed at wave 1, but only 50% of participants are assessed at wave 3. Consequently, an analysis that examines the influence of a predictor variable on the intercept would have very different power depending on whether the intercept was assigned to wave 1 or wave 3. If the goal is to maximize predictive power at wave 3, one option is to assign a larger proportion of the sample to the patterns with complete data at that assessment (e.g., patterns 2, 4, or 6). For convenience, we used an equal allocation strategy throughout the chapter, but this is certainly not necessary. Of course, adding, removing, or altering missing data patterns are also options. Fortunately, Monte Carlo simulations allow researchers to quickly audition different designs, and it is a good idea to explore the power for each of a study's major hypotheses.

Quadratic Growth Models

Planned missing data designs can also be employed for assessing quadratic growth. However, the designs tend to suffer from a slightly larger loss of power for detecting quadratic growth than for detecting linear growth. To demonstrate the effect of planned missingness on power to detect a quadratic effect, we ran Monte Carlo simulations for the three previous designs, keeping the total number of assessments fixed (i.e., scenario 1). All three designs were tested for their power to detect quadratic growth in a six-wave longitudinal study. The simulation's population parameters are based on results from Odgers and colleagues' (2009) study of antisocial behavior but with an added quadratic trend (the means from this study suggested that the developmental trajectory flattened somewhat over time). To illustrate the necessary changes to the Mplus code, Appendix 41.2 on *www.crmda.ku.edu/Guilford/HDRM* gives the syntax from one of the simulations.

The first design consisted of complete data for 1,000 participants (1,000 participants each given 6 assessments, for a total of 6,000 assessments). Note that we changed the sample size to 1,000 participants in order to achieve adequate power to detect the quadratic effect from the complete data design. This design correctly detected the quadratic effect in 85% of the 1,000 artificial data sets (i.e., the empirical power estimate was .85). Again, this value provides a useful benchmark for evaluating the planned missingness designs. The second design consisted of incomplete data for 1,500 participants (1,500 participants each given 4 assessments, for a total of 6,000 assessments). Consistent with Table 41.3, every combination of two assessments missing was represented equally across participants. This design correctly detected the quadratic effect 81% of the time, for a roughly 5% decrease in power relative to the complete data design. The final design also consisted of incomplete data for 1,500 participants (1,500 participants each given 4 assessments, for a total of 6,000 assessments). However, the first and last assessments were complete for all participants (see Table 41.4). This design was included because it proved to be the most powerful design for detecting linear effects. Consistent with the linear model simulations, this design actually increased power, correctly detecting the linear effect 87% of the time.

We next ran Monte Carlo simulations for the same three designs but kept the total number of cases fixed at 1,000 (i.e., scenario 2). Other than this change to the number of participants in each simulation, the designs are the same as those in Tables 41.3 and 41.4. As before, the complete data design detected the quadratic effect 85% of the time. The second design (i.e., every combination of two missing assessments was represented equally across participants) correctly detected the linear effect in 64% of the artificial data sets. Finally, the design in which the first and the last assessments were complete produced a power estimate of .71 for detecting the quadratic effect. As seen from these simulations, implementing a planned missing data design with the number of participants held constant leads to a decrease in power, but this loss in power can be minimized through choosing an appropriate design. In particular, the design with complete endpoints produced a relatively modest decrease in power. The same was true for the linear model simulations.

Growth Models with Predictor Variables

It is often of interest to examine the influence of predictor variables on longitudinal growth. These predictors may consist of qualitatively different subgroups for which theory predicts different developmental trajectories (e.g., males and females, treatment and control) or they may be continuous covariates. Predictor variables can easily be incorporated into a planned missing data power analysis in Mplus. They do not require any changes to the planned missing data portions of the power analysis (the PATMISS and PATPROBS commands in Mplus), so we present syntax for a planned missingness design with all combinations of two assessments missing to be consistent with the other examples.

To illustrate the inclusion of a predictor variable, suppose that we are interested in using Mplus to examine the power of a two-group intervention for reducing antisocial behavior. We chose to illustrate a categorical predictor because this is somewhat more difficult than incorporating a continuous covariate. Modeling the differences between a treatment and a control group requires only one new command, CUTPOINTS. In the MODEL POPULATION portion of Appendix 41.3 on *www.crmda.ku.edu/Guilford/HDRM*, the predictor is initially specified as a continuous variable named TXGROUP that has a mean of 0 and a variance of 1. Mplus subsequently categorizes the continuous variable using the threshold value given in parentheses on the CUTPOINTS command. For example, setting the threshold value to 0 implies that the cases falling above the mean will be classified into one group (i.e., TXGROUP = 1) and the cases falling below the mean will be classified into the second group (i.e., TXGROUP = 0). Although the classification process will vary from one sample to the next, participants will be equally distributed between the two groups, on average. Finally, note that, in order to generate a continuous predictor, you simply omit the CUTPOINTS command from the syntax.

Incorporating a binary predictor also necessitates a change to the estimates in the MODEL POPULATION portion of the syntax. The results from Odgers and colleagues' (2009) study of antisocial behavior readily serve as population estimates for our control group. For the treatment group, we needed to specify the amount by which its intercept and linear growth differ from the intercept and linear growth of the control group. For instance, we might assign a value of 0 to the difference between the intercepts because the groups should not differ at the beginning of the study in a randomized experiment. Under the belief that the treatment should lead to a more rapid decrease in antisocial behavior over time, we specified a value of –2 for the difference in linear growth between the groups to determine power for a range of effect sizes. In the absence of pilot data, it is a good idea to experiment with several values for this difference in order to determine power for a range of effect sizes.

Future Directions

To date, the methodological literature offers relatively little guidance on implementing longitudinal missing data designs. Despite their potential utility, a great deal of work remains to be done. As one example, existing literature on planned missing data designs has focused exclusively on linear growth models. We provided a cursory example of quadratic growth in this chapter, but the need for further study is underscored by the prevalence of quadratic and piecewise models in the developmental literature. Nonlinear models pose unique challenges and also have important limitations. For example, consider the complete endpoint design in Table 41.4. This design is not applicable to longitudinal studies with fewer than five waves because removing the middle two assessments for every participant in a four-wave study would result in a two-wave design rather than a four-wave design with planned missing data. Additionally, growth curve analyses fail to converge in five-wave planned missingness designs without making adjustments to the missing data patterns or to the analysis model. These convergence problems can be overcome by including a subset of cases with complete data at all assessments (e.g., a relatively small pattern composed of 5% of the total sample) or by constraining the residual variances to be equal over time. The shape of the growth form is also a unique challenge for implementing planned missingness designs, and the ideal distribution of the missing values likely depends on the location of the curvature. For example, a trajectory with rapid initial acceleration may require a different planned missingness pattern from one with acceleration at later assessments. We did not investigate this issue, but researchers should be aware of this nuance when planning their studies.

A second area that warrants further research is the application of planned missingness designs to multilevel data. Longitudinal studies frequently involve the collection of clustered data (children clustered within schools, siblings clustered within family, etc.). This adds a layer of complexity to designing a planned missing data study, as missingness can be added at the level of the cluster or at the level of the individual. To illustrate, consider a study of students clustered within schools. A planned missingness design could be implemented by randomly removing students (individual level) from one or more waves or by randomly removing schools (cluster level) from one or more waves. Implementing intentional missing data at the cluster level may lead to a greater drop in power than a design with missing data at the individual level, yet this strategy could be desirable for practical reasons. The trade-offs between and limitations of these designs (and possible combinations of the two) have yet to be examined.

References

Cohen, J. (1988). *Statistical power analysis for the behavioral sciences* (2nd ed.). Hillsdale, NJ: Erlbaum.

Cohen, J., Cohen, P., West, S. G., & Aiken, L. S. (2003). *Applied multiple regression/correlation analysis for the behavioral sciences* (3rd ed.). Mahwah, NJ: Erlbaum.

Duncan, S. C., Duncan, T. E., & Hops, H. (1996). Analysis of longitudinal data within accelerated longitudinal designs. *Psychological Methods, 1*, 236–248.

Enders, C. K. (2010a). *Applied missing data analysis*. New York: Guilford Press.

Enders, C. K. (2010b). *Selection models and pattern mixture models for latent growth curve analyses*. Manuscript submitted for publication.

Graham, J. W., Hofer, S. M., & MacKinnon, D. P. (1996). Maximizing the usefulness of data obtained with planned missing value patterns: An application of maximum likelihood procedures. *Multivariate Behavioral Research, 31*, 197–218.

Graham, J. W., Taylor, B. J., & Cumsille, P. E. (2001). Planned missing data designs in the analysis of change. In L. M. Collins & A. G. Sayer (Eds.), *New methods for the analysis of change* (pp. 335–353). Washington, DC: American Psychological Association.

Graham, J. W., Taylor, B. J., Olchowski, A. E., & Cumsille, P. E. (2006). Planned missing data designs in psychological research. *Psychological Methods, 11*, 323–343.

Little, R. J. A., & Rubin, D. B. (2002). *Statistical analysis with missing data* (2nd ed.). Hoboken, NJ: Wiley.

Muthén, L. K., & Muthén, B. O. (2002). How to use a Monte Carlo study to decide on sample size and determine power. *Structural Equation Modeling: A Multidisciplinary Journal, 9*, 599–620.

Muthén, L. K., & Muthén, B. O. (2010). *Mplus user's guide* (6th ed.). Los Angeles: Authors.

Nesselroade, J. R., & Baltes, P. B. (1979). *Longitudinal research in the study of behavior and development*. New York: Academic Press.

Odgers, C. L., Moffitt, T. E., Tach, L. M., Sampson, R. J., Taylor, A., Mathews, C. L., et al. (2009). The protective effects of neighborhood collective efficacy on British children growing up in deprivation: A developmental analysis. *Developmental Psychology, 45*, 942–957.

Paxton, P., Curran, P. J., Bollen, K. A., Kirby, J., & Chen, F. (2001). Monte Carlo experiments: Design and implementation. *Structural Equation Modeling: A Multidisciplinary Journal, 8*, 287–312.

Rubin, D. B. (1976). Inference and missing data. *Biometrika, 63*, 581–592.

Schafer, J. L. (1997). *Analysis of incomplete multivariate data*. Boca Raton, FL: Chapman & Hall.

Schafer, J. L., & Graham, J. W. (2002). Missing data: Our view of the state of the art. *Psychological Methods, 7*, 147–177.

Author Index

Subject Index

Page numbers followed by *f* indicate figure, *t* indicate table

About the Editors

Brett Laursen, PhD, is Professor of Psychology and Director of Graduate Training at Florida Atlantic University. He is also a Docent Professor of Social Developmental Psychology at the University of Jyväskylä, Finland. In 2008, Dr. Laursen received an honorary doctorate from Örebro University, Sweden. He is a Fellow of the American Psychological Association (Division 7, Developmental) and a Fellow and Charter Member of the Association for Psychological Science. In addition to his own research on parent–child and peer relationships, Dr. Laursen is a consultant and collaborator on several large longitudinal projects currently under way in North America and Europe. He is currently the Methods and Measures Editor at the *International Journal of Behavioral Development* and has edited or coedited six other books and monographs, the most recent being the *Handbook of Peer Interactions, Relationships, and Groups*.

Todd D. Little, PhD, is Professor of Psychology, Director of the Quantitative Training Program, and a member of the Developmental Training Program at the University of Kansas, where he is also Director of the Center for Research Methods and Data Analysis. Past president of the American Psychological Association's Division 5 (Evaluation, Measurement, and Statistics), Dr. Little organizes and teaches in the internationally renowned "Stats Camps" each June (see *www.Quant.KU.edu*) at the University of Kansas. Dr. Little has edited five books related to methodology and statistics, including the *Oxford Handbook of Quantitative Methods*. He is Series Editor for Guilford's Methodology in the Social Sciences series.

Noel A. Card, PhD, is Associate Professor in Family Studies and Human Development at the University of Arizona. His research centers around social development and quantitative methods, and especially the interaction of these disciplines. Dr. Card's developmental research focuses on aggression and peer relations during childhood and adolescence; his quantitative interests include longitudinal analyses, analysis of interdependent data, and meta-analysis. He is a recipient of the Society for Research in Child Development's Early Career Research Award. He serves as an associate editor for *Developmental Psychology* and for the *Journal of Early Adolescence* and the author of the book *Applied Meta-Analysis for Social Science Research*.

Contributors

Robert A. Ackerman, PhD, Department of Psychology, Michigan State University, East Lansing, Michigan

Lenneke R. A. Alink, PhD, Center for Child and Family Studies, Leiden University, Leiden, The Netherlands

Marian J. Bakermans-Kranenburg, PhD, Center for Child and Family Studies, Leiden University, Leiden, The Netherlands

William D. Barta, PhD, Center for Health/HIV Intervention and Prevention, University of Connecticut, Storrs, Connecticut

David F. Bjorklund, PhD, Department of Psychology, Florida Atlantic University, Boca Raton, Florida

Shelley A. Blozis, PhD, Department of Psychology, University of California, Davis, Davis, California

Jan Boom, PhD, Department of Methodology and Statistics, University of Utrecht, Utrecht, The Netherlands

James A. Bovaird, PhD, Department of Educational Psychology, University of Nebraska, Lincoln, Nebraska

Edmond P. Bowers, PhD, Institute for Applied Research in Youth Development, Tufts University, Boston, Massachusetts

Mara Brendgen, PhD, Department of Psychology, University of Quebec, Montreal, Quebec, Canada

William M. Bukowski, PhD, Center for Research in Human Development and Department of Psychology, Concordia University, Montreal, Quebec, Canada

Noel A. Card, PhD, Family Studies and Human Development, Norton School of Family and Consumer Sciences, University of Arizona, Tucson, Arizona

Heining Cham, MA, Department of Psychology, Arizona State University, Tempe, Arizona

Antonius H. N. Cillessen, PhD, Behavioral Science Institute, Radboud University Nijmegen, Nijmegen, The Netherlands

Charles E. Collyer, PhD, Department of Psychology, University of Rhode Island, Kingston, Rhode Island

David M. Condon, MA, Department of Psychology, Northwestern University, Evanston, Illinois

Rand D. Conger, PhD, Departments of Human and Community Development and Psychology, University of California, Davis, Davis, California

William L. Cook, PhD, Center for Psychiatric Research, Maine Medical Center, Portland, Maine

Pamela Davis-Kean, PhD, Institute for Social Research, University of Michigan, Ann Arbor, Michigan

Jaap Denissen, PhD, Institute of Psychology, Humboldt University of Berlin, Berlin, Germany

Christine DiStefano, PhD, Department of Educational Studies, University of South Carolina, Columbia, South Carolina

M. Brent Donnellan, PhD, Department of Psychology, Michigan State University, East Lansing, Michigan

Susan C. Duncan, PhD, Oregon Research Institute, Eugene, Oregon

Terry E. Duncan, PhD, Oregon Research Institute, Eugene, Oregon

Susan E. Embretson, PhD, School of Psychology, Georgia Institute of Technology, Atlanta, Georgia

Craig K. Enders, PhD, Department of Psychology, Arizona State University, Tempe, Arizona

E. Michael Foster, PhD, Departments of Maternal and Child Health and Health Policy and Management, School of Public Health, University of North Carolina at Chapel Hill, Chapel Hill, North Carolina

Matthew S. Fritz, PhD, Department of Psychology, Virginia Polytechnic Institute and State University, Blacksburg, Virginia

Lisa M. Gatzke-Kopp, PhD, Department of Human Development and Family Studies, Pennsylvania State University, University Park, Pennsylvania

Scott D. Gest, PhD, Department of Human Development and Family Studies, Pennsylvania State University, University Park, Pennsylvania

Alain Girard, PhD, Department of Psychology, University of Montreal, Montreal, Quebec, Canada

Richard Gonzalez, PhD, Department of Psychology, University of Michigan, Ann Arbor, Michigan

Andrea Follmer Greenhoot, PhD, Department of Psychology, University of Kansas, Lawrence, Kansas

Kevin J. Grimm, PhD, Department of Psychology, University of California, Davis, Davis, California

Silke Hertel, PhD, German Institute for International Educational Research, Frankfurt, Germany

Scott M. Hofer, PhD, Department of Psychology, University of Victoria, Victoria, British Columbia, Canada

Joop J. Hox, PhD, Department of Methodology and Statistics, University of Utrecht, Utrecht, The Netherlands

Ashley Anders Jackson, MA, Department of Human Development and Family Studies, Auburn University, Auburn, Alabama

Justin Jager, PhD, Section on Child and Family Research, National Institute of Child Health and Human Development, National Institutes of Health, Rockville, Maryland

Deborah A. Kashy, PhD, Department of Psychology, Michigan State University, East Lansing, Michigan

Margaret K. Keiley, EdD, Department of Human Development and Family Studies, Auburn University, Auburn, Alabama

Thomas A. Kindermann, PhD, Department of Psychology, Portland State University, Portland, Oregon

Cassandra Kirkland, MA, Department of Human Development and Family Studies, Auburn University, Auburn, Alabama

Julia Klug, DiplPsych, Institute for Psychology, Technische Universität Darmstadt, Darmstadt, Germany

Katja Kokko, PhD, Department of Psychology, University of Jyväskylä, Jyväskylä, Finland

Andrey Koval, MA, Department of Psychology, University of Oklahoma, Norman, Oklahoma

Brett Laursen, PhD, Department of Psychology, Florida Atlantic University, Fort Lauderdale, Florida

Ihno A. Lee, MA, Department of Psychology, University of Kansas, Lawrence, Kansas

Jacqueline V. Lerner, PhD, Department of Counseling, Developmental, and Educational Psychology, Lynch School of Education, Boston College, Boston, Massachusetts

Richard M. Lerner, PhD, Institute for Applied Research in Youth Development, Tufts University, Boston, Massachusetts

Todd D. Little, PhD, Department of Psychology, University of Kansas, Lawrence, Kansas

Lawrence L. Lo, BA, Department of Human Development and Family Studies, Pennsylvania State University, University Park, Pennsylvania

Kamala London, PhD, Department of Psychology, University of Toledo, Toledo, Ohio

David P. MacKinnon, PhD, Department of Psychology, Arizona State University, Tempe, Arizona

John J. McArdle, PhD, Department of Psychology, University of Southern California, Los Angeles, California

Roger E. Millsap, PhD, Department of Psychology, Arizona State University, Tempe, Arizona

Stephen A. Mistler, BS, Department of Psychology, Arizona State University, Tempe, Arizona

Peter C. M. Molenaar, PhD, Department of Human Development and Family Studies, Pennsylvania State University, University Park, Pennsylvania

Eun-Young Mun, PhD, Center of Alcohol Studies, Rutgers, The State University of New Jersey, New Brunswick, New Jersey

Daniel S. Nagin, PhD, Department of Statistics, Heinz College, Carnegie Mellon University, Pittsburgh, Pennsylvania

Jari-Erik Nurmi, PhD, Department of Psychology, University of Jyväskylä, Jyväskylä, Finland

Candice L. Odgers, PhD, Deartment of Psychology and Social Behavior, University of California, Irvine, Irvine, California

Andrea M. Piccinin, PhD, Department of Psychology, University of Victoria, Victoria, British Columbia, Canada

John Poggio, PhD, Department of Psychology and Research in Education, School of Education, University of Kansas, Lawrence, Kansas

Lea Pulkkinen, PhD, Department of Psychology, University of Jyväskylä, Jyväskylä, Finland

Nilam Ram, PhD, Department of Human Development and Family Studies, Pennsylvania State University, University Park, Pennsylvania

William Revelle, PhD, Department of Psychology, Northwestern University, Evanston, Illinois

Joseph Lee Rodgers, PhD, Department of Psychology, University of Oklahoma, Norman, Oklahoma

Michael J. Rovine, PhD, Department of Human Development and Family Studies, Pennsylvania State University, University Park, Pennsylvania

Bernhard Schmitz, PhD, Institute of Psychology, Technische University Darmstadt, Darmstadt, Germany

James P. Selig, PhD, Department of Individual, Family, and Community Education, University of New Mexico, Albuquerque, New Mexico

Leslie H. Shaw, MA, Buros Institute for Assessment Consultation and Outreach, University of Nebraska, Lincoln, Nebraska

Robert S. Stawski, PhD, Survey Research Center, Institute for Social Research, University of Michigan, Ann Arbor, Michigan

Christian Steglich, PhD, Department of Sociology, University of Groningen, Groningen, The Netherlands

Valgeir Thorvaldsson, PhD, Department of Psychology, University of Gothenburg, Gothenburg, Sweden

Russell B. Toomey, MA, Division of Family Studies and Human Development, Norton School of Family and Consumer Sciences, University of Arizona, Tucson, Arizona

Paul van Geert, PhD, Heymans Institute, University of Groningen, Groningen, The Netherlands

Marinus H. van IJzendoorn, PhD, Center for Child and Family Studies, Leiden University, Leiden, The Netherlands

René Veenstra, PhD, Interuniversity Center for Social Science Theory and Methodology, University of Groningen, Groningen, The Netherlands

Ana Maria Velásquez, PhD, Centro de Investigación y Formación en Educación, Universidad de los Andes, Bogotá, Colombia; Department of Psychology, Concordia University, Montreal, Quebec, Canada

Frank Vitaro, PhD, Department of Educational Psychology, University of Montreal, Montreal, Quebec, Canada

Brenda Volling, PhD, Department of Psychology, University of Michigan, Ann Arbor, Michigan

Alexander von Eye, PhD, Department of Psychology, Michigan State University, East Lansing, Michigan

Theodore A. Walls, PhD, Department of Psychology, University of Rhode Island, Kingston, Rhode Island

Joshua Wilt, MA, Department of Psychology, Northwestern University, Evanston, Illinois

Daniel B. Wright, PhD, Department of Psychology, Florida International University, Boca Raton, Florida

Tianyi Yu, PhD, Center for Family Research, University of Georgia, Athens, Georgia

Ali Zaremba, MS, Department of Human Development and Family Studies, Auburn University, Auburn, Alabama